FOUNDATIONS OF
Orthopedic
Physical Therapy

FOUNDATIONS OF
Orthopedic
Physical Therapy

Editors

Harvey W. Wallmann, PT, DSc, AT Ret, CSCS

Robert Donatelli, PT, PhD
Las Vegas Physical Therapy Orthopedic and Sports
Las Vegas, Nevada

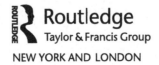

Routledge
Taylor & Francis Group

NEW YORK AND LONDON

First published 2024 by SLACK Incorporated

Published 2024 by Routledge
605 Third Avenue, New York, NY 10158

and by Routledge
4 Park Square, Milton Park, Abingdon, Oxon, OX14 4RN

Routledge is an imprint of the Taylor & Francis Group, an informa business

Library of Congress Cataloging-in-Publication Data

Names: Wallmann, Harvey W., editor. | Donatelli, Robert, editor.
Title: Foundations of orthopedic physical therapy / [edited by] Harvey W.
  Wallmann, Robert Donatelli.
Other titles: Orthopedic physical therapy
Description: Thorofare, NJ : SLACK Incorporated, [2024] | Includes
  bibliographical references and index.
Identifiers: LCCN 2022015862 (print) | ISBN
  9781630911676 (hardcover) |
Subjects: MESH: Musculoskeletal Diseases--therapy | Physical Therapy
  Modalities
Classification: LCC RM701 (print) | NLM WE 140 | DDC
  615.8/2--dc23/eng/20220525
LC record available at https://lccn.loc.gov/2022015862

Cover Artist: Katherine Christie

ISBN: 9781630911676 (pbk)
ISBN: 9781003524212 (ebk)

DOI: 10.4324/9781003524212

DEDICATION

I would like to dedicate this book to all the students, faculty, and clinicians with whom I have had the pleasure to work.

—Harvey W. Wallmann, PT, DSc, AT Ret, CSCS

This book is dedicated to my children, Rachel, Robby, and Briana Donatelli.

—Robert Donatelli, PT, PhD

Contents

ACKNOWLEDGMENTS

I would like to thank Dr. Bob Donatelli and SLACK Incorporated for allowing me to assist in the editing of this book. Also, a special thank you to all of the contributing authors who have given up countless hours in sharing their contributions with us.

—*Harvey W. Wallmann, PT, DSc, AT Ret, CSCS*

I would like to thank Dr. Harvey W. Wallmann and SLACK Incorporated for helping in the editing of this book.

Also, a special thank you to all of the gifted clinicians, educators, and specialists who have given their time and expertise in sharing their contributions with us.

—*Robert Donatelli, PT, PhD*

ABOUT THE EDITORS

Harvey W. Wallmann, PT, DSc, AT Ret, CSCS, has extensive teaching, research, and administrative experience in physical therapy as he served in academia for 24 years. He graduated with a master of science in physical therapy from the University of Indianapolis, Krannert Graduate School of Physical Therapy in 1989, and a doctor of science from Loma Linda University (Loma Linda, California) in 2000. His prior credentials include a bachelor of arts in movement and sports science and a master of science in exercise physiology, both from Purdue University (West Lafayette, Indiana). Dr. Wallmann holds certification as a Certified Strength Conditioning Specialist (CSCS) and previously held certifications as a Certified Athletic Trainer (ATC) and as a Board-Certified Sports Clinical Specialist (SCS).

Dr. Wallmann began his physical therapy academic career at the University of Nevada, Las Vegas, in Las Vegas, Nevada, in 1997, where he was founding Director of the program. He was also the founding Director/Department Head of the doctor of physical therapy program at Western Kentucky University (WKU) from 2011 to 2018, and served as professor and Department Chair/Program Director at the University of Findlay in Ohio from 2018 to 2021.

At the national level, he completed a term serving as the Chair of the Sports Specialty Council for the American Board of Physical Therapy Specialties, while prior to that serving as the Sports Certification Item Bank Coordinator as well as item writer/reviewer. He has collaborated with researchers from many disciplines besides physical therapy, including nursing, kinesiology, athletic training, engineering, and nutrition. Currently, he has more than 65 peer-reviewed publications, including articles and book chapters as well as dozens of poster and platform presentations and abstracts. Most of his research focuses on the areas of balance, gait training, and the effects of stretching on human performance. Dr. Wallmann was the guest editor for the Balance monograph published in *Orthopaedic Physical Therapy Clinics of North America*. He also served as the associate editor for North America for the international journal *Physical Therapy in Sport* for 7 years, served on the editorial boards for *Home Health Care Management & Practice* as well as the American College of Sports Medicine's *Health & Fitness Journal*, and served as a manuscript reviewer for 12 different professional journals.

Robert Donatelli, PT, PhD, is an adjunct faculty at Touro University (New York City, New York) for the Physical Therapy Department. Dr. Donatelli was the therapist for the University of Nevada, Las Vegas hockey team in 2016 and 2017. His responsibilities included the development of a postconcussion program and assessment and treatment of injuries. Dr. Donatelli worked with the Las Vegas Lights professional soccer team as well. From 2010–2011, Dr. Donatelli was asked to work with the Chinese Olympic Teams at the Chinese Olympic Center in Beijing, China. Dr. Donatelli worked directly with the Olympic athletes in the evaluation and treatment of injuries. Since May of 2001 to 2008, Dr. Donatelli has been the physical therapist working with Andy Roddick—ranked in the top 10 on the Association for Tennis Professionals (ATP) tour for 10 years. Dr. Donatelli worked as the physical therapist for the Jimmy Connors Champions Tennis Tour. Dr. Donatelli was also the physical therapist for the ATP tour, Mexico City and the Lipton ATP tennis tournaments in 1996, Germany Open in 1997, AT&T Challenge in Atlanta 1985–1999. From January 2004, Dr. Donatelli has worked on tour with the Professional Golfer's Association (PGA) for 6 months and worked individually with several professional golfers including Natalie Gublis, Amy Hung, Kim Hall, and Fred Funk. Dr. Donatelli served as a member of the PBATS (Professional Baseball Athletic Trainers Society) Research Committee from 1996–2001, and worked as a consultant for Montreal Expos, Philadelphia Phillies, and Milwaukee Brewers baseball teams.

Dr. Donatelli has published 4 textbooks: *Physical Therapy of the Shoulder, Fifth Edition*; *Orthopaedic Physical Therapy, Fourth Edition*; *Biomechanics of the Foot and Ankle, Second Edition*; and *Sports-Specific Rehabilitation*. Dr. Donatelli has published more than 35 articles in peer-reviewed journals. Dr. Donatelli has published 13 books (including new editions), and he has written numerous chapters within his 13 published books.

Dr. Donatelli lectures throughout the United States, Canada, England, Israel, Iceland, Italy, Greece, Ireland, Brazil, Russia, China, Scotland, Australia, Sweden, Spain, Romania, Poland, and Portugal.

CONTRIBUTING AUTHORS

Kristi M. Angelopoulou, PT, DPT, OCS, MCMT, Cert.MSKUS (Chapters 4 and 8)
Associate Professor
Emory & Henry College
Marion, Virginia

Charles Baycroft, MD (Chapter 11)

Bill Boissonnault, PT, DHSc, DPT (Chapter 3)
University of Wisconsin–Madison
Madison, Wisconsin

Benjamin S. Boyd, PT, DPTSc (Chapter 2)
Adjunct Associate Professor
Department of Physical Therapy
College of Health Sciences
Samuel Merritt University
Oakland, California

Blair Bundy, PT, DPT, SCS (Chapter 6)
Milwaukee Brewers
Phoenix, Arizona

Kenji Carp, PT, OCS, ATC (Chapter 18)
Cooperative Performance & Rehabilitation, LLC
Eugene, Oregon

Charles Clark, PT, DPT, MHS, MTC, CSCS, CDNT (Chapter 17)
Results Physiotherapy
Louisville, Kentucky

Jena Cleary, PT, DPT, OCS (Chapter 13)
Oxford, Mississippi

Michel W. Coppieters, PT, PhD (Chapter 2)
Menzies Foundation Professor of Allied Health Research
Menzies Health Institute Queensland
Griffith University
Brisbane & Gold Coast, Australia
Amsterdam Movement Sciences
Faculty of Behavioural and Movement Sciences
Vrije Universiteit Amsterdam
Amsterdam, The Netherlands

Georgeta Donatelli, PT, MS (Chapters 5, 11, and 12)

Mary Beth Geiser, PT, DPT, OCS (Chapter 13)
Senior Staff Physical Therapist
Aurora Sports Health
Mequon, Wisconsin
President
SCORE Advantage LLC
Belgium, Wisconsin

Ola Grimsby, PT (Chapter 15)
CEO
David G. Simons Academy
Winterthur, Switzerland

Christian Gröbli, PT (Chapter 20)
David G. Simons Academy
Winterthur, Switzerland

Chad Hanson, MD (Chapter 9)
Desert Orthopaedic Center
Las Vegas, Nevada

Corbin Hedt, PT, DPT, SCS, CSCS (Chapter 6)
Houston Methodist
Houston, Texas

Matthew L. Holland, PT, SCS, CSCS (Chapter 6)
Houston Methodist
Houston, Texas

Shain I. Howard, DO (Chapter 5)

Alec Kay, PT, DMT, ATC, OCS (Chapter 15)
Fellowship Program Director
Instructor
Ola Grimsby Institute
United Physical Therapy
Anchorage, Alaska

Tyler Kent, MD (Chapter 9)
Orthopedic Surgeon
Davis Orthopedics and Sports Medicine
Layton, Utah

Steven L. Kraus, PT, OCS Emeritus, MTC, CCTT, CODN (Chapter 14)
Division of Physical Therapy
Department of Rehabilitation Medicine
Emory University of Medicine
Horizon Physical Therapy LLC
Atlanta, Georgia

Kevin J. Lawrence, PT, MS, DHS, OCS (Chapter 7)
Tennessee State University
Nashville, Tennessee

Graham Linck, PT, DPT, cert DN (Chapter 3)
Advanced Spine and Posture
Las Vegas, Nevada

Tammy Luttrell, PhD, PT, CWS (Chapter 1)
Burn and Reconstructive Centers of America
Sunrise Hospital
Las Vegas, Nevada

Johnson McEvoy, BSc, MSc, DPT, MISCP, PT (Chapter 20)
United Physiotherapy Clinic
Limerick, Ireland
David G. Simons Academy
Winterthur, Switzerland
University College Dublin
Guest Lecturer
Athletic Therapy Department
Dublin City University
Dublin, Ireland

James M. McKivigan, PT (Chapter 19)
Touro University Nevada
Henderson, Nevada

Robert J. Nee, PT, PhD, MAppSc (Chapter 2)
Professor
Department of Physical Therapy
College of Health Sciences
Samuel Merritt University
Oakland, California

Beth Stone Norris, PhD, PT, OCS, E-RYT 500 (Chapters 10, 16, and 21)
Doctor of Physical Therapy Program
Western Kentucky University
Bowling Green, Kentucky

William H. O'Grady, PT, DPT, OCS, MA, FAPTA, FAAOMPT (Chapter 12)
Baylor University (retired)
Waco, Texas

Johnny G. Owens, MPT (Chapter 23)
Owens Recovery Science, Inc
San Antonio, Texas

Jeevan Pandya, PT, PhD, DPT, MHS, OCS, COMT (Chapter 13)
Hendricks Regional Health
Plainfield, Indiana

Janette Powell, PT, MHSC, OCS, SCS (Chapter 9)
University of Washington Medical Center
Seattle, Washington

Mohini Rawat, DPT, MS, ECS, OCS, RMSK (Chapter 22)
American Academy of MSK Ultrasound
New York, New York

Rodrigo Miguel Ruivo, PhD, MsC (Chapter 5)
Clinica das Conchas
Lisbon, Portugal

Mike Russell, DPT, CSCS (Chapter 12)
Henderson Physical Therapy
Henderson, Nevada

William R. VanWye, PT, DPT, PhD (Chapters 4, 8, and 23)
Board-Certified Clinical Specialist in Cardiovascular and Pulmonary Physical Therapy
Associate Professor
Florida Southern College
School of Physical Therapy
Lakeland, Florida

Sharon Wang-Price, PT, PhD, OCS (Chapter 16)
School of Physical Therapy
Texas Woman's University
Denton, Texas

Alyssa M. Weatherholt, PhD (Chapter 23)
University of Southern Indiana
Evansville, Indiana

Sonia N. Young, PT, DPT, EdD, MSCS (Chapter 17)
Western Kentucky University
Bowling Green, Kentucky

INTRODUCTION

The study of orthopedics and musculoskeletal impairments incorporates a wide range of concepts. A major form of nonsurgical management of musculoskeletal pathology incorporates physical and manual therapy and utilizes a thorough system based upon sound biomechanical principles of assessment as well as a patient's clinical response to pain and movement. The intent of this textbook is to provide information relevant to the needs of the practicing physical therapist who intends to work with the orthopedic population in the treatment and intervention of injuries, pathologies, and disorders. It was designed to provide a contemporary evidence-based approach to the topics that influence the clinician's decisions regarding rehabilitation and exercise program development. Additionally, this text will apprise the reader of the latest professional literature on current topics of interest, providing a tool for students, educators, and clinicians to enhance and apply their knowledge of orthopedic assessment and treatment. Several experienced clinicians and educators have contributed to this text with a number of them having extensive clinical experience in the area of orthopedics.

This text addresses 5 main areas. In Part I, the reader is taken through the Foundations of Orthopedic Rehabilitation, which comprise Chapters 1 through 3. Topics examined include areas such as soft tissue inflammation and healing, muscle physiology, reflex testing, and screening for medical conditions. Part II addresses the Upper Extremity and consists of Chapters 4 through 7, covering screening, dysfunction, evaluation, and treatment of the shoulder, elbow, and wrist and hand. Part III focuses on the Lower Extremity with Chapters 8 through 12 covering screening, dysfunction, evaluation, and treatment of the hip, knee, and foot and ankle, as well as an introduction to soft tissue mobilization and manual therapy. Part IV, consisting of Chapters 13 through 17, covers the Spinal Column and addresses diagnoses and treatment of temporomandibular disorders and head and orofacial pain; diagnosis and treatment of the cervical, thoracic, lumbar spine, and pelvis areas to include manual therapy and mobilizations; and evaluation and rehabilitation of spinal stability. Part V deals with Special Topics in Orthopedic Rehabilitation that address increasing areas of interest in orthopedic rehabilitation; it examines areas such as improving motor performance, electomyography analysis, dry needling, yoga, diagnostic imaging, and blood flow restriction training.

Another essential component of this textbook involves illustrative case studies in nearly every chapter. The reader will be presented with unique and diverse patients who require specific interventions related to their orthopedic issues. Each author will guide the reader with comments focusing on their perception of an effective patient intervention, providing evidence-based support for their decisions.

Clearly, the depth of understanding of orthopedics has increased within the past decade. As science evolves, more precise understanding and rehabilitation program development will provide a crucial element in helping expedite patient care. It is our intention that this book will provide clinicians with the necessary tools from which they can initiate treatment and rehabilitation of their patients. We would like to thank all of the authors who played a significant role in writing and contributing their expertise to the culmination of this book and who shared our vision and mission. Additionally, we are also indebted to the publishing team at SLACK Incorporated for their kind help in bringing this project to a successful completion.

PART I

Foundations of Orthopedic Rehabilitation

1

Trauma and Inflammation of Soft Tissue

Rehabilitation and Wound Healing and Remodeling of Collagen

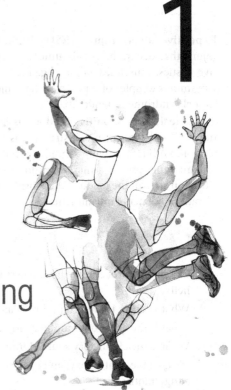

Tammy Luttrell, PhD, PT, CWS

KEY TERMS

Autocrine: Cell signaling in which the cell secretes a signaling molecule that binds to the receptors on the same cell, cell of origin, causing a change in that cell.

Chemokine: A specific class of cytokines, which are small proteins, that attract cells to a specific site. An example is the attraction of white blood cells (WBCs) to a site of infection by interleukin (IL)-1.

Cytokine: One of a variety of substances including growth factors or interferon that have an effect on neighboring cells.

Exosomes: A vesicle excreted by cells that contains chemokines, cytokines, proteins, and microRNA, which are involved in cell-to-cell communication.

Fibroblast: Most common cells found in connective tissue. Fibroblasts produce collagen and all precursors of all of the components of the extracellular matrix (ECM). These fibers include collagen, glycosaminoglycans (GAGs), and elastic and reticular fibers. Together these fibres form ground substance. Fibroblasts also are known to be early participants in initiation of the inflammatory response.

Ground substance: Ground substance is not granulation tissue. Rather, it is the gel-like substance found in the ECM. It has all of the components of the ECM except for the fiber-like tissues including collagen, elastin, and lamin. Ground substance is used by the resident cells for cellular support, water storage (as a medium for intercellular exchange [recall extravasation of leukocytes]), and perhaps most importantly, a binding site. In addition, ground substance provides lubrication around the collagen and elastin fibers found in the ECM, allowing for freer movement.

Paracrine: Cell signaling in which the cell secretes a signaling molecule that binds to the receptors on a neighboring or distant cell, causing a change in the recipient cell.

Proteoglycan (PG): A foundational component of granulation tissue and the ECM. PGs are unique in that they have a protein at their core with multiple GAGs attached via a serine residue. The GAG is joined to the core protein via a tetrasaccharide bridge (chondroitin sulfate). The chains formed are long linear carbohydrate polymers that are negatively charged. The negative charge provides a means for the PGs to attach to hyaluronic acid, water, cations (sodium, potassium, calcium), and cytokines and chemokines, thereby serving as a reservoir for growth factors. PGs and collagen form cartilage.

Wallmann HW, Donatelli R, eds. *Foundations of Orthopedic Physical Therapy* (pp 3-47).
© 2024 Taylor & Francis Group.

Repetitive stress injury (RSI): Painful musculoskeletal injury that occurs by small cumulative trauma to connective tissues, muscles, tendons, ligaments, nerves, or joints. Common examples of repetitive strain injury include carpal tunnel syndrome or tendonitis.

Tendonosis vs tendonitis: Tendonosis is a chronic condition where the collagen of a structure is not inflamed (as in tendonitis) but is actually degrading. Tendonitis is an acute inflammatory process, whereas tendonosis is a chronic deterioration state of the tendon. The "-osis" suffix refers to deterioration, not acute inflammation.

CHAPTER QUESTIONS

1. Explain the process of collagen formation and the triple helix.
2. What vitamin is important for collagen formation?
3. What is the effect of immobilization on water?
4. What is the circulatory source for tendons/ligaments?
5. What is the relative oxygen consumption for ligaments and tendons?
6. True or False—The inflammatory/repair process is purely serial (A happens then B happens).
7. Are the phases of repair totally separate and distinct from one another?
8. What is the function of cytokines? Chemokines?
9. Are cytokines/chemokines proteins?
10. Can a macrophage be both pro- and anti-inflammatory?
11. How do repair and regeneration differ?
12. What are exosomes? Could they be referred to as the *language of the cells*?
13. Is the etiology of tendon rupture precisely known?
14. Compare and contrast the differences between tendonitis and tendonosis.
15. What are the differences in tissues that are involved in chronic overuse vs healthy tissue?
16. True or False—Tenocytes cultured outside the body from areas of tendonosis continue to produce abnormal collagen.
17. True or False—Repetitive motion increases growth factor production resulting in tissue hypertrophy.
18. True or False—Abnormal levels of proteolytic enzymes can prolong healing.
19. True or False—Therapies can change the chemical environment and by doing so improve healing rates.
20. Define tendonosis.

INTRODUCTION: WHAT IS TRAUMA?

What is trauma? Trauma is a Greek word for injury, wound, pierce, damage, or deadly force. Although trauma can and often does cause a breech in the protective epithelial barrier, that is not always the case. Just as mechanisms of trauma vary, so do the resultant soft tissue injuries.[1] Injury and soft tissue integumentary damage occur either through a high velocity forceful event (eg, a kick, motor vehicle accident, collision, fracture) or through overuse (ie, repetitive action causing micro-tears and soft tissue disruption).

Trauma is often part of the experience of living. The good news is that the body has robust, sometimes duplicative processes,[1-8] designed to heal with the creation of a healing environment. Our role as health care professionals is to assist in the creation of that healing environment to effect an expedient return to function for our patients.

Resulting in either an open wound or a closed injury, trauma disrupts the epithelium and the underlying structures, or both. The skin and underlying structures, vascular, ECM, tendons, ligaments, and muscles can all be involved to various degrees depending on the force and the time over which the trauma occurs.[9-18] Whether the wound is open, the skin/epidermis is disrupted, or closed as found in a sprain, crush injury, tendinopathy, tendonitis, or strain, the progression from trauma through healing to restoration of the function follows similar pathways modulated by common cytokines, chemokines, cells, and cell signaling.[19,20]

This review will identify and draw parallels in healing based on the resolution of inflammation, promotion of the healing process, rate of collagen synthesis, biochemical processes, and cell talk that are ongoing and orchestrated to restore function.[21-23] The goal of rehabilitation is to facilitate a targeted, rapid, durable, and adaptable regimen to assist the body with creating the environment to heal and an expedient return to function. Achieving this requires an understanding of the structure of the tissues, down to the cellular, elastin, and collagen components and their interaction and interplay.[24-26]

Fiber content, function, and structure of the ECM, skin, tendons, and ligaments will be explored. Similarities in macro-structure include the following: relative avascularity, the reliance of these tissues on osmosis and diffusion for nutrition, maintenance, and repair.[3] A further review of the micro-structure, cells, fibers, adhesins, histological structures, dermis, hypodermis, collagen types, tendons, ligaments, and vasculature will be elucidated. Both normal and repair pathways will be identified and explained, including cell signaling and associated cytokines and chemokines. The active fluid state of cell transit into and out of the area of injury will be explained in response to normal mechanical force and abnormal forces seen in trauma.[27] The ECM is a common structure and has long been discussed as a static entity; however, science is now providing the information to demonstrate the ECM is anything but static.[28-30] Collagen in its various forms is the backbone of the ECM.[5,30-32]

Collagen formation, deposition, and exchange (ie, replacing one type of collagen with another) is paramount for the healing of wounds of the epidermis, dermis, and connective tissues including ligaments and tendons. It is well established that synthesis of collagen is required for restoration of physical strength of a cutaneous wound, as well as tendons and ligaments, and the whole of the soft tissue integumentary.[20,33-37] An understanding of the central role of collagen in the wound-integumentary-trauma-healing process requires information on the rate of collagen synthesis, type of collagen, quantity of collagen, and the balance of deposition and reabsorption occurring during the healing process.[38] Biosynthesis of collagen requires specific biochemical processes including the hydroxylation of proline to hydroxyproline.[37]

This chapter illustrates and identifies 3 important principles in healing:

1. Recognition of the pervasiveness of collagen, in the integument, tendons, and ligaments along with collagen's biosynthesis, reabsorption, and remodeling
2. The molecular and biochemical parallels of tissue healing for open wounds, soft tissue, tendon, and ligament injury
3. How the practitioner can effect a positive bias for healing

As the processes are elucidated, the clinician will obtain a cellular and physiological understanding to apply practical techniques to modify the phases of the healing environment to facilitate the patient's return to function.

STRUCTURES

What Is Collagen?

Collagens are the major proteins of connective tissue giving dynamic and static strength to the structure of tissues including bones, tendons, cartilage, ligaments, vertebral disks, skin, and blood vessels.[39-42] These tissues all contain collagen; however, the collagen type varies as does the proportion, depending on the functional characteristics and requirements of the tissues. It is estimated that 25% to 35% of total body protein is collagen in its various forms. Researchers have identified more than 20 kinds of collagen.[39-42] The more common collagen types are demarcated by Roman numerals and listed in Table 1-1. The main collagens found in connective tissue are types I, II, and III; these collagens form fibers that give tensile strength to tissues. In general, tendons, ligaments, skin, and bone are largely composed of type I collagen, and cartilage is mostly composed of type II collagen. Some collagen types (II, III, V) form fibrils by virtue of lateral crosslinking of the triple helix. These collagens form the major portion of connective tissue in the healing response and are responsible for scar formation. Crosslinking is a result of a covalent bond catalyzed by the enzyme lysyl-oxidase. This process depends on Vitamin C.[43-47]

At least 50 collagen genes have been identified with the majority responsible for the encoding of procollagens. For example, the colIA1 gene encodes the alpha1 chain for type I collagen, known as *alpha1(I)*, and the colIA2 gene encodes the alpha2 chain for type I collagen, known as *alpha2(I)*. Defects in the collagen genes can cause the collagen to be constructed incorrectly (with abnormal quantity or quality),

leading to weak tissue and various collagen diseases (see Table 1-1).[9,33,48-53]

Collagen Molecular Structure

As mentioned previously, a typical collagen molecule consists of 3 subunits called *alpha (α) chains*. In the case of a molecule of type I collagen, it has 2 α1 chains and 1 α2 chain. Each molecule of type III collagen has 3 α1 chains. The collagen molecule, composed of 3 α chains, is called a tripeptide. The α chains are composed of combinations of amino acids, the basic building blocks of proteins. The most abundant amino acids in collagen are glycine, proline, and lysine.

The process of collagen maturation begins within the fibroblast cells' endoplasmic reticulum, where tropocollagen (the precursor to all collagen types) is formed. In the endoplasmic reticulum, the tropocollagen has its proline and lysine hydroxylated. Once hydroxylated, the sulfur bonds allow 3 tropocollagen strands to form a helix; the triple helix is procollagen. The procollagen is secreted into the extracellular space, passing through the cell wall, where peptidases in the fibroblast Golgi bodies cleave the terminal peptide chains, creating a collagen fibril (Figure 1-1). Finally, the tropocollagen assembles into collagen fibrils, which then assemble into collagen fibers.[52-58]

Where Is Collagen Found?

Collagen is the glue that holds us together! It is found in literally every structure to varying degrees, in varying quantities and types. The epidermis, dermis, tendons, ligaments fascial bone, and joint components all have collagen as a key component. Globally, the function of collagen is a derivative of the type, location, synthesis, and cross section. Because trauma often involves the epidermis, as well as underlying integument and structures, the relationship of collagen to the epidermis, dermis, and ECM in normal skin will serve as a base for comparison of healing in skin, ligament, and tendon injury.

THE EXTRACELLULAR MATRIX

The ECM of the dermis is composed of collagen (mostly type I), elastic fibers, and ground substances such as GAGs and PGs (Figure 1-2). The ECM is a very dynamic structure and not a static structure as it is often portrayed. The ECM is also a reservoir of growth factors, chemokines, and cytokines, positioned to be released and activated in the event of injury. The ECM structure has PG, which are protein/polysaccharide complexes that trap water and directly correlate to the viscoelastic properties of the tissue. Essentially, the PG forms a gel that is highly compressible while providing resilience and lubrication, helping the tissue resist compressive forces. PGs consist of a proteinaceous core with attached GAGs. The uppermost surface of the dermis is reticular and interdigitates with the ridges of the epidermis; the structures

Table 1-1

COLLAGEN TYPES, SYNTHESIS, LOCATION, AND FUNCTION

	SYNTHESIZED	TISSUE	FUNCTION	STRUCTURE
TYPE I	Fibroblasts, osteoblasts, small muscle cells, chondroblasts, and chondrocytes	Dermis, tendons, bone, skin, tendon, muscles, cornea, and walls of blood vessels; fibrocartilage, ligaments, bone, dentin	Resist strain, force tension, and stretch	Fibers
TYPE II	Retinal cells, chondroblasts, and chondrocytes	Vitreous body of the eye, hyaline, and elastic cartilage intervertebral disks	Resist compression	Fibrils
TYPE III	Fibroblasts, smooth muscle, Schwann cells, liver cells, and endothelium	Support networks for soft tissues, reticular laminae of basement membrane in skin, papillary layer of dermis, and blood vessels	Structural support and elasticity and wound repair	Fine fibers and reticular fibers
TYPE IV	Sheet former, epithelial cells, muscle cells, Schwann cells, endothelial cells, and lens capsule of the eye	Lamina densa of basal/external lamina, capillary, and lens fiber	Support and filtration Also known as *perlecan* and can link to laminin	Does not form fibers or fibrils, form sheets
TYPE V	Fibroblasts, bone, and smooth muscle	Fetal membrane and placenta	Fibril forming; basement membrane of skin	Cornea, ECM, placenta, and hair cell surfaces
TYPE VI	Beaded filaments and fibroblasts	Connective tissue, blood vessels, skin, uterus, liver, kidney, and periodontal	Attach cells to connective tissue	Matrix association
TYPE VII	Anchoring fibrils, fibroblasts, and keratinocytes	Epithelial basement membrane anchoring fibrils	Attach cells to connective tissue	Links
TYPE VIII	Sheet former and corneal fibroblasts	Cornea	Stabilize cellular phenotype and maintain cellular integrity	Sheets
TYPE X	Fibroblasts	Endochondral growth plate formation, skeleton calcification, and cartilage	Component of reticular dermis	Facilitate removal of hypertrophic cartilage and cartilage to bone
TYPE XII	Fibroblasts	Reticular dermal integrity	Component of reticular dermis	Anchors

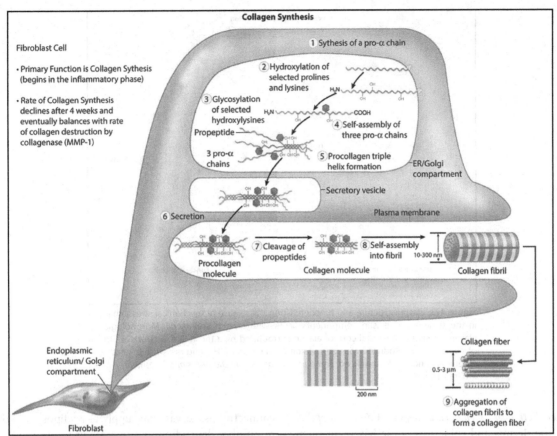

Figure 1-1. Collagen synthesis: Collagen synthesis occurs primarily in the fibroblast. This figure illuminates both the intracellular and extracellular steps required to produce collagen fibers, which are an integral part of the ECM. (ER = endoplasmic reticulum.) (Reproduced with permission from Luttrell T. Healing response in acute and chronic wounds. In: Hamm R, ed. *Text and Atlas of Wound Diagnosis and Treatment.* 2nd ed. McGraw Hill; 2019.)

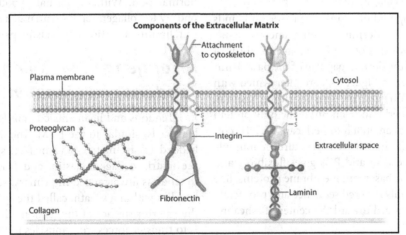

Figure 1-2. Components of the ECM: The ECM is complex and intimately involved in healing by regulating growth factor activation, cell signaling, and cell-to-matrix signaling. This figure illustrates the intricate positioning and connections for the glycoproteins, integrins, and PGs that compose the ECM. It serves as the scaffolding upon which the body builds replacement tissue. (Reproduced with permission from Luttrell T. Healing response in acute and chronic wounds. In: Hamm R, ed. *Text and Atlas of Wound Diagnosis and Treatment.* 2nd ed. McGraw Hill; 2019.)

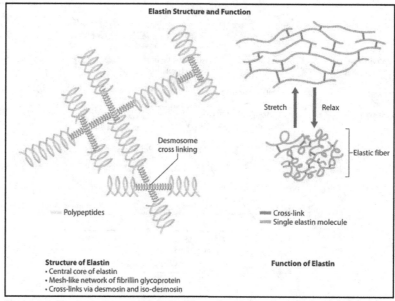

Figure 1-3. Elastin structure and function: Upon the release of mechanical stress, changes in the structure of elastin components occur with stretch and recoil. Morphologically, elastin consists of a central core of elastin surrounded by a mesh-like network of fibrillin glycoprotein. (Reproduced with permission from Luttrell T. Healing response in acute and chronic wounds. In: Hamm R, ed. *Text and Atlas of Wound Diagnosis and Treatment.* 2nd ed. McGraw Hill; 2019.)

are termed *Rete pegs* or *epidermal pegs* and *dermal papillae.* Between the dermis and epidermis is the basement membrane, consisting of the basal lamina and the reticular lamina. In addition to joining the 2 layers, the basement membrane allows the nutrients from the dermis vasculature to pass through to the avascular epidermis.[12,20,53,56-59]

The dermis is composed of connective tissue and binds the epidermis to the hypodermis or subcutaneous tissue. Acellular dermal components of the ECM, anchor fibrils of type IV collagen, form the dermal papillae of the basal lamina. Elastin fibers, as seen in Figure 1-3, are intertwined with other collagen fibers (VII) and proteins including laminin, entactins, and the PG, perlecan. Laminin is the only protein in the basal lamina that can attach to perlecan, type IV collagen, and entactin. The interwoven structure of multiple types of collagen with elastin and PGs gives flexibility and elasticity to the skin. The basement membrane proteins, like laminin, appear in a highly ordered sequence and proliferate from wound margins inward toward the center of a healing wound (Figure 1-4).[60]

The papillary layer contains the fibroblasts, mast cells, and macrophages, as well as some extravasated leukocytes.[1] The reticular layer is composed of dense, mainly type I collagen, and contains the vasculature, nerve endings, glands, hair follicles, and more elastic fibers.

Hypodermis

The hypodermis, or subcutaneous layer, is not anatomically part of the skin; however, it is the structure that binds the skin to the underlying structures. It is composed of loose connective tissue, vascular supply, and adipose cells that vary in number depending on the areas of the body. The hypodermis allows the skin to move freely over the underlying structures, thereby facilitating movement muscle and joint movement as seen in Figure 1-5, a graphic representation of normal skin. Without normal hypodermal excursion secondary to collagen repair, scarring and contractures can result, limiting function and causing pain.

Arrangement of Collagen in Tendons and Ligaments

Tendons and ligaments contain PGs, elastin, and fibroblast cells, similar to the ECM. The fibroblast cells are embedded in the matrix, and in fact, synthesize and secrete the matrix collagen, elastin, and PGs. The collagen fibers in tendons are arranged in primary, secondary, and tertiary bundles within a sheath, called the *epitenon,* that surrounds the exterior surface of the tendon. The function of tendons is to transfer forces from muscles to their bony attachments to produce joint movement. Ligaments further guide and restrict movement, maintain optimum joint alignment, and maximize the transfer of muscular force.

Just as the engineers for the San Francisco Bay Bridge employed various cables and intertwined bundles to provide incredible dynamic, light-weight support to traverse the San Francisco Bay, collagen in tendons and ligaments is arranged either in bundles or parallel fibers, giving tendons and ligaments a rope-like structure. Collagen sheets, as found in fascia, provide parallel strength. Fiber bundles in tendons and ligaments run parallel to the lines of force. Niu et al[61] has

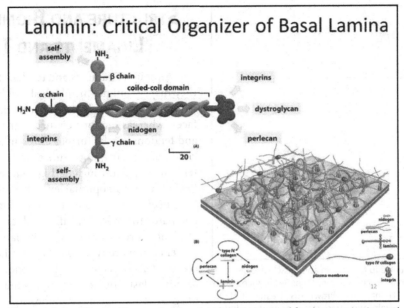

Figure 1-4. Basal lamina: The structural protein laminin is critical for the organization and assembly of the basal lamina. Laminin has specific attachments that orient perlecan, type IV collagen, and entactin. (Reproduced with permission from Luttrell T. Healing response in acute and chronic wounds. In: Hamm R, ed. *Text and Atlas of Wound Diagnosis and Treatment.* 2nd ed. McGraw Hill; 2019.)

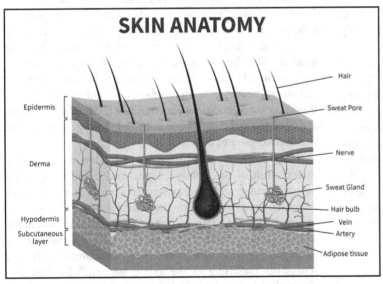

Figure 1-5. Normal intact skin: Normal intact and uninjured skin showing the layers of epidermis, dermis, and hypodermis. The appropriate and significant cells are illustrated in the corresponding layer of skin as observed in uninjured skin. (MicroOne/Shutterstock.com.)

demonstrated that keratinocyte fibroblasts line up and orient to the tension place on tissues; moreover, they morph in phenotype in response to tissue stress.[31,61,62] Collagen cross-links, perpendicular to the bundles of parallel fibers, add strength to the structure. Collagen in cartilage appears as a net mesh with a large amount of gel-like substance interdigitating between the collagen fibers, making the structure of cartilage more like a sponge. The characteristics of collagen-containing tissues are not homogeneous. The type and amount of collagen varies with the structure of the tissue, based on location and function; for example, tendons and ligaments have different types and ratios of collagen at the point of insertion to the bone as compared to the middle of the tendon or ligament.[25,63-65]

Tenocytes and tenoblasts lie between the collagen fibers along the long axis of the tendon.[11] The dry mass of human tendons is approximately 30% of the total tendon mass with water accounting for the remaining 70%. Collagen type I accounts for 65% to 80% and elastin accounts for approximately 2% of the dry mass of tendons.[66]

The PG/water component of tendon, ligament, and cartilage tissue is often referred to as *ground substance*. Predominantly, PGs are classified as *decorin* or *aggrecan*. Decorins are the most predominant PGs and work to regulate collagen fiber diameter. Typically, the length is 300 nm with a diameter of 1.5 nm. Decorin forms cross-links between collagen fibers and transfers or disperses the load or force between collagen fibers.[67,68] Aggrecan, which is associated with

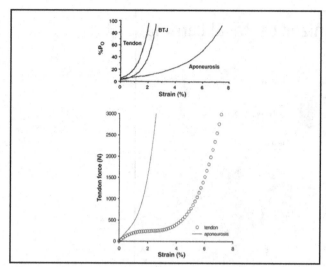

Figure 1-6. Load-strain relationship for tendon and muscle aponeurosis during passive and active muscle contraction. (Top: Reproduced with permission from Lieber RL, Leonard ME, Brown CG, Trestik CL. Frog semitendinosis tendon load-strain and stress-strain properties during passive loading. *Am J Physiol.* 1991;261[1]:C86-C92. Bottom: Reproduced with permission from Magnusson SP, Hansen P, Aagaard P, et al. Differential strain patterns of the human gastrocnemius aponeurosis and free tendon, in vivo. *Acta Physiol Scand.* 2003;177[2]:185-195.)

higher water content, is primarily found in areas of tendon compression.[69-71] Cartilage contains the greatest percentage of various PGs, and therefore, the highest amount of associated water molecules, resulting in a highly compressible, gel-like substance that provides cushioning for joints. Tendons contain a smaller percentage of water-loving PGs, and therefore, less associated water than cartilage. Elastin fibers, which can stretch and return to their original form, are interwoven with collagen fibers. The properties of memory, recoil, elasticity to the tendon, and resistance to tearing are illustrated in Figure 1-6. The elastin fibers form a network throughout the tissue, representing only 1% to 2% of tendon dry weight. Along with the associated water molecules, collagen represents 65% to 80% of the dry weight of tendon and is therefore the most abundant component of tendon.[69-71]

The Extracellular Matrix in Ligaments and Tendons

In tendon tissue, the fibroblasts work actively creating new collagen. When tissues are mature, the fibroblasts become less active and reside in the ECM of the tendon as fibrocytes. The fibrocytes do not actively create new tissue unless they are stimulated to return to a fibroblastic phenotype and repair damage or remodel old tissue. Morphologically, fibroblasts tend to look thicker, rounder, and larger than fibrocytes, which appear thin and linear. Fibrocytes found in tendons are called *tenocytes*. As a point of clarification, fibrocytes found in cartilage are called *chondrocytes* and fibrocytes found in bone are called *osteocytes*.[13,14,42,72-74]

STRUCTURE AND BIOMECHANICS OF LIGAMENTS AND TENDONS

Although ligaments and tendons have gross similarities, they display unique histological and biochemical characteristics. Functionally, ligaments articulate between bony surfaces, whereas tendons connect bone to muscle. Ligaments and tendons can be further differentiated based on their location and their unique function. In general, ligament and tendon properties include high mechanical strength, good flexibility, and an optimal level of elasticity.[21,42,74,75] Ligaments have been demonstrated to have a higher metabolic rate as compared to tendons, verified by higher DNA content, larger amounts of reducible cross-links, larger cell nuclei, and the presence of more type III collagen.[76] Ligaments also have increased GAGs as compared to tendons. In contrast, tendons are viscoelastic tissues, displaying the mechanical properties of stress/strain, force relaxation, and creep. These properties effectively transmit force generated by muscle to bone and simultaneously act as a buffer by absorbing external forces to limit muscle and skeletal damage.[77-80]

Tendons can be subdivided into 2 general classifications: (1) paratenon covered tendons and (2) sheathed tendons.[81-86] Paratenon covered tendons include the patellar and Achilles tendons. The paratenon covered tendons have a relatively rich vascular supply and typically heal better than sheathed tendons. Sheathed tendons, like those of the hand flexors, are less vascularized and typically receive nutrition through diffusion. Paratenon tendons often fail at either the myotendinous or osteotendinous junction (OTJ). Sheathed tendons are often injured due to laceration and are at greater risk for the development of adhesions.[81,85,86]

The biomechanical behavior of tendon collagen is a direct result of the number, types, and orientation of the intramolecular and intermolecular bonds. A stress-strain curve helps to demonstrate the behavior of the tendon (see Figure 1-6).[87-92] At rest, collagen fibers and fibrils display a crimped configuration.[37] The initial concave portion of the curve (toe region), where the tendon is strained up to 2%, represents flattening of the crimp pattern.[38] Beyond this point, the tendon deforms in a linear fashion due to intramolecular sliding of collagen triple helices, and the fibers become more parallel.[39] If the strain remains below 4%, the tendon behaves in an elastic fashion and returns to its original length when unloaded.[88-94]

The tensile strength of tendons relates both to the cross section of the tendon and the percentage and type of collagen present. X-ray diffraction studies have shown that collagen fibril elongation initially occurs due to molecular elongation. Microscopic failure occurs when the strain exceeds 4%, and beyond 8% to 10% strain, macroscopic failure occurs from intrafibril damage by molecular slippage.[91,93-96] Increasing stress enlarges the gap between molecules eventually leading to slippage of lateral adjoining molecules.[41] Complete failure occurs rapidly with the fibers recoiling into a tangled bud at the ruptured end.

To understand the elegance of the design and components, it is worth noting that a tendon with an area of 1 cm^2 is capable of bearing 500 to 1000 kg. Forces in tendons are highest during eccentric muscle contraction. Strenuous activities including eccentric activity, plyometrics, jumping, and weightlifting are most commonly associated with higher loads on tendons and ligaments. During running, forces in the Achilles tendon of 9 kiloNewton (kN), corresponding to 12.5 times body weight, have been recorded. These forces clearly exceed the single-load tensile strength of the tendon. Using noninvasive means, the mechanical properties of superficial tendons based on stress-strain curves can now be performed in humans in vivo. In review of the studies, tendons appear to be the most vulnerable for rupture if tension is applied quickly and obliquely.[91,97,98]

Physiological Responses

Observation of an increase in the cross section, weight, and tensile stiffness in both animals and humans who undergo an exercise or training program is well documented. These effects can be explained by an increase in collagen and ECM synthesis by tenocytes. Sparse data exist on the direct effect of exercise on human tendons, although intensively trained athletes are reported to have thicker Achilles tendons than control participants.[94,96,99,100]

Immobilization diminishes both the water and PG/glycoproteoglycan content of ligaments and tendons and increases the number of reducible collagen cross-links. Immobilization results in tendon atrophy, but these morphological changes occur slowly due in large part to the slow metabolism and sparsity of vasculature.[101,102]

With aging, tendon stiffness increases and overall biomechanical properties and associated function deteriorate in conjunction with muscle strength and power decline. One hypothesis is that a loss of collagen and its cross-linking results in increased tendon stiffness. Current studies demonstrate the ability of resistance training to partially reverse the effects of aging on tendon properties and function.[103]

It is important to remember that the position of comfort is often the position of contracture; however, immobilization is frequently required as a component of recovery. Consideration should be given to edema control, prevention of further soft tissue destruction, and where possible, maintenance of soft tissue/integument in a neutral position. In general, the timelines for the development of tissue restrictions are approximately as follows:

- Tendons and sheaths: 5 to 21 days
- Adaptive muscle shortening: 2 to 3 weeks
- Ligament and joint capsule: 1 to 3 months

Blood Supply

Ligaments, and to a lesser degree tendons, have a redundant vascular supply, receiving blood from 3 main sources: (1) the intrinsic systems at the OTJ and myotendinous junction (MTJ), (2) the extrinsic system via the paratenon, or (3) the synovial sheath. The ratio of blood supply from the intrinsic or extrinsic system varies depending on the location and the function of the ligament or tendon. As an example, the central third of the rabbit Achilles tendon receives 35% of its blood supply from the extrinsic system. At the MTJ, perimyseal vessels from the muscle continue between the fascicles of the tendon.[23] However, blood vessels originating from the muscle are unlikely to extend beyond the proximal third of the tendon. The blood supply for the OTJ is sparse and limited to the insertion zone of the tendon, although vessels from the extrinsic system communicate with periosteal vessels at the OTJ. In tendons enveloped by sheaths to reduce friction, branches from major vessels pass through the vincula (mesotenon) to reach the visceral sheet of the synovial sheath, where they form a plexus.[12] This plexus supplies the superficial part of the tendon, while some vessels from the vinculae penetrate the epitenon.

Ligament and tendon vascularity is compromised at junctional zones and sites of torsion, friction, or compression. In the Achilles tendon, angiographic injection techniques have demonstrated a zone of hypovascularity 2 to 7 cm proximal to the tendon insertion. However, laser Doppler flowmetry has demonstrated substantially reduced blood flow near the Achilles tendon insertion, with an otherwise even blood flow throughout the tendon. A similar zone of hypovascularity is present on the dorsal surface of the flexor digitorum profundus tendon subjacent to the volar plate within 1 cm of the tendon insertion. In general, tendon blood flow declines with increasing age and mechanical loading, and peak exercise peritendinous blood flow reaches only approximately 20% of the maximal blood flow capacity in that area.[104,105]

Innervation

Tendon and ligament innervation originates from cutaneous, muscular, and peritendinous nerve trunks. At the MTJ, nerve fibers cross and enter the endotenon septa. Nerve fibers form rich plexuses in the paratenon, and branches penetrate the epitenon. Most nerve fibers do not actually enter the main body of the tendon but terminate as nerve endings on its surface. Nerve endings of myelinated fibers function as specialized mechanoreceptors to detect changes in pressure or tension. These mechanoreceptors, the Golgi tendon organs, are most numerous at the MTJ. Golgi tendon organs are essentially a thin, delicate capsule of connective tissue that enclose a group of branches of large, myelinated nerve fibers. These fibers terminate with a spray of fiber endings between bundles of collagen fibers of the tendon. Unmyelinated nerve endings act as nociceptors and sense and transmit pain. Both sympathetic and parasympathetic fibers are present in tendon.[106-108]

Structure

Ligaments and tendons vary in form. Based on their location and function, they can appear as round cords, flat strap-like bands or ribbons. When healthy, they appear bright white and have a fibroelastic texture. Structurally, tendons are composed of tenoblasts and tenocytes, which lie in a network of ECM. Tenoblasts are immature tendon cells. They are spindle-shaped with numerous cytoplasmic organelles reflecting their high metabolic activity. With age, tenoblasts become elongated and transform into tenocytes.[5] Tenocytes have a lower nucleus-to-cytoplasm ratio than tenoblasts and correspondingly a decreased metabolic activity. Together, tenoblasts and tenocytes account for 90% to 95% of the cellular elements of tendons.[5] The remaining 5% to 10% of the cellular elements of tendons consists of chondrocytes at the bone attachment and insertion sites; synovial cells of the tendon sheath; and vascular cells, including capillary endothelial cells and smooth muscle cells of arterioles.[109]

Tenocytes synthesize collagen and all components of the ECM associated with the tendon and are active in energy generation. The tendon ECM or ground substance is integral to normal and injured tendon maintenance, repair, and function. The strongly hydrophilic (water loving) nature of PGs enable the rapid diffusion of water-soluble molecules and migration of cells. Adhesive glycoproteins, such as fibronectin and thrombospondin, participate in the repair and regeneration process. Tenascin-C is a glycoprotein expressed in the ECM of various tissue types including tendons. Tenascin-C is particularly abundant at the tendon body, OTJ, and MTJ.[110-116] Tenascin-C contains a series of repeating fibronectin type III domains and, following stress-induced unfolding of these domains, functions as an elastic protein. Importantly, the expression of tenascin-C is regulated by mechanical strain and is up-regulated in tendinopathy. Tenascin-C may also have a role in directing collagen fiber alignment and orientation.[110-116]

The epitenon is a delicate, loose, connective tissue sheath where the vascular, lymphatic, and nerve supply to the tendon envelopes the entire tendon, penetrating deep into the tertiary bundles and seamlessly becomes the endotenon. The endotenon, like the epitenon, is a reedy reticular network of connective tissue reaching into each tendon fiber. Superficially, the epitenon is surrounded by paratenon, a loose areolar connective tissue consisting of type I and III collagen fibrils, some elastic fibrils, and an inner lining of synovial cells.[117-121]

Synovial tendon sheaths are colocated where increased mechanical stress necessitates efficient lubrication, for example, in tendons of the hands and feet. Synovial sheaths consist of an outer fibrotic sheath and an inner synovial sheath, which consists of thin visceral and parietal sheets. The inner synovial sheath interlocks and interdigitates with the tendon body and functions as an ultrafiltration membrane to produce synovial fluid. The fibrous sheath forms anchors that function as pulley's and fulcrums to aid tendon biomechanical function.[19] At the MTJ, tendinous collagen fibrils are inserted into crevices formed by myocyte processes. The arrangement and specific ratio of collagens at the MTJ allow tension generated by intracellular contractile proteins of muscle fibers to be seamlessly transmitted to the collagen fibrils and move or stabilize the extremity with minimal loss

in force.[20] Complex fiber architecture decreases the tensile stress exerted during muscle contractions on the tendon. The MTJ is prone to injury as it is biomechanically the weakest point of the muscle-tendon unit.[117-119]

The OTJ is composed of 4 zones: a dense tendon zone, fibrocartilage, mineralized fibrocartilage, and bone. The specialized structure of the OTJ prevents collagen fiber bending, fraying, shearing, and failure.

Oxygen consumption by tendons and ligaments is 7.5 times lower as compared to skeletal muscles. Given their low metabolic rate and well-developed anaerobic energy generation capacity, tendons can maintain tension for long periods, carry sustained loads, and carry sustained loads with minimal energy requirements while simultaneously avoiding the risk of ischemia and subsequent necrosis. However, this is a double-edged sword. Normally, a small amount of energy is consumed as a result of the low cellular metabolic rate; however, the decreased metabolic rate also contributes to slow healing after injury, trauma, or wounding.[122]

THE HEALING RESPONSE: SOFT TISSUE REPAIR AND REGENERATION—A REVIEW

The inflammatory and repair processes are no longer thought of as simple, serial, straight-forward events. Rather, it is now known that this process is a very complicated, well-orchestrated cascade of cell processes running both in tandem and parallel. This review presents a brief overview of salient events associated with tissue repair, with an emphasis on the principal cells directing the process, the cell-to-cell signaling, the role of mechanical stress/strain, and some of the important cytokines and chemokines as opposed to the classical approach to wound healing. Herein, the healing process (repair) is demarcated into 4 broad stages, which are not mutually exclusive and overlap considerably. The 4 phases are presented here with slight modification from that typically seen, as function is incorporated. They are:

1. Hemostasis or bleeding
2. Inflammation, subdivided into 3 smaller phases
   ◦ Kill and contain the invader
   ◦ Debridement
   ◦ Angiogenesis
3. Proliferation
4. Remodeling

Overview of Healing Cascade

Figure 1-7 delves deeper into each of the phases and schematically illustrates some of the complexities of cell signaling and depicts the general timing of the phases. The phase delineations are largely a matter of convenience when discussing the cascade of well-orchestrated events occurring

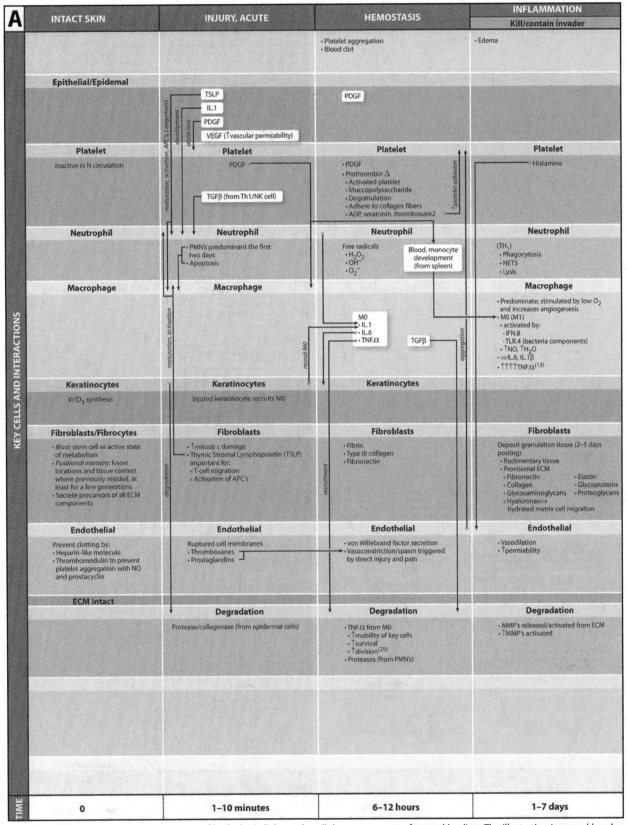

Figure 1-7. (A) The healing map is a summary of both the cellular and acellular components of wound healing. The illustration is parsed by phases of wound healing along the horizontal axis, while the primary cells of importance are along the vertical axis. The cytokines, chemokines, and growth factors important at each phase are depicted along with the directional impact exerted on healing by each of these components. (Reproduced with permission from Luttrell T. Healing response in acute and chronic wounds. In: Hamm R, ed. *Text and Atlas of Wound Diagnosis and Treatment.* 2nd ed. McGraw Hill; 2019.) *(continued)*

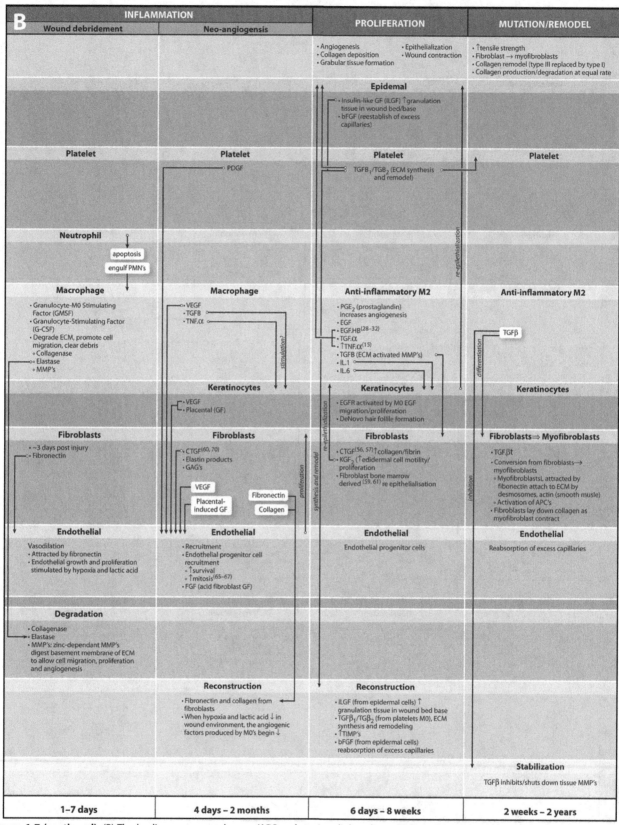

Figure 1-7 (continued). (B) The healing map second page. (ADP=adenosine diphosphate; APC=antigen presenting cell; bFGF=basic fibroblast growth factor; CTGF=connective tissue growth factor; EGF=epidermal growth factor; EGF.HB=epidermal growth factor.hemoglobulin; EGFR=epidermal growth factor receptor; GF=growth factor; H_2O_2=hydrogen peroxide; ILGF=insulin-like growth factor; KGF_2=keratinocyte growth factor-2; MMP=metallometallproteases; NETs=neutraphil extracellular trap; NK=natural killer; NO=nitric oxide; OH=hydroxide; O_2=dioxygen; PDGF=platelet-derived growth factor; PGE=prostaglandin E; PMN=polymorphonuclear leukocytes; $TGF\beta_2$=tansforming growth factor beta 2; $TGF\beta$=transforming growth factor-beta; THI=T helper cells 1; TIMP=tissue inhibitors of metalloproteinases; TNF=tumor necrosis factor; TSLP=thymic stromal lymphopoietin; $VITD_3$=vitamin D_3; VEGF=vascular endothelial growth factor.) (Reproduced with permission from Luttrell T. Healing response in acute and chronic wounds. In: Hamm R, ed. *Text and Atlas of Wound Diagnosis and Treatment.* 2nd ed. McGraw Hill; 2019.)

in response to tissue damage. Phases, although graphically represented as separate, actually overlap, interlink, and interrelate. The cells from one phase signaling to recruit the next flight of cells; all the while reliant on feedback loops that both inhibit and facilitate cell functions or encourage morphological changes in resident cells.

The injured area undergoes a healing process, which, for convenience, is divided into 4 broad but overlapping phases:

1. Hemostasis
2. Inflammation
3. Repair
4. Remodeling

Inflammation is further divided into 3 subphases: (1) kill and contain the invader, (2) debridement/removal of damaged cells, and (3) angiogenesis.

It is important that the therapist, in assisting the injured person to regain full function, understands the physiology unique to each of these phases or stages. As stated in the introduction, soft tissue damage may occur through a traumatic event involving high-velocity/high-force events, like a fall or an motor vehicle accident. Other trauma is the result of overstretching or cumulative repetitive overuse. An overuse or RSI develops over a period of hours, days, weeks, or years due to unaccustomed or excessive, repetitive activities that cause microtears and tissue deformation. In either forceful trauma or RSI, a level of disruption exists in the soft tissues: the skin, muscle, tendon, or ligament. Fibers are torn, blood vessels disrupted, and the epidermis breached. This leaves the way open for bacterial invasion at the injury site. In either case, whether open or closed wounding occurs, the healing cascade that ensues is similar for all integumentary tissue. Here, the healing phases will be presented in detail with description of the requisite activity at (1) the cellular, (2) the vascular, and (3) the cell-signaling level that occur in either regeneration or repair.[123-128]

1. Cellular events include the directed migration and accumulation of cells known to be necessary for wound healing (eg, neutrophils, macrophages) to the site of injury. These cells are able to morph in phenotype and function depending on the phase of healing, the surrounding stimuli, whether cytokine or chemokine, and the activation of the ECM.
2. Vascular events include hemostasis, transient vasoconstriction, and retrograde degradation of damaged capillaries or vessels. Transitions in endothelial differentiation, migration, and proliferation are also termed *neoangiogenesis*.
3. Cell signaling orchestrates healing by the mechanisms of cytokines, chemokines, growth factors, and receptor accessibility on target cells. Binding of chemical messengers to cell receptors displayed on the target cell surface activates or depresses target cell DNA transcription and ultimately protein translation of important activities performed by the target cell. These activities include the production of additional chemical messengers, a change in cell phenotype and, therefore, function, or

binding to adjacent ECM sites. Cell signaling occurs between the cell and ECM and between cells.[129-134]

PHASES OF REPAIR

Hemostasis Phase

This is a relatively short-lived phase and will occur following injury, trauma, or other insult when capillaries or larger vessels are disrupted. Following soft tissue injury, there may be macro- or micro-disruption, which results in bleeding into the tissues. The time for hemostasis to occur will vary with the nature and severity of the injury as well as the tissue insulted. The more vascular tissues (eg, muscle) will bleed for longer periods resulting in a larger blood loss, which permeates adjacent tissues. Relatively avascular tissues, including ligaments, tendons, or joint capsules will bleed less defined both in terms of duration and volume. The interval between injury and the conclusion of active bleeding is a matter of a few hours (4 to 6 hours is often quoted). Some tissues like muscle may continue to bleed for a significantly longer period, especially if the injured extremity is not immobilized properly.[135,136]

With the acute injury, the local blood vessels respond initially with vasoconstriction to stem further blood loss and tissue injury. Activated platelets adhere to the endothelium and eject adenosine diphosphate, which promotes the clumping of thrombocytes and furthers clot formation. The clot, or tissue plug, is composed of several cell types entwined in the fibrin fibers including red blood cells, WBCs, and platelets. Alpha granules containing platelet-derived growth factor (PDGF), platelet factor IV, and transforming growth factor-beta (TGF-β) are liberated from the platelets. Thrombocyte dense bodies release vasoactive amines, including histamine and serotonin. PDGF is chemotactic for fibroblasts and in coordination with TGF-β modulate the mitosis of fibroblasts, thereby increasing the number of resident fibroblasts near the wounded integumentary tissue. Fibrinogen is cleaved into fibrin, which undergirds the structural support for the completion of the coagulation process and further provides an active lattice for the important cellular components during the inflammatory phase.[137]

Inflammatory Phase: Overview

The inflammatory phase is an essential component of the tissue repair process. Clinically, inflammation presents as rubor (redness), tumor (swelling), calor (heat), and dolor (pain). Inflammation can either be acute, resolving in a timely manner (the 4 to 6 hours previously stated) or become chronic, lasting in some cases for years. There are numerous factors that initiate the inflammation cascade. Repetitive minor trauma, mechanical irritation, frank trauma, fracture, or open wounding all precipitate the inflammatory response in varying degrees. The inflammatory phase has a rapid onset (within a few hours) and increases in magnitude peaking at 1 to 3 days, before gradually resolving over the next couple of weeks.

Inflammation can result in several outcomes; however, it is essential and normal for tissue repair. The onset and resolution are swifter in more vascular tissues and occur more slowly in the relatively poorly vascularized tissues (tendons, ligaments, joint capsules, and skin). Initiation of inflammatory events include mechanical irritation, repeated minor trauma, excessive heating (burns), and cooling (frostbite), as well as infection and a wide range of autoimmune disorders.[138-142]

The triggered inflammatory events are essentially the same whichever "route" is the stimulus for initiation. In many instances, the final outcome of these combined events is the repair of damaged tissue with a scar, which is not a "like-for-like" replacement (regeneration) of the original, but does provide a functional, long-term repair enabling functional recovery from injury. Most patients move through this process without the need for drugs, therapy, or any outside intervention. Inflammation is designed to happen and robustly designed with redundancy. For those patients who have a problem with the resolution of inflammation or those in whom that magnitude of the damage is substantial, intervention may be required to facilitate the process. The body has an intricately complex and balanced sequence to modulate and progress through all of the phases of inflammation. However, it is possible intervention may be required in the event of an inhibited response, a delay in the cell reactions or repeated trauma, or on the background of multiple patient morbidities. In these cases, therapeutic intervention is of value.[137,138,143-146]

Normally, there is no need to alter or improve the normal process of tissue repair. Typically, the efficient system through which tissue repair is initiated and controlled leaves little to chance. The understanding of the normal healing processes will serve as the basis for the therapies intended to shorten the timeline for the complex patient's return to function. The creation of an environment conducive to healing is predicated on first understanding what is normal and identifying where in the process the patient is stalled, or whether the response is too robust or upregulated. In either case, the goal of treatment is to facilitate the progression through each phase to resolution by either repair or regeneration.

Kill and Contain the Invader

Within the first hours after injury, polymorphonuclear leukocytes (PMNs) or neutrophils flood the wound. TGF-β (released from platelets) directs PMN migration and extrusion from surrounding intact blood vessels to the interstitial wound space. PMNs are phagocytic cells, functioning to cleanse the wound of debris, including damaged tissue, necrotic cells, and pathogens. Approximately 24 to 48 hours after injury, the highest number of PMNs are observed. Normally, around 72 hours, PMNs are significantly reduced due to PMN programmed apoptosis and replacement of PMN by the more versatile macrophage. The programmed self-destruction of the PMNs is a signal for macrophage recruitment to the area. Neutrophils are noteworthy in the early phagocytosis of pathogens and in the recruitment of

macrophages through their programmed apoptosis. They are also capable of expelling a neutrophil extracellular trap that is composed of DNA and loosely aggregated chromatin. The neutrophil extracellular trap functions somewhat like fly paper, trapping would-be pathogens and increasing clearance of them by macrophages or other neutrophils recruited to the site of injury or infection.[147-149]

Mast cells are activated and become "sticky," adhering to the endothelial surface. Mast cells influence the local environment through the products they synthesize and release (eg, the degranulation of histamine). Histamine increases the permeability of endothelial cells and facilitates the extravasation of PMNs and macrophages.

Vascular Events/Angiogenesis

In addition to the vascular changes associated with bleeding, there are also marked changes in the state of the intact vessels. There are changes in the caliber of the blood vessels, in the vessel wall, and in the flow of blood through the vessels. Vasodilation follows an initial but brief vasoconstriction and persists for the duration of the inflammatory response. Flow increases through the main channels, and additionally, previously dormant capillaries are opened to increase the volume through the capillary bed.[150-156]

The cause of this dilation is primarily by chemical means (histamine, prostaglandins, complement cascade components C3 and C5, and many others), whilst the axon reflex and autonomic system may exert additional influences. There is an initial increase in velocity of the blood followed by a prolonged slowing of the stream. The PMNs marginate and the platelets adhere to the vessel walls and the endothelial cells.[157-161]

In addition to the vasodilation response, there is an increase in the vasopermeability of the local vessels (also mediated by numerous chemical mediators), and thus the combination of the vasodilation and vasopermeability response is that there is an increased flow through vessels that are more "leaky," resulting in an increased exudate production.[162,163]

The flow and pressure changes in the vessels allow fluid and the smaller solutes to pass into the tissue spaces. This can occur both at the arterial and venous ends of the capillary network as the increased hydrostatic pressure is sufficient to overcome the osmotic pressure of the plasma proteins. The vessels show a marked increase in permeability to plasma proteins. There are several phases to the permeability changes, but essentially, there is a separation of the endothelial cells, particularly in the venules, and an increased escape of protein-rich plasma to the interstitial tissue spaces. The chemical mediators responsible for the permeability changes include histamine, serotonin (5-HT), bradykinin, and leukotrienes together with a potentiating effect from the prostaglandins.[163]

The effect of the exudate is to dilute any irritant substances in the damaged area, and due to the high fibrinogen content of the fluid, a fibrin clot can form, providing an initial union between the surrounding intact tissues and a meshwork that can

Phase / Cell	Injury	Hemostasis	Inflammation-Early	Inflammation-Late	Degradation	Proliferative granulation, epithelialization contraction	Remodeling	Differentiation-Healed wound
Key Cells Arrival and Departure During Healing								
Time after Injury	Immed.	5-10 min	12 to 24 hours	24 hours	2-4 days	3-4 days; Lasts 15-16 days	~21 days	24-42 days
MΦ								
Dendritic cell	Sentinel							
γδT cell	Sentinel							
NK cell								
CD4+ Reg		Entering...				Leaving...		
B cells		Entering...	Antibodies produced - long distance "bombers"		Leaving...			
CD8 + T cells	Immed after..				Leaving...			
Macrophage		Migration	Increasing numbers				Remodeling clean up	
Neutrophil	Sentinel ...	Increasing in numbers			Leaving...			
Keratinocyte								
Fibroblast								

Figure 1-8. Timing of the arrival and departure of key cells during healing. (Reproduced with permission from Luttrell T. Healing response in acute and chronic wounds. In: Hamm R, ed. *Text and Atlas of Wound Diagnosis and Treatment.* 2nd ed. McGraw Hill; 2019.)

trap foreign particles and debris. The meshwork also serves as an aid to phagocytic activity. Mast cells in the damaged region release hyaluronic acid and other PGs, which bind with the exudate fluid and create a gel that limits local fluid flow and further traps various particles and debris.[164,165]

Cellular Events

The cellular components of the inflammatory response include the early emigration (within minutes) of the phagocytes (neutrophils; PMNs) from the vessels (Figure 1-8). This is followed by several other species leaving the main flow, including monocytes, lymphocytes, eosinophils, basophils,[163,166] and smaller numbers of red cells (though these leave the vessel passively rather than the active emigration of the white cells). Monocytes once in the tissue spaces become macrophages.[163,167-172] The main groups of chemical mediators responsible for chemotaxis are components of the complement cascade, lymphokines, factors released from the PMNs and peptides released from the mast cells in the damaged tissue. Although, these events are generally regarded as beneficial; the potential for detrimental effects of neutrophilia and macrophage dysregulation are observed in the hyper-proinflammatory response.[173-176]

The PMN escapees act as early debriders of the wound, and their apoptosis is a key signal to macrophages to move into the area and differentiate into wound-activated macrophages, which are proinflammatory. It is now known that these M_1, wound-activated, proinflammatory macrophages are central to the inflammatory response, orchestrating all of the cells, chemokines, and cytokines (Figure 1-9). Numerous chemical mediators have been identified as having a chemotactic role, for example, PDGF released from damaged platelets in the area. Components of the complement cascade (C3a and C5a), leukotrienes (released from a variety of white cells, macrophages, and mast cells), and lymphokines (released from polymorphs) have been identified.[173-176]

Therefore, the infiltration response results in a vascular response, cellular and fluid exudate, with resulting edema and phagocytic activation. The complex interaction of the chemical mediators not only stimulates various components of the inflammatory phase, but also signals the initiation of the proliferative phase. Lactic acid, one of the chemicals released due to phagocytosis, also stimulates the shift to proliferation and repair. The course of the inflammatory response will depend on the number of cells destroyed, the original causation of the process, and the tissue (ECM) condition at the time of insult.[144,156,168,177-179]

The chemical mediators or chemokines that make an active contribution to this process are ever increasing and are only now coming to light in terms of their number, interactions, and relevance. Some of the main chemokines are summarized in Table 1-2. Smith et al[141] provide a review of

Figure 1-9. Role of macrophage transition and differentiation in healing: Macrophages are central to wound healing and direct many of the cellular activities including the following: (1) production of growth factors, (2) phagocytosis, (3) wound debridement, (4) matrix synthesis, (5) cell activation and proliferation, and (6) cell recruitment. (GM-CSF = granulocyte macrophage colony stimulating factor; G-CSF = granulocyte colony stimulating factor; IFN = interferon; IGF = insulin growth factor.) (Reproduced with permission from Luttrell T. Healing response in acute and chronic wounds. In: Hamm R, ed. *Text and Atlas of Wound Diagnosis and Treatment.* 2nd ed. McGraw Hill; 2019.)

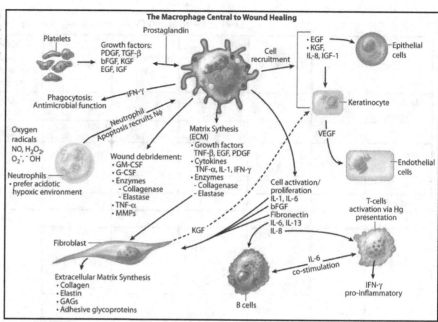

the mediators associated with muscle injury. Molloy et al[180] have specifically reviewed the role of these mediators in relation to ligament and tendon injury. Serhan[181] provides a very comprehensive review of the complement cascade in relation to growth and regeneration. Of note, many of the same chemokines and cytokines are involved in the entire spectrum of healing the integumentary system and restoring the appropriate tissue types (collagen) and function.

Outcomes of Inflammation

Resolution is a possible outcome at this stage on condition that less than a critical number of cells have been destroyed. For most patients that come to our attention, this is an unlikely scenario unless tissue irritation rather than overt damage is the initiator. There is some debate in the literature in regard to microinjury or microtrauma and whether it leads to a repair event or a resolution (Figure 1-10). This is of particular importance when considering RSI in ligaments and tendons and whether the injury will result in a microrepair or regeneration. If the microdamaged tissue fails to mount a repair response, the damage that piles up accumulates and may cause possible long-term issues. This debate continues and becomes more interesting with an ever-increasing depth and volume of evidence.[182-191]

Chronic inflammation does not necessarily imply inflammation of long duration. Rather, chronic inflammation may follow a transient or prolonged acute inflammatory stage or a truncated hemostasis response. The tissue is not completely restored to the original function and is therefore prone to reinjury. Essentially, there are 2 forms of chronic inflammation: (1) either the chronic reaction is delayed in relation to the acute reaction developing slowly with no acute phase or a failed initial acute phase (ab initio) or (2) the inflammatory bias never resolves, creating a churning environment.[192] Chronic inflammation ab initio can have

many causes including repetitive stress, local irritants, poor circulation, presence of some microorganisms, or immune disturbances. Chronic inflammation is usually more fibro-proliferative than exudative (ie, the result is the production of a greater amount of fibrous material than inflammatory exudate). This is true in the case of wounding to the integument, tendon injury, or ligamentous injury. Frequently, there is some tissue destruction, inflammation, and attempted healing occurring simultaneously.[181,193-196]

Healing/repair by fibrosis is the most common mechanism in the scenario of tissue repair. The fibrin deposits from the inflammatory stage will be partially removed by fibrinolytic enzymes (from the plasma and PMNs) and is gradually replaced by granulation tissue, which in turn, becomes organized to form scar tissue. Macrophages that have changed phenotype to M_2 (proliferative macrophages) are largely responsible for the removal of the fibrin, allowing capillary budding and fibroblastic activity to proceed (proliferation). The greater the volume of damaged tissue, the greater the extent and the density of the resulting scar tissue. Chronic inflammation is usually accompanied by some fibrosis even in the absence of significant tissue destruction.[140,197,198]

The effects of acute inflammation are largely beneficial. The fibrinogen forms fibrin clots providing a mechanical barrier, preventing the spread of microorganisms, and additionally assists with phagocytosis by trapping and containing invaders. Transportation of bacterial-invader–antigens to the lymphatic system stimulates a more robust immune response. During the proliferative state, vasodilatation and increased blood flow support increased cell metabolism that is necessary for the proliferative stage. Local oxygen content, necessary nutrients, and removal of waste products are all facilitated.

However, inflammation left unchecked may have negative effects. The increased local hydrostatic pressure from the

Table 1-2

SIGNALING MOLECULES

INTERLEUKINS AND CYTOKINES

- Which cell produces them?
- Primary activity

INTERLEUKINS	PRIMARY SOURCE	PRIMARY ACTIVITY	COMMENTS
IL-1α and IL-1β	Epithelial cells, fibroblast, platelets, macrophages, and other antigen presenting cells (APCs)	Costimulation of APCs and T cells, inflammation and host fever, hematopoiesis.	Acute phase response.
IL-2	Activated Th1 cells and natural killer (NK) cells	Proliferation of B cells and activated T cells, NK cell function. Regulate WBCs.	
IL-4	Th2 and mast cells Produced by CD4+ T cells in response to IL-18	B-cell proliferation, eosinophil and mast cell growth and function, immunoglobulin E and class II major histocompatibility class I and II (MHC) expression on B cells, inhibition of monkine production. Th0 differentiated to Th2 cells, Th2 cells produce increased IL-4. Promotes macrophage 0 to differentiate to M2 macrophage. The M2 macrophage phenotype is generally considered to be reparative or proliferative. The M2 phenotype when coupled with the secretion of IL-10 and TGF-β, results in decreased inflammation and diminution of pathological inflammation, creating an environment that favors neovascularization and granulation.	Broadly, regulate antibody production, hematopoiesis, and inflammation as well as effector T-cell development. Pleiotropic and anti-inflammatory.
IL-6	Activated Th2 cells, APCs, adipocytes, macrophages, and hepatocytes	Acute phase response, B-cell proliferation, thrombopoiesis. IL-6 works synergistically with IL-1β and TNF on T cells. Increased production of neutrophils in bone marrow.	Both pro- and anti-inflammatory. Also considered a myokine—produced in response to repetitive muscle contraction.
IL-8	Macrophages, epithelial, endothelial, and other somatic cells	Chemoattractant for neutrophils and T cells. Induces phagocytosis. IL-8 can be secreted by any cell with toll-like receptors that are involved in the innate immune response. Usually, it is the macrophages that "see" the invader first. Promotes angiogenesis.	Capable of crossing blood-brain barrier.
IL-10	Activated Th2 cells, CD8+, T and B cells, and macrophages	Inhibits cytokine production, promotes B-cell proliferation and antibody production, suppresses cellular immunity and mast cell growth.	

(continued)

Table 1-2 (continued) ───

SIGNALING MOLECULES

INTERLEUKINS	PRIMARY SOURCE	PRIMARY ACTIVITY	COMMENTS
IL-12	B cells, T cells, macrophages, and dendritic cells	Proliferation of NK cells. Increased cytotoxic activity of NK cells. Th0 to Th1. INF-γ production, promotes cell-mediated immune functions. Anti-angiogenesis via increased production of INF-γ.	Two different protein chains that form 3 distinct dimers: AA, AB, and BB.
IL-13	Th2 cells, B cells, and macrophages	Stimulates growth and proliferation of B cells, inhibits production of macrophage inflammatory cytokines. Induces MMPs. Induces immunoglobulin E secretion from activated B cells.	Central regulation of IgE synthesis. In the lungs, IL-13 is the central mediator of allergic asthma; where IL-13 regulates eosinophillic inflammation, mucus secretion and airway hyper-responsiveness.
IL-18	Macrophages	Increases NK cell activity and induces production of INF-γ. Induces cell mediated immunity. Stimulates NK and T cells to release INF-γ.	Proinflammatory. Also known as INF-γ inducing factory.
Interferons			
INFα, INF-β INF-γ	Macrophage, neutrophils	Antiviral effects, induction of class I MHC on all somatic cells, activation of NK cells and macrophages.	All 3 of these interferons impart viral resistance to cells.
INF-γ	Activated Th1 and NK cells, cytotoxic T cells	Induces expression of class I MHC on all somatic cells, induces class II MHC on APCs and somatic cells, activates macrophages, neutrophils, NK cells, promotes cell-mediated immunity, antiviral effects. Activates inducible nitric oxide synthesis. Increased production of IgG2g, IgG3 from activated plasma B cells. Increased MHC I and increased MHC II expression by APCs. Promotes adhesion binding for leukocyte migration.	Also called macrophage activating factor. Critical for both innate and adaptive immunity. Antiviral. INF-γ binds to GAG heparin sulfate at the cell surface. Binding, in general, inhibits biological activity.

(continued)

Table 1-2 (continued)

SIGNALING MOLECULES

INTERLEUKINS	PRIMARY SOURCE	PRIMARY ACTIVITY	COMMENTS
Adipocytokines			
C-reactive protein (CRP)	Hepatocytes, adipocytes Synthesized by the liver in response to factors released by macrophage and adipocytes (eg, IL-6)	CRP is a ligand binding protein (calcium dependent) that facilitates the interaction between complement and both foreign and damaged host cells. Enhances phagocytosis by macrophage. Modulates endothelial cell functions by inducing the expression of adhesion/"sticky" molecules (intercellular cell adhesion molecule-1 [ICAM-1], vascular cell adhesion molecule-1 [VCAM-1]). Attenuates nitric oxide production by down regulating nitric oxide synthase expression. CRP's level of expression is regulated by IL-6.	First pattern recognition receptor to be identified. Acute phase protein. Physiological role is to bind phosphocholine expressed on the surface of dead or dying cells and some types of bacteria to activate the complement system via C1Q complex; therefore, phagocytosis is enhanced. Opsonin-mediated phagocytosis helps amplify the early innate immune response.
Prostaglandin			
Considered to be hormone-like	Produced from the oxidation of a fatty acid, arachadonic acid, DGLA, or EPA by cyclooxygenases (COX-1 and COX-2) in combination with terminal PG synthases	Either constriction or dilation of vascular smooth muscle. Acts on platelets, endothelium, and mast cells. Causes aggregation or disaggregation of platelets. Regulates inflammatory mediation. Controls cell growth. Acts on thermoregulatory center of hypothalamus to produce fever.	PGs are potent but have a short half life before being activated or excreted. Therefore, send local signals; either autocrine (acting on the same cell from which it is synthesized) or paracrine (local adjacent cells). Stressors including trauma, tissue damage, infection, and illness can all trigger an increase in PG.

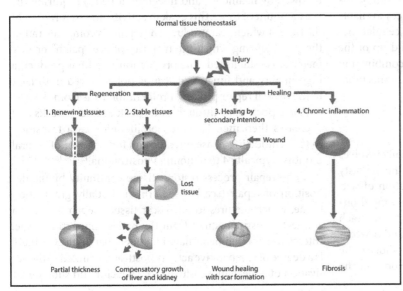

Figure 1-10. Healing vs regeneration—division of normal healing. The body responds to tissue injury in mechanisms that result in either tissue regeneration or restoration of structure and function. Four separate pathways exist: (1) regeneration, (2) compensatory growth, (3) renewal, and (4) fibrosis. When regeneration of epithelium or the underlying tissue fails to occur in a timely fashion, a state of chronic inflammation results. (Reproduced with permission from Luttrell T. Healing response in acute and chronic wounds. In: Hamm R, ed. *Text and Atlas of Wound Diagnosis and Treatment.* 2nd ed. McGraw Hill; 2019.)

Table 1-3

CYTOKINE ACTIVITY IN WOUND HEALING

CYTOKINE	CELL SOURCE	BIOLOGIC ACTIVITY
Proinflammatory Cytokines		
TNF-α	Macrophages	PMN margination and cytotoxicity, with or without collagen synthesis; provides metabolic substrate
IL-1	Macrophages Keratinocytes	Fibroblast and keratinocyte chemotaxis and collagen synthesis
IL-2	T lymphocytes	Increases fibroblast infiltration and metabolism
IL-6	Macrophages PMNs Fibroblasts	Fibroblast proliferation and hepatic acute phase protein synthesis
IL-8	Macrophages Fibroblasts	Macrophage and PMN chemotaxis and keratinocyte maturation
INF-γ	T lymphocytes Macrophages	Activates macrophages and PMNs, retards collagen synthesis and cross-linking, and stimulates collagenase activity
Anti-Inflammatory Cytokines		
IL-4	T lymphocytes Basophils Mast cells	Inhibition of TNF, IL-1, and IL-6 production; fibroblast proliferation and collagen synthesis
IL-10	T lymphocytes Macrophages Keratinocytes	Inhibition of TNF, IL-1, and IL-5 production; inhibition of macrophage and PMN activation

edema can restrict blood flow if the injured tissue space is limited (compartment syndrome is the extreme result of this phenomena). The reduction in blood flow reduces available oxygen for tissues in a state of repair and biases cellular metabolism toward anaerobic respiration. The build up of the byproducts of anaerobic cellular respiration in combination with inflammation produces pain and, therefore, limits function (Table 1-3)

Proliferative Phase

The proliferative phase (Figure 1-11) essentially involves the generation of the repair material, which for the majority of musculoskeletal injuries involves the production of scar (collagen) material. The proliferative phase has a rapid onset (24 to 48 hours) but takes considerably longer to reach its peak reactivity, which is usually between 2 and 3 weeks after injury. The more vascular the tissue, the shorter the time taken to reach peak proliferative production. On the

vascular continuum, tendons require the most time to heal, followed by ligaments, and integument (skin) requiring the least amount of time. This peak in activity does not represent the time at which scar production (repair) is complete, rather the phase during which the majority of the "patch" or scar material is established. The production of a final product, a high quality and functional scar, is not achieved until later in the overall repair process. Proliferation runs from the first day or 2 postinjury through to its peak at 2 to 3 weeks and decreases thereafter. However, proliferation as a transition to the remodeling phase often occurs for a period of several months (typically 4 to 6 months) posttrauma.[129,134,163,166,199-204]

The repair process restores tissue continuity by the deposition of repair (scar) tissue. This is initially granulation tissue, which matures to form scar tissue. Repair tissue is a connective tissue distinct from the native connective tissue. Interesting developments have identified that in muscle, there is a degree of regenerative activity posttrauma linked to the activation of a mechanosensitive growth factor and subsequent

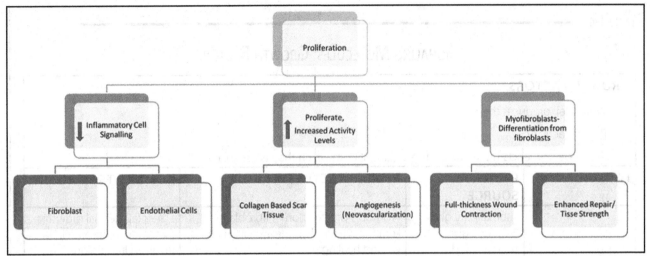

Figure 1-11. Proliferation schematic representation of the factors that affect healing outcomes.

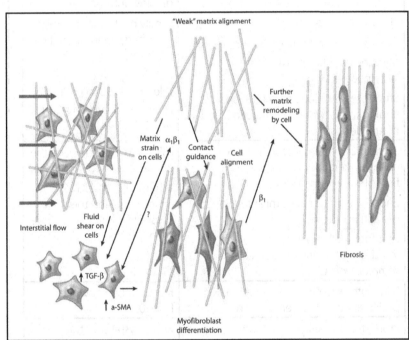

Figure 1-12. Transition of fibroblasts to myofibroblasts. Several mechanisms are known to influence the phenotypic change of fibroblasts to myofibroblasts. The known influencing mechanisms include chemical signaling and more recently mechanical stress. The presence of TGF-β1 and mechanical shear stress from interstitial fluid induces the production of a smooth muscle actin (αSMA) by fibroblasts, causing the phenotypic differentiation to myofibroblasts. Myofibroblasts drive matrix remodeling by facilitating ECM contraction and matrix alignment along the lines of stress. (Reproduced with permission from Luttrell T. Healing response in acute and chronic wounds. In: Hamm R, ed. *Text and Atlas of Wound Diagnosis and Treatment.* 2nd ed. McGraw Hill; 2019.)

activation of muscle satellite (stem) cells (Figure 1-12). The source of the majority of these proliferative-biased cytokines is the inflammatory phase, thus "turning off" or limiting the inflammatory events and simultaneously modulating the signal strength, stimulating these proliferative events.[205-209]

Two fundamental processes involved in the repair of integument, ligament, or tendon are fibroplasia and angiogenesis. The function of the fibroblast is to repair the connective tissue. Fibroblasts appear to migrate to the area from surrounding tissue. Fibroblastic activation is mediated largely by M_1 wound-activated, proinflammatory macrophages during the inflammatory stage. Fibroblasts migrate into the damaged area, upregulate their mitosis, and proliferate within the first few days after the tissue damage. Macrophage-derived growth factors (MDGFs) are a complex group of mediators responsible, at least in part, for the activation of fibroblasts.

Alongside the fibroblastic activation, capillaries in the region of the tissue damage bud and grow toward the repair zone. Loops and arcades are formed together with anastomoses, which reestablish a blood flow through the region, providing oxygen and nutrients whilst removing metabolic and repair waste products. Oxygen is critical for many of the reparative processes but especially for collagen production. A wide range of growth factors and chemical mediators have been identified that exert influences on the developing capillaries. A summary of these mediators are presented in Table 1-4. These include MDGFs, PDGFs, lactic acid, and fibroblast growth factor. Some of these mediators are produced during the inflammatory phase and serve as an essential transitional connection or link between the inflammatory and proliferative phases.

Table 1-4

SIGNALING MOLECULES: GROWTH FACTORS

GROWTH FACTORS

- Which cell produces them?
- Primary activity
- May have nomenclature based on the initial cell from which they were isolated

FACTOR	PRINCIPAL SOURCE	PRIMARY ACTIVITY	COMMENTS
EGF	Submaxillary gland, Brunner's gland, platelets, and macrophage	Promotes proliferation of fibroblast, keratinocyte, and epithelial cells in wound healing.	EGF-R (epidermal growth factor receptor) protein is involved in cell signaling pathways that control division and survival.
Fibroblast growth factor (FGF)	Wide range of cells including fibroblast, macrophage, mast cells, and endothelial cells Protein is associated with the ECM	Fibroblast proliferation. Chemotactic for fibroblasts. Mitogenic for fibroblasts and keratinocytes. Stimulates keratinocyte migration, angiogenesis, wound contraction, and matrix deposition.	Family of at least 18 family members, using distinct cell receptors. FGF family has diverse roles in regulating cell proliferation, migration, and differentiation.
Insulin growth factor (IGF-1 and IGF-2)	Macrophages and fibroblasts	Stimulates synthesis of sulfated PGs, collagen, keratinocyte migration, and fibroblast proliferation. Endocrine effects are similar to those of growth hormone. Promotes cell proliferation related to IGF-2 and proinsulin, also called *somatomedin C.*	IGF-1 and IGF-2 manage the effects of growth hormone. When IGF-1 and IGF-2 are disregulated they are associated with cancer and other proliferative diseases.
Keratinocyte growth factor	Fibroblasts	Stimulates keratinocyte migration, proliferation, and differentiation.	KGF-2 is also known as FGF-10.
PDGF	Platelets, endothelial cells, macrophage, keratinocytes, and placenta	Promotes proliferation of connective tissue and smooth muscle cells. Chemotactic for monocytes, PMNs, and fibroblasts. Activates PMNs, macrophages, and fibroblasts. Neoangiogenesis: mitogenic for fibroblasts and endothelial cells. Wound remodeling: stimulates production of MMPs, fibronectin, and hyaluronic acid.	X-ray crystal structure is very similar to that of VEGF.[76,77] Two different protein chains that form 3 distinct dimers: AA, AB, BB. SMALL molecule PDGF is active during the initial stages of hemostasis, whereas LARGE molecule PDGF is activated during the later stages of proliferation and remodeling.

(continued)

Table 1-4 (continued)

SIGNALING MOLECULES: GROWTH FACTORS

FACTOR	PRINCIPAL SOURCE	PRIMARY ACTIVITY	COMMENTS
TGF-β	Activated Th1 cells (T-helper), NK cells, platelets, macrophages, keratinocytes, and fibroblasts Leukocytes and multiple lineages of stromal cells	Anti-inflammatory (suppresses cytokine production and class II MHC expression) and promotes wound healing. Chemotactic for PMNs, macrophages, lymphocytes, and fibroblasts. Inhibits macrophage and lymphocyte proliferation.[7] Stimulates TIMP synthesis, keratinocyte migration, angiogenesis, and fibroplasia. Inhibits production of MMPs and keratinocyte proliferation. Induces TGF-β production.	Highly pleiotropic. More than 100 different family members. Promotes differentiation of fibroblast in to myofibroblast.[10] Functions as a tumor suppressor. Participates in angiogenesis and wound healing. When not regulated, leads to fibrosis. TGF-B is anti-inflammatory and a master regulator of the immune system.
TGF-α	Occurs in transformed cells Macrophage, T-lymphocytes, and keratin	Important for normal wound healing. Activates epithelial cell, facilitates epithelial proliferation, growth, and differentiation.	Related to EGF. In patients with systemic lupus erythromatosis, TNF-a is proinflammatory and TNF-b is anti-inflammatory.
VEGF	Keratinocytes	Increases vasopermeability, mitogenic for endothelial cells.	Angiogenesis. Neovascularization.

PATIENT INTERVENTION

In recent years, the identification of numerous cytokines and growth factors has led to several important discoveries and potential new treatment lines.[204,210-217] The effect of various therapies on the cytokine cascades is becoming more obvious with the increasing volume of research in this field.

If the tissue repair process is slowed, stalled, or delayed, the goal is to redirect tissues to the normal cascade sequence as supported by evidence-based intervention. For example, if the patient is having difficulty clearing the bacterial invader as part of the inflammatory response, the addition of antimicrobial dressings (eg, silver, iodine, hydrofera blue) can favorably alter the wound environment assisting with eradication of the bacterial invaders and allowing the patient to focus on moving forward through angiogenesis to proliferation. Mechanical irritation, thermal or chemical insult, and a wide variety of immune responses are some of the alternative initiators. For a wide range of patients experiencing an inflammatory response in the musculoskeletal tissues, these are commonly seen in the clinic; a brief summary is provided in Table 1-5.[218]

Granulation tissue invasion follows the demolition phase when autolytic or proteolytic enzymes are released from various cell types. The release and activation of these MMPs serve to liquefy the cellular environment, facilitating the movement and migration of cells. This includes the activation of fibroblasts and endothelial cells responsible for capillary budding. The combination of capillary budding and collagen production results in a site of hypervascularization. Initially, fibroblasts predominantly produce type III collagen, which will be replaced by type I collagen as the repair matures during remodeling. Fibroblasts also produce fibronectins and PGs, which are essential components of the ground substance (see Figure 1-5). Fibroblasts, activated by a variety of chemical mediators, alter their phenotype to become myofibroblasts and are responsible for full-thickness wound contraction and the early strength of the repair. Their ability to approximate the edges of the wound reduces the size of the final scar.[219-221]

Table 1-5

EFFECT OF MODALITIES ON HEALING

EXERCISE AND MECHANICAL STRESS

- Calatroni et al[399]—link between exercise and plasma GAG levels.[48-50]

- Heinemeier et al[400]—mechanical loading of tendon and muscle induces collagen expression, supporting a role for TGFβ-1 and IGF-1 as mediators.

- Hirose et al[401]—link between mechanical unloading and an increase in TNFα production with an associated decrease in type I collagen α-chain.[3]

- Kjaer[402]—extracellular matrix adaptation in tendon and skeletal muscle is depleted with unloading.

- Pedersen et al[403]—muscle disuse leads to IL-6 resistance with elevated circulating levels of IL-6, paralleling insulin resistance that is accompanied by hyperinsulinemia and leptin resistance.

- Jun Seok et al[404]—exercised induced myokines (IL-6, IL-15) play an anti-inflammatory role by inhibiting TNF-α and IL-15 may be important for modulation of glucose uptake/glucose tolerance.

- D'Urso[405]—mechanotransduction stimuli generates changes in cell phenotype and chemical signals (COX-2, IL-1β PGE-2, IL-8, physiological tissue regeneration and pathological fibrotic response.

ULTRASOUND (LOW-INTENSITY PULSED ULTRASOUND AND TRADITIONAL)

- Khanna et al[406]—LIPUS and a range of cytokine actions that promote healing in bone, cartilage, and intervertebral disk.

- Tsai et al[407]—ultrasound stimulates expression of type I and type III collagen likely mediated by the upregulation of TGF-β and is dose-dependent.

- Tsai et al[408]—dose-dependent increase in the cellularity of tendon cells by either, pulsed or continuous mode ultrasound mediated by upregulation of proliferating cell nuclear antigen (PCNA).

- Yeung[409]—increased tensile tendon strength with more regularly aligned and denser collagen fibers.

- Rego[410]—regenerative response ultrasound induced PGE2 production and COX-2 mRNA expression; having a positive effect on bone mineralization/cementum repair.

- Jung[411]—focused low intensity pulsed ultrasound (FLIPUS) aides in the healing of bone defects.

- Jia[412]—FLIPUS significantly increased ECM production mainly through decreasing cell apoptosis and lowering inflammatory mediators including nitric oxide (NO).

- Zhang[413]—LIPUS has positive osteogenic differentiation effects mediated through human adipose-derived stem cells (hASC) specifically up-regulating the protein levels of heat shock proteins (HSP70, HSP90) bone morphogenetic proteins (BMP-2 and BMP-7) in the hASCs.

(continued)

Granulation tissue matures with lymphatic development (in much the same way as capillary development), nerve fiber ingrowth, and mast cell invasion. Collagen fibers are oriented in response to local stress, thus providing tensile strength in parallel direction to the force vectors applied. As the granulation tissue matures, there is a process of devascularization with obliteration of the lumen of the vessels.[119,222-240]

Remodeling Phase: Overview

The remodeling phase (Figure 1-13) is an often-overlooked phase of repair in terms of its importance, especially in the context of therapy and rehabilitation. It is neither swift nor highly reactive, but does result in an organized, quality, and functional scar, which is capable of behaving in a similar way to the parent tissue (that which it is repairing or replacing). The remodeling phase has been widely quoted as starting at around the same time as the peak of the proliferative phase (2 to 3 weeks postinjury), but more recent evidence would support the proposal that the remodeling phase actually starts rather earlier than this, and it would be reasonable to consider the start point to be in the first week.[62,241]

Table 1-5 (continued)

EFFECT OF MODALITIES ON HEALING

LASER

- Bjordal[414]—LASER therapy reduced inflammatory musculoskeletal pain through reduction of PGE2.

- Laraia[415]—low level LASER therapy (LLLT) is an important modulator of inflammatory cytokines likely mediated through IL-10.

- Oliveira[416]—LLLT effectively reduces pulmonary inflammation in both pulmonary and extrapulmonary model of LPS-induced ARDS, decreasing inflammatory cytokines (IL-1β, IL-6 and TNF-α).

- Saygun et al[417]—LLLT increases the proliferation of osteoblast cells and stimulates the release of bFGF, IGF-I, and IGFBP3 from these cells. Biostimulatory effect of LLLT may be related to the enhanced production of the growth factors.

- Manoela[418]—LLLT resulted in higher expression of VEGF, increased levels of PMNs and mast cells with vasodilation.

OTHER THERAPIES

- Sakurai[419]—exposure to high magnetic field gradients induces secretion of PGE2 and COX-2 protein expression, mediated through nuclear factor kappa B (NF-κB) promoting osteoblast differentiation.

- Patruno[420]—extremely low frequency (ELF) electromagnetic fields (EMF) exposure enhanced keratinocyte proliferation and early NOS activities, decreases COX-2, PGE2 levels and O2, and induces activator protein-1 (AP-1) activation and nuclear translocation potentially elucidating a role of ELF-EMF in wound healing.

Remodeling Events

The remodeling phase primarily involves the refinement of the collagen and its associated ECM. The initial deposition of collagen produces relatively weak fibrils with random orientation with maturity; the collagen becomes more obviously oriented in line with local stresses. A proportion of the original fine (type III) collagen is reabsorbed (due to the action of collagenases) and is replaced with type I collagen with more cross-links and greater tensile strength. Collagen synthesis and lysis both occur at a greater rate in a normal wound compared with nonwounded tissue as old fibrous tissue is removed and new scar tissue is laid down. The maturing scar is, therefore, a dynamic system rather than a static one.

There are several influential factors during this long phase, including physical stress. This remodeling process is initiated during the proliferative stage proceeds, therefore providing a considerable overlap between the phases. Final remodeling will continue for months, and typically last for at least 1 year from the initial damage. The mechanism by which physical stress can influence cell and tissue behavior is elucidated by more recent papers linking mechanical stress and tissue repair. The strength of the final repair will not correlate to the preinjury strength.[155,242-246]

Arbitrarily, the factors known to delay healing are divided into general systemic and local.

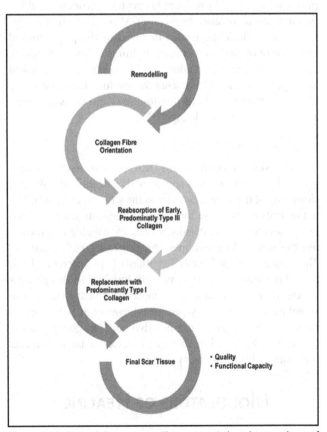

Figure 1-13. Remodeling process: This process is largely a resultant of the conversion of mechanical stress/force to specific cell signaling, which directs the changes in tissue, causing the move from immature collagen to mature tissue.

General Factors

- Age
- Protein deficiency
- Low vitamin C levels
- Steroids and nonsteroidal anti-inflammatory drugs (NSAIDs; inhibitory effect)
- Temperature (lower rate when colder)

Local Factors

- Poor blood supply/ischemia
- Adhesion to bone or other underlying tissue
- Prolonged inflammation
- Drying of the wound
- Excessive movement or mechanical stress (restarts inflammation)

Remodeling Responses

The histopathological process as the basis of the clinical manifestations of tendinopathy then can be viewed as a failure of cell matrix adaptation to a variety of stresses, due to an imbalance between matrix degeneration and synthesis.[102] Remodeling plays an important role in responding to microtrauma from repetitive loading. This repair mechanism is probably mediated by resident fibrocytes or tenocytes, which maintain a fine balance between ECM production and degradation. Remodeling is also involved in the physiological response of tendon to resistance training. In such situations, modeling adapts the tendon to the repetitive mechanical loads placed on it and prevents the tendons from incurring injuries. An increase in the tendon mass and cross-sectional area occurs during modeling.[245,246]

Regeneration

The skin is continuously regenerating itself through synthesis of new keratinocytes in the stratum basale and sloughing of the corneocytes from the stratum corneum. The major cells responsible for skin regeneration are the fibroblasts, located in the dermis, which are capable of producing the remodeling enzymes (eg, proteases, collagenases).[1] The collagen needed for cell synthesis is produced by both fibroblasts and myofibroblasts. Cells involved in this process are discussed in detail in this chapter as well as many of the signaling molecules they produce; however, it is important to realize that regeneration is a dynamic, on-going process that can be inhibited by disease processes or facilitated and upregulated by tissue injury.[178,247-251]

Modulators of Healing

Scarring

MMPs are important regulators of ECM remodeling, and their levels are altered during tendon healing.[70] In a rat flexor tendon laceration model, the expression of MMPs including MMP-9 and MMP-13 (collagenase-3) peaked between day 7 and 14. MMP-2, MMP-3, and MMP-14 (MT1-MMP) levels increased after surgery and remained high until day 28.[103] These findings suggest that MMP-9 and MMP-13 participate only in collagen degradation, whereas MMP-2, MMP-3, and MMP-14 participate in both collagen degradation and collagen remodeling. As mentioned earlier, wounding, trauma, and inflammation also provoke the release of growth factors and cytokines from platelets, PMNs, macrophages, and other inflammatory cells. These growth factors induce neovascularization and chemotaxis of fibroblasts and tenocytes and stimulate fibroblast and tenocyte proliferation and the associated synthesis of collagen.

Another signaling molecule, nitric oxide, a short-lived free radical with many biological functions. It is bactericidal, can induce apoptosis in inflammatory cells, and facilitate angiogenesis and vasodilation. Nitric oxide may play a role in several aspects of integumentary, ligamentous, or tendon healing. Nitric oxide synthase is responsible for synthesizing nitric oxide from L-arginine. Experimental studies have shown that levels of nitric oxide synthase peak after 7 days and return to baseline 14 days after tenotomy of rat Achilles tendons.[108] Inhibition of nitric oxide synthase reduced healing and resulted in decreased cross-sectional area as well as a decrease in the amount of load required to produce failure. In this study, the specific isoforms of nitric oxide synthase were not identified. However, more recently, the same group demonstrated a temporal expression of the 3 isoforms of nitric oxide synthase.[109] The inducible isoform peaks at day 4, the endothelial isoform peaks at day 7, and the neuronal isoform peaks at day 21. Interestingly, in a rat Achilles tendon rupture model, peak nerve fiber formation occurred between weeks 2 and 6, in concert with peak levels of the neuronal isoform of nitric oxide synthase.[110] These nerve fibers presumably deliver neuropeptides, which act as chemical messengers and regulators, and may play an important role in tendon healing and fiber directionality. Substance P and calcitonin gene-related peptide (CGRP) are both proinflammatory and cause vasodilation with protein extravasation. In addition, Substance P enhances cellular release of prostaglandins, histamines, and cytokines. Peak levels of substance P and CGRP occur during the proliferative phase, suggesting a possible role during this phase.[252-256]

Cell Signaling in Integumentary Repair and Regeneration

Tissue adaptation of the ECM, ligament, and tendon tissue occurs in response to mechanical loading or trauma. Figure 1-14 demonstrates the organization or the lack of organization that results from either appropriate tissue load or complete disarray with lack of tension and force.

Tissue healing (or *tissue repair*) refers to the body's replacement of injured, damaged, or destroyed tissue by living tissue. The process of healing can occur by 2 distinct pathways: regeneration or repair. The difference between the 2

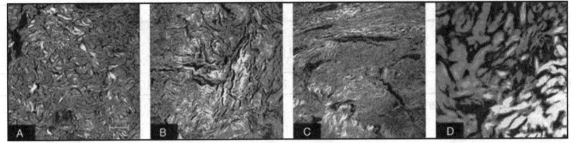

Figure 1-14. Aspect of the collagen architecture in normal skin and different scars by confocal microscopy. (A) Normal skin, (B) normotrophic scar, (C) hypertrophic scar, and (D) keloidal scar. The scale bar in (A) represents 100 μm and is also applicable to (B-D). (Reproduced with permission from Verhaegen PDHM, Van Zuijlen PPM, Pennings NM, et al. Differences in collagen architecture between keloid, hypertrophic scar, normotrophic scar, and normal skin: an objective histopathological analysis. *Wound Repair Regen.* 2009;17[5]:649-656. doi:10.1111/j.1524-475X.2009.00533.x)

pathways is identified by the tissue type produced as the end result. In regeneration, specialized tissues are replaced by the proliferation of surrounding undamaged specialized cells of the same type. Regeneration is the preferred pathway as the end result is the most similar in construct to the original tissues, both in function and structure.[109,247,257-273]

In repair, lost tissue is replaced by granulation tissue, which matures to form scar tissue that is different than the original tissue type. The advent of stem cell–based therapy in this field has seen the manifestation of the possibility of regeneration of the damaged tissue, which is clinically preferable. An example of this is seen in the treatment of large total body surface area burns that are now treated with the use of cultured epidermal autograft. The cultured epidermal autograft is grown in the lab and returned for patient application, approximately 6 weeks after collection of approximately 2 to 4 cm² of nonwounded epidermis. This technology has now moved regeneration from the laboratory bench to the bedside, a step forward in treatment.[109,247,257-285]

In the last 2 to 5 years advances in stem cell research have led to promising stem cell–based therapies for cartilage repair.[286,287] Mesenchymal stem cells (MSCs) are not always optimal for cartilage repair and they are limited by the local resident cells capacity for self-renewal, differentiation, proliferation, and maturation. Furthermore, increased understanding into the cellular attributes of human pluripotent stem cells and their mechanisms of extracellular communication via exosomes has opened an entirely new branch of study, that of extracellular secretory vesicles. Human pluripotent stem cells and their efficacy has been largely attributed to their paracrine secretion of trophic factors, exosomes, which are now known to be cell-secreted, bilipid membrane nanosized vesicles of 30 to 100 nm.[287-291] Zhang et al[290,291] have demonstrated the effect of MSC exosomes in a murine model in which the contralateral extremity served as the control over 12 weeks. Bilateral insults to the distal femoral chondral bone were made, the control side injected with phosphate buffered saline, while the experimental extremity was injected with MSC exosomes. After 12 weeks, the extremities were examined histopathologically. The experimental MSC exosome demonstrated complete restoration of cartilage and subchondral bone with hyaline cartilage and good surface continuity, including bonding to the adjacent cartilage and ECM.[290,291]

The importance of traditional therapy in conjunction with the cutting edge novel application of regenerative medicine will be revealed over time.

The Pathophysiology of Ligament and Tendon Injury

Tendon injuries can be acute or chronic and are caused by intrinsic or extrinsic factors, either alone or in combination. In acute trauma, extrinsic factors predominate, whereas in chronic cases, intrinsic factors also play a role. Ligament and tendon disorders are frequent and are responsible for a significant amount of morbidity both in sport and the workplace (Table 1-6).[292] Although the presence of degenerative changes does not always lead to symptoms, preexisting degeneration has been implicated as a risk factor for acute tendon or ligament injury and/or rupture. The term *tendinopathy* is a generic descriptor of the clinical conditions in and around tendons arising from repetitive trauma or overuse (Figure 1-15). The terms *tendinosis* and *tendinitis/tendonitis* should only be used after histopathological examination. In tendinopathy, healing is disorganized at best, and inflammation is usually absent. In acute injuries, the process of tendon healing is an indivisible process that can be categorized into overlapping phases, just as healing of the epithelium is described in wounding. Tendon healing can occur intrinsically, via proliferation of epitenon and endotenon tenocytes, or extrinsically, by invasion of cells from the surrounding sheath and synovium. Despite the induced repair or remodeling, the biochemical and mechanical properties of the repaired or healed ligament or tendon tissue never exactly match those of an intact, uninjured tendon. This is consistent with observations in wounding/repair of skin as well.[157,293-303]

Table 1-6

EFFECT OF MODALITIES ON HEALING

RISK FACTOR	POSSIBLE INTERVENTION
• Overuse and lack of recovery time (eg, hours of typing per day, per week, and per month as well as number of breaks per day)	• Preventative exercise program including stretching and ergonomics
• Genetics (eg, anything that makes the tendons more prone to injury, such as a higher initial type III/type I collagen ratio in the tendons or genetic defects in collagen)	• Early intervention • Joint protection • Dynamic and static splinting
• Ergonomics associated with repetitive motion activity (eg, awkward position, tools that cause vibration, improperly fitted tools or sports equipment, poor technique)	• Evaluate ergonomics and realign • On-site job evaluation • Use of protective equipment (antivibration gloves)
• Quality of medical care/advice that is received	• Comprehensive care, evaluation of the likely healing phase that the patient is experiencing
• Length of time the condition persists before the person seeks help and limits or corrects the activities that cause pain (this is often influenced by the person's awareness of RSI and the pressure the person feels to continue the injurious activity)	• Patient education • Splinting • Modified activities
• Age, level of fitness, and general health (chronic tendon degeneration is more common with age, with obesity and diabetes, and with poor fitness)	• Patient education • Nutritional consult • Lifestyle change incorporating nontraumatic aerobic exercise including aquatic therapy, pilates, or yoga

Figure 1-15. Structure of tendon tissue. Sections of tendon tissue. Top left: A transverse section of a tendon stained with hematoxylin and eosin. In the center of the section a fascicle with fibroblasts is seen surrounded by loose connective tissue endotenon (arrow). Top right: A confocal laser-scanning microscopy image of a transverse tendon section. High power view of a 3-dimensional reconstruction shows adjacent fibroblasts within a fascicle. It is notable that the cells have sheet-like processes toward each other. Bottom left and right: Transverse and longitudinal section, respectively, of a tendon stained with immunofluorescence labeling for the gap junction protein, connexin[43] (indicated by arrows on the longitudinal view, bottom right). Sections are counterstained with propidium iodide to indilsecate fibroblast nuclei. This indicates the gap junction coupling between tendon fibroblasts and supports the view of a communicative network of tendon cells. (Modified from Benjamin and co-workers and personal communication with M. Benjamin.) (Reproduced with permission from Kjær M. Role of extracellular matrix in adaptation of tendon and skeletal muscle to mechanical loading. *Physiol Rev.* 2004;84[2]:649-698.)

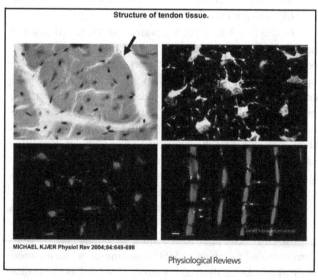

Structure of tendon tissue.

MICHAEL KJÆR Physiol Rev 2004;84:649-698

Physiological Reviews

Exploration of connective tissue in terms of basic cell biology is continuously being advanced (Figure 1-16). The addition of many of the relatively new tools in microbiology have increased understanding and elucidation of cellular biology for practitioners. Ideally, with the elucidation of cellular biology, clinicians will have increased insight and develop additional tools for successful management of ECM, epithelial, tendon, and ligament injury in the context of both function and cell science.

Understanding interaction between intrinsic and extrinsic factors is paramount. Intrinsic factors including histology, alignment, and biomechanical faults are reported as

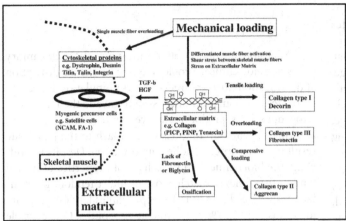

Figure 1-16. Intense loading of skeletal muscle and adaptive responses in ECM. Hypothetical interaction between ECM, cytoskeletal proteins, and skeletal muscle fibers in response to eccentric loading of the contracting musculature, whether they are trained or untrained. (FA-1 = fetal antigen-1; NCAM = neural cell adhesion molecule; PICP = procollagen type I C-terminal propeptide; PINP = procollagen 1 N-terminal propeptide.) (Reproduced with permission from Kjær M. Role of extracellular matrix in adaptation of tendon and skeletal muscle to mechanical loading. *Physiol Rev.* 2004;84[2]:649-698.)

causative factors in more than two-thirds of athletes with Achilles tendon disorders.[57] In particular, hyperpronation of the foot has been linked with an increased incidence of Achilles tendinopathy.[58] Excessive loading of tendons during vigorous physical training is hypothesized to be one of the primary pathological stimuli responsible for the initiation of a degeneration trajectory.[59] In the presence of intrinsic risk factors, excessive loading may carry a greater risk of inducing tendinopathy. Tendons respond to repetitive overload beyond physiological threshold by one of two mechanisms: (1) sheath inflammation or (2) degeneration of their body, or in some instances a combination of both.[60] Variation in stress or load appears to induce different responses. Damage due to fatigue weakens and eventually predisposes tendons and ligaments to rupture.[61] Tenocytes/fibroblasts and macrophages in residence within tendons, precisely balance ECM production and degradation, a state now known as *ECM dynamic reciprocity*. Tendon damage may result from stresses that are accepted as normal (those within the physiological boundaries). It is hypothesized that frequent microtrauma, within the bounds of normal forces, accumulates in the absence of sufficient time for repair. Microtrauma can also result from nonuniform stress within tendons, producing abnormal load concentrations and frictional forces between the fibrils, resulting in localized fiber damage. The etiology of tendinopathy remains unclear and many causes have been theorized. Hypoxia, ischemic damage, oxidative stress, hyperthermia, impaired apoptosis, inflammatory mediators, fluoroquinolones, and matrix metalloproteinase imbalance have all been implicated as mechanisms of tendon degeneration. Tendinopathy histology studies demonstrate disordered and haphazard collagen, evidence of the ongoing insufficient healing response. Inflammatory cells, including macrophage, are absent. The absence of these cells sets the stage for an insufficient healing response, including collagen degeneration, fiber disorientation, and overproduction of proteases resulting in thinning of existing tissues. This hypocellularity exists within a matrix of scattered and porous capillary growth and is combined with increased interfibrillar GAGs.[12] Macroscopically, the affected portions of the tendon lose their normal glistening white appearance

and become stringy, grey-brown, and amorphous.[287-297] "Tendinosis is often clinically silent, and its only manifestation may be a rupture, but it may also co-exist with symptomatic paratendinopathy."[157]

Tendon Rupture

The etiology of tendon rupture remains unclear.[10] Degenerative tendinopathy is the most common histological finding in spontaneous tendon ruptures. Garner and Whalen[304] first reported degenerative changes in all their patients with Achilles tendon rupture and hypothesized that these changes were due to intrinsic abnormalities present before the rupture.[157]

Tendon rupture is generally recognized as an acute injury, a result of the dominant extrinsic forces imposed. Achilles tendon rupture via an acceleration/deceleration mechanism has been reported in up to 90% of sports-related injuries. Malfunction of the normal protective inhibitory pathway of the musculotendinous unit may result in injury.

Kannus and Jozsa found degenerative changes in 865 of 891 (97%) spontaneous tendon ruptures, whilst degenerative changes were only seen in 149 of 445 (34%) of control tendons.[311] Tendon degeneration may lead to reduced tensile strength and a predisposition to rupture. Indeed, ruptured Achilles tendons have a histological picture of greater degeneration than chronic painful tendons from overuse injuries.[305-314]

Tendon Healing Following Acute Injuries

Tendon healing studies have predominantly been performed on transected animal tendons or ruptured human tendons, and their relevance to human tendinopathy with its associated healing failure response remains unclear. Tendon healing occurs in 3 overlapping phases. In the initial inflammatory phase, erythrocytes and inflammatory cells, particularly neutrophils, enter the site of injury. In the first 24 hours, monocytes and macrophages predominate, and phagocytosis of necrotic materials occurs. Vasoactive and chemotactic factors are released with increased vascular permeability, initiation of angiogenesis, stimulation of tenocyte proliferation, and recruitment of more inflammatory cells.[86] Tenocytes gradually migrate to the wound and type III collagen synthesis is initiated.[87] After a few days, the remodeling stage begins. Synthesis of type III collagen peaks during this stage, which lasts for a few weeks. Water content and GAG concentrations remain high during this stage.[87] After approximately 6 weeks, the modeling stage commences. During this stage, the healing tissue is resized and reshaped. A corresponding decrease in cellularity, collagen, and GAG synthesis occurs.

The modeling phase can be divided into consolidation and maturation stages. The consolidation stage commences at about 6 weeks and continues up to 10 weeks. In this period, the repair tissue changes from cellular to fibrous. Tenocyte metabolism remains high during this period, and tenocytes and collagen fibers become aligned in the direction of stress. A higher proportion of type I collagen is synthesized during this stage.[90] After 10 weeks, the maturation stage occurs, with gradual change of fibrous tissue to scar-like tendon tissue over the course of 1 year. During the latter half of this stage, tenocyte metabolism and tendon vascularity decline.[91] Tendon healing can occur intrinsically, via proliferation of epitenon and endotenon tenocytes, or extrinsically, by invasion of cells from the surrounding sheath and synovium. Epitenon tenoblasts initiate the repair process through proliferation and migration. Healing in severed tendons can be performed by cells from the epitenon alone, without relying on adhesions for vascularity or cellular support. Internal tenocytes contribute to the intrinsic repair process and secrete larger and more mature collagen than epitenon cells. Despite this, fibroblasts in the epitenon and tenocytes synthesize collagen during repair, and different cells probably produce different collagen types at different time points. Initially, collagen is produced by epitenon cells, with endotenon cells later synthesizing collagen. The relative contribution of each cell type may be influenced by the type of trauma sustained, anatomical position, presence of a synovial sheath, and the amount of stress induced by motion after repair has taken place. Tenocyte function may vary depending on the region of origin. Cells from the tendon sheath produce less collagen and GAG compared to epitenon and endotenon cells. However, fibroblasts from the flexor tendon sheath proliferate more rapidly. The variation in phenotypic expression of tenocytes has not been extensively investigated, and this information may prove useful for optimizing repair strategies. Intrinsic healing results in improved biomechanics and fewer complications. In particular, a normal gliding mechanism within the tendon sheath is preserved. In extrinsic healing, scar tissue results in adhesion formation, which disrupts tendon gliding. Different healing patterns may predominate in particular locations; for example, extrinsic healing tends to prevail in torn rotator cuffs.[263,305,306,312,313,315-317]

Limitations of Healing in Acute Tendon Injuries

Adhesion formation after intrasynovial tendon injury poses a major clinical problem. Synovial sheath disruption at the time of injury or surgery allows granulation tissue and tenocytes from surrounding tissue to invade the repair site. Exogenous cells predominate over endogenous tenocytes, allowing the surrounding tissues to attach to the repair site resulting in detrimental adhesion formation. Despite remodeling, the biochemical and mechanical properties of healed tendon tissue never match those of intact tendon. In spontaneously healed transected sheep Achilles tendons, rupture force was only 56.7% of normal at 12 months. One possible reason for this may be the absence of mechanical loading during the period of immobilization.[263,305,306,312,313,315-317]

Abnormal Collagen in Tendinosis/Tendinopathy

Normal tendons and ligaments consist mostly of type I collagen, with smaller amounts of type III collagen. When tendinosis develops some of the collagen is injured and undergoes remodeling and degrades. In chronic tendinosis, the body does not properly repair the ECM or collagens.

Tendinosis/tendinopathy injuries are not readily apparent from the outside, looking in. Swelling, heat, and redness are all symptoms of acute injury. However, chronic injury does not display any of these hallmarks of injury. Kjaer et al depicts the histology of the difference observed by the naked eye during surgery and microscopically.[91] The tissue that is injured appears dull, instead of glistening and white, and boggy as opposed to firm. Histologically, further analysis sheds light on the changes seen in chronically injured and inflamed tissue. In the example of patellar tendinopathy, there is an absence of cellular organization and absence of senescence of cells, resulting in poor and incomplete healing.[318-322]

Research has shown that chronic overuse injuries such as tendinosis (eg, Achilles, rotator cuff, lateral and medial elbow, posterior tibial, digital flexor, patellar), as well as carpal tunnel syndrome, and even temporomandibular joint disorders are associated with a failed healing response in which the body's fibroblasts produce abnormal tendon and ligament collagen. The composition and structure of the collagen is abnormal compared to uninjured tendon and ligament tissue. The following differences have been observed:

- The total amount of collagen is decreased (since breakdown exceeds repair).
- The amounts of PGs and GAGs are increased (possibly in response to increased compressive forces associated with the repetitive motion).
- The ratio of type III to type I collagen is abnormally high.
- The normal parallel bundled fiber structure is disturbed; the continuity of the collagen is lost with disorganized fiber structure and evidence of both collagen repair and collagen degeneration.

- Microtears and collagen fiber separations are seen. Many of the collagen fibers are thin, fragile, and separated from each other.

- The number of fibroblast cells is increased; the tenocytes look different, with a more blast-like morphology (the cells look thicker, less linear). These differences show that the cells are actively trying to repair the tissue.

- The vascularity is increased.

- Early studies found that inflammatory cells were not usually seen in the tendon but were sometimes seen in the synovium and peritendinous structures (the areas around the tendon). More recent studies have found some inflammatory cells in the tendon.

- Electronic microscopic observations have shown alterations in the size and shape of mitochondria in the nuclei of the tenocytes.

All of these changes have all been observed in tendon samples taken from sites of tendinosis. Researchers have also taken tenocytes (the tendon cells that make new collagen) from sites of tendinosis and cultured them. Astoundingly, the tenocytes removed from the tendinosis sites and cultured from tendinosis *continue* to produce abnormal collagen outside of the body. In addition, the tenocytes produced collagen with an abnormally high type III to type I ratios (as compared to collagen produced by tenocytes cultured from normal tendon). This is quite significant, as it demonstrates that the phenotype of the tenocytes has been altered. The tenocytes no longer produce normal collagen in the normal ratios with type I in higher concentration than type III. Instead, the altered phenotype tenocytes continue to produce abnormal collagen even when the repetitive motion is no longer present.[93,300,302,323-364]

Tendons and ligaments are similar structures; tendons connect muscle to bone, and ligaments connect bone to bone. Ligaments, as well as tendons, can develop chronic overuse injuries of failed healing. Ligaments injured through overuse show a similar kind of abnormal appearance under the microscope as tendons with tendinosis. One study showed that cells from the flexor retinaculum ligament of patients with carpal tunnel syndrome made collagen with an abnormally high type III to type I ratio just as has been observed with cells from tendons of patients with tendinosis. The carpal tunnel study also found that the injured ligament cells made collagen with a higher than normal ratio of alpha2(I) to alpha1.[318-322]

The Tendinosis Cycle

The tendinosis cycle begins when the state of dynamic reciprocity is disrupted; breakdown exceeds repair. Repetitive motion causes microinjuries that accumulate with time. Collagen breaks down and the tendon attempts to repair itself, but the cells produce new collagen with an abnormal structure and composition.

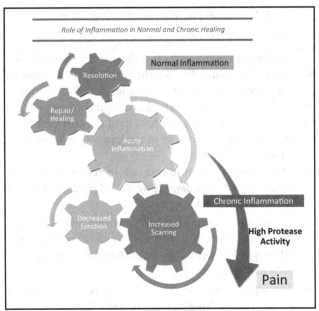

Figure 1-17. Normal vs abnormal inflammation and the resulting effects of high protease activity.

The new collagen has an abnormally high type III to type I ratio. Experiments show that the excess type III collagen at the expense of type I collagen weakens a tendon, making it prone to further degradation and injury. Part of the problem is the lack of collagen cross linking. The new collagen fibers are less organized into the normal parallel structure, making the tendon less able to withstand tensile stress along the direction of the tendon.[93,299,333-336,365-367]

Therefore, tendinosis is a slow accumulation of minor injuries that do not undergo proper repair and as a result leave the tendon vulnerable to yet more significant injury. This failed healing process is the reason many people with tendinosis do not completely heal. Moreover, they are unable to return to their previous level of activity. Once the tendinosis cycle starts, the tendon rarely heals back to its preinjury state.

Although rest is an essential part of the healing process for tendinosis, too much rest causes deconditioning of muscles and tendons. The weaker muscles and tendons leave the area more vulnerable to injury. Thus, the area becomes weaker on a large scale as well as on a cellular scale. This cycle of injury/rest/deconditioning/more injury can be difficult to break. Gradual, careful physical therapy exercises can help.

The pain from tendinosis probably comes partly from the physical injury itself (separation of collagen fibers and mechanical disruption of tissue) and partly from irritating biochemical substances that are produced as part of the injury process (Figure 1-17). The biochemical substances could irritate the pain receptors in the tendon and surrounding area. NSAIDs and cortisone injections may reduce the pain of tendinosis by reducing or blocking these biochemical substances and by interrupting any low-level inflammation.[295,297,301,302,336,368-372]

Risk Factors for Tendinosis and Tendinopathy

Tendinosis/tendinopathy is a chronic degenerative tendon injury that is usually brought on by repetitive motion. The repetitive motion is often associated with activities in the workplace or with sports. Microinjuries gradually accumulate faster than they can heal until the area eventually becomes painful. The severity of the injury is influenced by many factors, including:

- The amount of overuse and lack of recovery time (eg, hours of typing per day, per week, and per month as well as number of breaks per day)

- The person's genetics (eg, anything that makes the tendons more prone to injury, such as a higher initial type III to type I collagen ratio in the tendons or genetic defects in collagen)

- The ergonomics associated with the repetitive motion activity (eg, awkward position, tools that cause vibration, improperly fitted tools or sports equipment, poor technique)

- The person's age, level of fitness, and general health (chronic tendon degeneration is more common with age, with obesity and diabetes, and with poor fitness)

- The length of time the condition persists before the person seeks help and limits the activities that cause pain (this is often influenced by the person's awareness of RSI and the pressure the person feels to continue the injurious activity)

- The quality of medical care/advice that is received

People seem to vary in their susceptibility to tendinosis. Many people go through their entire lives without ever experiencing tendinosis. Some people experience mild tendon problems but recover. Others get chronic tendinosis from obvious overuse such as typing or sports. A few unlucky people get chronic tendon injuries in multiple places of the body, sometimes without obvious overuse. Dr. Leadbetter refers to this propensity for tendinosis as *mesenchymal syndrome*.[309] Even given the same ergonomics, different people have different levels of activity that constitute injury-producing overuse; the line between use and overuse varies with genetics. Any genetic variant that causes tendons to be weaker or slower to heal could make people more susceptible to tendinosis. If the reasons for differences in susceptibility can be better understood and elucidated, improved treatments for tendinosis may soon become a reality.[309]

Some people carry a propensity for tendinosis to the extreme and develop soft tissue problems in so many places and with such severity that it prevents them from leading a normal life. If a patient falls into this category, they may well have something systemic going on affecting the whole body, rather than simply a number of individual injuries to multiple body parts. They may need to be evaluated by a physician to rule out pathologies like autoimmune diseases and fibromyalgia.

POSSIBLE REASONS FOR THE FAILED HEALING

This list gives some of the possible explanations researchers have suggested for the abnormal collagen production associated with chronic overuse injuries. These 4 factors (the poor healing capacity of tendon, genetic variants in collagen, long-term exposure to growth factors, and abnormal levels of proteolytic enzymes) are just some of the possible reasons that have been suggested for the failed healing of collagen in tendinosis, but more research is needed to fully understand the tendinosis injury.

Tendon injuries give rise to substantial morbidity, and current understanding of the mechanisms involved in tendon injury and repair is limited. Further research is required to improve our knowledge of tendon healing. This will enable specific treatment strategies to be developed.

Poor Tendon Healing Capability and Changed Type I to III Collagen Ratio

Tendons and ligaments do not heal well, even when the injury does not become chronic. The strength of tendons and ligaments remains as much as 30% lower than normal, even months or years following an acute injury. Repair of acute injuries usually begins with the deposition of more type III collagen than type I collagen, and the site gradually returns to a more normal composition and structure with time. The site can have an abnormally high type III to type I collagen ratio even after a year and this abnormal collagen composition contributes to the weakness of the tissue. Possibly, some people with chronic injuries just never get past the initial phases of healing.

A team at the University of Glasgow (Glasgow, Scotland) is researching a possible way to correct the imbalance in types I and III collagen in tendinopathy. They discovered that a microRNA called *miR-29a* can up-regulate the production of type I collagen relative to type III to restore collagen to preinjury levels. Trials have been done in cultured cells and in mice, and horses will be next. One of their papers can be found here.[373]

Long-Term Exposure to Growth Factors

Another possible explanation for the abnormal collagen associated with chronic overuse injuries is that the fibroblasts could be damaged by long-term exposure to growth factors. The repetitive motion causes tissue breakdown, which stimulates growth factors to make repairs; if more injury is done before the repairs are complete, the tissue is continually exposed to growth factors for long periods of time. The repetitive motion itself could even stimulate production of growth factors. Some researchers suggest that this long exposure to growth factors could make the cells produce abnormal collagen and that this cell behavior can become permanent, even after the exposure to growth factors stops.[123,124,128,374,375]

In the previously mentioned study of carpal tunnel syndrome, cells were cultured from the wrist ligaments of injured patients and uninjured control patients.[91] The cells were exposed to 4 different growth factors, including TGF-β. The cells from injured patients produced abnormally high amounts of type III collagen and low amounts of type I collagen when exposed to the growth factors, as compared to cells from the control patients.[376]

The authors conclude that the cells in the injured patients had been altered by the injury so that the response to growth factors was different. They hypothesize that one explanation for this change in response to growth factors is the long exposure to growth factors while the injury was accumulating. Their study demonstrates that using growth factors to try to treat chronic overuse injuries is a tricky proposition because the growth factors could have different effects on the injured cells than you might expect based on their effects on healthy cells.

Growth factors have the potential to help tendons and ligaments heal, but sometimes they might actually hinder the process. More research is needed to sort out the effects of various growth factors and to investigate whether they can be used as treatments to promote collagen healing in tendinosis. One complication for this research is that growth factors can have completely different effects on cells in the body than on cells in the petri dish. Another complication is that many studies look at acute surgically-induced injuries rather than chronic overuse injuries, and the effects of growth factors could be very different in these 2 cases.

Genetic Variants in Collagen

Another possibility is that some people with chronic overuse injuries could have genetic differences that make their tendons and ligaments weaker and make them heal with abnormal collagen. Quite possibly, more than one genetic variant exists that causes tendons and ligaments to be prone to overuse injuries.

Many genetic collagen defects have already been discovered; some cause fairly rare collagen diseases, but some cause more common problems like osteoporosis, osteoarthritis, and vertebral disk herniations. A *colIA1* defect has been discovered to cause some cases of osteoporosis; the *colIA1* defect causes weaker type I collagen in the bones because of an abnormally high alpha1(I) to alpha2(I) ratio. A defect in type II collagen has been associated with osteoarthritis. A *colIXA2* defect is associated with an increased susceptibility to vertebral disk herniations (type IX collagen is found in small amounts in vertebral disks).[377-381]

The following list summarizes several observed collagen abnormalities that could contribute to the failed healing response of chronic overuse injuries. Perhaps we will soon discover the causes for these abnormalities.

Abnormal Alpha2(I) to Alpha1(I) Ratio

As mentioned earlier, one study found that the ligaments of carpal tunnel syndrome patients had abnormally high ratios of alpha2(I) to alpha1(I), just the opposite of the osteoporosis study. Perhaps people who are susceptible to carpal tunnel syndrome have a collagen defect that causes this abnormal ratio, or perhaps the repetitive motion itself somehow brings about the altered ratio. The end result is probably weaker, abnormal collagen that is more prone to overuse injuries like carpal tunnel syndrome.[48,382-384]

Abnormal Type III to Type I Ratio

The other collagen abnormality that has been associated with overuse injuries is a high type III to type I ratio. Perhaps some people have a genetic reason for a higher type III to type I collagen ratio in their tendons and ligaments, and this makes them more prone to chronic overuse injuries. Some studies have shown that people with chronic temporomandibular joint problems have higher than normal type III to type I collagen ratios in their skin, and these people are also more prone to tendon overuse problems in many areas of their bodies; a genetic variant in collagen seems a likely explanation for these observations.[385]

Gender may also play a role in connective tissue strength. Men seem less prone to chronic overuse injuries than women, and a few studies have found that men have higher total amounts of collagen in their tendons and lower type III to type I ratios. An abnormally high type III to type I ratio is a normal feature of the initial stages of tendon healing, but this ratio persists in tendinosis. If some people start out with higher than normal type III to type I ratios in their tendons because of a genetic difference, it would make them more prone to tendinosis because their tendons would be weaker. Once the tendinosis cycle starts, these people would develop even higher type III to type I ratios in the injured areas because that is how tendons heal. Perhaps these people develop more chronic cases of overuse injuries because they do not have any room to absorb the higher type III to type I ratio that automatically comes with injury. People with better initial type III to type I ratios might eventually heal to some threshold level that lets them function normally, but people with higher initial ratios might have a harder time reaching that threshold.[87,92,386,387]

Genetics will probably turn out to be an important piece of the tendinosis puzzle. Only one small study looked at the alpha2(I) to alpha1(I) ratio, so it might not be significant.[56,388,389] Many studies of all kinds of overuse injuries have observed the abnormally high type III to type I ratio so that observation is likely to be very significant.[87,387,390,391] Other collagen abnormalities might be discovered to be associated with overuse injuries as more research is done.

Abnormal Levels of Proteolytic Enzymes

Proteolytic enzymes are substances that help break down proteins; they are used to break down old tissue in order to repair it and also to break down new proteins in the various stages of building new collagen fibers. For example, enzymes are needed to remove the extra sequences at the ends of procollagen to make tropocollagen that can then assemble into types I, II, and III collagen fibers.

MMP-3, or stromelysin, is a proteolytic enzyme that is important in tissue remodeling. A study of Achilles tendinosis found that tendons with tendinosis had lower levels of MMP-3 mRNA than other tendons without tendinosis in the same patients.[392] Even more interesting, the "normal" tendons of patients with tendinosis had lower MMP-3 mRNA than tendons of control patients who had no tendinosis anywhere. This study implies that differences exist not only between tendons with and without tendinosis, but also between people who are and are not prone to tendinosis. Perhaps those prone to tendinosis start out with a lower rate of collagen turnover even before the injury cycle begins, possibly because of a down-regulation of proteolytic enzymes. This MMP-3 observation was made only in one small study, but it does illustrate that another factor to consider in the failed healing of tendinosis is the level of proteolytic enzymes available for tendon repair.

Of course, too high a level of proteolytic enzymes can also be a problem. It is not beneficial for the tissue to be broken down by the body so quickly that normal remodeling efforts cannot keep up. Tendinosis already involves an injury rate that exceeds the rate of repair. Ideally resolution results with slowing of the injury rate and acceleration of the repair process. The presence of a sufficient amount of proteolytic enzymes to enable repair of injured tissue, but not such a high concentration of proteolytic enzymes that uninjured tissue is broken down. Normally, the body maintains a balance between proteolytic enzymes and their inhibitors to achieve a balance between tissue breakdown and repair.[295,393,394]

INTERVENTION

Therapy Influences

Clearly, the effects of the whole range of therapies cannot be considered in any significant detail here, but in principle, a therapy that is beneficial to the repair events is a therapy that stimulates rather than "changes" the natural sequence. These therapies will be discussed in the additional chapters found within this text. Promoting or stimulating the inflammatory events is not intended to achieve a "bigger" inflammatory response but to maximize its efficiency. Similarly, if delivering therapy during the proliferative phase, there would be no benefit in simply creating a bigger volume of scar tissue. The advantage of appropriate intervention is that it stimulates a maximally efficient response, and therefore, the required repair material is generated with best quality and minimal time. In the remodeling phase, the refinement of the scar tissue is the aim and the use of therapy can have a significant effect, especially given the growing body of evidence relating the effects of mechanical stress and collagen behavior.

Inappropriate therapy at any stage is perfectly capable of inhibiting these events and therefore resulting in a less good repair—therapy is not guaranteed to be beneficial; one has to be mindful of the events needed and be selective of the most appropriate (evidenced) therapy at each stage.

The other interesting recent development is that there is an increasing body of knowledge that supports the idea that existing therapies have an effect on the chemical environment of the repairing tissue.[395] Exercise therapy, manual therapy, and various modalities in electrotherapy are now known to exert such effects (some examples having been provided earlier in this chapter). This need not replace the current explanations for the mode of action of therapy, but do offer an extended effects model in which there are mechanical, neurological, gross physiological, chemical, and bioelectric effects of therapy. The mode of action of those therapies, historically employed, is actually a lot more complex than was originally conceived and hitherto understood.

In addition to the "classic" modalities in this regard, it remains possible that small (endogenous) electric currents can exert an influence.[396-398] The application of microcurrent-based therapies is thought to enhance this component of the inflammatory/repair sequence,[396] and while most electrical stimulation modalities do not have a direct influence on the tissue repair sequence, microcurrent-based therapies do appear to be increasingly supported by the research evidence in this regard.

There are many aspects of the inflammatory events that can be influenced by therapeutic intervention, ranging from the mechanical to the biochemical. There is a growing body of evidence to support the effects of manual and exercise therapy on the "soup" of chemical mediators, cytokines, and growth factors.

CONCLUSION

Tissue healing is a complex and dynamic system that enables effective repair of damaged tissue. The repair control system and links between its various components are complex, and there is an ever-increasing volume of literature that continues to identify new mediators, cytokines, and variants. Whilst this knowledge base continues to expand, the links between the effects of therapy and these chemical control systems is also growing.

There is little doubt that appropriate therapy has the capacity to influence the process in a positive way, and the most logical and best-evidence approach to intervention is to stimulate or promote the normal events rather than trying to change them to something better. If repair is underway, then keep it moving. If it is delayed, then stimulate it to help get it back on track. Whilst there are myriad approaches, those that are most effective appear to follow this philosophy: Injuries cannot be made to heal faster than their natural speed. Without completion of any of the three phases, the scar tissue will not be adequate for normal function. Failure in any phase of the repair process may result in ineffectual healing, leading to chronic degenerative changes, repeated structural failure, or less than optimal tissue.

The key point is the body has evolved ways and means for dealing with injuries and insults to tissue. As therapists, we should not be trying to subvert the body's owns processes, but instead, attempt to work with and complement these processes to ensure the optimal outcome.

REFERENCES

1. Adams CS, Shapiro IM. Mechanisms by which extracellular matrix components induce osteoblast apoptosis. *Connective Tissue Research.* 2003;44(suppl 1):230-239.

2. Adams JC, Watt FM. Regulation of development and differentiation by the extracellular matrix. *Development.* 1993;117(4):1183-1198.

3. Cukierman E, Pankov R, Stevens DR, Yamada KM. Taking cell-matrix adhesions to the third dimension. *Science.* 2001;294(5547):1708-1712.

4. Gosselin LE, Adams C, Cotter TA, McCormick RJ, Thomas DP. Effect of exercise training on passive stiffness in locomotor skeletal muscle: role of extracellular matrix. *J Appl Physiol.* 1998;85(3):1011-1016.

5. Kim DJ, Christofidou ED, Keene DR, Hassan Milde M, Adams JC. Intermolecular interactions of thrombospondins drive their accumulation in extracellular matrix. *Mol Biol Cell.* 2015;26(14):2640-2654.

6. Krivacic KA, Levine AD. Extracellular matrix conditions T cells for adhesion to tissue interstitium. *J Immunol.* 2003;170:5034-5044.

7. Matsushita T, Oyamada M, Fujimoto K, et al. Remodeling of cell-cell and cell-extracellular matrix interactions at the border zone of rat myocardial infarcts. *Circ Res.* 1999;85(11):1046-1055.

8. McKay IA, Leigh IM. Epidermal cytokines and their roles in cutaneous wound healing. *Br J Dermatol.* 1991;124(6):513-518.

9. Andersen MB, Pingel J, Kjaer M, Langberg H. Interleukin-6: a growth factor stimulating collagen synthesis in human tendon. *J Appl Physiol.* 2011;110(6):1549-1554.

10. Chiu TC, Ngo HC, Lau LW, et al. An investigation of the immediate effect of static stretching on the morphology and stiffness of Achilles tendon in dominant and non-dominant legs. *PLoS One.* 2016;11(4):e0154443.

11. Gump BS, McMullan DR, Cauthon DJ, et al. Short-term acetaminophen consumption enhances the exercise-induced increase in Achilles peritendinous IL-6 in humans. *J Appl Physiol.* 2013;115(6):929-936.

12. Moerch L, Pingel J, Boesen M, Kjaer M, Langberg H. The effect of acute exercise on collagen turnover in human tendons: influence of prior immobilization period. *Eur J Appl Physiol.* 2013;113(2):449-455.

13. Pang BS, Ying M. Sonographic measurement of Achilles tendons in asymptomatic subjects: variation with age, body height, and dominance of ankle. *J Ultrasound Med.* 2006;25(10):1291-1296.

14. Siu WL, Chan CH, Lam CH, Lee CM, Ying M. Sonographic evaluation of the effect of long-term exercise on Achilles tendon stiffness using shear wave elastography. *J Sci Med Sport.* 2016;19(11):883-887.

15. Ying M, Yeung E, Li B, Li W, Lui M, Tsoi CW. Sonographic evaluation of the size of Achilles tendon: the effect of exercise and dominance of the ankle. *Ultrasound Med Biol.* 2003;29(5):637-642.

16. Yinger K, Mandelbaum BR, Almekinders LC. Achilles rupture in the athlete. Current science and treatment. *Clin Podiatr Med Surg.* 2002;19(2):231-250, v.

17. Edlich RF, Rodeheaver GT, Morgan RF, Berman DE, Thacker JG. Principles of emergency wound management. *Ann Emerg Med.* 1988;17(12):1284-1302.

18. Edlich RF, Rodeheaver GT, Thacker JG, Winn HR, Edgerton MT. Management of soft tissue injury. *Clin Plast Surg.* 1977;4(2):191-198.

19. Ben-Porath I, Weinberg RA. The signals and pathways activating cellular senescence. *Int J Biochem Cell Biol.* 2005;37(5):961-976.

20. Dalton SJ, Whiting CV, Bailey JR, Mitchell DC, Tarlton JF. Mechanisms of chronic skin ulceration linking lactate, transforming growth factor-beta, vascular endothelial growth factor, collagen remodeling, collagen stability, and defective angiogenesis. *J Invest Dermatol.* 2007;127(4):958-968.

21. Tohyama H, Yasuda K. The effects of stress enhancement on the extracellular matrix and fibroblasts in the patellar tendon. *J Biomech.* 2000;33(5):559-565.

22. Yasuda T, Kondo S, Homma T, Harris RC. Regulation of extracellular matrix by mechanical stress in rat glomerular mesangial cells. *J Clin Invest.* 1996;98(9):1991-2000.

23. Yudoh K, Matsui H, Kanamori M, Ohmori K, Yasuda T, Tsuji H. Characteristics of high and low laminin-adherent Dunn osteosarcoma cells selected by adhesiveness to laminin. Correlation between invasiveness through the extracellular matrix and pulmonary metastatic potential. *Tumour Biol.* 1996;17(6):332-340.

24. Frisen M, Magi M, Sonnerup L, Viidik A. Rheological analysis of soft collagenous tissue. Part II: experimental evaluations and verifications. *J Biomech.* 1969;2(1):21-28.

25. Viidik A. Functional properties of collagenous tissues. *Int Rev Connect Tissue Res.* 1973;6:127-215.

26. Viidik A. On the rheology and morphology of soft collagenous tissue. *J Anat.* 1969;105(Pt 1):184.

27. Noble WC. *The Skin Microflora and Microbial Skin Disease.* Cambridge University Press; 1993.

28. Dogic D, Eckes B, Aumailley M. Extracellular matrix, integrins and focal adhesions. *Curr Top Pathol.* 1999;93:75-85.

29. Eckes B, Kessler D, Aumailley M, Krieg T. Interactions of fibroblasts with the extracellular matrix: implications for the understanding of fibrosis. *Springer Semin Immunopathol.* 1999;21(4):415-429.

30. Krieg T, Aumailley M. The extracellular matrix of the dermis: flexible structures with dynamic functions. *Exp Dermatol.* 2011;20(8):689-695.

31. Ng CP, Hinz B, Swartz MA. Interstitial fluid flow induces myofibroblast differentiation and collagen alignment in vitro. *J Cell Sci.* 2005;118(Pt 20):4731-4739.

32. Sudbeck BD, Pilcher BK, Welgus HG, Parks WC. Induction and repression of collagenase-1 by keratinocytes is controlled by distinct components of different extracellular matrix compartments. *J Biol Chem.* 1997;272(35):22103-22110.

33. Adamson IY, King GM, Young L. Influence of extracellular matrix and collagen components on alveolar type 2 cell morphology and function. *In Vitro Cell Dev Biol.* 1989;25(6):494-502.

34. Axelrad TW, Deo DD, Ottino P, et al. Platelet-activating factor (PAF) induces activation of matrix metalloproteinase 2 activity and vascular endothelial cell invasion and migration. *FASEB J.* 2004;18(3):568-570.

35. Park HJ, Cho DH, Kim HJ, et al. Collagen synthesis is suppressed in dermal fibroblasts by the human antimicrobial peptide LL-37. *J Invest Dermatol.* 2009;129(4):843-850.

36. Pilcher BK, Dumin JA, Sudbeck BD, Krane SM, Welgus HG, Parks WC. The activity of collagenase-1 is required for keratinocyte migration on a type I collagen matrix. *J Cell Biol.* 1997;137(6):1445-1457.

37. Wu L, Gonzalez S, Shah S, et al. Extracellular matrix domain formation as an indicator of chondrocyte dedifferentiation and hypertrophy. *Tissue Eng Part C Methods*. 2014;20(2):160-168.

38. Ozbek S, Balasubramanian PG, Chiquet-Ehrismann R, Tucker RP, Adams JC. The evolution of extracellular matrix. *Mol Biol Cell*. 2010;21(24):4300-4305.

39. Bey MJ, Derwin KA. Measurement of in vivo tendon function. *J Shoulder Elbow Surg*. 2012;21(2):149-157.

40. Derwin KA, Baker AR, Spragg RK, Leigh DR, Iannotti JP. Commercial extracellular matrix scaffolds for rotator cuff tendon repair. Biomechanical, biochemical, and cellular properties. *J Bone Joint Surg Am*. 2006;88(12):2665-2672.

41. Derwin KA, Soslowsky LJ. A quantitative investigation of structure-function relationships in a tendon fascicle model. *J Biomech Engineering*. 1999;121(6):598-604.

42. Thomopoulos S, Parks WC, Rifkin DB, Derwin KA. Mechanisms of tendon injury and repair. *J Orthop Res*. 2015;33(6):832-839.

43. Czaker R. Extracellular matrix (ECM) components in a very primitive multicellular animal, the dicyemid mesozoan Kantharella antarctica. *Anat Rec*. 2000;259(1):52-59.

44. Sercu S, Zhang M, Oyama N, et al. Interaction of extracellular matrix protein 1 with extracellular matrix components: ECM1 is a basement membrane protein of the skin. *J Invest Dermatol*. 2008;128(6):1397-1408.

45. Sobel G, Szabo I, Paska C, et al. Changes of cell adhesion and extracellular matrix (ECM) components in cervical intraepithelial neoplasia. *Pathol Oncol Res*. 2005;11(1):26-31.

46. Tsushima Y, Tomino Y, Wang LN, et al. Immunofluorescent analysis of extracellular matrix (ECM) components in glomeruli of the hepatic glomerulosclerosis. *Nihon Jinzo Gakkai Shi*. 1993;35(8):949-955.

47. Wang X, Waldeck H, Kao WJ. The effects of TGF-alpha, IL-1beta and PDGF on fibroblast adhesion to ECM-derived matrix and KGF gene expression. *Biomaterials*. 2010;31(9):2542-2548.

48. Akhtar S, Meek KM, James V. Immunolocalization of elastin, collagen type I and type III, fibronectin, and vitronectin in extracellular matrix components of normal and myxomatous mitral heart valve chordae tendineae. *Cardiovasc Pathol*. 1999;8(4):203-211.

49. Amini R, Voycheck CA, Debski RE. A method for predicting collagen fiber realignment in non-planar tissue surfaces as applied to glenohumeral capsule during clinically relevant deformation. *J Biomech Eng*. 2014;136(3):031003.

50. Ayad S, Chambers CA, Berry L, Shuttleworth CA, Grant ME. Type VI collagen and glycoprotein MFPI are distinct components of the extracellular matrix. *Biochem J*. 1986;236(1):299-302.

51. Chagnot C, Agus A, Renier S, et al. In vitro colonization of the muscle extracellular matrix components by Escherichia coli O157:H7: the influence of growth medium, temperature and pH on initial adhesion and induction of biofilm formation by collagens I and III. *PLoS One*. 2013;8(3):e59386.

52. De Fougerolles AR, Sprague AG, Nickerson-Nutter CL, Chi-Rosso G, Rennert PD. Regulation of inflammation by collagen-binding integrins alpha1beta1 and alpha2beta1 in models of hypersensitivity and arthritis. *J Clin Invest*. 2000;105:721-729.

53. Ehrlich HP, Tarver H, Hunt TK. Effects of vitamin A and glucocorticoids upon inflammation and collagen synthesis. *Ann Surg*. 1973;177(2):222-227.

54. Barenberg SA, Filisko FE, Geil PH. Ultrastructural deformation of collagen. *Connect Tissue Res*. 1978;6(1):25-35.

55. Bashey RI, Martinez-Hernandez A, Jimenez SA. Isolation, characterization, and localization of cardiac collagen type VI. Associations with other extracellular matrix components. *Circ Res*. 1992;70(5):1006-1017.

56. Egeblad M, Shen HC, Behonick DJ, et al. Type I collagen is a genetic modifier of matrix metalloproteinase 2 in murine skeletal development. *Dev Dyn*. 2007;236(6):1683-1693.

57. Horacek MJ, Thompson JC, Dada MO, Terracio L. The extracellular matrix components laminin, fibronectin, and collagen IV are present among the epithelial cells forming Rathke's pouch. *Acta Anat (Basel)*. 1993;147(2):69-74.

58. Karttunen T, Alavaikko M, Apaja-Sarkkinen M, Autio-Harmainen H. Distribution of basement membrane laminin and type IV collagen in human reactive lymph nodes. *Histopathology*. 1986;10(8):841-849.

59. Chen R, Fu MG, Lu Y, Wang L, Ping P, Fan ZH. [Effects of antisense oligonucleotides on the expression of focal adhesion kinase gene and collagen synthesis in the cultured human fibroblasts of hypertrophic scar]. *Zhonghua Zheng Xing Wai Ke Za Zhi*. 2008;24(6):475-477.

60. Lawson MA, Purslow PP. Development of components of the extracellular matrix, basal lamina and sarcomere in chick quadriceps and pectoralis muscles. *Br Poult Sci*. 2001;42(3):315-320.

61. Niu J, Chang Z, Peng B, et al. Keratinocyte growth factor/fibroblast growth factor-7-regulated cell migration and invasion through activation of NF-kappaB transcription factors. *J Biol Chem*. 2007;282(9):6001-6011.

62. Ng CP, Swartz MA. Mechanisms of interstitial flow-induced remodeling of fibroblast-collagen cultures. *Ann Biomed Eng*. 2006;34(3):446-454.

63. Ng GY, Oakes BW, Deacon OW, McLean ID, Eyre DR. Long-term study of the biochemistry and biomechanics of anterior cruciate ligament-patellar tendon autografts in goats. *J Orthop Res*. 1996;14(6):851-856.

64. Ng KW, Wanivenhaus F, Chen T, et al. Differential cross-linking and radio-protective effects of genipin on mature bovine and human patella tendons. *Cell Tissue Bank*. 2013;14(1):21-32.

65. Pingel J, Langberg H, Skovgard D, et al. Effects of transdermal estrogen on collagen turnover at rest and in response to exercise in postmenopausal women. *J Appl Physiol*. 2012;113(7):1040-1047.

66. Chuen FS, Chuk CY, Ping WY, Nar WW, Kim HL, Ming CK. Immunohistochemical characterization of cells in adult human patellar tendons. *J Histochem Cytochem*. 2004;52(9):1151-1157.

67. Leask A. CCN2/decorin interactions: a novel approach to combating fibrosis? *J Cell Commun Signal*. 2011;5(3):249-250.

68. Pingel J, Fredberg U, Mikkelsen LR, et al. No inflammatory gene-expression response to acute exercise in human Achilles tendinopathy. *Eur J Appl Physiol*. 2013;113(8):2101-2109.

69. Abraham S, Riggs MJ, Nelson K, Lee V, Rao RR. Characterization of human fibroblast-derived extracellular matrix components for human pluripotent stem cell propagation. *Acta Biomater*. 2010;6(12):4622-4633.

70. Gagliano N, Menon A, Martinelli C, et al. Tendon structure and extracellular matrix components are affected by spasticity in cerebral palsy patients. *Muscles Ligaments Tendons J*. 2013;3(1):42-50.

71. Halper J, Kjaer M. Basic components of connective tissues and extracellular matrix: elastin, fibrillin, fibulins, fibrinogen, fibronectin, laminin, tenascins and thrombospondins. *Adv Exp Med Biol*. 2014;802:31-47.

72. Pingel J, Harrison A, Simonsen L, Suetta C, Bulow J, Langberg H. The microvascular volume of the achilles tendon is increased in patients with tendinopathy at rest and after a 1-hour treadmill run. *Am J Sports Med*. 2013;41(10):2400-2408.

73. Pingel J, Harrison A, Suetta C, Simonsen L, Langberg H, Bulow J. The acute effects of exercise on the microvascular volume of Achilles tendons in healthy young subjects. *Clin Physiol Funct Imaging*. 2013;33(4):252-257.

74. Thomopoulos S, Hattersley G, Rosen V, et al. The localized expression of extracellular matrix components in healing tendon insertion sites: an in situ hybridization study. *J Orthop Res*. 2002;20(3):454-463.

75. Tsuzaki M, Yamauchi M, Banes AJ. Tendon collagens: extracellular matrix composition in shear stress and tensile components of flexor tendons. *Connect Tissue Res*. 1993;29(2):141-152.

76. Amiel D, Akeson WH, Harwood FL, Frank CB. Stress deprivation effect on metabolic turnover of the medial collateral ligament collagen. A comparison between nine- and 12-week immobilization. *Clin Orthop Relat Res*. 1983;(172):265-270.

77. Ng GY, Fung DT. Combining therapeutic laser and herbal remedy for treating ligament injury: an ultrastructural morphological study. *Photomed Laser Surg*. 2008;26(5):425-432.

78. Ng GY, Oakes BW, McLean ID, Deacon OW, Lampard D. The long-term biomechanical and viscoelastic performance of repairing anterior cruciate ligament after hemitransection injury in a goat model. *The American Journal of Sports Medicine*. 1996;24(1):109-117.

79. Ohashi M, Ide S, Sawaguchi A, Suganuma T, Kimitsuki T, Komune S. Histochemical localization of the extracellular matrix components in the annular ligament of rat stapediovestibular joint with special reference to fibrillin, 36-kDa microfibril-associated glycoprotein (MAGP-36), and hyaluronic acid. *Med Mol Morphol*. 2008;41(1):28-33.

80. Ping A, Gu J, Wang X. [Reconstruction of anterior cruciate ligament by free autograft of middle one third of bone-patellar tendon-bone complex]. *Zhongguo Xiu Fu Chong Jian Wai Ke Za Zhi*. 2000;14(2):72-73.

81. Buda R, Castagnini F, Pagliazzi G, Giannini S. Treatment algorithm for chronic Achilles tendon lesions: review of the literature and proposal of a new classification. *J Am Podiatr Med Assoc*. 2017;107(2):144-149.

82. Chen CH, Chen CH, Chang CH, et al. Classification and analysis of pathology of the long head of the biceps tendon in complete rotator cuff tears. *Chang Gung Med J*. 2012;35(3):263-270.

83. Del Buono A, Chan O, Maffulli N. Achilles tendon: functional anatomy and novel emerging models of imaging classification. *Int Orthop*. 2013;37(4):715-721.

84. Guelfi M, Pantalone A, Mirapeix RM, et al. Anatomy, pathophysiology and classification of posterior tibial tendon dysfunction. *Eur Rev Med Pharmacol Sci*. 2017;21(1):13-19.

85. Noth U, Trojanowski M, Reichert JC, Rolf O, Rackwitz L. [Patellar tendon injuries after total knee arthroplasty: classification and management]. *Der Orthopade*. 2016;45(5):425-432.

86. Werd MB. Achilles tendon sports injuries: a review of classification and treatment. *J Am Podiatr Med Assoc*. 2007;97(1):37-48.

87. Aagaard P, Simonsen EB, Andersen JL, Magnusson SP, Halkjaer-Kristensen J, Dyhre-Poulsen P. Neural inhibition during maximal eccentric and concentric quadriceps contraction: effects of resistance training. *J Appl Physiol*. 2000;89(6):2249-2257.

88. Doessing S, Heinemeier KM, Holm L, et al. Growth hormone stimulates the collagen synthesis in human tendon and skeletal muscle without affecting myofibrillar protein synthesis. *J Physiol*. 2010;588(Pt 2):341-351.

89. Holm L, van Hall G, Rose AJ, et al. Contraction intensity and feeding affect collagen and myofibrillar protein synthesis rates differently in human skeletal muscle. *Am J Physiol Endocrinol Metab*. 2010;298(2):E257-E269.

90. Hansen P, Haraldsson BT, Aagaard P, et al. Lower strength of the human posterior patellar tendon seems unrelated to mature collagen cross-linking and fibril morphology. *J Appl Physiol*. 2010;108(1):47-52.

91. Kjaer M, Langberg H, Heinemeier K, et al. From mechanical loading to collagen synthesis, structural changes and function in human tendon. *Scand J Med Sci Sports*. 2009;19(4):500-510.

92. Couppe C, Hansen P, Kongsgaard M, et al. Mechanical properties and collagen cross-linking of the patellar tendon in old and young men. *J Appl Physiol*. 2009;107(3):880-886.

93. Langberg H, Ellingsgaard H, Madsen T, et al. Eccentric rehabilitation exercise increases peritendinous type I collagen synthesis in humans with Achilles tendinosis. *Scand J Med Sci Sports*. 2007;17(1):61-66.

94. Langberg H, Rosendal L, Kjaer M. Training-induced changes in peritendinous type I collagen turnover determined by microdialysis in humans. *J Physiol*. 2001;534(Pt 1):297-302.

95. Koskinen SO, Wang W, Ahtikoski AM, et al. Acute exercise induced changes in rat skeletal muscle mRNAs and proteins regulating type IV collagen content. *Am J Physiol Regul Integr Comp Physiol*. 2001;280(5):R1292-R1300.

96. Langberg H, Skovgaard D, Asp S, Kjaer M. Time pattern of exercise-induced changes in type I collagen turnover after prolonged endurance exercise in humans. *Calcif Tissue Int*. 2000;67(1):41-44.

97. Kjaer M, Langberg H, Miller BF, et al. Metabolic activity and collagen turnover in human tendon in response to physical activity. *J Musculoskelet Neuronal Interact*. 2005;5(1):41-52.

98. Magnusson SP, Heinemeier KM, Kjaer M. Collagen homeostasis and metabolism. *Adv Exp Med Biol*. 2016;920:11-25.

99. Miller BF, Hansen M, Olesen JL, et al. Tendon collagen synthesis at rest and after exercise in women. *J Appl Physiol*. 2007;102(2):541-546.

100. Olesen JL, Heinemeier KM, Gemmer C, Kjaer M, Flyvbjerg A, Langberg H. Exercise-dependent IGF-I, IGFBPs, and type I collagen changes in human peritendinous connective tissue determined by microdialysis. *J Appl Physiol*. 2007;102(1):214-220.

101. Maganaris CN, Baltzopoulos V, Tsaopoulos D. Muscle fibre length-to-moment arm ratios in the human lower limb determined in vivo. *J Biomech*. 2006;39(9):1663-1668.

102. Maganaris CN. Validity of procedures involved in ultrasound-based measurement of human plantarflexor tendon elongation on contraction. *J Biomech*. 2005;38(1):9-13.

103. Bayer ML, Schjerling P, Biskup E, et al. No donor age effect of human serum on collagen synthesis signaling and cell proliferation of human tendon fibroblasts. *Mech Ageing Dev*. 2012;133(5):246-254.

104. Narici MV, Maganaris C, Reeves N. Myotendinous alterations and effects of resistive loading in old age. *Scand J Med Sci Sports*. 2005;15(6):392-401.

105. Reeves ND, Maganaris CN, Narici MV. Plasticity of dynamic muscle performance with strength training in elderly humans. *Muscle Nerve*. 2005;31(3):355-364.

106. Ng EL, Wang Y, Tang BL. Rab22B's role in trans-Golgi network membrane dynamics. *Biochem Biophys Res Commun*. 2007;361(3):751-757.

107. Ng MM, Dippold HC, Buschman MD, Noakes CJ, Field SJ. GOLPH3L antagonizes GOLPH3 to determine Golgi morphology. *Mol Biol Cell*. 2013;24(6):796-808.

108. Want A, Gillespie SR, Wang Z, et al. Autophagy and mitochondrial dysfunction in tenon fibroblasts from exfoliation glaucoma patients. *PLoS One*. 2016;11(7):e0157404.

109. Zhang Q, Zhou J, Ge H, Cheng B. Tgif1 and SnoN modified chondrocytes or stem cells for tendon-bone insertion regeneration. *Med Hypotheses*. 2013;81(2):163-166.

110. Curzi D, Sartini S, Guescini M, et al. Effect of different exercise intensities on the myotendinous junction plasticity. *PLoS One*. 2016;11(6):e0158059.

111. Lionello G, Fognani R, Baleani M, Sudanese A, Toni A. Suturing the myotendinous junction in total hip arthroplasty: a biomechanical comparison of different stitching techniques. *Clin Biomech*. 2015;30(10):1077-1082.

112. Knudsen AB, Larsen M, Mackey AL, et al. The human myotendinous junction: an ultrastructural and 3D analysis study. *Scand J Med Sci Sports*. 2015;25(1):e116-e123.

113. Kinugasa R, Oda T, Komatsu T, Edgerton VR, Sinha S. Interaponeurosis shear strain modulates behavior of myotendinous junction of the human triceps surae. *Physiol Rep*. 2013;1(6):e00147.

114. Curzi D, Salucci S, Marini M, et al. How physical exercise changes rat myotendinous junctions: an ultrastructural study. *Eur J Histochem.* 2012;56(2):e19.

115. Charvet B, Ruggiero F, Le Guellec D. The development of the myotendinous junction. A review. *Muscles Ligaments Tendons J.* 2012;2(2):53-63.

116. Sharafi B, Ames EG, Holmes JW, Blemker SS. Strains at the myotendinous junction predicted by a micromechanical model. *J Biomech.* 2011;44(16):2795-2801.

117. Mendias CL, Gumucio JP, Bakhurin KI, Lynch EB, Brooks SV. Physiological loading of tendons induces scleraxis expression in epitenon fibroblasts. *J Orthop Res.* 2012;30(4):606-612.

118. Shepard ME, Lindsey DP, Chou LB. Biomechanical testing of epitenon suture strength in Achilles tendon repairs. *Foot Ankle Int.* 2007;28(10):1074-1077.

119. Xia CS, Hong GX, Dou RR, Yang XY. Effects of chitosan on cell proliferation and collagen production of tendon sheath fibroblasts, epitenon tenocytes, and endotenon tenocytes. *Chin J Traumatol.* 2005;8(6):369-374.

120. Mashadi ZB, Amis AA. Strength of the suture in the epitenon and within the tendon fibres: development of stronger peripheral suture technique. *J Hand Surg Br.* 1992;17(2):172-175.

121. Kleinau W, Loetzke HH. [Blood vessel supply of the tendon sheath and epitenon of the tendons of the peroneal group and the long deeply situated flexors in man]. *Gegenbaurs Morphol Jahrb.* 1968;112(4):565-593.

122. Kubo K, Ikebukuro T, Tsunoda N, Kanehisa H. Changes in oxygen consumption of human muscle and tendon following repeat muscle contractions. *Eur J Appl Physiol.* 2008;104(5):859-866.

123. Melo AS Jr. The risk of developing repetitive stress injury in seamstresses, in the clothing industry, under the perspective of ergonomic work analysis: a case study. *Work.* 2012;41(suppl 1):1670-1676.

124. Rietveld S, van Beest I, Kamphuis JH. Stress-induced muscle effort as a cause of repetitive strain injury? *Ergonomics.* 2007;50(12):2049-2058.

125. Lerner EJ. Computer as menace: repetitive stress injury. *N J Med.* 1998;95(4):69-70.

126. Frymoyer J. Repetitive stress injury. *J Bone Joint Surg Am.* 2001;83-A(1):137-141.

127. Amadio PC. Repetitive stress injury. *J Bone Joint Surg Am.* 2001;83-A(1):136-137; author reply 138-141.

128. Szabo RM, King KJ. Repetitive stress injury: diagnosis or self-fulfilling prophecy? *J Bone Joint Surg Am.* 2000;82(9):1314-1322.

129. Hyldig K, Riis S, Pennisi CP, Zachar V, Fink T. Implications of extracellular matrix production by adipose tissue-derived stem cells for development of wound healing therapies. *Int J Mol Sci.* 2017;18(6):1167.

130. Chang M. Restructuring of the extracellular matrix in diabetic wounds and healing: a perspective. *Pharmacol Res.* 2016;107:243-248.

131. Tracy LE, Minasian RA, Caterson EJ. Extracellular matrix and dermal fibroblast function in the healing wound. *Adv Wound Care.* 2016;5(3):119-136.

132. Briquez PS, Hubbell JA, Martino MM. Extracellular matrix-inspired growth factor delivery systems for skin wound healing. *Adv Wound Care.* 2015;4(8):479-489.

133. Asthana S, Goyal P, Dhar R, et al. Evaluation extracellular matrix-chitosan composite films for wound healing application. *J Mater Sci Mater Med.* 2015;26(8):220.

134. Xue M, Jackson CJ. Extracellular matrix reorganization during wound healing and its impact on abnormal scarring. *Adv Wound Care.* 2015;4(3):119-136.

135. Alfredson H, Pietila T, Ohberg L, Lorentzon R. Achilles tendinosis and calf muscle strength. The effect of short-term immobilization after surgical treatment. *Am J Sports Med.* 1998;26(2):166-171.

136. Christensen B, Dyrberg E, Aagaard P, Kjaer M, Langberg H. Short-term immobilization and recovery affect skeletal muscle but not collagen tissue turnover in humans. *J Appl Physiol.* 2008;105(6):1845-1851.

137. Anderson K, Hamm RL. Factors that impair wound healing. *J Am Coll Clin Wound Spec.* 2012;4(4):84-91.

138. Bharara M, Schoess J, Nouvong A, Armstrong DG. Wound inflammatory index: a "proof of concept" study to assess wound healing trajectory. *J Diabetes Sci Technol.* 2010;4(4):773-779.

139. Kohlgraf KG, Pingel LC, Dietrich DE, Brogden KA. Defensins as anti-inflammatory compounds and mucosal adjuvants. *Future Microbiol.* 2010;5(1):99-113.

140. Raghow R. The role of extracellular matrix in postinflammatory wound healing and fibrosis. *FASEB J.* 1994;8(11):823-831.

141. Smith C, Kruger MJ, Smith RM, Myburgh KH. The inflammatory response to skeletal muscle injury: illuminating complexities. *Sports Med.* 2008;38(11):947-969.

142. Zhang S, Li TS, Soyama A, et al. Up-regulated extracellular matrix components and inflammatory chemokines may impair the regeneration of cholestatic liver. *Sci Rep.* 2016;6:26540.

143. Al-Mulla F, Leibovich SJ, Francis IM, Bitar MS. Impaired TGF-beta signaling and a defect in resolution of inflammation contribute to delayed wound healing in a female rat model of type 2 diabetes. *Mol Biosyst.* 2011;7(11):3006-3020.

144. Maquart FX, Monboisse JC. Extracellular matrix and wound healing. *Pathol Biol.* 2014;62(2):91-95.

145. Rodero MP, Khosrotehrani K. Skin wound healing modulation by macrophages. *Int J Clin Exp Pathol.* 2010;3(7):643-653.

146. Schreml S, Szeimies RM, Prantl L, Landthaler M, Babilas P. Wound healing in the 21st century. *J Am Acad Dermatol.* 2010;63(5):866-881.

147. Brinkmann V, Zychlinsky A. Neutrophil extracellular traps: is immunity the second function of chromatin? *J Cell Biol.* 2012;198(5):773-783.

148. Mantovani A, Cassatella MA, Costantini C, Jaillon S. Neutrophils in the activation and regulation of innate and adaptive immunity. *Nat Rev Immunol.* 2011;11(8):519-531.

149. Minton K. Tumour immunology: neutrophils fight back in the final round. *Nat Rev Immunol.* 2011;11(10):640.

150. Deen S, Ball RY. Basement membrane and extracellular interstitial matrix components in bladder neoplasia—evidence of angiogenesis. *Histopathology.* 1994;25(5):475-481.

151. Hansen NU, Willumsen N, Sand JM, Larsen L, Karsdal MA, Leeming DJ. Type VIII collagen is elevated in diseases associated with angiogenesis and vascular remodeling. *Clin Biochem.* 2016;49(12):903-908.

152. Imamura M. [Extracellular matrix components and angiogenesis]. *Nihon Yakurigaku Zasshi.* 1996;107(3):153-160.

153. Kirkpatrick ND, Andreou S, Hoying JB, Utzinger U. Live imaging of collagen remodeling during angiogenesis. *Am J Physiol Heart Circ Physiol.* 2007;292(6):H3198-H3206.

154. Koch AE, Volin MV, Woods JM, et al. Regulation of angiogenesis by C-X-C chemokines interleukin-8 and epithelial neutrophil activating peptide 78 in the rheumatoid joint. *Arthritis Rheum.* 2001;44:31-40.

155. Mammoto A, Sero JE, Mammoto T, Ingber DE. Methods for studying mechanical control of angiogenesis by the cytoskeleton and extracellular matrix. *Methods Enzymol.* 2008;443:227-259.

156. Milch HS, Schubert SY, Hammond S, Spiegel JH. Enhancement of ischemic wound healing by inducement of local angiogenesis. *Laryngoscope.* 2010;120(9):1744-1748.

157. Dallaudiere B, Louedec L, Lenet MP, et al. The molecular systemic and local effects of intra-tendinous injection of platelet rich plasma in tendinosis: preliminary results on a rat model with ELISA method. *Muscles Ligaments Tendons J.* 2015;5(2):99-105.

158. Li N, Wallen NH, Savi P, Herault JP, Herbert JM. Effects of a new platelet glycoprotein IIb/IIIa antagonist, SR121566, on platelet activation, platelet-leukocyte interaction and thrombin generation. *Blood Coagul Fibrinolysis.* 1998;9(6):507-515.

159. Lounes KC, Ping L, Gorkun OV, Lord ST. Analysis of engineered fibrinogen variants suggests that an additional site mediates platelet aggregation and that "B-b" interactions have a role in protofibril formation. *Biochemistry.* 2002;41(16):5291-5299.

160. Monto RR. Platelet rich plasma treatment for chronic Achilles tendinosis. *Foot Ankle Int.* 2012;33(5):379-385.

161. Leask RL, Johnston KW, Ojha M. Hemodynamic effects of clot entrapment in the TrapEase inferior vena cava filter. *J Vasc Interv Radiol.* 2004;15(5):485-490.

162. Roberts WG, Palade GE. Increased microvascular permeability and endothelial fenestration induced by vascular endothelial growth factor. *J Cell Sci.* 1995;108(Pt 6):2369-2379.

163. Murphy K, ed. *Janeway's Immunobiology.* 7th ed. Garland Science, Taylor & Francis Group, LLC; 2007.

164. Bastian OW, Koenderman L, Alblas J, Leenen LP, Blokhuis TJ. Neutrophils contribute to fracture healing by synthesizing fibronectin+ extracellular matrix rapidly after injury. *Clin Immunol.* 2016;164:78-84.

165. Bordon Y. Antibody responses: neutrophils zone in to help B cells. *Nat Rev Immunol.* 2012;12(2):73.

166. Lorena D, Uchio K, Costa AM, Desmouliere A. Normal scarring: importance of myofibroblasts. *Wound Repair Regen.* 2002;10(2):86-92.

167. Fort MM, Cheung J, Yen D, et al. IL-25 induces IL-4, IL-5, and IL-13 and Th2-associated pathologies in vivo. *Immunity.* 2001;15(6):985-995.

168. Hammerle CH, Giannobile WV. Working Group 1 of the European Workshop on Periodontology. Biology of soft tissue wound healing and regeneration--consensus report of Group 1 of the 10th European Workshop on Periodontology. *J Clin Periodontol.* 2014;41(suppl 15):S1-S5.

169. Hubner G, Brauchle M, Smola H, Madlener M, Fassler R, Werner S. Differential regulation of pro-inflammatory cytokines during wound healing in normal and glucocorticoid-treated mice. *Cytokine.* 1996;8(7):548-556.

170. Humpert PM, Bartsch U, Konrade I, et al. Locally applied mononuclear bone marrow cells restore angiogenesis and promote wound healing in a type 2 diabetic patient. *Exp Clin Endocrinol Diabetes.* 2005;113(9):538-540.

171. Kim MH, Liu W, Borjesson DL, et al. Dynamics of neutrophil infiltration during cutaneous wound healing and infection using fluorescence imaging. *J Invest Dermatol.* 2008;128(7):1812-1820.

172. Martin JM, Zenilman JM, Lazarus GS. Molecular microbiology: new dimensions for cutaneous biology and wound healing. *J Invest Dermatol.* 2010;130(1):38-48.

173. Lawrence T, Natoli G. Transcriptional regulation of macrophage polarization: enabling diversity with identity. *Nat Rev Immunol.* 2011;11(11):750-761.

174. Martinez FO, Helming L, Gordon S. Alternative activation of macrophages: an immunologic functional perspective. *Annu Rev Immunol.* 2009;27:451-483.

175. Ploeger DT, van Putten SM, Koerts JA, van Luyn MJ, Harmsen MC. Human macrophages primed with angiogenic factors show dynamic plasticity, irrespective of extracellular matrix components. *Immunobiology.* 2012;217(3):299-306.

176. St Pierre BA, Tidball JG. Macrophage activation and muscle remodeling at myotendinous junctions after modifications in muscle loading. *Am J Pathol.* 1994;145(6):1463-1471.

177. Hammond MA. Moist wound healing: breaking down the dry barrier. *Nurs Mirror.* 1979;149(18):38-40.

178. Martin JM, Zenilman JM, Lazarus GS. Molecular microbiology: new dimensions for cutaneous biology and wound healing. *J Invest Dermatol.* 2010;130(1):38-48.

179. Olczyk P, Mencner L, Komosinska-Vassev K. The role of the extracellular matrix components in cutaneous wound healing. *Biomed Res Int.* 2014;2014:747584.

180. Molloy T, Wang Y, Murrell G. The roles of growth factors in tendon and ligament healing. *Sports Med.* 2003;33(5):381-394.

181. Serhan CN. Novel lipid mediators and resolution mechanisms in acute inflammation: to resolve or not? *Am J Pathol.* 2010;177(4):1576-1591.

182. Rompe JD, Furia J, Maffulli N. Eccentric loading versus eccentric loading plus shock-wave treatment for midportion Achilles tendinopathy: a randomized controlled trial. *Am J Sports Med.* 2009;37(3):463-470.

183. Rompe JD, Furia JP, Maffulli N. Mid-portion Achilles tendinopathy--current options for treatment. *Disabil Rehabil.* 2008;30(20-22):1666-1676.

184. Rompe JD, Furia J, Maffulli N. Eccentric loading compared with shock wave treatment for chronic insertional achilles tendinopathy. A randomized, controlled trial. *J Bone Joint Surg Am.* 2008;90(1):52-61.

185. Chandra P, Lai K, Sung HJ, Murthy NS, Kohn J. UV laser-ablated surface textures as potential regulator of cellular response. *Biointerphases.* 2010;5(2):53-59.

186. Frick MA, Murthy NS. Imaging of the elbow: muscle and tendon injuries. *Semin Musculoskelet Radiol.* 2010;14(4):430-437.

187. Farrow LD, Mahoney AJ, Stefancin JJ, Taljanovic MS, Sheppard JE, Schickendantz MS. Quantitative analysis of the medial ulnar collateral ligament ulnar footprint and its relationship to the ulnar sublime tubercle. *Am J Sports Med.* 2011;39(9):1936-1941.

188. Taljanovic MS, Adam RD. Musculoskeletal coccidioidomycosis. *Semin Musculoskelet Radiol.* 2011;15(5):511-526.

189. Taljanovic MS, Goldberg MR, Sheppard JE, Rogers LF. US of the intrinsic and extrinsic wrist ligaments and triangular fibrocartilage complex--normal anatomy and imaging technique. *Radiographics.* 2011;31(1):e44.

190. Taljanovic MS, Nisbet JK, Hunter TB, Cohen RP, Rogers LF. Humeral avulsion of the inferior glenohumeral ligament in college female volleyball players caused by repetitive microtrauma. *Am J Sports Med.* 2011;39(5):1067-1076.

191. Wise JN, Daffner RH, Weissman BN, et al. ACR Appropriateness Criteria(R) on acute shoulder pain. *J Am Coll Radiol.* 2011;8(9):602-609.

192. Hurley MC, Fox IH. Human placental nucleoside kinase activities. *Ann N Y Acad Sci.* 1985;451:42-53.

193. Siebenhaar F, Magerl M, Peters EM, Hendrix S, Metz M, Maurer M. Mast cell-driven skin inflammation is impaired in the absence of sensory nerves. *J Allergy Clin Immunol.* 2008;121(4):955-961.

194. Atsumi T, Cho YR, Leng L, et al. The proinflammatory cytokine macrophage migration inhibitory factor regulates glucose metabolism during systemic inflammation. *J Immunol.* 2007;179(8):5399-5406.

195. Metz M, Grimbaldeston MA, Nakae S, Piliponsky AM, Tsai M, Galli SJ. Mast cells in the promotion and limitation of chronic inflammation. *Immunol Rev.* 2007;217:304-328.

196. Metz R, Kerkhoffs GM, Verleisdonk EJ, van der Heijden GJ. Acute Achilles tendon rupture: minimally invasive surgery versus non operative treatment, with immediate full weight bearing. Design of a randomized controlled trial. *BMC Musculoskelet Disord.* 2007;8:108.

197. Leask A, Denton CP, Abraham DJ. Insights into the molecular mechanism of chronic fibrosis: the role of connective tissue growth factor in scleroderma. *J Invest Dermatol.* 2004;122(1):1-6.

198. Leask A, Holmes A, Abraham DJ. Connective tissue growth factor: a new and important player in the pathogenesis of fibrosis. *Curr Rheumatol Rep.* 2002;4(2):136-142.

199. Adzick NS, Longaker MT. Scarless wound healing in the fetus: the role of the extracellular matrix. *Prog Clin Biol Res.* 1991;365:177-192.

200. Foolen J, Wunderli SL, Loerakker S, Snedeker JG. Tissue alignment enhances remodeling potential of tendon-derived cells - Lessons from a novel microtissue model of tendon scarring. *Matrix Biol.* 2018;65:14-29.

201. Lam MT, Nauta A, Meyer NP, Wu JC, Longaker MT. Effective delivery of stem cells using an extracellular matrix patch results in increased cell survival and proliferation and reduced scarring in skin wound healing. *Tissue Eng Part A.* 2013;19(5-6):738-747.

202. Leask A. Scar wars: is TGFbeta the phantom menace in scleroderma? *Arthritis Res Ther.* 2006;8(4):213.

203. Winn HR, Jane JA, Rodeheaver G, Edgerton MT, Edlich RF. Influence of subcuticular sutures on scar formation. *Am J Surg.* 1977;133(2):257-259.

204. Sun M, He Y, Zhou T, Zhang P, Gao J, Lu F. Adipose extracellular matrix/stromal vascular fraction gel secretes angiogenic factors and enhances skin wound healing in a murine model. *Biomed Res Int.* 2017;2017:3105780.

205. Boursinos LA, Karachalios T, Poultsides L, Malizos KN. Do steroids, conventional non-steroidal anti-inflammatory drugs and selective Cox-2 inhibitors adversely affect fracture healing? *J Musculoskelet Neuronal Interact.* 2009;9(1):44-52.

206. Bird L. Inflammation: directions from the matrix. *Nat Rev Immunol.* 2011;11(1):6.

207. Bordon Y. Immunotherapy: leukadherins get a grip on inflammation. *Nat Rev Immunol.* 2011;11(10):638.

208. Buckley CD, Gilroy DW, Serhan CN, Stockinger B, Tak PP. The resolution of inflammation. *Nat Rev Immunol.* 2013;13(1):59-66.

209. Chawla A, Nguyen KD, Goh YP. Macrophage-mediated inflammation in metabolic disease. *Nat Rev Immunol.* 2011;11(11):738-749.

210. Baum P, Hermann W, Verlohren HJ, Wagner A, Lohmann T, Grahmann F. Diabetic neuropathy in patients with "latent autoimmune diabetes of the adults" (LADA) compared with patients with type 1 and type 2 diabetes. *J Neurol.* 2003;250(6):682-687.

211. Cardona ID, Goleva E, Ou LS, Leung DY. Staphylococcal enterotoxin B inhibits regulatory T cells by inducing glucocorticoid-induced TNF receptor-related protein ligand on monocytes. *J Allergy Clin Immunol.* 2006;117(3):688-695.

212. Chouhan D, Chakraborty B, Nandi SK, Mandal BB. Role of non-mulberry silk fibroin in deposition and regulation of extracellular matrix towards accelerated wound healing. *Acta Biomater.* 2017;48:157-174.

213. Chouhan D, Janani G, Chakraborty B, Nandi SK, Mandal BB. Functionalized PVA-silk blended nanofibrous mats promote diabetic wound healing via regulation of extracellular matrix and tissue remodeling. *J Tissue Eng Regen Med.* 2018;12(3):e1559-e1570.

214. Fox LT, Mazumder A, Dwivedi A, Gerber M, du Plessis J, Hamman JH. In vitro wound healing and cytotoxic activity of the gel and whole-leaf materials from selected aloe species. *J Ethnopharmacol.* 2017;200:1-7.

215. Kunkemoeller B, Kyriakides TR. Redox signaling in diabetic wound healing regulates extracellular matrix deposition. *Antioxid Redox Signal.* 2017;27(12):823-838.

216. Mir-Mari J, Benic GI, Valmaseda-Castellon E, Hammerle CHF, Jung RE. Influence of wound closure on the volume stability of particulate and non-particulate GBR materials: an in vitro cone-beam computed tomographic examination. Part II. *Clin Oral Implants Res.* 2017;28(6):631-639.

217. Spater T, Frueh FS, Menger MD, Laschke MW. Potentials and limitations of Integra(R) flowable wound matrix seeded with adipose tissue-derived microvascular fragments. *Eur Cell Mater.* 2017;33:268-278.

218. Rodeheaver GT, Gentry S, Saffer L, Edlich RF. Topical antimicrobial cream sensitivity testing. *Surg Gynecol Obstet.* 1980;151(6):747-752.

219. Desmouliere A, Geinoz A, Gabbiani F, Gabbiani G. Transforming growth factor-beta 1 induces alpha-smooth muscle actin expression in granulation tissue myofibroblasts and in quiescent and growing cultured fibroblasts. *J Cell Biol.* 1993;122(1):103-111.

220. Gabbiani G. The myofibroblast in wound healing and fibrocontractive diseases. *J Pathol.* 2003;200(4):500-503.

221. Meyer-ter-Vehn T, Han H, Grehn F, Schlunck G. Extracellular matrix elasticity modulates TGF-beta-induced p38 activation and myofibroblast transdifferentiation in human tenon fibroblasts. *Invest Ophthalmol Vis Sci.* 2011;52(12):9149-9155.

222. Serpooshan V, Zhao M, Metzler SA, et al. The effect of bioengineered acellular collagen patch on cardiac remodeling and ventricular function post myocardial infarction. *Biomaterials.* 2013;34(36):9048-9055.

223. Sherman-Baust CA, Weeraratna AT, Rangel LB, et al. Remodeling of the extracellular matrix through overexpression of collagen VI contributes to cisplatin resistance in ovarian cancer cells. *Cancer Cell.* 2003;3(4):377-386.

224. Shin JM, Kong SJ, Shin YA, et al. Possible role of tropomyosin-receptor kinase fused gene on skin collagen remodeling. *J Dermatol Sci.* 2017;88(3):375-377. doi:10.1016/j.jdermsci.2017.08.010.

225. Simionescu DT, Lu Q, Song Y, et al. Biocompatibility and remodeling potential of pure arterial elastin and collagen scaffolds. *Biomaterials.* 2006;27(5):702-713.

226. Simon DD, Murtada SI, Humphrey JD. Computational model of matrix remodeling and entrenchment in the free-floating fibroblast-populated collagen lattice. *Int J Numer Method Biomed Eng.* 2014;30(12):1506-1529.

227. Skovgaard D, Kjaer A, Heinemeier KM, Brandt-Larsen M, Madsen J, Kjaer M. Use of cis-[18F]fluoro-proline for assessment of exercise-related collagen synthesis in musculoskeletal connective tissue. *PLoS One.* 2011;6(2):e16678.

228. Sluijter JP, Smeets MB, Velema E, Pasterkamp G, de Kleijn DP. Increase in collagen turnover but not in collagen fiber content is associated with flow-induced arterial remodeling. *J Vasc Res.* 2004;41(6):546-555.

229. Soares AL, Stekelenburg M, Baaijens FP. Remodeling of the collagen fiber architecture due to compaction in small vessels under tissue engineered conditions. *J Biomech Eng.* 2011;133(7):071002.

230. Song YH, Shon SH, Shan M, Stroock AD, Fischbach C. Adipose-derived stem cells increase angiogenesis through matrix metalloproteinase-dependent collagen remodeling. *Integr Biol (Camb).* 2016;8(2):205-215.

231. Steplewski A, Kasinskas A, Fertala A. Remodeling of the dermal-epidermal junction in bilayered skin constructs after silencing the expression of the p.R2622Q and p.G2623C collagen VII mutants. *Connect Tissue Res.* 2012;53(5):379-389.

232. Swasdison S, Mayne R. In vitro attachment of skeletal muscle fibers to a collagen gel duplicates the structure of the myotendinous junction. *Exp Cell Res.* 1991;193(1):227-231.

233. Tamariz E, Grinnell F. Modulation of fibroblast morphology and adhesion during collagen matrix remodeling. *Mol Biol Cell.* 2002;13(11):3915-3929.

234. Tang Y, Ballarini R, Buehler MJ, Eppell SJ. Deformation micromechanisms of collagen fibrils under uniaxial tension. *J R Soc Interface.* 2010;7(46):839-850.

235. Tian L, Lammers SR, Kao PH, et al. Impact of residual stretch and remodeling on collagen engagement in healthy and pulmonary hypertensive calf pulmonary arteries at physiological pressures. *Ann Biomed Eng.* 2012;40(7):1419-1433.

236. Tornero-Esteban P, Hoyas JA, Villafuertes E, et al. Efficacy of supraspinatus tendon repair using mesenchymal stem cells along with a collagen I scaffold. *J Orthop Surg Res.* 2015;10:124.

237. Wilson W, Driessen NJ, van Donkelaar CC, Ito K. Prediction of collagen orientation in articular cartilage by a collagen remodeling algorithm. *Osteoarthritis Cartilage.* 2006;14(11):1196-1202.

238. Wolf J, Carsons S. Synovial extracellular matrix: partial characterization of matrix components and identification of type VI collagen molecular forms. *Clin Exp Rheumatol.* 1991;9(1):51-54.

239. Xu J, Zutter MM, Santoro SA, Clark RA. A three-dimensional collagen lattice activates NF-kappaB in human fibroblasts: role in integrin alpha2 gene expression and tissue remodeling. *J Cell Biol.* 1998;140(3):709-719.

240. Yajima T. Collagen remodeling in wound healing by gingival fibroblasts in vitro. *Adv Dent Res.* 1988;2(2):228-233.

241. Schiller M, Javelaud D, Mauviel A. TGF-beta-induced SMAD signaling and gene regulation: consequences for extracellular matrix remodeling and wound healing. *J Dermatol Sci.* 2004;35(2):83-92.

242. Luo Y, Xu X, Lele T, Kumar S, Ingber DE. A multi-modular tensegrity model of an actin stress fiber. *J Biomech.* 2008;41(11):2379-2387.

243. Xia N, Thodeti CK, Hunt TP, et al. Directional control of cell motility through focal adhesion positioning and spatial control of Rac activation. *FASEB J.* 2008;22(6):1649-1659.

244. Cavanaugh JT, Killian SE. Rehabilitation following meniscal repair. *Curr Rev Musculoskelet Med.* 2012;5(1):46-58.

245. Killian ML, Cavinatto L, Galatz LM, Thomopoulos S. The role of mechanobiology in tendon healing. *J Shoulder Elbow Surg.* 2012;21(2):228-237.

246. Killian ML, Cavinatto L, Galatz LM, Thomopoulos S. Recent advances in shoulder research. *Arthritis Res Ther.* 2012;14(3):214.

247. Metcalfe AD, Ferguson MW. Tissue engineering of replacement skin: the crossroads of biomaterials, wound healing, embryonic development, stem cells and regeneration. *J R Soc Interface.* 2007;4(14):413-437.

248. Ayello EA. 20 years of wound care: where we have been, where we are going. *Adv Skin Wound Care.* 2006;19(1):28-33.

249. Barrientos S, Stojadinovic O, Golinko MS, Brem H, Tomic-Canic M. Growth factors and cytokines in wound healing. *Wound Repair Regen.* 2008;16(5):585-601.

250. Lazarus GS, Cooper DM, Knighton DR, et al. Definitions and guidelines for assessment of wounds and evaluation of healing. *Arch Dermatol.* 1994;130(4):489-493.

251. Martin JM, Zenilman JM, Lazarus GS. Molecular microbiology: new dimensions for cutaneous biology and wound healing. *J Invest Dermatol.* 2010;130(1):38-48.

252. Walker JT, McLeod K, Kim S, Conway SJ, Hamilton DW. Periostin as a multifunctional modulator of the wound healing response. *Cell and Tissue Research.* 2016;365(3):453-465.

253. Johnson MS, Sarkisian SR Jr. Using a collagen matrix implant (Ologen) versus mitomycin-C as a wound healing modulator in trabeculectomy with the Ex-PRESS mini glaucoma device: a 12-month retrospective review. *J Glaucoma.* 2014;23(9):649-652.

254. Siriwardena D, Khaw PT, King AJ, et al. Human antitransforming growth factor beta(2) monoclonal antibody--a new modulator of wound healing in trabeculectomy: a randomized placebo controlled clinical study. *Ophthalmology.* 2002;109(3):427-431.

255. Vesaluoma M, Teppo AM, Gronhagen-Riska C, Tervo T. Platelet-derived growth factor-BB (PDGF-BB) in tear fluid: a potential modulator of corneal wound healing following photorefractive keratectomy. *Curr Eye Res.* 1997;16(8):825-831.

256. Chung SI, Lee SY, Ryogin U, Kamemitsu K. Affects of F XIII in wound-healing--fibrin stability in tissues and cross linking of angiogenesis modulator, osteonectin to fibrin. *Rinsho Byori.* 1997;(suppl 104):50.

257. Chattopadhyay A, Galvez MG, Bachmann M, et al. Tendon regeneration with tendon hydrogel-based cell delivery: a comparison of fibroblasts and adipose-derived stem cells. *Plast Reconstr Surg.* 2016;138(3):617-626.

258. Chen L, Jiang C, Tiwari SR, et al. TGIF1 gene silencing in tendon-derived stem cells improves the tendon-to-bone insertion site regeneration. *Cell Physiol Biochem.* 2015;37(6):2101-2114.

259. Christgau M, Caffesse RG, Schmalz G, D'Souza RN. Extracellular matrix expression and periodontal wound-healing dynamics following guided tissue regeneration therapy in canine furcation defects. *J Clin Periodontol.* 2007;34(8):691-708.

260. Crowe CS, Chiou G, McGoldrick R, Hui K, Pham H, Chang J. Tendon regeneration with a novel tendon hydrogel: in vitro effects of platelet-rich plasma on rat adipose-derived stem cells. *Plast Reconstr Surg.* 2015;135(6):981e-989e.

261. de Luca AC, Lacour SP, Raffoul W, di Summa PG. Extracellular matrix components in peripheral nerve repair: how to affect neural cellular response and nerve regeneration? *Neural Regen Res.* 2014;9(22):1943-1948.

262. Gantus MA, Nasciutti LE, Cruz CM, Persechini PM, Martinez AM. Modulation of extracellular matrix components by metalloproteinases and their tissue inhibitors during degeneration and regeneration of rat sural nerve. *Brain Research.* 2006;1122(1):36-46.

263. Jozsa L, Balint BJ, Reffy A. Regeneration of human tendons after homologous tendon-graft transplantation. A morphological study of 25 cases. *Arch Orthop Trauma Surg.* 1987;106(5):268-273.

264. Lamme EN, de Vries HJ, van Veen H, Gabbiani G, Westerhof W, Middelkoop E. Extracellular matrix characterization during healing of full-thickness wounds treated with a collagen/elastin dermal substitute shows improved skin regeneration in pigs. *J Histochem Cytochem.* 1996;44(11):1311-1322.

265. Lee CH, Lee FY, Tarafder S, et al. Harnessing endogenous stem/progenitor cells for tendon regeneration. *J Clin Invest.* 2015;125(7):2690-2701.

266. Litwiniuk M, Krejner A, Speyrer MS, Gauto AR, Grzela T. Hyaluronic acid in inflammation and tissue regeneration. *Wounds.* 2016;28(3):78-88.

267. Liu W, Yin L, Yan X, et al. Directing the differentiation of parthenogenetic stem cells into tenocytes for tissue-engineered tendon regeneration. *Stem Cells Transl Med.* 2017;6(1):196-208.

268. Martin P. Wound healing--aiming for perfect skin regeneration. *Science.* 1997;276(5309):75-81.

269. Martini R. Expression and functional roles of neural cell surface molecules and extracellular matrix components during development and regeneration of peripheral nerves. *J Neurocytol.* 1994;23(1):1-28.

270. Ode A, Duda GN, Glaeser JD, et al. Toward biomimetic materials in bone regeneration: functional behavior of mesenchymal stem cells on a broad spectrum of extracellular matrix components. *J Biomed Mater Res A.* 2010;95(4):1114-1124.

271. Park GY, Kwon DR, Lee SC. Regeneration of full-thickness rotator cuff tendon tear after ultrasound-guided injection with umbilical cord blood-derived mesenchymal stem cells in a rabbit model. *Stem Cells Transl Med.* 2015;4(11):1344-1351.

272. Ramdass B, Koka PS. Ligament and tendon repair through regeneration using mesenchymal stem cells. *Curr Stem Cell Res Ther.* 2015;10(1):84-88.

273. Simon S, Hammoudeh J, Low C, Nathan N, Armstrong M, Thaller S. Complex wound management with an artificial dermal regeneration template. *Wounds.* 2008;20(11):299-302.

274. Barillo DJ, Nangle ME, Farrell K. Preliminary experience with cultured epidermal autograft in a community hospital burn unit. *J Burn Care Rehabil.* 1992;13(1):158-165.

275. Chiba T, Ishida N, Kohda F, Furue M. Air exposure may be associated with the histological differentiation of a cultured epidermal autograft (JACE). *Australas J Dermatol.* 2018;59(3):e244-e246.

276. Haith LR Jr., Patton ML, Goldman WT. Cultured epidermal autograft and the treatment of the massive burn injury. *J Burn Care Rehabil.* 1992;13(1):142-146.

277. Hayashi M, Muramatsu H, Nakano M, et al. Changes in the dermal structure during cultured epidermal autograft engraftment process. *Plast Reconstr Surg Glob Open.* 2016;4(9):e870.

278. Herndon DN, Rutan RL. Comparison of cultured epidermal autograft and massive excision with serial autografting plus homograft overlay. *J Burn Care Rehabil.* 1992;13(1):154-157.

279. Lopez Gutierrez JC, Ros Z, Vallejo D, Perdiguero M, Soto C, Tovar J. Cultured epidermal autograft in the management of critical pediatric burn patients. *Eur J Pediatr Surg.* 1995;5(3):174-176.

280. Matsumura H, Gondo M, Imai R, Shibata D, Watanabe K. Chronological histological findings of cultured epidermal autograft over bilayer artificial dermis. *Burns.* 2013;39(4):705-713.

281. Matsumura H, Matsushima A, Ueyama M, Kumagai N. Application of the cultured epidermal autograft "JACE((R)")" for treatment of severe burns: results of a 6-year multicenter surveillance in Japan. *Burns.* 2016;42(4):769-776.

282. Munster AM. Use of cultured epidermal autograft in ten patients. *J Burn Care Rehabil.* 1992;13(1):124-126.

283. Odessey R. Addendum: multicenter experience with cultured epidermal autograft for treatment of burns. *J Burn Care Rehabil.* 1992;13(1):174-180.

284. Shinkuma S, Sawamura D, Fujita Y, et al. Long-term follow-up of cultured epidermal autograft in a patient with recessive dystrophic epidermolysis bullosa. *Acta Derm Venereol.* 2014;94(1):98-99.

285. Theopold C, Eriksson E. The need for aggressive follow-up after cultured epidermal autograft-grafted full-thickness burn. *Plast Reconstr Surg.* 2006;117(2):708.

286. Zhang S, Chu WC, Lai RC, Lim SK, Hui JH, Toh WS. Exosomes derived from human embryonic mesenchymal stem cells promote osteochondral regeneration. *Osteoarthritis Cartilage.* 2016;24(12):2135-2140.

287. Toh WS, Foldager CB, Pei M, Hui JH. Advances in mesenchymal stem cell-based strategies for cartilage repair and regeneration. *Stem Cell Rev Rep.* 2014;10(5):686-696.

288. Toh ML, Bonnefoy JY, Accart N, et al. Bone- and cartilage-protective effects of a monoclonal antibody against colony-stimulating factor 1 receptor in experimental arthritis. *Arthritis Rheumatol.* 2014;66(11):2989-3000.

289. Toh WS, Cao T. Derivation of chondrogenic cells from human embryonic stem cells for cartilage tissue engineering. *Methods Mol Biol.* 2014;1307:263-279.

290. Zhang B, Yin Y, Lai RC, Tan SS, Choo AB, Lim SK. Mesenchymal stem cells secrete immunologically active exosomes. *Stem Cells Dev.* 2014;23(11):1233-1244.

291. Zhang HG, Grizzle WE. Exosomes: a novel pathway of local and distant intercellular communication that facilitates the growth and metastasis of neoplastic lesions. *Am J Pathol.* 2014;184(1):28-41.

292. Ng TK. Descriptive occupational morbidity statistics. World health statistics quarterly. *Rapport trimestriel de statistiques sanitaires mondiales.* 1988;41(3-4):200-208.

293. Stenson JF, Reb CW, Daniel JN, Saini SS, Albana MF. Predicting failure of nonoperative treatment for insertional Achilles tendinosis. *Foot Ankle Spec.* 2018;11(3):252-255.

294. Dupley L, Charalambous CP. Platelet-rich plasma injections as a treatment for refractory patellar tendinosis: a meta-analysis of randomised trials. *Knee Surg Relat Res.* 2017;29(3):165-171.

295. Charnoff J, Naqvi U. *Tendinosis (Tendinitis).* StatPearls; 2017.

296. Startzman AN, Fowler O, Carreira D. Proximal hamstring tendinosis and partial ruptures. *Orthopedics.* 2017;40(4):e574-e582.

297. Brockmeyer M, Haupert A, Kohn D, Lorbach O. Surgical technique: jumper's knee-arthroscopic treatment of chronic tendinosis of the patellar tendon. *Arthrosc Tech.* 2016;5(6):e1419-e1424.

298. Mohamadi A, Chan JJ, Claessen FM, Ring D, Chen NC. Corticosteroid injections give small and transient pain relief in rotator cuff tendinosis: a meta-analysis. *Clin Orthop Relat Res.* 2017;475(1):232-243.

299. Werber B. Amniotic tissues for the treatment of chronic plantar fasciosis and Achilles tendinosis. *J Sports Med (Hindawi Publ Corp).* 2015;2015:219896.

300. Jawahar A, Lu Y, Okur G, Kliethermes S, Lomasney L. Gastrocnemius tendinosis--a frequent finding on MRI knee examination. *Eur J Radiol.* 2015;84(12):2579-2585.

301. Retraction. Skin-derived fibroblasts for the treatment of refractory Achilles tendinosis: preliminary short-term results by H. Obaid, A. Clarke, P. Rosenfeld, C. Leach, and D. Connell. J Bone Joint Surg Am. 2012 Feb 1;94(3):193-200. *J Bone Joint Surg Am.* 2015;97(8):667.

302. Lopez RG, Jung HG. Achilles tendinosis: treatment options. *Clin Orthop Surg.* 2015;7(1):1-7.

303. Rigby RB, Cottom JM, Vora A. Early weightbearing using Achilles suture bridge technique for insertional Achilles tendinosis: a review of 43 patients. *J Foot Ankle Surg.* 2013;52(5):575-579.

304. Garner HW, Whalen JL. Acute calcific tendinosis of the flexor hallucis brevis: case report. *Foot Ankle Int.* 2013;34(10):1451-1455.

305. Jarvinen TA, Jozsa L, Kannus P, et al. Mechanical loading regulates the expression of tenascin-C in the myotendinous junction and tendon but does not induce de novo synthesis in the skeletal muscle. *J Cell Sci.* 2003;116(Pt 5):857-866.

306. Paavola M, Kannus P, Jarvinen TA, Jarvinen TL, Jozsa L, Jarvinen M. Treatment of tendon disorders. Is there a role for corticosteroid injection? *Foot and Ankle Clinics.* 2002;7(3):501-513.

307. Jarvinen TA, Kannus P, Paavola M, Jarvinen TL, Jozsa L, Jarvinen M. Achilles tendon injuries. *Curr Opin Rheumatol.* 2001;13(2):150-155.

308. Jozsa L, Kannus P. Histopathological findings in spontaneous tendon ruptures. *Scand J Med Sci Sports.* 1997;7(2):113-118.

309. Jarvinen M, Jozsa L, Kannus P, Jarvinen TL, Kvist M, Leadbetter W. Histopathological findings in chronic tendon disorders. *Scand J Med Sci Sports.* 1997;7(2):86-95.

310. Jarvinen M, Jozsa L, Johnson RJ, et al. Effect of anterior cruciate ligament reconstruction with patellar tendon or prosthetic ligament on the morphology of the other ligaments of the knee joint. An experimental study in dogs. *Clin Orthop Relat Res.* 1995;(311):176-182.

311. Kannus P, Jozsa L. Histopathological changes preceding spontaneous rupture of a tendon. A controlled study of 891 patients. *J Bone Joint Surg Am.* 1991;73(10):1507-1525.

312. Lehto M, Jozsa L, Kvist M, Jarvinen M, Balint BJ, Reffy A. Fibronectin in the ruptured human Achilles tendon and its paratenon. An immunoperoxidase study. *Ann Chir Gynaecol.* 1990;79(2):72-77.

313. Jozsa L, Lehto M, Kannus P, et al. Fibronectin and laminin in Achilles tendon. *Acta Orthop Scand.* 1989;60(4):469-471.

314. Jozsa L, Lehto M, Kvist M, Balint JB, Reffy A. Alterations in dry mass content of collagen fibers in degenerative tendinopathy and tendon-rupture. *Matrix.* 1989;9(2):140-146.

315. Jozsa L, Balint BJ, Reffy A. [Reorganization of homologous tendon grafts in man]. *Morphol Igazsagugyi Orv Sz.* 1985;25(1):28-34.

316. Jozsa L, Balint BJ, Vandor E, Reffy A, Demel Z. Recapillarization of tenotomized skeletal muscles after delayed tendon suture. I. Experimental study. *Res Exp Med (Berl).* 1985;185(2):163-168.

317. Kvist M, Jozsa L, Jarvinen M. Vascular changes in the ruptured Achilles tendon and paratenon. *Int Orthop.* 1992;16(4):377-382.

318. Mauney J, Olsen BR, Volloch V. Matrix remodeling as stem cell recruitment event: a novel in vitro model for homing of human bone marrow stromal cells to the site of injury shows crucial role of extracellular collagen matrix. *Matrix Biol.* 2010;29(8):657-663.

319. Cross VL, Zheng Y, Won Choi N, et al. Dense type I collagen matrices that support cellular remodeling and microfabrication for studies of tumor angiogenesis and vasculogenesis in vitro. *Biomaterials.* 2010;31(33):8596-8607.

320. Baaijens F, Bouten C, Driessen N. Modeling collagen remodeling. *J Biomech.* 2010;43(1):166-175.

321. Karamichos D, Brown RA, Mudera V. Collagen stiffness regulates cellular contraction and matrix remodeling gene expression. *J Biomed Mater Res A.* 2007;83(3):887-894.

322. Abraham LC, Dice JF, Lee K, Kaplan DL. Phagocytosis and remodeling of collagen matrices. *Exp Cell Res.* 2007;313(5):1045-1055.

323. James SL, Ali K, Pocock C, et al. Ultrasound guided dry needling and autologous blood injection for patellar tendinosis. *Br J Sports Med.* 2007;41(8):518-521; discussion 522.

324. Jayaseelan DJ, Magrum EM. Eccentric training for the rehabilitation of a high level wrestler with distal biceps tendinosis: a case report. *Int J Sports Phys Ther.* 2012;7(4):413-424.

325. Johansson FR, Skillgate E, Adolfsson A, et al. Asymptomatic elite adolescent tennis players' signs of tendinosis in their dominant shoulder compared with their nondominant shoulder. *J Athl Train.* 2015;50(12):1299-1305.

326. Johnson KW, Zalavras C, Thordarson DB. Surgical management of insertional calcific achilles tendinosis with a central tendon splitting approach. *Foot Ankle Int.* 2006;27(4):245-250.

327. Kaeding C, Best TM. Tendinosis: pathophysiology and nonoperative treatment. *Sports Health.* 2009;1(4):284-292.

328. Kaeding CC, Pedroza AD, Powers BC. Surgical treatment of chronic patellar tendinosis: a systematic review. *Clin Orthop Relat Res.* 2007;455:102-106.

329. Khan KM, Bonar F, Desmond PM, et al. Patellar tendinosis (jumper's knee): findings at histopathologic examination, US, and MR imaging. Victorian Institute of Sport Tendon Study Group. *Radiology.* 1996;200(3):821-827.

330. Khan KM, Cook JL, Taunton JE, Bonar F. Overuse tendinosis, not tendinitis part 1: a new paradigm for a difficult clinical problem. *Phys Sportsmed.* 2000;28(5):38-48.

331. Kingzett-Taylor A, Tirman PF, Feller J, et al. Tendinosis and tears of gluteus medius and minimus muscles as a cause of hip pain: MR imaging findings. *AJR Am J Roentgenol.* 1999;173(4):1123-1126.

332. Kirkley A, Litchfield RB, Jackowski DM, Lo IK. The use of the impingement test as a predictor of outcome following subacromial decompression for rotator cuff tendinosis. *Arthroscopy.* 2002;18(1):8-15.

333. Knobloch K. Eccentric rehabilitation exercise increases peritendinous type I collagen synthesis in humans with Achilles tendinosis. *Scand J Med Sci Sports.* 2007;17(3):298-299.

334. Krahe MA, Berlet GC. Achilles tendon ruptures, re rupture with revision surgery, tendinosis, and insertional disease. *Foot Ankle Clin.* 2009;14(2):247-275.

335. Kraushaar BS, Nirschl RP. Tendinosis of the elbow (tennis elbow). Clinical features and findings of histological, immunohistochemical, and electron microscopy studies. *J Bone Joint Surg Am.* 1999;81(2):259-278.

336. Lai Wei Hong S, Tang Qian Ying C, Thwin L, Thevendran G. Return to sport and physical activity after calcaneoplasty for insertional Achilles tendinosis. *J Foot Ankle Surg.* 2016;55(6):1190-1194.

337. Leumann A, Merian M, Valderrabano V. [Ossification in chronic Achilles tendinosis: a third calf bone]. *Der Orthopade.* 2008;37(5):481-484.

338. Lin CH, Chao HL, Chiou HJ. Calcified plaque resorptive status as determined by high-resolution ultrasound is predictive of successful conservative management of calcific tendinosis. *Eur J Radiol.* 2012;81(8):1776-1781.

339. Lin JT, Adler RS, Bracilovic A, Cooper G, Sofka C, Lutz GE. Clinical outcomes of ultrasound-guided aspiration and lavage in calcific tendinosis of the shoulder. *HSS J.* 2007;3(1):99-105.

340. Lin YH, Chiou HJ, Wang HK, Lai YC, Chou YH, Chang CY. Management of rotator cuff calcific tendinosis guided by ultrasound elastography. *J Chin Med Assoc.* 2015;78(10):603-609.

341. Lind B, Ohberg L, Alfredson H. Sclerosing polidocanol injections in mid-portion Achilles tendinosis: remaining good clinical results and decreased tendon thickness at 2-year follow-up. *Knee Surg Sports Traumatol Arthrosc.* 2006;14(12):1327-1332.

342. Loew M, Jurgowski W. [Initial experiences with extracorporeal shockwave lithotripsy (ESWL) in treatment of tendinosis calcarea of the shoulder]. *Zeitschrift fur Orthopadie und ihre Grenzgebiete.* 1993;131(5):470-473.

343. Loew M, Jurgowski W, Thomsen M. [Effect of extracorporeal shockwave therapy on tendinosis calcarea of the shoulder. A preliminary report]. *Der Urologe Ausg A.* 1995;34(1):49-53.

344. Lorbach O, Diamantopoulos A, Paessler HH. Arthroscopic resection of the lower patellar pole in patients with chronic patellar tendinosis. *Arthroscopy.* 2008;24(2):167-173.

345. Lorbach O, Diamantopoulos A, Passler HH. [Arthroscopic treatment of chronic tendinosis of the patellar tendon (Jumper's Knee): surgical technique]. *Sportverletz Sportschaden.* 2008;22(1):58-61.

346. Low SC, Tan SC. Ectopic insertion of the pectoralis minor muscle with tendinosis as a cause of shoulder pain and clicking. *Clin Radiol.* 2010;65(3):254-256.

347. Lui TH. Minimally invasive flexor hallucis longus transfer in management of acute Achilles tendon rupture associated with tendinosis: a case report. *Foot Ankle Spec.* 2012;5(2):111-114.

348. Lundin AC, Aspenberg P, Eliasson P. Trigger finger, tendinosis, and intratendinous gene expression. *Scand J Med Sci Sports.* 2014;24(2):363-368.

349. Lundin AC, Eliasson P, Aspenberg P. Trigger finger and tendinosis. *J Hand Surg Eur Vol.* 2012;37(3):233-236.

350. Maffulli N, Cook JL, Khan KM. Re: Recalcitrant patellar tendinosis in elite athletes: surgical treatment in conjunction with aggressive postoperative rehabilitation. *Am J Sports Med.* 2006;34(8):1364; author reply 1364-1365.

351. Maffulli N, Kenward MG, Testa V, Capasso G, Regine R, King JB. Clinical diagnosis of Achilles tendinopathy with tendinosis. *Clin J Sport Med.* 2003;13(1):11-15.

352. Mafi N, Lorentzon R, Alfredson H. Superior short-term results with eccentric calf muscle training compared to concentric training in a randomized prospective multicenter study on patients with chronic Achilles tendinosis. *Knee Surg Sports Traumatol Arthrosc.* 2001;9(1):42-47.

353. Maier M, Durr HR, Kohler S, Staupendahl D, Pfahler M, Refior HJ. [Analgesic effect of low energy extracorporeal shock waves in tendinosis calcarea, epicondylitis humeri radialis and plantar fasciitis]. *Zeitschrift fur Orthopadie und ihre Grenzgebiete.* 2000;138(1):34-38.

354. Maier M, Maier-Bosse T, Refior HJ, Schulz CU. [Roentgen morphologic evaluation of tendinosis calcarea of the shoulder is interobserver judgment dependent]. *Zeitschrift fur Orthopadie und ihre Grenzgebiete.* 2003;141(2):126-127.

355. Mangone G, Veliaj A, Postiglione M, Viliani T, Pasquetti P. Radial extracorporeal shock-wave therapy in rotator cuff calcific tendinosis. *Clin Cases Miner Bone Metab.* 2010;7(2):91-96.

356. Mardh A, Lund I. High power laser for treatment of Achilles tendinosis - a single blind randomized placebo controlled clinical study. *J Lasers Med Sci.* 2016;7(2):92-98.

357. Martin RL, Manning CM, Carcia CR, Conti SF. An outcome study of chronic Achilles tendinosis after excision of the Achilles tendon and flexor hallucis longus tendon transfer. *Foot Ankle Int.* 2005;26(9):691-697.

358. Maxwell NJ, Ryan MB, Taunton JE, Gillies JH, Wong AD. Sonographically guided intratendinous injection of hyperosmolar dextrose to treat chronic tendinosis of the Achilles tendon: a pilot study. *AJR Am J Roentgenol.* 2007;189(4):W215-W220.

359. McCormack R. Effectiveness of a single corticosteroid injection for chronic rotator cuff tendinosis. *Clinical Journal of Sport Medicine.* 2006;16(1):88-89.

360. McGarvey WC, Palumbo RC, Baxter DE, Leibman BD. Insertional Achilles tendinosis: surgical treatment through a central tendon splitting approach. *Foot Ankle Int.* 2002;23(1):19-25.

361. McShane JM, Nazarian LN, Harwood MI. Sonographically guided percutaneous needle tenotomy for treatment of common extensor tendinosis in the elbow. *J Ultrasound Med.* 2006;25(10):1281-1289.

362. Meknas K, Johansen O, Steigen SE, Olsen R, Jorgensen L, Kartus J. Could tendinosis be involved in osteoarthritis? *Scand J Med Sci Sports.* 2012;22(5):627-634.

363. Meloni F, Milia F, Cavazzuti M, et al. Clinical evaluation of sodium hyaluronate in the treatment of patients with sopraspinatus tendinosis under echographic guide: experimental study of periarticular injections. *Eur J Radiol.* 2008;68(1):170-173.

364. Milch H. Patellar tendinosis. *Bull Hosp Joint Dis.* 1955;16(2):125-128.

365. Alfredson H, Lorentzon M, Backman S, Backman A, Lerner UH. cDNA-arrays and real-time quantitative PCR techniques in the investigation of chronic Achilles tendinosis. *J Orthop Res.* 2003;21(6):970-975.

366. Fedorczyk JM, Barr AE, Rani S, et al. Exposure-dependent increases in IL-1beta, substance P, CTGF, and tendinosis in flexor digitorum tendons with upper extremity repetitive strain injury. *Journal of Orthopaedic Research.* 2010;28(3):298-307.

367. Willberg L, Sunding K, Ohberg L, Forssblad M, Fahlstrom M, Alfredson H. Sclerosing injections to treat midportion Achilles tendinosis: a randomised controlled study evaluating two different concentrations of Polidocanol. *Knee Surg Sports Traumatol Arthrosc.* 2008;16(9):859-864.

368. Swiontkowski MF, Tolo VT. Update to the retraction of "Skin-derived fibroblasts for the treatment of refractory Achilles tendinosis: preliminary short-term results" by H. Obaid, A. Clarke, P. Rosenfeld, C. Leach, and D. Connell. J Bone Joint Surg Am. 2012 Feb 1;94(3):193-200. *J Bone Joint Surg Am.* 2015;97(12):1011.

369. Chang YJ, Kulig K. The neuromechanical adaptations to Achilles tendinosis. *J Physiol.* 2015;593(15):3373-3387.

370. Ford RD, Schmitt WP, Lineberry K, Luce P. A retrospective comparison of the management of recalcitrant lateral elbow tendinosis: platelet-rich plasma injections versus surgery. *Hand.* 2015;10(2):285-291.

371. Dallaudiere B, Zurlinden O, Perozziello A, et al. Combined intra-tendinous injection of platelet rich plasma and bevacizumab accelerates and improves healing compared to platelet rich plasma in tendinosis: comprehensive assessment on a rat model. *Muscles Ligaments Tendons J.* 2014;4(3):351-356.

372. Seo JB, Yoo JS, Ryu JW. Sonoelastography findings of biceps tendinitis and tendinosis. *J Ultrasound.* 2014;17(4):271-277.

373. Millar NL, Gilchrist DS, Akbar M, et al. MicroRNA29a regulates IL-33-mediated tissue remodelling in tendon disease. *Nat Commun.* 2015;6:6774.

374. MacEoin F, Robinson P. Repetitive stress-related injury of the proximal metacarpus in a seven-year old thoroughbred racehorse with emphasis on diagnostic analgesia of the proximopalmar metacarpus. *Ir Vet J.* 2014;67(1):26.

375. Wong E, Lee G, Zucherman J, Mason DT. Successful management of female office workers with "repetitive stress injury" or "carpal tunnel syndrome" by a new treatment modality--application of low level laser. *Int J Clin Pharmacol Ther.* 1995;33(4):208-211.

376. Saito K, Shimizu F, Sato T, Oite T. Modulation of human mesangial cell behaviour by extracellular matrix components--the possible role of interstitial type III collagen. *Clin Exp Immunol.* 1993;91(3):510-515.

377. Lim VF, Khoo JK, Wong V, Moore KH. Recent studies of genetic dysfunction in pelvic organ prolapse: the role of collagen defects. *Aust N Z J Obstet Gynaecol.* 2014;54(3):198-205.

378. Palma E, Tiepolo T, Angelin A, et al. Genetic ablation of cyclophilin D rescues mitochondrial defects and prevents muscle apoptosis in collagen VI myopathic mice. *Hum Mol Genet.* 2009;18(11):2024-2031.

379. Sugimoto H, Mundel TM, Sund M, Xie L, Cosgrove D, Kalluri R. Bone-marrow-derived stem cells repair basement membrane collagen defects and reverse genetic kidney disease. *Proc Natl Acad Sci USA.* 2006;103(19):7321-7326.

380. Prockop DJ. Genetic defects of collagen. *Hosp Pract (Off Ed).* 1986;21(2):125-129, 133-125, 138-140.

381. Eyre DR. Collagen defects in genetic disorders of connective tissue. *Dev Med Child Neurol.* 1974;16(4):531-533.

382. Barascuk N, Vassiliadis E, Larsen L, et al. Development and validation of an enzyme-linked immunosorbent assay for the quantification of a specific MMP-9 mediated degradation fragment of type III collagen--A novel biomarker of atherosclerotic plaque remodeling. *Clin Biochem.* 2011;44(10-11):900-906.

383. Horslev-Petersen K. Circulating extracellular matrix components as markers for connective tissue response to inflammation. A clinical and experimental study with special emphasis on serum amino-terminal type III procollagen peptide in rheumatic diseases. *Dan Med Bull.* 1990;37(4):308-329.

384. Miedel EL, Brisson BK, Hamilton T, et al. Type III collagen modulates fracture callus bone formation and early remodeling. *J Orthop Res.* 2015;33(5):675-684.

385. Ping FY, Yan FG, Cheng J. [Use of 3-D cranial model in the treatment of bilateral TMJ ankylosis with microsomia by distraction osteogenesis]. *Zhonghua Kou Qiang Yi Xue Za Zhi.* 2008;43(3):185-186.

386. Hansen P, Kovanen V, Holmich P, et al. Micromechanical properties and collagen composition of ruptured human Achilles tendon. *Am J Sports Med.* 2013;41(2):437-443.

387. Aagaard P, Simonsen EB, Andersen JL, Magnusson P, Dyhre-Poulsen P. Neural adaptation to resistance training: changes in evoked V-wave and H-reflex responses. *J Appl Physiol.* 2002;92(6):2309-2318.

388. Coussens LM, Fingleton B, Matrisian LM. Matrix metalloproteinase inhibitors and cancer: trials and tribulations. *Science.* 2002;295(5564):2387-2392.

389. DeClerck YA, Mercurio AM, Stack MS, et al. Proteases, extracellular matrix, and cancer: a workshop of the path B study section. *Am J Pathol.* 2004;164(4):1131-1139.

390. Aagaard P. Training-induced changes in neural function. *Exerc Sport Sci Rev.* 2003;31(2):61-67.

391. Aagaard P, Simonsen EB, Andersen JL, Magnusson P, Dyhre-Poulsen P. Increased rate of force development and neural drive of human skeletal muscle following resistance training. *J Appl Physiol.* 2002;93(4):1318-1326.

392. Tanigawa S, Aida Y, Kawato T, et al. Interleukin-17F affects cartilage matrix turnover by increasing the expression of collagenases and stromelysin-1 and by decreasing the expression of their inhibitors and extracellular matrix components in chondrocytes. *Cytokine.* 2011;56(2):376-386.

393. Bass E. Tendinopathy: why the difference between tendinitis and tendinosis matters. *Int J Ther Massage Bodywork.* 2012;5(1):14-17.

394. Beischer AD, Beamond BM, Jowett AJ, O'Sullivan R. Distal tendinosis of the tibialis anterior tendon. *Foot Ankle Int.* 2009;30(11):1053-1059.

395. Korniejewska A, McKnight AJ, Johnson Z, Watson ML, Ward SG. Expression and agonist responsiveness of CXCR3 variants in human T lymphocytes. *Immunology.* 2011;132(4):503-515.

396. Poltawski L, Edwards H, Todd A, Watson T, Lees A, James CA. Ultrasound treatment of cutaneous side-effects of infused apomorphine: a randomized controlled pilot study. *Mov Disord.* 2009;24(1):115-118.

397. Roach KE, Ally D, Finnerty B, et al. The relationship between duration of physical therapy services in the acute care setting and change in functional status in patients with lower-extremity orthopedic problems. *Phys Ther.* 1998;78(1):19-24.

398. Poltawski L, Johnson M, Watson T. Microcurrent therapy in the management of chronic tennis elbow: pilot studies to optimize parameters. *Physiother Res Int.* 2012;17(3):157-166.

399. Calatroni A, Avenoso A, Ferlazzo AM, Lindner A, Campo GM. Transient increase with strenuous exercise of plasma levels of glycosaminoglycans in humans and horses. *Connect Tissue Res.* 2008;49(6):416-425. doi:10.1080/03008200802324949

400. Heinemeier KM, Olesen JL, Haddad F, Langberg H, Kjær M, Baldwin KM, Schjerling P. Expression of collagen and related growth factors in rat tendon and skeletal muscle in response to specific contraction types. *J Physiol.* 2007:582(Pt 3):1303-1316

401. Hirose T, Nakazato K, Song H, Ishii N. TGF-beta1 and TNF-alpha is involved in the transcription of type I collagen alpha2 gene in soleus muscle atrophied by mechanical unloading. *J Appl Physiol.* 2007;104(1):170-177.

402. Kjær M. Role of extracellular matrix in adaptation of tendon and skeletal muscle to mechanical loading. *Physiol Rev.* 2004;84(2): 649-698.

403. Pedersen B, Febbraio M. Muscles, exercise and obesity: skeletal muscle as a secretory organ. *Nat Rev Endocrinol.* 2012;8(8):457-465. doi:10.1038/nrendo.2012.49

404. Son JS, Chae SA, Testroet ED, Du M, Jun H-P. Exercise-induced myokines: a brief review of controversial issues of this decade. *Expert Rev Endocrinol Metab.* 2018;13(1): 51-58. doi:10.1080/17446651.2018.1416290

405. D'Urso M, Kurniawan NA. Mechanical and physical regulation of fibroblast-myofibroblast transition: from cellular mechanoresponse to tissue pathology. *Front Bioeng Biotechnol.* 2020;8:609653. doi:10.3389/fbioe.2020.609653

406. Khanna A, Nelmes RTC, Gougoulias N, Maffulli N, Gray J. The effects of LIPUS on soft-tissue healing: a review of literature. *Br Med Bull.* 2009;89:169-182. doi:10.1093/bmb/ldn040

407. Tsai W-C, Pang J-HS, Hsu C-C, Chu N-K, Lin M-S, Hu C-F. (2006), Ultrasound stimulation of types I and III collagen expression of tendon cell and upregulation of transforming growth factor beta. *J Orthop Res.* 2006;24(6):1310-1316. doi:10.1002/jor.20130

408. Tsai W-C, Hsu C-C, Tang F-T, Chou S-W, Chen Y-J, Pang J-HS. Ultrasound stimulation of tendon cell proliferation and upregulation of proliferating cell nuclear antigen. *J Orthop Res.* 2005;23:970-976. doi:10.1016/j.orthres.2004.11.013

409. Yeung CK, Guo X, Ng YF. Pulsed ultrasound treatment accelerates the repair of Achilles tendon rupture in rats. J Orthop Res. 2006;24(2):193-201. doi:10.1002/jor.20020

410. Rego EB, Inubushi T, Kawazoe A, et al. Ultrasound stimulation induces PGE(2) synthesis promoting cementoblastic differentiation through EP2/EP4 receptor pathway. *Ultrasound Med Biol.* 2010;36(6):907-915. doi:10.1016/j.ultrasmedbio.2010.03.008

411. Jung YJ, Kim R, Ham HJ, et al. Focused low-intensity pulsed ultrasound enhances bone regeneration in rat calvarial bone defect through enhancement of cell proliferation. *Ultrasound Med Biol.* 2015;41(4):999-1007.

412. Jia L, Chen J, Wang Y, Zhang Y Chen W. Focused low-intensity pulsed ultrasound affects extracellular matrix degradation via decreasing chondrocyte apoptosis and inflammatory mediators in a surgically induced osteoarthritic rabbit model. *Ultrasound Med Biol.* 2016;42(1):208-219. doi:10.1016/j.ultrasmedbio.2015.08.010.

413. Zhang Z, Ma Y, Guo S, He Y, Bai G, Zhang W. Low-intensity pulsed ultrasound stimulation facilitates in vitro osteogenic differentiation of human adipose-derived stem cells via up-regulation of heat shock protein (HSP)70, HSP90, and bone morphogenetic protein (BMP) signaling pathway. *Biosci Rep.* 2018;38(3). doi:10.1042/BSR20180087

414. Bjordal JM, Iversen V, Lopes-Martins RAB. Low level laser therapy reduces inflammation in activated Achilles tendinitis, Proc. SPIE 6140, Mechanisms for Low-Light Therapy, 61400G (28 February 2006). doi:10.1117/12.645516

415. Laraia EMS, Silva IS, Pereira DM, et al. Effect of low-level laser therapy (660 nm) on acute inflammation induced by tenotomy of Achilles tendon in rats. Photochem Photobiol. 2012;88:1546-1550. doi:10.1111/j.1751-1097.2012.01179.x

416. Oliveira MC, Greiffo FR, Rigonato-Oliveira NC, et al. Low level laser therapy reduces acute lung inflammation in a model of pulmonary and extrapulmonary LPS-induced ARDS. *J Photochem Photobiol B.* 2014;134:57-63. doi:10.1016/j.jphotobiol.2014.03.021

417. Saygun I, Nizam N, Uğur Ural A, Abdülkadir Serdar M, Avcu F, Fikret Tözüm T. Low-level laser irradiation affects the release of basic fibroblast growth factor (bFGF), insulin-like growth factor-I (IGF-I), and receptor of IGF-I (IGFBP3) from osteoblasts. *Photomed Laser Surg.* 2012;30(3):149-154.

418. Pereira MCMC, Bacellar de Pinho C, Ribeiro Peixoto Medrado A, de Araújo Andrade Z, Regina de Almeida Reis S. Influence of 670 nm low-level laser therapy on mast cells and vascular response of cutaneous injuries. *J Photochem Photobiol B.* 2010;98(3):188-192. doi:10.1016/j.jphotobiol.2009.12.005

419. Sakurai T, Terashima S, Miyakoshi J. Enhanced secretion of prostaglandin E2 from osteoblasts by exposure to a strong static magnetic field. *Bioelectromagnetics.* 2008;29(4):277-283. doi:10.1002/bem.20392

420. Patruno A, Amerio P, Pesce M, et al. Extremely low frequency electromagnetic fields modulate expression of inducible nitric oxide synthase, endothelial nitric oxide synthase and cyclooxygenase-2 in the human keratinocyte cell line HaCat: potential therapeutic effects in wound healing. *Br J Dermatol.* 2010;162(2):258-266. doi:10.1111/j.1365-2133.2009.09527.x

Peripheral and Central Nervous System Reflex Testing

Neurodynamic Testing and Treatment for the Spine and Extremities

Robert J. Nee, PT, PhD, MAppSc; Benjamin S. Boyd, PT, DPTSc; and Michel W. Coppieters, PT, PhD

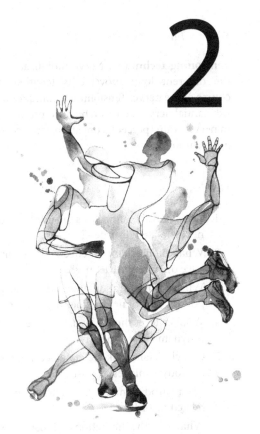

KEY TERMS

Kappa statistic: Quantifies the reliability of a categorical measure by correcting for agreement that could occur by chance. Higher values indicate higher levels of agreement beyond what would be expected by chance.

Negative likelihood ratio (-LR): The change in odds of a patient having the target condition of interest when the clinical test is negative. -LRs less than 0.2 reflect potentially important decreases in the patient's odds of having the target condition when the clinical test is negative.

Nerve mobilization exercises: Active or passive movements that create movement between sensitized neural tissues and surrounding structures. They aim to normalize the altered homeostasis in and around the nervous system to reduce nerve mechanosensitivity. They can be categorized as *sliding* or *tensioning techniques*.

Neurodynamic test: A series of spine and limb movements that aim to detect increased nerve mechanosensitivity by applying mechanical forces to part of the nervous system. Neurodynamic tests apply different types of mechanical forces to nerves because test movements lengthen the anatomical course of the nerve.

Positive likelihood ratio (+LR): The change in odds of a patient having the target condition of interest when the clinical test is positive. +LRs greater than 5.0 reflect potentially important increases in the patient's odds of having the target condition when the clinical test is positive.

Sliding technique: Nerve mobilization exercise where a joint movement that lengthens the anatomical course of the nerve is simultaneously counterbalanced by another joint movement that shortens the anatomical course of the nerve. Sliding techniques produce significant amounts of nerve excursion with relatively minimal increases in nerve strain (percent elongation).

Smallest detectable difference (SDD; or minimal detectable change): Quantifies the absolute reliability of a continuous measure. It is the threshold for the difference between 2 measurements that is not likely to be due to error. An SDD of 20 degrees means that a difference between 2 measurements greater than 20 degrees suggests a "true" difference.

Standardized mean difference: Quantifies the size of a treatment effect. Expresses the difference between group means as a proportion of the standard deviation for the entire sample. If the difference between group means is 5 points and the standard deviation for the sample is 10 points, the standardized mean difference is 0.5.

Wallmann HW, Donatelli R, eds. *Foundations of Orthopedic Physical Therapy* (pp 49-79).
© 2024 Taylor & Francis Group.

Tensioning technique: Nerve mobilization exercise where the different joint movements lengthen the anatomical course of the nerve. Tensioning techniques may still produce substantial nerve excursion but also produce larger increases in nerve strain (percent elongation) than corresponding sliding techniques.

CHAPTER QUESTIONS

1. Are neurodynamic tests plausible tests for detecting nerve-related disorders?

2. What biomechanical effects do neurodynamic tests have on neural structures?

3. What is structural differentiation and why is it an important part of neurodynamic testing?

4. What criteria should be used to decide whether a neurodynamic test is positive?

5. Can clinicians make reliable decisions about whether a neurodynamic test is positive?

6. Are neurodynamic tests accurate for detecting nerve-related disorders?

7. What are the limitations of using electrodiagnostic testing as the reference standard for judging the accuracy of neurodynamic tests for detecting nerve-related disorders?

8. Does a positive neurodynamic test indicate where along the nerve the problem is located?

9. Why might it be useful clinically to change the order of movement of a neurodynamic test?

10. Does a positive neurodynamic test mean that nerve movement is restricted?

11. Is it important to consider psychosocial factors when interpreting the findings from a neurodynamic test?

12. What are the 3 broad treatment approaches that attempt to reduce nerve mechanosensitivity?

13. What is the primary goal of pain biology education and why is it an important part of treating patients who have increased nerve mechanosensitivity?

14. What is the evidence for neurodynamic treatment effects?

15. What are the potential mechanisms behind neurodynamic treatment effects?

16. Does a positive neurodynamic test mean that nerve mobilization exercises need to be part of the intervention program?

17. What differences are there in the biomechanical effects of "sliding" techniques and "tensioning" techniques?

18. Which type of nerve mobilization exercises are better: sliding techniques or tensioning techniques?

19. What factors should clinicians consider when making decisions about the dosage of neurodynamic treatment techniques (eg, provocation of symptoms, frequency each day, number of repetitions)?

20. Are neurodynamic treatment techniques safe?

INTRODUCTION

Neurodynamics employs movement and education to evaluate and treat nervous system related disorders.[1-3] Historically, neurodynamics focused on musculoskeletal nerve-related conditions such as radicular pain and peripheral nerve entrapment syndromes. However, more recent discussion has proposed that neurodynamics may also have a role in the management of systemic conditions such as diabetes mellitus[4,5] and central nervous system (CNS) disorders such as stroke,[6,7] acquired brain injury,[8] and cerebral palsy.[9] This chapter focuses on the application of neurodynamics in musculoskeletal rehabilitation.

In musculoskeletal rehabilitation, an important feature of nerve-related disorders that neurodynamics tries to address is increased mechanosensitivity.[1-3] Specific combinations of spine and limb movements can be used to detect increased nerve mechanosensitivity (neurodynamic tests).[1,2,10-12] Movements can alternatively be designed to restore homeostasis in and around the nervous system, reduce nerve mechanosensitivity, and restore symptom-free function (neurodynamic treatment techniques).[1,13,14] Educational messages help patients understand the purpose and results of neurodynamic tests and the rationale for neurodynamic treatment techniques.[1,15]

It is important to remember that patients who may have radicular pain or peripheral nerve entrapment syndromes are not the only candidates for neurodynamic testing and treatment. Neurodynamics can also be applied to other conditions that sometimes have a component of increased nerve mechanosensitivity such as lateral elbow pain, Achilles tendinopathy, plantar heel pain, and intramuscular hamstring injury.[1,15] This chapter provides an evidence-informed review of neurodynamics for patients who have nerve-related musculoskeletal conditions.

NEURODYNAMIC TESTING

Neurodynamic tests try to detect increased nerve mechanosensitivity by using a series of spine and limb movements to apply mechanical forces to part of the nervous system.[1,10-12] Neurodynamic tests also apply forces to nonneural tissues. Distinguishing neural from nonneural tissue responses to a neurodynamic test can be potentially achieved through structural differentiation. Structural differentiation involves moving a proximal or distal body part that further loads or unloads the nervous system, but does not change the load on relevant nonneural tissues, and monitoring its effect on the neurodynamic test response.[1,2,10-12] An abnormal test response that changes with structural differentiation is thought to reflect increased nerve sensitivity as long as central pain mechanisms are not making the primary contribution to the patient's pain experience.[1,2,10-12,16] For example, dorsiflexing the ankle to change low back and buttock pain provoked in a straight leg raise (SLR) test position suggests a neural tissue response to this neurodynamic test. Standard neurodynamic tests and associated structural differentiation maneuvers are summarized in Tables 2-1 and 2-2, and the end positions for these tests are illustrated in Figures 2-1 and 2-2.

According to expert clinicians, neurodynamic tests are important for diagnosing nerve-related disorders.[20] Guidelines also recommend that neurodynamic tests be part of the clinical examination of patients who have spine or limb symptoms.[21-26] It is therefore important to understand the validity of neurodynamic tests for diagnosing nerve-related disorders. Neurodynamic test validity can be assessed by answering 4 questions[27-31]:

1. Are neurodynamic tests plausible tests for detecting nerve-related disorders?

2. What criteria should be used to define a positive neurodynamic test?

3. Can clinicians make reliable decisions about a positive neurodynamic test?

4. Are neurodynamic tests accurate for detecting nerve-related disorders (concurrent validity)?

Plausibility of Neurodynamic Tests

Biomechanical and experimental pain data suggest that neurodynamic tests are plausible tests for detecting nerve-related disorders. Biomechanical studies (cadaver and in vivo) consistently show that spine,[32-37] upper limb,[17,18,31,38-46] and lower limb[39,45,47-63] movements involved in neurodynamic tests produce strain, tension, and excursion in neural tissues. Strain (percent elongation) and tension increase because neurodynamic test movements lengthen the anatomical course of the corresponding nerve. Excursion involves longitudinal and transverse sliding of nerves relative to surrounding structures. Longitudinal sliding of a nerve segment will be toward the moving joint as the anatomical course of the nerve is lengthened and away from the moving joint as the anatomical course of the nerve is shortened,[64] but the direction of transverse sliding is more variable.

A neurodynamic test applies more load to its corresponding nerve than to other major nerves in the limb, especially in the distal part of the limb. For example, mechanical loading of the radial and ulnar nerves in the upper arm near the axilla is greatest with the radial and ulnar nerve neurodynamic tests, respectively.[17,41] Another study, however, did not find these differences to be statistically significant.[65] Data consistently show that mechanical loading of the median nerve at the elbow and wrist is greatest with the median nerve upper limb neurodynamic test (ULNT1$_{MEDIAN}$).[66,67] Collectively, these data suggest that testing for increased nerve mechanosensitivity in the limb, especially the distal part of the limb, may be best achieved by using the neurodynamic test thought to target that nerve. Examples include combining ankle dorsiflexion and inversion with passive SLR to assess sural nerve mechanosensitivity near the Achilles tendon,[56] or using ankle plantarflexion and inversion during the slump test to assess deep fibular nerve mechanosensitivity in patients who have symptoms related to an inversion ankle sprain.[68] However, neurodynamic tests cannot selectively test the mechanosensitivity of individual spinal nerves or nerve roots.[40,49,52,65,69]

In the biomechanical studies cited earlier, strain, tension, and excursion generated by a joint movement are greatest in nerve segments that are closest to the moving joint. However, the biomechanical effects of a joint movement performed at the end of a neurodynamic test may spread along the entire nerve.[31,51,54,70,71] These findings support the concept of structural differentiation because the spread of biomechanical effects along the nerve is a plausible explanation for why sensory responses provoked at the end of a neurodynamic test can change with movement of a proximal or distal body part.[31]

Transmission of strain and tension through fascial networks in the neck, trunk, and limbs could also explain why movement of a proximal or distal body part changes a neurodynamic test response.[72-76] However, studies are still needed to determine whether strain and tension produced by a structural differentiation maneuver at the end of a neurodynamic test are transmitted over multiple joints involved in the corresponding fascial network as has been shown for the nervous system.[31]

Neurodynamic test movements also increase pressure within and around nerves. Increased strain and tension are accompanied by increased intraneural pressure.[77-82] There are several examples of neurodynamic test movements that increase pressure around nerves. Wrist extension increases pressure around the median nerve in the carpal tunnel[83-85]; the combination of elbow flexion and wrist extension increases pressure around the ulnar nerve at the elbow[86,87]; the combination of elbow extension, forearm pronation, and wrist flexion increases pressure around the deep branch of the radial nerve in the radial tunnel[88,89]; and the combination of ankle dorsiflexion and eversion increases pressure around the tibial nerve in the tarsal tunnel.[90]

Table 2-1

SUMMARY OF NEURODYNAMIC TESTS FOR THE UPPER LIMB WITH ASSOCIATED MANEUVERS FOR STRUCTURAL DIFFERENTIATION[1,10]

TEST	STANDARD SEQUENCE*	TYPICAL STRUCTURAL DIFFERENTIATION MANEUVERS
ULNT1$_{MEDIAN}$ (emphasis shoulder abduction)	• Shoulder girdle stabilization • Shoulder abduction • Wrist/finger extension • Forearm supination • Shoulder external rotation • Elbow extension	• Cervical side-bending • Release wrist extension
ULNT2$_{MEDIAN}$ (emphasis shoulder girdle depression)	• Shoulder girdle depression • Elbow extension • Shoulder external rotation and forearm supination • Wrist/finger extension • Shoulder abduction	• Cervical side-bending • Release shoulder girdle depression • Release wrist extension
ULNT$_{RADIAL}$	• Shoulder girdle depression • Elbow extension • Shoulder internal rotation and forearm pronation • Wrist/finger flexion • Shoulder abduction	• Cervical side-bending • Release shoulder girdle depression • Release wrist flexion
ULNT$_{ULNAR}$	• Wrist/finger extension • Forearm pronation • Elbow flexion • Shoulder external rotation† • Shoulder girdle depression • Shoulder abduction	• Cervical side-bending • Release shoulder girdle depression • Release wrist extension

* Although standard sequences have been recommended to increase test reliability, clinicians are encouraged to adjust the order of movement to match an individual patient's presentation.

† Shoulder internal rotation may also be an option.[17,18,19]

Table 2-2

SUMMARY OF NEURODYNAMIC TESTS FOR THE LOWER LIMB AND TRUNK WITH ASSOCIATED MANEUVERS FOR STRUCTURAL DIFFERENTIATION[1,11,12,16,34,47,91-93]

TEST	STANDARD SEQUENCE*	TYPICAL STRUCTURAL DIFFERENTIATION MANEUVERS
PNF[†]	• Upper cervical flexion ("head on neck" flexion) • Lower cervical flexion ("neck on shoulder" flexion)	• None[‡]
SLR	• Pre-position with knee extended • Hip flexion	• Ankle DF • Hip ADD or ABD • Hip IR or ER • Neck flexion[§]
Slump	• Trunk flexion • Neck flexion • Ankle DF • Knee extension	• Release neck flexion
PKB	• Knee flexion	• None[‖]
Side-lying slump ("femoral slump")	• Pre-position in side lying with trunk and neck flexed; tested limb in 90-degree knee flexion • Hip extension • Knee flexion	• Release neck flexion

* Although standard sequences have been recommended to increase test reliability, clinicians are encouraged to adjust the order of movement to match an individual patient's presentation.

† May be performed in supine or sitting.[16,34]

‡ Focus on reproduction of symptoms in the lumbar region.[16,34]

§ Data suggest that neck flexion rarely changes SLR response (< 20%).[16,47]

‖ Focus on reproduction of symptoms consistent with nerve sensitivity.[93]

ABD = abduction; ADD = adduction; DF = dorsiflexion; ER = external rotation; EV = eversion; INV = inversion; IR = internal rotation; PKB = prone knee bend; PF = plantarflexion; PNF = passive neck flexion.

These biomechanical data suggest that neurodynamic tests are plausible tests for detecting nerve-related disorders. Strain, tension, and pressure from neurodynamic test movements will likely provoke mechanically sensitive neural tissues in patients who have nerve-related disorders.[94-99] Additionally, proximal or distal joint movements applied at the end of a neurodynamic test (structural differentiation) can likely help determine whether a test response is related to nerve mechanosensitivity because their biomechanical effects spread along the entire nerve.

Experimental pain studies also support the plausibility of neurodynamic tests. Experimental pain induced by injecting hypertonic saline into the thenar or calf muscles is not changed by applying structural differentiation maneuvers associated with the ULNT1$_{MEDIAN}$ or the SLR and slump tests, respectively.[100,101] Similarly, experimental pain induced by injecting hypertonic saline into the medial infrapatellar fat pad is not changed by neck movements performed at the end of the side-lying slump test (femoral slump test).[102] These data suggest that neurodynamic tests can potentially distinguish pain related to irritation of nonneural tissues from pain related to irritation of neural tissues.[31] Even though biomechanical and experimental pain data support using neurodynamic tests to detect nerve-related problems, plausibility is the lowest level of test validity.[28]

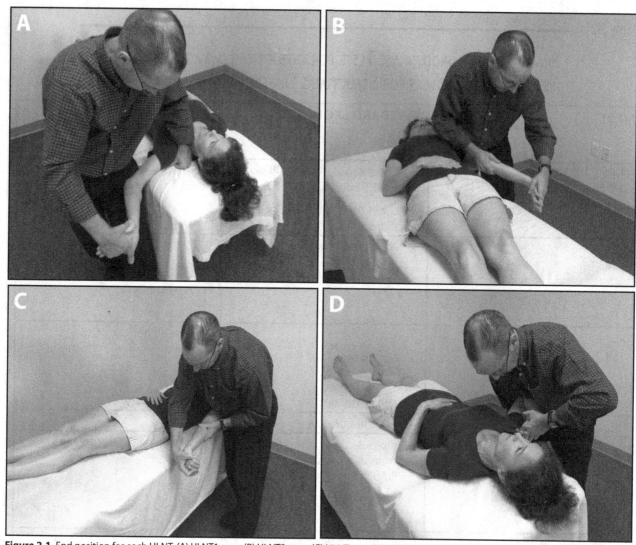

Figure 2-1. End position for each ULNT. (A) ULNT1$_{MEDIAN}$. (B) ULNT2$_{MEDIAN}$. (C) ULNT$_{RADIAL}$. (D) ULNT$_{ULNAR}$.

Criteria for a Positive Neurodynamic Test

Criteria for a positive neurodynamic test need to discriminate patients who have nerve-related disorders from asymptomatic individuals, and patients who have nerve-related disorders from patients who have competing diagnoses (concurrent validity).[30] Clinicians have been encouraged to assess sensory responses, resistance to movement, and range of motion (ROM) during a neurodynamic test to judge whether a patient has signs of increased nerve mechanosensitivity.[1,10] The ability of these components of a neurodynamic test response to discriminate patients who have nerve-related disorders from asymptomatic individuals forms the rationale behind proposed criteria for a positive neurodynamic test.[31] Concurrent validity is addressed later in this chapter.

Most asymptomatic individuals (greater than or equal to 80%) report sensory responses at the end of a neurodynamic test that change with structural differentiation.[19,31,91,103-108] Common descriptors include stretch, ache, pain, burning, and tingling.[19,31,91,103-109] Asymptomatic individuals, therefore, appear to have a certain level of nerve mechanosensitivity. The range of sensory responses reported by asymptomatic individuals makes it important to specify which sensory responses qualify as a positive neurodynamic test in symptomatic populations. A neurodynamic test is most likely identifying a patient with increased nerve mechanosensitivity when the test reproduces at least part of the patient's symptoms and the symptoms change with structural differentiation.[31]

Resistance to movement and ROM are not likely to discriminate patients who have nerve-related disorders from asymptomatic individuals. Different examiners cannot reliably identify the onset of resistance to elbow extension during ULNT1$_{MEDIAN}$.[110,111] The SDD between examiners at a 95% confidence level (SDD$_{95}$)[112] for measuring the onset of resistance to elbow extension is 28 degrees.[31] Studies quantifying the onset of resistance during the SLR and slump tests have only reported intra-examiner reliability.[113,114] Large measurement error between examiners suggests that onset of resistance is not likely to be sensitive enough to discriminate

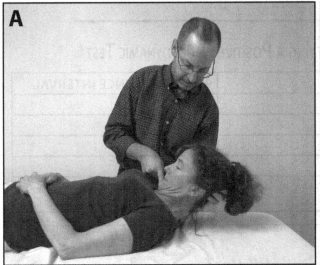
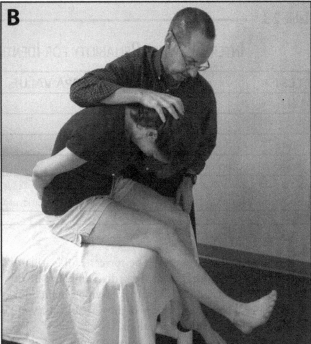
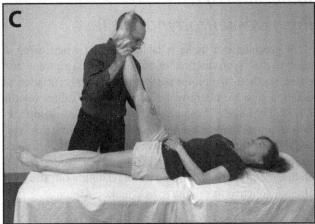
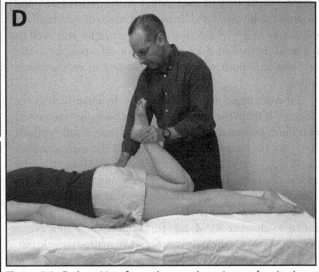
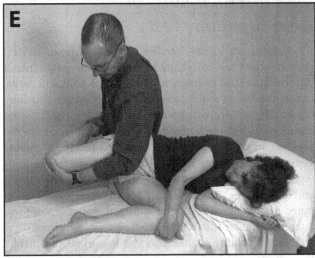

Figure 2-2. End position for each neurodynamic test for the lower limbs and trunk. (A) PNF. (B) Slump. (C) SLR. (D) PKB. (E) Side-lying slump ("femoral slump").

patients who have nerve-related disorders from asymptomatic individuals. Therefore, resistance to movement is unlikely to be useful for defining a positive neurodynamic test.[31]

Neurodynamic test ROM is most commonly measured at pain onset or pain tolerance during the last component of the test.[31] Examples include elbow extension during $ULNT1_{MEDIAN}$ or elbow flexion for $ULNT_{ULNAR}$, shoulder abduction during $ULNT_{RADIAL}$, hip flexion during SLR, and

knee extension during the slump test. As with resistance to movement, there are relatively large errors between examiners for measuring neurodynamic test ROM at pain onset. SDDs (SDD_{95}) between examiners for measuring ROM at pain onset are approximately 15 to 20 degrees for the $ULNT1_{MEDIAN}$,[111,115,116] $ULNT_{ULNAR}$,[117] SLR,[118-120] and slump[120] tests (calculated from reported data).

Table 2-3

INTER-EXAMINER RELIABILITY FOR IDENTIFYING A POSITIVE NEURODYNAMIC TEST*

TEST	KAPPA VALUE	95% CONFIDENCE INTERVAL
ULNTs[130]†	0.45	0.27, 0.63
SLR[120,131-133]	≥0.49	0.14, 1.00
Slump[120,134]	≥0.71	0.33, 0.97
Side-lying slump[92] (femoral slump)	0.71	0.33, 1.00

* Positive test defined as at least partial reproduction of the patient's symptoms and changing these symptoms with structural differentiation.

† Collective estimate for the median, radial, and ulnar nerve neurodynamic tests.

Even if reliability issues could be corrected, it is still unlikely that neurodynamic test ROM can discriminate patients who have nerve-related disorders from asymptomatic individuals. Neurodynamic test ROM is highly variable in asymptomatic and symptomatic populations.[31,104,107,109,114,117,118,120-125] There is also a lot of overlap in neurodynamic test ROM between asymptomatic and symptomatic individuals, and between the involved and uninvolved limbs of symptomatic individuals.[31,120,123-125] Because of this variability and overlap, it is unlikely that an absolute ROM cut-off would be useful for defining a positive neurodynamic test in an individual patient.

Neurodynamic test ROM can also be quantified as the deficit in ROM in the involved limb relative to the uninvolved limb (limb asymmetry). Asymptomatic individuals typically have 5 to 10 degree differences in ROM between limbs for ULNT1$_{MEDIAN}$,[126-129] ULNT$_{ULNAR}$,[117] and SLR[122] tests. It is still unclear if a certain amount of limb asymmetry in neurodynamic test ROM can discriminate patients who have nerve-related disorders from asymptomatic individuals. Therefore, similar to absolute ROM, it seems unlikely that limb asymmetry in ROM can help define a positive neurodynamic test.

Current evidence does not support using resistance to movement or ROM to define a positive neurodynamic test because of the previously described problems with measurement error and lack of discriminatory cut-off values. At this point, the recommended criteria for a positive neurodynamic test include at least partial reproduction of the patient's symptoms *and* a change in these symptoms with structural differentiation.[31] Reproducing the patient's symptoms helps distinguish the patient's response from sensory responses to neurodynamic tests that are typical for asymptomatic individuals. Changing the patient's symptoms with structural differentiation makes it more likely that these symptoms are at least partly related to increased nerve mechanosensitivity.

Reliability of a Positive Neurodynamic Test

Clinicians can make reliable decisions when using at least partial reproduction of the patient's symptoms and changing these symptoms with structural differentiation to define a positive neurodynamic test. Kappa values for the ULNTs,[130] SLR,[120,131-133] slump,[120,134] and side-lying slump[92] reflect adequate inter-examiner reliability for making this "yes" or "no" decision about a positive test (Table 2-3). Although kappa values between 0.41 and 0.60 suggest moderate reliability,[135] clinical tests with moderate reliability can still have enough concurrent validity to help make a diagnosis.[29,136]

Concurrent Validity of Neurodynamic Tests

Concurrent validity studies use results from a reference standard test to quantify the diagnostic performance of the clinical test of interest.[29,30] Radicular pain and carpal tunnel syndrome are the nerve-related disorders that have been addressed in concurrent validity studies on neurodynamic tests. Reference standard tests used to establish the presence of these nerve-related disorders include a grading system for diagnosing neuropathic pain,[137] electrodiagnosis (eg, nerve conduction studies, needle electromyography), and imaging (eg, magnetic resonance imaging [MRI], computed tomography scans). Strengths and limitations of these reference standards affect the conclusions drawn from these concurrent validity studies. It is also important to consider the criteria used to define a positive neurodynamic test.[138] This section focuses on studies where criteria for a positive neurodynamic test made it likely that symptoms were at least partly related to increased nerve mechanosensitivity.

Table 2-4

DIAGNOSTIC ACCURACY OF THE
STRAIGHT LEG RAISE AND SLUMP TESTS FOR LUMBAR RADICULAR PAIN*

TEST	REFERENCE STANDARD	SENSITIVITY (95% CI)	SPECIFICITY (95% CI)	POSITIVE LR (95% CI)	NEGATIVE LR (95% CI)
SLR[140†‡]	Imaging or EDX	0.19 to 0.97	0.10 to 0.89	1.1 to 4.7	0.27 to 0.96
SLR[142]	Imaging§	0.59 (0.41, 0.75)	0.53 (0.41, 0.64)	1.26 (0.84, 1.87)	0.77 (0.47, 1.28)
SLR[142]	Imaging‖	0.93 (0.66, 1.00)	0.57 (0.45, 0.67)	2.1 (1.6, 2.8)	0.13 (0.02, 0.84)
SLR[142]	Imaging	0.32 (0.17, 0.52)	0.43 (0.33, 0.55)	0.56 (0.31, 1.03)	1.55 (1.08, 2.29)
SLR[143†]	EDX	0.63 (0.58, 0.69)	0.46 (0.39, 0.53)	1.2 (1.0, 1.5)	0.80 (0.64, 0.98)
Slump[139]	Imaging	0.84 (0.74, 0.90)	0.83 (0.73, 0.90)	4.9 (2.7, 9.0)	0.19 (0.11, 0.36)
Slump[142]	Imaging§	0.78 (0.59, 0.89)	0.36 (0.26, 0.48)	1.2 (0.93, 1.6)	0.61 (0.29, 1.3)
Slump[142]	Imaging‖	1.00 (0.77, 1.00)	0.38 (0.27, 0.49)	1.6 (1.4, 1.9)	0 (0.0, 0.0)
Slump[142]	Imaging¶	0.48 (0.29, 0.69)	0.26 (0.16, 0.37)	0.7 (0.42, 0.99)	2.0 (1.2, 3.5)
Slump[141]	Grading system#	0.91 (0.62, 0.98)	0.70 (0.40, 0.89)	3.0 (1.2, 8.0)	0.13 (0.02, 0.88)
Slump[141**]	Grading system#	0.55 (0.28, 0.79)	1.00 (0.72, 1.00)	11.9 (0.76, 188)	0.48 (0.26, 0.90)

* Unless noted otherwise, a positive test is defined as at least partial reproduction of the patient's symptoms and changing these symptoms with structural differentiation.

† Positive SLR was reproduction of patient's symptoms below the knee.

‡ Range of values reported from this systematic review.

§ MRI confirmed disk extrusion.

‖ MRI confirmed "high-grade" subarticular nerve root compression (obliteration of periradicular cerebrospinal fluid and fat).

¶ MRI confirmed high-grade foraminal nerve root compression.

Location and history of symptoms consistent with lumbar radicular pain *and* sensory signs present in areas consistent with lumbar radicular pain. Imaging findings could contribute to the diagnosis of lumbar radicular pain but were not required.[137,141]

** Positive slump test involved reproduction of patient's symptoms below the knee and changing these symptoms with structural differentiation.

CI = confidence interval; EDX = electrodiagnosis; LR = likelihood ratio.

Lumbar Radicular Pain

It appears that the slump test is more useful than SLR for diagnosing lumbar radicular pain, even when a positive SLR focuses on reproduction of symptoms below the knee (Table 2-4).[139-143] SLR results do not make clinically important changes in the odds of a patient having lumbar radicular pain because +LRs are consistently below 5.0 and -LRs are consistently above 0.2.[140,142-144] In contrast, both positive and negative slump test results are more commonly associated with clinically important changes in the odds of having this nerve-related disorder.[139,141,142,144] A positive slump test is particularly useful if it reproduces the patient's symptoms below the knee.[141] It appears, however, that diagnostic performance may vary according to the specific imaging finding used as the reference standard for radicular pain (eg, disk extrusion, subarticular nerve root compression, foraminal nerve root compression; see Table 2-4).[142]

One exception to the poor diagnostic performance of the SLR for detecting lumbar radicular pain is the crossed SLR. When SLR of the uninvolved limb reproduces symptoms in the involved limb (a positive crossed SLR), the patient is much more likely to have lumbar radicular pain related to lumbar disk herniation.[145] However, a positive crossed SLR is a relatively rare clinical finding.

Although SLR of the involved limb does not perform well as an isolated test, it may help detect lumbar radicular pain when combined with other clinical information. Two diagnostic decision tools suggest that provocation of a patient's typical leg symptoms during the SLR can help detect lumbar radicular pain when combined with other clinical information such as the distribution of the patient's symptoms and positive findings on a clinical neurological examination (ie, myotomes, reflexes, dermatomes).[146,147] However, the performance of these diagnostic decision tools needs to be confirmed in separate samples of patients before they can be recommended for use in clinical practice.[148]

Table 2-5

DIAGNOSTIC ACCURACY OF THE PRONE KNEE BEND AND SIDE-LYING SLUMP TESTS FOR LUMBAR RADICULAR PAIN AFFECTING THE L2 THROUGH L4 NERVE ROOTS*

TEST	REFERENCE STANDARD	SENSITIVITY (95% CI)	SPECIFICITY (95% CI)	POSITIVE LR (95% CI)	NEGATIVE LR (95% CI)
PKB[93]†	Imaging	0.50 (0.31, 0.69)	1.00 (0.88, 1.00)	∞‡	0.50 (0.34, 0.75)
Side-lying slump[92]§ (femoral slump)	Imaging	1.00 (0.40, 1.00)	0.83 (0.52, 0.98)	6.0 (1.6, 19.4)	0.0 (0.0, 0.6)
Side-lying slump[142] (femoral slump)	Imaging‖	0.43 (0.16, 0.75)	0.64 (0.36, 0.85)	1.2 (0.37, 3.8)	0.90 (0.41, 2.0)
Side-lying slump[142] (femoral slump)	Imaging¶	1.0 (0.21, 1.00)	0.65 (0.41, 0.83)	2.8 (1.5, 5.4)	0.0 (0.0, 0.0)
Side-lying slump[142] (femoral slump)	Imaging#	0.17 (0.03, 0.56)	0.50 (0.25, 0.75)	0.33 (0.05, 2.2)	1.67 (0.85, 3.3)

* Unless noted otherwise, a positive test is defined as at least partial reproduction of the patient's symptoms and changing these symptoms with structural differentiation.

† Reproduction of patient's lower limb symptoms only because no structural differentiation for PKB.

‡ Not able to calculate +LR value because specificity was 100%.

§ Patients in sample with upper/mid lumbar nerve root involvement only had problems at L4; none had L2 or L3 nerve root involvement.

‖ MRI confirmed disk extrusion.

¶ MRI confirmed high-grade subarticular nerve root compression (obliteration of periradicular cerebrospinal fluid and fat).

MRI confirmed high-grade foraminal nerve root compression.

CI = confidence interval; LR = likelihood ratio.

The PKB and side-lying slump neurodynamic tests may help identify radicular pain affecting the L2 through L4 nerve roots (Table 2-5).[92,93,142] Reproducing low back-related leg pain during a PKB makes it more likely that upper/mid lumbar nerve root involvement is contributing to the patient's pain experience, but a negative PKB does not significantly reduce the odds of upper/mid lumbar nerve root involvement.[93] Both positive and negative findings from the side-lying slump test make clinically important changes in a patient's odds of having L2 through L4 nerve root involvement.[92,142] However, similar to the slump test, diagnostic performance of the side-lying slump test appears to vary depending on the specific imaging finding used as the reference standard for radicular pain at these lumbar nerve root levels (see Table 2-5).[142]

Additional research with larger samples is needed so that estimates of diagnostic performance of the PKB, slump, and side-lying slump tests can be more precise.[92,93,141,142] Future research on the diagnostic performance of the SLR should consistently incorporate structural differentiation into the definition of a positive test.[140]

Cervical Radicular Pain

The median and ulnar nerve neurodynamic tests can help diagnose cervical radicular pain (Table 2-6).[149,150] A positive ulnar nerve test is associated with a clinically important increase in the patient's odds of having cervical radicular pain. A negative median nerve test (ULNT1$_{MEDIAN}$) significantly decreases the patient's odds of having this condition. It is important to note that shoulder girdle depression and shoulder abduction of at least 100 degrees were the first 2 movements for both the median and ulnar nerve tests in this study.[149] These 2 movements apply tensile forces throughout the brachial plexus,[17,65] so it makes sense biomechanically that the median and ulnar nerve tests help diagnose cervical radicular pain when performed in this manner. Confidence in these findings will increase if they are replicated in a separate sample of patients.

Other published data suggest that ULNT1$_{MEDIAN}$ can help diagnose cervical radicular pain.[151] However, a positive test did not require both reproduction of symptoms and a change in symptoms with structural differentiation. It is

Table 2-6

DIAGNOSTIC ACCURACY OF NEURODYNAMIC TESTS FOR CERVICAL RADICULAR PAIN[149]*†

TEST	SENSITIVITY (95% CI)	SPECIFICITY (95% CI)	POSITIVE LR‡ (95% CI)	NEGATIVE LR‡ (95% CI)
ULNT1$_{MEDIAN}$	0.88 (0.66, 0.93)	0.75 (0.48, 0.93)	3.3 (1.4, 7.8)	0.23 (0.1, 0.5)
ULNT2$_{MEDIAN}$	0.66 (0.48, 0.81)	0.75 (0.48, 0.93)	2.6 (1.1, 6.3)	0.46 (0.3, 0.8)
ULNT$_{RADIAL}$	0.43 (0.26, 0.61)	0.75 (0.48, 0.93)	1.7 (0.7, 4.3)	0.76 (0.5, 1.1)
ULNT$_{ULNAR}$	0.71 (0.54, 0.85)	0.87 (0.62, 0.98)	5.7 (1.5, 21.2)	0.33 (0.2, 0.6)

* Positive test is defined as at least partial reproduction of the patient's symptoms and changing these symptoms with structural differentiation.

† Reference standard for diagnosing cervical radicular pain involved patient history, clinical neurological examination, Spurling test, and MRI.

‡ Calculated by reconstructing 2 x 2 contingency tables from reported data.

CI = confidence interval.

Table 2-7

DIAGNOSTIC ACCURACY OF THE MEDIAN NERVE NEURODYNAMIC TEST (ULNT1$_{MEDIAN}$) FOR CARPAL TUNNEL SYNDROME*†

TEST	SENSITIVITY (95% CI)	SPECIFICITY (95% CI)	POSITIVE LR (95% CI)	NEGATIVE LR (95% CI)
Vanti et al[152]	0.29 (0.16, 0.45)	0.82 (0.69, 0.91)	1.6 (0.9, 2.8)	0.87 (0.5, 1.5)
Bueno-Gracia et al[153]	0.58 (0.45, 0.71)	0.84 (0.72, 0.96)	3.7 (1.7, 7.9)	0.50 (0.4, 0.7)

* Positive test is defined as at least partial reproduction of the patient's symptoms and changing these symptoms with structural differentiation (contralateral side-bending of the neck).

† Reference standard for diagnosing carpal tunnel syndrome was electrodiagnosis with nerve conduction studies.

CI = confidence interval.

therefore unclear whether a positive neurodynamic test was at least partly related to increased nerve mechanosensitivity. The accompanying diagnostic clinical prediction rule that included ULNT1$_{MEDIAN}$ has not been validated, so it cannot yet be recommended for clinical practice.[148]

Carpal Tunnel Syndrome

The median nerve neurodynamic test (ULNT1$_{MEDIAN}$) might not help diagnose carpal tunnel syndrome (Table 2-7).[150,152,153] ULNT1$_{MEDIAN}$ results do not make clinically important changes in the odds of a patient having carpal tunnel syndrome because +LRs are consistently below 5.0 and -LRs are consistently above 0.2.[144,152,153] These findings support other data showing low correlation between ULNT1$_{MEDIAN}$ results and electrodiagnostically confirmed carpal tunnel syndrome.[154] Despite these data, neurodynamic testing may still be relevant for patients suspected to have carpal tunnel syndrome. The prevalence of cervical radicular pain in patients who have carpal tunnel syndrome is much higher than in the general population.[155] Including neurodynamic testing as part of a comprehensive examination may help determine whether a patient suspected to have carpal tunnel syndrome has coexisting cervical radicular pain.

Potential for Bias in Concurrent Validity Studies

In concurrent validity studies, it is important that the intent of the reference standard test matches the intent of the clinical test.[29] There is a mismatch between the intent of neurodynamic tests (identifying increased nerve mechanosensitivity) and the reference standard tests used in published concurrent validity studies. Electrodiagnostic tests have limitations as a reference standard because they focus on loss of function in large-diameter nerve fibers.[156,157] These tests cannot detect irritation of small-diameter afferents[94,95,97,157-159] or increased excitability in nociceptors innervating neural connective tissues[160-162] that can contribute to increased nerve mechanosensitivity. This explains why some patients who have radicular pain[163] or carpal tunnel syndrome[164] have increased nerve mechanosensitivity even when electrodiagnostic tests are normal. Patients with a nerve-related disorder who have increased nerve mechanosensitivity but no loss of large-diameter nerve fiber function may therefore be misclassified by an electrodiagnostic reference standard as not having a nerve-related disorder. Misclassification of patients may also occur when imaging is the reference standard because there is often no strong correlation between imaging findings and nerve-related pain.[165] Misclassification of patients by these reference standards will bias estimates of the diagnostic accuracy of neurodynamic tests, or any other clinical test, for detecting nerve-related disorders.[166]

The difficulty in quantifying the concurrent validity of neurodynamic tests is that there is no agreed upon reference standard for establishing that an individual patient has increased nerve mechanosensitivity.[167] Until a reference standard for increased nerve mechanosensitivity can be agreed upon, using neurodynamic tests for diagnostic purposes will often be based on lower level evidence from previously described biomechanical and experimental pain studies.[168] Lateral elbow pain is a good example of this situation. A significant proportion of patients who have lateral elbow pain exhibit increased nerve mechanosensitivity with the radial nerve neurodynamic test ($ULNT_{RADIAL}$).[169-171] Lack of a reference standard for nerve mechanosensitivity means that the diagnostic validity of these $ULNT_{RADIAL}$ findings has not been quantified. Nevertheless, positive $ULNT_{RADIAL}$ findings should be monitored to make sure that nerve mechanosensitivity improves with interventions for lateral elbow pain. If nerve mechanosensitivity does not improve after evidence-based interventions such as eccentric exercise and mobilization with movement at the elbow,[172,173] neurodynamic treatment techniques may be indicated.

The mismatch between the intent of electrodiagnostic and neurodynamic tests also highlights the limitations of neurodynamic testing. The focus on nerve mechanosensitivity means that neurodynamic tests cannot capture changes in large-diameter (light touch, strength, reflexes) and small-diameter (pin prick, thermal) nerve fiber function that can be part of nerve-related problems.[137,157,174-177] A comprehensive examination, therefore, requires clinical neurological testing of nerve fiber function complemented by neurodynamic testing.

Test Application

Neurodynamic tests, like most orthopedic physical therapy examination techniques, are psychophysical tests because they require a patient to report the response to a physical stimulus. Cooperation from the patient is also required for proper execution of the test. The psychophysical and cooperative aspects of neurodynamic testing mean that patient-related factors may influence the test response and, therefore, diagnostic performance. Patients' pain cognitions, pain catastrophizing, and expectations of pain prior to testing influence neurodynamic test responses.[178-181] Clinicians should keep this in mind when explaining the purpose of neurodynamic testing to a patient. It may be best initially to describe a neurodynamic test as a general test of mobility or tolerance to movement and not a specific test of nerve sensitivity. If initially described as a test of nerve sensitivity, the patient's thoughts on whether or not the problem is nerve related may bias the response to the neurodynamic test and associated structural differentiation maneuvers.[182]

The spread of biomechanical effects along a nerve mean that a positive neurodynamic test by itself cannot identify the location of the problem.[1,15] It seems intuitive that nerve palpation could help identify the location of the problem. However, clinical observations suggest that tenderness to palpation can spread throughout the length of a sensitized nerve.[2] If present, tenderness to nerve palpation helps build a case for increased mechanosensitivity,[2,94,167,183] but it is not necessarily a good indication of the location of the problem.

Neurodynamic test sequencing has been proposed as a method to help identify the location of a nerve problem.[1] Sequencing is partly based on the belief that different orders of movement can apply different levels of strain to a particular nerve segment at the end of a neurodynamic test.[1] However, cadaveric data show that when joints are moved through similar ROM, different orders of movement do not change nerve strain at the end of a neurodynamic test.[46,55] Joints likely move through different ROM, however, when different neurodynamic test sequences are applied clinically. These potential differences between sequences in the amount of motion that occurs at each joint are more likely to affect nerve biomechanics at the end of a neurodynamic test than any specific effects from the order of movement.[46] It still needs to be determined whether different sequences can improve the diagnostic performance of a neurodynamic test.

Even if sequencing does not ultimately improve neurodynamic test performance, applying a test with different orders of movement may still be useful clinically.[168] A joint movement is not likely to reach full ROM when performed near the end of a neurodynamic test.[184] Clinicians can use this knowledge to modify a neurodynamic test when examining a patient with a sensitive or stiff body part. If a patient has a sensitive or stiff shoulder, neurodynamic testing of the median nerve may be best achieved with a sequence where shoulder abduction would be the last movement. Moving the shoulder last applies less mechanical load to the non-neural tissues in the shoulder but still applies adequate nerve strain, tension, and pressure to provoke sensitized neural tissues. Options for median nerve neurodynamic testing where shoulder abduction would be the last movement include performing $ULNT1_{MEDIAN}$ in a distal-to-proximal sequence or $ULNT2_{MEDIAN}$ in the standard sequence.

Different orders of movement can also help with structural differentiation. If a patient has plantar heel pain, performing ankle dorsiflexion and eversion prior to hip flexion during the SLR can help differentiate increased sensitivity originating from the tibial and plantar nerves from increased sensitivity originating from the plantar fascia. Ankle dorsiflexion and eversion apply strain to the plantar fascia and tibial and plantar nerves simultaneously.[51] Subsequent hip flexion further increases strain on the tibial and plantar nerves without changing strain on the plantar fascia.[51] This modified SLR test sequence could help the clinician determine whether there is a nerve-related component to the patient's heel symptoms. Lastly, clinicians have always been encouraged to change the order of movement to match a patient's aggravating activities, especially in situations where results from standard neurodynamic tests are inconclusive.[1,10,11]

Educational Messages

Based on data available at this time, interpretation and explanation of a positive neurodynamic test should focus on increased mechanosensitivity, rather than restricted nerve movement or increased nerve stiffness. Even though nerve excursion is reduced in a significant proportion of patients who have carpal tunnel syndrome[185-187] or diabetes mellitus,[4] it does not appear to be reduced in patients who have neck-arm pain with signs of increased nerve mechanosensitivity.[188] For patients who have low back–related leg pain with signs of increased nerve mechanosensitivity, spinal cord movement may be reduced,[189] but there are no apparent restrictions in sciatic nerve movement in the posterior thigh.[60] Although sciatic nerve movement may not be restricted, preliminary data from a small sample suggest that patients who have low back–related pain greater than 6 months duration have increased sciatic nerve stiffness as measured by ultrasound shear-wave elastography.[190] Before concepts about altered nerve biomechanics can have a larger effect on the interpretation of a positive neurodynamic test, clinically feasible methods to determine whether an individual patient has altered nerve biomechanics need to be developed. Clinical trials also need to show that changes in nerve biomechanics are necessary for improvements in patients' nerve-related symptoms and activity levels.

The focus on nerve mechanosensitivity is consistent with the previous discussion on describing a neurodynamic test as a test of tolerance to movement. It is also consistent with helping patients who have a positive neurodynamic test understand why symptoms were changed by movement of a proximal or distal body part during structural differentiation. Explaining structural differentiation to patients provides an opportunity to describe the physical continuity of the nervous system and how different combinations of spine and limb movements apply more mechanical load to neural tissues than nearby nonneural tissues.[1,15] Connecting these concepts to aggravating activities can help patients better understand how increased nerve mechanosensitivity contributes to their symptoms.

A complete understanding and explanation of a patient's nerve-related disorder, including its location, can only come from synthesizing results from the entire examination (eg, distribution of symptoms, patient history, physical examination of nonneural tissues, neurological examination).[15,137,191,192] Discussing relevant impairments from the examination with a patient sets a foundation for implementing a variety of interventions to reduce nerve mechanosensitivity.

NEURODYNAMIC TREATMENT

Neurodynamic treatment tries to reduce nerve mechanosensitivity by restoring homeostasis in and around the nervous system so that the patient can return to full activity without symptoms.[1,15] In musculoskeletal rehabilitation, there are 3 broad approaches that attempt to reduce nerve mechanosensitivity: (1) nerve mobilization exercises that move neural tissues relative to surrounding structures and can be described as sliding or tensioning techniques[13,193,194]; (2) contralateral cervical lateral glide (CCLG)[14,195] and side-lying lumbar foraminal opening[196] techniques that conversely mobilize structures around sensitized neural tissues[2]; and (3) interventions directed at other (nonneural) musculoskeletal impairments.[1,15] Regardless of the approach(es) used, education about the pain biology underlying the nerve-related disorder can improve outcomes[197,198] and may help the patient better understand the rationale for movement-based interventions.[1,15,199]

Nerve Mobilization Exercises

Nerve mobilization exercises are passive or active techniques that try to reduce nerve mechanosensitivity by moving neural tissues relative to surrounding structures.[13,193,194] Historically, nerve mobilization exercises were based on neurodynamic test movements where one or more joints were moved in a way that lengthened the anatomical course of the nerve (Figure 2-3).[168] These are now referred to as *tensioning techniques*[13,193,194] because while they do create excursion of the nerve relative to surrounding tissues, they also create significant increases in nerve strain.[13,59,60,193,194] However, different combinations of joint movements have markedly different effects on nerve biomechanics. When a joint movement that lengthens the anatomical course of the nerve is simultaneously offset by another movement that shortens the anatomical course of the nerve (see Figure 2-3), there are 2.5 to 5 times greater amounts of nerve excursion without significant increases in nerve strain.[13,59,193,194] The emphasis on nerve excursion over strain is why these movement combinations are referred to as *sliding techniques*.[13,193,194]

Despite different biomechanical effects, it is impossible to state that one type of nerve mobilization exercise is clinically superior to the other.[13] There are conflicting data on whether sliding or tensioning techniques have larger immediate hypoalgesic effects in asymptomatic individuals.[200-202] Additionally, there are no data to date comparing the effects of sliding and tensioning techniques in symptomatic populations over longer follow-up. Technique selection needs to

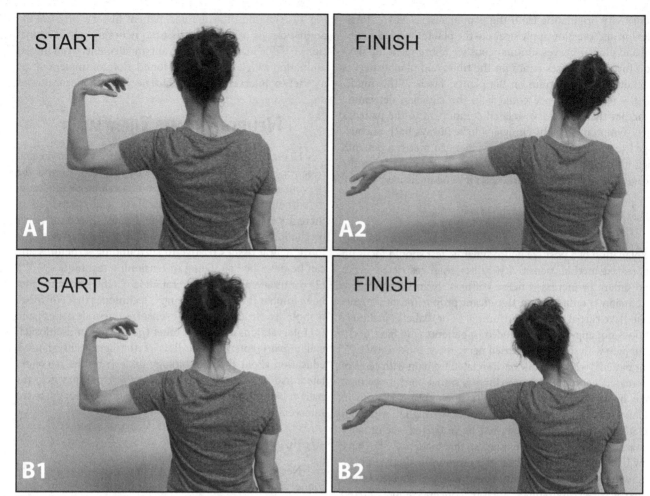

Figure 2-3. Examples of active nerve mobilization exercises for the cervical nerve roots and median nerve. (A) Tensioning technique where contralateral neck side-bending, elbow extension, and wrist extension lengthen the anatomical course of the nerve. (B) Sliding technique where elbow and wrist extension movements that lengthen the anatomical course of the nerve are offset by ipsilateral neck side-bending that shortens the anatomical course of the nerve.

be based on sound clinical reasoning that takes into account the movement requirements of the patient's activities. Sliding techniques are less vigorous biomechanically and, therefore, may be indicated when the patient's symptoms are more reactive or irritable, assuming that a movement-based intervention is deemed appropriate.[203-205] Tensioning techniques may be appropriate for less irritable conditions or when the patient's tolerance for movements that lengthen the anatomical course of the nerve has not been restored with other interventions.

Mobilizing Structures Around Sensitized Neural Tissues

Mobilizing structures around sensitized neural tissues is another approach that tries to reduce mechanosensitivity by creating movement between nerves and surrounding structures.[2,14] The CCLG technique, originally described by Elvey,[14] is the most commonly studied example of this type of neurodynamic treatment technique (Figure 2-4). It has shown immediate hypoalgesic effects in a variety of conditions such as nerve-related neck and arm pain,[206,207] lateral epicondylalgia,[208] and whiplash-associated disorder.[209] Furthermore, the CCLG technique in isolation[210] or as part of a neurodynamic treatment program[211,212] can improve the short-term natural history of nerve-related neck and arm pain. An analogous technique in the lumbar region is a side-lying foraminal opening technique where the affected lumbar spine motion segments are laterally flexed away from the symptomatic limb (Figure 2-5).[196] Observational[196] and clinical trial[213] data suggest that this technique may be helpful for patients who have low back–related leg pain with signs of increased nerve mechanosensitivity. When reassessment shows that the patient's rate of improvement has slowed or plateaued, a progression of these techniques would be to perform them with the limb positioned to pre-load the affected neural tissues (see Figures 2-4 and 2-5).[14]

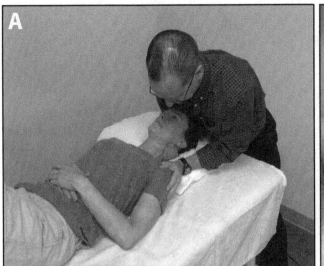
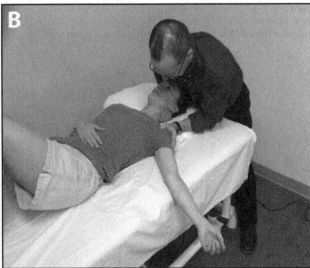

Figure 2-4. CCLG technique. (A) The head and neck are translated in the frontal plane away from the symptomatic arm so that there is minimal rotation or side-bending of the cervical spine. The hand on the shoulder girdle helps the clinician monitor resistance to movement. (B) The technique can be progressed by positioning the limb to pre-load the upper extremity neural tissues. The illustrated upper extremity position would pre-load the median nerve and associated neural tissues.

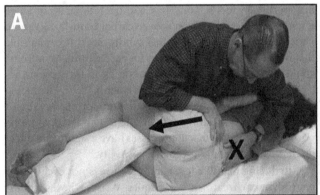
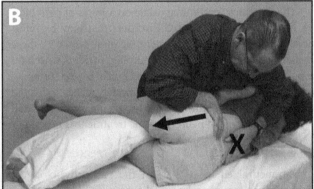

Figure 2-5. Lumbar foraminal opening technique. (A) Lumbar lateral flexion away from the symptomatic limb is created by moving the pelvis (arrow shows direction of force) while stabilizing the spinous process of the superior vertebra of the affected segment (X). (B) The technique can be progressed by positioning the limb to pre-load the lower extremity neural tissues.

Interventions Directed at Other (Nonneural) Musculoskeletal Impairments

Even though they do not try to create movement between neural tissues and surrounding structures, interventions targeting relevant nonneural musculoskeletal impairments can also be used to decrease nerve mechanosensitivity.[1,15] Examples include clinical trials for carpal tunnel syndrome[214,215] and a trial protocol for nerve-related neck and arm pain[216] where soft tissue techniques are applied at places along the nerve that can often be associated with increased mechanosensitivity (eg, scalenes, pectoralis minor, medial aspect of the upper arm, pronator teres, palmar aponeurosis). Case studies provide examples of a commonly observed clinical phenomenon where manual therapy applied to the spine (or extremities) is associated with immediate improvements in neurodynamic test findings.[217,218] The intensity of these manual therapy techniques can also be increased if necessary by using limb position to pre-load the affected neural tissues (Figure 2-6).[217,218] Therapeutic exercise targeting nonneural structures is another intervention that can reduce nerve mechanosensitivity. For example, in a patient who has clinical signs of glenohumeral instability,[219,220] associated problems with nerve mechanosensitivity may be reduced by therapeutic exercise targeting the rotator cuff and scapulothoracic musculature (Case Study One). The key clinical message is that patients who have symptoms related to increased nerve mechanosensitivity do not always have to receive nerve mobilization exercises as part of their intervention.

Figure 2-6. Example of progressing a manual therapy technique (lumbar central posterior-anterior mobilization) by placing the limb in a partial SLR position to pre-load the lumbosacral nerve roots and sciatic tract.

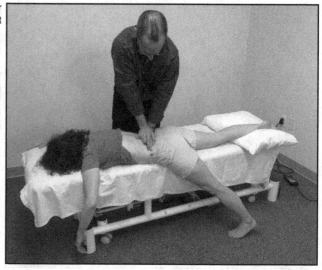

Potential Mechanisms of Neurodynamic Treatment

There are now preliminary data on aspects of pain biology involved in nerve-related disorders that may be influenced by neurodynamic treatment techniques.[13,168,199] These mechanistic studies have usually enrolled patients who have carpal tunnel syndrome (a common clinical model for nerve compression) or employed animal models of nerve-related pain. Although initial findings are promising, more research on the mechanisms of neurodynamic treatment is needed.[168]

Reduction of Edema and Pressure

Intraneural edema is part of the pathophysiology of nerve root and peripheral nerve disorders.[221-224] It reflects an inflammatory response to mechanical and chemical stimuli that compromise intraneural circulation.[222-224] Removing intraneural edema is difficult because nerve roots and peripheral nerves do not have a lymphatic system.[225,226] Persistent edema increases pressure inside nerve fascicles, creating a miniature compartment syndrome that perpetuates the problem.[221,225] Persistent intraneural edema also provides an environment for the development of fibrosis and can contribute to degradation of myelin and axon loss.[223]

Preliminary data suggest that neurodynamic treatment techniques can potentially reduce intraneural edema. A 1-week program of nerve mobilization exercises reduces MRI evidence of intraneural edema in patients who have carpal tunnel syndrome, something not observed in those who receive advice to remain active.[227] Cadaveric data show that tensioning techniques have immediate mechanical effects that produce dispersion of intraneural fluid in nerve roots and peripheral nerves.[80-82] Although limitations in applying cadaveric data to the clinical setting must be acknowledged, the authors hypothesized that these mechanical effects could help reduce intraneural edema.[80-82]

Edema around nerves and the associated increased pressure can contribute to some nerve-related disorders such as carpal tunnel syndrome[228] and radicular pain.[229,230] Although not specifically focused on nerve gliding, brief bouts of active wrist flexion and extension reduce carpal tunnel pressure in patients who have carpal tunnel syndrome.[231] It is plausible that nerve mobilization exercises for carpal tunnel syndrome could also have this effect because they can incorporate active wrist flexion and extension movements.[193,227,232] Reducing edema and pressure around nerves is important because it may help improve intraneural circulation and axonal transport. These 2 physiological processes have a significant effect on nerve function and mechanosensitivity.[95,226,233,234]

Reducing neural edema and pressure is not exclusive to neurodynamic treatment techniques. Wrist orthoses (splinting) can also reduce MRI evidence of intraneural edema in patients who have carpal tunnel syndrome.[227] The rationale for night splinting to prevent extremes of elbow flexion in patients who have cubital tunnel syndrome is to reduce strain and pressure applied to the ulnar nerve.[235] However, splinting may not be necessary when patients are educated on the pathomechanics of cubital tunnel syndrome and advised to avoid aggravating positions.[236]

Dispersal of Inflammatory Chemicals

Animal models of mild nerve injury have shown that the inflamed portion of the nerve can be extremely sensitive to stretch and pressure even when nerve conduction is largely unaffected.[94,95,98,99] The development of mechanosensitivity and associated behavioral signs indicative of nerve-related pain are partly due to the interruption of axonal transport.[95,97,99] Impaired axonal transport allows for accumulation of inflammatory and other chemical mediators that increase mechanosensitivity at the inflamed site of the nerve.[95,97,237]

The ability for nerve mobilization exercises to disperse intraneural fluid in cadaver studies[80-82] suggests that these techniques may also be able to disperse inflammatory mediators related to mechanosensitivity.[13] However, this hypothesis needs to be tested. Techniques directed at nonneural tissues also have the potential to disperse inflammatory mediators involved in nerve-related disorders. In an animal model of nerve-related pain where inflammatory chemicals were placed within the L5 intervertebral foramen, spinal manipulation significantly decreased inflammation and neuronal hyperexcitability in the dorsal root ganglion, and decreased mechanical and thermal hyperalgesia in the hind paw when compared to no intervention.[238] The authors proposed that faster reductions in inflammation, hyperexcitability, and hyperalgesia could be related to spinal manipulation improving blood supply and nutrition to the affected dorsal root ganglion.

Impact on Neuroimmune Responses

Immune cell activation contributes to the neuroinflammatory response at the site of the nerve problem and in corresponding dorsal root ganglia.[239,240] These immune cell responses spread to the dorsal horn of the spinal cord (eg, the side contralateral to the nerve injury) and higher centers in the CNS when there are greater amounts of axon loss.[199,241] Neuroimmune responses throughout the nervous system contribute to increased mechanosensitivity and help explain why nerve-related disorders often present with symptoms and signs outside of the expected innervation territory.[199,241] For example, patients who have radicular pain[163,242,243] or carpal tunnel syndrome[244-247] often have symptoms outside of the expected dermatome or median nerve distribution, respectively.

Nerve mobilization exercises have beneficial effects on neuroimmune responses in animal models of nerve injury. Levels of nerve growth factor and myelin protein 0 increased at the site of sciatic nerve injury after a nerve mobilization intervention.[248] These changes were associated with faster rates of myelin and axon regeneration and lower amounts of intraneural fibrosis.[248] The same nerve mobilization intervention reduced levels of nerve growth factor and substance P in the dorsal root ganglion; increased expression of opioid receptors in the dorsal root ganglion; reduced expression of brain-derived neurotrophic factor in the thalamus and midbrain; and reduced glial cell activation in the dorsal root ganglion, spinal cord, thalamus, and midbrain.[249-251] Importantly, these changes were associated with decreased pain sensitivity as measured by hind paw withdrawal to mechanical and thermal stimuli.[249] Similar to cadaveric data, applying results from animal studies to the clinical setting must be done with caution.

Facilitation of Descending Modulation

Neurodynamic treatment techniques may help reduce nerve-related symptoms by facilitating descending modulation. Nerve mobilization exercises facilitate endogenous analgesic mechanisms within the CNS in an animal model of sciatic nerve injury.[252] In patients who have lateral elbow pain, CCLG applied with the upper limb positioned to preload the radial nerve produces immediate hypoalgesia that is specific to mechanical, rather than thermal, stimuli and is associated with sympathoexcitation.[208,253] This pattern of hypoalgesia is thought to be related to activation of descending nociceptive inhibitory pathways that project from higher centers in the CNS to the spinal cord.[254-256] A tensioning technique increases endogenous analgesia (conditioned pain modulation) in patients with neck pain[257] and reduces temporal summation from a thermal stimulus in patients who have carpal tunnel syndrome.[258] Reduced temporal summation suggests a decrease in dorsal horn excitability that can be related to activation of spinal and descending nociceptive inhibitory mechanisms.[258] However, these hypoalgesic effects can also be elicited when other manual therapy techniques are applied to patients who have various musculoskeletal conditions.[255,256,259-263] Therefore, it seems likely that neurodynamic treatment techniques share similar neurophysiological mechanisms with other manual therapy interventions. More work is needed to determine whether these immediate neurophysiological effects are still present at longer term follow-up and whether they correspond to patient-reported outcomes.[255,264]

It has been hypothesized that benefits from progressive mechanical loading with exercise may be partly due to reductions in CNS sensitivity involved in the patient's pain experience.[265] Appropriate progressive mechanical loading can help the patient perform previously symptomatic tasks with minimal to no pain. These experiences enable the conscious and nonconscious parts of the patient's nervous system to learn that the previously painful area can be used without exacerbating symptoms.[265-267] This learning process can reduce the level of perceived threat of these symptoms, which in theory, can decrease CNS sensitivity.[265-267] Nerve mobilization exercises, particularly active sliding and tensioning techniques, can be presented to the patient as a form of progressive mechanical loading of sensitized neural tissues. It is therefore conceivable that benefits from nerve mobilization exercises could be related to reductions in the perceived threat of the symptoms and associated decreases in CNS sensitivity. This hypothesis also needs to be tested. Attempting to reduce the perceived threat of the symptoms through progressive mechanical loading is consistent with principles of pain biology education discussed in the next section of this chapter.[197]

Educational Messages

The basis for education as part of intervention is that helping patients understand the biology underlying their pain experience can reduce pain[197,198] and, importantly, create a context within which movement-based interventions (eg, neurodynamic treatment) can be more effective.[1,15,197,266,268-270] The primary goal of pain biology education is to help patients understand that pain is a reflection of the perceived need to protect body tissues, rather than a reflection of tissue damage.[197] Pain biology education is consistent with a biopsychosocial approach because it discusses how biological, psychological, and social factors can interact and contribute to the perceived need to protect body tissues.[197] Patients can understand pain biology when presented in lay terminology.[271]

Similar to principles for explaining a positive neurodynamic test, resources for educating patients about the pain biology involved in nerve-related disorders emphasize nerve mechanosensitivity over altered nerve biomechanics.[1,197,230,269,272-274] Biomechanical information, however, still has an important role in the educational process. It can help reassure patients that their neural tissues are well designed to handle the mechanical forces that accompany spine and limb movements, which may help reduce the perceived threat of the symptoms.[1,15] It can also help them understand how neurodynamic treatment techniques produce mechanical stimuli that can impact biological processes (eg, intraneural edema, neuroimmune responses) involved in their nerve-related disorder. Making a connection between pain biology and potential neurodynamic treatment effects is important. Patients who receive pain biology education state it is important for them to see how educational messages are relevant to their current pain experience.[275,276] Linking pain biology to potential neurodynamic treatment effects may help increase the patient's perception of relevance.

Clinical Trial Evidence

Clinical trials measuring neurodynamic treatment effects have most commonly studied lumbar radicular pain and carpal tunnel syndrome. Other nerve-related disorders addressed in these trials include cervical radicular pain, cubital tunnel syndrome, and tarsal tunnel syndrome.

Patients who have lumbar radicular pain do better when SLR or slump tensioning techniques are added to a program of lumbar mobilization and exercise.[277-283] Lumbar radicular pain was most commonly defined as reproduction of symptoms with SLR or slump testing, no neurological signs, and no centralization of symptoms with repeated movements. Intervention typically lasted 3 to 4 weeks (6 to 8 visits). Standardized mean differences (reported or calculated from reported data) for pain and self-reported disability at the end of intervention consistently showed moderate (greater than or equal to 0.6 but less than 1.2)[284] to large (greater than or equal to 1.2 but less than 2.0)[284] effects favoring neurodynamic treatment. However, neurodynamic treatment may not be helpful after lumbar surgery.[285]

Neurodynamic treatment is better than advice to remain active in patients who have cervical radicular pain.[210,212,282,286] Cervical radicular pain was defined as reproduction of symptoms with ULNT1$_{MEDIAN}$ and, depending on the study, provocation of symptoms with Spurling test, alleviation of symptoms with cervical distraction, or less than 2 abnormal neurological signs at the same nerve root level.[210,212,286] When CCLG[210] or a median nerve mobilization technique[286] were

applied in isolation, there were very large (greater than or equal to 2.0)[284] standardized mean differences for pain and self-reported disability that favored neurodynamic treatment at the end of a 6-week intervention. However, these trials involved 30 treatment sessions with the clinician, which is not feasible for most settings. Beneficial effects can still be achieved with a more feasible intervention program.[212] Neurodynamic treatment included brief education, manual therapy with CCLG and shoulder girdle oscillation techniques, and a home program of active sliding and tensioning techniques for the cervical nerve roots and median nerve.[211,212] Intervention was administered over 2 weeks (4 visits) and neurodynamic treatment techniques were applied so as not to provoke patients' symptoms. Standardized mean differences for pain (0.7 to 0.9) and self-reported function (0.6 to 0.9) at 3- to 4-week follow-up showed moderate effects favoring neurodynamic treatment.[212] More work is needed to determine whether neurodynamic treatment is beneficial for cervical radicular pain when compared to or combined with other interventions over a longer follow-up.

Except for carpal tunnel syndrome, there are relatively few published trials on neurodynamic treatment effects for nerve-related disorders originating in the upper or lower limb. Nerve mobilization exercises appear to be better than no treatment for patients who have carpal tunnel syndrome, but they are not better than other interventions such as wrist orthoses (splinting).[282,287-290] Furthermore, combining nerve mobilization exercises with other interventions such as wrist orthoses or tendon gliding exercises does not improve pain or self-reported disability.[287,290,291] These findings are consistent regardless of whether nerve mobilization exercises focus on moving just the wrist and hand or involve moving the entire upper limb. Additional high-quality research on neurodynamic treatment effects for carpal tunnel syndrome is needed. Future studies should try to blind participants to intervention where possible, blind outcome assessors, and measure short- and long-term outcomes, including the need for surgery.[287]

We are aware of only single trials that have investigated neurodynamic treatment effects in patients who have cubital tunnel syndrome[236] or tarsal tunnel syndrome.[292] One trial on patients who have cubital tunnel syndrome showed that adding nerve mobilization exercises to education about the pathomechanics of the condition and advice to avoid aggravating positions did not improve pain or self-reported function at 6-month follow-up.[236] These results need to be interpreted cautiously because nearly 30% of participants did not complete follow-up and were not accounted for in the statistical analysis. A single clinical trial on patients who have tarsal tunnel syndrome showed that adding neurodynamic treatment to nonsurgical management may not be helpful.[292] Nonsurgical management included ice, gastrocnemius stretching, lower extremity strengthening, shoe inserts for those who had low medial arches or overpronation, and bandaging for patients who had ankle edema. Neurodynamic treatment involved a slump tensioning technique. The only difference between groups after the 6-week intervention was that significantly fewer participants who received neurodynamic treatment still had a positive Tinel's sign at the tibial nerve below the medial malleolus (risk difference calculated from reported data = 0.54, 95% confidence interval 0.31 to 0.93). There were no differences between groups for pain, combined talocrural and subtalar ROM, foot muscle strength, or the number of participants whose symptoms were provoked with the ankle dorsiflexion eversion test for the tibial nerve (knee flexed). No firm conclusions for or against neurodynamic treatment for a particular nerve-related disorder can be made on the basis of a single clinical trial.

Additional high-quality research on neurodynamic treatment effects is needed, particularly for cervical radicular pain and nerve-related disorders originating in the limbs. As with any clinical trial, clear enrollment criteria are needed.[293] Given that neurodynamic treatment tries to reduce nerve mechanosensitivity, it seems logical that participants should have a positive neurodynamic test with or without increased sensitivity to nerve palpation. This has not always been the case in previous research.[236,292,294] Parameters of neurodynamic treatment (and other interventions) need to be clearly described as recommended by recent guidelines.[295] Credible "sham" neurodynamic treatment techniques should be used when possible and when appropriate for the research question.[258] It is also important for future studies to more consistently look at long-term outcomes that extend beyond the completion of the intervention.

Future research on neurodynamic treatment effects should also expand to conditions other than radicular pain and peripheral nerve entrapment syndromes. As mentioned previously, lateral elbow pain often has a component of increased nerve mechanosensitivity based on a positive $ULNT_{RADIAL}$.[169-171] Despite case study evidence suggesting that nerve mobilization exercises might have a role in treating nerve-related lateral elbow pain,[296] there are currently no clinical trial data on neurodynamic treatment effects for this population. Plantar heel pain is another musculoskeletal problem that can have a component of increased nerve mechanosensitivity.[297] As with lateral elbow pain, there is case study evidence[298] suggesting that nerve mobilization exercises might help with treating nerve-related plantar heel pain (Case Study Two). A published clinical trial included a tensioning technique as part of the intervention for patients who have plantar heel pain.[299] Unfortunately, the study design did not allow conclusions to be made about the contribution of neurodynamic treatment to the observed outcomes. Intramuscular hamstring injury is a musculoskeletal problem that can have a component of increased nerve mechanosensitivity identified during slump testing.[300,301] A small clinical trial showed that adding nerve mobilization in a slump position to a hamstring rehabilitation program resulted in a faster return to competition for Australian rules football players.[302] Additional trials need to determine if these results can be replicated in other groups of patients who have intramuscular hamstring injuries with increased nerve mechanosensitivity.

Patient Selection

Identifying characteristics that can help select patients who will respond to an intervention has consistently been a research priority.[303,304] Decision-making tools have been proposed to select patients with spine-related limb pain[196,305] and anterior knee pain[306] who will do well with neurodynamic treatment. It is still unclear whether these decision-making tools identify patients who do well regardless of the intervention (prognosis) or patients who respond better to neurodynamic treatment than to alternate interventions (treatment effect modifiers).[307,308] These decision-making tools, therefore, cannot yet be recommended for clinical practice.[148]

In the absence of validated decision-making tools, the following principles can help clinicians decide whether a patient may be a good candidate for neurodynamic treatment[10,137]:

- Distribution, behavior, and history of symptoms are consistent with a nerve-related disorder or a musculoskeletal condition that can have a component of increased nerve mechanosensitivity (eg, lateral elbow pain)

- Presence of increased nerve mechanosensitivity evidenced by a positive neurodynamic test with or without increased sensitivity to nerve palpation

- Additional physical examination findings support that symptoms are consistent with a musculoskeletal condition and potentially amenable to physical therapy intervention

Clinicians should also be aware of any impairments in large-diameter (light touch, strength, reflexes) or small-diameter (pin-prick, thermal) nerve fiber function. Significant impairments from the neurological examination mean that neurodynamic treatment techniques should be applied more cautiously.[1] These principles are consistent with the enrollment criteria in many of the previously discussed clinical trials that showed benefits from neurodynamic treatment.

Additional Considerations

There are minimal data to guide dosage parameters for neurodynamic treatment. Neurodynamic treatment techniques should probably be applied in a nonprovocative fashion initially. When symptoms are not provoked and the strongest sensory response allowed is a gentle stretching or pulling sensation that settles immediately,[211] these techniques are likely to be safe. Patients with nerve-related neck and arm pain who received this type of neurodynamic treatment over 4 visits experienced only mild adverse events (mainly temporary posttreatment soreness) that did not detract from positive outcomes.[212]

There are conflicting results on the potential safety of nerve mobilization exercises when physiological measures of nerve function are used. In patients with carpal tunnel syndrome, sensory axon excitability decreased after one session of a nonprovocative passive nerve mobilization exercise, even though nerve conduction velocity did not change.[309]

There were no changes in sensory axon excitability when the same intervention was applied to asymptomatic individuals. It is unclear whether these were transient or more long-standing changes because nerve function was only measured immediately after treatment. Additionally, the nerve mobilization exercise was applied in 2-minute bouts for a total of 15 minutes in this single treatment session, which is much longer than the 30- to 60-second bouts for a total of 3 to 8 minutes that have typically been used in published clinical trials.[211,212,277,279] In contrast, one session of a passive SLR tensioning technique (60-second bouts for a total of 3 minutes) did not have any detrimental effects on vibration thresholds in patients with nerve-related low back and leg pain.[310] Further research on the potential safety of neurodynamic treatment techniques is clearly needed. These studies should monitor both patient-reported and physiological outcomes over multiple sessions of neurodynamic treatment to help better inform clinical practice.

As with passively applied techniques, there is no known optimal dosage for active nerve mobilization exercises in terms of repetitions per session and number of sessions per day. Given that neurodynamic treatment tries to reduce nerve mechanosensitivity, it probably makes the most sense for nerve mobilization exercises to be performed at multiple sessions spread throughout the day. Patients should be given guidelines for self-monitoring and whether to modify or stop the exercises. For example, clear instructions on the sensory responses allowed during and after each nerve mobilization exercise are important. Patients should also have some type of movement that can be used as a "measuring stick" to monitor the effects after each session. The movement could be a functional task that is consistently symptomatic or an active neurodynamic test. Examples of active neurodynamic tests include active shoulder abduction while keeping the elbow and wrist extended to simulate a median nerve test or an active slump test. If there is potential worsening of the condition, patients should be instructed on whether to decrease the dosage or stop the home program. These ideas are consistent with principles for using reassessment to guide decision making[203,311,312] and increasing adherence with home programs.[313,314]

Although ROM is not helpful for defining a positive neurodynamic test, it may be worth monitoring during treatment. Changes in neurodynamic test ROM are thought to reflect changes in nerve mechanosensitivity and could help clinicians gauge the response to intervention (ie, increased neurodynamic test ROM suggests reduced nerve mechanosensitivity). Clinical studies often use ROM to quantify changes in nerve mechanosensitivity after neurodynamic treatment.[5,206,315,316] However, there are currently no data on how much change in neurodynamic test ROM reflects a clinically important change in the patient's condition. Clinicians need to judge the importance of changes in neurodynamic test ROM by looking at whether they correspond to changes in other physical examination impairments and patient-reported outcomes.

As with any physical therapy intervention, the importance of the patient–clinician relationship must be acknowledged. A stronger therapeutic alliance between patient and clinician is associated with better outcomes for patients who have musculoskeletal[317] or nerve-related[318,319] disorders. Understanding the patient's perspective about the pain experience, discussing and acknowledging the effect of psychosocial issues, providing clear explanations about diagnosis and treatment, and collaborating with the patient on decision making are examples of factors that strengthen the therapeutic alliance.[317,320-323] These approaches to strengthening the therapeutic alliance mesh well with principles of pain biology education[197] and using clinical reasoning to tailor treatment (eg, neurodynamic treatment) to the individual patient's presentation.[1,15,203]

Conclusion

In musculoskeletal rehabilitation, neurodynamics combines movement and education to address the increased mechanosensitivity that can accompany nerve-related disorders. Neurodynamic tests are plausible tests for identifying increased nerve mechanosensitivity and can be applied reliably in the clinic. A positive test should at least partly reproduce the patient's symptoms, and these symptoms should change with structural differentiation. Existing evidence suggests that neurodynamic tests can help diagnose radicular pain but might not help diagnose carpal tunnel syndrome. However, existing evidence on neurodynamic test performance needs to be interpreted cautiously because there is no agreed upon reference standard for increased nerve mechanosensitivity in an individual patient. The lack of an agreed upon reference standard also makes it difficult to quantify the diagnostic validity of neurodynamic tests in musculoskeletal conditions that can have a component of increased nerve mechanosensitivity such as lateral elbow pain, Achilles tendinopathy, plantar heel pain, and intramuscular hamstring injury. Nevertheless, neurodynamic test findings should be monitored when treating these conditions.

Neurodynamic treatment techniques create movement between sensitized neural tissues and surrounding structures. The aim is to normalize the altered homeostasis in and around the nervous system to reduce nerve mechanosensitivity. Clinical trial evidence to date suggests that neurodynamic treatment is beneficial for radicular pain, especially lumbar radicular pain, but may not be better than other nonsurgical interventions for carpal tunnel syndrome, such as wrist orthoses (splinting). Neurodynamic treatment techniques likely share similar neurophysiological mechanisms with other manual therapy interventions and are likely to be safe when applied in a nonprovocative fashion. More research on neurodynamic treatment effects is needed. This research should expand to musculoskeletal conditions that can have a component of increased nerve mechanosensitivity such as lateral elbow pain, Achilles tendinopathy, plantar heel pain, and intramuscular hamstring injury.

Educational messages about neurodynamic testing and treatment should emphasize nerve mechanosensitivity over altered nerve biomechanics. Focusing on nerve mechanosensitivity fits well with incorporating pain biology education into the intervention program. It also facilitates linking pain biology underlying the nerve-related disorder to potential mechanisms of neurodynamic treatment, which in turn may increase the patient's perception of the relevance of this information.

There are currently no validated decision-making tools to select patients with nerve-related disorders who are likely to have a preferential response to neurodynamic treatment. There are also no data to recommend an optimal neurodynamic treatment dosage. Therefore, clinicians should use sound clinical reasoning that synthesizes findings from the patient interview and physical examination to tailor treatment to the patient's presentation. Clinicians should also cultivate a strong therapeutic alliance with the patient to maximize outcomes.

CASE STUDIES

Case Study One

A 25-year-old female graduate student and ballerina for the metropolitan dance company reported right shoulder pain and apprehension along with pain and tingling in the ulnar forearm and hand. Symptoms were aggravated by longitudinal traction/pulling forces through the right upper extremity with the elbow extended. Examples included carrying groceries with the arm at her side ("briefcase style") and ballet movements with her partner that required pulling through her upper extremity. Shoulder symptoms woke her at night if she slept with her arm overhead. She worried that she would not be able to continue the rehearsal schedule required for a ballet performance taking place in 4 weeks.

The shoulder symptoms started 5 weeks ago when rehearsals began for the aforementioned ballet performance. The routine required her to be lifted in the air by her partner, and she had experienced multiple falls during the first week of practice. She reported that, after breaking each fall with her hands, she ended up in a face-down position with her arms overhead. Shoulder pain started immediately after the falls but the apprehension feeling started 1 week later. Forearm and hand symptoms started 2 weeks after the initial falls. She had not missed any rehearsals and reported that all symptoms were gradually worsening each week. The patient had not received treatment and did not have any previous shoulder, upper extremity, or neck problems.

The patient reported mild forearm and hand tingling when standing with arms at her sides. The right scapula was in a downwardly rotated position, and reducing this downward rotation with manual repositioning alleviated the tingling. Active shoulder movements were unremarkable except for provocation of shoulder pain and apprehension with overpressure to shoulder flexion. There was, however, reduced upward rotation of the right scapula during active shoulder elevation. The apprehension-relocation test was positive on the right for shoulder apprehension and pain. The apprehension part of this test also provoked forearm and hand tingling that was alleviated with the relocation part of the test. The sulcus test for the glenohumeral joint provoked shoulder apprehension and forearm and hand tingling. The patient exhibited moderate rotator cuff and scapulothoracic muscle weakness. The ulnar nerve neurodynamic test was positive for the patient's forearm and hand tingling. The ulnar nerve on the right was also more sensitive to palpation in the upper arm and at the elbow. Neurological examination revealed increased sensitivity to light touch and pin-prick testing in the ulnar distribution of the forearm and hand. There were no signs of cervical spine involvement.

Intervention involved McConnell taping for multidirectional instability of the glenohumeral joint. The technique theoretically approximates the humeral head into the glenoid by applying rigid tape in a distal-to-proximal direction over the anterior, lateral, and posterior aspects of the deltoid. This alleviated the forearm and hand tingling that was present when standing with the arms at the sides. It also markedly reduced the apprehension and tingling provoked with the sulcus test. The patient received a progressive strengthening and endurance program for the rotator cuff and scapulothoracic musculature. This program progressed to dynamic stabilization activities in increasing amounts of shoulder elevation and external rotation according to the patient's tolerance.

The forearm and hand symptoms and signs of increased nerve mechanosensitivity with neurodynamic testing and nerve palpation were alleviated after 2 weeks of treatment. Shoulder pain and apprehension were 85% improved after 4 weeks of treatment, which was when the ballet performance took place. The patient completed the entire ballet rehearsal and performance schedule and reported her shoulder was fully recovered 3 weeks after completing the ballet performance.

Case Study Two

A 42-year-old male computer software engineer reported left plantar heel pain that limited his half-marathon training. His pain was worse with the first steps after getting out of bed each morning and also prevented him from running longer than 2 miles.

The symptoms started gradually 8 weeks ago after increasing his running from 15 to 30 miles a week. There were no other changes in his training or footwear. He continued running the first 3 weeks but the pain increased. For the past 5 weeks, he ran only 10 miles a week and bicycled or swam for additional training. Self-treatment with ice, calf stretching, and massaging his plantar fascia with a golf ball had no effect. He reported no previous lower extremity or low back problems. His initial score on the Activities of Daily Living subscale of the Foot and Ankle Ability Measure (FAAM) was 68% (57/84).[324]

Physical examination revealed pronated feet bilaterally. The Foot Posture Index was +9 on the left and +6 on the right (more pronated on left).[325] Windlass testing in bilateral stance provoked his left heel pain. Single-leg calf raise was weaker on the left (15 repetitions compared to 25 on the right) but painfree. Ankle dorsiflexion in subtalar neutral on the left was 5 degrees less than the right. Posterior glide of the talus on the left was moderately stiff and painfree. Other mobility testing of the rearfoot was unremarkable. The patient was tender to palpation at the left medial calcaneal tubercle, especially in a Windlass test position.

A modified SLR suggested a nerve-related component to the patient's heel pain. Ankle dorsiflexion and eversion did not provoke symptoms, but additional hip flexion to 45 degrees provoked his heel pain. Modified SLR testing on the right provoked pulling in the posterior calf at 65 degrees. There were no clinical signs of a lumbar problem.

Initial treatment involved changing the stretching program. Gastrocnemius and soleus stretching were modified by placing a folded towel under the medial side of the entire foot. This inverted the rearfoot to emphasize mobility in the talocrural joint and ankle plantarflexors during stretching. A nonweightbearing plantar fascia–specific stretch was added by passively dorsiflexing the toes with the ankle dorsiflexed. A strengthening program of unilateral calf raises with a small towel roll placed under the toes to increase toe dorsiflexion was added 1 week later.[326] The patient continued running so that changes in symptoms could more likely be attributed to treatment.

After 2 weeks the patient reported a 50% decrease in pain with first steps in the morning and the FAAM score increased to 72% (61/84). However, the modified SLR on the left was unchanged. A tensioning technique involving repeated ankle dorsiflexion plus knee extension in a slump position was added to the treatment program. Two weeks later (4 weeks after the initial visit), the patient reported an 85% reduction in pain with first steps in the morning compared to baseline. The FAAM score had increased to 83% (70/84) which exceeded the minimal clinically important change of 9 points relative to baseline.[324] The modified SLR suggested that nerve sensitivity had decreased. The reported intensity of symptoms provoked by this neurodynamic test was markedly less than initially and hip flexion had increased to 60 degrees.

The patient continued his stretching, strengthening, and nerve mobilization exercises and was educated in a progressive running program. Total mileage and the duration of his long run were increased by no more than 10% each week,[327] even though there is limited evidence for nominating a specific threshold of change in weekly training load that reduces the risk of running-related injury.[328,329] It was mutually decided to reschedule the half-marathon to later in the year so that the patient could follow the recommended running program.

REFERENCES

1. Butler D. *The Sensitive Nervous System*. Noigroup Publications; 2000.

2. Hall T, Elvey R. Nerve trunk pain: physical diagnosis and treatment. *Man Ther*. 1999;4(2):63-73.

3. Shacklock M. Neurodynamics. *Physiotherapy*. 1995;81(1):9-16.

4. Boyd B, Dilley A. Altered tibial nerve biomechanics in patients with diabetes mellitus. *Muscle Nerve*. 2014;50:216-223. doi:10.1002/mus.24155

5. Boyd B, Nee R, Smoot B. Safety of lower extremity neurodynamic exercises in adults with diabetes mellitus: a feasibility study. *J Man Manip Ther*. 2017;25:30-38. doi:10.1080/10669817.2016.1180772

6. Godoi J, Kerppers I, Rossi L, et al. Electromyographic analysis of biceps brachii muscle following neural mobilization in patients with stroke. *Electromyogr Clin Neurophysiol*. 2010;50:55-60.

7. Cha H, Cho H, Choi J. Effects of nerve mobilization technique on lower limb function in patients with poststroke hemiparesis. *J Phys Ther Sci*. 2014;26:981-983.

8. Díez Valdés S, Vega J, Martinez-Pubil J. Upper limb neurodynamic test 1 in patients with acquired brain injury: a cross-sectional study. *Brain Inj*. 2019;33(8):1039-1044. doi:10.1080/02699052.02692019.01606441

9. Marsico P, Tal-Akabi A, van Hedel H. The relevance of nerve mobility on function and activity in children with cerebral palsy. *BMC Neurology*. 2016;16:194. doi:10.1186/s12883-016-0715-z

10. Elvey R. Physical evaluation of the peripheral nervous system in disorders of pain and dysfunction. *J Hand Ther*. 1997;10:122-129.

11. Maitland G. Negative disc exploration: positive canal signs. *Aust J Physiother*. 1979;25(3):129-134.

12. Maitland G. The slump test: examination and treatment. *Aust J Physiother*. 1985;31(6):215-219.

13. Coppieters M, Butler D. Do 'sliders' slide and 'tensioners' tension? An analysis of neurodynamic techniques and considerations regarding their application. *Man Ther*. 2008;13(3):213-221. doi:10.1016/j.math.2006.12.008

14. Elvey R. Treatment of arm pain associated with abnormal brachial plexus tension. *Aust J Physiother*. 1986;32:225-230.

15. Nee R, Butler D. Management of peripheral neuropathic pain: integrating neurobiology, neurodynamics, and clinical evidence. *Physical Therapy in Sport*. 2006;7:36-49. doi:10.1016/j.ptsp.2005.10.002

16. Troup J. Straight-leg-raising (SLR) and the qualifying tests for increased root tension: their predictive value after back and sciatic pain. *Spine*. 1981;6:526-527.

17. Manvell N, Manvell J, Snodgrass S, Reid S. Tension of the ulnar, median, and radial nerves during ulnar nerve neurodynamic testing: observational cadaveric study. *Physical Therapy*. 2015;95:891-900. doi:10.2522/ptj.20130536

18. Gugliotti M, Futterman B, Ahrens T, et al. Impact of shoulder internal rotation on ulnar nerve excursion and strain in embalmed cadavers. A pilot study. *J Man Manip Ther*. 2016;24:111-116. doi:10.1179/2042618614Y.0000000093

19. Gugliotti M, Cohen D, Hernandez A, Hinrichs K, Osmundsen N. Impact of shoulder internal rotation on normal sensory response during ulnar nerve-biased neurodynamic testing of asymptomatic individuals. *J Man Manip Ther*. 2017;25:39-46. doi:10.1080/10669817.2016.1173317

20. Smart K, Blake C, Staines A, Doody C. Clinical indicators of 'nociceptive', 'peripheral neuropathic' and 'central' mechanisms of musculoskeletal pain. A Delphi survey of expert clinicians. *Man Ther*. 2010;15:80-87. doi:10.1016/j.math.2009.07.005

21. American Physical Therapy Association. *Guide to Physical Therapist Practice 3.0*. 2014. Accessed August 29, 2022 http://guidetoptpractice.apta.org.

22. Childs J, Cleland J, Elliott J, et al. Neck pain: clinical practice guidelines linked to the International Classification of Functioning, Disability, and Health from the Orthopaedic Section of the American Physical Therapy Association. *J Orthop Sports Phys Ther*. 2008;38(9):A1-A34. doi:10.2519/jospt.2008.0303

23. Delitto A, George S, Van Dillen L, et al. Low back pain: clinical practice guidelines linked to the International Classification of Functioning, Disability, and Health from the Orthopaedic Section of the American Physical Therapy Association. *J Orthop Sports Phys Ther*. 2012;42(4):A1-A57. doi:10.2519/jospt.2012.0301

24. Martin R, Davenport T, Reischl S, et al. Heel pain - plantar fasciitis: Revision 2014 Clinical Practice Guidelines Linked to the International Classification of Functioning, Disability and Health from the Orthopaedic Section of the American Physical Therapy Association. *J Orthop Sports Phys Ther*. 2014;44:A1-A23. doi:10.2519/jospt.2014.0303

25. Blanpied P, Gross A, Elliott J, et al. Neck pain: Revision 2017 Clinical Practice Guidelines linked to the International Classification of Functioning, Disability, and Health from the Orthopaedic Section of the American Physical Therapy Association. *J Orthop Sports Phys Ther*. 2017;47(7):A1-A83. doi:10.2519/jospt.2017.0302

26. Oliveira C, Maher C, Pinto R, et al. Clinical practice guidelines for the management of non-specific low back pain in primary care: an updated overview. *Eur Spine J*. 2018;27:2791-2803. doi:10.1007/s00586-018-5673-2

27. Krebs D. Measurement theory. *Phys Ther*. 1987;67(12):1834-1839.

28. Sim J, Arnell P. Measurement validity in physical therapy research. *Phys Ther*. 1993;73(2):102-115.

29. Fritz J, Wainner R. Examining diagnostic tests: an evidence-based perspective. *Phys Ther*. 2001;81(9):1546-1564.

30. Sackett D, Haynes R. Evidence base of clinical diagnosis: the architecture of diagnostic research. *British Medical Journal*. 2002;324:539-541. doi:10.1136/bmj.324.7336.539

31. Nee R, Jull G, Vicenzino B, Coppieters M. The validity of upper-limb neurodynamic tests for detecting peripheral neuropathic pain. *J Orthop Sports Phys Ther*. 2012;42:413-424. doi:10.2519/jospt.2012.3988

32. Breig A, Marions O. Biomechanics of the lumbosacral nerve roots. *Acta Radiol Diagn (Stockh)*. 1963;1:1141-1160.

33. Louis R. Vertebroradicular and vertebromedullar dynamics. *Anatomia Clinica*. 1981;3:1-11.

34. Troup J. Biomechanics of the lumbar spinal canal. *Clin Biomech (Bristol, Avon)*. 1986;1:31-43.

35. Rossitti S. Biomechanics of the pons-cord tract and its enveloping structures: an overview. *Acta Neurochir (Wien)*. 1993;124:144-152.

36. Muhle C, Wiskirchen J, Weinert D, et al. Biomechanical aspects of the subarachnoid space and cervical cord in healthy individuals examined with kinematic magnetic resonance imaging. *Spine*. 1998;23(5):556-567.

37. Shum G, Attenborough A, Marsden J, Hough A. Tibial nerve excursion during lumbar spine and hip flexion measured with diagnostic ultrasound. *Ultrasound Med Biol*. 2013;39:784-790. doi:10.1016/j.ultrasmedbio.2012.11.023

38. Patel W, Heidenreich F, Bindra R, Yamaguchi K, Gelberman R. Morphologic changes in the ulnar nerve at the elbow with flexion and extension: a magnetic resonance imaging study with 3-dimensional reconstruction. *J Shoulder Elbow Surg*. 1998;7:368-374.

39. Silva A, Manso A, Andrade R, Domingues V, Brandao M, Silva A. Quantitative in vivo longitudinal nerve excursion and strain in response to joint movement: a systematic literature review. *Clin Biomech*. 2014;29:839-847. doi:10.1016/j.clinbiomech.2014.07.006

40. Lohman C, Gilbert K, Sobczak S, et al. 2015 Young Investigator Award Winner: cervical nerve root displacement and strain during upper limb neural tension testing. Part 1: a minimally invasive assessment in unembalmed cadavers. *Spine*. 2015;40:793-800. doi:10.1097/BRS.0000000000000686

41. Manvell J, Manvell N, Snodgrass S, Reid S. Improving the radial nerve neurodynamic test: an observation of tension of the radial, median and ulnar nerves during upper limb positioning. *Man Ther*. 2015;20:790-796. doi:10.1016/j.math.2015.03.007

42. Meng S, Reissig L, Beikircher R, Tzou C, Grisold W, Weninger W. Longitudinal gliding of the median nerve in the carpal tunnel: ultrasound cadaveric evaluation of conventional and novel concepts of nerve mobilization. *Arch Phys Med Rehabil*. 2015;96:2207-2213. doi:10.1016/j.apmr.2015.08.415

43. Ochi K, Horiuchi Y, Horiuchi K, Iwamoto T, Morisawa Y, Sato K. Shoulder position increases ulnar nerve strain at the elbow of patients with cubital tunnel syndrome. *J Shoulder Elbow Surg*. 2015;25:1380-1385. doi:10.1016/j.jse.2015.01.014

44. Kasehagen B, Ellis R, Mawston G, Allen S, Hing W. Assessing the reliability of ultrasound imaging to examine radial nerve excursion. *Ultrasound Med Biol*. 2016;42:1651-1659. doi:10.1016/j.ultrasmedbio.2016.02.013

45. Greening J, Dilley A. Posture-induced changes in peripheral nerve stiffness measured by ultrasound shear-wave elastography. *Muscle Nerve*. 2017;55:213-222. doi:10.1002/mus.25245

46. Nee R, Yang C, Liang C, Tseng G, Coppieters M. Impact of order of movement on nerve strain and longitudinal excursion: a biomechanical study with implications for neurodynamic test sequencing. *Man Ther*. 2010;15(4):376-381. doi:10.1016/j.math.2010.03.001

47. Breig A, Troup J. Biomechanical considerations in the straight-leg-raising test: cadaveric and clinical studies of the effects of medial hip rotation. *Spine*. 1979;4(3):242-250.

48. de Peretti F, Micalef J, Bourgeon A, Argenson C, Rabischong P. Biomechanics of the lumbar spinal nerve roots and first sacral root within the intervertebral foramina. *Surgical and Radiologic Anatomy*. 1989;11:221-225.

49. Smith S, Massie J, Chesnut R, Garfin S. Straight leg raising: anatomical effects on the spinal nerve root without and with fusion. *Spine*. 1993;18(8):992-999.

50. Kobayashi S, Suzuki Y, Asai T, Yoshizawa H. Changes in nerve root motion and intraradicular blood flow during intraoperative femoral nerve stretch test. Report of four cases. *J Neurosurg*. 2003;99:298-305.

51. Coppieters M, Alshami A, Babri A, Souvlis T, Kippers V, Hodges P. Strain and excursion of the sciatic, tibial, and plantar nerves during a modified straight leg raising test. *J Orthop Res*. 2006;24:1883-1889. doi:10.1002/jor.20210

52. Ko H, Park B, Park J, Shin Y, Shon H, Lee H. Intrathecal movement and tension of the lumbosacral roots induced by straight-leg raising. *Am J Phys Med Rehabil*. 2006;85:222-227. doi:10.1097/01.phm.0000200386.28819.6a

53. Gilbert K, Brismee J, Collins D, et al. 2006 Young Investigator Award Winner: lumbosacral nerve root displacement and strain. Part 2. A comparison of 2 straight leg conditions in unembalmed cadavers. *Spine*. 2007;32:1521-1525. doi:10.1097/BRS.0b013e318067dd72

54. Alshami A, Babri A, Souvlis T, Coppieters M. Strain in the tibial and plantar nerves with foot and ankle movements and the influence of adjacent joint positions. *J Appl Biomech*. 2008;24(4):368-376.

55. Boyd B, Topp K, Coppieters M. Impact of movement sequencing on sciatic and tibial nerve strain and excursion during the straight leg raise test in embalmed cadavers. *J Orthop Sports Phys Ther*. 2013;43(6):398-403. doi:10.2519/jospt.2013.4413

56. Coppieters M, Crooke J, Lawrenson P, Khoo S, Skulstad T, Bet-Or Y. A modified straight leg raise test to differentiate between sural nerve pathology and Achilles tendinopathy. A cross-sectional cadaver study. *Man Ther*. 2015;20:587-591. doi:10.1016/j.math.2015.01.013

57. Rade M, Shacklock M, Könönen M, et al. Part 3: developing methods of in vivo MRI measurement of spinal cord displacement in the thoracolumbar region of asymptomatic subjects with unilateral and bilateral straight leg raise tests. *Spine*. 2015;40:935-941. doi:10.1097/BRS.0000000000000914

58. Rade M, Kononen M, Marttila J, et al. In vivo MRI measurement of spinal cord displacement in the thoracolumbar region of asymptomatic subjects with unilateral and sham straight leg raise tests. *PLoS One*. 2016;11:e0155927. doi:10.1371/journal.pone.0155927

59. Coppieters M, Andersen L, Johansen R, et al. Excursion of the sciatic nerve during nerve mobilization exercises: an in vivo cross-sectional study using dynamic ultrasound imaging. *J Orthop Sports Phys Ther*. 2015;45:731-737. doi:10.2519/jospt.2015.5743

60. Ridehalgh C, Moore A, Hough A. Sciatic nerve excursion during a modified passive straight leg raise test in asymptomatic participants and participants with spinally referred leg pain. *Man Ther*. 2015;20:564-569. doi:10.1016/j.math.2015.01.003

61. Andrade R, Nordez A, Hug F, et al. Non-invasive assessment of sciatic nerve stiffness during human ankle motion using ultrasound shear wave elastography. *J Biomech*. 2016;49:326-331. doi:10.1016/j.jbiomech.2015.12.017

62. Rade M, Shacklock M, Könönen M, et al. Normal multiplanar movement of the spinal cord during unilateral and bilateral straight leg raise: quantification, mechanisms, and overview. *J Orthop Res*. 2017;35:1335-1342. doi:10.1002/jor.23385

63. Sierra-Silvestre E, Bosello F, Fernandez-Carnero J, Hoozemans M, Coppieters M. Femoral nerve excursion with knee and neck movements in supine, sitting, and side-lying slump: an in vivo study using ultrasound imaging. *Musculoskelet Sci Pract*. 2018;37:58-63. doi:10.1016/j.msksp.2018.06.007

64. Topp K, Boyd B. Structure and biomechanics of peripheral nerves: nerve responses to physical stress and implications for physical therapist practice. *Phys Ther*. 2006;86(1):92-109. doi:10.1093/ptj/86.1.92

65. Kleinrensink G, Stoeckart R, Mulder P, et al. Upper limb tension tests as tools in the diagnosis of nerve and plexus lesions: anatomical and biomechanical aspects. *Clin Biomech*. 2000;15(1):9-14.

66. Byl C, Puttlitz C, Byl N, Lotz J, Topp K. Strain in the median and ulnar nerves during upper-extremity positioning. *J Hand Surg Am*. 2002;27A(6):1032-1040.

67. Kleinrensink G, Stoeckart R, Vleeming A, Snijders C, Mulder P. Mechanical tension in the median nerve. The effects of joint positions. *Clin Biomech*. 1995;10(5):240-244.

68. Pahor S, Toppenberg R. An investigation of neural tissue involvement in ankle inversion sprains. *Man Ther*. 1996;1(4):192-197.

69. Gilbert K, Brismee J, Collins D, et al. 2006 Young Investigator Award Winner: lumbosacral nerve root displacement and strain; Part 1. A novel measurement technique during straight leg raise in unembalmed cadavers. *Spine*. 2007;32:1513-1520. doi:10.1097/BRS.0b013e318067dd55

70. Brochwicz P, von Piekartz H, Zalpour C. Sonography assessment of the median nerve during cervical lateral glide and lateral flexion. Is there a difference in neurodynamics of asymptomatic people? *Man Ther*. 2013;18:216-219. doi:10.1016/j.math.2012.10.001

71. Boyd B, Gray A, Dilley A, Wanek L, Topp K. The pattern of tibial nerve excursion with active ankle dorsiflexion is different in older people with diabetes mellitus. *Clin Biomech*. 2012;27:967-971. doi:10.1016/j.clinbiomech.2012.06.013

72. Barker P, Briggs C. Attachments of the posterior layer of lumbar fascia. *Spine*. 1999;24(17):1757-1764.

73. Smith D, Mitchell D, Peterson G, Will A, Mera S, Smith L. Medial brachial fascial compartment syndrome: anatomic basis of neuropathy after transaxillary arteriography. *Radiology*. 1989;173:149-154.

74. Stecco C, Gagey O, Macchi V, et al. Tendinous muscular insertions onto the deep fascia of the upper limb. First part: anatomical study. *Morphologie*. 2007;91:29-37. doi:10.1016/j.morpho.2007.05.001

75. Huijing P. Epimuscular myofascial force transmission: a historical review and implications for new research. International society of biomechanics Muybridge award lecture, Taipei, 2007. *J Biomech*. 2009;42(1):9-21. doi:10.1016/j.jbiomech.2008.09.027

76. Willard F, Vleeming A, Schuenke M, Danneels L, Schleip R. The thoracolumbar fascia: anatomy, function and clinical considerations. *J Anat*. 2012;221:507-536. doi:10.1111/j.1469-7580.2012.01511.x

77. Pechan J, Julis I. The pressure measurement in the ulnar nerve. A contribution to the pathophysiology of cubital tunnel syndrome. *J Biomech*. 1975;8:75-79.

78. Millesi H, Zoch G, Reihsner R. Mechanical properties of peripheral nerves. *Clin Orthop Relat Res*. 1995;314:76-83.

79. Gelberman R, Yamaguchi K, Hollstein S, et al. Changes in interstitial pressure and cross-sectional area of the cubital tunnel and of the ulnar nerve with flexion of the elbow. *J Bone Joint Surg Am*. 1998;80:492-501.

80. Brown C, Gilbert K, Brismee J, Sizer P, James C, Smith M. The effects of neurodynamic mobilization on fluid dispersion within the tibial nerve at the ankle: an unemablmed cadaveric study. *J Man Manip Ther*. 2011;19(1):26-34. doi:10.1179/2042618610Y.0000000003

81. Gilbert K, Smith M, Sobczak S, James C, Sizer P, Brismee J. Effects of lower limb neurodynamic mobilization on intraneural fluid dispersion of the fourth lumbar nerve root: an unemblamed cadaveric investigation. *J Man Manip Ther*. 2015;23:239-245. doi:10.1179/2042618615Y.0000000009

82. Boudier-Revéret M, Gilbert K, Allégue D, et al. Effect of neurodynamic mobilization on fluid dispersion in median nerve at the level of the carpal tunnel: a cadaveric study. *Musculoskelet Sci Pract*. 2017;31:45-51. doi:10.1016/j.msksp.2017.07.004

83. Weiss N, Gordon L, Bloom T, So Y, Rempel D. Position of the wrist associated with the lowest carpal tunnel pressure: implications for splint design. *J Bone Joint Surg*. 1995;77A(11):1695-1699.

84. Werner R, Armstrong T, Bir C, Aylard M. Intracarpal canal pressures: the role of finger, hand, wrist and forearm position. *Clin Biomech*. 1997;12(1):44-51.

85. Coppieters M, Schmid A, Kubler P, Hodges P. Description, reliability and validity of a novel method to measure carpal tunnel pressure in patients with carpal tunnel syndrome. *Man Ther*. 2012;17:589-592. doi:10.1016/j.math.2012.03.005

86. Macnicol M. Extraneural pressures affecting the ulnar nerve at the elbow. *Hand*. 1982;14(1):5-11.

87. Werner C, Ohlin P, Elmqvist D. Pressures recorded in ulnar neuropathy. *Acta Orthop Scand*. 1985;56:404-406.

88. Erak S, Day R, Wang A. The role of supinator in the pathogenesis of chronic lateral elbow pain: a biomechanical study. *J Hand Surg Br*. 2004;29B(5):461-464.

89. Links A, Graunke K, Wahl C, Green J, Matsen F. Pronation can increase the pressure on the posterior interosseous nerve under the arcade of Frohse: a possible mechanism of palsy after two-incision repair for distal biceps rupture - clinical experience and a cadaveric investigation. *J Shoulder Elbow Surg*. 2009;18:64-68. doi:10.1016/j.jse.2008.07.001

90. Kinoshita M, Okuda R, Morikawa J, Jotoku T, Abe M. The dorsiflexion-eversion test for diagnosis of tarsal tunnel syndrome. *J Bone Joint Surg*. 2001;83A(12):1835-1839.

91. Lai W, Shih Y, Lin P, Chen W, Ma H. Normal neurodynamic responses to the femoral slump test. *Man Ther*. 2012;17:126-132. doi:10.1016/j.math.2011.10.003

92. Trainor K, Pinnington M. Reliability and diagnostic validity of the slump knee bend neurodynamic test for upper/mid lumbar nerve root compression: a pilot study. *Physiotherapy*. 2011;97:59-64. doi:10.1016/j.physio.2010.05.004

93. Suri P, Rainville J, Katz J, et al. The accuracy of the physical examination for the diagnosis of midlumbar and low lumbar nerve root impingement. *Spine*. 2011;36:63-73.

94. Dilley A, Lynn B, Pang S. Pressure and stretch mechanosensitivity of peripheral nerve fibres following local inflammation of the nerve trunk. *Pain*. 2005;117:462-472. doi:10.1016/j.pain.2005.08.018

95. Dilley A, Bove G. Disruption of axoplasmic transport induces mechanical sensitivity in intact rat C-fiber nociceptive axons. *J Physiol.* 2008;586:593-604. doi:10.1113/jphysiol.2007.144105

96. Dilley A, Bove G. Resolution of inflammation-induced axonal mechanical sensitivity and conduction slowing in C-fiber nociceptors. *J Pain.* 2008;9:185-192. doi:10.1016/j.jpain.2007.10.012

97. Dilley A, Richards N, Pulman K, Bove G. Disruption of fast axonal transport in the rat induces behavioral changes consistent with neuropathic pain. *J Pain.* 2013;14:1437-1449. doi:10.1016/j.jpain.2013.07.005

98. Govea R, Barbe M, Bove G. Group IV nociceptors develop axonal chemical sensitivity during neuritis and following treatment of the sciatic nerve with vinblastine. *J Neurophysiol.* 2017;118(4):2103-2109. doi:10.1152/jn.00395.2017

99. Satkeviciute I, Goodwin G, Bove G, Dilley A. Time course of ongoing activity during neuritis and following axonal transport disruption. *J Neurophysiol.* 2018;119:1993-2000. doi:10.1152/jn.00882.2017

100. Coppieters M, Kurz K, Mortensen T, et al. The impact of neurodynamic testing on the perception of experimentally induced muscle pain. *Man Ther.* 2005;10(1):52-60. doi:10.1016/j.math.2004.07.007

101. Coppieters M, Alshami A, Hodges P. An experimental pain model to investigate the specificity of the neurodynamic test for the median nerve in the differential diagnosis of hand symptoms. *Arch Phys Med Rehabil.* 2006;87(10):1412-1417. doi:10.1016/j.apmr.2006.06.012

102. Lai W, Shih Y, Lin P, Chen W, Ma H. Specificity of the femoral slump test for the assessment of experimentally induced anterior knee pain. *Arch Phys Med Rehabil.* 2012;93:2347-2351. doi:10.1016/j.apmr.2012.06.003

103. Walsh J, Flatley M, Johnston N, Bennett K. Slump test: sensory responses in asymptomatic subjects. *J Man Manip Ther.* 2007;15(4):231-238.

104. Boyd B, Wanek L, Gray A, Topp K. Mechanosensitivity of the lower extremity nervous system during straight-leg raise neurodynamic testing in healthy individuals. *J Orthop Sports Phys Ther.* 2009;39(11):780-790. doi:10.2519/jospt.2009.3002

105. Martinez M, Cubas C, Girbes E. Ulnar nerve neurodynamic test: study of the normal sensory response in asymptomatic individuals. *J Orthop Sports Phys Ther.* 2014;44:450-456. doi:10.2519/jospt.2014.5207

106. Leoni D, Falla D, Heitz C, et al. Test-retest reliability in reporting the pain induced by a pain provocation test: further validation of a novel approach for pain drawing acquisition and analysis. *Pain Pract.* 2017;17:176-184. doi:10.1111/papr.12429

107. Sierra-Silvestre E, Torres Lacomba M, de la Villa Polo P. Effect of leg dominance, gender and age on sensory responses to structural differentiation of straight leg raise test in asymptomatic subjects: a cross-sectional study. *J Man Manip Ther.* 2017;25:91-97. doi:10.1080/10669817.2016.1200216

108. Lin P, Shih Y, Chen W, Ma H. Neurodynamic responses to the femoral slump test in patients with anterior knee pain syndrome. *J Orthop Sports Phys Ther.* 2014;44:350-357. doi:10.2519/jospt.2014.4781

109. Bueno-Gracia E, Malo-Urriés M, Borrella-Andrés S, et al. Neurodynamic test of the peroneal nerve: study of the normal response in asymptomatic subjects. *Musculoskelet Sci Pract.* 2019;43:117-121. doi:10.1016/j.msksp.2019.1006.1005.

110. Hines T, Noakes R, Manners B. The upper limb tension test: intertester reliability for assessing the onset of passive resistance R1. *J Man Manip Ther.* 1993;1(3):95-98.

111. Vanti C, Conteddu L, Guccione A, et al. The upper limb neurodynamic test I: intra- and intertester reliability and the effect of several repetitions on pain and resistance. *J Manip Physiol Ther.* 2010;33(4):292-299. doi:10.1016/j.jmpt.2010.03.003

112. Eliasziw M, Young S, Woodbury M, Fryday-Field K. Statistical methodology for the concurrent assessment of interrater and intrarater reliability: using goniometric measurements as an example. *Phys Ther.* 1994;74(8):777-788.

113. Hall T, Zusman M, Elvey R. Adverse mechanical tension in the nervous system? Analysis of straight leg raise. *Man Ther.* 1998;3(3):140-146.

114. Herrington L, Bendix K, Cornwell C, Fielden N, Hankey K. What is the normal response to structural differentiation within the slump and straight leg raise tests? *Man Ther.* 2008;13(4):289-294. doi:10.1016/j.math.2007.01.013

115. Coppieters M, Stappaerts K, Janssens K, Jull G. Reliability of detecting 'onset of pain' and 'submaximal pain' during neural provocation testing of the upper quadrant. *Physiother Res Int.* 2002;7(3):146-156.

116. van der Heide B, Bourgoin C, Ellis G, Garnevall B, Blackmore M. Test-retest reliability and face validity of a modified neural tissue provocation test in patients with cervicobrachial pain syndrome. *J Man Manip Ther.* 2006;14(1):30-36.

117. Tong M, Liu V, Hall T. Side-to-side range of movement variability in an ulnar neurodynamic test sequence variant in asymptomatic people. *Hong Kong Physiother J.* 2018;38(2):133-139. doi:10.1142/S1013702518500117

118. Boland R, Adams R. Effects of ankle dorsiflexion on range and reliability of straight leg raising. *Aust J Physiother.* 2000;46(3):191-200.

119. Dixon J, Keating J. Variability in straight leg raise measurements. *Physiotherapy.* 2000;86(7):361-370.

120. Walsh J, Hall T. Agreement and correlation between the straight leg raise and slump tests in subjects with leg pain. *J Manip Physiol Ther.* 2009;32(3):184-192. doi:10.1016/j.jmpt.2009.02.006

121. Johnson E, Chiarello C. The slump test: the effects of head and lower extremity position on knee extension. *J Orthop Sports Phys Ther.* 1997;26(6):310-317.

122. Boyd B, Villa P. Normal inter-limb differences during the straight leg raise neurodynamic test: a cross sectional study. *BMC Musculoskelet Disord.* 2012;13:245. doi:10.1186/1471-2474-13-245

123. Lopez-de-Uralde-Vallanueva I, Beltran-Alacreu H, Fernandez-Carnero J, Gil-Martinez A, La Touche R. Differences in neural mechanosensitivity between patients with chronic nonspecific neck pain with and without neuropathic features. A descriptive cross-sectional study. *Pain Med.* 2016;17(1):136-148. doi:10.1111/pme.12856

124. Ekedahl K, Jönsson B, Frobell R. Validity of the fingertip-to-floor test and straight leg raising test in patients with acute and subacute low back pain: a comparison by sex and radicular pain. *Arch Phys Med Rehabil.* 2010;91(8):1243-1247. doi:10.1016/j.apmr.2010.05.002

125. Ekedahl H, Jönsson B, Frobell R. Fingertip-to-floor and straight leg raising test: validity, responsiveness, and predictive value in patients with acute/subacute low back pain. *Arch Phys Med Rehabil.* 2012;93:2210-2215. doi:10.1016/j.apmr.2012.04.020

126. Covill L, Petersen S. Upper extremity neurodynamic tests: range of motion asymmetry may not indicate impairment. *Physiother Theory Pract.* 2011;28(7):535-541. doi:10.3109/09593985.2011.641198

127. Boyd B. Common interlimb asymmetries and neurogenic responses during upper limb neurodynamic testing: implications for test interpretation. *J Hand Ther.* 2012;25(1):56-64. doi:10.1016/j.jht.2011.09.004

128. Van Hoof T, Vangestel C, Shacklock M, Kerckaert I, D'Herde K. Asymmetry of ULNT1 elbow extension range-of-motion in a healthy population: consequences for clinical practice and research. *Phys Ther Sport.* 2012;13(3):141-149. doi:10.1016/j.ptsp.2011.09.003

129. Stalioraitis V, Robinson K, Hall T. Side-to-side range of movement variability in variants of the median and radial neurodynamic test sequences in asymptomatic people. *Man Ther.* 2014;19:338-342. doi:10.1016/j.math.2014.03.005

130. Schmid A, Brunner F, Luomajoki H, et al. Reliability of clinical tests to evaluate nerve function and mechanosensitivity in the upper limb peripheral nervous system. *BMC Musculoskelet Disord.* 2009;10:11. doi:10.1186/1471-2474-10-11

131. Strender L, Sjöblom A, Sundell K, Ludwig R, Taube A. Interexaminer reliability in physical examination of patients with low back pain. *Spine.* 1997;22:814-820.

132. Bertilson B, Bring J, Sjöblom A, Sundell K, Strender L. Interexaminer reliability in the assessment of low back pain (LBP) using the Kirkaldy-Willis classification (KWC). *Eur Spine J.* 2006;15(11):1695-1703. doi:10.1007/s00586-005-0050-3

133. Billis E, McCarthy C, Gliatis J, Gittins M, Papandreou M, Oldham J. Inter-tester reliability of discriminatory examination items for sub-classifying non-specific low back pain. *J Rehabil Med.* 2012;44(10):851-857. doi:10.2340/16501977-0950

134. Philip K, Lew P, Matyas T. The inter-therapist reliability of the slump test. *Aust J Physiother.* 1989;35(2):89-94.

135. Landis J, Koch G. The measurement of observer agreement for categorical data. *Biometrics.* 1977;33(1):159-174.

136. Wainner R. Reliability of the clinical examination: how close is "close enough"? *J Orthop Sports Phys Ther.* 2003;33(9):488-491.

137. Finnerup N, Haroutounian S, Kamerman P, et al. Neuropathic pain: an updated grading system for research and clinical practice. *Pain.* 2016;157:1599-1606. doi:10.1097/j.pain.0000000000000492

138. Whiting P, Rutjes A, Westwood M, et al. QUADAS-2: a revised tool for the quality assessment of diagnostic accuracy studies. *Ann Intern Med.* 2011;155(8):529-536. doi:10.7326/0003-4819-155-8-201110180-00009

139. Majlesi J, Togay H, Unalan H, Toprak S. The sensitivity and specificity of the slump and the straight leg raising tests in patients with lumbar disc herniation. *J Clin Rheumatol.* 2008;14(2):87-91. doi:10.1097/RHU.0b013e31816b2f99

140. Scaia V, Baxter D, Cook C. The pain provocation-based straight leg raise test for diagnosis of lumbar disc herniation, lumbar radiculopathy, and/or sciatica: a systematic review of clinical utility. *J Back Musculoskelet Rehabil.* 2012;25(4):215-223. doi:10.3233/BMR-2012-0339

141. Urban L, MacNeil B. Diagnostic accuracy of the slump test for identifying neuropathic pain in the lower limb. *J Orthop Sports Phys Ther.* 2015;45:596-603. doi:10.2519/jospt.2015.5414

142. Ekedahl H, Jönsson B, Annertz M, Frobell R. Accuracy of clinical tests in detecting disk herniation and nerve root compression in subjects with lumbar radicular symptoms. *Arch Phys Med Rehabil.* 2018;99(4):726-735. doi:10.1016/j.apmr.2017.11.006

143. Homayouni K, Jafari S, Yari H. Sensitivity and specificity of modified Bragard test in patients with lumbosacral radiculopathy using electrodiagnosis as a reference standard. *J Chiropr Med.* 2018;17(1):36-43. doi:10.1016/j.jcm.2017.10.004

144. Jaeschke R, Guyatt G, Sackett D. Users' guides to the medical literature. III. How to use an article about a diagnostic test. B. What are the results and will they help me in caring for my patients? *JAMA.* 1994;271(9):703-707.

145. van der Windt D, Simons E, Riphagen I, et al. Physical examination for lumbar radiculopathy due to disc herniation in patients with low back pain. *Cochrane Database Syst Rev.* 2010;Issue 2:CD007431. doi:10.1002/14651858.CD007431.pub2

146. Genevay S, Courvoisier D, Konstantinou K, et al. Clinical classification criteria for radicular pain caused by lumbar disc herniation: the radicular pain caused by disc herniation (RAPIDH) criteria. *Spine J.* 2017;17(10):1464-1471. doi:10.1016/j.spinee.2017.05.005

147. Stynes S, Konstantinou K, Ogollah R, Hay E, Dunn K. Clinical diagnostic model for sciatica developed in primary care patients with low back-related leg pain. *PLoS One.* 2018;13:e0191852. doi:10.1371/journal.pone.0191852

148. McGinn T, Guyatt G, Wyer P, Naylor C, Stiell I, Richardson W. Users' guides to the medical literature. XXII: How to use articles about clinical decision rules. *JAMA.* 2000;284(1):79-84.

149. Apelby-Albrecht M, Andersson L, Kleiva I, Kvale K, Skillgate E, Josephson A. Concordance of upper limb neurodynamic tests with medical examination and magnetic resonance imaging in patients with cervical radiculopathy: a diagnostic cohort study. *J Manip Physiol Ther.* 2013;36(9):626-632. doi:10.1016/j.jmpt.2013.07.007

150. Koulidis K, Veremis Y, Anderson C, Heneghan N. Diagnostic accuracy of upper limb neurodynamic tests for the assessment of peripheral neuropathic pain: a systematic review. *Musculoskelet Sci Pract.* 2019;40:21-33. doi:10.1016/j.msksp.2019.01.001

151. Wainner R, Fritz J, Irrgang J, Boninger M, Delitto A, Allison S. Reliability and diagnostic accuracy of the clinical examination and patient self-report measures for cervical radiculopathy. *Spine.* 2003;28(1):52-62.

152. Vanti C, Bonfiglioli R, Calabrese M, Marinelli F, Violante F, Pillastrini P. Relationship between interpretation and accuracy of the upper limb neurodynamic test 1 in carpal tunnel syndrome. *J Manipulative Physiol Ther.* 2012;35(1):54-63. doi:10.1016/j.jmpt.2011.09.008

153. Bueno-Gracia E, Tricas-Moreno J, Fanlo-Mazas P, et al. Validity of the upper limb neurodynamic test 1 for the diagnosis of carpal tunnel syndrome. The role of structural differentiation. *Man Ther.* 2016;22:190-195. doi:10.1016/j.math.2015.12.007

154. Baselgia L, Bennett D, Silbiger R, Schmid A. Negative neurodynamic tests do not exclude neural dysfunction in patients with entrapment neuropathies. *Arch Phys Med Rehabil.* 2017;98(3):480-486. doi:10.1016/j.apmr.2016.06.019

155. Schmid A, Coppieters M. The double crush syndrome revisited - A Delphi study to reveal current expert views on mechanisms underlying dual nerve disorders. *Man Ther.* 2011;16:557-562. doi:10.1016/j.math.2011.05.005

156. Lee D, Claussen G, Oh S. Clinical nerve conduction and needle electromyography studies. *J Am Acad Orthop Surg.* 2004;12(4):276-287.

157. Schmid A, Hailey L, Tampin B. Entrapment neuropathies: challenging common beliefs with novel evidence. *J Orthop Sports Phys Ther.* 2018;48(2):58-62. doi:10.2519/jospt.2018.0603

158. Eliav E, Benoliel R, Tal M. Inflammation with no axonal damage of the rat saphenous nerve trunk induces ectopic discharge and mechanosensitivity in myelinated axons. *Neurosci Lett.* 2001;311(1):49-52.

159. Bove G, Ransil B, Lin H, Leem J. Inflammation induces ectopic mechanical sensitivity in axons of nociceptors innervating deep tissues. *J Neurophysiol.* 2003;90(3):1949-1955.

160. Asbury A, Fields H. Pain due to peripheral nerve damage: an hypothesis. *Neurology.* 1984;34:1587-1590.

161. Kallakuri S, Cavanaugh J, Blagoev D. An immunohistochemical study of innervation of lumbar spinal dura and longitudinal ligaments. *Spine.* 1998;23(4):403-411.

162. Sauer S, Bove G, Averbeck B, Reeh P. Rat peripheral nerve components release calcitonin gene-related peptide and prostaglandin E2 in response to noxious stimuli: evidence that nervi nervorum are nociceptors. *Neuroscience.* 1999;92(1):319-325.

163. Slipman C, Plastaras C, Palmiter R, Huston C, Sterenfeld E. Symptom provocation of fluoroscopically guided cervical nerve root stimulation: are dynatomal maps indentical to dermatomal maps? *Spine.* 1998;23(20):2235-2242.

164. Witt J, Hentz J, Stevens J. Carpal tunnel syndrome with normal nerve conduction studies. *Muscle Nerve.* 2004;29(4):515-522. doi:10.1002/mus.20019

165. Beith I, Kemp A, Kenyon J, Prout M, Chestnut T. Identifying neuropathic back and leg pain: a cross-sectional study. *Pain.* 2011;152:1511-1516. doi:10.1016/j.pain.2011.02.033

166. Reitsma J, Rutjes A, Khan K, Coomarasamy A, Bossuyt P. A review of solutions for diagnostic accuracy studies with an imperfect or missing reference standard. *J Clin Epidemiol.* 2009;62(8):797-806. doi:10.1016/j.jclinepi.2009.02.005

167. Walsh J, Hall T. Reliability, validity and diagnostic accuracy of palpation of the sciatic, tibial and common peroneal nerves in the examination of low back-related leg pain. *Man Ther.* 2009;14:623-629. doi:10.1016/j.math.2008.12.007

168. Coppieters M, Nee R. Neurodynamic management of the peripheral nervous system. In: Jull G, Moore A, Falla D, Lewis J, McCarthy C, Sterling M, eds. *Grieve's Modern Musculoskeletal Physiotherapy.* 4th ed. Elsevier; 2015:287-297.

169. Yaxley G, Jull G. Adverse tension in the neural system: a preliminary study of tennis elbow. *Aust J Physiother.* 1993;39(1):15-22.

170. Berglund K, Persson B, Denison E. Prevalence of pain and dysfunction in the cervical and thoracic spine in persons with and without lateral elbow pain. *Man Ther.* 2008;13:295-299. doi:10.1016/j.math.2007.01.015

171. Coombes B, Bisset L, Vicenzino B. Bilateral cervical dysfunction in patients with unilateral lateral epicondylalgia without concomitant cervical or upper limb symptoms: a cross-sectional case-control study. *J Manipulative Physiol Ther.* 2014;37(2):79-86. doi:10.1016/j.jmpt.2013.12.005

172. Cullinane F, Boocock M, Trevelyan F. Is eccentric exercise an effective treatment for lateral epicondylitis? A systematic review. *Clin Rehabil.* 2014;28(1):3-19. doi:10.1177/0269215513491974

173. Coombes B, Bisset L, Vicenzino B. Management of lateral elbow tendinopathy: one size does not fit all. *J Orthop Sports Phys Ther.* 2015;45:938-949. doi:10.2519/jospt.2015.5841

174. Freynhagen R, Rolke R, Baron R, et al. Pseudoradicular and radicular low-back pain - a disease continuum rather than different entities? Answers from quantitative sensory testing. *Pain.* 2008;135:65-74. doi:10.1016/j.pain.2007.05.004

175. Tampin B, Slater H, Hall T, Lee G, Briffa N. Quantitative sensory testing somatosensory profiles in patients with cervical radiculopathy are distinct from those in patients with nonspecific neck-arm pain. *Pain.* 2012;153:2403-2414. doi:10.1016/j.pain.2012.08.007

176. Schmid A, Bland J, Bhat M, Bennett D. The relationship of nerve fibre pathology to sensory function in entrapment neuropathy. *Brain.* 2014;137:3186-3199. doi:10.1093/brain/awu288

177. Konstantinou K, Dunn K, Ogollah R, Vogel S, Hay E. Characteristics of patients with low back and leg pain seeking treatment in primary care: baseline results from the ATLAS cohort study. *BMC Musculoskelet Disord.* 2015;16:332. doi:10.1186/s12891-015-0787-8

178. McCracken L, Gross R, Sorg P, Edmands T. Prediction of pain in patients with chronic low back pain: effects of inaccurate prediction and pain anxiety. *Behav Res Ther.* 1993;31(7):647-652.

179. Moseley G. Evidence for a direct relationship between cognitive and physical change during an education intervention in people with chronic low back pain. *Eur J Pain.* 2004;8(1):39-45.

180. Beneciuk J, Bishop M, George S. Pain catastrophizing predicts pain intensity during a neurodynamic test for the median nerve in healthy participants. *Man Ther.* 2010;15:370-375. doi:10.1016/j.math.2010.02.008

181. Lloyd D, Helbig T, Findlay G, Roberts N, Nurmikko T. Brain areas involved in anticipation of clinically relevant pain in low back pain populations with high levels of pain behavior. *J Pain.* 2016;17(5):577-587. doi:10.1016/j.jpain.2016.01.470

182. Coppieters M, Hodges P. Beliefs regarding the pathobiological basis of pain influence the level of pain during a clinical provocation test. Research report platform presentation. World Confederation of Physical Therapy Congress 2007. Vancouver, Canada. *Physiotherapy.* 2007;93(suppl 1):S133.

183. Jepsen J, Laursen L, Hagert C, Kreiner S, Larsen A. Diagnostic accuracy of the neurological upper limb examination II: relation to symptoms of patterns of findings. *BMC Neurol.* 2006;6:10. doi:10.1186/1471-2377-6-10

184. Coppieters M, van de Velde M, Stappaerts K. Positioning in anesthesiology: toward a better understanding of stretch-induced perioperative neuropathies. *Anesthesiology.* 2002;97(1):75-81.

185. Erel E, Dilley A, Greening J, Morris V, Cohen B, Lynn B. Longitudinal sliding of the median nerve in patients with carpal tunnel syndrome. *J Hand Surg.* 2003;28B(5):439-443.

186. Hough A, Moore A, Jones M. Reduced longitudinal excursion of the median nerve in carpal tunnel syndrome. *Arch Phys Med Rehabil.* 2007;88(5):569-576.

187. Korstanje J, Scheltens-de-Boer M, Blok J, et al. Ultrasonographic assessment of longitudinal median nerve and hand flexor tendon dynamics in carpal tunnel syndrome. *Muscle Nerve.* 2012;45:721-729. doi:10.1002/mus.23246

188. Dilley A, Odeyinde S, Greening J, Lynn B. Longitudinal sliding of the median nerve in patients with non-specific arm pain. *Man Ther.* 2008;13:536-543. doi:10.1016/j.math.2007.07.004

189. Rade M, Pesonen J, Kononen M, et al. Reduced spinal cord movement with the straight leg raise test in patients with lumbar intervertebral disc herniation. *Spine.* 2017;42:1117-1124. doi:10.1097/BRS.0000000000002235

190. Neto T, Freitas S, Andrade R, et al. Noninvasive measurement of sciatic nerve stiffness in patients with chronic low back related leg pain using shear wave elastography. *J Ultrasound Med.* 2019;38(1):157-164. doi:10.1002/jum.14679

191. Jepsen J, Laursen L, Kreiner S, Larsen A. Neurological examination of the upper limb: a study of construct validity. *Open Neurol J.* 2009;3:54-63. doi:10.2174/1874205X00903010054

192. Smart K, Blake C, Staines A, Doody C. The discriminative validity of "nociceptive", "peripheral neuropathic", and "central sensitization" as mechanisms-based classifications of musculoskeletal pain. *Clin J Pain.* 2011;27:655-663. doi:10.1097/AJP.0b013e318215f16a

193. Coppieters M, Alshami A. Longitudinal excursion and strain in the median nerve during novel nerve gliding exercises for carpal tunnel syndrome. *J Orthop Res.* 2007;25(7):972-980. doi:10.1002/jor.20310

194. Coppieters M, Hough A, Dilley A. Different nerve gliding exercises induce different magnitudes of median nerve longitudinal excursion. An in vivo study using dynamic ultrasound imaging. *J Orthop Sports Phys Ther.* 2009;39(3):164-171. doi:10.2519/jospt.2008.2913

195. Vicenzino B, Neal R, Collins D, Wright A. The displacement, velocity and frequency profile of the frontal plane motion produced by the cervical lateral glide treatment technique. *Clin Biomech.* 1999;14:515-521.

196. Schäfer A, Hall T, Muller G, Briffa K. Outcomes differ between subgroups of patients with low back and leg pain following neural manual therapy: a prospective cohort study. *Eur Spine J.* 2011;20:482-490. doi:10.1007/s00586-010-1632-2

197. Moseley G, Butler D. Fifteen years of explaining pain: the past, present and future. *J Pain.* 2015;16(9):807-813. doi:10.1016/j.jpain.2015.05.005

198. Louw A, Zimney K, Puentedura E, Diener I. The efficacy of pain neuroscience education on musculoskeletal pain: a systematic review of the literature. *Physiother Theory Pract.* 2016;32(5):332-355. doi:10.1080/09593985.2016.1194646

199. Schmid A, Nee R, Coppieters M. Reappraising entrapment neuropathies - mechanisms, diagnosis and management. *Man Ther.* 2013;18:449-457. doi:10.1016/j.math.2013.07.006

200. Beltran-Alacreu H, Jimenez-Sanz L, Carnero J, La Touche R. Comparison of hypoalgesic effects of neural stretching vs neural gliding: a randomized controlled trial. *J Manipulative Physiol Ther.* 2015;38(9):644-652. doi:10.1016/j.jmpt.2015.09.002

201. Martins C, Pereira R, Fernandes I, et al. Neural gliding and neural tensioning differently impact flexibility, heat and pressure pain thresholds in asymptomatic subjects: a randomized, parallel and double-blind study. *Phys Ther Sport*. 2019;36:101-109. doi:10.1016/j.ptsp.2019.01.008

202. Gamelas T, Fernandes A, Magalhães I, Ferreira M, Machado S, Silva A. Neural gliding versus neural tensioning: effects on heat and cold thresholds, pain thresholds and hand grip strength in asymptomatic individuals. *J Bodyw Mov Ther*. 2019;23(4):799-804. doi:10.1016/j.jbmt.2019.1004.1011.

203. Maitland G. *Vertebral Manipulation*. 5th ed. Butterworths; 1986.

204. Barakatt E, Romano P, Riddle D, Beckett L. The reliability of Maitland's irritability judgments in patients with low back pain. *J Man Manip Ther*. 2009;17(3):135-140.

205. Barakatt E, Romano P, Riddle D, Beckett L, Kravitz R. An exploration of Maitland's concept of pain irritability in patients with low back pain. *J Man Manip Ther*. 2009;17:196-205.

206. Coppieters M, Stappaerts K, Wouters L, Janssens K. The immediate effects of a cervical lateral glide treatment technique in patients with neurogenic cervicobrachial pain. *J Orthop Sports Phys Ther*. 2003;33:369-378. doi:10.2519/jospt.2003.33.7.369

207. Coppieters M, Stappaerts K, Wouters L, Janssens K. Aberrant protective force generation during neural provocation testing and the effect of treatment in patients with neurogenic cervicobrachial pain. *J Manipulative Physiol Ther*. 2003;26(2):99-106. doi:10.1067/mmt.2003.16

208. Vicenzino B, Collins D, Wright A. The initial effects of a cervical spine manipulative physiotherapy treatment on the pain and dysfunction of lateral epicondylalgia. *Pain*. 1996;68(1):69-74.

209. Sterling M, Pedler A, Chan C, Puglisi M, Vuvan V, Vicenzino B. Cervical lateral glide increases nociceptive flexion reflex threshold but not pressure or thermal pain thresholds in chronic whiplash associated disorders: a pilot randomised controlled trial. *Man Ther*. 2010;15:149-153. doi:10.1016/j.math.2009.09.004

210. Rodriguez-Sanz D, Calvo-Lobo C, Unda-Solano F, Sanz-Corbalan I, Romero-Morales C, Lopez-Lopez D. Cervical lateral glide neural mobilization is effective in treating cervicobrachial pain: a randomized waiting list controlled clinical trial. *Pain Med*. 2017;18(12):2492-2503. doi:10.1093/pm/pnx011

211. Nee R, Vicenzino B, Jull G, Cleland J, Coppieters M. A novel protocol to develop a prediction model that identifies patients with nerve-related neck and arm pain who benefit from the early introduction of neural tissue management. *Contemp Clin Trials*. 2011;32(5):760-770. doi:10.1016/j.cct.2011.05.018

212. Nee R, Vicenzino B, Jull G, Cleland J, Coppieters M. Neural tissue management provides immediate clinically relevant benefits without harmful effects for patients with nerve-related neck and arm pain: a randomised trial. *J Physiother*. 2012;58(1):23-31. doi:10.1016/S1836-9553(12)70069-3

213. Ferreira G, Stieven F, Araujo F, et al. Neurodynamic treatment did not improve pain and disability at two weeks in patients with chronic nerve-related leg pain: a randomised trial. *J Physiother*. 2016;62:197-202. doi:10.1016/j.jphys.2016.08.007

214. Fernández-de-Las Peñas C, Ortega-Santiago R, de la Llave-Rincón A, et al. Manual physical therapy versus surgery for carpal tunnel syndrome: a randomized parallel-group trial. *J Pain*. 2015;16:1087-1094. doi:10.1016/j.jpain.2015.07.012

215. Fernández-de-Las-Peñas C, Cleland J, Palacios-Ceña M, Fuensalida-Novo S, Pareja J, Alonso-Blanco C. The effectiveness of manual therapy versus surgery on self-reported function, cervical range of motion, and pinch grip force in carpal tunnel syndrome: a randomized clinical trial. *J Orthop Sports Phys Ther*. 2017;47:151-161. doi:10.2519/jospt.2017.7090

216. Basson C, Stewart A, Mudzi W. The effect of neural mobilisation on cervico-brachial pain: design of a randomised controlled trial. *BMC Musculoskelet Disord*. 2014;15:419. doi:10.1186/1471-2474-15-419

217. Klingman R. The pseudoradicular syndrome: a case report implicating double crush mechanisms in peripheral nerve tissue of the lower extremity. *J Man Manip Ther*. 1999;7:81-91. doi:10.1179/106698199790811735

218. Petersen S, Scott D. Application of a classification system and description of a combined manual therapy intervention: a case with low back related leg pain. *J Man Manip Ther*. 2010;18:89-96. doi:10.1179/106698110X12640740712572

219. Kelley M, Shaffer M, Kuhn J, et al. Shoulder pain and mobility deficits: adhesive capsulitis. Clinical practice guidelines linked to the International Classification of Functioning, Disability, and Health from the Orthopaedic Section of the American Physical Therapy Association. *J Orthop Sports Phys Ther*. 2013;43(5):A1-A31. doi:10.2519/jospt.2013.0302

220. McClure P, Michener L. Staged approach for rehabilitation classification: shoulder disorders (STAR-Shoulder). *Phys Ther*. 2015;95:791-800. doi:10.2522/ptj.20140156

221. Parke W, Whalen J. The vascular pattern of the human dorsal root ganglion and its probable bearing on a compartment syndrome. *Spine*. 2002;27(4):347-352.

222. Takahashi N, Yabuki S, Aoki Y, Kikuchi S. Pathomechanisms of nerve root injury caused by disc herniation: an experimental study of mechanical compression and chemical irritation. *Spine*. 2003;28:435-441. doi:10.1097/01.BRS.0000048645.33118.02

223. Rempel D, Diao E. Entrapment neuropathies: pathophysiology and pathogenesis. *J Electromyogr Kinesiol*. 2004;14:71-75. doi:10.1016/j.jelekin.2003.09.009

224. Kobayashi S, Yoshizawa H, Yamada S. Pathology of lumbar nerve root compression. Part 1: intraradicular inflammatory changes induced by mechanical compression. *J Orthop Res*. 2004;22(1):170-179. doi:10.1016/S0736-0266(03)00131-1

225. Lundborg G, Myers R, Powell H. Nerve compression injury and increased endoneurial fluid pressure: a "miniature compartment syndrome." *J Neurol Neurosurg Psychiatry*. 1983;46(12):1119-1124.

226. Lundborg G. Intraneural microcirculation. *Orthop Clin North Am*. 1988;19(1):1-12.

227. Schmid A, Elliott J, Strudwick M, Little M, Coppieters M. Effect of splinting and exercise on intraneural edema of the median nerve in carpal tunnel syndrome - an MRI study to reveal therapeutic mechanisms. *J Orthop Res*. 2012;30:1343-1350. doi:10.1002/jor.22064

228. Bland J. Carpal tunnel syndrome. *BMJ*. 2007;335:343-346. doi:10.1136/bmj.39282.623553.AD

229. Farmer J, Wisneski R. Cervical spine nerve root compression: an analysis of neuroforaminal pressures with varying head and arm positions. *Spine*. 1994;19(16):1850-1855.

230. Gifford L. Acute low cervical nerve root conditions: symptom presentation and pathobiological reasoning. *Man Ther*. 2001;6:106-115. doi:10.1054/math.2000.0386

231. Seradge H, Jia Y, Owens W. In vivo measurement of carpal tunnel pressure in the functioning hand. *J Hand Surg*. 1995;20A:855-859. doi:10.1016/S0363-5023(05)80443-5

232. Totten P, Hunter J. Therapeutic techniques to enhance nerve gliding in thoracic outlet syndrome and carpal tunnel syndrome. *Hand Clin*. 1991;7(3):505-520.

233. Kirkcaldie M, Collins J. The axon as a physical structure in health and acute trauma. *J Chem Neuroanat*. 2016;76(Pt A):9-18. doi:10.1016/j.jchemneu.2016.05.006

234. Lopez-Leal R, Alvarez J, Court F. Origin of axonal proteins: is the axon-Schwann cell unit a functional syncytium? *Cytoskeleton*. 2016;73:629-639. doi:10.1002/cm.21319

235. Shah C, Calfee R, Gelberman R, Goldfarb C. Outcomes of rigid night splinting and activity modification in the treatment of cubital tunnel syndrome. *J Hand Surg*. 2013;38A:1125-1130. doi:10.1016/j.jhsa.2013.02.039

236. Svernlöv B, Larrson M, Rehn K, Adolfsson L. Conservative treatment of the cubital tunnel syndrome. *J Hand Surg.* 2009;34E:201-207. doi:10.1177/1753193408098480

237. Costigan M, Scholz J, Woolf C. Neuropathic pain: a maladaptive response of the nervous system to damage. *Ann Rev Neurosci.* 2009;32:1-32. doi:10.1146/annurev.neuro.051508.135531

238. Song X, Gan Q, Cao J, Wang Z, Rupert R. Spinal manipulation reduces pain and hyperalgesia after lumbar intervertebral foramen inflammation in the rat. *J Manipulative Physiol Ther.* 2006;29(1):5-13. doi:10.1016/j.jmpt.2005.10.001

239. Schmid A, Coppieters M, Ruitenberg M, McLachlan E. Local and remote immune-mediated inflammation after mild peripheral nerve compression in rats. *J Neuropathol Exp Neurol.* 2013;72(7):662-680. doi:10.1097/NEN.0b013e318298de5b

240. Albrecht D, Ahmed S, Kettner N, et al. Neuroinflammation of the spinal cord and nerve roots in chronic radicular pain patients. *Pain.* 2018;159:968-977. doi:10.1097/j.pain.0000000000001171

241. Cohen S, Mao J. Neuropathic pain: mechanisms and their clinical implications. *BMJ.* 2014;348:f7656. doi:10.1136/bmj.f7656

242. Murphy D, Hurwitz E, Gerrard J, Clary R. Pain patterns and descriptions in patients with radicular pain: does the pain necessarily follow a specific dermatome? *Chiropr Osteopat.* 2009;17:9. doi:10.1186/1746-1340-17-9

243. Furman M, Johnson S. Induced lumbosacral radicular symptom referral patterns: a descriptive study. *Spine J.* 2019;19:163-170. doi:10.1016/j.spinee.2018.05.029

244. Nora D, Becker J, Ehlers J, Gomes I. Clinical features of 1039 patients with neurophysiological diagnosis of carpal tunnel syndrome. *Clin Neurol Neurosurg.* 2004;107(1):64-69. doi:10.1016/j.clineuro.2004.08.003

245. Caliandro P, La Torre G, Aprile I, et al. Distribution of paresthesias in carpal tunnel syndrome reflects the degree of nerve damage at wrist. *Clin Neurophysiol.* 2006;117(1):228-231. doi:10.1016/j.clinph.2005.09.001

246. Zanette G, Cacciatori C, Tamburin S. Central sensitization in carpal tunnel syndrome with extraterritorial spread of sensory symptoms. *Pain.* 2010;148:227-236. doi:10.1016/j.pain.2009.10.025

247. Mansiz-Kaplan B, Akdeniz-Leblecicier M, Yagci I. Are extramedian symptoms associated with peripheral causes in patient with carpal tunnel syndrome? Electrodiagnostic and ultrasonographic study. *J Electromyogr Kinesiol.* 2018;38:203-207. doi:10.1016/j.jelekin.2017.08.003

248. da Silva J, Santos F, Giardini A, et al. Neural mobilization promotes nerve regeneration by nerve growth factor and myelin protein zero increased after sciatic nerve injury. *Growth Factors.* 2015;33(1):8-13. doi:10.3109/08977194.2014.953630

249. Santos F, Silva J, Giardini A, et al. Neural mobilization reverses behavioral and cellular changes that characterize neuropathic pain in rats. *Mol Pain.* 2012;8:57. doi:10.1186/1744-8069-8-57

250. Gardini A, Dos Santos F, da Silva J, de Oliveira M, Martins D, Chacur M. Neural mobilization treatment decreases glial cells and brain-derived neurotrophic factor expression in the central nervous system in rats with neuropathic pain induced by CCI in rats. *Pain Res Manag.* 2017;2017:Article ID:7429761. doi:10.1155/2017/7429761

251. Santos F, Silva J, Rocha I, Martins D, Chacur M. Non-pharmacological treatment affects neuropeptide expression in neuropathic pain model. *Brain Res.* 2018;1687:60-65. doi:10.1016/j.brainres.2018.02.034

252. Santos F, Grecco L, Pereira M, et al. The neural mobilization technique modulates the expression of endogenous opioids in the periaqueductal gray and improves muscle strength and mobility in rats with neuropathic pain. *Behav Brain Funct.* 2014;10:19. doi:10.1186/1744-9081-10-19

253. Vicenzino B, Collins D, Benson H, Wright A. An investigation of the interrelationship between manipulative therapy-induced hypoalgesia and sympathoexcitation. *J Manipulative Physiol Ther.* 1998;21(7):448-453.

254. Schmid A, Brunner F, Wright A, Bachmann L. Paradigm shift in manual therapy? Evidence for a central nervous system component in the response to passive cervical joint mobilisation. *Man Ther.* 2008;13:387-396. doi:10.1016/j.math.2007.12.007

255. Bishop M, Torres-Cueco R, Gay C, Lluch-Girbes E, Beneciuk J, Bialosky J. What effect can manual therapy have on a patient's pain experience. *Pain Manag.* 2015;5(6):455-464. doi:10.2217/pmt.15.39

256. Lascurain-Aguirrebeña I, Newham D, Critchley D. Mechanism of action of spinal mobilizations: a systematic review. *Spine.* 2016;41:159-172. doi:10.1097/BRS.0000000000001151

257. Fernández-Carnero J, Sierra-Silvestre E, Beltran-Alacreu H, Gil-Martinez A, La Touche R. Neural tension technique improves immediate conditioned pain modulation in patients with chronic neck pain: a randomized clinical trial. *Pain Med.* 2019;20:1227-1235. doi:10.1093/pm/pny115

258. Bialosky J, Bishop M, Price D, Robinson M, Vincent K, George S. A randomised sham-controlled trial of a neurodynamic technique in the treatment of carpal tunnel syndrome. *J Orthop Sports Phys Ther.* 2009;39:709-723. doi:10.2519/jospt.2009.3117

259. Paungmali A, O'Leary S, Souvlis T, Vicenzino B. Hypoalgesic and sympathoexcitatory effects of mobilization with movement for lateral epicondylalgia. *Phys Ther.* 2003;83(4):374-383.

260. Bialosky J, Bishop M, Robinson M, Zeppieri G, George S. Spinal manipulative therapy has an immediate effect on thermal pain sensitivity in people with low back pain: a randomized controlled trial. *Phys Ther.* 2009;89:1292-1303. doi:10.2522/ptj.20090058

261. Kingston L, Claydon L, Tumilty S. The effects of spinal mobilizations on the sympathetic nervous system: a systematic review. *Man Ther.* 2014;19:281-287. doi:10.1016/j.math.2014.04.004

262. Voogt L, de Vries J, Meeus M, Struyf F, Meuffels D, Nijs J. Analgesic effects of manual therapy in patients with musculoskeletal pain: a systematic review. *Man Ther.* 2015;20:250-256. doi:10.1016/j.math.2014.09.001

263. Wirth B, Gassner A, de Bruin E, et al. Neurophysiological effects of high velocity and low amplitude spinal manipulation in symptomatic and asymptomatic humans: a systematic literature review. *Spine.* 2019;44:E914-E926. doi:10.1097/BRS.0000000000003013

264. Bialosky J, Beneciuk J, Bishop M, et al. Unraveling the mechanisms of manual therapy: modeling an approach. *J Orthop Sports Phys Ther.* 2018;48:8-18. doi:10.2519/jospt.2018.7476

265. Littlewood C, Malliaras P, Bateman M, Stace R, May S, Walters S. The central nervous system - An additional consideration in 'rotator cuff tendinopathy' and a potential basis for understanding response to loaded therapeutic exercise. *Man Ther.* 2013;18:468-472. doi:10.1016/j.math.2013.07.005

266. Moseley G. A pain neuromatrix approach to patients with chronic pain. *Man Ther.* 2003;8(3):130-140.

267. Smith B, Hendrick P, Bateman M, et al. Musculoskeletal pain and exercise - challenging existing paradigms and introducing new. *Br J Sports Med.* 2019;53(14):907-912. doi:10.1136/bjsports-2017-098983

268. Shacklock M. Central pain mechanisms: a new horizon in manual therapy. *Aust J Physiother.* 1999;45:83-92.

269. Louw A, Nijs J, Puentedura E. A clinical perspective on a pain neuroscience education approach to manual therapy. *J Man Manip Ther.* 2017;25:160-168. doi:10.1080/10669817.2017.1323699

270. Marris D, Theophanous K, Cabezon P, Dunlap Z, Donaldson M. The impact of combining pain education strategies with physical therapy interventions for patients with chronic pain: a systematic review and meta-analysis of randomized controlled trials. *Physiother Theory Pract.* 2021;37(4):461-472. doi:10.1080/095939 85.09592019.01633714

271. Moseley G. Unraveling the barriers to reconceptualization of the problem in chronic pain: the actual and perceived ability of patients and health professionals to understand the neurophysiology. *J Pain.* 2003;4(4):184-189.

272. Butler D, Moseley G. *Explain Pain.* 2nd ed. Noigroup Publications; 2013.

273. Louw A, Puentedura E. *Therapeutic Neuroscience Education.* Orthopedic Physical Therapy Products; 2013.

274. Louw A, Zimney K, O'Hotto C, Hilton S. The clinical application of teaching people about pain. *Physiother Theory Pract.* 2016;32:385-395. doi:10.1080/09593985.2016.1194652

275. Robinson V, King R, Ryan C, Martin D. A qualitative exploration of people's experiences of pain neurophysiological education for chronic pain: the importance of relevance for the individual. *Man Ther.* 2016;22:56-61. doi:10.1016/j.math.2015.10.001

276. Watson J, Ryan C, Cooper L, et al. Pain neuroscience education for adults with chronic musculoskeletal pain: a mixed-methods systematic review and meta-analysis. *J Pain.* 2019;20(10):1140.e1-1140.e22. doi:10.1016/j.jpain.2019.1002.1011.

277. Cleland J, Childs J, Palmer J, Eberhart S. Slump stretching in the management of non-radicular low back pain: a pilot clinical trial. *Man Ther.* 2006;11:279-286. doi:10.1016/j.math.2005.07.002

278. Adel S. Efficacy of neural mobilization in treatment of low back dysfunctions. *Journal of American Science.* 2011;7(4):566-573.

279. Nagrale A, Patil S, Gandhi R, Learman K. Effect of slump stretching versus lumbar mobilization with exercise in subjects with non-radicular low back pain: a randomized clinical trial. *J Man Manip Ther.* 2012;20:35-42. doi:10.1179/2042618611Y.0000000015

280. Ahmed N, Tufel S, Khan M, Khan P. Effectiveness of neural mobilization in the management of sciatica. *J Musculoskel Res.* 2013;16(3). doi:10.1142/S0218957713500127

281. Jeong U, Kim C, Park Y, Hwang-Bo G, Nam C. The effects of self-mobilization techniques for the sciatic nerves on physical functions and health of low back pain patients with lower limb radiating pain. *J Phys Ther Sci.* 2016;28:46-50. doi:10.1589/jpts.28.46

282. Basson A, Olivier B, Ellis R, Coppieters M, Stewart A, Mudzi W. The effectiveness of neural mobilization for neuro-musculoskeletal conditions: a systematic review and meta-analysis. *J Orthop Sports Phys Ther.* 2017;47:593-615. doi:10.2519/jospt.2017.7117

283. Pourahmadi M, Hesarikia H, Keshtkar A, et al. Effectiveness of slump stretching on low back pain: a systematic review and meta-analysis. *Pain Med.* 2019;20:378-396. doi:10.1093/pm/pny208

284. Hopkins W. A new view of statistics. 2011. Accessed August 29, 2022. www.sportsci.org/resource/stats/index.html

285. Scrimshaw S, Maher C. Randomized controlled trial of neural mobilization after spinal surgery. *Spine.* 2001;26(24):2647-2652.

286. Rodriguez-Sanz D, Lopez-Lopez D, Unda-Solano F, et al. Effects of median nerve mobilization in treating cervicobrachial pain: a randomized waiting list-controlled clinical trial. *Pain Pract.* 2018;18(4):431-442. doi:10.1111/papr.12614

287. Page M, O'Connor D, Pitt V, Massy-Westropp N. Exercise and mobilisation interventions for carpal tunnel syndrome (Review). *Cochrane Database Syst Rev.* 2012;Issue 6:Art. No.:CD009899. doi:10.1002/14651858.CD009899

288. Ballestero-Perez R, Plaza-Manzano G, Urraca-Gesto A, et al. Effectiveness of nerve gliding exercises on carpal tunnel syndrome: a systematic review. *J Manipulative Physiol Ther.* 2017;40(1):50-59. doi:10.1016/j.jmpt.2016.10.004

289. Wolny T, Linek P. Is manual therapy based on neurodynamic techniques effective in the treatment of carpal tunnel syndrome? A randomized controlled trial. *Clin Rehabil.* 2019;33(3):408-417. doi:10.1177/0269215518805213

290. Huissstede B, Hoogvliet P, Franke T, Randsdorp M, Koes B. Carpal tunnel syndrome: effectiveness of physical therapy and electrophysical modalities. An updated systematic review of randomized controlled trials. *Arch Phys Med Rehabil.* 2018;99(8):1623-1634. e1623.doi:10.1016/j.apmr.2017.08.482

291. Sim S, Gunasagaran J, Goh K, Ahmad T. Short-term clinical outcome of orthosis alone vs combination of orthosis, nerve, and tendon gliding exercises and ultrasound therapy for treatment of carpal tunnel syndrome. *J Hand Ther.* 2019;32(4):411-416. doi:10.1016/j.jht.2018.1001.1004

292. Kavlak Y, Uygur F. Effects of nerve mobilization exercise as an adjunct to the conservative treatment for patients with tarsal tunnel syndrome. *J Manipulative Physiol Ther.* 2011;34:441-448. doi:10.1016/j.jmpt.2011.05.017

293. Chan A, Tetzlaff J, Gotzsche P, et al. SPRIT 2013 explanation and elaboration: guidance for protocls of clinical trials. *BMJ.* 2013;346:e7586. doi:10.1136/bmj.e7586

294. Heebner M, Roddey T. The effects of neural mobilization in addition to standard care in persons with carpal tunnel syndrome from a community hospital. *J Hand Ther.* 2008;21:229-241. doi:10.1197/j.jht.2007.12.001

295. Hoffmann T, Glasziou P, Boutron I, et al. Better reporting of interventions: template for intervention description and replication (TIDieR) checklist and guide. *BMJ.* 2014;348:g1687. doi:10.1136/bmj.g.1687

296. Ekstrom R, Holden K. Examination of and intervention for a patient with chronic lateral elbow pain with signs of nerve entrapment. *Phys Ther.* 2002;82(11):1077-1086.

297. Alshami A, Souvlis T, Coppieters M. A review of plantar heel pain of neural origin: differential diagnosis and management. *Man Ther.* 2008;13:103-111. doi:10.1016/j.math.2007.01.014

298. Meyer J, Kulig K, Landel R. Differential diagnosis and treatment of subcalcaneal heel pain: a case report. *J Orthop Sports Phys Ther.* 2002;32:114-124. doi:10.2519/jospt.2002.32.3.114

299. Saban B, Deutscher D, Ziv T. Deep massage to posterior calf muscles in combination with neural mobilization exercises as a treatment for heel pain: a pilot randomized clinical trial. *Man Ther.* 2014;19:102-108. doi:10.1016/j.math.2013.08.001

300. Turl S, George K. Adverse neural tension: a factor in repetitive hamstring strain? *J Orthop Sports Phys Ther.* 1998;27(1):16-21.

301. Heiderscheit B, Sherry M, Silder A, Chumanov E, Thelen D. Hamstring strain injuries: recommendations for diagnosis, rehabilitation, and injury prevention. *J Orthop Sports Phys Ther.* 2010;40:67-81. doi:10.2519/jospt.2010.3047

302. Kornberg C, Lew P. The effect of stretching neural structures on grade one hamstring injuries. *J Orthop Sports Phys Ther.* 1989;10:481-487.

303. Goldstein M, Scalzitti D, Craik R, et al. The revised research agenda for physical therapy. *Phys Ther.* 2011;91:165-174. doi:10.2522/ptj.20100248

304. Foster N, Hill J, O'Sullivan P, Hancock M. Stratified models of care. *Best Pract Res Clin Rheumatol.* 2013;27(5):649-661. doi:10.1016/j.berh.2013.10.005

305. Nee R, Vicenzino B, Jull G, Cleland J, Coppieters M. Baseline characteristics of patients with nerve-related neck and arm pain predict the likely response to neural tissue management. *J Orthop Sports Phys Ther.* 2013;43(6):379-391. doi:10.2519/jospt.2013.4490

306. Huang B, Shih Y, Chen W, Ma H. Predictors for identifying patients with patellofemoral pain syndrome responding to femoral nerve mobilization. *Arch Phys Med Rehabil.* 2015;96(5):920-927. doi:10.1016/j.apmr.2015.01.001

307. Hancock M, Herbert R, Maher C. A guide to interpretation of studies investigating subgroups of responders to physical therapy interventions. *Phys Ther.* 2009;89(7):698-704. doi:10.2522/ptj.20080351

308. Kent P, Keating J, Leboeuf-Yde C. Research methods for subgrouping low back pain. *BMC Med Res Methodol.* 2010;10:62. doi:10.1186/1471-2288-10-62

309. Ginanneschi F, Cioncoloni D, Bigliazzi J, Bonifazi M, Lore C, Rossi A. Sensory axons excitability changes in carpal tunnel syndrome after neural mobilization. *Neurol Sci.* 2015;36(9):1611-1615. doi:10.1007/s10072-015-2218-x

310. Ridehalgh C, Moore A, Hough A. The short term effects of straight leg raise neurodynamic treatment on pressure pain and vibration thresholds in individuals with spinally referred leg pain. *Man Ther.* 2016;23:40-47. doi:10.1016/j.math.2015.12.013

311. Cook C, Showalter C, Kabbaz V, O'Halloran B. Can a within/between-session change in pain during reassessment predict outcome using manual therapy intervention in patients with mechanical low back pain? *Man Ther.* 2012;17:325-329. doi:10.1016/j.math.2012.02.020

312. Cook C, Lawrence J, Michalak K, et al. Is there preliminary value to a within- and/or between-session change for determining short-term outcomes of manual therapy on mechanical neck pain? *J Man Manip Ther.* 2014;22(4):173-180. doi:10.1179/2042618614Y.0000000071

313. Elvén M, Hochwälder J, Dean E, Soderlund A. A clinical reasoning model focused on clients' behaviour change with reference to physiotherapists: its multiphase development and validation. *Physiother Theory Pract.* 2015;31(4):231-243. doi:10.3109/09593985.2014.994250

314. Peek K, Sanson-Fisher R, Mackenzie L, Carey M. Interventions to aid patient adherence to physiotherapist prescribed self-management strategies: a systematic review. *Physiotherapy.* 2016;102:127-135. doi:10.1016/j.physio.2015.10.003

315. Hall T, Hardt S, Schäfer A, Wallin L. Mulligan bent leg raise technique - a preliminary randomized trial of immediate effects after a single intervention. *Man Ther.* 2006;11:130-135. doi:10.1016/j.math.2005.04.009

316. Hanney R, Ridehalgh C, Dawson A, Lewis D, Kenny D. The effects of neurodynamic straight leg raise treatment duration on range of hip flexion and protective muscle activity at P1. *J Man Manip Ther.* 2016;24:14-20. doi:10.1179/2042618613Y.0000000049

317. Kinney M, Seider J, Beaty A, Coughlin K, Dyal M, Clewley D. The impact of therapeutic alliance in physical therapy for chronic musculoskeletal pain: a systematic review of the literature. *Physiother Theory Pract.* 2020;36(8):886-898. doi:10.1080/09593985.0959201 8.01516015.

318. Ong B, Konstantinou K, Corbett M, Hay E. Patients' own accounts of sciatica. *Spine.* 2011;36:1251-1256. doi:10.1097/BRS.0b013e318204f7a2

319. Hopayian K, Notley C. A systematic review of low back pain and sciatica patients' expectations and experiences of health care. *Spine J.* 2014;14:1769-1780. doi:10.1016/j.spinee.2014.02.029

320. Pinto R, Ferreira M, Oliveira V, et al. Patient-centred communication is associated with positive therapeutic alliance: a systematic review. *J Physiother.* 2012;58(2):77-87.

321. Peersman W, Rooms T, Bracke N, Van Waelvelde H, De Maeseneer J, Cambier D. Patients' priorities regarding outpatient physiotherapy care: a qualitative and quantitative study. *Man Ther.* 2013;18:155-164. doi:10.1016/j.math.2012.09.007

322. O'Keeffe M, Cullinane P, Hurley J, et al. What influences patient-therapist interactions in musculoskeletal physical therapy? Qualitative systematic review and meta-synthesis. *Phys Ther.* 2016;96:609-622. doi:10.2522/ptj.20150240

323. Miciak M, Mayan M, Brown C, Joyce A, Gross D. A framework for establishing connections in physiotherapy practice. *Physiother Theory Pract.* 2019;35:40-56. doi:10.1080/09593985.2018.1434707

324. Martin R, Irrgang J, Burdett R, Conti S, van Swearingen J. Evidence of validity for the foot and ankle ability measure (FAAM). *Foot Ankle Int.* 2005;26(11):968-983.

325. Redmond A, Crosbie J, Ouvrier R. Development and validation of a novel rating system for scoring standing foot posture: the Foot Posture Index. *Clin Biomech.* 2006;21:89-98. doi:10.1016/j.clinbiomech.2005.08.002

326. Rathleff M, Molgaard C, Fredberg U, et al. High-load strength training improves outcome in patients with plantar fasciitis: a randomized controlled trial with 12-month follow-up. *Scand J Med Sci Sports.* 2015;25(3):e292-e300. doi:10.1111/sms.12313

327. Nielsen R, Parner E, Nohr E, Sorensen H, Lind M, Rasmussen S. Excessive progression in weekly running distance and risk of running-related injuries: an association which varies according to type of injury. *J Orthop Sports Phys Ther.* 2014;44:739-742. doi:10.2519/jospt.2014.5164

328. Damsted C, Glad S, Nielsen R, Sørensen H, Malisoux L. Is there evidence for an association between changes in training load and running-related injuries? A systematic review. *Int J Sports Phys Ther.* 2018;13(6):931-942. doi:10.26603/ijspt20180931

329. Damsted C, Parner E, Sørensen H, Malisoux L, Hulme A, Nielsen R. The association between changes in weekly running distance and running-related injury: preparing for a half marathon. *J Orthop Sports Phys Ther.* 2019;49:230-238. doi:10.2519/jospt.2019.854

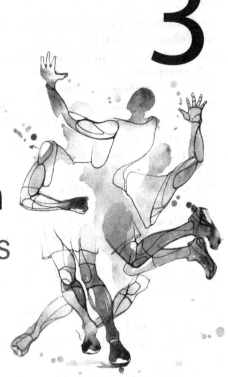

Symptom Investigation
Screening for Medical Conditions

Graham Linck, PT, DPT, cert DN
and Bill Boissonnault, PT, DHSc, DPT

KEY TERMS

Boa's sign: Hypersensitivity in the right scapular region that may indicate potential gall bladder pathology.

Cardiac tamponade: A medically emergent condition in which fluid fills the pericardial sac putting excessive pressure on the heart and leading to decreased ventricular filling and abnormal heart function.

Cauda equina syndrome: A medical emergency in which the lumbar plexus below the termination of the spinal cord is compromised, resulting in severe low back pain (LBP), saddle anesthesia, bowel/bladder/sexual dysfunction, decreased lower extremity strength/reflexes, and gait disturbances.

Cholecystitis: Inflammation of the gall bladder due to blockage of the cystic duct.

Claudication: Painful cramping in the lower extremities as a result of decreased arterial blood flow. It occurs with prolonged standing and walking and resolves with rest.

Clonus: Series of involuntary rhythmic muscle contractions and relaxations. It indicates an upper motor neuron lesion (eg, cerebral palsy, stroke, multiple sclerosis).

Complex regional pain syndrome (CRPS; reflex sympathetic dystrophy): A regional, posttraumatic neuropathic pain condition that usually occurs in an arm/or leg following a previous injury; the pain is usually out of proportion to the actual extent of the injury.

Deep vein thrombosis (DVT): A blood clot that forms in the deep veins of the body, most commonly in the legs. It is characterized by pain, swelling, erythema, and tenderness.

Differential diagnosis: The distinguishing of one condition/ disease from others that present with similar signs/symptom.

Ivory white vertebrae: Increased opacity of the vertebrae while still retaining its normal size and contours and with no change in opacity of adjacent vertebrae.

Metastasis: The spread of cancer cells from one part of the body to another.

Murphy's sign: Palpation of subcostal space/liver border with inhalation that may indicate pathology/inflammation in the gall bladder.

Pneumothorax: Also known as a *collapsed lung*, occurs when an abnormal collection of air is present in the pleural space between the lung and chest wall.

Pulmonary embolus: A blockage of an artery in the lungs; most commonly caused by a blood clot/DVT.

Wallmann HW, Donatelli R, eds. *Foundations of Orthopedic Physical Therapy* (pp 81-104).
© 2024 Taylor & Francis Group.

Pyelonephritis: A kidney infection that usually results due to an obstruction in the urinary tract.

Raynaud's disease: An avascular disorder in which spasms of blood vessels, usually in the fingers and toes, result in possible pain, numbness, and paresthesia.

Red flags: Prognostic variables for serious pathology that may be found during an initial physical therapy examination that warrant immediate referral to physician.

Referred pain: Pain perceived at a site other than the actual origin of the painful stimuli.

Stable angina: Chest pain that occurs in a predictable manner in response to exercise/activity.

Unstable angina: Chest pain that occurs without a predictable manner or response to exercise/activity.

Chapter Questions

1. What is an ivory white vertebrae sign and how can it be detected?

2. What are the differences between stable and unstable angina?

3. What lumbar spine condition may mimic the symptoms of intermittent claudication?

4. What is a red flag/medically emergent condition characterized by saddle anesthesia and loss of bowel/bladder control?

5. Describe different symptom presentations for kidney stones vs gall stones.

6. What are the 5 clinical signs of compartment syndrome?

7. In what body region (eg, head, thorax, extremities) is referred pain most common?

8. Name 2 cervical ligament instability tests and describe how to perform them.

9. What are the 3 types of meningitis, and which is potentially the most fatal?

10. Which carpal bone is involved and what wrist motion is most painful, when a Colles fracture is present?

11. Describe 4 peripheral upper extremity nerve presentations and what scapular muscles will be most affected with each.

12. What lung condition must a therapist be aware of immediately following a traumatic blow to the chest?

13. What is the most common incomplete spinal cord injury and what are 2 patient risk factors that may contribute to this condition?

14. What are some differences between Raynaud's disease and CRPS?

15. What are 2 juvenile hip conditions that a therapist must be aware of in the treatment of juvenile hip pain?

16. Describe the process of osteonecrosis and give 3 potential risk factors for this condition?

17. What diagnostic medical tests can be used to confirm the presence of ankylosing spondylitis?

18. What other medical event may occur with pericarditis?

19. What are 3 red flags for pancreatic cancer?

20. Describe Boa's and Murphy's sign and what condition these referred pain patterns may suggest.

Introduction

As physical therapists strive to become more accepted as first-contact providers within the direct access model,[1] the importance of thorough symptom investigation during the initial physical therapy examination is paramount. This chapter will help identify and describe what history and physical examination/test and measures findings may constitute a red flag that requires a referral to a physician. It will review common musculoskeletal and nonmusculoskeletal examination findings that may present during an initial physical therapy encounter and discuss the pertinent medical screening questionnaires that can be used to aide in the decision-making process for the clinician. Symptom investigation includes deducing the location, onset, and behavior of symptoms to assist in the differential diagnosis of a patient's condition.

The vision statement adopted in 2013 by the American Physical Therapy Association House of Delegates identifies several key principles, which if achieved, would allow physical therapists "to engage with consumers to reduce preventable health care costs and overcome barriers to participation in society."[2] A few of these key principles—Quality, Collaboration, Value, Advocacy, and Access/Equity—directly relate to including a comprehensive initial examination that incorporates a review of systems to result in the best possible patient outcomes. Quality care is an expectation within the profession made up of evidence-based practitioners. Physical therapists will adopt best practice standards in order to make sound clinical judgement about the best course of treatment for any patient. There are some conflicting findings in the research regarding the safety/efficacy of physical therapists' ability to properly manage patients within a direct access model. A robust study by Moore et al[3] in 2005, found no adverse events in a 40-month period, with physical therapists providing direct access care in military health care facilities. In contrast a recent survey study, by Laderia, revealed that physical therapists' proposed clinical management of red/yellow flag conditions associated with LBP had only a combined success rate of 41% when managing 3 different cases of lower back symptom presentation.[4] Collaboration with other health care providers, in the event that a red flag or an atypical symptom presentation is found, is an essential responsibility in order for physical therapists to be recognized as a valuable contributor in primary care settings.[5] The value of physical therapists being able to correctly and efficiently determine when a patient needs care outside of their scope of practice is not only in the patient's best interest, but also provides a financial benefit to the health care economy and reinforces the altruistic nature of the profession. Patient advocacy and empowerment that come with knowledge of their condition and the best course of action to address their needs actually reinforces the therapists' value to patients and society as a whole. The initial examination should address the patients' primary complaints and functional limitations, along with identification of other possible underlying health issues that may contribute to their condition. Following the patient examination, the therapist should conclude that either physical therapy is appropriate, the patient needs to be referred to another medical provider in combination with physical therapy, or that physical therapy is not indicated and this condition needs to be managed by another medical professional.

Many different motivations drive patients to seek physical therapy. Most common orthopedic issues include lower back, knee, and shoulder pathology[6] and can exist as a result of trauma, poor posture/body mechanics, repetitive strain, or an arthritic condition, but a small percentage of these types of patients may also be experiencing more serious medical conditions of a nonmusculoskeletal origin (eg, cancer, infection).[7] When patients decide to undergo a physical therapy examination, their first communication with the therapist usually comes from filling out necessary intake forms: previous medical history, pain diagrams, and functional indexes. These forms can be extremely beneficial in helping the therapist potentially identify certain risk factors before the examination even begins. For example, an older male patient presents with lower back/hip pain and lists that he previously had colon cancer that resolved with treatments more than 5 years ago. A pertinent follow-up question to this finding on his intake forms would be, when was the last time the patient saw his oncologist?

After reviewing the patient's medical history, the therapist then needs to review the pain diagram along with the symptom description. One would expect to find a localized region of symptoms with a consistent behavior pattern of symptoms that is predictably altered by some position, activity, or event decreasing the likelihood of finding potential red flag conditions. This may be difficult because some patients may not be able to provide the desired details when describing their condition on their initial intake forms. On the other hand, there are patients who may present with multiple complex medical conditions (eg, chronic pain, fibromyalgia, CRPS; Figure 3-1), which may make communicating the severity and intensity of their symptoms or condition difficult. The intake forms provide initial clues of where therapists may need to delve further with their examination questioning to discern the true source of a patient's complaints.

During the initial chart review, a great number of potential red flag prognosticators can be found by thoroughly examining a patient's information. For example, Deyo and Diehl[8] listed 4 common red flag findings: age greater than 50 years, a history of cancer, unexplained weight loss, or failure

of conservative treatment to relieve a condition, but this also caused a false alarm rate of 40%. In fact, in a recent review in the *British Journal of Sports Medicine*, Cook et al[9] suggested that red flag screening by a physical therapist is not consistent with best practice guidelines in the management of LBP due to "lack of support for their diagnostic capacity." Red flags have historically been developed by clinical observation and retrospective analyses leading to a large amount of listed and overlapping findings. It should be recognized that no red flag finding achieved 100% agreement and that many of the guidelines developed have relied on secondary citations as noted by Henscke and Maher[10] and Klaber-Moffet et al.[11] Nearly all of this demographic patient data can be collected prior to the initial patient contact while reviewing the patient's intake forms. It should be noted that there have been more than 100 subjective and 40 objective findings that have been reported as potential red flags in the literature when clinical guidelines for the physical therapy management of LBP were released by the Chartered Society of Physiotherapy in 2007.[12] This is why red flag screening can be difficult and confusing, especially to novice but even to experienced clinicians, due to the wide variability of patients' responses to examination questions. Roberts et al[13] reported that these 11 common red flag findings were found in more than 50% of the papers reviewed: weight loss, previous history of cancer, night pain, greater than 50 years of age, violent trauma, fever, saddle anesthesia, difficulty with urination, intravenous (IV) drug use, progressive neurology, and systemic steroids.

In discussing symptom location, an important phenomenon of which all practitioners should be cognizant is referred pain. Referred pain has a neurological basis as tremendous amounts of sensory input converge into the central nervous system (CNS) and then proceed up to the higher brain centers for perception. Due to this large amount of information converging into the sensory system and other latent neural connections, the brain can either be confused as to the proper location of nociceptive stimulus or the stimulus is not significant enough to generate an action potential to register the true source of nociception to the brain.[14] The most common example of referred pain seen in most medical literature is increased left shoulder/arm pain associated with a myocardial infarction (MI). Since this is a medical emergency and commonly known phenomenon, therapists will also have to be more aware of other visceral structures (eg, organs), which may cause local or referred pain and the locations of these abnormal sensations to help to differentially diagnose the source of the patient's symptoms. Since the visceral organs are located in the abdomen/trunk, these regions are the most common sites of referred pain (Figure 3-2), which can also mimic many sources of musculoskeletal pathologies found in the trunk (eg, low back/thoracic pain; Table 3-1).

Once therapists have reviewed the intake forms, they should then proceed to take an extensive verbal history in

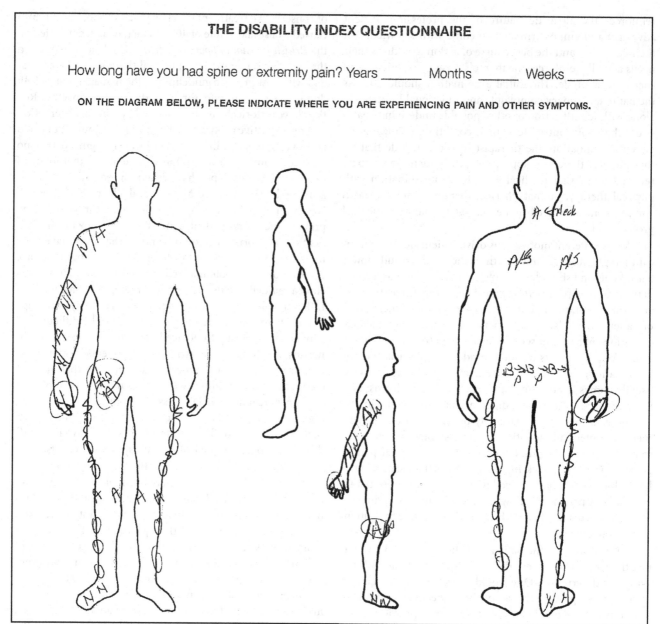

Figure 3-1. Body diagram.

which they follow up on any abnormal findings on their intake forms. It is also during this time that therapists need to ask more detailed questions regarding symptom behavior and history. The first question to address with the patient is the primary complaint and when did their symptoms onset? What led to coming into the clinic to undergo a physical therapy examination? Is this a recent injury, chronic, or an exacerbation of a chronic condition? Most common etiologies for musculoskeletal impairments are a traumatic incident, repetitive overuse, sustained postural strain, or recent change in intensity/frequency of physical activity. In some occasions, the patient may not be able to relate the onset of the condition to any incident and this is where the therapist's

history taking and examination skills can be beneficial. More attention and further examination need to be given to chronic conditions, such as osteoarthritis in the spine, that may have recently returned suddenly, as the patient may just think this is my "old/normal" issue returning and may not give credence to the thought that a new underlying pathology may be driving the return of symptoms. It is the responsibility of the therapist during the initial examination to determine the true source of dysfunction based on the patient's history, symptom location, and symptom description.

After the onset of the current condition has been investigated, further questions to determine how the patient's symptoms respond to various stimulus throughout the

Referred Pain Diagram

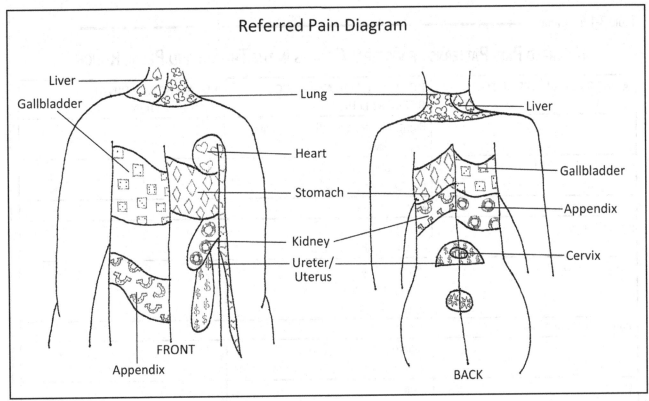

Figure 3-2. Referred pain locations from visceral organs.

Table 3-1

REFERRED PAIN PATTERNS OF VISCERAL ORGANS IN THE THORAX AND PELVIC REGIONS

ANATOMICAL STRUCTURE	POSSIBLE LOCATIONS OF REFERRED PAIN	SEGMENTAL SPINAL INNERVATION
Cardiopulmonary System		
Heart	Anterior cervical	T1-T5
	Upper thorax	
	Left upper extremity	
Lungs and bronchi	Ipsilateral thoracic spine	T5-T6
	Cervical spine (if diaphragm involved)	
Diaphragm	Cervical spine	C3-C5
Digestive System		
Esophagus	Substernal and upper abdomen	T4-T6
Stomach	Upper abdomen	T6-T10
	Middle/lower thoracic spine	
Pancreas	Upper abdomen	T10
	Lower thoracic	
	Upper lumbar spine	
Gall bladder	Right upper abdomen	T7-T9
	Right middle/lower thoracic	
	Spine	
	Scapula	*(continued*

Table 3-1 (continued)

REFERRED PAIN PATTERNS OF VISCERAL ORGANS IN THE THORAX AND PELVIC REGIONS

ANATOMICAL STRUCTURE	POSSIBLE LOCATIONS OF REFERRED PAIN	SEGMENTAL SPINAL INNERVATION
Liver	Right middle/lower thoracic spine Right cervical spine	T7-T9
Common bile duct	Upper abdomen Middle thoracic spine	T8-T10
Small intestine	Middle thoracic spine	T7-T10
Large intestine	Lower abdomen Middle lumbar spine	T11-L1
Sigmoid colon	Upper sacrum Suprapubic region Left lower abdomen	T11-T12
Retroperitoneal Region		
Kidney	Ipsilateral lumbar spine Upper/lower abdomen	T10-L1
Ureter	Groin Medial/proximal thigh Upper abdomen Suprapubic region Thoracic/lumbar spine	T11-L2, S2-S4
Urinary bladder	Sacral apex Suprapubic region Thoracic/lumbar spine	T11-L2, S2-S4
Prostate gland	Sacrum Testes Thoracic/lumbar spine	T11-S1, S2-S4
Pelvic Organs		
Uterus (including ligaments)	Sacrum Lumbosacral junction Thoracic/lumbar spine	T11-L1 S2-S4
Ovaries/testes	Lower abdomen Sacrum	T10-T11

normal course of a day can help to determine the source of a patient's concerns. Knowing common symptoms of various body systems can help to determine which tissue may be contributing to the condition. For example, vascular symptoms are described as throbbing, pulsating, and pounding, whereas neurological symptoms may be described as burning, tingling, and weakness. A list of common symptoms related to various body systems can be found in Table 3-2. It is also important to recognize certain common local and

systemic functions that may be driving a patient's condition. For example, common findings when one may have a fracture include pain/swelling/bruising/tenderness at local site of injury, bony deformity, pain with weight bearing/axial loading, and weakness/pain with activity. Red flags for vertebral fracture reported in a 2016 study included age greater than 75 years old, trauma, osteoporosis, back pain intensity score of 7 or greater, and thoracic pain were associated with a higher chance of the patient having a vertebral fracture as

Table 3-2

TISSUE-BASED SYMPTOM DESCRIPTION

- Vascular: Ischemia leads to a feeling of aching pain, heaviness, weakness, or numbness/tingling
- Neurological: Burning, numbness, tingling, weakness, hypersensitivity, or impaired proprioception
- Bone: Dull, deep, boring, and aching, more common at night; acute fracture: sharp/stabbing with extreme tenderness/swelling
- Myofascial/soft tissue: Sharp, stabbing, tightness/spasming, weakness/fatigue; active/latent trigger occasionally referred pain
- Visceral: Diffuse/poorly defined, pallor, profuse sweating, nausea, gastrointestinal disturbances; referred pain and changes in autonomic responses (body temperature, blood pressure, heart rate)

the source of their lower back pain.[15] Another source of a patient's symptoms, especially if they have been recently hospitalized,[16] could possibly be an infection. Infection symptoms may include[17] fever, chills/sweats, diarrhea, vomiting, abdominal/rectal pain, redness/soreness/swelling in an area (especially around surgical sites), change in cough/new cough, sore throat or new mouth sore, shortness of breath, nasal congestion, stiff neck, burning/painful urination, increased urination, or vaginal irritation/unusual discharge.

Asking what activities/positions aggravate and ease their condition/symptoms can give the therapist more insight into the origin of the patient's condition. A patient who reports lower back symptoms that are aggravated by sitting longer than 1 hour, are worse at the end of the day, and are worse with bending and lifting activities of daily life is demonstrating a normal mechanical pattern of a flexion-based pathology in the lower back; this contrasts with a patient who reports their symptoms as constant and low-level without any significant change in activity or position. After hearing this subjective report, during the orthopedic and physical examination, the therapist should be actively trying to alter the patient's symptoms with certain range of motion (ROM), strength, coordination, and special tests to determine if there is a mechanical cause/contribution to their condition. In general, most patients will receive some mild or temporary relief of symptoms from certain modalities, such as moist heat, cryotherapy, soft tissue mobilization/massage, and/or resting whether in a supine or seated position. However, a patient report that absolutely nothing will relieve the symptoms should be an alarming finding to the therapist and reason to look more in depth during the physical/orthopedic examination.

The frequency, duration, and change in symptoms over a defined period can also help the therapist potentially identify abnormal findings, which would help in potentially identifying if the patient is a true candidate for physical therapy treatment. Depending on the nature of the condition, the time frames to be examined can vary. Usually, a description of their symptoms over the course of a normal 24-hour day is an excellent barometer of how symptoms may change in relation to a variety of stimuli. However, if the patient also suffers from more chronic degenerative conditions, the therapist may have to look at a much longer time frame (ie, 3 to 6 months) to get a better appreciation of how the symptom pattern is contributing to the patient's condition and limiting function. One commonly known red flag that has been associated with both cancer and infection is that of night pain. Night pain is described as symptoms that wake someone from sleep.[18-21] While the presence of night pain should put therapists on alert, they must also realize that a great number of orthopedic conditions may also generate night pain, such as degenerative joint disease/arthritis in the lumbar, shoulder, and knee regions.[6] Follow-up questions on the presence of night pain should include the following:

- Do you wake up at a consistent time nightly?
- Do you find yourself in a certain position each time you wake?
- How many nights per week do you wake?
- Are you able to get back to sleep once you have woken up?

After further investigation of the source of a patient's night pain, the therapist should be more concerned if the patient reported the most intense/bothersome symptoms as night pain or that the evening symptoms were becoming more intense and/or frequent.

Symptom investigation is a complex and vital process during the physical therapy examination for the therapist to determine if the patient is a candidate for therapy or requires referral for further medical investigation. Use of initial intake forms, including a previous medical history, pain diagrams, and functional indices, in combination with detailed symptom and follow-up questioning can help the therapist identify if the patient's condition is appropriate for a musculoskeletal condition or if findings may be more suggestive of a possible nonmusculoskeletal origin.

Table 3-3

OBJECTIVE EXAMINATION FINDINGS FOR LOW BACK CASE STUDY

OBJECTIVE

- 34 scored on General Disability Index

- 21 scored on Oswestry Low Back Disability Questionnaire

- Posture screen: Right iliac crest elevated vs left. Left acromioclavicular joint elevated vs right; right posterior pelvic and left posterior thoracic rotations noted

LUMBAR RANGE OF MOTION

- 55 degrees ROM flexion

- 30 degrees ROM extension

- 30 degrees ROM left lateral flexion

- 35 degrees ROM right lateral flexion

HIP RANGE OF MOTION

- Left hip flexion: 100 degrees

- Right hip flexion: 100 degrees, with painful arc demonstrated through ROM and increased pain at end range

- Left hip: Active straight leg raise (SLR): 65 degrees ROM/passive SLR to 75 degrees

- Right hip: Active SLR: 55 degrees ROM/passive SLR to 60 degrees with pain at end range

- Left hip external rotation/internal rotation/FABER (flexion, abduction, and external rotation; Patrick's) test: Grossly within normal limits

- Right hip internal rotation: 20 degrees with pain during movement and pain at end range

- Right hip external rotation: 45 degrees

- Right FABER (Patrick's) test: decreased ROM with pain

KNEE RANGE OF MOTION

- Bilateral knees: Extension: 0 degrees; flexion: 135 degrees

(continued)

REGIONAL PAIN PATTERNS AND ASSOCIATED DISEASES/CONDITIONS

Low Back Pain and Pelvic, Hip, and Thigh Disorders

LBP has been found to be the leading cause of disability and work absence in the world[22] and that upward of 31 million Americans can suffer from it at any given time.[23] Due to the prevalence in society, therapists need to perform a complete examination, and ruling out any potential red flags for patients presenting with this common complaint is essential to continuing to progress the American Physical Therapy Association vision statement.

Case Study

A 43-year-old man presented for physical therapy with the primary complaints of lower back, right hip, and bilateral knee pain. He stated his lower back symptoms were due to his career in the military for the past 15 years. He reported his knee symptoms had been present intermittently over the past 8 years. He also relayed that he was diagnosed with right hip trochanteric bursitis and underwent cortisone injections and anti-inflammatory treatments within the past year. He reports that his hip responded well initially to his anti-inflammatory treatment, but that he still used his medication as needed to manage his symptoms when they become exacerbated. He reported his lumbar and right hip symptoms were recently exacerbated about 4 months before, after a long cross-country car trip, which led him to seek medical attention from his primary care physician (Table 3-3).

Table 3-3 (continued)

OBJECTIVE EXAMINATION FINDINGS FOR LOW BACK CASE STUDY

LOWER EXTREMITY MANUAL MUSCLE TESTS

- Left iliopsoas/quadriceps: 5/5
- Right iliopsoas/right quadriceps/bilateral hamstrings: 4+/5
- Right gluteus maximus/piriformis: 3+/5, tenderness to palpation with moderate trigger points/ fascial restrictions noted
- Left gluteus maximus/medius/piriformis: 4/5, holds test position against moderate pressure
- Right glutes medius: 4-/5- moderate pain (6/10), tenderness to palpation with moderate trigger points/ fascial restrictions noted
- Bilateral tibialis anterior, gastrocnemius/soleus: 5/5

SENSATION

- Normal sensation L2, L3, L4, L5, and S1 dermatomes

PALPATION

- Tenderness to palpation: Right L5-S1 facet joints, L5-S1 spinal processes, right sacroiliac joint, and right pelvic crest
- Tenderness to palpation: Right greater trochanter and iliotibial tract/tensor fascia lata
- Tenderness to palpation: Bilateral patellar tendon and inferior patellar pole

FUNCTIONAL RESTRICTIONS

- Patient experiences severe pain (8/10) while sitting for longer than 30 minutes
- Patient experiences severe pain (8/10) and difficulty/pain with transitional movements (ie, sitting to standing)
- Patient experiences severe pain (8/10) and difficulty with bending and lifting activities of daily life
- Patient experiences moderate pain (6/10) in bilateral knees and right hip with navigating stairs
- Patient experiences moderate pain (6/10) with recreational activities (eg, playing sports, squatting, exercising, running)

After reviewing the initial intake forms, taking a subjective history, and performing a physical examination, the therapist determined that the patient demonstrated symptoms consistent with lumbar/knee arthritis, right hip bursitis, and potentially lumbar radiculopathy. Despite his presentation, which demonstrated typical mechanical patterns of symptomology for knee/hip osteoarthritis and hip bursitis, more detailed follow-up questioning during the examination was warranted to screen for more serious pathology. The therapist should be aware of the 4 most common nonmusculoskeletal conditions that may present as LBP: spinal infection, vertebral fracture, cauda equina syndrome, or tumor.[18] Other medical conditions that could mimic symptoms of the patient's hip condition may include pathological hip fracture, osteonecrosis, and cancer/tumor.

To rule out any of these more serious conditions the therapist should ask appropriate screening questions, which may help to detect if something more sinister could be driving his condition. Questions that can help to detect a possible spinal infection such as osteomyelitis include the following:

- Does your pain ease when you rest in a comfortable position?
- Have you recently had a fever?
- Have you recently taken any antibiotics or other medications to treat an infection?
- Have you ever been diagnosed with an immunosuppressive disorder?

The patient denied having a recent fever, taking any anti-infection medications, or being diagnosed with any immunosuppressive disorder, which significantly reduced the likelihood that he had a spinal infection.

Table 3-4

DIAGNOSTIC CRITERIA FOR ANKYLOSING SPONDYLITIS: NEW YORK CRITERIA

MOTION DEFICITS	PAIN LOCATION	CHEST EXPANSION	RADIOLOGY FINDINGS
Decreased lumbar ROM—all planes	Pain in lumbar or thoracolumbar junction	Decreased chest expansion of 1 inch	Bilateral sacroiliitis—grade 2+ or unilateral sacroiliitis—grade 3+

Table 3-5

COMMON FINDINGS OF A PATHOLOGICAL FEMUR FRACTURE

- History of a FALL from standing position
  - Sudden/painful "SNAP" or "giving way"
- Metabolic bone disease (eg, osteoporosis/Paget's disease)
  - Women more than men
  - Greater than 50 years old
- Acute groin/anteromedial thigh pain
- Shortened appearance on the fractured extremity
- Fractured extremity held in external rotation

Ankylosing spondylitis is another inflammatory back condition that should be considered as a potential source of his symptoms (Table 3-4). Ankylosing spondylitis is characterized by onset in the third decade of life and is 66% more common in men.[24] The pathogenesis of this immune-mediated inflammatory condition is poorly understood, but the initial symptoms are dull often bilateral buttock and/or lower lumbar pain along with morning stiffness. Patients will present with a significant limitation of spinal mobility along with bony tenderness to their lumbar and other peripheral joints due to the autoimmune nature of this condition. Ankylosing spondylitis symptoms will improve with activity and return with periods of inactivity, with their worst symptoms being reported at night.[24] Confirmation of this condition includes positive spinal x-ray, usually indicating inflammation or possible fusion of the sacroiliac joints. Other laboratory findings, such as blood or genetic tests to identify the presence of the *HLA-B27* gene, increased C-reactive protein levels, or an elevated erythrocyte sedimentation rate, can indicate the presence of ankylosing spondylitis.

The patient had already undergone x-ray imaging of his lumbar spine, which revealed no issues at his sacroiliac joints, and he demonstrated mild restrictions in his lumbar mobility during his physical examination. He did report that sitting/laying down will help to temporarily decrease his hip and back symptoms, which is opposite to the normal symptom pattern of ankylosing spondylitis and more suggestive of a mechanical origin for his condition.

To rule out a potential spinal and/or hip fracture, the 43-year-old patient was asked if he had any recent trauma such as a slip/fall or a motor vehicle collision, which he denied. Another screening question that might help detect a possible spinal/hip fracture would be if he has ever been told that he has osteoporosis or any other medical condition that might cause his bones to weaken. Other medical conditions that might cause compromised bone density include hyperparathyroidism, renal failure, chronic gastrointestinal disorders, and long-term use of corticosteroids. Pathological fractures of the proximal femoral neck often occur as a result of disease and in the absence of trauma (Table 3-5).[25] He reported that based on previous x-ray imaging studies of his lumbar spine and right hip, no fracture, osteoporosis, or osteopenia have been detected. The patient denied any recent significant trauma/fall or any medical condition that might cause weakened bones. This decreases the suspicion that he may have a spinal and/or femoral fracture.

Osteonecrosis, or avascular/aseptic necrosis, results from an insufficient arterial supply to the head of the femur. Osteonecrosis of the femur is usually associated with trauma (ie, fracture/dislocation), sickle cell disease, or long-term corticosteroid use (ie, patients on medication for lupus, rheumatoid arthritis, or asthma). Due to the ischemia, the bony tissue in the hip joint dies and osteoarthritis pain/symptoms increases to the point that the patient will require a hip replacement procedure to address this issue so he can return to normal daily function without significant restrictions. (A famous case of this involved Bo Jackson, a professional football and baseball player, who dislocated his hip resulting in arterial disruption of blood flow to the femoral head. He later became the first professional athlete to undergo and return to sport following a total hip replacement.) Due to the 43-year-old patient's lack of trauma and no history of medication/blood disorders, the chance that his symptoms are due to osteonecrosis are relatively small, and the therapist can proceed to rule out other sources for the patient's condition.

In addition, the 43-year-old patient's age decreased his chance of demonstrating Legg-Calve-Perthes disease or a slipped capital femoral epiphysis. To quickly review these more juvenile conditions, Legg-Calve-Perthes disease usually occurs in men, ages 5 to 8 years, as a result of an idiopathic blood loss to the femoral head. Children will present with complaints of groin, thigh, and knee pain that increases with prolonged weight-bearing activities. The examination findings would demonstrate an antalgic gait pattern with/following prolonged weight-bearing activities, decreased/painful internal rotation and abduction of the involved hip,[26] and possible shortening of the involved lower extremity. Slipped capital femoral epiphysis occurs in slightly older, more overweight, children during adolescence and is a result of the progressive displacement of the femoral head through the growth plate. The description of their symptoms is a diffuse vague pain in their groin, thigh, or knee along with the physical examination findings of an antalgic gait, the involved lower extremity held in a more externally rotated position, and limited hip internal rotation on the involved side.

Cauda equina syndrome occurs most frequently following a large central lumbar disk herniation, prolapse, or sequestration or by smaller prolapses if the patient also has spinal stenosis.[27] To effectively screen for cauda equina syndrome, the therapist needs to complete both the subjective history and clinical examination before eliminating this serious medical emergency. Possible red flags for a patient presenting with cauda equina syndrome include the following:

- Severe LBP
- Sciatica—Leg pain—Often bilateral (sometimes absent), especially at L5/S1
- Saddle and/or genital sensory disturbance
- Bladder, bowel, and sexual dysfunction (reduced anal tone, urinary retention, incontinence)[28]

The patient had no positive findings related to the red flags of cauda equina during his physical examination or medical history, severely decreasing the possibility that he was suffering from cauda equina syndrome.

Since this patient was only 43 years old, but had been experiencing these symptoms chronically, and the symptoms had been progressively worsening and responding only temporarily to his current medication regimen, the therapist attempted to detect any potential red flags that might suggest the patient possibly had cancer or a tumor. Colon cancer is the third most common cancer among both sexes and results from malignancies that develop in the large intestine.[29] As this type of cancer is a gradually developing pathology, therapists should encourage their older patients to be vigilant with routine screening examinations, such as colonoscopies. These diagnostic tests can detect polyps, which are precursors to the cancerous lesions and may be removed surgically if found, preventing them from further developing.

This patient has a family history of cancer as reported on his initial intake forms. The patient was also questioned about any unexplained weight loss or any change in bowel habits, such as bloody or black stools. Therapists should also be aware that colon cancer will metastasize most frequently to the thoracic spine and rib cage and that those regions should be investigated as well to determine if any positive red flag findings are present upon evaluation.[30]

During the patient's physical examination, severe tenderness was noted at and inferior to his right greater trochanteric region. The patient reported his most severe hip pain occurred with prolonged walking, transitional activities, and stair climbing. He stated that his symptoms decrease temporarily with anti-inflammatory medication, but that they seemed to be progressively increasing in intensity. At that point, the therapist used their clinical judgement skills to determine that further investigation of his hip presentation was warranted, based on the patient's failure to respond to treatment. Further imaging of the man's right hip by his primary care physician was initiated. In situations like this, if treatment proceeds prior to undergoing further diagnostic imaging and any malignancies are found later, the therapist might have placed the patient and themself at unnecessary risk.

The 43-year-old male patient returned to his primary care physician and underwent magnetic resonance imaging (MRI), which revealed a right femoral shaft chondrosarcoma without metastasis. The patient underwent surgical removal of the chondrosarcoma, in addition to partial right hip replacement, and returned for his postoperative therapy a few months later.

Knee, Lower Leg, and Ankle/Foot Pain and Disorders

The lower leg screening for potential red flag conditions should include evaluation for potential DVT, compartment syndrome, peripheral artery disease, stress fracture, septic arthritis, and cellulitis. DVTs and compartment syndrome both typically relate to the after effects of a prior injury in the lower extremity. Due to increased inflammation and swelling and the resultant decrease in mobility, patients experience a higher risk for developing either DVTs, compartment syndrome, or both. DVTs are characterized by a spontaneous obstruction of the popliteal vein in the lower leg. Compartment syndrome, in contrast, is characterized by an abnormal rise in pressure in the fascial compartments of the leg, which can be a medical emergency due to the potential for vascular compromise and nerve entrapment. DVTs are more common due to prolonged immobilization following an injury, pregnancy, or sometimes with prolonged seated positioning, as in a long plane ride or car trip. Conversely, compartment syndrome is usually more acute in nature following a blunt or crush injury to the lower leg or a significant increase in unaccustomed exercise, such as increased running while training for an upcoming race.

Case Study

Consider a 47-year-old man who presented for physical therapy evaluation and treatment following a right knee arthroscopy due to a meniscus tear. He presented 1 week following his procedure, ambulating with a mild antalgic gait and demonstrating mild joint effusion and restricted end ranges of flexion and extension. He reported his average pain as a 3/10 and his worst as a 5/10. After completing the

Table 3-6

THE 5 "P" CLINICAL SIGNS OF COMPARTMENT SYNDROME

1. Pain
2. Palpable tenderness
3. Paresthesias
4. Paresis
5. Pulselessness

examination, treatment was initiated and included passive ROM by the therapist along with cryotherapy and electrical stimulation to his lower extremity. The patient was shown his home exercise program, including ankle, calf, and knee mobility; muscle activation; and gait retraining exercises. Upon returning for his follow-up appointment 2 days later, the patient's symptoms had worsened; he now reported his pain level as an 8/10 and reported increased joint stiffness along with popliteal swelling and tenderness. The patient's gait pattern had become more antalgic, and he also reported increased throbbing/aching in his calf with prolonged dependent positioning. The therapist found increased calf tenderness and warmth. A positive Homan's sign was detected, pain with passive and rapid dorsiflexion of the ankle. The therapist suspected that a DVT might be present and discontinued all treatment. He contacted the patient's orthopedic surgeon, and the patient underwent venous imaging (diagnostic ultrasound). A DVT was found and the patient was placed on anticoagulation medication. To continue physical therapy, the patient had to be medically cleared to resume therapy by his surgeon.

The therapist would have suspected compartment syndrome if the patient had been more active prior to the onset of his symptoms, but since he was recovering from surgery, his activity level was decreased. During the physical examination for compartment syndrome, one would expect to find swelling, palpable tension (ie, hardness), and exquisite tenderness. The increase in fascial pressure might cause nerve entrapment and compression resulting in paresthesia and paresis to the surrounding regions. Vascular compromise is also a possibility, which would result in decreased peripheral pulses (Table 3-6).

Peripheral arterial occlusive disease, or peripheral vascular disease, results from the atherosclerosis of the arterial walls below the abdominal aorta. The risk factors, which are highly prevalent in today's society and include diabetes mellitus, smoking, and sedentary lifestyle, make this disease suspect with any patient presenting with heart disease (Table 3-7). The classic distinguishing feature of this disease is intermittent claudication, which is described as an aching pain in the thigh, buttock, or calf that increases with walking or other lower extremity aerobic exercise and disappears with rest. Physical examination findings would be decreased foot pulses, coolness in the involved extremity, and wounds/sores on the toes/foot. Clinical tests that are beneficial in the confirmation of peripheral vascular disease include the ankle-to-arm systolic pressure, also known as the *ankle/brachial index (ABI)*, and the reactive hyperemia test. The ABI is performed by comparing the highest systolic blood pressure at the ankle and dividing it by the highest systolic blood pressure from the brachial artery (arm). Any ABI result of less than 0.97 indicates the presence of peripheral vascular disease.[31] The reactive hyperemia test assesses the integrity of the vascular system in reperfusing blood following postural changes. To perform the test, the patient is supine, and the therapist performs a passive SLR to 45 degrees and maintains this for 1 to 3 minutes or until the color of the foot/ankle/lower leg is blanched/pale. Then, the therapist lowers the limb and measures the amount of time required for the limb to turn pink. Normal venous filling time is 1 to 2 seconds. Anything greater than 20 seconds is a positive confirmation of peripheral vascular disease. The recommended therapy for this condition is supervised aerobic exercise such as a progressive walking program. As this disease indicates ischemic heart disease, medical referral is required for the patient to undergo cardiac exercise stress tests and possible pharmacological management.

Another potential lower extremity condition that may onset following a recent increase in activity would be a stress fracture. Stress fractures are partial or incomplete fractures that occur due to repeated local stress to the bone or weakening the outer surface of the bone.[32] Although not a medical emergency, a suspected stress fracture should be confirmed via a bone or computed tomography scan so a patient can recover more quickly. A proper rehabilitation program includes a cyclic process of activity and rest to allow for the remodeling process of the bone. There are 2 types of stress fractures: fatigue and insufficiency fractures. Fatigue fractures occur due to repeated local mechanical stress from increased training intensity, hard training surface, inappropriate footwear, or poor anatomical alignment of the feet.[33] Insufficiency fractures are most prevalent in patients who have also been identified to have a nutrient deficiency, osteoporosis, or rheumatoid arthritis. Symptoms are described as pain and localized tenderness/swelling that worsens with activity and resolves with rest. If left unaddressed, pain will begin to onset earlier during activity, and as the injury progresses, lead to more persistent symptoms and night pain.

Septic arthritis is a result of a bacterial infection causing increased inflammation in the joint; it most commonly affects the knee in approximately 50% of cases.[34] Patients will complain of a constant throbbing ache and/or throbbing pain and swelling in a joint. Risk factors for septic arthritis include preexisting joint diseases, overlying skin infection over a prosthetic joint, previous joint surgery, and patients who may be immunosuppressed. Different types of preexisting

Table 3-7

RISK FACTORS FOR HEART DISEASE, SYMPTOMS OF PERIPHERAL ARTERY DISEASE AND INTERMITTENT CLAUDICATION, AND OTHER CONDITIONS WITH SIMILAR PRESENTATION TO PHYSICAL THERAPY

HEART DISEASE RISK FACTORS	SYMPTOMS OF PERIPHERAL ARTERY DISEASE/ INTERMITTENT CLAUDICATION	OTHER CONDITIONS THAT MAY MIMIC SYMPTOMS OF PERIPHERAL ARTERY DISEASE

• High blood pressure
• High cholesterol
• Hyperlipidemia
• Renal insufficiency
• Diabetes/prediabetic*
• Smoking*
• Unhealthy diet
• Sedentary lifestyle
• Family history
	• Cramping/muscle pain along with paresthesias/weakness in the lower extremities
	• Increases with walking
	• Relieved with short rest period (10 minutes or less)
	• Cool skin
	• Weak/absent distant pulses in lower extremities
		• Neurological
		  ◦ Spinal stenosis (ie, pseudoclaudication)
		  ◦ Nerve compression (ie, radiculopathy, disk herniation)
		  ◦ Peripheral neuropathies (ie, diabetic/alcohol)
		  ◦ Nerve entrapment
		• Musculoskeletal
		  ◦ Arthritis
		  ◦ Overuse injuries (ie, muscle strain, medial tibial stress syndrome)
		  ◦ Compartment syndrome
		  ◦ Baker's cyst when symptomatic
		• Vascular
		  ◦ DVT
		  ◦ Compartment syndrome
		  ◦ Venous insufficiency
		  ◦ Popliteal artery entrapment
		  ◦ Vasculitis

* Highest relative risk factors for developing lower extremity peripheral artery disease.

joint diseases include joint arthritis in its various forms, such as rheumatoid arthritis, osteoarthritis, and psoriatic arthritis. Septic arthritis is usually a result of local or distant site infections or any recent invasive medical procedure including surgery or an intra-articular injection. Identifying the type of infection is crucial in prompt antibiotic management of the infection, as cartilage can be destroyed within days.[34,35] Immunosuppression may be due to a wide array of reasons including prolonged corticosteroid use, renal failure, alcohol abuse, diabetes mellitus, IV drug use, organ transplantation, AIDs, or collagen vascular disease.

Cellulitis is an infection in the superficial tissues that usually occurs after a recent skin trauma, such as an ulceration or abrasion,[36] and is classified by pain, skin swelling, warmth, and an advancing, irregular margin of erythema or reddish streaks of discoloration. Patients may also report other classic signs of infection as discussed earlier, such as fever, chills, fatigue, and weakness. Common medical conditions that are known to be risk factors for developing cellulitis include congestive heart failure, diabetes mellitus, renal failure, liver cirrhosis, lower extremity venous insufficiency, and advanced age. Another rare but potentially fatal infection that is sometimes mistaken for cellulitis is necrotizing fasciitis, an infection of the subcutaneous tissue and fascia. It is also known as the *flesh-eating disease* and only early diagnosis and aggressive surgical management reduce morbidity and mortality.[37]

Table 3-8

TYPES OF ANGINA: STABLE VERSUS UNSTABLE

STABLE	UNSTABLE
Predictable pattern (ie, following exercise/exertion)	Unpredictable pattern; occurs without a precipitating exertional event
Substernal chest pain/pressure with possible referred pain to left upper extremity	Substernal squeezing/pressure, referred pain into bilateral upper extremities, shortness of breath, pallor, diaphoresis, lasting longer than 30 minutes
Alleviated by decreasing exertional output (ie, resting or administering sublingual nitroglycerin)	NOT alleviated by rest/sublingual nitroglycerin; treated with aspirin, heparin, beta-blockers, or primary angioplasty
Benign if managed correctly	Fatal if mismanaged

Thoracic/Trunk Pain: Cardiac, Pulmonary, and Gastrointestinal Disorders

The thoracic spine and rib cage, due to their proximity to many visceral organs, are common for local and referred pain when these organ systems are pathological. In fact, a common manifestation of metastatic bone disease in the thoracic spine is a pathological fracture of the thoracic vertebrae and ribs.[21] Cardiac conditions that may require referral due to their red flag presentation include angina (unstable/stable) or MI. Pulmonary disorders that may present with thoracic pain are lung or other visceral organ cancer, pulmonary embolus, pneumothorax, pneumonia, and pleurisy. Potential gastrointestinal disorders that may present with thoracic pain and will be reviewed are pyelonephritis, kidney/gall stones, peptic ulcer, and cholecystitis.

Chest pain, or angina, is often most associated with MI, which is an acute blockage of a coronary artery that results in necrosis to a portion of the heart muscle tissue and has a high mortality rate. The cardinal feature of MI is angina, with symptoms described as discomfort, pressure, tightness, or squeezing in the chest with potential for referral pain into the arm, neck, or jaw.[38] Women usually have a more atypical presentation when compared to men, having more pain in their right shoulder, epigastric, and midthoracic spine regions. It should be noted that half of patients diagnosed with MI do not complain of angina.[39] Other symptoms that may be a result of MI include cardiac arrest, dyspnea, palpations, syncope, and nausea/vomiting. When addressing a patient with angina, the therapist should differentiate whether the patient is presenting with stable or unstable angina. Stable angina is described as substernal chest pain/pressure that occurs with predictable exertion or precipitating events; for example, exercise/exertion at higher-than-normal levels. Stable angina is relieved by decreasing activity (ie, rest) or by self-administered sublingual nitroglycerin. Unstable angina does not present with a typical pattern or respond to nitroglycerin. Due to the variation of symptoms, which may include substernal squeezing/crushing pressure, shortness of breath, pallor, diaphoresis, or any of these symptoms lasting longer than 30 minutes, a person exhibiting them should be transported for emergency medical attention as quickly as possible. The survival rate for an MI improves significantly with early detection and the patient having access to life saving therapies such as angioplasty, aspirin, beta-blockers, and heparin (Table 3-8).[39]

An interesting case observed personally by the author involved a complicated 63-year-old female patient being treated after knee surgery. The patient had a previous medical history including anxiety, depression, bipolar disorder, and chronic neck and lumbar degeneration, along with a history of transient ischemic attacks. She had been progressing with her therapy slowly because of her multiple comorbidities following knee arthroscopy. She presented to the clinic using a walker. As she was checking with the front office, she began experiencing severe left chest pain along with pain into her left shoulder and fell to the ground in a controlled fashion by the time the therapist was alerted. Emergency medical attention was contacted and she was rushed to the emergency room. Upon stabilizing her, the emergency room staff performed a differential diagnosis and determined the patient had an esophageal spasm. Although an MI was ruled out due to the patient's presentation, emergency referral was warranted to ensure that no potentially life-threatening condition was causing her symptoms.

Another source of angina may be due to a possible infection surrounding the heart, known as *pericarditis*. Infection from bacterial or viral pathogens or systemic disease, such as kidney failure, lupus, rheumatoid disease, heart failure, or increased fluid around the heart due to a leaking aortic aneurysm, may be the cause. This condition is characterized by chest pain that refers pain into the left shoulder, possibly down the left arm, and is accompanied by a fever. The patient's symptoms will increase with supine position, inhalation, or coughing and will be alleviated with a forward lean while sitting. The excess pressure around the heart due to inflammation causes decreased heart expansion and thus less decreased stroke volume or blood leaving the heart. To accommodate for this loss of stroke volume, the heart will beat faster, and if unable to compensate for the deficiency, the patient may breathe heavily, demonstrate increased distention of the neck veins, and have significant decreases in blood pressure during inhalation. When this sequence of events occurs, the patient is experiencing cardiac tamponade and will need to be seen for emergency medical attention to decrease the pressure surrounding the heart and normalize their heart rate and cardiac output.[40]

Pulmonary embolus, a blood clot in the pulmonary artery around the heart, may also cause angina-like pain. If suspected by the therapist during the examination, this is another medical emergency. Pain is usually substernal but can be anywhere in the thorax depending on the location of the embolus. Patients may also complain of abdominal or referred shoulder pain. They will demonstrate dyspnea, wheezing, and a marked drop in blood pressure. Risk factors for a pulmonary embolus are similar to those of DVTs in the lower extremities, such as immobilization following trauma, a prolonged trip, or a recent surgery.

Pneumothorax is another condition that will produce chest/thoracic pain with inspiration due to increased air being present in the thoracic cage. This condition can be spontaneous but is usually associated with disruption to the wall of the lung lining. The rupture will prevent the lungs from maintaining negative pressure during normal respiration movement by the diaphragm and thoracic cage. Examination findings will include difficulty of the chest to rise on the affected side, reduced breath sounds, and hyperresonance of the affected area with percussion. Small pneumothoraxes' can occur spontaneously, following a bout of extreme coughing or extreme physical activity and may resolve within a couple of days without medical intervention. A large pneumothorax, however, will require aspiration of the increased air surrounding the lung to alleviate symptoms (Table 3-9). A tension pneumothorax is a medical emergency and occurs following trauma to the chest region, such as a blow to the chest during a motor vehicle collision or with contact sports. These symptoms are usually more intense and will include extreme shortness of breath, distended neck veins, tachycardia, hypotension, hyperresonance with percussion, and tracheal deviation. The patient will require medical attention as a chest tube with a seal or Heimlich valve will help to decrease air present in the thoracic cavity.

Pleurisy and pneumonia are inflammatory conditions that may also cause chest and thoracic pain. Pleurisy is an irritation of the pleural membranes that make up the lining between the lungs and inner surface of the rib cage. The chest pain is often sharp and stabbing and increases with deep and forceful inspiration (ie, coughing). Passive mobility testing of the ribs and thoracic cage may produce pain as well. Pleurisy can be caused by a variety of causes such

Table 3-9 ———————————————
PREDISPOSING FACTORS FOR PNEUMOTHORAX
• Asthma
• Chronic obstructive pulmonary disease
• Cystic fibrosis
• Lung cancer
• Menstruation in young people

as tumor, viral infection, or rheumatoid diseases. A "pleural rub" sound can be detected with auscultation over the thorax. Pneumonia, a viral or bacterial infection of the lungs, can also cause chest pain and is distinguished by a productive cough of sputum of varying coloration. Typical signs of infection should also be present, including chills, fever, malaise, nausea, vomiting, and possibly pleuritic type pain as described above. Occasionally the fever will be absent in older patients who may also present with gradually progressing mental confusion.[41]

Potential gastrointestinal disorders that may present in conjunction with thoracic and/or abdominal pain include abdominal aortic aneurysm (AAA), gastric/peptic ulcer disease, appendicitis, and cholecystitis. AAAs are unfortunately mostly asymptomatic; undetectable on physical examination, they are often confirmed by radiographic diagnostic studies for other reasons. Ultrasound is the preferred method of screening and surgical repair is indicated if the aneurysm becomes larger than 5.5 cm in diameter or grows more than 0.6 to 0.8 cm per year.[42] However, the symptomatic presentation of AAA has been described as back, abdominal, buttock, groin, testicular, or leg pain. These patients require immediate medical attention because a complete rupture of the abdominal aorta will result in rapid blood loss (Table 3-10).

Ulcers are described based on their anatomic location and occur when digestive acids become corrosive to the lining of the digestive tract. Symptoms are described as a dull, gnawing, or burning pain in the epigastric, midthoracic (T6-T10), or supraclavicular regions. These ulcers are common in patients who have used nonsteroidal anti-inflammatory drugs (NSAIDs; eg, aspirin, ibuprofen, naproxen) for a prolonged duration, and the clinician should be sure to question those who report using NSAIDs to manage their symptoms. Therapists should focus on dosage, frequency, and duration of use when questioning these patients. Since appendicitis is the most common abdominal emergency, it is important to recognize the known presentation, which is the complaint of colicky periumbilical abdominal pain that intensifies during the first 24 hours and becomes more constant and sharper while migrating to the right iliac fossa. The patient may also report loss of appetite, constipation, or nausea.[43]

Table 3-10

POTENTIAL RED FLAGS IN THE THORACIC/ABDOMINAL REGIONS: CLASSIFIED BY REGION/SYSTEM

CARDIAC	PULMONARY	ABDOMINAL
• MI	• Pulmonary embolus	• Cholecystitis
• Stable/unstable angina	• Pneumothorax	• Nephrolithiasis
• Pericarditis	• Pneumonia	• Pyelonephritis
	• Pleurisy	

Cholecystitis, or inflammation of the gall bladder, is most commonly due to a blockage of the cystic duct by a gall stone and is characterized by pain in the right upper abdominal quadrant or referred pain into the interscapular or right scapular (Boas' sign) regions.[44] Murphy's sign, which is pain during palpation of the right upper abdominal quadrant, presents in more than 50% of patients presenting with the disorder.[44] The pain with cholecystitis has been described as severe enough to cause severe nausea and vomiting.

Kidney disorders that may result in pain presenting in the posterolateral aspect of the thoracic cage include renal stones or pyelonephritis. Renal stones, or more commonly known as *kidney stones*, can occur either in the kidney, which is known as *nephrolithiasis*, or anywhere in the urinary tract, referred to as *urolithiasis*. The stones are formed by salts that precipitate from the urine when it becomes oversaturated with a particular, usually mineral, substance. Most stones are derived from calcium, but other stones may be a result of uric acid, cysteine, or struvite. Women are 4 times more likely to develop kidney stones when compared to men. Also, White men are 3 times as likely to develop kidney stones when compared to Black men. Predictive risk factors are previous episodes of kidney stones (50% recurrence rate),[45] leukemia or other similar diseases that result in high cell turnover,[46] or living in a warm, humid climate (Table 3-11). Pyelonephritis is a kidney infection, either viral or bacterial, that may be caused by conditions that obstruct urine flow, such as renal stones or benign prostate hyperplasia.[47] These infections are most commonly located in the ascending urinary tract.

Lastly, the clinician must eliminate potential malignancies in the thorax and abdominal cavity that could be producing pain in those regions (Figure 3-3).[48] A 73-year-old woman presented to physical therapy for midscapular and lower cervical pain. She reported her pain had been a constant low-level dull ache over the past 8 or 9 months with increased pain when reaching/lifting activities overhead and increased stiffness/tightness in her painful areas. During her history review, she reported being previously diagnosed with pancreatic cancer, which had been in remission for the past 4 years. Pancreatic cancer has the worst survival rate for any cancer due to its late detection. Red flags for pancreatic cancer include abdominal pain, unexplained weight/appetite loss, or abdominal distension.[49] She reported she now

has semi-annual examinations with her oncologist to monitor her condition. The patient had been previously treated by the therapist for a lower back condition the previous year. Her physical examination revealed abnormal posture consistent with upper crossed syndrome. She also demonstrated decreased/painful cervical/thoracic and right shoulder mobility along with weakness in her scapular and spinal stabilizing musculature. She demonstrated tenderness in her pericervical and scapular musculature, but denied any upper extremity paresthesia. Despite all of these findings, which are consistent with normal musculoskeletal presentation, during and following the evaluation, the patient reported that none of the examination truly reproduced or changed her symptoms. Before proceeding with physical therapy treatment, the patient was referred back to her oncologist for further examination. X-ray imaging later revealed an ivory vertebrae, an area of bone that will appear whiter in appearance, on her T2 and T3 vertebral bodies (see Figure 3-3). This finding, which detects increased lucency in the vertebrae, is indicative of metastatic cancer, in her case from her previous pancreas cancer. The red flags that should have alerted the clinician to the possible presence of a tumor/cancer were her previous history of cancer and the inability to reproduce or change her symptoms during the physical examination of her thoracic spine.

Lung cancer is another cancer the clinician must consider when a patient presents with thoracic pain. Lung cancer is responsible for more deaths than any other type of cancer worldwide, and it alone accounts for more deaths than breast, prostate, or colon cancer combined.[50] Lung cancer can metastasize to virtually any bone, but is most common in the axial skeleton or proximal portion of long bones. The patient may complain of bony pain in the region of metastasis and possible pleuritic pain if the ribs are involved. The patient may also report recent weight loss, cough, dyspnea, fatigue, chest infections, or hemoptysis during the subjective history.[51] A special type of lung cancer to be aware of is a Pancoast's tumor, which is a malignant tumor located in the upper lung apices. However, the most common initial presentation of this tumor is shoulder pain instead of thoracic/trunk pain. Patients will complain of nagging pain in the shoulder and along the medial border of the scapula due to irritation of the parietal pleura. The pain will progressively

Table 3-11

KIDNEY STONES VERSUS GALL STONES

	KIDNEY	GALL BLADDER
PAIN LOCATION	Posterolateral aspect of thoracic and upper lumbar spines (ie, flank)	Right upper abdominal quadrant or right scapular region
SYMPTOMS	Severe pain (renal colic), chills, fever, nausea, and vomiting	Severe pain (biliary colic—positive Murphy's sign), nausea, vomiting, worsens with eating fatty food, not relieved by rest or increase in activity
CONSIST OF	Solidified masses of salts, calcium, uric acid (gout), cystine, or struvite	Solidified deposits of cholesterol, salt, or bilirubin
PATHOGENESIS	Urine is oversaturated with substance and the stone blocks renal ducts (nephrolithiasis) or urinary tract (urolithiasis)	Stone blocks the cystic duct
TREATMENT	Dietary modification Increase: Hydration Decrease • Oxalate-rich foods • Sodium/protein intake Small stone • Pain relievers • Alpha blocker to relax muscles in ureter and help stone pass • Ca+—thiazide • Uric acid—allopurinol • Struvite—long-term, small dose antibiotics • Cystine—tiopronin Large stone • Extracorporeal shock wave lithotripsy • Nephrolithotomy • Ureteroscope	Nonsurgical options Dietary/lifestyle modification • Decrease fat intake • Extracorporeal shock wave lithotripsy Medication options • Ursodeoxycholic acid to help dissolve stones Surgical options • Cholecystectomy • Endoscopic retrograde cholangiopancreatography

become more burning and extend down into the ulnar nerve distribution of the involved upper extremity. Atrophy of the intrinsic hand muscles on the involved side may occur as the tumor grows. At later stages, occlusion of the subclavian vein may occur, which will cause venous distention and increased swelling into the involved arm. As with any potential metastasis, early identification is key and may aid in life-saving treatment being initiated before the disease progresses to mortal levels.

Cervical, Cranial/Facial, and Shoulder Pain

Patients presenting with cervical and shoulder complaints are quite common in the outpatient orthopedic physical therapy population.[6] The cervical spine is a much less common location for metastases compared to other regions of the axial skeleton,[21] which lessens the suspicion of cancer in patients who present with upper quadrant symptomology.

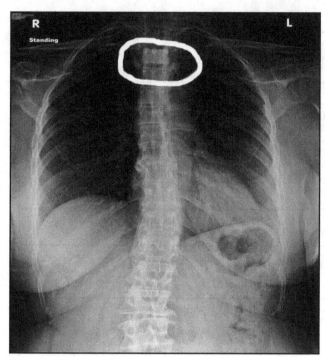

Figure 3-3. Ivory white vertebrae. Notice the increased lucency of the upper thoracic vertebrae.

Other medical conditions that should be screened for during the evaluation of a patient with cervical and/or shoulder pain include ligamentous instability, central cord syndromes, trigeminal neuralgia, and brachial plexus neuropathies.

Following a trauma such as a slip/fall or motor vehicle collision, cervical ligamentous injury must be screened. Ligamentous instability can cause neurological and cardiovascular compromise resulting in tingling, numbness, weakness, or burning pain in the pericervical or scapular regions and either unilateral or bilateral upper extremity paresthesia. Bilateral upper extremity paresthesia and dizziness, nystagmus, or vertigo with head movements would lead the therapist to suspect possible compromise of the spinal cord and need for medical referral. Patients with a history of rheumatoid arthritis, ankylosing spondylitis, Down syndrome, or use of oral contraceptives may be more prone to developing cervical ligament instability. Clinical tests that may be performed by the therapist during the physical examination include the Sharp-Purser, the alar ligament stress test, assessing clonus, and the Babinski reflex (Table 3-12). If ligament instability is suspected, referral for diagnostic imaging such as x-ray, digital motion x-ray, computed tomography scan, or MRI is necessary. Confirming the presence of this pathology is essential to identify which ligamentous structures may be involved and to ensure that treatment progression may not exacerbate underlying instability. For example, performing a grade V joint mobilization to the upper cervical spine with ligament instability places the patient at increased risk for a potential neurological injury and is contraindicated. Central cord syndromes are the most common incomplete spinal cord injury and frequently present in older adults with cervical spondylosis who sustain hyperextension injuries (ie,

whiplash in a motor vehicle collision) that results in injury to the medial portion of the lateral corticospinal tract in the cervical spine.[52]

Brachial plexus neuropathies can be classified into 3 categories: sensory, motor, and mixed. These neuropathies are normally related to more normal pathogenesis of musculoskeletal conditions such as repetitive overuse, postural strain, or trauma. Pain produced by motor neuropathies has been described as present at rest, not well localized, and having a retrograde distribution. The affected muscles supplied by the nerve being suspected may be atrophied and tender to palpation, along with a positive Tinel's sign. When assessing for brachial plexus neuropathies, bilateral reflex, dermatomal, and myotomal investigation must be completed to accurately detect any potential abnormal neurological findings (Table 3-13).

Craniofacial conditions that may present to a therapist may include temporomandibular joint dysfunction, Bell's palsy, trigeminal neuralgia, stroke, or any back/neck condition that could alert the therapist of the possible presence of meningitis, potential brain tumor, or a subarachnoid hemorrhage. Meningitis is an infection of either bacterial, viral, or fungal origin that occurs in the meningeal membranes that line the skull/vertebral canal and encase the brain and spinal cord. It is most common in children or in populations of people living in close proximity. There are 3 types of meningitis: bacterial, viral, and fungal. Bacterial is the most serious and can cause death within hours, viral is the least serious, and fungal is most common in patients who are immunosuppressed, such as HIV patients (Table 3-14). The slump test places strain on the meninges and may aid in the detection of this condition. Other common symptoms of infection may be present, including fever, seizures, mental confusion, fatigue, and vomiting/nausea, along with a headache, photophobia, and complaints of a stiff neck. To confirm the diagnosis of meningitis, medical referral is required, and the patient must undergo a spinal tap to analyze the cerebrospinal fluid for potential inflammatory markers.

An interesting presentation of trigeminal neuralgia may occur following a flare up of shingles. Shingles is caused by the Herpes zoster virus, which causes chicken pox in childhood and is a result of the reactivation of the virus. It leads to severe pain, itchy skin with a rash and/or blisters, and possible fever. An example of this is a patient who presented to physical therapy following a motor vehicle collision complaining of cervical, right shoulder, and facial pain. He reported that 6 months prior to his accident he had a bout of shingles affecting his facial nerve. After the resolution of his shingles, his facial pain/paresthesia remained leading to the diagnosis of trigeminal neuralgia. Classic pathogenesis of trigeminal neuralgia is due to neurovascular compression of the facial nerve. The patient describes the pain as shock-like in the distribution of the trigeminal nerve unilaterally. If the patient describes bilateral symptoms, abnormal neurological findings, lack of triggered pain, and an absence of a refractory period, these factors may be clues to look for a secondary cause of their symptoms, such as multiple sclerosis.[53]

Table 3-12

SPECIAL TESTS FOR CERVICAL INSTABILITY AND UPPER MOTOR NEURON LESIONS

Sharp-purser: To assess the stability of the atlanto-axial, most specifically the integrity of the transverse ligament.

Procedure: Patient is seated. One hand on forehead, the other index finger on the spinous process of C2. Patient is then asked to perform slight cervical flexion as the therapist applies a posterior force to the forehead.

Alar ligament stress test: To assess the upper cervical stability of the alar ligaments that resist lateral flexion and rotation.

Procedure: Patient is supine. One hand on the occiput and the other on the spinous process of C2. Then side-bend or rotate the head to one side. The spinous process should move to the opposite side.

Babinski reflex: To assess for possible upper motor neuron lesion/damage to the corticospinal tract.

Procedure: The lateral plantar aspect of the foot is stimulated with a blunt instrument from the heel to the base of the metatarsals in a lateral to medial fashion. Normal response is flexion of the first toe.

Clonus: To assess presence of possible upper motor neuron lesion.

Procedure: Most commonly assessed at ankle by moving the joint into either dorsiflexion or plantarflexion. Involuntary, rhythmic series of muscle contraction follows the provoking movement, also usually accompanied by spasticity.

Table 3-13

UPPER EXTREMITY PERIPHERAL NERVE ENTRAPMENT PRESENTATIONS

UPPER EXTREMITY NERVE	PRESENTATION	POTENTIAL MECHANISMS OF INJURY
Spinal accessory	Weakness of shoulder abduction and inability to shoulder shrug, dull aching pain, paralysis of trapezius (shoulder droop), and scapular winging	Blunt trauma to posterior neck triangle, traction injury: Depressed shoulder with head laterally flexed to opposite side, following cervical surgery
Axillary	Weakness of shoulder abduction, flexion, and external rotation; numbness sometimes present	Shoulder dislocation that tractions nerve or directly landing on shoulder
Long thoracic nerve	Weakness/atrophy of serratus anterior: Shoulder girdle pain, decreased active shoulder motion, and scapular winging	Excessive shoulder use, trauma to lateral chest wall, or prolonged traction to nerve
Suprascapular	Weakness/atrophy of supraspinatus or infraspinatus: Decreased abduction/ external rotation and diffuse/deep shoulder pain	Repetitive microtrauma associated with poor scapular stability, distal blunt trauma to shoulder—fall on outstretched arm

---

Table 3-14

TYPES OF MENINGITIS

	SEVERITY/PREVALENCE	TREATMENT
BACTERIAL	Most fatal: MEDICAL EMERGENCY!	Hospitalization required to monitor treatments with anti-bacterial medications
FUNGAL	Least common type, usually found in immunocompromised (ie, HIV/cancer) *Cryptococcus neoformans*	Anti-fungal medications: will require hospitalization for treatment management
VIRAL	Most common type Enterovirus, HIV, West Nile, herpes	Most cases will self-resolve, some with higher risk factors (ie, old/young/immunocompromised) still will require hospitalization

---

Table 3-15

POTENTIAL SYMPTOMS OF PRIMARY BRAIN TUMOR

- Ataxia
- Sensory abnormalities
- Visual disturbances
- Seizures
- Nausea/vomiting
- Speech deficits

A primary brain tumor occurs relatively infrequently as its prevalence is 6 to 9 people per 100,000.[54] However, the CNS is a common site of metastases from either lung, skin (melanoma), or breast cancers, which may also metastasize to the brain. Once patients have reported a previous history of these more common cancers, the therapist needs to be thorough in screening for potential red flag symptoms. Headache is a normal/common complaint, but those with brain tumors usually have more neurological symptoms presenting during the initial and middle stages of the disorder (Table 3-15).[55]

A subarachnoid hemorrhage usually occurs by a rupture of an intracranial aneurysm, a rupture of an arteriovenous malformation, or following head trauma. This condition shares a similar presentation to both meningitis and a potential brain tumor but is most often reported as "the worst headache" of the patient's life. If this condition is suspected, emergency medical attention is required to identify the location of the rupture and stop the bleeding to attempt to decrease the pressure that will be building on the CNS.

Elbow, Wrist, and Hand Pain Conditions

Many typical orthopedic injuries of the upper extremity lead patients to seek physical therapy evaluation, including infections, fractures, sprains/strains, or Raynaud's disease, and CRPS (also known as *reflex sympathetic dystrophy*). As discussed earlier, the red flag symptoms for fractures in other body regions are bony and/or angular deformity, severe joint tenderness, pain with both active/passive motion, axial loading/weight bearing, and muscle testing. The therapist should be aware of these potential upper extremity fractures (Table 3-16) that may present after blunt trauma, a slip/fall, or in patients with decreased bone density (ie, osteoporosis/osteopenia).

Raynaud's disease, or Raynaud's phenomenon, is a disorder that may affect both the hands or feet. The patient's digits when exposed to cold or a severe emotional disturbance will blanch, become cyanotic, and turn red. During the rubor stage, which lasts approximately 15 to 20 minutes, the patient will complain of increased pain and paresthesia as the blood returns to the digits. Raynaud's is more common in patients with rheumatoid arthritis, occlusive vascular disease, or a history of smoking or taking beta-adrenergic medications used to treat migraine, angina, or hypertension. CRPS has a variable presentation but always occurs following a previous injury to the distal extremities of the arm or leg. Any orthopedic injury may result in this condition, but those who also experience neurological symptoms may be more prone to developing the following symptoms characterized by a lag period between the original injury and the onset of severe aching, stinging, boring, or cutting pain that is out of proportion to the mechanical nature of the injury, surgery, or healing tissue. Hypersensitivity, swelling, warmness, and redness are noted in the involved limb and treatment is usually targeted by desensitization exercises and slow/gentle progression with active and resistive therapies.

Table 3-16

SEVERAL TYPES OF WRIST FRACTURES

FRACTURE TYPE	MECHANISM OF INJURY	CLINICAL FINDINGS
Radial head	Fall on outstretched arm in supination	• Anterolateral elbow pain/tenderness • Unable to pronate/supinate
Colles—distal radius	Fall on outstretched arm with wrist in extension	• Wrist swelling • Pain with wrist extension
Scaphoid	Fall on outstretched arm	• Wrist swelling • Pain in anatomical snuff box
Lunate	Fall on outstretched arm	• Generalized wrist pain/swelling • Diffuse synovitis • Decreased motion all planes • Decreased grip strength

CONCLUSION

The investigation of symptoms during the physical therapy examination process is imperative in determining if physical therapy treatment is warranted or may possibly be contraindicated. Using the information gathered from the initial intake forms and patient history (the location, onset, and behavior of their symptoms) can help the physical therapist make the appropriate clinical decision for determining the best course of treatment. Therapists should be aware of common and atypical symptom presentations, referred pain, unresponsiveness to conservative treatment, and other prognostic risk factors which may help identify patients presenting with red flags who would require medical referral and management.

DIFFERENTIAL DIAGNOSIS AND CLINICAL RATIONALE CASE STUDIES

Case Study One

The patient is a 30-year-old female runner who is familiar to the therapist as she was previously being treated for neck pain. She presents to the clinic for recent onset of severe bilateral calf pain. She reports she recently began increasing her training volume as she is preparing for a half marathon in the coming months. Her recent increase in training volume is a clinically significant finding in determining the

source of her new bilateral calf symptoms.[56] She reports she had what she would consider normal soreness following her longer training runs, but that recently her soreness has become more painful and would require more rest time in between her runs to recover.[57] She reports that after her last run of 8 miles 2 days ago, her pain has increased significantly in intensity and that she has had increased pain, weakness, heaviness, and some numbness into her bilateral: right greater than left ankles/feet regions. She has come to the therapist by direct access and has not had any other medical provider contact at the time of her evaluation. Based on her history and clinical presentation please choose what you think may be the best possible differential diagnoses.

Objective Findings

- Antalgic gait pattern, pain with weight bearing on right more than left lower extremities; decreased heel strike; increase fore foot contact and knee flexion during stance phase
- Visual Analog Scale: 8-9/10 pain in right more than left calf
- Active ROM
  - Decreased active dorsiflexion to neutral (0 degrees); noted increased pain with passive dorsiflexion
  - Plantarflexion: 50 degrees with pain at end range
  - Inversion: 35 degrees
  - Eversion: 10 degrees

- Manual muscle tests
  - Tibialis anterior: 3/5
  - Gastrocnemius/soleus: 3/5 with pain unable to complete full active range with standing calf raise due to pain
  - Peroneals: 4-/5 with pain
  - Tibialis posterior: 4/5
- Absent dorsalis pedal pulse on right, faint on left
- Sensation: Decreased light touch to lateral/dorsal aspects of right more than left feet
- Negative orthopedic special tests: Thompson test bilaterally, anterior drawer; left bump test
- Positive orthopedic special tests: Homan's and right bump tests

Differential Diagnosis of Bilateral Calf Pain in Adult Woman

1. Shin splints/medial tibial stress syndrome: characterized by increased repetitive stress to the medial or anterior soft tissue structures of the calves[58,59]
2. Stress fracture/bone marrow edema: characterized by an area of bony weakness due to increased repetitive stress
3. Acute exertional compartment syndrome: characterized by an increase in lower leg compartment pressure that may cause muscle/nerve damage usually in the peripheral extremities[60-62]
4. DVT: blood clots that usually occur in lower extremities due to periods of inactivity/disuse

After considering the patient's symptom presentation and examination findings, a DVT was ruled out since she has been physically active, despite having a positive Homan's sign. She was referred to urgent care/emergency room for further diagnostic consultation due to increased severity/intensity of her symptoms. The most significant clinical findings were her subjective history, severity of her weakness, and her increased vascular/neurological symptoms warranting the therapist to appropriately refer her to her local hospital for emergency medical consultation.[63,64] She was found to have exertional compartment syndrome and had to undergo emergency fasciotomy to relieve her symptoms. She was then referred for physical therapy following her decompression procedure; she was able to return to running after recovering and going through a graded/progressive running program to ensure she did not overload these tissues repetitively.

Case Study Two

The patient is a 16-year-old adolescent girl who was previously being treated for lower back pain. She presents to the clinic reporting recent increase in right medial knee pain after a fall at home, approximately 2 months ago. She reports she has had intermittent knee pain over the past year, prior to her fall, but that within the past 2 months her symptoms

have become more intense and constant. She reports she did consult with her pediatric orthopedist and was given a referral for medial knee pain and chondromalacia issues. She reports her symptoms increase with weight-bearing activities (eg, standing, walking, stair climbing). She reports that she now has low-level pain when resting and that her symptoms occasionally disturb her sleep, but that cryotherapy gives her some mild temporary relief. She also reports she has had a myriad of other joint/muscle/skin issues throughout her life, as she was born with neurofibromatosis, a rare genetic disorder.[65,66] She has begun treatment and progressed with her therapeutic exercise program over the past month, but her symptoms have unfortunately not decreased, which has led to referral back to her pediatric orthopedist for further diagnostic imaging. Based on her history and current objective findings, please select what differential diagnosis may best explain her continued symptoms.

Objective Findings

- Active knee ROM: 0 to 125 degrees, with pain at end-range flexion
- Manual muscle tests
  - Hip flexor/hamstring: 4+/5
  - Quadriceps: 4/5 with pain
  - Gluteus medius/maximus: 4/5
  - Hip external rotators: 4-/5 with pain
  - Hip internal rotators 4/5 with pain
- Gait analysis: Noted hip internal rotation during stance with overpronation bilaterally, right more than left
- Visual Analog Scale: 6 to 7/10 at worst when exacerbated
- Balance: Tandem 1 minute without loss of balance eyes open/closed—Single leg: Right 15 vs left 20
- Positive orthopedic special tests: Clarke's sign/patellar grind; positive valgus stress, Apley's compression, Mcmurray's, Thessaly
- Negative orthopedic special tests: Varus, posterior drawer, Apley's distraction

Differential Diagnosis of Medial Knee Pain in Adolescent Girl

1. Chondromalacia of medial patella: Her objective findings (ie, gait analysis and special tests) indicate that this may be a possible cause of her symptoms.
2. Medial meniscus tear: Her prolonged duration of symptoms and positive special tests may indicate possible pathology contributing to her condition.
3. Fibroma of distal medial femoral shaft: Her medial history of neurofibromatosis and the prolonged duration of her symptoms make this a possible cause of her knee symptoms.
4. Osteochondral defect of medial femoral condyle: Her report of increased pain with prolonged weight bearing and positive orthopedic special tests make this a possible diagnosis.

After undergoing MRI the patient was found to have a nonossifying fibroma in her posterior/medial region of her distal femoral shaft.[67-69] Imaging also showed some chondromalacia of the medial patella along with active inflammation/bursitis around her medial knee structures; however, she was not found to have any ligament/chondral pathology despite having a number of clinical positive special tests for those findings. This is an example that despite having a number of positive clinical findings to help direct the differential diagnoses process, her prolonged symptom duration and nonresponse to conservative treatments warranted medical imaging to better assist in the treatment of her symptoms. After her imaging findings, therapy was deferred until after the patient had a biopsy and subsequent surgical removal of the fibroma. She then returned for physical therapy following her surgical debridement of the fibroma.

REFERENCES

1. Boissonnault WG, Badke MB, Powers JM. Pursuit and implementation of hospital-based outpatient direct access to physical therapy services: an administrative case report. *Phys Ther.* 2010;90(1):100-109.

2. Bellamy J. Vision statement for the physical therapy profession and guiding principles to achieve the vision. 2013. www.apta.org/vision/

3. Moore JH, McMillan DJ, Rosenthal MD, et al. Risk determination for patients with direct access to physical therapy in military care health care facilities. *J Orthop Sports Phys Ther.* 2005;35(10):674-678.

4. Laderia CE. Physical therapy clinical specialization and management of red and yellow flags in patients with low back pain in the United States. *J Man Manip Ther.* 2018;26(2):66-77.

5. Jette DU, Ardleigh K, Chandler K, et al. Decision-making ability of physical therapists: physical therapy intervention or medical referral. *Phys Ther.* 2006;86:1619-1629.

6. DiFabio RP, Boissonnault W. Physical therapy and health-related outcomes for patients with common orthopaedic diagnoses. *J Orthop Sports Phys Ther.* 1998;27(3):219-230.

7. Jarvik JG Deyo RA. Diagnostic evaluation of low back pain with emphasis on imaging. *Ann Intern Med.* 2002;137(7):586-597.

8. Deyo RA, Diehl AK. Cancer as a cause of back pain: frequency, clinical presentation, and diagnostic strategies. *J Gen Intern Med.* 1988;3(3):230-238.

9. Cook CE, George SZ, Reiman MP. Red flag screening for low back pain: nothing to see here, move along: a narrative review. *Br J Sports Med.* 2018;52(8):493-496.

10. Henscke N, Maher C. Red flags need more evaluation. *Rhuematology.* 2006;45:920-921.

11. Klaber-Moffet J, McClean S, Roberts L. Red flags need more evaluation: reply. *Rheumatology.* 2006;45:921.

12. Chartered Society of Physiotherapy. *Clinical Guidelines for the Effective Physiotherapy Management of Persistent Low Back Pain.* Charted Society of Physiotherapy; 2007.

13. Roberts L, Fraser F, Murphy EA. In: *What is a Red Flag, 15th International WCPT Congress,* Vancouver; 2007.

14. Murray G. Referred Pain. *J Appl Oral Sci.* 2009;17(6):i.

15. Enthoven WT, Geuze J, Scheele J, et al. Prevalence and "red flags" regarding specified causes of back pain in older adults presenting in general practice. *Phys Ther.* 2016;96(3):305-312.

16. Lobdell KW, Stamou S, Sanchez JA. Hospital-acquired infections. *Surg Clin North Am.* 2012;92(1):65-77.

17. Division of Cancer Prevention and Control, Centers of Disease Control and Prevention. Know the signs and symptoms of infection. Reviewed November 10, 2020. Accessed November 10, 2021. https://www.cdc.gov/cancer/preventinfections/symptoms.htm

18. Bigos S, Bowyer O, Braen G, et al. Acute lower back problems in adults: clinical practice guidelines. No. 14, AHCPR publication no 95-0642; Agency for Health Care Policy and Research, Public Health Service, US Department of Health and Human Services; 1994.

19. Schofferman L, Shofferman J, Zuckerman J, et al. Occult infection causing persistent low back pain. *Spine.* 1989;14:417-419.

20. Vanharanta H, Sachs BJ, Spivey M, et al. A comparison of CT discography, pain response and radiographic disc height. *Spine.* 1998;13:321-324.

21. Weinstein JN, Mclain RF. Primary tumors of the spine. *Spine.* 1987;12:843-851.

22. Delitto A, George S, Van Dillen L, et al. Clinical practice guidelines linked to the International Classification of Functioning, Disability, and Health from the Orthopaedic Section of the American Physical Therapy Association. *JOSPT.* 2012;42(4):A1-A5.

23. Jensen M, Brant Zawadzki M, Obuchowski N, et al. Magnetic resonance imaging of the lumbar spine in people without back pain. *N Engl J Med.* 1994;331:69-73.

24. Sieper J, Braun J, Rudwaleit M, et al. Ankylosing spondylitis: an overview. *Ann Rheum Dis.* 2002;61(suppl III):iii8-iii18.

25. Tronzo RG: Femoral neck fractures. In: Steinburg ME, ed, *The Hip and Its Disorders.* Saunders; 1991:247-279.

26. Wenger DR, Ward WT, Herring JA. Current concepts review: Legg-Clave-Perthes disease. *J Bone Joint Surg.* 1991;73:778-788.

27. Gardner A, Gardner E, Morley T. Cauda equine syndrome: a review of current clinical and medico-legal position. *Eur Spine J.* 2011;20(5):690-697.

28. Dionne N, Adefolarin A, Kunzelman D, et al. What is the diagnostic accuracy of red flags related to cauda equina syndrome (CES), when compared to magnetic resonance imaging (MRI)? A systematic review. *Musculoskelet Sci Pract.* 2019;42:125-133.

29. Jemal A, Murray T, Samuels A, et al. Cancer statistics, 2003, CA. *Cancer J Clin.* 2003;53:5-26.

30. Deyo RA, Rainville J, Kent DL. What can the history and physical examination tell us about lower back pain? *JAMA.* 1992;268:760-765.

31. Bojko EJ, Ahroni JH, Davignon D, et al. Diagnostic utility of the history and physical examination for peripheral vascular disease among patients with diabetes mellitus. *J Clin Epidemiol.* 1997;50:659-668.

32. Rizzone KH, Ackerman KE, Roos KG, Dompier TP, Kerr ZY. Epidemiology of stress fractures in collegiate student-athletes, 2004-2005 through 2013-2014 academic years. *J Athl Train.* 2017;52(10):966-975.

33. Romani WA, Gieck JH, Perrin D, et al. Mechanisms and management of stress fractures in physically active persons. *J Athl Train.* 2002;37(3):306-314.

34. Carpenter CR, Schuur JD, Everett, et al. Evidence-based diagnostics: adult septic arthritis. *Acad Emerg Med.* 2011;18(8):781-796.

35. Gupta MN, Sturrock RD, Field MA. prospective 2-year study of 75 patients with adult-onset septic arthritis. *Rheumatology.* 2001;40(1):24-30.

36. Bailey E, Kroshinsky D. Cellulitis: diagnosis and management. *Dermatol Ther.* 2011;24(2):229-39.

37. Voros D, Pissiotis C, Georgantas D, Katsaragakis S, Antoniou S, Papadimitriou J. Role of early and extensive surgery in the treatment of severe necrotizing soft tissue infection. *Br J Surg.* 1993;80(9):1190-1191

38. Malik MA, Alam Khan S, Safdar S, Taseer IU. Chest Pain as a presenting complaint in patients with acute myocardial infarction (AMI). *Pak J Med Sci.* 2013;29(2):565-568.

39. Canto JG, Shiplak MG, Rogers WJ, et al. Prevalence, clinical characteristics, and mortality among patients with myocardial infarction presenting without chest pain. *JAMA.* 2000;283:3223-3229.

40. Ariyarajah V, Spodick DH. Cardiac tamponade revisited: a postmortem look at a cautionary case. *Tex Heart Inst J.* 2007;34(3):347-351.

41. Hoare Z, Lim WS. Pneumonia: update on diagnosis and management. *BMJ.* 2006;332(7549):1077-1079.

42. Upchurch GR Jr, Schaub TA. Abdominal aortic aneurysm. *Am Fam Physician.* 2006;73(7):1198-1204.

43. Humes DJ, Simpson J. Acute appendicitis. *BMJ.* 2006;333(7567):530-534.

44. BE Njeze. Gallstones. *Niger J Surg.* 2013;19(2):49-55.

45. Saklayen M. Medical management of nephrolithiasis. *Med Clin North Am.* 1997;81:785-799.

46. Wells K. Nephrolithiasis with unusual initial symptoms. *J Manipulative Physiol Ther.* 2000;23:196-203.

47. Ramakrishnan K, Scheid DC. Diagnosis and management of acute pyelonephritis in adults. *Am Fam Physician.* 2005;71(5):933-942.

48. Weiner SL. *Differential Diagnosis of Acute Body Pain by Region.* McGraw-Hill; 1993:532, 542, 616, 645, 678, 680.

49. Hippisley-Cox J, Coupland C. Identifying patients with suspected pancreatic cancer in primary care: derivation and validation of an algorithm. *Br J Gen Pract.* 2012;62(594):e38-e45.

50. Jemal A, Siegel R, Ward E, et al. Cancer statistics, 2008, CA. *Cancer J Clin.* 2008;58(2):71-96.

51. Buccheri G, Ferrigno D. Lung cancer: clinical presentation and specialist referral time. *Eur Respir J.* 2004;24:898-904.

52. Jimenez O, Marcillo A, Levi AD. A histopathological analysis of the human cervical spinal cord in patients with acute traumatic central cord syndrome. *Spinal Cord.* 2000;38:532-537.

53. Montano N, Conforti G, Di Bonaventura R, et al. Advances in the diagnosis and treatment of trigeminal neuralgia. *Ther Clin Risk Manag.* 2015;11:289-299.

54. Synder H, Robinson K, Shah D, et al. Signs and symptoms of patient with brain tumors presenting in the emergency department. *J Emerg Med.* 1993;11:253-258.

55. Issacs ER, Bookhout MR. Screening for pathological origins of head and facial pain. In: Boissonnault WG, ed. *Examination on Physical Therapy Practice: Screening for Medical Disease.* 2nd ed. Churchill Linvingstone; 1995:181-182.

56. Craig DI. Medial tibial stress syndrome: evidence-based prevention. *J Athl Train.* 2008;43(3):316-8.

57. Choi HJ, Cho HM. Multiple stress fractures of the lower extremity in healthy young men. *J Orthop Traumatol.* 2012:13(2):105-110.

58. Schulze C, Finze S, Bader R, Lison A. Treatment of medial tibial stress syndrome according to the fascial distortion model: a prospective case control study. *Scientific WorldJournal.* 2014;2014:790626.

59. Galbraith RM, Lavallee ME. Medial tibial stress syndrome: conservative treatment options. *Curr Rev Musculoskelet Med.* 2009;2(3):127-133.

60. Tucker AK. Chronic exertional compartment syndrome of the leg. *Curr Rev Musculoskelet Med.* 2010;3(1-4):32-37.

61. Wilder RP, Magrum E. Exertional compartment syndrome. *Clin Sports Med.* 2010;29(3):429-435.

62. Schubert AG. Exertional compartment syndrome: review of the literature and proposed rehabilitation guidelines following surgical release. *Int J Sports Ther.* 2011;6(2):126-141.

63. Moran DS, Evans RK, Hadad E. Imaging of lower extremity stress fracture injuries. *Sports Med.* 2008;38(4):345-356.

64. Robertson GA, Wood AM. Lower limb stress fractures in sport: optimising their management and outcome. *World J Orthop.* 2017;8(3):242-255.

65. Gerber PA, Antal AS, Neumann NJj, et al. Neurofibromatosis. *Eur J Med Res.* 2009;14(3):102-105.

66. Boyd KP, Korf BR, Theos A. Neurofibromatosis type 1. *J Am Acad Dermatol.* 2009;61(1):1-14.

67. Rosenbaum T, Wimmer K. Neurofibromatosis type 1 (NF1) and associated tumors. *Klin Pediatr.* 2014;226(6-7):309-315.

68. Karajannis MA, Ferner RE. Neurofibromatosis-related tumors: emerging biology and therapies. *Curr Opin Pediatr.* 2015;27(1):26-33.

69. Hatori M, Hosaka M, Watanabe M, et al. Osteosarcoma in a patient with neurofibromatosis type 1: a case report and review of the literature. *Tohoku J Exp Med.* 2006;208(4):343-348.

PART II

Upper Extremity

4

Upper Quarter Systems Review and Referred Pain Patterns

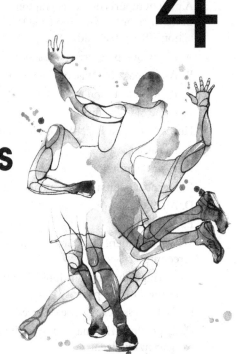

William R. VanWye, PT, DPT, PhD
and Kristi M. Angelopoulou, PT, DPT, OCS, MCMT, Cert.MSKUS

KEY TERMS

Patient/Client Management Model: Conceptual model developed by the American Physical Therapy Association (APTA) to guide the physical therapist examination.

Radicular pain: Pain due to direct irritation of a nerve root.

Referred pain: Pain perceived in an area of the body separate from the location of the actual source.

Systems review: A hands-on, brief scan examination focusing on the 5 systems deemed most related to physical therapist practice: (1) communication, (2) cardiovascular/pulmonary, (3) integumentary, (4) musculoskeletal, and (5) neuromuscular.

Upper extremity gross functional screen: Application of forces in functional patterns to assess the gross musculoskeletal integrity of the patient's upper extremities.

CHAPTER QUESTIONS

1. A patient presents with weakness of wrist flexion and elbow extension. Which nerve root should you *most* suspect?

   A. C5

   B. C6

   C. C7

   D. C8

2. You assess the upper trapezius muscle with resisted shoulder shrug. You find it to be weak on the right compared to the left. Which cranial nerve (CN) should you suspect?

   A. CN X

   B. CN XII

   C. CN IX

   D. CN XI

Wallmann HW, Donatelli R, eds. *Foundations of Orthopedic Physical Therapy* (pp 107-125).
© 2024 Taylor & Francis Group.

3. A patient reports onset of symptoms with cervical rotation active range of motion (AROM). What is your next action? (See Case Study One.)

    A. Apply overpressure and assess end-feel.

    B. Assess passive range of motion (PROM).

    C. Perform tests and measures.

    D. None of the above.

4. How do you assess CN VII (facial nerve)?

    A. Facial sensation

    B. Facial symmetry

    C. Sternocleidomastoid manual muscle testing (MMT)

    D. All of the above

    E. A and B

5. Which statement is accurate regarding upper quadrant screening?

    A. During palpation, any lump found must be reported to the patient's primary care physician.

    B. Gait assessment can be deferred.

    C. A positive Hoffmann test indicates lower motor neuron involvement.

    D. Palpation should be assessed by going from superficial to deeper structures

6. Which components are part of the subjective examination?

    A. Medical history

    B. Patient interview

    C. Review of systems

    D. All of the above

7. Which is a component of the musculoskeletal systems review?

    A. Balance

    B. Orthopedic special tests

    C. Gross symmetry

    D. MMT

8. Which tests or signs, when clustered together, are known to increase the likelihood of a patient having cervical myelopathy? (See Case Study Two.)

    A. Sharp Purser, upper extremity reflex testing, age greater than 40 years

    B. Gait deviation, Hoffmann reflex, inverted supinator sign

    C. Hoffmann reflex, limited cervical rotation, age greater than 45 years

    D. Spurling, distraction, upper limb tension testing

9. You evaluate a patient and find a positive flip sign. What should this *most* likely indicate?

    A. Rotator cuff weakness

    B. Accessory nerve injury

    C. Dorsal scapular nerve injury

    D. Long thoracic nerve injury

10. Which deep tendon reflex (DTR) grade is considered normal?

    A. 4

    B. 3

    C. 2

    D. 1

    E. 0

11. A patient presents with significant scapular winging during a wall push-up, which nerve should you *most* likely suspect is injured?

    A. Axillary

    B. Long thoracic

    C. Suprascapular

    D. Musculocutaneous

12. Which visceral structure is *most* likely to refer pain to the cervical and/or shoulder region?

    A. Liver

    B. Uterus

    C. Kidney

    D. Stomach

13. You are referred a patient with neck and shoulder pain. Which test/finding would help you rule out radiculopathy?

    A. Upper limb tension test A (ULTT-A)

    B. Spurling test

    C. Distraction test

    D. Cervical rotation range of motion (ROM)

14. _____ is good for ruling out the facet joint as the cause of the patient's pain.

    A. The upper limp tension test

    B. Manual spinal extension

    C. The extension-rotation test

    D. Palpation for segmental tenderness (PST)

15. Which structure below is *not* considered a structure that produces somatic referred pain?

    A. Nerve root

    B. Facet joints

    C. Intervertebral disks (IVDs)

    D. Muscle tissue

16. Which of the following sequences is the correct integration of the systems review?

    A. Observation, vitals, palpation, ROM, neurological, tests and measures, gross functional screen

    B. Vitals, palpation, ROM, neurological, tests and measures, gross functional screen

    C. Observation, vitals, gross functional screen, ROM, neurological, tests and measures, palpation

    D. Vitals, observation, gross functional screen, ROM, neurological, palpation, tests and measures

17. The ABCDEF acronym to screen for skin cancer stands for which of the following?

    A. Active growth, bluish, color, dullness, evaluation

    B. Asymmetry, borders, color, diameter, evolving, funny looking

    C. Asymmetry, burn, condition, degree, event

    D. Assessment, borders, condition, dullness, evolving

18. Which of the following systems, according to the APTA Patient/Client Model to guide the physical therapist examination, is *not* one of the 5 systems most related to physical therapist practice?

    A. Communication

    B. Immunological

    C. Musculoskeletal

    D. Neuromuscular

    E. Integumentary

19. Palpation should be performed _____.

    A. Before tests and measures to warm up the tissue

    B. During passive motion and overpressure

    C. During observation to save time

    D. Later in the examination to avoid irritating the tissue

20. Physical therapists are responsible for taking vitals as part of the cardiovascular and pulmonary systems review _____.

    A. Every visit for all patients

    B. Only if the patient has a history of cardiovascular disease

    C. At a minimum, during the initial examination

    D. Only if the patient is symptomatic

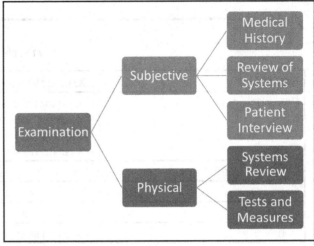

Figure 4-1. APTA conceptual model.

Introduction

As musculoskeletal experts, physical therapists must first screen to determine whether the patient's pain is coming from a potentially serious or life-threatening disorder (Chapter 2). If this is the case, then referral is warranted. However, if the physical therapist determines that the patient's condition is appropriate for physical therapist treatment, then the examination transitions to determining where the individual's pain arises, and, holistically, what has caused the condition to develop and persist.[1] It is therefore essential for physical therapists to use a dedicated examination approach to thoroughly screen and avoid being misled by the patient's location of pain.

Examination Purpose

The APTA *Guide to Physical Therapist Practice* provides a Patient/Client Management Model to guide the physical therapist examination (Figure 4-1).[2] Examination is divided into a subjective portion and a physical portion. The components of the subjective examination include the medical history, review of systems, and patient interview. The physical examination has 2 components: the systems review and tests and measures. Tests and measures (eg, orthopaedic special tests) are selected based on the findings during the subjective examination and systems review. These tests are typically more precise and are used judiciously to rule in or out the cause of the patient's chief complaint.

The systems review is a hands-on brief scan examination focusing on the 5 systems deemed most related to physical therapist practice: (1) communication, (2) cardiovascular/pulmonary, (3) integumentary, (4) musculoskeletal, and (5) neuromuscular (Table 4-1). The authors of this chapter suggest viewing the systems review as the aforementioned holistic approach for collecting the data to determine the cause of the chief complaint, not only from the area of concern, but from the system as a whole. Although the systems review may seem like additional work in the examination process, it is designed to prevent overlooking important information, and ultimately, along with the subjective examination, help guide the use of test and measures and arrive at an accurate physical therapist diagnosis. An exception to routine use of the systems review is a patient with a known, acute injury. For these cases, the focus should be on the area of concern with the remaining components being completed over subsequent visits.

Overall, the systems review is a necessary step for an autonomous practitioner, including doctors of physical therapy. This chapter focuses on the upper quarter (UQ; occiput to T12 and the upper extremities) systems review process for musculoskeletal physical therapists. The authors provide a suggested sequence for the UQ examination, detailing the use of the systems review and giving additional considerations to help guide the selection and integration of tests and measures.

Table 4-1	
SYSTEMS REVIEW	
SYSTEM	**EXAMINATION DATA**
Communication	Communication ability, affect, cognition, language, ability to make needs known, consciousness, orientation, expected emotional/behavioral responses, as well as learning style, potential learning barriers, and education needs
Cardiovascular/pulmonary	Heart rate (HR), respiratory rate (RR), blood pressure (BP), and edema
Integumentary	Pliability (texture), presence of scar formation, skin color, and skin integrity
Musculoskeletal	Gross symmetry, gross ROM, gross strength, and height and weight
Neuromuscular	Balance, gait, transfers, motor control, and motor learning

Adapted from American Physical Therapy Association. *Guide to Physical Therapist Practice 3.0.* 2014. Accessed August 29, 2022. http://guidetoptpractice.apta.org/

Table 4-2

INTEGRATION OF THE UPPER QUARTER SYSTEMS REVIEW

- Observation, including posture and gross symmetry
- Cardiovascular/pulmonary
- Gross functional screen, including gait and balance
- Gross ROM
  - AROM
  - PROM including overpressures
- Neurological
- Tests and measures*
- Palpation

* Not part of the systems review, but included to show its position in the sequence.

UPPER QUARTER SYSTEMS REVIEW

For an overview of the sequence, see Table 4-2.

Observation

Patient Position: Variable

Observation begins as soon as you greet the patient and continues throughout the examination and treatment. Also, observe for possible cognitive impairment throughout the examination and if a more detailed examination is required (eg, Mini-Mental State Examination).

At the beginning of the physical examination, after taking vitals, observe the patient's posture in standing from the anterior, posterior, and lateral positions, documenting any gross asymmetries of soft tissues (eg, atrophy, tendon rupture) or bony structures. Refer to Chapter 8 for more in-depth information regarding posture examination.

Examination of the integumentary system includes observation of the skin, hair, and nails. Observe skin contour, color, and condition, as well as noting any rashes, ulcers, scars, or swelling. Also, a useful screen for skin cancer is the ABCDEF method.[3] The addition of F helps improve the sensitivity of the screening tool as F stand for "funny looking," accounting for the "ugly duckling sign" (ie, spot unlike the others). Any abnormal finding should be brought to the patient's attention along with follow-up questioning to determine whether the change is new, if the patient's physician is aware of the change, and if it is worsening.[4]

- A—Asymmetry
- B—Borders
- C—Color
- D—Diameter
- E—Evolving
- F—Funny looking

Cardiovascular and Pulmonary Screen

Patient Position: Seated, Feet Supported

It is essential for physical therapists to screen for underlying cardiovascular conditions. At a minimum, during the initial examination the patient's HR, RR, and BP should be assessed, as well as observation for the presence of edema. If a patient has a history of cardiovascular disease, these values should be checked each session. These values should be assessed prior to any physical activity, preferably after sitting quietly for at least 5 minutes, in order to achieve resting values.[5]

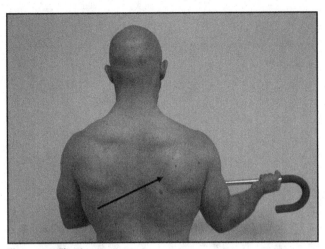

Figure 4-2. Flip sign.

Additional Considerations

- During the initial examination height and weight should be assessed, which also allows for calculation of body mass index (height and weight are part of the musculoskeletal systems review).

- Patients with a history of heart failure should monitor their weight daily using the same scale, time of day, and similar clothing as a screening tool to detect the potential onset of acute heart failure. A weight change of more than 2 to 3 pounds (lbs) is considered abnormal.[6]

- Auscultation of heart sounds is indicated for patients with a history of heart failure. The presence of an S3 sound or "gallop" is abnormal and indicates exacerbation of the patient's condition. Urgent referral to their physician is warranted.[6]

- In addition to HR, RR, and BP, patients with known lung disease should have their oxygen saturation (SpO$_2$) assessed each session. In addition, lung sounds should be assessed during the initial examination and again if the patient presents with known lung disease or increased shortness of breath.

- Postoperative patients should have their temperature assessed as well.

Gross Functional Screen

Patient Position: Standing

The gross functional screen includes aspects from the musculoskeletal and neuromuscular systems review. Gait and balance are essential components of the UQ systems review.

Although the patient's chief complaint may be located within the UQ, observation of gait and balance may aid differential diagnosis.[7] Balance can be screened by assessing the patient standing in each of the following positions, first with eyes open then with eyes closed: feet together, tandem stance, and single leg stance. Observe for gait deviations by viewing the patient from the anterior, posterior, and lateral positions.

Assessment of gross UQ ROM begins by asking the patient to make a fist with each hand (thumbs inside the fist), placing one shoulder in flexion, abduction, and external rotation (elbow flexed), and then placing the other shoulder in extension, adduction, and internal rotation (elbow flexed). Assess bilaterally for symmetry and change in symptoms.[8] Next, perform a clearing maneuver by having the patient reach their hand to the opposite shoulder and then attempt to take their elbow up toward the ceiling. Assess for symmetry and change in symptoms.[8] Gross strength can be assessed via myotome testing, which is detailed later.

Also, gross strength of the UQ can be assessed by having the patient perform a wall push-up (minimum of 10 repetitions). Multiple repetitions may reveal dysfunction due to muscular fatigue not otherwise seen with a single repetition. Observe for the scapular flip sign (Figure 4-2), which is evident by displacement of the scapula's medial border off the thorax due to the unopposed pull of the external rotators, indicating middle and lower trapezius weakness or spinal accessory nerve injury. Furthermore, note if there is scapular winging (Figure 4-3), representing serratus anterior weakness or long thoracic nerve injury.[9]

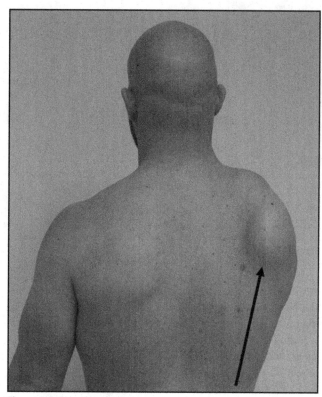

Figure 4-3. Scapular winging.

Additional Considerations

- AROM
  - Patient position: Seated, feet supported
    - Use visual observation AROM to note any gross asymmetries and if found, more detailed test and measures (eg, goniometry, tape measure) are indicated. In addition, observe and note the quality of motion and if symptoms are altered by the motion. Begin by assessing cervical spine AROM flexion, extension, lateral flexion, rotation, protraction, and retraction. Next, assess the thoracic spine by having the patient hug themselves and squeeze a pillow between their thighs and then perform AROM flexion, extension, lateral flexion, and rotation. Progress to assessing AROM of the extremities.
- PROM including overpressures
  - Patient position: Seated, feet supported
    - After assessing active motions, perform PROM of the UQ and add overpressure to assess end-feels

Neurological Examination

The neuromuscular systems review includes assessment of balance, gait, transfers, motor control, and motor learning. However, the subjective examination and systems review may reveal the need to utilize neuromuscular tests and measures, especially if a patient's chief complaint is head or neck pain. If the patient's chief complaint is head or neck pain the examination should include assessment of dermatomes, myotomes, and DTRs. In addition, assessment of CNs in patients with head or neck pain is strongly recommended. Additional neurological tests and measures that can assist with UQ screening include neural tension tests and upper motor neuron tests.

- Dermatomes[10]
  - Patient position: Seated, feet supported
  - Assess sensation to light touch for levels C2-T10 (Figure 4-4)
- Myotomes[10]
  - Patient position: Seated, feet supported
  - Assess gross motor function of C1-T1 nerve roots. Assess bilaterally, grade as either within normal limits (WNL) or diminished. If a deficiency is noted, more detailed tests and measures (eg, MMT, dynamometry) are indicated.
  - C1-C2 neck flexion (Figure 4-5)
  - C3 neck lateral flexion (Figure 4-6)
  - C4 shoulder elevation/shrug (Figure 4-7)
  - C5 shoulder abduction (Figure 4-8)
  - C5-C6 elbow flexion (Figure 4-9)
  - C6 wrist extension (Figure 4-10)
  - C7 elbow extension, wrist flexion (Figure 4-11)
  - C8 thumb extension (Figure 4-12)
  - T1 finger abduction (Figure 4-13)
- DTR[11]
  - Patient position: Seated, feet supported
  - Lower motor neuron: Assess the following DTR: Biceps (Figure 4-14), brachioradialis (Figure 4-15), and triceps (Figure 4-16)
    - DTR grade
      - Very brisk (4+)
      - Brisk (3+)
      - Normal (2+)
      - Diminished (1+)
      - Absent (0)

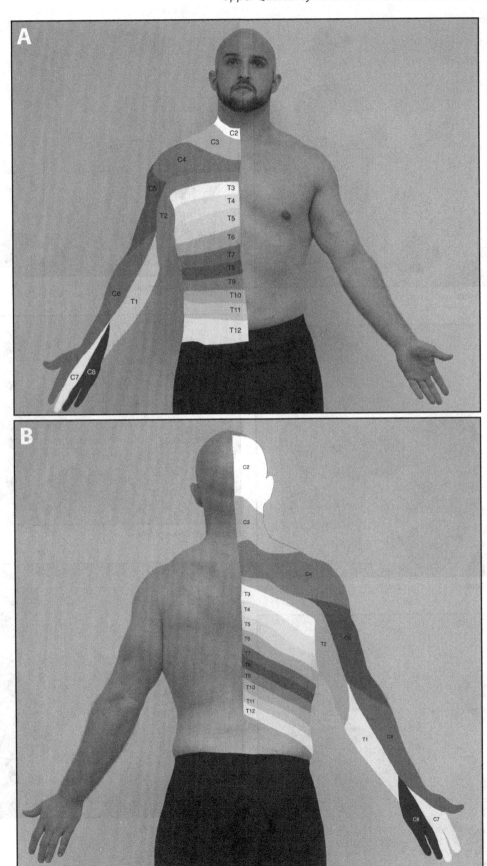

Figure 4-4. Dermatomes.

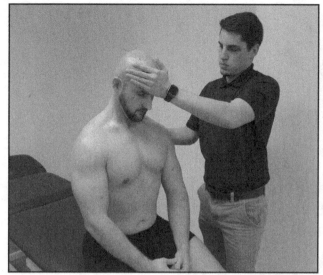

Figure 4-5. C1-C2 myotomes.

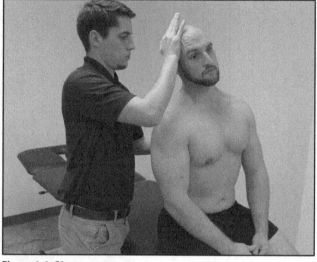

Figure 4-6. C3 myotome.

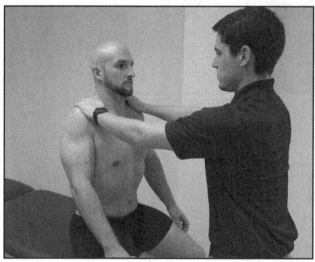

Figure 4-7. C4 myotome.

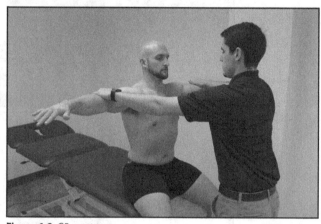

Figure 4-8. C5 myotome.

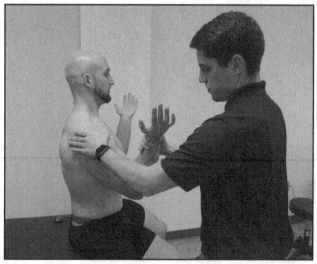

Figure 4-9. C5-C6 myotomes.

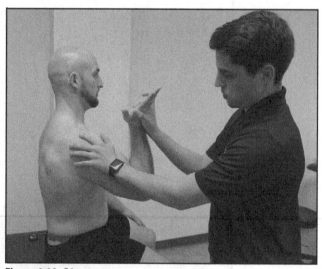

Figure 4-10. C6 myotome.

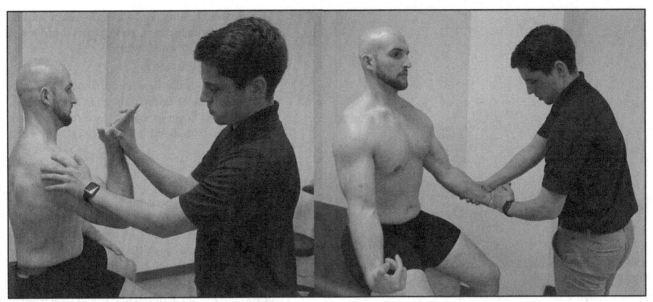

Figure 4-11. C7 myotome.

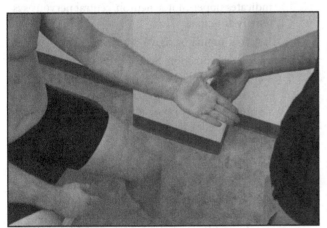

Figure 4-12. C8 myotome.

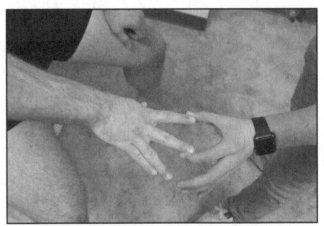

Figure 4-13. T1 myotome.

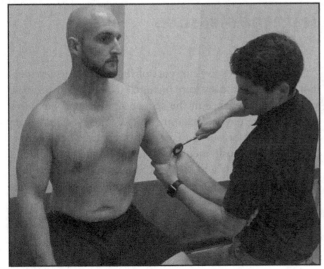

Figure 4-14. Biceps DTR.

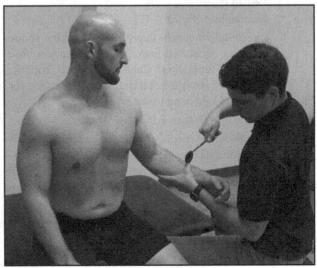

Figure 4-15. Brachioradialis DTR.

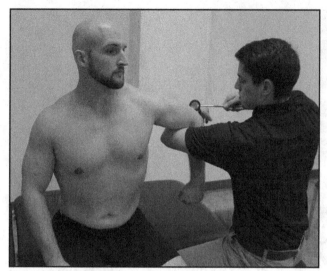

Figure 4-16. Triceps DTR.

- CN examination (Table 4-3)
  - Patient position: Seated, feet supported
  - This examination should be performed if the patient's symptoms are inconsistent with a musculoskeletal condition. For example:
    - Change in vision, hearing, speech, or taste
    - Head or neck trauma
    - History of neurological condition (eg, stroke)
    - Sensory change that does not fit a peripheral nerve or spinal nerve root pattern
- Upper limb tension testing[12]
  - Patient position: Supine
  - Median bias (Figure 4-17)
    - Shoulder girdle depression, shoulder abduction, wrist and finger/thumb extension, forearm supination, shoulder external rotation, elbow extension, cervical side-bend away, cervical side-bend toward
  - Radial bias (Figure 4-18)
    - Shoulder girdle depression, shoulder extension, elbow extension, whole arm internal rotation (shoulder internal rotation, forearm pronation), wrist and finger/thumb flexion

(further tensing via ulnar deviation and/or shoulder abduction), cervical side-bend away, cervical side-bend toward
  - Ulnar bias (Figure 4-19)
    - Shoulder girdle depression, shoulder abduction, shoulder external rotation, elbow flexion, wrist and finger extension, forearm pronation, cervical side-bend away, cervical side-bend toward
- Upper motor neuron tests
  - Hoffmann reflex (Figure 4-20) as abnormal (present) or normal (absent). The Hoffmann reflex is assessed with the patient seated, head in neutral. The therapist stabilizes the third (middle) digit of the patient's hand and then flicks the distal phalange into flexion. A positive (abnormal) finding is flexion of the first (thumb) interphalangeal joint, with or without flexion of the second (index) distal interphalangeal joint.[13] Presence of the Hoffmann reflex indicates upper motor neuron/central nervous system dysfunction.
  - Inverted supinator sign[14]
    - Patient position: Seated, feet supported
    - Clinician places patient's forearm in slight pronation and applies series of strikes near the styloid process of the radius, similar to brachioradialis reflex testing
  - Babinski test[14]
    - Patient position: Supine
    - Clinician supports the foot in neutral, uses the blunt end of the reflex hammer, and applies a stroking stimulation to the plantar surface of the foot, lateral to medial from heel to metatarsals

Tests and Measures

Patient Position: Variable

Although they are not part of the systems review, certain test and measures were included to show their position and explain relevance in the sequence. Tests and measures are part of the physical examination as a means of gathering data to rule in or out the cause of the patient's chief complaint. As previously mentioned, tests and measures should be used judiciously and selected based on the findings during the subjective examination and systems review. Tests and

Table 4-3

CRANIAL NERVE EXAMINATION

NERVE	FUNCTION	TEST PROCEDURE	SIGNIFICANT FINDINGS
I Olfactory	Smell	Odor recognition (eg, coffee, orange, vanilla)	Loss of smell
II Optic	Visual acuity	Snellen or Rosenbaum eye chart	Partial or complete vision loss
II Optic III Oculomotor	Pupillary light reflex	Place ulnar side of hand with fingers extended on bridge of patient's nose (block contralateral eye from light). Shine light to ipsilateral eye and (1) observe for pupil constriction, and (2) observe contralateral eye for consensual response; repeat for other eye.	Absent pupil constriction or consensual response to light
III Oculomotor IV Trochlear VI Abducens	Extraocular eye movements	(1) 12 to 18 inches from patient's eyes, perform "H" movement with finger.* Patient asked to follow with eyes only (head stationary). (2) 12 to 18 inches from patient's eyes, hold up 2 widely spaced targets* (eg, one finger from each hand). Ask patient to take eyes quickly from one finger to the other.	Abnormal gaze, nystagmus, or uncoordinated eye movement
V Trigeminal	Facial sensation	Assess sensation with cotton to facial areas V1, V2, and V3	Absent or asymmetrical
VII Facial	Facial expression symmetry	Ask patient to wrinkle (forehead), wink, whistle, and wince	Absent or asymmetrical
VIII Vestibulocochlear	Hearing, balance	Eyes closed, therapist rubs fingers near patient's ear	Absent or asymmetrical
IX Glossopharyngeal X Vagus	Gag reflex, swallowing, and uvula symmetry	Use a tongue depressor to stimulate the back of the throat Ask the patient to say "ah" and observe the uvula	Absent gag reflex Deviated uvula
XI Accessory	Head, neck motion	MMT trapezius and sternocleidomastoid	Weakness
XII Hypoglossal	Tongue movement	Tongue protrusion	Deviation to affected side

* Keep fingers in patient's midcervical spine ROM to prevent end-point (normal) nystagmus.

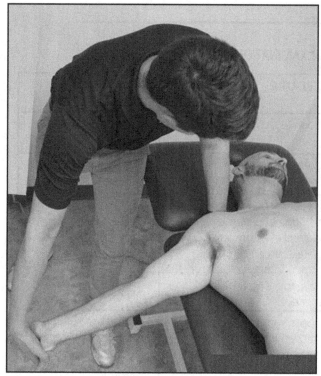

Figure 4-17. Upper limb tension testing median bias.

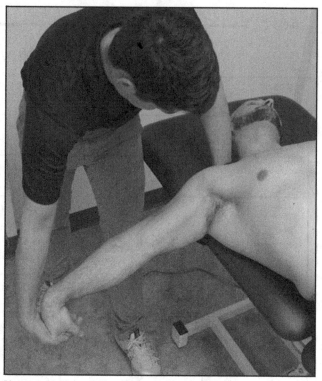

Figure 4-18. Upper limb tension testing radial bias.

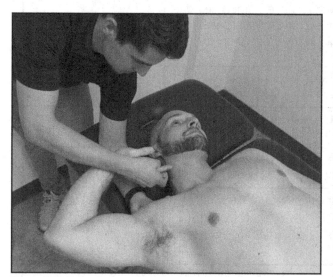

Figure 4-19. Upper limb tension testing ulnar bias.

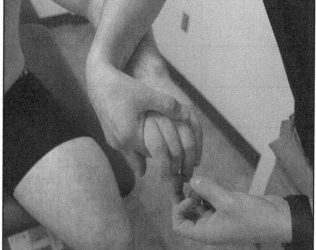

Figure 4-20. Hoffmann reflex.

measures help confirm or reject a hypothesis and/or support clinical decisions regarding diagnosis, prognosis, and the plan of care. The following is from a list of test and measure categories for the *Guide to Physical Therapist Practice*[2]:

- Aerobic Capacity/Endurance
- Balance
- Cranial and Peripheral Nerve Integrity
- Joint Integrity and Mobility
- Mental Functions
- Mobility (Including Locomotion)
- Motor Function
- Muscle Performance (Including Strength, Power, Endurance, and Length)
- Posture
- ROM
- Reflex Integrity
- Sensory Integrity
- Skeletal Integrity

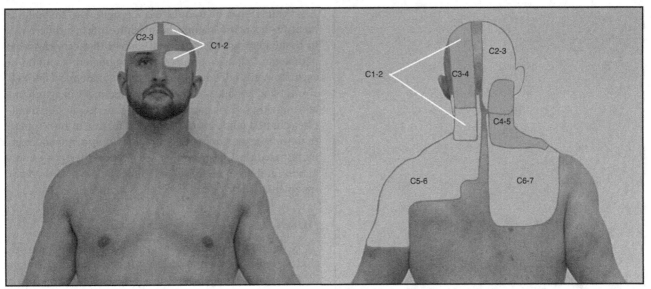

Figure 4-21. Facet joint referral patterns.

Palpation

Patient Position: Variable

Various texts recommend performing palpation early in the physical examination sequence. However, from clinical experience, early palpation can cause irritation, possibly altering the results of the remaining physical examination components. Regardless, layer palpation should be performed, which means the examiner works from superficial to deeper tissues. Any change in contour (ie, lump, bump, or lesion) should be brought to the patient's attention. Follow-up questions include determining whether their physician is aware of the lump and if there has been any change to it. Palpate in a systematic fashion the UQ soft tissues and bony structures. Knowledge of UQ lymph nodes and arteries is also important. In general, during palpation ask the patient if there is any discomfort or change in symptoms. The grading scale below can be used to quantify palpation.

- Grade 1 = Tenderness
- Grade 2 = Tenderness with flinch
- Grade 3 = Severe tenderness, withdrawal
- Grade 4 = Hyperalgesia

UPPER QUARTER REFERRAL PATTERNS

For the purposes of this chapter and inconsistent use of definitions regarding referral patterns, it is important to begin by defining relevant terminology.[15,16] Referred pain can be either somatic or viscerogenic and is defined as pain perceived in an area of the body separate from the location of the actual source.[17] Common somatic pain generators include facet (zygapophyseal) joints, IVDs, and muscle tissue. Viscerogenic referred pain is believed to be a result of multisegmental innervation and direct pressure/shared pathways.[16]

Radicular pain is due to a direct irritation of the nerve root and is not considered a type of referred pain.

Referred Pain—Facet Joints

Facet joints are innervated spinal synovial joints and a known structure to produce somatic referred pain (Figure 4-21). Facet joints as a pain generator is common with more than 50% of patients with cervical spine pain and more than 40% of patients with thoracic spine pain having at least one symptomatic facet joint.[18,19] Referral of pain beyond the upper arm, especially below the elbow, would likely rule out facet joint as a cause of the patient's pain.[18]

Published evidence to best distinguish facet joint pain from other causes from subjective examination findings is lacking.[20] A review of the literature concluded that the clinical presentation of cervical facet joint pain is similar to other axial neck pain etiologies with the main clinical feature being pain, which may radiate to the occiput, the shoulders, or midscapular region.[20] From clinical experience, patients are typically older (50 years or older), describe pain as worse in end-range extension, and abolished in flexion.

A clinical decision guide (CDG)[21] has been developed, which can help rule in or out cervical facet joint as the cause of symptoms for patients with a chief complain of neck pain. The CDG includes the following physical examination findings:

- PST: Reproduction of familiar pain/tenderness with palpation of segmental musculature (patient in prone)
- Manual spinal extension: Reproduction of familiar pain with a posterior to anterior force (patient in prone)
- Extension-rotation test: Reproduction of familiar pain with active end-range extension, followed by rotation (patient seated)

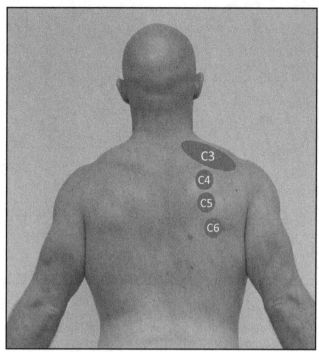

Figure 4-22. IVD referral patterns.

If each test is positive, the CDG increases the posttest probability from 42% to 78%. Conversely, the negative result for PST is good for ruling out the facet joint as the cause of the patient's pain due to its low negative likelihood ratio (0.08 [95% confidence interval (CI), 0.03 to 0.24]). That is, a negative result for the PST reduces the posttest probability of a diagnosis of facet joint pain from 42% to 5%. Although this CDG was developed for patients with neck pain, it may be plausible to adapt this guide for patients with thoracic spine pain; however, it is important to note that this CDG has yet to be validated in any population.[21]

Referred Pain—Intervertebral Disk

Referral of pain from IVDs (also known as the *Cloward sign*) is well documented. Mapping of cervical IVD referral patterns is established (Figure 4-22), and although referral patterns of thoracic IVD have not been mapped, it is believed to be a pain generator.[22-24] It is important to note this is somatic referred pain from the IVD itself, not impingement upon the nerve root (ie, radiculopathy).[15]

Somatic structures, such as facet joints and IVD, which are innervated by the same spinal segment, result in neural convergence of afferent nociception, making differentiation between structures difficult.[17] Therefore, because the goal of the examination is to make a physical therapist diagnosis and begin treatment, if it is determined that the source of the patient's symptoms is appropriate for physical therapist intervention (ie, musculoskeletal), then differentiating the anatomical source of pain is not required.

While it may be useful from a prognosis standpoint to identify the pathoanatomical structure due to differences in tissue healing time, it is well known that cervical spine pathological changes observed on imaging are common in asymptomatic individuals, making pathoanatomical findings suspect and less likely to help guide treatment in symptomatic individuals.[25] As musculoskeletal experts, physical therapists can best guide examination and treatment by response to movement and/or loading, which is congruent with treatment-based classifications that use physical therapist examination findings to establish and guide the physical therapist treatment plan.[26,27]

Referred Pain—Muscular

Common terminology to describe muscular pain includes *myofascial pain*, *myofascial trigger points*, or simply *trigger point*. A trigger point is a palpable tender spot in a taut band of skeletal muscle that produces pain in a predictable referral pattern and a local twitch response.[28,29] Unfortunately, the definition of a trigger point is inconsistent, therefore making comparisons in the literature regarding diagnostic criteria difficult.[29] In addition, locating trigger points via palpation, the main tool advocated for identifying these structures, has been found to have marginal to poor reliability, even after training.[30,31]

Although the authors of this chapter are speculating, trigger points may be a sign of nervous system irritability, similar to neural tension testing, as opposed to a local tissue issue. It appears palpation of the irritable tissue may refer pain consistent with its innervation. For example, the purported infraspinatus muscle trigger point referral pattern is consistent with the C5-C6 dermatome distribution.[28] The infraspinatus is innervated by the suprascapular nerve, which arises from the superior trunk of the brachial plexus, consisting of C5 and C6.[10]

Referred Pain—Viscerogenic

Although the abdomen is often associated with the lower quarter examination, abdominal structures must be included as a potential source of UQ pain due to referral patterns. Viscerogenic referred pain is believed to be a result of 3 mechanisms. First, embryologic development is believed to play a role. For example, during human embryonic development, the pericardium is formed in the gut, which may help explain why a myocardial infarction can refer pain to the abdomen.[16] Second, there is multisegmental innervation of viscera, resulting in overlap with somatic structures that share the same spinal afferent pathway, a concept known as *visceral-organ cross-sensitization*.[16] Last, viscerogenic referred pain can be caused by direct pressure of an inflamed visceral structure on the respiratory diaphragm.[16] The respiratory diaphragm is innervated by the phrenic nerve (C3-C5), which shares common innervation with the shoulder. Refer to Figure 4-23 for common viscerogenic referral sites.

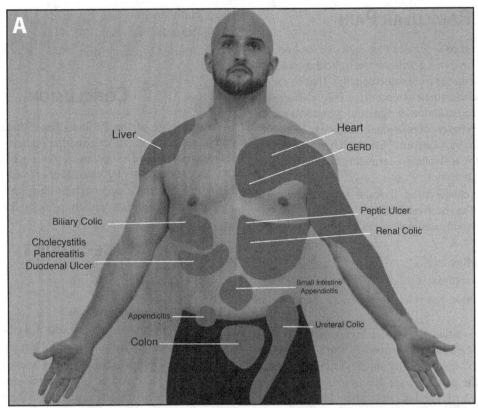

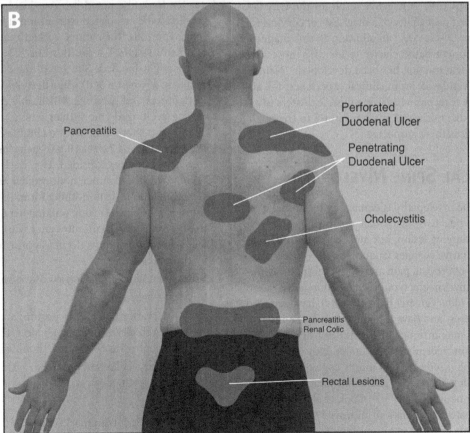

Figure 4-23. Viscerogenic.

RADICULAR PAIN

It is important to recognize that radicular and referred pain are not synonymous. Furthermore, radicular pain must be further differentiated from radiculopathy. That is, radicular pain is limited to a single symptom (ie, pain), whereas radiculopathy is a constellation of signs and symptoms including diminished reflexes, dermatomal numbness, myotomal weakness, and can include pain.[15] Sensory change associated with radiculopathy will follow a dermatomal pattern, whereas radicular pain does not.[15,32]

A diagnostic cluster using clinical tests to identify cervical radiculopathy has been established.[33] The cluster includes the following physical examination findings:

- Positive ULTT-A
- Positive Spurling test
- Positive distraction test
- Cervical rotation less than 60 degrees to the ipsilateral side

If all 4 are positive, the cluster increases the posttest probability from 23% to 90%. Conversely, the ULTT-A (median bias) is a good test for ruling out cervical radiculopathy as the cause of the patient's pain due to its high sensitivity (.97 [95% CI, 0.9 to 1]) and small negative likelihood ratio (.12 [95% CI, .01 to 1.9]). A negative result for the ULTT-A reduces the posttest probability of a diagnosis of cervical radiculopathy from 23% to 3%.[33] In addition to this diagnostic cluster, a treatment-based cluster to identify those who benefit from cervical traction has been developed.[34] Neither cluster has been validated. From clinical experience, the authors of this chapter recommend using these 2 clusters to aid your differential diagnosis and guide response to treatment if cervical radiculopathy is suspected.

CERVICAL SPINE MYELOPATHY

Cervical spine myelopathy is damage to the spinal cord via compression due to spinal canal narrowing (stenosis) from a space-occupying lesion, but most commonly associated with degenerative changes (spondylosis).[35] When compared to all cases of cervical pain and dysfunction, individuals with cervical myelopathy typically have a longer duration of symptoms, are older (greater than 45 years), have reduced quality of life scores, and have a higher body mass index.[36] Possible findings may include chief complaint of neck stiffness; shoulder pain; radicular signs; upper extremity weakness and/or atrophy; reduced fine motor control; as well as lower extremity deficits such as gait abnormality, weakness, and upper motor neuron signs.[13,37,38] Cook et al[36] found that the following cluster combination improved the ability to identify those with cervical spine myelopathy (3 of 5 present = positive likelihood ratio of 30.9; [95% CI, 5.5 to 181.8]):

- Age great than 45 years
- Gait deviation
- + Hoffmann test
- + Babinski test
- + Inverted supinator sign

CONCLUSION

Knowledge of the Patient/Client Management Model and its subcomponents can assist clinicians with organizing their examination. The systems review is a basic examination that all patients seen by physical therapists should receive. Using this systematic approach can help the physical therapist avoid missing a pain pattern associated with pathology.

CASE STUDIES

Case Study One

Patient: 27-year-old woman

Chief complaint: 3-month history of elbow pain

- Subjective examination—Medical history: Unremarkable
- Subjective examination—Patient interview: The patient was seen via direct access with the chief complaint of right elbow pain (patient pointed to the common extensor tendon). She noted it began insidiously and that it seemed to be associated with sitting at her desk for prolonged periods. The patient worked as an office associate at a dentist's office, a position she has held for 3 years, and is right-handed. She rated her current pain 0/10 and pain at worst a 6/10 while describing her symptoms as tightness and burning, which only occurred at work during prolonged (more than 1 hour) sitting. Position change or a short walk used to eliminate her symptoms; however, the past 2 weeks it has been closer to 1 hour before her symptoms subsided. Two weeks ago, she began taking over-the-counter nonsteroidal anti-inflammatories, which do little to nothing for managing her symptoms. Her hobbies include walking her 6-month-old son in his stroller for 30 minutes after work and gardening. Her current symptoms do not appear to be aggravated by these activities.
- Subjective examination—Review of systems: Unremarkable
- Physical examination
  - ° Observation, including posture and gross symmetry: Well-developed female, no visible asymmetries or atrophy. Head forward, shoulders rounded.
  - ° Cardiovascular and pulmonary: Unremarkable
  - ° Gait and balance: Unremarkable
  - ° Gross ROM
    - AROM: Unremarkable
    - PROM including overpressures: Unremarkable

- ◦ Neurological
  - ▪ Dermatomes: WNL
  - ▪ Myotomes: WNL
  - ▪ Reflexes
    - ◻ DTR
      - ➤ Biceps: 2
      - ➤ Brachioradialis: 2
      - ➤ Triceps: 2
    - ◻ Upper motor neuron
      - ➤ Hoffmann reflex: Normal (absent)
  - ▪ Upper limb tension testing: Positive radial bias on right, reproducing the patient's symptoms
  - ▪ CN examination: Not tested
  - ◦ Palpation: Unremarkable, including the right common extensor tendon and muscle bellies
- Physical examination—Additional tests and measures
  - ◦ MMT: Upper extremities 5/5, strong and painless bilaterally
  - ◦ Accessory motion: Cervical spine posterior to anterior mobilizations revealed hypomobility and increased tenderness of C5-C6. All other joints were unremarkable.

Discussion

- What is the differential diagnosis in this case?
  - ◦ Lateral epicondylitis (tennis elbow)
  - ◦ Radial nerve neural tension
- What factors in the patient history and physical examination led the clinician to the previous differential diagnoses?
  - ◦ Lateral epicondylitis (tennis elbow): Location of symptoms, possible association with repetitive work
  - ◦ Radial nerve neural tension: Reproduction of symptoms with radial nerve bias neural tension test, hypomobility, and pain with C5-C6 accessory motion testing, and poor sitting posture
- What is the plan of action for this patient (clinical decision-making process)?
  - ◦ Treat
- Why?
  - ◦ The patient does not present with red flags that would prevent initiating treatment. It was hypothesized that the patient's symptoms were due to cervical spine hypermobility and neural tension. The radial nerve travels laterally along the elbow, deep to the common extensor tendon. Radial nerve bias neural tension testing reproduced the patient's symptoms. The patient has a history of work that involves prolonged sitting; positive findings with cervical spine accessory motion testing and observation revealed poor sitting posture. Treatment included cervical spine mobilizations to C5-C6,

including mobilization with the patient positioned in the same manner used to test radial nerve neural tension.[39] Also, home exercise plan of neural tension mobilizations as described by Butler, as well as posture correction education.[12]

Case Study Two

Patient: 57-year-old man

Chief complaint: 6-month history of neck and right shoulder pain

- Subjective examination—Medical history: High BP, managed by medication
- Subjective examination—Patient interview: The patient reported his primary care physician diagnosed him with osteoarthritis, confirmed by radiographs, and referred him for physical therapist evaluation. He is left-handed and works as a business executive. He reported an insidious onset but has no history of neck and/or shoulder pain. His pain is located along the right lower cervical spine and right shoulder diffusely. He rated his current pain 3/10 and his pain at worst an 8/10. He noted the last few weeks his left shoulder has been painful in the morning as well, at worst a 2/10. He described his symptoms as a dull pain with stiffness in the morning. The stiffness is abolished after about 30 minutes, but the pain remains throughout the workday. He has difficulty sleeping due to the pain but sleeps through the night once he falls asleep. He is taking a prescription opioid (Tramadol). His hobbies were walking up to 5 miles per day, golfing, and swimming. Due to his chief complaint, he had to decrease his walking to 1 to 2 miles and he stopped golfing.
- Subjective examination—Review of systems: Change in balance
- Physical examination
  - ◦ Observation, including posture and gross symmetry: Head forward, shoulders rounded, and increased upper thoracic kyphosis
  - ◦ Cardiovascular and pulmonary: Unremarkable
  - ◦ Gait: Patient ambulated independently, wide base of support. Further questioning reveals a change in balance and numerous near falls over the past 6 months. The patient did not report this during the review of systems.
  - ◦ Gross ROM
    - ▪ AROM
      - ◻ Global limitations of cervical spine, most significant in extension
      - ◻ Bilateral upper extremities within functional limits and symmetrical

- PROM including overpressures
  - PROM with overpressure into neck extension reproduced patient's neck and shoulder pain
  - Bilateral upper extremities within functional limits and symmetrical
- Neurological
  - Dermatomes: Decreased sensation to light touch C4 and C5 bilaterally
  - Myotomes: Diminished strength C5 and C6 bilaterally
  - Reflexes
    - DTR
      - Biceps: 3
      - Brachioradialis: 3
      - Triceps: 2
    - Upper motor neuron
      - Hoffmann reflex: Abnormal (present)
  - Upper limb tension testing: Median bias positive bilaterally
  - CN exam: Normal
- Palpation: Diffuse cervical spine grade I tenderness
- Physical examination—Additional tests and measures
  - Upper extremity MMT
    - Deltoid: 4-/5 bilaterally
    - Biceps: 4-/5 bilaterally
  - Cluster due to suspicion for cervical radiculopathy
    - Positive ULTT-A: Positive
    - Positive Spurling test: Positive for neck pain
    - Positive distraction test: Positive for relief of neck pain
    - Cervical rotation less than 60 degrees to the ipsilateral side: Positive
  - Cluster due to suspicion for cervical myelopathy
    - Age more than 45 years: Positive
    - Gait deviation: Positive
    - + Hoffmann test: Positive
    - + Babinski test: Not tested
    - + Inverted supinator sign: Not tested

Discussion

- What is the differential diagnosis in this case?
  - Cervical spine and shoulder osteoarthritis
  - Cervical radiculopathy
  - Cervical myelopathy

- What factors in the patient history and physical examination led the clinician to the previous differential diagnoses?
  - Cervical spine and shoulder osteoarthritis: Age, morning stiffness improved within 60 minutes of awakening
  - Cervical radiculopathy
    - Cluster for suspicion of cervical radiculopathy revealed 3 of the 4 tests as positive
    - Dermatomes: Decreased sensation to light touch C5 bilaterally
    - Myotomes: Diminished strength C5 and C6 bilaterally
  - Cervical myelopathy
    - Cluster for suspicion of cervical myelopathy revealed 3 of the 5 tests as positive
- What is the plan of action for this patient (clinical decision-making process)?
  - Refer
- Why?
  - Although the patient had signs and symptoms of osteoarthritis and cervical radiculopathy, his presentation is most consistent with cervical myelopathy. Cervical myelopathy is damage to the spinal cord via compression due to spinal canal narrowing (stenosis), which due to the patient's age, was most likely caused by degeneration (spondylosis). This most likely explains why the patient presented with morning stiffness that improved within 60 minutes of awakening and that he had relief with the distraction test. However, due to the positive upper motor neuron signs, the patient needs to be evaluated by a neurosurgeon or orthopedic surgeon prior to physical therapist intervention. If the patient is cleared for conservative care, then the physical therapist can initiate treatment. Recommended treatments for this condition include intermittent cervical traction, thoracic spine high-velocity, low-amplitude manipulation, posture education, balance training, and therapeutic exercise.[40,41]

REFERENCES

1. Murphy DR, Hurwitz EL. A theoretical model for the development of a diagnosis-based clinical decision rule for the management of patients with spinal pain. *BMC Musculoskelet Disord*. 2007;8:75. doi:10.1186/1471-2474-8-75

2. American Physical Therapy Association. *Guide to Physical Therapist Practice 3.0*. 2014. Accessed November 12, 2021. http://guidetoptpractice.apta.org/

3. Jensen JD, Elewski BE. The ABCDEF rule: combining the "ABCDE rule" and the "ugly duckling sign" in an effort to improve patient self-screening examinations. *J Clin Aesthetic Dermatol*. 2015;8(2):15.

4. VanWye WR, Boissonnault WG. Primary Care for the Physical Therapist: Examination and Triage. 3rd ed. Elsevier/Saunders; 2020.

5. Liguori G, Feito Y, Fountaine C, Roy BA, eds; American College of Sports Medicine. *ACSM's Guidelines for Exercise Testing and Prescription*. 11th ed. Wolters Kluwer Health/Lippincott Williams & Wilkins; 2021.

6. Hillegass E. *Essentials of Cardiopulmonary Physical Therapy*. 5th ed. Elsevier; 2022.

7. Jordan CL, Rhon DI. Differential diagnosis and management of ankylosing spondylitis masked as adhesive capsulitis: a resident's case problem. *J Orthop Sports Phys Ther*. 2012;42(10):842-852. doi:10.2519/jospt.2012.4050

8. Cook G, Burton L, Hoogenboom B. Pre-participation screening: the use of fundamental movements as an assessment of function—part 2. *N Am J Sports Phys Ther*. 2006;1(3):132-139.

9. Kibler WB, Sciascia A, Wilkes T. Scapular dyskinesis and its relation to shoulder injury. *J Am Acad Orthop Surg*. 2012;20(6):364-372. doi:10.5435/JAAOS-20-06-364

10. Moore KL, Dalley AF, Agur AMR. *Clinically Oriented Anatomy*. 7th ed. Wolters Kluwer Health/Lippincott Williams & Wilkins; 2014.

11. Jarvis C. *Physical Examination & Health Assessment*. 7th ed. Elsevier; 2016.

12. Butler DS. *The Sensitive Nervous System*. Noigroup Publications; 2000.

13. Cook CE, Hegedus E, Pietrobon R, Goode A. A pragmatic neurological screen for patients with suspected cord compressive myelopathy. *Phys Ther*. 2007;87(9):1233-1242. doi:10.2522/ptj.20060150

14. Cook C, Roman M, Stewart KM, Leithe LG, Isaacs R. Reliability and diagnostic accuracy of clinical special tests for myelopathy in patients seen for cervical dysfunction. *J Orthop Sports Phys Ther*. 2009;39(3):172-178. doi:10.2519/jospt.2009.2938

15. Bogduk N. On the definitions and physiology of back pain, referred pain, and radicular pain. *PAIN*. 2009;147(1-3):17-19. doi:10.1016/j.pain.2009.08.020

16. Heick J, Lazaro RT. *Goodman and Snyder's Differential Diagnosis for Physical Therapists: Screening for Referral*. 7th ed. Elsevier; 2022.

17. International Association for the Study of Pain. *Classification of Chronic Pain, Second Edition (Revised)*. Updated 2011. Accessed November 12, 2021. http://www.iasp-pain.org/PublicationsNews/Content.aspx?ItemNumber=1673

18. Cooper G, Bailey B, Bogduk N. Cervical zygapophysial joint pain maps. *Pain Med*. 2007;8(4):344-353. doi:10.1111/j.1526-4637.2006.00201.x

19. Manchikanti L, Boswell MV, Singh V, Pampati V, Damron KS, Beyer CD. Prevalence of facet joint pain in chronic spinal pain of cervical, thoracic, and lumbar regions. *BMC Musculoskelet Disord*. 2004;5:15. doi:10.1186/1471-2474-5-15

20. Kirpalani D, Mitra R. Cervical facet joint dysfunction: a review. *Arch Phys Med Rehabil*. 2008;89(4):770-774. doi:10.1016/j.apmr.2007.11.028

21. Schneider GM, Jull G, Thomas K, et al. Derivation of a clinical decision guide in the diagnosis of cervical facet joint pain. *Arch Phys Med Rehabil*. 2014;95(9):1695-1701. doi:10.1016/j.apmr.2014.02.026

22. Cloward RB. Cervical diskography: a contribution to the etiology and mechanism of neck, shoulder and arm pain. *Ann Surg*. 1959;150(6):1052-1064.

23. Manchikanti L, Dunbar EE, Wargo BW, Shah RV, Derby R, Cohen SP. Systematic review of cervical discography as a diagnostic test for chronic spinal pain. *Pain Physician*. 2009;12(2):305-321.

24. Schellhas KP, Pollei SR, Dorwart RH. Thoracic discography. A safe and reliable technique. *Spine*. 1994;19(18):2103-2109.

25. Nakashima H, Yukawa Y, Suda K, Yamagata M, Ueta T, Kato F. Abnormal findings on magnetic resonance images of the cervical spines in 1211 asymptomatic subjects. *Spine*. 2015;40(6):392-398. doi:10.1097/BRS.0000000000000775

26. Childs JD, Fritz JM, Piva SR, Whitman JM. Proposal of a classification system for patients with neck pain. *J Orthop Sports Phys Ther*. 2004;34(11):686-700. doi:10.2519/jospt.2004.34.11.686

27. Fritz JM, Brennan GP. Preliminary examination of a proposed treatment-based classification system for patients receiving physical therapy interventions for neck pain. *Phys Ther*. 2007;87(5):513-524. doi:10.2522/ptj.20060192

28. Simons DG, Travell JG, Simons LS, Travell JG. *Travell & Simons' Myofascial Pain and Dysfunction: The Trigger Point Manual*. Williams & Wilkins; 1999.

29. Tough EA, White AR, Richards S, Campbell J. Variability of criteria used to diagnose myofascial trigger point pain syndrome--evidence from a review of the literature. *Clin J Pain*. 2007;23(3):278-286. doi:10.1097/AJP.0b013e31802fda7c

30. Hsieh CY, Hong CZ, Adams AH, et al. Interexaminer reliability of the palpation of trigger points in the trunk and lower limb muscles. *Arch Phys Med Rehabil*. 2000;81(3):258-264.

31. Myburgh C, Larsen AH, Hartvigsen J. A systematic, critical review of manual palpation for identifying myofascial trigger points: evidence and clinical significance. *Arch Phys Med Rehabil*. 2008;89(6):1169-1176. doi:10.1016/j.apmr.2007.12.033

32. Murphy DR, Hurwitz EL, Gerrard JK, Clary R. Pain patterns and descriptions in patients with radicular pain: does the pain necessarily follow a specific dermatome? *Chiropr Osteopat*. 2009;17:9. doi:10.1186/1746-1340-17-9

33. Wainner RS, Fritz JM, Irrgang JJ, Boninger ML, Delitto A, Allison S. Reliability and diagnostic accuracy of the clinical examination and patient self-report measures for cervical radiculopathy. *Spine*. 2003;28(1):52-62. doi:10.1097/01.BRS.0000038873.01855.50

34. Raney NH, Petersen EJ, Smith TA, et al. Development of a clinical prediction rule to identify patients with neck pain likely to benefit from cervical traction and exercise. *Eur Spine J*. 2009;18(3):382-391. doi:10.1007/s00586-008-0859-7

35. Kong L-D, Meng L-C, Wang L-F, Shen Y, Wang P, Shang Z-K. Evaluation of conservative treatment and timing of surgical intervention for mild forms of cervical spondylotic myelopathy. *Exp Ther Med*. 2013;6(3):852-856. doi:10.3892/etm.2013.1224

36. Cook C, Brown C, Isaacs R, Roman M, Davis S, Richardson W. Clustered clinical findings for diagnosis of cervical spine myelopathy. *J Man Manip Ther*. 2010;18(4):175-180. doi:10.1179/106698110X12804993427045

37. Bednarik J, Kadanka Z, Dusek L, et al. Presymptomatic spondylotic cervical myelopathy: an updated predictive model. *Eur Spine J*. 2008;17(3):421-431. doi:10.1007/s00586-008-0585-1

38. Harrop JS, Hanna A, Silva MT, Sharan A. Neurological manifestations of cervical spondylosis: an overview of signs, symptoms, and pathophysiology. *Neurosurgery*. 2007;60(1 suppl 1):S14-S20. doi:10.1227/01.NEU.0000215380.71097.EC

39. Vicenzino B, Collins D, Wright A. The initial effects of a cervical spine manipulative physiotherapy treatment on the pain and dysfunction of lateral epicondylalgia. *Pain*. 1996;68(1):69-74.

40. Browder DA, Erhard RE, Piva SR. Intermittent cervical traction and thoracic manipulation for management of mild cervical compressive myelopathy attributed to cervical herniated disc: a case series. *J Orthop Sports Phys Ther*. 2004;34(11):701-712. doi:10.2519/jospt.2004.34.11.701.

41. Almeida GPL, Carneiro KKA, Marques AP. Manual therapy and therapeutic exercise in patient with symptomatic cervical spondylotic myelopathy: a case report. *J Bodyw Mov Ther*. 2013;17(4):504-509. doi:10.1016/j.jbmt.2013.03.009.

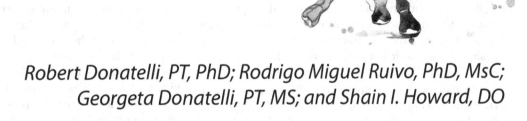

Normal Mechanics, Dysfunction, Evaluation, and Treatment of the Shoulder

Robert Donatelli, PT, PhD; Rodrigo Miguel Ruivo, PhD, MsC;
Georgeta Donatelli, PT, MS; and Shain I. Howard, DO

KEY TERMS

Arthrokinematics: Is the roll, spin, and slide of the convex joint surface on a concave joint surface

Force couple: Is a biomechanical term where by 2 or more muscles are acting in different directions causing a rotation movement. When the forces are of equal magnitude and in opposite directions, the limb will rotate around its long axis.

Linear joint: Is a joint that moves in a straight line (eg, the knee joint moves in a straight line of flexion and extension).

Osteokinematics: Is the movement of the bone in different body planes

Plane of the scapula (POS): Is movement of the shoulder into abduction that is 30 degrees anterior to the frontal plane.

CHAPTER QUESTIONS

1. What are the mechanics of shoulder elevation?
2. What is a linear joint?
3. What is a force couple?
4. What are the force couples in the shoulder?
5. What does dynamic stabilization mean?
6. What is the POS and what is its clinical significance?
7. What are the arthrokinematics of the glenohumeral (GH) joint?
8. What are the 7 rotation tests?
9. What are the stages of adhesive capsulitis?
10. What is the etiology of adhesive capsulitis?
11. What is the recommended treatment for adhesive capsulitis?
12. What muscles make-up the scapula force couple?
13. What muscles make-up the GH force couple?
14. What is the treatment to restore shoulder mobility in an adhesive capsulitis patient?
15. What are the surgical considerations for postoperative rotator cuff tears (RCTs)?
16. What is the recommended treatment approach to post-operative rotator cuff surgery?
17. What is the recommended treatment approach to post-operative shoulder instability surgery?
18. What exercises isolate the rotator cuff and scapula rotators?
19. What is a superior labral anterior to posterior (SLAP) lesion?
20. What is a Bankart lesion?

Wallmann HW, Donatelli R, eds. *Foundations of*
Orthopedic Physical Therapy (pp 127-151).
© 2024 Taylor & Francis Group.

FUNCTIONAL ANATOMY AND MECHANICS: EVALUATION AND PATHOPHYSIOLOGY OF THE SHOULDER

The shoulder joint is one of the most misunderstood and mistreated joints in the body. Restoring passive and active elevation is the major goal in rehabilitation of the shoulder. To restore mobility of the shoulder, the rehabilitation specialist must have an in-depth understanding of the shoulder joint mechanics, muscle function, and be able to perform a detailed evaluation in order to develop an effective treatment program. This chapter describes the relevant functional anatomy and mechanics of the shoulder complex and how it relates to improving functional activities and dynamic stability. The chapter also includes a review of the stiff and painful shoulder and surgical intervention in the case of RCTs and instability. This chapter is not a traditional chapter in that it is a clinical chapter written by clinicians. Therefore, the detailed biomechanical discussions will emphasize a clinical application, not necessarily detailed joint mechanics. For example, the most important biomechanical principal of the shoulder is that it is a rotation joint, which has 2 force couples.

The shoulder joint complex is described as a series of articulations moving together to allow normal shoulder function. Most authors, when describing the shoulder joints, include the acromioclavicular (AC) joint, sternoclavicular (SC) joint, scapulothoracic, and GH joint.[1-4] Dempster relates the integrated and harmonious roles of all of the links are necessary for full normal mobility.[5] The GH joint sacrifices stability for mobility. The shoulder is capable of moving in more than 16,000 planes of elevation if we differentiated 1 degree per plane in a normal person because of the inherit laxity of the GH joint.[6] The static stabilizers of the shoulder are often insufficient in providing restraints to prevent and control excessive movements at the joint. In light of this inherit laxity, the shoulder relies on dynamic stabilization for stability throughout all shoulder movements. The term *Dynamic stabilization* is defined in this chapter as the synchronized firing of muscles that surround the scapula and GH joint during all shoulder movements. The normal forces that are created around the shoulder joint during active movement include shearing, distractive, and compressive forces. The forces that are most important in establishing dynamic stabilization are the compressive forces that hold the head of the humerus on the glenoid. These compressive forces are a result of a coordinated contraction of the rotator cuff muscles and the scapula rotators, which help to stabilize the scapula allowing a precise centering of the humeral head within the glenoid fossa.[7]

As the shoulder moves into elevation, the compressive forces that pull the head of the humerus into the glenoid joint surface are an important part of normal joint mechanics. These forces counteract the shearing and distractive forces, which can cause impingement and instability. Unlike other joints where compressive forces are considered to enhance degenerative changes, the shoulder relies on compressive forces for dynamic stabilization and normal function.

The rotator cuff muscles have been described as primary dynamic stabilizers of the GH joint; the contraction of the rotator cuff muscles generates a compression force between the glenoid fossa and the humeral head.[8,9] The subscapularis, supraspinatus, infraspinatus, and teres minor muscles work to pull the humeral head into the glenoid and have significantly higher muscle activity during shoulder elevation, which might reflect their greater role as a humeral head stabilizer.[10]

ARTHROKINEMATIC MOVEMENT

The small surface area of the glenoid requires that the head of the humerus implement arthrokinematic movements, of which there are 3 types: rolling, gliding, and spinning. These movements of the humeral head are motions that are necessary for the large humeral head to take advantage of the small glenoid articular surface.[11] Effective arthrokinematic movements are achieved by the dynamic action of the rotator cuff muscles that actually create the arthrokinematic movements. There is a 1.5-mm movement of the humeral head in superior/inferior directions with a rotation (spin) of 3 mm.[12]

> ### Clinical Note
>
> The large humeral head articulates on a small glenoid through proper arthrokinematics, which is a rolling, sliding, and spinning of the humeral head. The normal arthrokinematics are generated by the action of the rotator cuff muscles along with good extensibility of the capsule.

OSTEOKINEMATIC MOVEMENT

Analysis of shoulder movement traditionally emphasizes the synchronized movement of 4 joints: the GH, scapulothoracic, SC, and AC joints.[2,4,11,13] Osteokinematics are traditionally described as movement of the arm occurring in 1 of 4 traditional body planes: the frontal plane (abduction), sagittal plane (flexion), transverse plane (horizontal abduction/adduction), and elevation in the POS (30 degrees anterior to the frontal plane).[11,13]

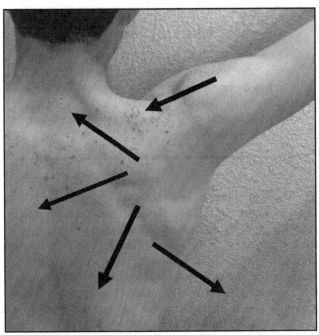

Figure 5-1. Force couple of the scapula.

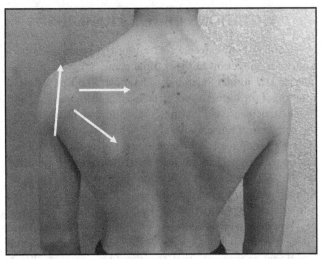

Figure 5-2. Force couple of the GH joint.

Plane of the Scapula

Scaption-Abduction

The most functional movement of the shoulder into elevation is the POS, which is part of all functional movements overhead. Abduction of the shoulder in the frontal or coronal plane has been extensively researched.[4,11,12,14-19] Poppen and Walker[18] and Johnston[14] advocate that the true plane of shoulder abduction is in the POS. The POS is defined as elevation of the shoulder in a range between 30 and 45 degrees anterior to the frontal plane.[14] For the purposes of this chapter, we define the POS as 30 degrees anterior to the frontal plane. Several authors have demonstrated that the POS is clinically significant because the length-tension relationship of the external rotators is optimum in this plane.[14,20] Maximum tension within a normal muscle is developed when the muscle length is approximately 90% of its maximum.[21] Conversely, when the muscle is fully shortened, the tension developed is minimal.[21,22] Therefore, the optimal lengthened position of the muscle will facilitate peak muscle contraction. The rotator cuff muscles are dependent on length tension, which is an essential component to the development of muscle strength.[23]

Several studies have compared the torque production of different shoulder muscle groups when tested in POS vs other body planes.[23-25] Soderberg and Blaschak[24] and Hellwig and Perrin[15] demonstrated no significant differences in the peak torque of the GH rotators between POS and 45 degrees anterior to the frontal plane, the sagittal plane, in neutral (adducted position), and at 90 degrees of abduction. The results indicated that there was no significant difference in

the strength of the rotator cuff. However, Greenfield and Donatelli reported greater torque production of the external rotators when tested in the POS, 30 degrees anterior to the frontal plane vs the coronal plane.[20] Furthermore, Tata and colleagues[25] reported higher ratios of external to internal torque when tested in the POS, 35 degrees anterior to the frontal plane.

In addition to optimal muscle length-tension relationship in the POS, the capsular fibers of the GH joint are under no strain.[14] If the capsule is under less strain in the POS, mobilization and low-load prolonged stretch (LLPS) in the POS may be tolerated better than in other planes. Clinically, the POS may be an advantageous plane for mobilization, LLPS, and strengthening of the GH joint.

THE MECHANICS OF SHOULDER ELEVATION

One of the most important biomechanical principles of shoulder elevation is that the shoulder is not a linear joint. *Linear motion*, also referred to as *rectilinear motion*, is a motion along a straight line and can therefore be described mathematically using only one spatial dimension.[26] An example of linear motion is an athlete running 500 m along a straight track.[26] There is no one muscle in the shoulder that can elevate the arm in the linear motion of elevation. Shoulder elevation is dependent upon 2 force couples, which are surrounding the scapula and GH joint.

A force couple is a biomechanical principle "whereby two or more muscles acting in different directions influence the rotation of a joint in a specific direction. When the forces are of equal magnitude and in opposite directions, the limb will rotate about its long axis."[26] There are 2 force couples in the shoulder: the scapula (Figure 5-1) and the GH joint (Figure 5-2).

ROTATIONS OF THE HUMERUS

Concomitant external rotation of the humerus is necessary for abduction in the coronal plane.[4,11,12,17,20] Using cadaveric GH joints, Rajendran[27] demonstrated that external rotation of the humerus occurred even in the absence of soft tissue structures such as the coracohumeral ligament and the rotator cuff muscles. An et al[28] used a magnetic tracking system to monitor the 3-dimensional movement of the humerus with respect to the scapula. Ludewig et al[29] reported greater GH joint external rotation with increased humeral thoracic elevation, and that the angle of external rotation of humerus during abduction was larger than that of flexion.

For the purposes of this chapter, restoring external and internal rotation in all planes is necessary for the normal functional movements that the shoulder complex allows. Therefore, loss of external and internal rotation could result in significant functional disability.

Clinical Note

When treating patients with limited passive and active elevation, the clinician should avoid pushing the joint into painful elevation movements. When elevation of the shoulder is limited in any plane, restoring passive external and internal rotation is a safe and effective way of restoring extensibility to the capsule and enhancing active elevation of the shoulder without pain and trauma to the soft tissues.

STATIC STABILIZERS OF THE GLENOHUMERAL JOINT

The static stability of the GH joint also contributes to the stability of the joint. Several soft tissue structures such as the labrum, GH ligaments, and capsular ligaments add to the stability of the GH joint.[30]

The head of the humerus is large in relation to the glenoid fossa. The labrum increases the joint surface of the glenoid 9 mm in the superior-inferior direction and 5 mm in the anteroposterior direction.[31] The GH joint has been described by Matsen and colleagues[32] as a "suction cup" because of the seal of the labrum and glenoid to the humeral head. Compression of the head into the socket, created by the compressive forces of the rotator cuff muscles, expels the synovial fluid to create a suction that resists distraction.

Clinical Note

The head of the humerus needs to sit in a central position on the glenoid. If the head of the humerus is not in a central position, it will reduce dynamic stability by altering the length-tension of the rotator cuff muscles creating a less forceful contraction and poor arthrokinematics.

The coracohumeral ligament is the strongest supporting ligament of the GH joint on the superior aspect of the joint from the coracoid process to the head of the humerus. The rotator cuff interval, the region of the capsule between the border of the supraspinatus and the subscapularis muscle, is reinforced by the coracohumeral ligament.[32,33] The superior GH ligament and the coracohumeral ligament limit external rotation and abduction of the humerus and are important stabilizers in the inferior direction from 0 to 50 degrees abduction.[33,34]

The superior GH ligament forms an anterior cover around the long head of the biceps (LHB) tendon and is also part of the rotator cuff interval.[32] The middle GH ligament blends with portions of the subscapularis. The middle GH ligament has been shown to become taut at 45 degrees abduction, and 10 degrees extension and external rotation, providing anterior stability between 45 degrees and 60 degrees abduction.[33,34]

The inferior GH ligament complex is a hammock-like structure with attachments to the glenoid. The inferior GH ligament complex was found to be the most important stabilizer against anteroinferior shoulder dislocation.[32,34]

The capsule attaches around the glenoid rim and forms a sleeve around the head of the humerus, attaching on the anatomical neck. A functional interdependence exists between the anterior and posterior, and superior and inferior portions of the capsule. This interconnection is referred to as the *circle theory*, which indicates that excessive translation in one direction may produce damage to the capsule on the same and opposite sides of the joint.[35]

Guanche and associates[36] studied the synergistic action of the capsule and the shoulder muscles. A reflex arch was described from mechanoreceptors within the GH capsule to muscles crossing the joint. Stimulation of the anterior and inferior axillary articular nerves elicited electromyographic (EMG) activity in the biceps, subscapularis, supraspinatus, and infraspinatus muscles. Stimulation of the posterior axillary articular nerve elicited EMG activity in the acromio-deltoid muscle. In the early stages of repair, as in a rotator cuff repair, gentle oscillations are capable to stimulate important muscle activation early in rehabilitation.

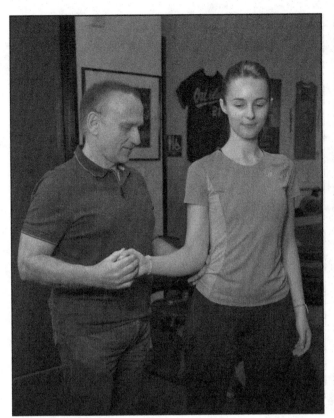

Figure 5-3. Adducted frontal plane.

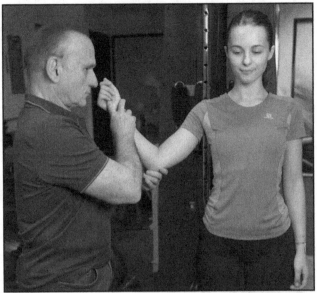

Figure 5-4. 45 degrees of abduction frontal plane.

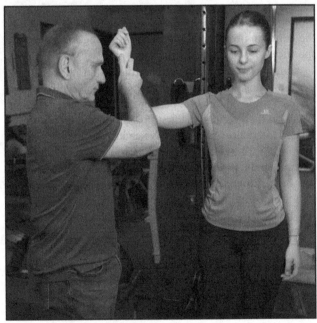

Figure 5-5. 90 degrees of abduction.

DONATELLI SEVEN PASSIVE GLENOHUMERAL ROTATION TESTS

Soft Tissue Restraints and Assessment of Shoulder Mobility

Based on clinical evidence and 4 dissection studies, the senior author on this chapter has developed 7 passive rotation tests to determine soft tissue limitations at the GH joint. Once the capsular and ligamentous restrictions are identified, LLPS and mobilization into the barrier can be more specific.

It is difficult to make a differential soft tissue diagnosis by gross movements of the shoulder overhead. Cadaver dissection is often used as a model to examine soft tissue responses to loads.[37] Several cadaver studies have calculated the mechanical strain on soft tissue structures surrounding the GH joint during passive rotation. Based on several cadaver studies, passive external rotation of the GH joint increases tension on the coracohumeral ligament,[38] the pectoralis major, the LHB,[39] and the subscapularis.

Turkel et al[40] reported that during passive external rotation of the GH joint in the frontal plane at 0 degrees of abduction, the subscapularis muscle is the most important stabilizer of the GH joint (Figure 5-3). At 45 degrees of abduction in the frontal plane, a portion of the subscapularis and the middle GH ligament are the most stabilizing

mechanisms to the anterior capsule (Figure 5-4). At 90 degrees of abduction, the most stabilizing structure of the anterior capsule is the inferior GH ligamentous complex (Figure 5-5). Furthermore, Turkel et al[40] described the inferior GH ligament as the thickest and most consistent structure.

Muraki et al[41] studied the strain on the 3 bellies of the subscapularis muscle during passive external rotation in the POS. Their results demonstrated that passive external rotation in the POS (30 degrees anterior to the frontal plane; Figure 5-6) created a large muscle strain on the upper, middle, and lower fibers of the subscapularis muscle. The previous dissection studies can be useful for clinical application in the assessment of passive rotation range of

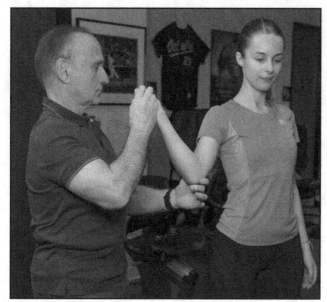

Figure 5-6. POS 30 degrees anterior to the frontal plane.

motion (ROM) restrictions. The assessment may help guide the clinician's treatment approach providing insight of the specificity of soft tissue restrictions.

Izumi et al[42] demonstrated in a dissection study that various positions with the GH joint passively internally rotated placed a strain on different portions of the posterior capsule. Based on their results, the first position of the shoulder was rotated internally at 30 degrees of abduction and in the POS (Figure 5-7). This position was determined to provide a significant strain to the posterior capsule. Then the shoulder was moved into extension with internal rotation causing a significant strain to the posterior capsule (Figure 5-8).

Itoi et al[43] concluded that the LHB and short head of the biceps have similar functions as anterior stabilizers of the GH joint with the arm in abduction and external rotation. Furthermore, the role of the LHB and short head of the biceps increased with shoulder instability. Lastly, Borstad and Dashottar[44] demonstrated in a cadaver study that the most strain to the posterior capsule was with passive internal rotation and flexion at 60 degrees (Figure 5-9). An interesting finding pointed out in both cadaver studies that measure posterior capsular strain was that flexion at 90 degrees and internal rotation did not produce a significant strain on the posterior capsule. At 90 degrees of flexion and internal rotation is referred to as the *sleeper stretch* and is designed to stretch the posterior capsule. This position is also the Hawkins impingement test position, which is positive for pain. Therefore, a better stretch position would be internal rotation at 60 degrees of flexion.

Scapula, Acromioclavicular, and Sternoclavicular Joints

The major muscles that act on the GH joint and the scapulothoracic articulation may be grouped into the

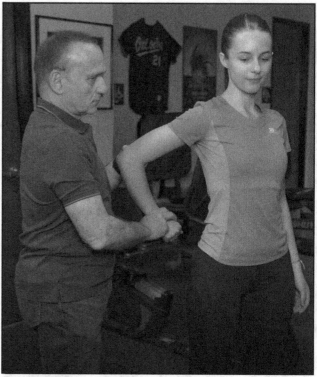

Figure 5-7. Internal rotation and extension.

scapulohumeral muscles, which are the rotator cuff muscles that originate on the scapula and insert on the humerus. The axiohumeral and axioscapular muscles include the muscles of the scapulothoracic area of the shoulder.[45] We have already discussed the role of the rotator cuff and the importance of providing dynamic stabilization to the GH joint. It is important to include the deltoid and the scapula rotators' role in the dynamic stabilization of the shoulder.

The deltoid muscle makes up a large percent of the scapulohumeral muscle mass. The deltoid is a multipennate and fatigue-resistant muscle. This could explain why the deltoid is rarely involved in shoulder pathologic conditions. The deltoid and the rotator cuff muscles produce shearing and compressive forces that vary as the muscle alignment changes.

The scapula is not a synovial joint; it is primarily stabilized by muscles. As noted previously, the muscles around the scapula constitute a true force couple. The importance of the scapula rotators has been established as an essential ingredient to GH mobility and stability. Scapula rotation is described as upward and downward rotation or protraction and retraction. The muscles that are activated to achieve these movements include the upper trapezius and lower digitations of the serratus anterior to form an upper component of the force couple and the lower trapezius a lower component of a force couple, producing upward rotation of the scapula. Similarly, rhomboids, levator scapulae, and upper digitations of the serratus anterior form an upper component, and pectoralis major/minor form a lower component of a force couple, producing downward rotation of the scapula.[45]

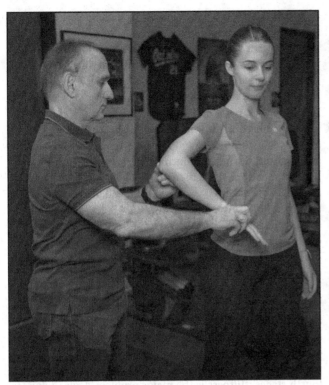

Figure 5-8. Internal rotation in the POS.

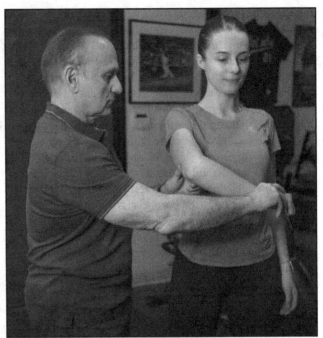

Figure 5-9. Internal rotation in 60 degrees of flexion.

In summary, the scapula moves in 3 spatial planes,[46] which can change the orientation of the arm completely.[19] In addition to the scapula, shoulder muscles also change their activation level according to the speed and ROM of flexion or abduction.[47]

Rotation of the Clavicle

Axial rotation of the clavicle occurs between 70 and 90 degrees of arm elevation and at the end range of overhead motion. Axial rotation of the clavicle is part of the important rotation movements that the shoulder allows. The lateral aspect of the clavicle elevation is coupled with upward scapula elevation. If the clavicle does not rotate at the distal end, it could cause a limitation in scapula rotation resulting in limited arm elevation.[48] Essentially, rotation of the clavicle is initiated at the SC joint and elevation of the clavicle occurs at the AC articulation. There are no muscles that are considered to be rotators of the clavicle; 2 major ligaments, the conoid and trapezoid, collectively called the coracoclavicular ligament, translate scapula rotational movement to the clavicle. Clinically, to improve clavicular mechanics, the scapula needs to rotate via muscular coordinated action. The rotation of the clavicle is the major movement at the AC joint and is more stabilized at the SC joint.

Conclusion

Patients with shoulder dysfunction are routinely sent to be treated in a physical therapy clinic. Too often, the therapist treats the shoulder as a linear joint forcing it into

elevation movements. As noted earlier, the shoulder consists of 2 force couples; therefore, restoring rotation should be an important part of the rehabilitation.

Treatment should be directed toward restoring mobility, providing stability, or a combination of the 2. The shoulder relies on various stabilizing mechanisms, including shapes of joint surfaces, ligaments, and muscles to prevent excessive motion. Almost 20 muscles act on this joint complex in some manner and at various times they can be both prime movers and stabilizers. Harmonious actions of these muscles are necessary for the full function of this joint.

THE STIFF AND PAINFUL SHOULDER— ADHESIVE CAPSULITIS

Historic Review

Duplay,[49,50] in 1896, was the first investigator to recognize pathologic disorders of extra-articular tissues as possible reasons for stiff and painful shoulders. It was his belief that an inflammatory process of the subacromial bursa was the causative agent producing this syndrome. He termed the clinical entity of frozen shoulder as *periarthritis scapulohumeral*, attributing the condition to inflammation of the subacromial bursa. The term *periarthritis of the shoulder* was then used by others, both as a diagnosis and to explain the pathology.[51]

Later, in 1934, Codman[52] called the same disorder *frozen shoulder syndrome* and related the dysfunction to uncalcified tendinitis of the rotator cuff. Based on his observations, he stated that although the "condition was difficult to define, difficult to treat, and difficult to explain from the point of view of pathology," the disorder would almost certainly resolve. Soon after Codman's findings, Neviaser, in 1945, introduced the concept of *adhesive capsulitis* when he discovered a tight, thickened capsule that stuck to the humerus.[53] He described an inflammatory reaction that led to adhesions, specifically in the axillary fold and in the attachment of the capsule at the anatomic neck of the humerus. Later evidence suggested that thickening and contracture of the GH joint capsule was associated with frozen shoulder, without adhesions to the humerus.[54] Capsular adhesions have also not been reported in other investigations, which infers that the term adhesive capsulitis appears not to appropriately describe the condition and should be abandoned.[55] The term *frozen shoulder* emerged and became predominant.[56] Recently, based in a study by Bunker[57] that recommended using the term *contracture of the shoulder*, Lewis[50] proposed the term *frozen shoulder contracture syndrome (FSCS)*. Lewis[50] advocated that the inclusion of the word contracture best incorporated the clinical and histological presentation of this condition, yet preserved the association of this condition with restriction and pain.

Definition, Epidemiology, and Clinical Presentation

For the purposes of this chapter, we are going to use the term *FSCS*. This term describes a pathological condition of the shoulder complex associated with a clinical manifestation of signs and symptoms altering normal motion and pain free function of the affected upper extremity. This pathologic condition is associated with thickening and fibrosis of the rotator interval, obliteration and scarring of the subscapular recess, increased cytokine concentrations, proliferation of fibroblasts and myofibroblasts, reduced joint volume and fibrosis, scarring and contracture of the capsuloligamentous complex,[58] and inflammation of the joint capsule and synovium.[59] Regarding the capsuloligamentous changes, they result in global loss of both passive and active ROM of the GH joint, with external rotation usually being the most restricted physiologic movement.[60,61] Abnormal shoulder kinematics are also associated with less scapula posterior tipping and upward rotation during arm elevation.[62] Recent published data suggest FSCS occurs in 2% to 5% of the population, being reported to affect women slightly more than men, and usually seen between the ages of 40 and 60 years old with 14% of all cases being bilateral.[63,64]

FSCS is a medical diagnosis and can be divided into 2 categories: primary, in which there are no obvious causes, but where there is an idiopathic onset; and secondary onset, where a cause is identified (from history, clinical examination, and radiographic appearances), like a trauma or forced inactivity following trauma or surgery to the affected upper extremity prior to their shoulder symptomology. The terms *primary* and *secondary frozen shoulder* were first introduced by Lundberg (1969).[56]

Risk factors for FSCS appear to include diabetes, prolonged shoulder immobility (trauma, overuse injuries, or surgery), genetic predisposition, or systemic diseases (hyperthyroidism, hypothyroidism, cardiovascular disease, or Parkinson disease).[65-68]

FSCS can be described as involving 3 stages: (1) Inflammation, pain, and freezing. In this stage, there is an insidious onset of pain increasing in severity, ranging from a few weeks to 36 weeks.[67] The pain is initially felt mostly at night and during certain movements (eg, brushing hair, hand into back pocket), then pain usually progresses to constant pain at rest and it is aggravated by all movements of the shoulder. Both active and passive ROM is restricted. There is a characteristic loss of movement of external rotation > abduction > internal rotation). (2) Frozen or stiffness. The pain begins to abate, leaving global stiffness (4 to 9/12 months); clinically, the shoulder movement is still very restricted and there is some pain. Additionally, there is reduced capsular volume. (3) Thawing or recovery phase. In this phase, pain is almost nonexistent and movement is restricted, but returning to normal (5 to 26 months).[67] Other authors describe 4 stages, like Neviaser and Hannafin[60] who report that in the first 2 stages, pain is the predominant problem, and in the third and fourth stages, stiffness is the major problem. Lewis[50] divides the condition clinically into 2 stages: (1) more pain than stiffness and (2) more stiffness than pain. Patients suffering from shoulder FSCS face months to years of progressive pain, stiffness, and disability with the average duration being 30.1 months (range: 12 to 42 months).[69,70] Although Codman[52] stated that recovery will occur and should be expected, this may not be correct, with 50% of people diagnosed with FSCS experiencing pain and/or stiffness at an average 7 years post onset.

Diagnosis

There is no definitive gold standard test to diagnose FSCS, and diagnosis is based upon the patient's history and clinical examination. Inside the physical examination, the key feature is the presence of reduced active and passive external rotation and the presence of a normal GH radiograph. Radiographs are required to exclude other pathologies and conditions such as locked dislocations, metastatic neoplasms, arthritis, fractures, or avascular necrosis that may painfully restrict movement and masquerade as FSCS. In gathering all this information together, a consensus and simple clinical diagnostic criterion involves an equal restriction of active and passive GH external rotation and an essentially normal shoulder radiograph[57] with the exception of osteopenia of the humeral head and calcific tendinosis.[71] Other diagnostic considerations that can be taken into account are the fasting blood sugar (diabetes) and thyroid stimulating hormone levels (hyperthyroidism).[72]

Management

After the establishment of the diagnosis and the determination of the phase of the disease, an evidence-based approach is needed. In what concerns the diminishment of pain and restoration of motion in patients with FSCS, no therapeutic intervention is currently universally accepted as the most effective. There is no consensus for interventions for patients with FSCS and it is not yet fully understood.[60,73,74] This chapter presents an evidence-based overview on the effectiveness of interventions for FSCS. Treatment options documented in the literature include the following: steroid injections; physical therapy including different modalities such as stretching, exercise, and mobilization; acupuncture; arthroscopic capsular release; manipulation under anesthesia; and distension arthrography.[75-79]

Steroid Injections

Intra-articular corticosteroid injections are a commonly used intervention in treating shoulder pain in general. Corticosteroids may be injected into the GH joint by an anterior, lateral, and/or posterior approach, into the subacromial space, tendon sheaths, or locally into trigger or tender points.[80] Several randomized controlled trials[81-83] compared steroid injections with placebo. All found significant differences in favor of intra-articular steroids for pain $P = .02$ (standard error of the mean 36.7.5 [5.1] vs 18.9 [5.1]) in the short and midterm (95% confidence interval 11.6 [0.4 to 22.8]) and no significant differences were found with ROM (95% confidence interval 5.5 [-1.7 to 12.8]).

Laser Therapy

Laser therapy has been cited as a safe and effective modality to accelerate pain relief and healing.[83,84] To be more precise, laser therapy is a modality treatment used to facilitate recovery by attempting to promote a healing response at the cellular level.[85,86] Several authors suggest that laser therapy with a high power level of impulse or biphasic dose response has the capacity to drive photons (light energy) to the target tissue at depths of up to 10 to 13 cm. These proposed healing effects are possible due to an improvement of microcirculation at an adequate depth of penetration to reach the targeted soft tissue structures and increase cell metabolism.[85] This may assist in returning the damaged cells to a healthy, stable state.[85] For example, in a study comparing a placebo group with an experimental group, laser therapy recorded higher improvement in the shoulder pain after 15 treatment sessions.[87] In short, due to the effects outlined previously, laser therapy is very often used, in conjunction with other modalities, in the FSCS treatment plan. For instance, combined with home exercises, laser therapy was shown to be beneficial when administered over 12 weeks in 12 treatment sessions.[88]

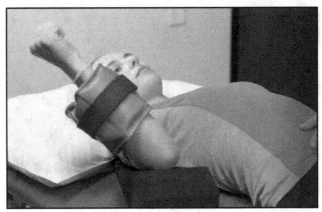

Figure 5-10. LLPS into external rotation of the GH joint at 30 degrees of abduction in the POS.

Stretching and Strengthening Exercises

Stretching and strengthening exercises appear to be beneficial for pain relief and functional improvement.[89-91] In addition to a LLPS, strengthening of the scapular stabilizers and rotator cuff muscles is beneficial to the rehabilitation of a stiff and painful shoulder. LLPS (Figure 5-10) has historically been utilized in physical therapy as an effective means to induce lengthening of soft tissue.[58] As previously discussed, the shoulder is not a linear joint, therefore, the authors of this chapter support that restoring shoulder elevation is accomplished by restoring external and internal rotation. Therefore, the low-load stretching technique is performed into the restricted rotation ranges, which attempts to apply end-range tensile stress to the capsule, extracapsular ligaments, and tendons of the rotator cuff in an effort to gain greater extensibility of the restricting periarticular structure and allowing increased ROM over the course of time, and has been shown to make improvements in the mobility of a stiff shoulder.[58,92] The shoulder is held at the end ROM in the scapular plane, stretching an external rotated or internal rotated position, and placing the scarred or contracted tissue under strain. The joint displacement is incrementally increased with the expectation that remodeling of the periarticular connective tissues will improve the active and passive ROM.[93] It has been shown that force applied to the tissue, accompanied by a progressively increased load, will produce a plastic deformation.[94] Vermeulen et al[95] reported that end-range mobilization techniques were effective in restoring permanent changes in passive and active overhead movements in patients with adhesive capsulitis. LLPS was implemented at the onset of treatment to promote tissue lengthening without inducing pain. In treating joint stiffness, the amount of tensile stress applied to the periarticular tissues should be adjusted until the clinicians and physical therapists can achieve a therapeutic result (increased ROM). An insufficient amount of stress will have no therapeutic effect, whereas an excessive dose will produce complications such

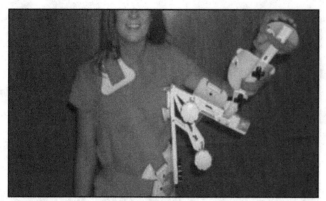

Figure 5-11. Joint Active Systems Shoulder Rotation Device.

as pain and inflammation. When calculating the prescribed amount of force delivered to soft tissues, 3 factors must be considered: intensity, duration, and frequency. In regard to these variables, Bonutti et al[96] reported motion gains with the use of 30-minute sessions up to 3 times per day as tolerated. Other authors also recommended a 30-minute treatment protocol daily.[88,96] Intensity, which is the amount of force applied, is usually limited by the patient's pain tolerance. Mahmoud et al[97] reported significant improvements in elevation by restoring rotation using the Joint Active System shoulder device (Figure 5-11). The recommended protocol, as noted earlier, was 30-minute sessions 3 times daily. Use of a static progressive stretch orthosis compared to physical therapy alone demonstrated a significantly greater mean improvement in all ROM categories.

Manual Therapy

Manual therapy can include trigger point therapy and mobilization techniques. Trigger point therapy can be effectively used to alleviate any soft tissue restrictions present within different muscles and to aid in adhesive capsulitis treatment.[98] For example, Fergunson[99] reported 3 cases of frozen shoulder that he successfully treated using trigger point therapy techniques. Trigger point therapy can be beneficial in the treatment of the subscapularis muscle, infraspinatus, teres minor, and/or upper trapezius. The subscapularis, among other soft tissues such as coracohumeral ligament and the pectoralis major can limit shoulder external rotation.[86,99] Jewell et al[69] demonstrated in a study that the combination of joint mobilization and exercise was associated with better outcomes than the ultrasound and massage in patients with FSCS. In another study, 100 people diagnosed with FSCS receiving an average of 20 treatments over 12 weeks, both high- and low-grade GH inferior, anterior, and posterior mobilization techniques, demonstrated significant improvements over 12 months with a trend for greater improvement (pain and movement) in the high-grade group.[76] Noten et al[100] indicated the benefits of manual therapy and exercise in the treatment of frozen shoulder. Several other studies indicate the benefits of physical therapy intervention in the treatment

of patients with frozen shoulder.[100,101] Further definitions of mobilization techniques, indications, contraindications, and examples of various mobilization techniques can be found in Chapter 12.

Arthroscopic Capsular Release

When conservative treatment fails, other options such as arthroscopic capsular release are taken into account. Nowadays, arthroscopic capsular release has become increasingly commonplace.[102] This technique requires general anesthesia and an examination under anesthesia to document the preoperative ROM. Standard posterior and anterior portals are made, a diagnostic arthroscopy is performed to confirm the diagnosis, and a synovectomy of the rotator interval is done. The capsular release starts with excision of the rotator interval to the undersurface of the conjoint tendon; the release is extended inferiorly posterior to the tendon of the subscapularis down to the 5 o'clock position. The superior release is then extended to reach the LHB and is continued to release the coracohumeral ligament in the plane between the superior glenoid and supraspinatus.[102] Postoperatively, the immediate improvements in symptoms and motion are readily perceived by the patient, which reinforces the patient's commitment to the rehabilitation process. Although many authors support and list the several advantages of arthroscopic capsular release,[102,103] others still mention that further research is required to better understand the clinical benefit of capsular release as the quality of the evidence supporting this practice is currently low.[104]

Treatment Objectives

Various forms of treatment are effective in reducing pain and increasing ROM in patients with FSCS. After careful assessment and physical examination to confirm the diagnosis of FSCS, and the determination of the current phase of the condition, physical therapists must be prepared to design an individual treatment program based on their assessment (Table 5-1). The physician, in conjunction with the physical therapist, should direct each case to determine if physical therapy is to be used alone or with other medical or surgical treatment.[59] During the painful phases the main goal is to relieve pain. A combination of medical pharmaceutical management and exercise with certain modalities may help accomplish this objective.[104] Intra-articular corticosteroids may provide rapid pain relief, mainly in the short-term period.[104]

Bal et al[74] evaluated the effect of intra-articular corticosteroids on home exercise program outcomes in patients with FSCS. Eighty patients were randomly assigned to 2 groups; group 1 received intra-articular corticosteroid, group 2 received intra-articular serum physiologic, and both groups underwent a 12-week comprehensive home exercise program. Outcome measures were night pain, passive ROM, and Shoulder Pain and Disability Index end-result scores; group 1 achieved significantly better scores in all outcomes

Table 5-1

FROZEN SHOULDER CONTRACTURE SYNDROME ASSESSMENT AND MANAGEMENT OPTIONS

ASSESSMENT	MANAGEMENT OPTIONS
• Full patient interview and physical examination • Equal restriction of active and passive external rotation • Normal GH radiograph • May consider screening for diabetes or other related health conditions • Fully inform patient about condition and management options	*Stage I to Early Stage II—Focus on Pain Reduction* • Guided intra-articular injection • Laser therapy • Soft tissue massage • Gentle mobilizations and exercise program that promotes ROM in the pain-free range • Passive movements
	Late Stage II to Stage III—Focus on Pain Reduction and Increasing Range of Motion • LLPS • Mobilizations • Exercise program involving regular active movements, self-assisted active movements, and stretching • Consider surgery for non-responders

Data Source: Lewis J. Frozen shoulder contracture syndrome—aetiology, diagnosis and management. *Man Ther [Internet]*. Elsevier Ltd; 2014:1-8.

measured at week 2. However, no significant differences between the groups were noted at week 12. The investigation concluded intra-articular steroids provided rapid pain relief in the first weeks of an exercise program, which is really helpful for patients with predominant pain symptoms. In the freezing phase, combined with these relieving agents, the patient should be encouraged to use their arm as the condition allows. An exercise program should be recommended that promotes ROM in the pain-free range, especially in external and internal rotation. The patient should be educated about GH elevation within a range to prevent impingement and compensatory scapular motion. Some gentle mobilizations can be performed by the physical therapist to promote accessory joint motion. At 6 weeks to 9 months after onset, restricted ROM is predominant. During the stiff or frozen and thawing phases, treatment objectives should focus on pain reduction and in increasing ROM. LLPS, exercise prescription (eg, isometric and isotonic activities), and manual therapy should take place. Target-specific mobilization should be performed and the patient's capsular restrictions must be carefully assessed to determine the most effective technique. At this phase, when designing a treatment program, the patient alignment, movement impairments, and muscular balance must be taken into account. Very often, the patient will benefit from strengthening the rotator cuff rather than just exclusively strengthening the deltoid and/or upper trapezius.[105]

Conclusion

The condition of FSCS can be painful and debilitating to many patients. To optimize recovery time, physical therapists have to understand the typical presentation of the FSCS and the literature supporting the various treatment approaches. The chosen treatment interventions should depend on the stage at presentation for treatment and the failure of previous treatments. Often times, a combination of different treatment approaches is advisable.

CASE STUDY

Patient History

A 54-year-old woman presented with left shoulder pain and ROM restriction. Pain had started insidiously in the left shoulder 4 months before the first clinical assessment. At that time, she saw her family physician who prescribed anti-inflammatory medications and injected corticosteroid into her left shoulder. Despite the reduction of pain symptoms for the first 3 weeks, this relief was only transitory and she continued to have pain and left shoulder movement restriction that got progressively worse; she then saw an orthopedic surgeon who injected her left shoulder with cortisone and recommended physical therapy. At this time, the patient presented to the clinic with a 4-month history of dull and achy

Table 5-2				
IMPROVEMENT OF THE PATIENT'S LEFT SHOULDER ACTIVE AND PASSIVE RANGE OF MOTION WITH TREATMENT				
RANGE OF MOTION	**TYPE OF MOVEMENT**	**ABDUCTION/POS/FRONTAL (DEGREES)**	**FLEXION (DEGREES)**	**EXTERNAL ROTATION (DEGREES) PASSIVE**
Initial	Active	65/45	90	0
	Passive	70/50	90	0
At 4 weeks	Active	70/60	120	45
	Passive	80	135	60
At 13 weeks	Active	150	158	72
	Passive	168	170	80
At 16 weeks	Active	Full	Full	Full
	Passive	Full	Full	Full

pain in the left shoulder without being able to identify a specific traumatic situation. She also complained of not being able to move her left arm and having difficulty doing most of her daily activities. The pain was aggravated by some movements of the left arm and lying on the left arm; she was also awakened at night when she rolled onto the affected arm. Diagnostic ultrasound results suggested incipient heterogeneity of the left supraspinatus tendon and incipient tenosynovitis of the left biceps. The patient's self-report section of American Shoulder and Elbow Surgeons Standardized Shoulder Assessment form was completed at the initial evaluation, and the patient scored 45 points.

Examination

Examination of the patient's left shoulder demonstrated GH joint active—active elevation ROM was:

The opposite extremity was measured for comparison and was found to be within normal limits in both active and passive ROM. Manual muscle testing of the left shoulder indicated significant weakness of the rotator cuff. Manual muscle testing of the supraspinatus in the "full can" position and the subscapularis while performing the lift-off test was difficult, and pain and stiffness did not allow for an accurate test. Trigger points were identified upon palpation of the superior and inferior lateral aspect on the anterior surface of the subscapularis muscle belly with the patient positioned in supine with the humerus supported in an abducted and externally rotated position. Trigger points were also noted in the infraspinatus, teres minor, upper trapezius, and in pectoralis minor. At the conclusion of the physical examination, the identifying signs and symptoms led to the clinical diagnosis of the left shoulder adhesive capsulitis (Table 5-2).

Treatment Plan and Outcomes

Following the examination, the patient began physical therapy treatment. Sessions were performed twice a week, approximately 1 hour, with the supervision of a qualified shoulder specialist. The focus of treatment was relieving pain, regaining active and passive ROM, and then reestablishing scapulohumeral coordination by improving strength and mobility of the shoulder complex allowing the patient to return to daily activities. In general, we divided the protocol treatment in the protocol for the first FSCS phase, where the patient still had pain, and a protocol for the second and third phases, characterized for more stiffness than pain (Table 5-3).

In the first phase during the first month, the physical therapy aims were to diminish pain symptoms, begin ROM restoration and stimulate appropriate muscle activation, and promote muscular endurance. Treatment consisted of LLLT, LLPS-duration (see Figure 5-11), stretching into external rotation, soft tissue mobilization of the subscapularis and upper trapezius, manual scapular tilt distraction, passive movements, sleeper stretch exercise, and a progressive resistive exercise program to address weakness and postural adaptations of the rotator cuff and scapula rotator muscles. In this initial phase, therapeutic exercises were initiated using high repetitions (12 to 15 x 2 to 3 sets) and moderate to light weight with an emphasis on pain-free motion. Specific exercises of the rotator cuff and scapular rotators that elicited high EMG activity of the targeted musculature were performed.

Table 5-3

PHASED INTERVENTION DURING THE TREATMENT OF THE PARTICIPANT IN THE CASE STUDY

PHYSICAL THERAPY TREATMENT	PHASE I (WEEK 1 TO 4) PAIN > STIFF PHASE	PHASE II (WEEK 5 TO 13) STIFF > PAIN PHASE	PHASE III (WEEK 14 TO 16) STIFF > PAIN PHASE
Low-level laser therapy (LLLT) with sustained pressure	8 minutes (moderate pressure on trigger points) 0 degrees abduction	8 minutes (moderate pressure on trigger points) 0 degrees abduction and 30 degrees abduction in POS	4 minutes (moderate pressure on trigger points) 30 degrees abduction and 30 degrees abduction in POS
Ultrasound 1,6 w/cm², t-4′	5 minutes		
Scapular tilt and distraction	5 minutes manual scapular distraction	5 minutes manual scapular distraction	
Trigger points therapy	5 minutes in subscapularis infraspinatus, teres minor, upper trapezius, and pectoralis minor	5 minutes in subscapularis infraspinatus, teres minor, upper trapezius, and pectoralis minor	When necessary
Fulcrum technique	8 minutes	5 minutes	
LLPS	15 minutes 1 kg weight 0 degrees abduction	12 minutes 2 kg weight 0 degrees abduction and 30 degrees abduction in the POS	12 minutes 2 kg weight 0 degrees abduction and 30 degrees abduction in the POS
Intelligent pendulum exercise	2*8 1 kg dumbell	2*8 2 kg dumbell	2*8 2 kg dumbell
Push Swiss ball against the wall	2*12-15	3*12-15	***
External rotation at 0 degrees abduction	3*15 light tube	3*8-12 tube or 5 kg pulley	3*6-8 tube or 8 kg pulley
Prone extension	3*15	3*8-12 1 kg dumbbell	3*6-8 2 kg dumbbell
Belly exercise	2*15	3*12-15	
Low row	3*15 tube	3* 8-12 tube or 15 kg weight machine	3*6-18 20 kg weight machine
Sleeper stretch	6 minutes 3*(1′ON+1OFF)	6 minutes 3*(1′ON+1OFF)	6 minutes 3*(1′ON+1OFF)
Dynamic hug		3*12-15 10 kg pulley	3*8-12 15 kg pulley
Prone horizontal abduction with external rotation below 90 degrees abduction		3*8-15	3*8-12 15 1 kg dumbbell
Scaption		2*12	3*12 1kg dumbbell
Lift-off exercise		2*12	3*12 manual resistance

(continued)

Table 5-3 (continued)

PHASED INTERVENTION DURING THE TREATMENT OF THE PARTICIPANT IN THE CASE REPORT

PHYSICAL THERAPY TREATMENT	PHASE I (WEEK 1 TO 4) PAIN > STIFF PHASE	PHASE II (WEEK 5 TO 13) STIFF > PAIN PHASE	PHASE III (WEEK 14 TO 16) STIFF > PAIN PHASE
Subscapularis internal rotation diagonal exercise		3*8-12 10 kg pulley	3*8-12 15 kg pulley
Push-up plus			Body weight push-up with arms on an elevated surface
Core exercises		Wall plank (2*10 seconds) Lift 2*15 1 kg dumbbell (2*12) tube	Plank and side plank with knees (3*10 seconds) Lift 2*12 2 kg dumbbell Pallof press (3*10) tube
Hip exercises for the medium and maximum gluteus		Wall squat Swiss ball (3*12)	Total-body resistance exercise squat and single leg squat (3*12)

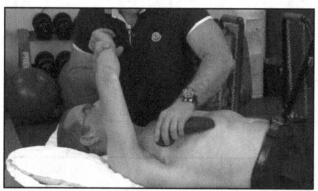

Figure 5-12. LASER probe into the subscapularis muscle belly (Radiance Medical).

Manual mobilization of the scapula and the fulcrum technique was utilized in phase I and II (a picture of this technique can be found in Chapter 12). The physical therapist, who is posterior to the patient with the inner hand thread under the involved extremity and supporting the anterior GH joint, grasps the vertebral border and tilts the scapula away from the thoracic wall. This technique is used in cases of restriction in external rotation. In the fulcrum technique, used to mobilize the posterior capsule, the patient is lying prone and the therapist puts the closest forearm under the anterior part of the GH joint while the other hand is placed just proximal to the elbow. Then, while pushing up on the patient's GH joint with the forearm, the therapist also pulls down on the elbow to create a stretch on the posterior aspect off the GH joint (a picture of this technique can be found in Chapter 12). In addition, the use of the LLLT, LLPS, and the sleeper stretch exercise can be used to increase soft tissue extensibility. In conjunction with

LLLT, the laser is used with deep sustained pressure to relieve trigger points in the subscapularis muscle belly.[106] In addition, soft tissue mobilization of the subscapularis can be achieved using a LASER with a probe (Radiance Medical). The probe is pushed into the belly of the subscapularis as seen in Figure 5-12. Furthermore, LLPS into GH external rotation was applied continuously for 15, 12, and 8 minutes in phases I, II, and III, respectively. The patient was positioned in the supine position with the shoulder supported on a foam wedge in 0 degrees of abduction (phase I) or with 30 degrees of abduction in the POS (phases II to III), allowing gravity to produce the intended stretch into external rotation. The sleeper stretch exercise was also used in the 3 phases and is considered to have a beneficial effect in the increasing of the ROM.

By the end of the fourth week of treatment, the patient demonstrated better active external rotation and ROM in all directions. The active external rotation, forward flexion, and abduction improved to 45 degrees, 120 degrees, and 70 degrees, respectively; whereas, for passive ROM, an increase of 25 degrees in passive external rotation and 25 degrees of forward flexion were measured. In phase II, with a less painful and stiff shoulder, the aims were to almost fully achieve the normal ROM, to continue stimulating appropriate muscle activation, and to promote muscular strength. We performed the same exercises using increased weight with fewer repetitions (8 to 12 repetitions × 3 sets) in order to emphasize more on muscular strengthening of the shoulder complex. New exercises were added, such as scaption, targeting the supraspinatus, the push-up plus, and exercises like the dynamic hug and the subscapularis internal rotation diagonal exercise that highly elicit the subscapularis muscle activity.[103] At the same time, taking into consideration a total body approach concept, core and hip exercises were also performed. By the end of the 13th week (end of phase II), the patient had 90% of the ROM in all movement directions. In the final phase from the 14th to 16th week, the goals are to achieve active and passive ROM in all planes, achieve normal strength of the scapula and GH rotators, and return function of the shoulder to allow symptom free daily activities. The resistance of the therapeutic exercise targeting the rotator cuff and scapular rotators was increased according to the patient's tolerance and ability to demonstrate proper technique throughout the exercise. We prescribed low repetition exercise (6 to 8 repetitions x 3 sets) with higher resistance. In the end, the patient had full active elevation without evidence of compensatory movement patterns, symmetrical scapulae, pain free grades of 5/5 during manual muscle testing of the rotator cuff and scapular rotator musculature, improved passive ROM to 85 degrees of external rotation at 0 degrees of abduction. The American Shoulder and Elbow Surgeons questionnaire was completed again, and the patient scored 88 points. Table 5-3 identifies the prescription of therapeutic exercise and the phase in which specific therapeutic interventions were implemented in relation to this case study.

It must be outlined that the patient had 3 guided treatment sessions per week and she had to perform a twice-a-week at-home exercise program with the strengthening and stretching exercises specific for each phase and that she used in the treatment sessions. The exercises and weight selection were the responsibility of the physical therapist, as was confirmation as to proper technique in the execution of the exercises every week in the guided sessions.

Summary of the Case Study

This case study demonstrated the effectiveness of a multi-approach intervention for the primary FSCS in a 54-year-old woman. At the end of the 16-week period, the patient's shoulder ROM was full and pain free.

ROTATOR CUFF TEARS/SURGERY

Etiology

Rotator cuff syndrome is a spectrum of disease encompassing disorders from impingement and tendonitis to rotator cuff arthropathy. Rotator cuff disorders are the most common cause of disability related to the shoulder.[107] The rotator cuff is the primary dynamic stabilizer of the GH joint, and RCTs can develop from a wide variety of causes including, but not limited to, impingement, eccentric overload, chronic tendinitis, scapular dyskinesis, trauma, and/or dislocation.

Different injury patterns and mechanisms are associated with certain patient demographics. Older patients are more likely to have chronic, degenerative tears, whereas the younger athlete is more likely to sustain an injury within their sport.[108,109] Several mechanisms have been proposed particularly in the overhead athlete who is susceptible to repetitive microtrauma. These include primary impingement, primary overload, or secondary impingement from GH instability. Trauma to the rotator cuff can also be sustained through high impact to the shoulder or GH dislocation, characteristically with the arm abducted and externally rotated.

Patient factors such as age, smoking, hypercholesterolemia, and family history have been shown to predispose individuals to RCTs, with age being a strong determinant of healing after repair.[107] Additionally, tear size and number of tendons that are torn will significantly and negatively affect outcomes.[110]

Several studies have investigated the prevalence through cadaveric[111,112] magnetic resonance imaging (MRI) and ultrasonography. Full-thickness tears ranged from 6% to 17% in cadaveric studies and from 4% to 28% in asymptomatic patients less than 60 years old. Although studies have shown significantly varied results, prevalence of tears increases dramatically with age more than 60 years old. Partial-thickness RCTs range from 13% to 32% in cadaveric studies, while one MRI study of asymptomatic individuals showed overall prevalence of 20%.[107,111]

Diagnosis

As with any musculoskeletal injury, the diagnosis should start with the foundation of a history and thorough physical examination. While pain is the most common symptom for partial-thickness RCTs, they may also have painful arc of motion, crepitus, weakness, and positive impingement signs. The examination should include both active and passive ROM as well as sensory and motor examinations. The patient's position, posture, tissue texture, and quality of movement may provide subtle information regarding the chronicity and severity of the injury. There are many special tests that can be implemented to aid in the diagnosis of RCTs. More than 30 tests have been documented and many more are used clinically. Problems with their accuracy are owed to many factors including difference in technique, inability for the patient to tolerate positioning, lack of reproducibility, and lack of validation. While none is entirely pathognomonic for RCTs, their combination improves their diagnostic value.[113] The external rotation lag sign and drop arm sign are 2 well-known tests that may be used in the diagnosis of RCTs, but their accuracy depends on a very subtle difference in degrees of motion. The impingement tests, such as Hawkins-Kennedy and Jobe's tests, have been well studied, proving their sensitivity to be better than their specificity. The lift-off test and resisted internal rotation provided the best sensitivity and specificity for subscapularis pathology with the least bias.

These special tests are combined with imaging to guide treatment. MRI, magnetic resonance arthrography (MRA), and ultrasonography have all been found to be useful in detecting full-thickness RCTs.[114] Although the accuracy of ultrasonography evaluation of RCTs is very much operator dependent,[114] ultrasonography is a reliable and cost-effective tool in the accurate detection of full-thickness RCTs.[115,116]

MRA, however, remains the imaging modality of choice. Its high mean sensitivity (85.9%) and specificity (96.0%) place it superior to other imaging modalities.[117,118] Drawbacks are that MRA is more expensive, time-consuming, and invasive than MRI.[117] For these reasons, MRI remains the most commonly used imaging modality for RCT assessment, both before and after surgery.

RCTs lead to degeneration of the cuff muscles and fatty infiltration that generally correlates with the size of the tear. More than 25 different classifications systems for the MRI evaluation of RCT have been proposed. Many of them are centered on the degree of fatty infiltration or muscle loss, which has been found to have a low inter- and intra-observer reliability. The mechanism underlying fatty infiltration is not clearly understood, and hypotheses range from complex gene activation by peroxisome proliferator-activated receptor gamma to denervation, as there have been examples of infraspinatus infiltration in the setting of isolated supraspinatus tears.[111] Operative treatment of this shoulder pathology should be pursued after failure of nonoperative treatment and can be performed open or arthroscopically. This discussion will forego nonoperative treatment as well as open surgical repair.

Arthroscopic Evaluation

Arthroscopy is both diagnostic and therapeutic for intra-articular GH pathology and subacromial pathology. Although the diagnostic imaging modalities described earlier are helpful, there is no substitute for directly visualizing the anatomy. Indications for GH arthroscopy include biceps tears, labral tears, subscapularis tears, chondral injuries, loose bodies, adhesive capsulitis, and shoulder instability. Indications for subacromial arthroscopy include RCTs, subacromial bursitis/impingement, and AC osteoarthritis. Shoulder arthroscopy is contraindicated during active infection, especially involving the skin in the surgical field.[119]

Operative Treatment

Shoulder arthroscopy is performed under general anesthesia, and regional anesthesia such as an interscalene block may be performed to help with postoperative pain and analgesia requirements.[120] Positioning is largely surgeons' preference as both of the following positions are acceptable for shoulder arthroscopy and each have their advantages and disadvantages. Beach chair position offers ease of access to the subacromial space as well as conversion to an open procedure but carries the risk of possible cerebral hypoperfusion.[121,122] The lateral decubitus position gives good access to the posterior shoulder and carries a small risk of traction neuropraxia.[123] Injecting the GH joint with 30 to 40 mL saline helps distract the joint before making incisions and inserting the cannulas. While the posterior and anterior portals are generally made for every shoulder arthroscopy, there are a wide variety of accessory portals used to help with instrumentation and repair. Once portals have been created and the arthroscope is inserted, diagnostic arthroscopy begins.

All intracapsular structures are then examined systematically in the order the surgeon chooses, but this generally begins with identification of the LHB as it attaches to the superior aspect of the glenoid labrum. Any fraying or separation of the biceps from its attachment is in immediate view, and, along with the labrum, it can be probed to assess its integrity. Manipulation of the arm to put the subscapularis on stretch along with careful probing and use of the arthroscopes obliquity can provide excellent visualization of the tendon. As with any of these structures, switching the arthroscope into alternative portals, such as the anterior portal, can provide an alternate view and improve visualization. Continuing anteriorly, the GH complex can be evaluated for any abnormalities. Retracting the arthroscope posterior superiorly past the LHB provides an intra-articular view of the rotator cuff, which can be followed to its insertion the greater tuberosity. The distalmost, crescent-shaped portions of the supraspinatus and infraspinatus just before they attach to the greater tuberosity is the rotator crescent. This thin cuff of tissue that is prone to injury is protected by the rotator cable, which is a thickening of fibers that runs perpendicular and just proximal to the rotator crescent. The rotator cable runs from the biceps anteriorly to infraspinatus posteriorly.[124] The arthroscope can then be directed inferiorly to evaluate the remainder of the posterior labrum, humeral head, and bare area. Lastly, the capsular attachments and inferior gutter, which can be a site for loose bodies, can also be evaluated here.[111]

Diagnostic arthroscopy is continued in the subacromial space. A lateral incision is usually made from which to enter the subacromial space to evaluate the bursal aspect of the rotator cuff, coracoacromial ligaments, and the morphology of the acromion. Indications for rotator cuff repair generally include bursal-sided tears that extend more than 3 mm or 25% of the depth of the cuff and articular-sided tears that extend more than 7 mm or 50% of the thickness of the cuff. Arthroscopic subacromial decompression may be anticipated based on clinical examination and imaging, but the final decision is made under direct visualization. Many factors should be considered in the decision to repair the cuff. For example, the likelihood of healing decreases dramatically with age greater than 60 years old and multiple tendon involvement.[125,126] Also, the greater the size of the tear, the less likely it is to heal; additionally, most failures occur between 12 and 26 weeks postoperatively.[127]

Although we understand that the natural course of this injury pattern is for tears to progress and likely become symptomatic, there is a place for conservative management particularly in older patient populations with isolated tears.[108,128,129] Many aspects of the repair technique such as number of anchors, sutures, and configuration of repair show discrepancy between biomechanical and clinical outcomes and continue to be areas of research and debate.[129] As with any surgical procedure, however, the benefits should be carefully weighed against the risks with patient's expectations in mind.

TRAUMATIC GLENOHUMERAL INSTABILITY AND LABRAL PATHOLOGY

Etiology

The shoulder has the greatest ROM of any joint in the body; however, with that increased arc of motion, comes increased risk of dislocation. The shoulder is the most commonly dislocated large joint in the body, with incidence of shoulder dislocation documented at 24 per 100,000 persons per year.[130,131] The GH joint position is maintained through a series of static and dynamic stabilizers. The dynamic stabilizers consist of the surrounding musculotendinous structures such as the rotator cuff, LHB tendon, deltoid, and periscapular musculature. The static stabilizers consist of bony and cartilaginous structures that confer stability to the GH joint such as the glenoid fossa, coracoid, acromion, labrum, and capsuloligamentous structures. The glenoid labrum is a cartilaginous structure that lines the glenoid. As noted previously, with joint compression, the labrum increases the joint surface area, thereby increasing the joint stability. Instability of the GH articulation can be from a variety of different injury patterns depending on the mechanism of abnormal forces applied to it.[132]

SLAP tears can occur as isolated lesions or be associated with internal impingement, RCTs, or instability. SLAP tears are commonly seen in throwing athletes, and it is thought that tightness of the posterior aspect of the inferior GH ligament shifts the GH contact point posterosuperior and increases the shear force on the superior aspect of the labrum.[133-135]

An anteriorly directed force with the arm in abducted and externally rotated position predisposes to GH dislocation. There are variety of injury patterns associated with this classic anterior-inferior dislocation. The Bankart lesion, which is an avulsion of the anterior labrum and anterior band of the inferior GH ligament from the anterior-inferior glenoid, is most commonly seen and has very inferior shoulder dislocations and is present in up to 80% to 90% of patients with shoulder dislocation.[136] The same injury mechanism can present with a bony Bankart lesion, as a segment of the anterior-inferior glenoid bone shears off along with the labrum. A Hill-Sachs defect can also be seen as an impaction injury to the posterior-superior aspect of the humerus as it contacts the anteroinferior aspect of the glenoid during dislocation. This can be present in up to 80% of patients with shoulder dislocation and can cause cartilaginous defects or engaging bony defects.[137,138] A variety of other labral and cartilaginous lesions can be sustained with traumatic dislocation of the GH joint. These include, but are not limited to, humeral avulsion of the GH ligament, anterior labral periosteal sleeve avulsion, glenoid labral articular defects, and other fracture patterns including greater and lesser tuberosity fractures that are far beyond the scope of this discussion.

Diagnosis

The diagnosis of cartilaginous injury of the glenoid labrum begins with a thorough history and physical examination. In cases of traumatic unilateral GH joint dislocation, this is usually straightforward. In prospective trials, intra-articular block with lidocaine has also shown to be very effective for analgesia and capable of producing equivalent success of reduction as compared to sedation.[139] Orthogonal postreduction films will not only show adequate reduction of the GH joint, but may also show evidence of bony injury such as a bony Bankart or Hill-Sachs lesion mentioned earlier. Patients should be immobilized in a sling for approximately 3 to 4 weeks and may begin passive ROM, limiting external rotation past neutral and abduction past 90 degrees.

On reevaluation of symptomatic patients in the clinic, likely positive physical examination findings would be an apprehension sign, in which the patient is placed in the supine position with the arm at the 90-90 position and slowly externally rotated; this elicits immediate pain and discomfort as the humeral head shifts off the center of the glenoid. The patient may also have a relocation sign, which is a decrease in apprehension with an anterior force applied to the shoulder during this maneuver.[140] In severe cases, the patient may display a sulcus sign, which is simply observed as a depression just superior to the humeral head with the patient in a resting, seated/standing position.

Diagnosis of SLAP lesions similarly starts with a thorough history and physical examination; however, the eliciting event may not be as clear. In addition, SLAP lesions are seen with coexisting shoulder pathology in up to 88% of cases. The patient may have a history of repetitive throwing activities or may just present with any injury mechanism that places increased shear or tension on the LHB tendon. They will usually complain of a deep, difficult to describe shoulder pain, and possibly associated mechanical symptoms such as popping and clicking. Physical examination may include the O'Brien's test, in which the arm is held in 90 degrees forward flexion and adducted to midline with the arm in a fully pronated position. An inferiorly directed force by the clinician is then resisted by the patient with production of pain being a positive finding.[141] Diagnosis of a SLAP tear is further supported by performing this same maneuver with the arm in a fully supinated position and finding significantly less pain. The Mayo shear test can also be used, particularly in the overhead athlete, by placing them in an abducted and externally rotated position similar to the late cocking position during the throwing motion. An inferior shear force is then applied, and the arm is moved from slight internal to external rotation, with positive findings being pain or mechanical symptoms. The examination of labral pathology undoubtedly requires thorough evaluation of the biceps-labrum complex, and the 3-pack examination has shown promising inter- and intra-observer reliability in a prospective study by Taylor et al.[142] The 3-pack examination focuses on the intra-articular, junctional, and bicipital tunnel regions and has been shown an excellent means to rule out hidden extra-articular bicipital tunnel disease with a negative predictive value of 93% to 96%. Examination includes minimum of 3 components: active compression, throwing test, and bicipital tunnel palpation, each focused on their respective regions of the biceps-labrum complex.[143]

Imaging follows a thorough physical examination and usually starts with a complete series of shoulder x-rays, which includes the anterior-posterior, axillary, and scapular Y views. A computed tomography scan can be helpful for the evaluation of bony structures in a traumatic dislocation. MRI is the best imaging test for visualization of a labral tear and can be used as an adjunct in the diagnosis of SLAP tears, with a reported sensitivity of approximately 50% and specificity of 90%.[144]

CLASSIFICATION

Snyder et al[145] were among the first to create a classification system for SLAP tears, and the original description contained 4 types:

1. Superior labral fraying and local degeneration.
2. Detachment of the superior labrum and biceps anchor from the superior glenoid. These lesions are the most common and usually show hypermobility of the anchor complex.
3. Bucket handle tears with an intact biceps anchor.
4. Bucket handle tears that extend into and involve the biceps tendon but maintain superior labral attachment.

TREATMENT

Treatment of traumatic unilateral anterior shoulder dislocations varies depending on the patient, as the physiologic status determines their risk of redislocation as well as concomitant soft tissue injuries. Patients younger than 20 years of age have a significantly higher rate of redislocation as compared to older patients, whereas patients older than 60 years of age have a significantly increased risk of RCT with traumatic unilateral shoulder dislocation.[146] Though the initial management of first time dislocation is controversial, surgical management of a first time traumatic dislocation in an athlete under 20 years old is recommended, particularly in competitive athletes performing high contact sports.[147]

The size of the Bankart and Hill-Sachs lesion can also help determine the need for and type of operative management. Engaging Hill-Sachs lesions and those more than 25% of humeral head should be considered for surgical management with remplissage or similar procedure, which is insetting the infraspinatus into the Hill-Sachs lesion.[145] Bony

Bankart lesions with significant bone loss of more than 20% and those that have failed soft tissue repairs will likely require more advanced procedures. These patients are candidates for tricortical iliac crest graft or coracoid transfers such as the Latarjet procedure. The Latarjet procedure involves taking a piece of the coracoid process with the tendons attached and attaching it to the defective glenoid, thereby increasing the joint surface area of the glenoid.[148]

First-line treatment of the SLAP lesion on the other hand includes conservative physical therapy and nonsteroidal anti-inflammatory drugs (NSAIDs). Therapy should be directed to address GH internal rotation deficiency, scapular dyskinesia, and the rotator cuff. Arthroscopic repair is unnecessary for incidental SLAP tears found in patients greater than 50 years old, as it is associated with stiffness and poor outcomes.[149] Additionally, anatomic variants such as the Buford complex should be recognized and not repaired surgically. The Buford complex is a cord-like middle GH ligament and absent anterosuperior labrum that will lead to stiffness and pain if repaired to the glenoid.[148]

Surgery is indicated in patients with severe symptoms that have failed nonoperative treatment for several months. The earlier-mentioned 3-pack examination can also help guide surgical planning with absence of extra-articular pain suggesting SLAP or a proximal biceps tenodesis.

Arthroscopic Evaluation

Although imaging studies are helpful as an adjunct to the physical examination and can be helpful with preoperative planning, diagnosis is confirmed intraoperatively through diagnostic arthroscopy. The biceps anchor and glenoid labrum can be thoroughly evaluated with probes and other instruments. The biceps load test should also be performed at the labrum with 90 degrees of external rotation and abduction.[149] Erythema on the undersurface of the labrum is more suggestive of a tear than labral recess/variant.

Operative Treatment

Arthroscopic debridement is recommended for type I SLAP tears. For type II SLAP tears, patient factors such as age, activity, and goals are taken into account to determine whether SLAP repair, biceps tenotomy, or biceps tenodesis is most appropriate. In the younger and more active patient, a knotless suture anchor repair is indicated.[150] Older and lower demand patients with more significant degenerative bicep changes do well with biceps tenotomy or tenodesis. Type III tears may usually be managed by arthroscopic resection of the bucket handle portion with the anchor addressed as previously stated. Type IV lesions should be assessed for the amount of biceps involvement and can be resected if there is less than 50% involvement.

Patient Case One: Subacromial Impingement

A 41-year-old man with a longstanding history of right shoulder pain and multiple dislocations throughout the last few years presents to the clinic for evaluation. He is a recreational athlete who notices pain with overhead activities like weightlifting or even throwing a ball with his son. Clinical examination revealed pain and mild crepitus with motion as well as mild bicipital tenderness, positive Neers test, and positive Hawkins test. Shoulder x-rays show mild AC and GH arthritis. An MRI is ordered, and the patient is given a right shoulder subacromial injection of cortisone along with oral anti-inflammatories. When seen back in the clinic 2 weeks later, he reports minimal relief with anti-inflammatories and injection, and his MRI shows GH osteoarthritis, a spinoglenoid notch cyst, and AC arthritis with osteophytes. The patient is scheduled for right shoulder arthroscopy with subacromial decompression. At the time of arthroscopy, the biceps tendon is found to be intact and the superior labrum to be well attached circumferentially with minimal discontinuity at the anteroinferior border. Moderate GH arthritis with several chondral lesions was noted. Upon entering the subacromial space, a large amount of adhesions and inflamed bursa filled a narrow subacromial space. Clearing of bursa and adhesions revealed minor tearing of the bursal aspect of the rotator cuff accounting for less than 10% of the tendon depth as well as a downsloping type II acromion with a prominent osteophyte. Subacromial decompression was then performed, and the patient was placed in a sling. At the first postoperative visit 10 days later, the sutures were removed, sling discontinued, and the patient began ROM exercises. At the 6-week follow-up, the patient reported a decrease in pain with ROM and better tolerance with light overhead activities.

Patient Case Two: Shoulder Chronic Dislocation-Instability

A 30-year-old man was seen in clinic for evaluation of right shoulder pain. He explains that he first dislocated his right shoulder approximately 10 years ago while throwing a football as hard as he could. Since that time, he has dislocated his shoulder frequently, most recently about once every few months. He states that he feels instability simply reaching out in front of him to pick things up. The patient was noted to have shoulder instability with a positive load shift test and positive apprehension sign on physical examination. He also had a painful arc of motion, negative empty can test, and tenderness at the origin of the LHB. MRI arthrogram was ordered and the patient was given Norco (hydrocodone/acetaminophen) 5/325 as well as a topical NSAID. On a follow-up visit, the patient's MRI showed evidence of prior shoulder dislocation with a remote Hill-Sachs lesion, labroligamentous Bankart lesion, and a chronic anterior labral tearing from the 1 o'clock to the 5 o'clock position. After thorough discussion about risks, benefits, and complications of shoulder arthroscopy, the patient agreed to and was scheduled for surgery. He was placed in the lateral decubitus position. The patient had significant bursitis of the subacromial space, an impinging bone spur, and a grade IV engaging lesion on the humerus. A partial undersurface tearing of the supraspinatus with no bursal-sided tearing was noted. Chronic injury to the anterior aspect of the glenoid with grade II changes was also noted. Four anchors with Arthrex push locks were sequentially placed. An arthroscopic liberator was used to free the anterior aspect of the labrum and an arthroscopic shaver was then used to remove enough bone to stimulate bleeding in the area.

Patient Case Three: Traumatic Rotator Cuff Tear and Superior Labral Anterior-to-Posterior Lesion

A 31-year-old man presented with right shoulder pain and deformity following a mechanical fall while attempting to jump a BMX bicycle. On removal of the sling he brought from home, swelling and ecchymosis was noted over the anterior and anterolateral aspect of the right shoulder. The patient was unwilling to actively range the right shoulder and passive ROM produced mild crepitus and was limited secondary to pain. An x-ray showed a 100% displaced distal clavicle fracture, and the patient was sent home with Norco and an order for a right shoulder MRI. On follow-up, the MRI showed a SLAP tear and a partial coracoacromial ligament tear. The patient was counseled on his diagnosis and surgery was recommended. At the time of surgery, the beach chair position was used to allow for open reduction and internal fixation of the right clavicle as well as right shoulder arthroscopy. An incision was made over the fracture site and the fracture was reduced. The fracture was then fixed with a superiorly placed plate with 3 bicortical screws on each end of the fracture site. The subacromial space was then entered arthroscopically and grade III AC separation was confirmed. Dog bone suture was placed through the clavicle plate and coracoid to complete the AC reconstruction. After closing the incision over the clavicle with Ethibond suture (Ethicon), arthroscopy revealed minimal degenerative joint disease, an RCT, and a SLAP tear. Probing of the labrum showed a peel back sign and confirmed a type II SLAP tear, which was then fixed with 2 arthroscopic anchors. The bursal-sided RCT was noted to be slightly less than half the thickness of the cuff and was repaired with a single, triple-loaded arthroscopic anchor. The patient was maintained in a sling until 6 weeks after surgery, at which point he initiated physical therapy.

POSTOPERATIVE REHABILITATION

There is a great deal of controversy about when to start rehabilitation following a surgical repair of the rotator cuff.

The general goals of rehabilitation are to restore the extensibility, tensile strength, and muscle strength of the repaired rotator cuff. The rehabilitation should be dictated by

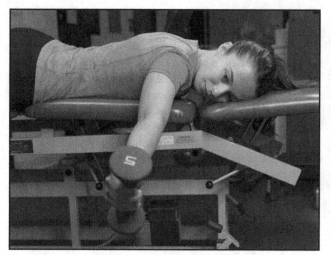

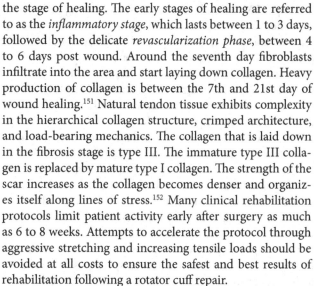

Figure 5-13. Horizontal abduction thumb up at 90 degrees of abduction.

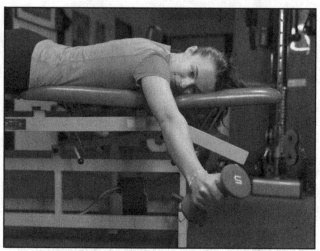

Figure 5-14. Horizontal abduction at 45 degrees of abduction.

the stage of healing. The early stages of healing are referred to as the *inflammatory stage*, which lasts between 1 to 3 days, followed by the delicate *revascularization phase*, between 4 to 6 days post wound. Around the seventh day fibroblasts infiltrate into the area and start laying down collagen. Heavy production of collagen is between the 7th and 21st day of wound healing.[151] Natural tendon tissue exhibits complexity in the hierarchical collagen structure, crimped architecture, and load-bearing mechanics. The collagen that is laid down in the fibrosis stage is type III. The immature type III collagen is replaced by mature type I collagen. The strength of the scar increases as the collagen becomes denser and organizes itself along lines of stress.[152] Many clinical rehabilitation protocols limit patient activity early after surgery as much as 6 to 8 weeks. Attempts to accelerate the protocol through aggressive stretching and increasing tensile loads should be avoided at all costs to ensure the safest and best results of rehabilitation following a rotator cuff repair.

The following 2 studies provide more specific guidelines for early rehabilitation following a rotator cuff repair. Peltz et al[153] reported immediate postoperative passive motion was found to be detrimental to passive shoulder mechanics. They speculate that early motion results in increased scar formation in the subacromial space, thereby resulting in decreased ROM and increased joint stiffness. The group that was immobilized for 2 weeks and then started passive and then active mobilization demonstrated the best results. Uhthoff et al[154] reported the initial period of rehabilitation should include passive movements followed by active ROM exercises with no resistance to allow optimal reformation of tendon insertion into the bone. Subsequently, gradual increases in active resistive exercises are necessary to reverse the effects of disuse atrophy of the subchondral bone and to strengthen the supraspinatus insertion and the muscle. Finally, Lee et al[155] reported early postoperative rotator cuff repairs demonstrated significant improvement in passive external and internal rotation and elevation, compared to Group B that

was limited in early passive ROM. Furthermore, exercise is a necessary treatment to enhance soft tissue healing. Eccentric loading is essential. While the mechanism of action of eccentric exercise is poorly understood, it is theorized that eccentric exercise loads the tendon to a greater magnitude compared with concentric contraction, thereby stimulating a more effective repair response. Furthermore, eccentric exercise may facilitate remodeling by increasing the number of collagen cross-linkages.[156] Stanish et al[157] suggested that eccentric exercises prepare patients for return to functional, sports-related activities better than those that emphasize concentric muscle strengthening.

Based on the previous studies for the purposes of this chapter, we have recommendations for treatment of postoperative rotator cuff repairs. Protocols for treatment of postoperative rotator cuff repairs are not specific to the patient. The treating therapist needs to evaluate the patients' progress and decide what is the best treatment approach on a daily basis. The following are recommendations, not a rigid protocol for the treatment of postoperative rotator cuff repairs, postoperative SLAP lesions, and Bankart surgical repairs.

First Two Weeks

No passive movement for the first 2 weeks.

Phase One

Recommended Two to Four Weeks

- LLPS heat—no pain—10 to 20 minutes (see Figure 5-11)
- Trigger points treatment to subscapularis—infraspinatus—supraspinatus (see Figure 5-12). Use of LASER probe (Multi-Radiance Medical)
- Eccentric strengthening to uninvolved limb in the prone position (Figures 5-13 and 5-14)
- External rotation strengthening—eccentric loading in the POS (Figure 5-15)

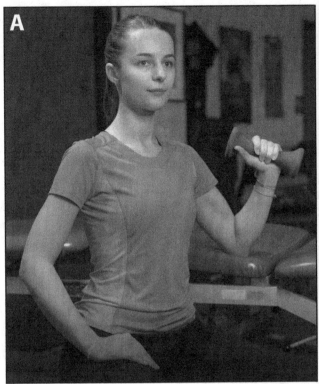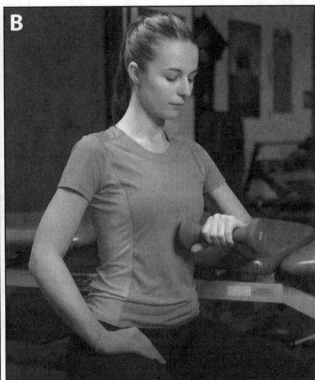

Figure 5-15. (A) External rotation in the POS starting position. (B) Eccentric loading external rotation.

- Russian current to the external rotators and lower middle fibers of trapezius
- Scapula exercises—Protraction—Retraction
- Rib facet restrictions—Manual therapy
- Cervical spine manual therapy of restricted segments

Phase Two

Recommended Four to Six Weeks

- Mobilization of the restricted portions of joint capsule
- LLPS: External rotation NO PAIN—10 minutes with heat (see Figure 5-10)
- Pressure wave and LASER to trigger points
- Subscapularis soft tissue techniques (see Chapter 15); pressure wave into the subscapularis trigger points
- Pulley exercises—biceps/triceps, GH extensions—rows—light-weight high repetitions 3 sets/20 repetitions
- Passive rotation device
- Free weights in pendulum position—horizontal abduction at 90 degrees, 145 degrees, rows, extensions, retractions; light weight—high repetitions—progress to heavier weights

Phase Three

Recommended Six to Eight Weeks Progression With No Pain

- More aggressive mobilization to capsular restrictions
- LLPS continue with heat 15 to 20 minutes—Joint Active Systems device at home
- Increase free weights in all positions—Small increments
- Dynamic hug, 90/90 lower trapezius, bench with reach, latissimus dorsi pulls, scapular depressions
- Scapular mobilization—Subscapularis
- Trigger point treatment with pressure over area with use of laser
- Weight training during this phase should be 60% to 80% of 1 repetition maximum, or find a weight that allows 3 sets/6 to 8 repetitions, then progress to 3 sets/12 to 15 repetitions

Phase Four

Recommended 8 to 12 Weeks and Beyond

- Increase weights to tolerance in all exercises
- Continue to perform manual therapy = mobilization
- LLPS, soft mobilization

REFERENCES

1. Kent BE. Functional anatomy of the shoulder complex: a review. *Phys Ther.* 1971;51(8):947.

2. Lucas D. Biomechanics of the shoulder joint. *Arch Surg.* 1973;107:425-432.

3. Sarrafian SK. Gross and functional anatomy of the shoulder. *Clin Orthop Rel Res.* 1983;173:11-19.

4. Inman VT, Saunders M, Abbott LC. Observations on the function of the shoulder joint. *J Bone Joint Surg.* 1944;26A:1.

5. Dempster WT. Mechanism of shoulder movement. *Arch Phys Med Rehabil.* 1965;46:49-70.

6. Moseley JB Jr, Jobe FW, Pink M, Perry J, Tibone J. EMG analysis of the scapular muscles during a shoulder rehabilitation program. *Am J Sports Med.* 1992;20(2):128-134.

7. Matsen FA, Lippitt SB, Slidles JA, et al. Stability. In Matson FA, Lippitt SB, Slides JA, et al, eds. *Practical Evaluation and Management of the Shoulder.* WB Saunders; 1993.

8. Alpert SW, Pink MM, Jobe FW, McMahon PJ, Mathiyakom W. Electromyographic analysis of deltoid and rotator cuff function under varying loads and speeds. *J Shoulder Elbow Surg.* 2000;9:47-58.

9. Hawkes DH, Alizadehkhaiyat O, Fisher AC, Kemp GJ, Roebuck MM, Frostick SP. Normal shoulder muscular activation and co-ordination during a shoulder elevation task based on activities of daily living: an electromyographic study. *J Orthop Res.* 2012;30:53-60.

10. Wickham J, Pizzari T, Balster S, Ganderton C, Watson L. The variable roles of the upper and lower subscapularis during shoulder motion. *Clin Biomech.* 2014;29:885-891.

11. Saha AK. *Theory of Shoulder Mechanism: Descriptive and Applied.* Thomas; 1961.

12. Warwick R, Williams P, eds. *Gray's Anatomy*, British ed 35. WB Saunders; 1973.

13. Bechtol CO. Biomechanics of the shoulder. *Clin Orthop.* 1980;146:37-41.

14. Johnston TB. Movements of the shoulder joint: plea for use of "plane of the scapula" as plane of reference for movements occurring at humero-scapular joint. *Br J Surg.* 1937;25(98):252-260.

15. Hellwig EV, Perrin DH. A comparison of two positions for assessing shoulder rotator peak torque: the traditional frontal plane versus the plane of the scapula. *Isokin Exerc Sci.* 1991;1:1-5.

16. Doody SG, Freedman L, Waterland JC. Shoulder movements during abduction in the scapular plane. *Arch Phys Med Rehabil.* 1970;51(10):595-604.

17. Saha AK. Mechanics of elevation of glenohumeral joint. *Acta Orthop Scand.* 1973;44(6):668-678.

18. Poppen NK, Walker PS. Forces at the glenohumeral joint in abduction. *Clin Orthop.* 1978;135:165-170.

19. Poppen NK, Walker PS. Normal and abnormal motion of the shoulder. *J Bone Joint Surg.* 1976;58(2):195-201.

20. Greenfield BH, Donatelli R, Wooden MJ, Wilkes J. Isokinetic evaluation of shoulder rotational strength between the plane of the scapula and the frontal plane. *Am J Sports Med.* 1990;18:124-128.

21. Williams PE, Goldspink G. Changes in sarcomere length and physiological properties in immobilized muscle. *J Anat.* 1978;127(Pt 3):459-468.

22. Tardieu C, Huet de la Tour E, Bret MD, Tardieu G. Muscle hypoextensibility in children with cerebral palsy: I. Clinical and experimental observations. *Arch Phys Med Rehabil.* 1982;63(3):97-102.

23. Soderberg GJ, Blaschak MJ. Shoulder internal and external rotation peak torque production through a velocity spectrum in differing positions. *J Orthop Sports Phys Ther.* 1987;8(11):518-524.

24. Hellwig EV, Perrin DH. A comparison of two positions for assessing shoulder rotator peak torque: the traditional frontal plane versus the plane of the scapula. *Isokin Exerc Sci.* 1991;1:1-5.

25. Tata EG, Ng L, Kramer JF. Shoulder antagonistic strength ratios during concentric and eccentric muscle actions in the scapular plane. *J Orthop Sports Phys Ther.* 1993;18(6):654-660.

26. Halliday D, Resnick R, Jeral W. *Fundamentals of Physics.* 10th ed. Wiley and Sons; 2014.

27. Rajendran K. The rotary influence of articular contours during passive glenohumeral abduction. *Singapore Med J.* 1992;33(5):493-495.

28. An KN, Browne AO, Korinek S, Tanaka S, Morrey BF. Three-dimensional kinematics of glenohumeral elevation. *J Orthop Res.* 1991;9(1):143-149.

29. Ludewig PM, Phadke V, Braman JP, Hassett DR, Cieminski CJ, LaPrade RF. Motion of the shoulder complex during multiplanar humeral elevation. *J Bone Joint Surg Am.* 2009;91(2):378-389.

30. Bigliani L, Kelkar R, Faltow E, Pollock RG, Mow VC. Glenohumeral stability: biomechanical properties of passive and active stabilizers. *Clin Orthop Rel Res.* 1996;330:13-30.

31. Bowen MK, Russell FW. Ligamentous control of shoulder stability based on selective cutting and static translation experiments. *Clin Sports Med.* 1991;10(4):757-782.

32. Matsen FA, Lippitt SB, Slidles JA, et al. Stability. In: Matson FA, Lippitt SB, Slides JA, et al, eds. *Practical Evaluation and Management of the Shoulder.* WB Saunders;1993.

33. Burkart A, Debski R. Anatomy and function of the glenohumeral ligaments in anterior shoulder instability. *Clin Orthop Rel Res.* 2002;1:32-39.

34. Kapanji IA. *The Physiology of the Joints & Upper Limb.* Churchill Livingstone; 1970.

35. Abboud J, Soslowsky L. Interplay of the static and dynamic restraints in glenohumeral instability. *Clin Orthop Rel Res.* 2002;1:48-57.

36. Guanche C, Knatt T, Solomonow M, Lu Y, Baratta R. The synergistic action of the capsule and the shoulder muscles. *Am J Sports Med.* 1995;23(3):301-306.

37. Borstad JD, Dashottar A. Quantifying strain on posterior shoulder tissues during 5 stimulated clinical tests: a cadaver study. *J Orthop Sports Phys Ther.* 2011;41(2):90-99.

38. Izumi T, Aoki M, Tanaka Y, et al. Stretching positions for the coracohumeral ligament: strain measurement during passive motion using fresh/frozen cadaver shoulders. *Sports Med Arthrosc Rehabil Ther Technol.* 2011;3(1):2.

39. McGahan PJ, Patel H, Dickinson E, Leasure J, Montgomery W. The effect of biceps adhesions on glenohumeral range of motion: a cadaveric study. *J Shoulder Elbow Surg.* 2013;22(5):658-665.

40. Turkel SJ, Panio MW, Marshall JL, Girgis FG. Stabilizing mechanisms preventing anterior dislocation of the glenohumeral joint. *J Bone Joint Surg Am.* 1981;63(8):1208-1217.

41. Muraki T, Aoki M, Uchiyama E, Takasaki H, Murakami G, Miyamoto S. A cadaveric study of strain on the subscapularis muscle. *Arch Phys Med Rehabil.* 2007;88(7):941-946.

42. Izumi T, Aoki M, Muraki T, Hidaka E, Miyamoto S. Stretching positions for the posterior capsule of the glenohumeral joint: strain measurement using cadaver specimens. *American J Sports Med.* 2008;36(10):2014-2022.

43. Itoi E, Kuechle DK, Newman SR, Morrey BF, An KN. Stabilizing function of the biceps in stable and unstable shoulders. *J Bone Joint Surg.* 1992;75(4):546-550.

44. Borstad JD, Dashottar A. Quantifying strain on posterior shoulder tissues during 5 simulated clinical tests: a cadaver study. *J Orthop Sports Phys Ther.* 2011;41(2):90-99.

45. McClure PW, Michener LA, Sennett BJ, Karduna AR. Direct 3-dimensional measurement of scapular kinematics during dynamic movements in vivo. *J Shoulder Elbow Surg.* 2001;10(3):269-277.

46. Van den Noort JC, Wiertsema SH, Hekman KMC, Schönhuth CP, Dekker J, Harlaar J. Reliability and precision of 3D wireless measurement of scapular kinematics. *Med Biol Eng Comput.* 2014;52(11):921-931.

47. Castillo-Lozano R, Cuesta-Vargas A, Gabel CP. Analysis of arm elevation muscle activity through different movement planes and speeds during in-water and dry-land exercise. *J Shoulder Elbow Surg.* 2014;23(2):159-165.

48. Ludewig SA, Behrens SM, Meyer SM, Spoden LA, Wilson LA. Three-dimensional clavicular motion during arm elevation: reliability and descriptive data. *J Orthop Sports Phys Ther.* 2004;34(3):140-149.

49. Duplay S. De la periarthrite scapulo-humerale. *Rev Frat d Trav de Med.* 1896;53:226; translated, M Week. 1896;4:253. On Scapulo-Humeral Periarthritis. M Press. 1900;59:571.

50. Lewis J. Frozen shoulder contracture syndrome—aetiology, diagnosis and management. *Man Ther.* 2015;20(1):2-9.

51. Dickson J, Crosby E. Periarthritis of the shoulder: an analysis of two hundred cases. *JAMA.* 1932;99(27):2252-2257.

52. Codman EA. Tendinitis of the short rotators. In: *The Shoulder: Rupture of the Supraspinatus Tendon and Other Lesions in or About the Subacromial Bursa.* Thomas Todd; 1934:216-224.

53. Neviaser J. Adhesive capsulitis of the shoulder: a study of the pathological findings in periarthritis of the shoulder. *J Bone Joint Surg.* 1945;27:211-222.

54. Wiley A. Arthroscopic appearance of frozen shoulder. *Arthrosc J Arthrosc Relat Surg.* 1991;7:138-143.

55. Bunker TD, Anthony PP. The pathology of frozen shoulder. A Dupuytren-like disease. *J Bone Joint Surg Br.* 1995;77(5):677-683.

56. Lundberg BJ. The frozen shoulder: clinical and radiographical observations the effect of manipulation under general anesthesia structure and glycosaminoglycan content of the joint capsule local bone metabolism. *Acta Orthop Scand Suppl.* 1969;40(Suppl 119):1-59.

57. Bunker T. Time for a new name for frozen shoulder-contracture of the shoulder. *Shoulder Elb.* 2009;1:4-9.

58. Donatelli R, Ruivo RM, Thurner M, Ibrahim MI. New concepts in restoring shoulder elevation in a stiff and painful shoulder patient. *Phys Ther Sport.* 2014;15(1):3-14. doi:10.1016/j.ptsp.2013.11.001

59. Uppal HS, Evans JP, Smith C. Frozen shoulder: a systematic review of therapeutic options. *World J Orthop.* 2015;6(2):263-268. doi:10.5312/wjo.v6.i2.263

60. Neviaser AS, Hannafin JA. Adhesive capsulitis: a review of current treatment. *Am J Sports Med.* 2010;38(11):2346-2356.

61. Uhthoff HK, Boileau P. Primary frozen shoulder: global capsular stiffness versus localized contracture. *Clin Orthop Relat Res.* 2007;456(456):79-84.

62. Yang J, Jan M-H, Chang C, Lin J. Effectiveness of the end-range mobilization and scapular mobilization approach in a subgroup of subjects with frozen shoulder syndrome: a randomized control trial. *Man Ther.* 2012;17(1):47-52.

63. Wong PL, Tan HC. A review on frozen shoulder. *Singapore Med J.* 2010;51(9):694-697. doi:pubmed/23413793

64. Smith CD, Hamer P, Bunker TD. Arthroscopic capsular release for idiopathic frozen shoulder with intra-articular injection and a controlled manipulation. *Ann R Coll Surg Engl.* 2014;96(1):55-60.

65. Hirschhorn P, Schmidt JM. Frozen shoulder in identical twins. *Joint Bone Spine.* 2000;67(1):75-76.

66. Hakim AJ, Cherkas LF, Spector TD, MacGregor AJ. Genetic associations between frozen shoulder and tennis elbow: a female twin study. *Rheumatology (Oxford).* 2003;42(6):739-742.

67. Smith CD, White WJ, Bunker TD. The associations of frozen shoulder in patients requiring arthroscopic release. *Shoulder Elbow.* 2012;4(2):87-89.

68. Wang K, Ho V, Hunter-Smith DJ, Beh PS, Smith KM, Weber AB. Risk factors in idiopathic adhesive capsulitis: a case control study. *J Shoulder Elbow Surg.* 2013;22(7):e24-e29.

69. Jewell DV, Riddle DL, Thacker LR. Interventions associated with an increased or decreased likelihood of pain reduction and improved function in patients with adhesive capsulitis: a retrospective cohort study. *Phys Ther.* 2009;89(5):419-429.

70. Shaffer B, Tibone JE, Kerlan RK. Frozen shoulder. A long-term follow-up. *J Bone Joint Surg.* 1992;74(5):738-746.

71. Zuckerman D, Rokito A. Frozen shoulder: a consensus definition. *J Shoulder Elbow Surg.* 2011;20:322-325.

72. Reeves B. The natural history of the frozen shoulder syndrome. *Scand J Rheumatol.* 1975;4(4):193-196.

73. Buchbinder R, Youd JM, Green S, et al. Efficacy and cost-effectiveness of physiotherapy following glenohumeral joint distension for adhesive capsulitis: a randomized trial. *Arthritis Rheum.* 2007;57(6):1027-1037.

74. Bal A, Eksioglu E, Gulec B, Aydog E, Gurcay E, Cakci A. Effectiveness of corticosteroid injection in adhesive capsulitis. *Clin Rehabil.* 2008;22(6):503-512.

75. Castellarin G, Ricci M, Vedovi E, et al. Manipulation and arthroscopy under general anesthesia and early rehabilitative treatment for frozen shoulders. *Arch Phys Med Rehabil.* 2004;85(8):1236-1240.

76. Vermeulen HM, Rozing PM, Obermann WR, le Cessie S, Vliet Vlieland TPM. Comparison of high-grade and low-grade mobilization techniques in the management of adhesive capsulitis of the shoulder: randomized controlled trial. *Phys Ther.* 2006;86(3):355-368.

77. Yang J-L, Chang C-W, Chen S-Y, Wang S-F, Lin J-J. Mobilization techniques in subjects with frozen shoulder syndrome: randomized multiple-treatment trial. *Phys Ther.* 2007;87(10):1307-1315.

78. Maund E, Craig D, Suekarran S, et al. Management of frozen shoulder: a systematic review and cost-effectiveness analysis. *Heal Technol Assess.* 2012;16(11):1-264.

79. Kivimäki J, Pohjolainen T, Malmivaara A, et al. Manipulation under anesthesia with home exercises versus home exercises alone in the treatment of frozen shoulder: a randomized, controlled trial with 125 patients. *J Shoulder Elb Surg.* 2007;16(6):722-726.

80. Buchbinder R, Green S, Youd JM. Corticosteroid injections for shoulder pain. *Cochrane Database Syst Rev.* 2003;2003(1):CD004016.

81. Calis M, Demir H, Ulker S, Kirnap M, Duygulu F, Calis HT. Is intraarticular sodium hyaluronate injection an alternative treatment in patients with adhesive capsulitis? *Rheumatol Int.* 2006;26(6):536-540.

82. Ryans I, Montgomery A, Galway R, Kernohan WG, McKane R. A randomized controlled trial of intra-articular triamcinolone and/or physiotherapy in shoulder capsulitis. *Rheumatology.* 2005;44(4):529-535.

83. Carette S, Moffet H, Tardif J, et al. Intraarticular corticosteroids, supervised physiotherapy, or a combination of the two in the treatment of adhesive capsulitis of the shoulder: a placebo-controlled trial. *Arthritis Rheum.* 2003;48(3):829-838.

84. Thurner MS, Donatelli RA, Bascharon R. Subscapularis syndrome: a case report. *Int J Sports Phys Ther.* 2013;8(6):871-882.

85. Huang Y, Chen AC-H, Carroll JD, Hamblin MR. Biphasic dose response in low level light therapy. *Dose Response.* 2009;7(4):358-383.

86. Kneebone W. Laser therapy. Deep penetration therapeutic laser. *Pract Pain Manag.* 2007;7(4):54-56.

87. Taverna E, Parrini M, Cabitza P. Laser therapy versus placebo in the treatment of some bone and joint pathology. *Minerva Ortop E Traumatol.* 1990;41:631-636.

88. Stergioulas A. Low-power laser treatment in patients with frozen shoulder: preliminary results. *Photomed Laser Surg.* 2008;26:99-105.

89. Geraets J, Goossens ME, de Groot IJ, et al. Effectiveness of a graded exercise therapy program for patients with chronic shoulder complaints. *Aust J Physiother.* 2005;51(2):87-94.

90. Hand C, Clipsham K, Rees JL, Carr AJ. Long-term outcome of frozen shoulder. *J Shoulder Elbow Surg.* 2008;17(2):231-236.

91. Levine WN, Kashyap CP, Bak SF, Ahmad CS, Blaine TA, Bigliani LU. Nonoperative management of idiopathic adhesive capsulitis. *J Shoulder Elb Surg.* 2007;16(5):569-573.

92. Kelley MJ, Shaffer MA, Kuhn JE, et al. Shoulder pain and mobility deficits: adhesive capsulitis. *J Orthop Sports Phys Ther.* 2013;43(5):A1-A31. doi:10.2519/jospt.2013.0302

93. Mcclure PW, Michener LA, Andrew R. Research report shoulder function and 3-dimensional scapular kinematics in people with and without shoulder impingement syndrome. *Phys Ther.* 2006;86(8):1075-1090.

94. Bonutti PM, McGrath MS, Ulrich SD, McKenzie SA, Seyler TM, Mont MA. Static progressive stretch for the treatment of knee stiffness. *Knee.* 2008;15(4):272-276. doi:10.1016/j.knee.2008.04.002

95. Vermeulen HM, Obermann WR, Burger BJ, Kok GJ, Rozing PM, van Den Ende CH. End-range mobilization techniques in adhesive capsulitis of the shoulder joint: a multiple-subject case report. *Phys Ther.* 2000;80(12):1204-1213.

96. Bonutti PM, Windau JE, Ables BA, Miller BG. Static progressive stretch to reestablish elbow range of motion. *Clin Orthop Relat Res.* 1994;303:128-134.

97. Mahmoud I, Johnson AJ, Pivec R, Issa K, Naziri Q, Kapadia BH, Mont MA. Treatment of adhesive capsulitis of the shoulder with a static progressive stretch device: a prospective, randomized study. *J Long Term Eff Med Implants.* 2012;22(4):281-291.

98. Ulrich SD, Bonutti PM, Seyler TM, Marker DR, Morrey BF, Mont MA. Restoring range of motion via stress relaxation and static progressive stretch in posttraumatic elbow contractures. *J Shoulder Elbow Surg.* 2010;19(2):196-201. doi:10.1016/j.jse.2009.08.007

99. Fergunson L. Treating shoulder dysfunction and a frozen shoulder. *Chirop Tech.* 1995;7(3):73-81.

100. Noten S, Meeus M, Stassijns G, Van Glabbeek F, Verborgt O, Struyf F. Efficacy of different types of mobilization techniques in patients with primary adhesive capsulitis of the shoulder: a systematic review. *Arch Phys Med Rehabil.* 2015;97(5):815-825. doi:10.1016/j.apmr.2015.07.025

101. Jain TK, Sharma NK. The effectiveness of physiotherapeutic interventions in treatment of frozen shoulder/adhesive capsulitis: a systematic review. 2014;27:247-273. doi:10.3233/BMR-130443

102. Hsu JE, Anakwenze OA, Warrender WJ, Abboud JA. Current review of adhesive capsulitis. *J Shoulder Elbow Surg.* 2011;20(3):502-514.

103. Arce G. Capsular Release. *Arthrosc Tech.* 2016;4(6):e717-e720. doi:10.1016/j.eats.2015.06.004

104. Warzczykowskim M, Polguj M, Fabis J. The impact of arthroscopic capsular release in patients with primary frozen shoulder on shoulder muscle strength. *Biomed Res Int.* 2014;2014:834283. doi:10.1155/2014/834283

105. Favejee MM, Huisstede BM, Koes BW. Frozen shoulder: the effectiveness of conservative and surgical interventions—systematic review. *Br J Sports Med.* 2011;45:49-56. doi:10.1136/bjsm.2010.071431

106. Bjordal JM, Couppe C, Ljunggren AE. Low level laser therapy for tendinopathy: evidence of a dose-response pattern. *Phys Ther Rev.* 2001;6:91-99.

107. Donatelli R. *Physical Therapy of the Shoulder.* 5th ed. Churchill Livingstone; 2012

108. Tashjian RZ. Epidemiology, natural history, and indications for treatment of rotator cuff tears. *Clin Sports Med.* 2012;31(4):589-604. doi:10.1016/j.csm.2012.07.001

109. Kukkonen J, Joukainen A, Lehtinen J, et al. Treatment of non-traumatic rotator cuff tears: a randomized controlled trial with two years of clinical and imaging follow-up. *J Bone Joint Surg Am.* 2015;97(21):1729-1737.

110. Kim HM, Dahiya N, Teefey SA, et al. Location and initiation of degenerative rotator cuff tears: an analysis of three hundred and sixty shoulders. *J Bone Joint Surg Am.* 2010;92(5):1088-1096.

111. Mall NA, Tanaka MJ, Choi LS, Paletta GA Jr. Factors affecting rotator cuff healing. *J Bone Joint Surg Am.* 2014;96(9):778-788.

112. Chakravarty K, Webley M. Shoulder joint movement and its relationship to disability in the elderly. *J Rheumatol.* 1993;20:1359-1361.

113. Sher JS, Uribe JW, Posada A, Murphy BJ, Zlatkin MB. Abnormal findings on magnetic resonance images of asymptomatic shoulders. *J Bone Joint Surg Am.* 1995;77(1):10-15.

114. Tennent TD, Beach WR, Meyers JF. A review of the special tests associated with shoulder examination. Part I: the rotator cuff tests. *Am J Sports Med.* 2003;31(1):154-160.

115. Ok J-H, Kim Y-S, Kim J-M, Yoo T-W. Learning curve of office-based ultrasonography for rotator cuff tendons tears. *Knee Surg Sports Traumatol Arthrosc.* 2013;21:1593-1597.

116. Teefey SA, Middleton WD, Payne WT, Yamaguchi K. Detection and measurement of rotator cuff tears with sonography: analysis of diagnostic errors. *AJR Am J Roentgenol.* 2005;184(6):1768-1773.

117. Wiener SN, Seitz WH Jr. Sonography of the shoulder in patients with tears of the rotator cuff: accuracy and value for selecting surgical options. *AJR Am J Roentgenol.* 1993;160(1):103-107.

118. Saccomanno MF, Cazzato G, Fodale M, Sircana G, Milano G. Magnetic resonance imaging criteria for the assessment of the rotator cuff after repair: a systematic review. *Knee Surg Sports Traumatol Arthrosc.* 2015;23(2):423-442.

119. Dominique L, Samagh SP, Liu X, Kim HT, Feeley BT. Muscle degeneration in rotator cuff tears. *J Shoulder Elbow Surg.* 2012;21(2):164-174.

120. Burkhart SS, Lo IKY. Arthroscopic rotator cuff repair. *J Am Acad Orthop Surg.* 2006;14:333-346.

121. Singh A, Kelly C, O'Brien T, Wilson J, Warner JJP. Ultrasound-guided interscalene block anesthesia for shoulder arthroscopy: a prospective study of 1319 patients. *J Bone Joint Surg Am.* 2012;94(22):2040-2046.

122. Gillespie R, Shishani Y, Streit J, et al. The safety of controlled hypotension for shoulder arthroscopy in the beach-chair position. *J Bone Joint Surg Am.* 2012;94(14):1284-1290.

123. Moen TC, Rudolph GH, Caswell K, Espinoza C, Burkhead WZ Jr, Krishnan SG. Complications of shoulder arthroscopy. *Am Acad Orthop Surg.* 2014;22:410-419.

124. Paxton ES, Backus J, Keener J, Brophy RH. Shoulder arthroscopy: basic principles of positioning, anesthesia, and portal anatomy. *J Am Acad Orthop Surg.* 2013;21:332-342.

125. Burkhart SS, Esch JC, Jolson RS. The rotator crescent and rotator cable: an anatomic description of the shoulder's "suspension bridge." *Arthroscopy.* 1993;9(6):611-616. Published correction appears in *Arthroscopy.* 1994;10(2):239. doi:10.1016/S0749-8063(05)80104-5

126. Nho SJ, Shindle MK, Adler RS, Warren RF, Altchek DW, MacGillivray JD. Prospective analysis of arthroscopic rotator cuff repair: subgroup analysis. *J Shoulder Elbow Surg.* 2009;18(5):697-704.

127. Tashjian RZ, Hollins AM, Kim HM, et al. Factors affecting healing rates after arthroscopic double-row rotator cuff repair. *Am J Sports Med.* 2010;38(12):2435-2442.

128. Iannotti JP, Deutsch A, Green A, et al. Time to failure after rotator cuff repair. *J Bone Joint Surg Am.* 2013;95(11):965-971.

129. Moosmayer S, Tariq R, Stiris M, Smith H. The natural history of asymptomatic rotator cuff tears: a three-year follow-up of fifty cases. *J Bone Joint Surg Am.* 2013;95(14):1249-1255.

130. Cho NS, Rhee YG. The factors affecting the clinical outcome and integrity of arthroscopically repaired rotator cuff tears of the shoulder. *Clin Orthop Surg.* 2009;1(2):96-104.

131. Charousset C, Bellaïche L, Kalra K, Petrover D. Arthroscopic repair of full-thickness rotator cuff tears: is there tendon healing in patients aged 65 years or older? *Arthroscopy*. 2010;26(3):302-309.

132. Jost PW, Khair MM, Chen DX, Wright TM, Kelly AM, Rodeo SA. Suture number determines strength of rotator cuff repair. *J Bone Joint Surg Am*. 2012;94(14):e100.

133. Zacchilli MA, Owens BD. Epidemiology of shoulder dislocations presenting to emergency departments in the United States. *J Bone Joint Surg Am*. 2010;92(3):542-549.

134. Egol KA, Koval KJ, Zuckerman JD, eds. *Handbook of Fractures*. 4th ed. Lippincott Williams & Wilkins; 2010.

135. Cooper DE, Arnoczky SP, O'Brien SJ, Warren RF, DiCarlo E, Allen AA. Anatomy, histology, and vascularity of the glenoid labrum: an anatomical study. *J Bone Joint Surg Am*. 1992;74:46-52.

136. Andrews JR, Carson WG Jr, McLeod WD. Glenoid labrum tears related to the long head of the biceps. *Am J Sports Med*. 1985;13:337-341.

137. Pradhan RL, Itoi E, Hatakeyama Y, Urayama M, Sato K. Superior labral strain during the throwing motion: a cadaveric study. *Am J Sports Med*. 2001;29:488-492.

138. Pradhan RL, Itoi E, Hatakeyama Y, Urayama M, Sato K. Superior labral strain during the throwing motion: a cadaveric study. *Am J Sports Med*. 2001;29:488-492.

139. Rowe CR, Patel D, Southmayd WW. The Bankart procedure: a long-term end-result study. *J Bone Joint Surg Am*. 1978;60(1):1-16.

140. Robinson CM, Shur N, Sharpe T, Ray A, Murray IR. Injuries associated with traumatic anterior glenohumeral dislocations. *J Bone Joint Surg Am*. 2012;94(1):18-26.

141. Provencher MT, Frank RM, Leclere LE, et al. The Hill-Sachs lesion: diagnosis, classification, and management. *J Am Acad Orthop Surg*. 2012;20(4):242-252.

142. Taylor SA, Newman AM, Dawsom C, et al. The "3-pack" examination is critical for comprehensive evaluation of the biceps-labrum complex and the bicipital tunnel: a prospective study. *Arthroscopy*. 2017;33(1):28-38.

143. Miller SL, Cleeman E, Auerbach J, Flatow EL. Comparison of intra-articular lidocaine and intravenous sedation for reduction of shoulder dislocations: a randomized, prospective study. *J Bone Joint Surg Am*. 2002;84(12):2135-2139.

144. Lo IK, Nonweiler B, Woolfrey M, Litchfield R, Kirkley A. An evaluation of the apprehension, relocation, and surprise tests for anterior shoulder instability. *Am J Sports Med*. 2004;32:301-307.

145. Snyder SJ, Karzel RP, Del Pizzo W, Ferkel RD, Friedman MJ. SLAP lesions of the shoulder. *Arthroscopy*. 1990;6:274-279.

146. O'Brien SJ, Pagnani MJ, Fealy S, McGlynn SR, Wilson JB. The active compression test: a new and effective test for diagnosing labral tears and acromioclavicular joint abnormality. *Am J Sports Med*. 1998;26:610-613.

147. Jee WH, McCauley TR, Katz LD, Matheny JM, Ruwe PA, Daigneault JP. Superior labral anterior posterior (SLAP) lesions of the glenoid labrum: reliability and accuracy of MR arthrography for diagnosis. *Radiology*. 2001;218:127-132.

148. Ahmed I, Ashton F, Robinson CM. Arthroscopic Bankart repair and capsular shift for recurrent anterior shoulder instability: functional outcomes and identification of risk factors for recurrence. *J Bone Joint Surg Am*. 2012;94(14):1308-1315.

149. Ahmed I, Ashton F, Robinson CM. Arthroscopic Bankart repair and capsular shift for recurrent anterior shoulder instability: functional outcomes and identification of risk factors for recurrence. *J Bone Joint Surg Am*. 2012;94(14):1308-1315.

150. Burkhart SS, De Beer JF, Barth JR, Cresswell T, Roberts C, Richards DP. Results of modified Latarjet reconstruction in patients with anteroinferior instability and significant bone loss. *Arthroscopy*. 2007;23(10):1033-1041.

151. Lynch JR, Clinton JM, Dewing CB, Warme WJ, Matsen FA III. Treatment of osseous defects associated with anterior shoulder instability. *J Shoulder Elbow Surg*. 2009;18(2):317-328.

152. Williams MM, Snyder SJ, Buford D Jr. The Buford complex—the "cord-like" middle glenohumeral ligament and absent anterosuperior labrum complex: a normal anatomic capsulolabral variant. *Arthroscopy*. 1994;10(3):241-247.

153. Galloway MT, Lalley AI, Shearn JT. Current concepts review. The role of mechanical loading in tendon. Development, maintenance, injury and repair. *J Bone Joint Surg Am*. 2013;95:1620-1628.

154. Peltz CD, Dourte LM, Kuntz AF, et al. The effect of postoperative passive motion on rotator cuff healing in a rat model. *J Bone Joint Surg A*. 2009;91(10):2421-2429.

155. Uhthoff HK, Seki M, Backman DS, Trudel G, Himori K, Sano H. Tensile strength of the supraspinatus after reimplantation into a bony trough: an experimental study in rabbits. *J Shoulder Elbow Surg*. 2002;11(5):504-509.

156. Lee BG, Cho NS, Rhee YG. Effect of two rehabilitation protocols on range of motion and healing rates after arthroscopic rotator cuff repair: aggressive versus limited early passive exercises. *Arthroscopy*. 2012;28(1):34-42.

157. Stanish WD, Rubinovich RM, Curwin S. Eccentric exercise in chronic tendinitis. *Clin Orthop Relat Res*. 1986;(208):65-68.

6

Dysfunction, Evaluation, and Treatment of the Elbow

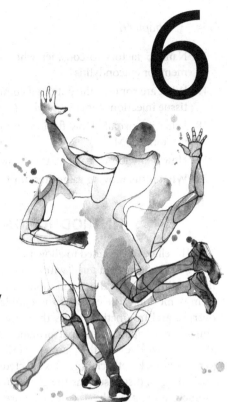

Matthew L. Holland, PT, SCS, CSCS; Corbin Hedt, PT, DPT, SCS, CSCS; and Blair Bundy, PT, DPT, SCS

KEY TERMS

Elbow: The joint connecting the upper and lower arm, consisting of the humerus, ulna, and radius.

Kinetic chain: A concept relating human movement characteristics to the multiregional demands of associated body parts.

Overhead athlete: Amateur or professional athlete who participates in overhead-specific activities (eg, throwing, pulling, swimming, racquet sports).

Overuse injuries: Injuries encountered by means of repetitive trauma and stress.

Throwing: The act of propelling an object through the air by movement of the upper extremities.

CHAPTER QUESTIONS

1. What is the angular velocity at the elbow during throwing?
2. What 2 phases of throwing are of particular importance to understanding throwing-related injuries?
3. What is the normal carrying angle of the elbow?

4. What is Little League elbow?
5. What are the main overuse injuries in the elbow?
6. What is the role of eccentric exercise in treating chronic epicondylitis?
7. How long is a patient immobilized following a distal biceps rupture repair?
8. How long should a young athlete rest from throwing with medial epicondylar apophysitis?
9. Why is it important to use an interval throwing program following ulnar collateral ligament (UCL) reconstruction in the elbow?
10. How long after UCL reconstruction does a patient have to wait to begin throwing?
11. What is valgus extension overload (VEO)?
12. What are the typical sports that result in osteochondral defects in the elbows of youth athletes?
13. What are the types/classification of radial head fractures?
14. Why is it important for early rehabilitation following elbow dislocation?
15. What is the general timeline for return to play following UCL reconstruction in the elbow of a baseball player?

Wallmann HW, Donatelli R, eds. *Foundations of Orthopedic Physical Therapy* (pp 153-167).
© 2024 Taylor & Francis Group.

16. Name 5 factors to consider when determining treatment for epicondylitis?

17. What are some of the potential complications with soft tissue injections for epicondylitis?

18. What is normal elbow flexion and extension range of motion (ROM)?

19. How many joints make up the elbow complex?

20. What is the moving valgus test for the elbow?

INTRODUCTION

The elbow is designed to allow for shortening or lengthening of the arm combined with forearm rotation, providing stability for skilled hand motions and forceful upper extremity motions. The elbow is susceptible to both repetitive overuse and traumatic injuries that can severely impair an athlete's participation and performance in sport. We must also acknowledge that the elbow is a critical link in the upper extremity kinetic chain and is affected by structures both proximal and distal, such as the glenohumeral and scapulothoracic joints, as well as the musculature of the forearm and various bony articulations at the wrist and hand. As such, we would be remiss to not include and emphasize the importance of assessing structures that contribute to dynamic stabilization of the upper extremity kinetic chain as well as the muscles and joints of the elbow itself in the comprehensive evaluation of the athletic elbow. This chapter discusses how to best identify and treat elbow injuries in the athlete and provides evidence-based treatment progressions for both repetitive overuse as well as traumatic elbow injuries.

After reading this chapter, the reader will be able to:

- Discuss anatomy and biomechanics of the elbow in regard to various athletic endeavors.

- Effectively assess the pathologic elbow and upper quarter and implement key examination strategies to identify ligamentous, musculoskeletal, and neurological injury.

- Discuss special concerns regarding the skeletally immature athlete.

- Identify both tendinous and muscular overuse pathologies in the elbow and appropriately manage the patient's rehabilitation, with an emphasis on return to sport.

- Explain how to properly manage a patient who has undergone UCL reconstruction.

- Introduce and progress an interval-throwing program in both operative and nonoperative patients.

- Differentiate the common causes of various elbow fractures and dislocations and how to manage both operative and nonoperative care.

- Identify and differentiate VEO from olecranon stress fractures in throwing athletes and determine an appropriate course of rehabilitation.

- Discuss the management of osteochondritis dissecans (OCD) lesions in overhead athletes.

ANATOMY

The distal humerus articulates with the radius and ulna, providing for 2 degrees of freedom with elbow flexion and extension as well as forearm pronation and supination. The elbow is comprised of 3 different joints surrounded by a common joint capsule and works in conjunction with the wrist and shoulder to provide increased versatility and durability.[1] The humeroulnar joint is the junction of the trochlear notch of the ulna articulating with the trochlear groove of the humerus. The humeroulnar joint, a simple hinge joint, allows for elbow flexion and extension. The head of the radius articulates with the capitellum of the humerus, creating a ball and socket joint known as the *humeroradial joint*. Finally, the proximal radioulnar joint is a pivot joint made up of the head of the radius and radial notch of the ulna, and allows for both pronation and supination.

Both ligaments and muscles span the elbow joint, providing components of static and dynamic stability during athletic activity. The UCL (medial) is a thick triangular band beginning at the medial epicondyle of the elbow that unites the distal humerus with the proximal aspect of the ulna at both the olecranon and coronoid process. The anterior band resists valgus stress between 30 and 120 degrees of elbow flexion and is most often injured, the posterior band contributes to valgus stress resistance at elbow flexion angles greater than 90 degrees, and the transverse band runs from the olecranon process to the coronoid process of the elbow and does not articulate with the humerus. The radial (lateral) collateral ligament spans between the lateral epicondyle of the humerus and the annular ligament, and resists varus stress. The annular ligament encircles the head of the radius, preventing dislocation and allowing for pronation and supination of the radial head.[1]

The primary contributors to elbow flexion are the brachialis, biceps brachii, and brachioradialis, while the extensors are composed of the triceps brachii and anconeus muscles. The brachialis originates low on the anterior side of the humerus and is inserted into the tuberosity of the ulna. The biceps brachii originate via 2 heads proximally at the shoulder, and insert with a common tendon at the radial tuberosity and lacertus fibrosis to origins of the forearm flexors. The biceps brachii contributes to both elbow flexion and forearm supination. The brachioradialis originates at the lateral supracondylar ridge distally on the humerus and inserts distally on the radius at the styloid process, helping with flexion and forearm supination/pronation. The triceps brachii originate with 2 heads posteriorly on the humerus and with its long head on the scapula just below the shoulder joint, inserting posteriorly on the olecranon process of the ulna. The anconeus originates on the posterior surface of the lateral epicondyle of the humerus and inserts distally on the posterior surface of the ulna, providing a negligible contribution to extension of the elbow. The muscles responsible for pronation and supination of the forearm include the pronator teres and supinator. The pronator teres originates from the medial supracondylar ridge of the humerus at the common flexor tendon and at the coronoid process of the ulna and inserts along the middle lateral surface of the radius. It helps pronate the forearm and provides dynamic resistance to valgus force. The supinator originates from the supinator crest of the ulna, lateral epicondyle of humerus, radial collateral ligament, and annular radial ligament, and inserts along the lateral proximal radial shaft. It functions to supinate the forearm at the elbow. The median, radial, ulnar, and musculocutaneous nerves and their respective branches provide innervations to these muscles.[1]

BIOMECHANICS OF THE ELBOW

The elbow is a vital contributor to participating in sports and is subject to very high levels of stress through various movement patterns, particularly overhead throwing. Angular velocities at the elbow have been measured at more than 3000 degrees per second during the acceleration phase of throwing, and varus torque measurements have been shown to be between 64 and 100 Newton-meters (Nm) at the elbow when the shoulder is in a maximally externally rotated position during the throwing motion.[2] The 2 critical instances of elbow stress during the throwing motion are at the elbow cocking and deceleration phases, where large forces must be absorbed through the musculature in order to avoid overloading the underlying static stabilizers.[3] According to Morrey and An,[4] the UCL provides up to 54% of static varus torque at the elbow, and DiGiovine[5] showed that the flexor-pronator muscle mass generates a dynamic varus torque to resist valgus stress at the elbow, unloading the UCL and radiocapitellar joint. During the deceleration phase of throwing, biceps, triceps, and wrist flexor and extensor muscle activity all increase tremendously to further dissipate forces from the violent motion, further sparing static structures from forces with which they are not prepared to handle alone.

EXAMINATION OF THE ELBOW

A thorough evaluation of the elbow includes the accurate measurement of both distal and proximal joint ROM, muscular strength assessment, radiographic examination (if indicated), and selected use of several special tests. It should be noted that in the unilaterally dominant individual, adaptive changes can occur in the dominant arm; therefore, careful inspection of the contralateral upper extremity can give the clinician a better understanding of if and how these adaptive changes are contributing to an individual's injury. These differences can often be seen by visual inspection of the carrying angle of the elbow, seen by having the patient stand in front of you while assuming the anatomical position, or seen

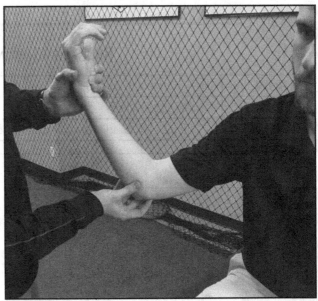

Figure 6-1. Elbow examination.

by having them raise the arms in front of their body to 90 degrees flexion with their elbows fully extended and palms in full supination. Overhead athletes subjected to the repetitive valgus stress associated with throwing can present with 11 to 14 degrees of valgus in men (13 to 16 degrees in women) and carrying angles in excess of 15 degrees.[6] Starting with palpation, the clinician should take the elbow through its complete ROM passively (Figure 6-1), carefully noting for crepitus, localized discomfort, or any impedance to full ROM. Normative values for the elbow and wrist are referenced in Table 6-1. The examiner should take care to assess the radial head for either tenderness or crepitus by passively rotating the forearm into both pronation and supination while palpating the radial head at its most prominent aspect.

A thorough examination of the muscles immediately surrounding the elbow as well as the muscles above and below the elbow (Figures 6-2 and 6-3) is crucial in identifying soft tissue pathologies, and care should be taken to look at ROM in the wrist and glenohumeral joint as well (Figure 6-4), as the elbow is merely one link in the upper extremity kinetic chain. Ellenbecker et al[7] also recommend a static and dynamic assessment of the scapulothoracic joint, as they have found "a high association of scapular and rotator cuff weakness with elbow overuse injuries in the throwing athlete." Assessment of the glenohumeral joint should include a measurement of the athlete's shoulder internal rotation (Figure 6-5), external rotation, and cross-body shoulder adduction (Figure 6-6), as Dines et al[8] have found a correlation between shoulder internal rotation ROM loss and UCL injuries in baseball players. It is also recommended to obtain strength measurements of shoulder external and internal rotation, as this ratio has been shown to play a role in the development of lateral epicondylalgia.[9]

Table 6-1

RANGE OF MOTION NORMATIVE DATA

ELBOW	Extension/flexion	0 degrees/145 degrees
FOREARM	Pronation/supination	70 degrees/85 degrees
WRIST	Flexion/extension/radial deviation/ulnar deviation	70 degrees/75 degrees/20 degrees/35 degrees

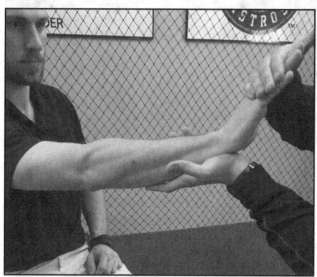

Figure 6-2. Wrist strength testing.

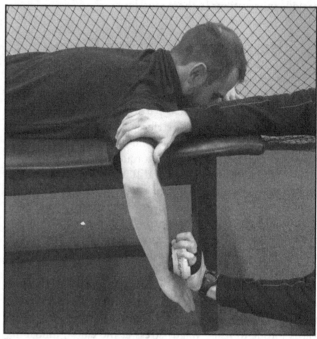

Figure 6-3. Shoulder strength testing.

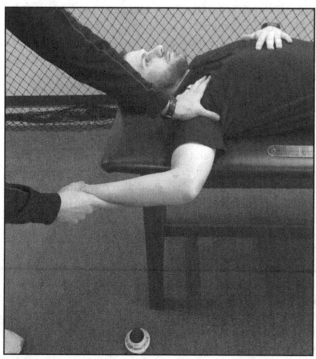

Figure 6-4. Shoulder ROM.

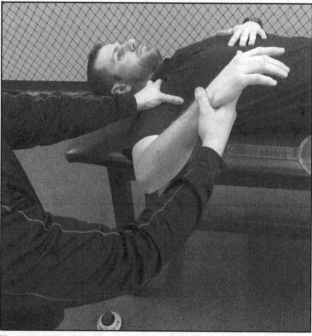

Figure 6-5. Shoulder internal ROM.

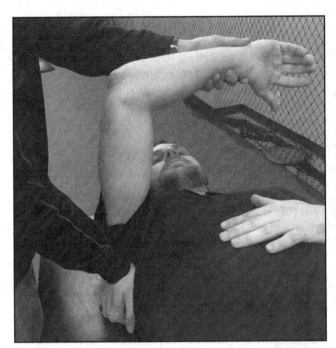

Figure 6-6. Cross-body adduction.

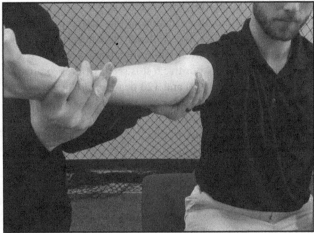

Figure 6-7. Valgus stress test.

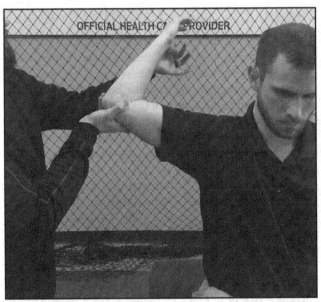

Figure 6-8. Milking test.

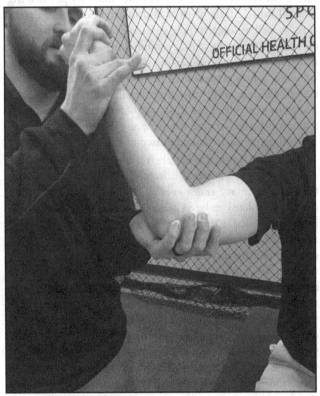

Figure 6-9. Moving valgus stress test.

A variety of special tests currently exist for examination of the elbow, such as Tinel's test, varus/valgus stress test (Figure 6-7), VEO test, milking test (Figure 6-8), moving valgus stress test (Figure 6-9), and muscular provocation tests. Tinel's test is performed by having the examiner tap the ulnar nerve as it runs through the cubital tunnel retinaculum in the medial elbow. Reproduction of paresthesias along the course of the nerve indicates a positive test.[10] Valgus stress testing assesses the integrity of the UCL and is performed with the elbow in 15 to 25 degrees of elbow flexion with the forearm in supination, where maximum stress can be imparted to the UCL by administering a valgus stress at the elbow joint.

Even in unilaterally dominant athletes, symmetrical elbow laxity should be expected when the UCL is intact.[7] Varus stress testing is performed in the same elbow position, with a varus stress imparted at the elbow joint to assess the integrity of the radial (lateral) collateral ligament.[4] The VEO test is used to determine whether posterior elbow pain is caused by an osteophyte abutting the medial margin of the trochlea and the olecranon fossa. Placing the affected elbow in full flexion, a valgus stress is imparted to the elbow while moving the elbow into full extension, reproducing the stress seen in the acceleration phase of throwing or serving.[11] The moving valgus stress test is another test to assess UCL integrity and is performed by placing the affected upper extremity into 90 degrees of shoulder abduction in the frontal plane, with the elbow fully flexed. The clinician then moves the elbow into an extended position while imparting a valgus stress through the elbow. A positive test is seen with reproduction of symptoms between 70 and 120 degrees of elbow flexion. This best represents the shear seen at the elbow during the "late cocking" phase of throwing, and has been shown to be both highly sensitive and specific.[12] Another test for UCL integrity is the milking sign, which the patient can perform on themselves by placing the elbow into 90 degrees of flexion, with the opposite arm reaching underneath and grabbing the thumb on the affected extremity and pulling laterally. This maneuver imparts a valgus stress and can better assess the integrity of the posterior band of the UCL.[4] Lastly, flexor and extensor muscular provocation tests should be performed to screen the muscle tendon units of the elbow. By performing manual muscle tests of wrist and finger flexion and extension, as well as forearm pronation and supination, the clinician can provoke the muscle tendon unit at either the medial or lateral epicondyle, indicating a possible overload/overuse muscular injury at these sites. Reproduction of medial or lateral elbow pain with resisted testing in the aforementioned positions would lead to a diagnosis of humeral epicondylitis, a flexor-pronator muscle strain, or an extensor muscle strain depending on the location of discomfort.[13]

Special care should be taken when examining the skeletally immature patient. Distinguishing between a muscle-tendon unit injury and a growth plate injury in the young throwing athlete can be a challenging diagnosis; therefore, it is recommended to rule out any potential osteochondral injuries prior to determining a treatment strategy. Growth plates, or an epiphyseal plate or physis, are the last sites of the bone to ossify, and can remain open and active for up to 16 years of age.[14] Dotter first described Little League shoulder in the literature in 1953,[15] and Heyworth et al[16] postulated the condition stems from chronic, repetitive microtraumatic shear, torque, or traction forces imposed on the unossified cartilage of the proximal humeral physis in the growing arm. Unfortunately, we have seen an increase in prevalence and diagnosis of this condition over the past 10 years.[16] The medial epicondylar apophysis is also suspect to overuse injuries through repetitive valgus stresses in a condition known as *Little League elbow*. Rather than rupture the UCL, repeated stress to the apophysis can result in apophyseal widening and result in a traction apophysitis or even an avulsion fracture. These unossified growth plates represent a weak link in the upper extremity kinetic chain in the adolescent athlete and are particularly vulnerable to the repeated forceful muscular contractions associated with the acceleration phase of throwing and the overhead serving motion in tennis.[17,18] Apophysitis will be addressed in further detail later in this chapter.

ELBOW OVERUSE INJURIES

Medial and lateral elbow tendon complications are often due to repetitive overload of the proximal attachments of the forearm flexor or extensor muscle groups. These pathologies are dichotomized based on the laterality of the associated tendon group: tennis elbow (forearm extensors) and golfer's elbow (forearm flexors).

Lateral Epicondylitis (Tennis Elbow)

Lateral epicondylitis is a pathology defined as gradual onset pain and tenderness over the lateral aspect of the forearm and elbow. Resisted wrist extension and third finger extension is often painful with a tender point just distal to the lateral epicondyle of the humerus. Most cases are unilateral and of the dominant upper extremity. Pain can be elicited by performing movements that use the extensor muscles, such as closing a jar, tennis backhand, repetitive heavy lifting or use of heavy tools, or precision forearm movements (eg, using a screwdriver). Thus, at-risk populations for this disorder include manual laborers and tennis players.[19,20]

Medial Epicondylitis (Golfer's Elbow)

Medial epicondylitis is commonly identified as pain and tenderness over the medial epicondyle of the humerus, radiating into the forearm musculature and is aggravated by wrist flexion and pronation. A dull ache is prominent along this region and is gradual in nature. Shaking hands, opening a jar, swinging a golf club (dominant arm), or bowling will usually exacerbate pain the most. It is not uncommon to experience symptoms of neuropathy in the ulnar nerve distribution as well, including paresthesias (numbness or tingling) in the fourth and fifth fingers as well as weakness in gripping. This is due to the anatomical proximity of the ulnar nerve and the medial epicondyle. Careful attention should be given to differential diagnoses that could present as similar conditions.[21]

Treatment for medial and lateral epicondylitis can vary widely based on the practitioner and patient presentation. There is a lack of ultimate consensus on best treatment for either disorders, propagating as a source of frustration for patients and clinicians.[22] However, many studies suggest that treatment approaches should be multifactorial and not necessarily implement a one-size-fits-all model.[23] Factors to consider when determining treatment interventions include the following[23]:

- Advanced tendon pathology (chronicity of biophysical changes)
- Severity of pain
- Neck or shoulder complications
- Associated neurological impairments
- Work-related task requirements

Typically, patients will undergo conservative (nonsurgical) therapy before considering more invasive procedures.[24] The initial focus of care for medial or lateral epicondylitis is to reduce pain and inflammation of the affected area.[25] Nonsteroidal anti-inflammatory drugs (NSAIDs) are a common mainstay of treatment, although evidence for their efficacy is limited.[21,26] Splinting or taping techniques are also commonly used to help alleviate pain and discomfort; however, caution should be used to avoid prolonged immobilization and subsequent joint stiffness or muscle atrophy. Corticosteroid injections are typically reserved for later in the rehabilitation process if general NSAIDs and other conservative measures are ineffective. There is strong evidence that corticosteroid injections provide short-term relief of symptoms (2 to 12 weeks) but leads to no long-term benefit. There are also increased iatrogenic risks associated with corticosteroids, including tendon weakening, nerve injury, or muscle atrophy. Therefore, injections are usually not indicated as a first-line treatment measure.[25,26] As an individual begins to progress past the initial phases of pain and inflammation, they are able to incorporate further physical therapy approaches such as exercise and manual therapy. These treatments are central to the management of medial or lateral epicondylitis.[25] Initial goals in physical therapy include restoration of ROM and flexibility in the flexor/pronator or extensor muscle masses. Manual therapy, including passive stretching and joint mobilization, provides high levels of successful relief of pain-producing movements. If impairments in the spinal or shoulder regions are also present and addressed, manual therapy can provide additional clinical benefit as part of a multiregional approach. Exercise may be introduced early in the rehabilitation process but should be closely monitored by skilled therapists. Strengthening should focus on the affected muscle groups and low loads may be implemented initially, gradually increasing as tolerated. Global activities can be added to improve shoulder and postural strength, generally improving overall upper extremity performance and efficiency. General guidelines indicate that optimal frequency, intensity, and type of exercise may differ between patients. Isometric activities are typically initiated first and progressed to concentric and eccentric, respectively.

Eccentric exercise has been studied in depth for medial and lateral epicondylitis along with other tendinous pathology.[25-27] Typically, eccentrics are indicated to improve healing parameters for the affected tendon and musculature. Conflicting evidence exists on appropriate time frames for eccentric loading as well as volume. However, multiple studies indicate that a combination of concentric and eccentric activities for those with degenerative tendinopathy is beneficial for long-term improvement in symptoms.[25]

Overall, professional expertise and judgement will guide treatment. Utilization of current evidence-based concepts is paramount to achieve optimal outcomes. Emerging research trends are evaluating further treatment approaches including extracorporeal shockwave therapy, blood-flow restriction training, platelet-rich plasma injections, ultrasound, and electrical stimulation techniques. Caution should be taken when considering these approaches as their efficacy has not been fully evaluated.[25,26]

DISTAL BICEPS/TRICEPS PATHOLOGY

Complications of the distal tendons in the biceps/triceps muscle groups are relatively uncommon. Tendonitis/tendonosis is rare in this region,[26] and clinicians will more often see partial or complete ruptures of the tendon complex.

Distal Biceps Rupture

Biceps ruptures are often acute injuries occurring in conjunction with a large eccentric contraction.[26] The biceps tendon avulses from the radial tuberosity, leading to immediate pain and loss of function. Reported risk factors are prior distal biceps rupture, hand dominance, tobacco use, and anabolic steroid use. A painful "pop" is commonly reported along with immediate weakness of elbow flexion and/or supination. Examination should include palpation of the affected area, which may reveal a void in the antecubital fossa. Visual deformity may also be present with proximal retraction causing a reverse "Popeye deformity." Diffuse ecchymosis and edema will likely persist following the injury. Magnetic resonance imaging scans are used to confirm tears and delineate between partial and complete ruptures.

Surgical repair of a distal biceps tendon rupture often results in the greatest return of function.[28] There are several different reported techniques for repair, but postoperative rehabilitation is fairly uniform. Typically, patients are immobilized at 90 degrees of elbow flexion with initial restrictions to limit passive or active extension to protect surgical integrity. Forearm passive pronation supination and pronation are allowed day 1 postoperative. Progressive elbow extension is allowed up to week 6, with a goal of full ROM at postoperative week 6. Gradual strengthening may be incorporated at this time under a skilled rehabilitation professional.

Distal Triceps Rupture

Triceps tendon pathology is often the least common type of elbow tendinopathy.[26] True triceps tendonitis may occur in overhead athletes who perform rapid, repetitive, extension-based activities. Typically, triceps ruptures occur more often in young, active men who experience a traumatic, forced elbow flexion—often when falling onto an outstretched hand.[29] Rupture usually occurs in conjunction with avulsion from the olecranon process. Examination will reveal edema and ecchymosis at the posterior elbow along with a palpable void proximal to the olecranon. Partial tears may lead to a preservation of some active elbow extension, but weakness and pain will persist. X-ray imaging will indicate if an avulsion is present. Magnetic resonance imaging or ultrasonography can also be used to examine the extent of muscular damage.

Patients with triceps tendonitis often respond well to activity modification, NSAIDs, and physical therapy.[29] Resolution occurs over weeks to months. Incomplete tears may be managed conservatively as well but are often immobilized in a 30-degree flexion splint for up to 4 weeks.[29] They will then progress through stretching and strengthening exercises to regain full function. Complete thickness tears and avulsion cases are often repaired surgically. Immobilization is then provided for up to 6 weeks before strengthening and ROM are initiated. Surgical triceps repair often yields good results with proper compliance.[29]

APOPHYSEAL INJURY

Medial apophyseal complications occur far more than lateral apophysis injury. Generally, the apophysis of the medial side of the elbow is subject to high tensile loads from the flexor muscle complex during throwing or rapid overhead movements. The repetitive stress from these associated muscles and tendons leads to inflammation of the apophyseal junction, including cartilage within the growth plate. Over time, this structure may be compromised and result in avulsion, fracture, or general inflammation. This can lead to debilitating pain and loss of function.[29]

Treatment of Epicondylar Apophysitis

Treatment of medial epicondyle apophysitis generally consists of a period of rest from throwing for a minimum of 4 to 8 weeks.[29] We have seen an increase in these injuries due to the early sports specialization with young athletes performing more game and practice repetitions than their immature musculoskeletal system can withstand. Oftentimes the parents of these athletes will hear only the 4- to 8-week rest period and assume full return to play immediately after that time frame. In our experience, the rest should be followed by a period of time that the athlete performs a progressive interval throwing program to re-introduce gradual stress back to the medial elbow in a controlled manner to decrease the likelihood of re-injury.

ULNAR COLLATERAL LIGAMENT INJURY

In the skeletally mature athlete, the UCL is placed under significant load with throwing. In the cocking phase, the UCL is placed under a great deal of stress, and with the repetitive nature of throwing, the ligament is subjected to high repetitive load with an incomplete time of recovery between bouts of throwing. Over time, this repetitive microtrauma can lead to attenuation or tearing of the ligament, which may lead to insufficiency of the ligament to provide valgus stability during cocking.

Treatment of Ulnar Collateral Ligament Tears

For treatment of UCL tears, typically, nonoperative treatment is attempted first, but the long-term outcomes and limited studies have not provided promising results.[30] For partial tears, a period of rest is usually prescribed that includes at least 8 to 12 weeks of no throwing. During this time, the athlete should undergo a thorough rehabilitation program that includes treatment of postural deficits and strength training of the shoulder and elbow with special attention to the posterior shoulder musculature. The athlete should also be examined for loss of internal rotation ROM (see Figure 6-5) or cross-body horizontal adduction (see Figure 6-6) ROM, as well as hip and core strengthening. Balance retraining should also be addressed. Following the rest period, a progressive interval throwing program should be utilized that will gradually progress the athlete back to competition. Many previous studies have examined the beneficence of interval-based return-to-sport progressions.[31-34] In our experience, the throwing program is a critical component and lack of gradual progression may lead to failure in the nonoperative rehabilitation process. Available literature supports that programs should be customized based on age, gender, position, level of play, and injury type to allow for a structured and specific means of graduated activity progression.[31-40] Proper throwing mechanics must also be addressed by the rehabilitation professional or coach to decrease the likelihood of re-injury.

UCL reconstruction has become commonplace in baseball. There have been advances in the technique used to repair the UCL, and these have been shown to be equal in regard to biomechanics and clinical outcomes.[30]

Postoperative rehabilitation for UCL reconstruction is similar between the various types of repair. Phase 1 (weeks 0 to 3) typically involves protection of the elbow and gentle ROM exercises to prevent postoperative stiffness. Phase 2 (weeks 3 to 6) involves initiation of light strength exercises for the shoulder and elbow while avoiding any valgus stress to elbow. At week 6, the postoperative brace is generally discontinued and the athlete should have normal or near normal ROM. If an extension lag is present, the athlete should use low-load long duration stretching to achieve normal extension ROM. During weeks 6 to 12, progressive strengthening exercises are used, and from weeks 14 to 16, plyometric exercises are initiated starting with 2 hand drills and progressing to unilateral activities. A progressive throwing program is initiated no sooner than 16 weeks postoperative, and athletes will typically take 4 to 8 months of interval throwing program to return to their respective position in game play. Most players return to game play from 10 to 18 months postoperative.[30]

VALGUS EXTENSION OVERLOAD

Dugas[41] describes VEO as a "syndrome of symptoms and physical findings" caused by impingement of the posteromedial tip of the olecranon process along the medial wall of the olecranon fossa. When assessing the overhead athlete, the clinician must take care to differentiate between olecranon stress fractures and VEO, as their symptoms can overlap. A key finding in the diagnosis of VEO in the overhead athlete is posterior elbow pain at ball release. Olecranon stress fractures can result from repeated abutment of the olecranon into the olecranon fossa in combination with valgus forces and traction stress from eccentric triceps activity during the deceleration phase of throwing.

Olecranon stress fractures can be divided into 2 types: transverse and oblique. Transverse fractures occur when triceps traction and extension forces predominate, whereas oblique fractures are caused by valgus and extension forces, resulting in olecranon contact on the medial wall of the olecranon fossa.[42] Pain can be elicited with resistive triceps activity and forced elbow extension, mimicking ball release during the throwing motion, or possibly during valgus stress testing. Upon examination, an athlete with an olecranon stress fracture may present with tenderness to palpation more distal and lateral on the proximal shaft of the olecranon compared with the posteromedial olecranon seen during VEO. It can be difficult to distinguish VEO from an olecranon stress fracture, as both conditions can present with tenderness during forced elbow extension.

Initially, both olecranon stress fractures and VEO should be treated with a course of active rest from throwing, while therapy should focus on rotator cuff and scapular strengthening and addressing any soft tissue dysfunction around the elbow and shoulder that could be limiting ROM or promoting aberrant movement patterns. A plyometric program should be initiated when the athlete is pain-free at rest, has negative provocative tests and radiographic resolution with any stress fracture, appropriate shoulder/elbow ROM, and adequate shoulder internal/external rotation strength ratios. After completion of a plyometric program that first incorporates bilateral motions before progressing to unilateral motions, an interval-throwing program should be implemented to allow for a step-wise return to competition. In the case of return to sport with an olecranon stress fracture, the initial treatment requires rest from throwing. The clinician should note that return to competition can be delayed up to 6 months, secondary to the slower rate of healing of olecranon stress fractures when compared with regular fracture healing.[42]

OSTEOCHONDRAL DEFECTS OF THE ELBOW

OCD is a lesion or injury to the subchondral bone and may involve the integrity of the surrounding articular cartilage. The close relationship between OCD and adjacent cartilage carries with it the risk for injury and disruption that can lead to premature arthritis.[43] OCD lesions are primarily seen in pediatric/adolescent athletes, typically between the ages of 10 and 12 years, are more common in boys than girls, and are often seen in sports such as gymnastics, cheerleading, and sports involving overhead throwing. A patient with a suspected OCD lesion of the elbow will often describe a history of overuse, repetitive impact, or participation in overhead sports. Due to increased involvement in competitive, unilaterally dominant, year-round sport, capitellar OCD lesions are rising in prevalence.[44,45] During the acceleration phase of throwing, excess valgus forces place undue stress across the capitellum; these stresses are magnified with repetitive activity, resulting in added compressive and shear forces. As the elbow is compressed, immature bones are forced together, which can result in the underlying cartilage or subchondral bone damage. The pain associated with an OCD lesion can often subside if the athlete rests from the offending activity for a few weeks, giving them a false sense of security in the health of their elbow. An athlete with an OCD lesion typically presents with insidious onset of activity-related pain, tenderness to palpation along the posterolateral joint line, edema, possible ROM limitations (particularly loss of terminal elbow extension), and a positive VEO test with pain over the *lateral* aspect of the elbow. This pain over the lateral aspect of the elbow is a key differentiator between a possible OCD lesion and an overuse injury on the medial side of the elbow. High-resolution imaging may be warranted to further rule out other joint conditions, such as a physeal stress injury or Panner disease.[44]

OCD lesions can be classified as stable or unstable. Stable lesions show an open physes, normal elbow ROM, and flattening of the subchondral bone, whereas unstable lesions are characterized by a mature capitellum with a closed physes, bone fragments within the joint space, and restricted elbow ROM. Stable lesions are most often managed nonoperatively with good outcomes, whereas unstable lesions typically show poorer outcomes with nonoperative care and are best managed surgically.[46] If the clinician determines that a nonoperative course of treatment is in the athlete's best interest, the immediate goal of treatment should be to decrease pain, restore ROM at both the elbow and possibly the shoulder, and reduce edema. During this early phase, patient and family education regarding activity avoidance and modification is vital to prevent further disease progression. It is currently unclear at this time as to how long an appropriate period of rest from the offending activity is, with current literature showing anywhere from 6 weeks to 6 months.[43] Education to both the athlete and parent is vital during the initial phases of rehabilitation, as Mihara and Bain[47] found that 75% of patients who showed radiographic evidence of lesion progression upon reexamination had gone against medical advice and continued throwing.[47] This underscores the importance of adherence to a strict schedule of rest from throwing in order to obtain a positive outcome.

During the initial phase of nonoperative treatment, any incidences of increased elbow pain, loss of elbow ROM, or mechanical symptoms such as locking, clicking, or catching warrant a referral to a physician to evaluate for potential lesion progression.[43,47] Passive modalities (eg, cryotherapy, electrical stimulation) combined with passive and active ROM exercises are ideal for the acute phase of treatment to best address pain and restore the athlete's full elbow ROM. Isometric and proprioceptive exercises should be included to minimize the negative effects of inactivity and further inhibit pain. To best avoid excess shear and compressive forces, the authors recommend early rehabilitation exercises be performed in an open-chain environment.[43]

Isotonic strengthening can be introduced once the athlete is ready to progress to the intermediate phase of nonoperative rehabilitation, and progressive resistive exercise at the shoulder and wrist may be advanced. The authors continue to recommend open-chain exercise strategies during this phase of rehabilitation. It is also during this phase that the athlete can begin using the upper body ergometer for conditioning. The athlete should display at least 80% of shoulder and elbow strength on the involved side compared to the noninvolved side to progress to the advanced stage of rehabilitation.

During the advanced stage of nonoperative rehabilitation, activities in both the open- and closed-chain environment should be introduced, progressive resistance exercises should be further progressed, and plyometric exercises should be included to best acclimatize the affected extremity to the demands of sport. Paterno et al[43] recommend that the athlete demonstrate at least 90% of shoulder and elbow strength on the affected extremity compared to the unaffected extremity, be able to bear weight through the affected extremity, and perform pain-free unilateral plyometric exercise with the affected extremity to progress to the return-to-sport phase of rehabilitation.[43] Current evidence suggests that an interval-throwing program for return to overhead sport should begin at approximately 3 to 4 months.[31-34]

For patients with unstable lesions, surgical correction has been correlated with the best outcomes. Initial goals of the acute phase of a postoperative rehabilitation program should include elimination of postoperative pain and discomfort, increase elbow ROM, and minimize the effects of inactivity. Clinicians should consider the use of manual therapy strategies to address joint and scar mobility, and isometric elbow

exercises should be initiated. During this phase, proximal strengthening can be performed as tolerated.

In order to progress to the intermediate phase of postoperative rehabilitation, pain and edema should have fully subsided and full elbow ROM should be present. Progression from isometric to isotonic exercise should be encouraged. Patients undergoing a surgical correction should anticipate up to 12 weeks of rehabilitation prior to being able to progress to the return-to-sport phase, as well as show at least 90% or greater strength at the involved limb compared to the uninvolved limb, be able to bear weight through the affected extremity, and perform pain-free unilateral plyometric exercises prior to being cleared for the return-to-sport phase of rehabilitation. Paterno et al[43] recommend delaying progression to full sports participation until a minimum of 3 to 4 months after a microfracture surgery and up to 6 months after undergoing a structural repair.

FRACTURES OF THE ARM/ELBOW

Radial Head Fractures

Athletes commonly fracture their radius by falling on an outstretched arm, resulting in axial, valgus, or posterolateral rotational loading patterns across the elbow. Radial head fractures account for one-third of all elbow fractures, making them the most common type of fracture seen at the elbow. Radial head fractures are classified according to the amount of displacement and by the presence of a mechanical block to motion.[48,49] Athletes presenting with a radial head fracture will often have pain and/or tenderness to palpation at the lateral elbow, likely supination/pronation ROM limitations, increased joint crepitus, and possible bony blocks to elbow motion.[48] The examiner should take careful note of blocks to motion, and a thorough neurovascular examination is warranted (Table 6-2).

Mason type I fractures are classified as minimally displaced fractures with no mechanical blocks to motion and commonly handled nonoperatively with initial sling immobilization and initiation of active ROM exercise within the first week as pain subsides.[48] The athlete's elbow ROM should slowly improve with conservative treatment, ideally returning to preinjury levels between 6 and 12 weeks. There is currently a debate as to whether Mason type II fractures are best treated surgically vs nonsurgically. A Mason type II fracture shows greater than 2 mm of displacement at the fracture site with possible mechanical blocks to elbow motion. Kodde et al[48] has demonstrated no clear standard of care for a type II fracture. Mason type III fractures are addressed either via arthroplasty or open reduction internal fixation (ORIF), although no surgical option has been shown to be superior at this time.[48] Active, active-assisted, and passive motion are initiated in the first few days following surgical intervention, with the goal of achieving full elbow ROM by 6 weeks. Isometric exercises should begin prior to

Table 6-2	
MASON CLASSIFICATION OF RADIAL HEAD FRACTURES[48]	
TYPE I	Minimally displaced fracture with no mechanical block to motion
TYPE II	Greater than 2 mm displaced fracture with possible mechanical block to motion
TYPE III	Comminuted and displaced fracture with mechanical block to motion

6 weeks, progressing to isotonic progressive resistive exercise between 6 and 8 weeks after surgery, ideally in an open-chain environment. After 12 weeks, higher intensity isotonic exercise can begin in both open- and closed-chain environments, and plyometric exercise should be initiated in the absence of any remaining functional deficits.[50,51] Complications after surgical correction of a radial head fracture include stiffness, malunion, avascular necrosis, and painful hardware, with postoperative stiffness being the most likely complication.[48]

Distal Humerus Fractures

Fractures of the distal humerus are commonly the result of high-energy trauma in younger men and low-energy trauma sustained from falls in an older adult population, with a distal intercondylar fracture pattern being the most prevalent.[49] Upon presentation, an athlete with a distal humerus fracture will often have gross elbow instability. A thorough neurovascular examination is of supreme importance, as both Nauth et al[49] and Pollock et al[52] have shown a greater incidence of incomplete ulnar neuropathy at the time of injury with bicolumnar distal humerus fractures.

Rarely are distal humerus fractures managed nonoperatively in an athletic population—the amount of time needed for casted immobilization can lead to nonunion or malunion and a high rate of posttraumatic elbow stiffness. In the event the athlete suffered a nondisplaced fracture with adequate stability to allow for early elbow ROM, nonoperative management may be appropriate.[52] Surgical management of a distal humerus fracture is addressed either with arthroplasty or ORIF. The importance of achieving optimal stability of the fracture to allow for early elbow mobilization and prevention of stiffness or posttraumatic arthritis has been shown numerous times in the literature.[49,52] Early ROM exercise is initiated within the first week of postoperative care to minimize the chance for posttraumatic elbow stiffness or heterotopic ossification formation.[53] Isometric and isotonic exercises should commence at 6 weeks, with the goal of full elbow ROM and at least 80% elbow flexion/extension strength compared to the nonaffected extremity by 12 weeks. Initiation of a high-intensity return-to-sport program can commence only after these levels of strength and motion are present, along with the absence of pain on provocative tests.

Olecranon Fractures

Accounting for roughly 10% of adult elbow fractures, olecranon fractures are often the result of direct trauma that drives the proximal ulna into the distal humerus, such as during a fall while landing on the posterior tip of the olecranon, or indirectly as the result of high amounts of eccentric triceps tension, causing an avulsion of the olecranon at the triceps insertion.[54,55] Olecranon fractures are classified according to 3 variables: level of displacement, joint stability, and comminution. Type I fractures are nondisplaced, type II fractures are displaced but stable, and type II fractures are displaced and unstable. Each fracture type can be further subdivided into noncomminuted and comminuted.[54,55] An athlete presenting with an olecranon fracture will often complain of localized posterior elbow pain, edema, and an inability to extend the elbow against gravity, indicating a disruption of the triceps mechanism. As mentioned previously, a thorough neurovascular examination is imperative.[55]

Nondisplaced olecranon fractures are often treated with conservative care, with the elbow immobilized in 45 to 90 degrees of flexion for up to 4 weeks. Passive motion can begin at week 1 through a protected ROM, and active and active-assisted ROM exercise should commence around 4 weeks while avoiding elbow flexion greater than 90 degrees until radiographic healing has been demonstrated, usually between 6 and 8 weeks.[55] Postoperative care will be determined by the approach, either surgical repair or fixation. Typical postoperative rehabilitation begins with gentle active-assisted and passive ROM exercise within 5 to 7 days of surgery, and the athlete is initially splinted in full elbow extension to minimize tension across the fracture site. The initial phase of rehabilitation seeks to minimize stress and tension at the site of injury, so passive motion is typically emphasized until healing is confirmed via radiographs, usually between 8 and 12 weeks. At this time, progressive resistance exercise should be initiated and advanced in both speed and intensity, varying between open- and closed-chain environments. A removable brace may be warranted for patients participating in closed-chain athletic endeavors.[54,55]

Capitellum Fractures

Capitellum fractures are rare and typically result from a fall on an outstretched arm, resulting in excess compressive forces to the capitellum imparted by the radial head. Upon examination, an athlete with an isolated capitellum fracture can present with lateral elbow pain and tenderness, joint swelling, and a possible mechanical block to elbow flexion and extension.[56,57]

Nonoperative management of an athlete with an isolated capitellum fracture with minimal displacement should include posterior splint immobilization for no more than 3 weeks to avoid the likelihood of increased elbow stiffness. Early passive ROM should be introduced immediately, with the goal to regain full elbow flexion, extension, and pronation/supination by 6 weeks. Operative care can include ORIF, fragment excision, and arthroplasty, depending on the amount of displacement and the presence of large fragments. Postoperative care for capitellum fractures is similar to other fractures discussed in this chapter, with emphasis on early, protected motion to minimize joint stiffness and introduction of progressive resistance exercise at 6 weeks. Trinh et al[57] showed no difference in outcomes between patients undergoing surgical care and those treated conservatively.

ELBOW DISLOCATION

Elbow dislocations occur more frequently in men than women, and 90% of all elbow dislocations are either posterior or posterolateral. The highest incidence of elbow dislocation can be seen in athletes between the ages of 10 and 19 years of age, with person-to-person contact being the most common mechanism of injury (46.9%) followed by contact with a playing surface (46.0%). Loss of terminal elbow extension has been reported in up to 60% of cases, demonstrating the importance for early rehabilitation.[58-61] Athletes with an elbow joint dislocation often present with swelling and marked joint deformity. A thorough neurovascular examination must be completed both prior to and after any attempts at joint reduction, as ulnar and median nerve injuries can occur. Following reduction, the clinician should assess elbow ROM, noting any crepitus or blocks to motion, as this could be indicative of a fracture fragment.[59,60]

Neurovascular injury, compartment syndrome, heterotropic ossification, elbow flexion and extension contractures, and posttraumatic arthritis are all noted complications associated with elbow dislocation injuries. Calcification of soft tissues is relatively common following a dislocation, and although it has been reported in up to 75% of cases,[62] it rarely limits the athlete's motion.[60,61] Dislocations can be classified as simple, with no accompanying fracture, or complex, which typically involves a fracture of the coronoid process, radial head, or the olecranon. An elbow dislocation combined with a radial head and coronoid process fracture has been described as "the terrible triad," and is often associated with poor outcomes.[61]

Nonoperative management of an elbow dislocation in the athlete begins with an assessment of stability. As previously mentioned in this chapter with regard to different elbow fractures, immobilization for greater than 3 weeks is associated with a higher incidence of posttraumatic stiffness. Simple dislocations should be splinted in 45 to 90 degrees of elbow flexion for up to 1 week, and any joint swelling or soft tissue pain can be managed with passive modalities such as compression and cryotherapy. Active ROM exercise between 30 and 90 degrees of flexion should be initiated after 1 week of rest, allowing for 10 to 15 degrees of increased motion per week. Passive ROM should be avoided in the acute phase, as it can increase tissue irritation and inflammation. The clinician can expect full elbow flexion ROM to return between 6 and 12 weeks; however, elbow extension progress can take much longer, slowly improving for up to 5 months after dislocation. Progressive resistance exercises can be initiated between 4 and 8 weeks, and return-to-sport programs should only be initiated when the athlete has near full ROM, no pain with provocative testing, and no apprehension with higher-level activities.[59,61] Complex elbow dislocations tend to be managed surgically with closed joint reduction, ORIF of fractures, ligament reconstruction, and/or dynamic external fixation. Extended periods of immobilization in the postoperative recovery period increase the likelihood for postoperative stiffness and poor outcomes. The pace of rehabilitation for complex elbow dislocations is determined by the postreduction stability of the affected joint.[60]

CONCLUSION

A joint as dynamic as the elbow often will receive a lot of attention when concerning athletes and injuries. As a prime link in the upper extremity kinetic chain, we can expect an elbow undergoing powerful, repetitive movements to be at risk for chronic degradation and acute trauma. Certain sports, such as baseball, place large loads of force across the structures of the elbow and can lead to injuries that hinder an athlete's competitive potential or even reduce career viability. Thus, it is paramount to understand how the biomechanics and kinetic forces involved in upper extremity movements play a role in injury and how we can best prevent the deleterious effects of these repetitious movements. Furthermore, an efficacious rehabilitation program will target progressive loads to the injured structures with a goal in managing the athlete as a whole rather than just the affected joint.

CASE STUDIES

Case Study One

A 17-year-old high school baseball pitcher is referred for physical therapy for a right elbow UCL partial tear. Upon initial evaluation, his primary question is "how long will it be before I can pitch in a game?" Examination of his right elbow reveals normal ROM; right shoulder ROM reveals internal rotation deficit of 25 degrees and cross-body adduction deficit of 20 degrees. Strength of the right shoulder with hand-held dynamometer reveals 20% deficit of supraspinatus and external rotation. The rehabilitation plan includes initial rest from throwing for 8 to 12 weeks. During this initial rest time, the athlete will perform rotator cuff and scapular stabilization exercises with a special emphasis on eccentric external rotator strengthening, hip and core stability exercises, and single leg balance activities to promote improved dynamic stability during pitching. He will also perform self-stretching and receive manual therapy for his internal rotation deficit and decreased cross-body adduction ROM. At week 8 to 12 if strength, balance, and ROM are at least 90% of uninvolved side, he will begin an interval throwing program. Progression through the throwing program will take 10 to 12 weeks to ramp back up and get back into game shape; so, barring any setbacks during the rehabilitation, he will require 5 to 6 months of time, at a minimum, to return to play. Throughout the throwing program, he will work on his throwing mechanics and work to eliminate faults that increase stress on the ligament, including opening up his front side too soon, landing with an open front leg, or throwing with a dropped elbow position. As previously discussed, there are limited studies and evidence to show that conservative treatment will be successful. In cases where an athlete spends 5 to 6 months attempting to avoid surgery and then eventually undergoes surgery and needs another 12 months to recover, this would most likely mean they miss 2 full seasons of high school baseball, which may be the entirety of their varsity career. In the author's experience, often these athletes will opt for surgery sooner to avoid missing 2 seasons.

Case Study Two

A 20-year-old left-handed collegiate pitcher presents with complaints of elbow pain after pitching 3 innings in his previous game. His pain is worst during follow-through, but the acceleration phase of throwing has also recently become painful. He notes tenderness with palpation to the olecranon process and is unable to fully extend his elbow without significant discomfort. The VEO test is positive, and the patient has no pain with resisted triceps testing. Imaging is warranted in this case to rule out an olecranon stress fracture. X-rays showed no osteophytes and computed tomography imaging was also negative for osseous pathology. In this case, the athlete is diagnosed to have VEO.

The first line of conservative treatment for VEO should be rest from offending activity (ie, pitching). This period can last anywhere from 2 to 6 weeks, depending on severity of symptoms, patient's age, and previous medical history or episodes of VEO. Rotator cuff and scapular exercises should be emphasized during this period of active rest, while encouraging the athlete to discontinue any exercise or activity that aggravates this condition. In light of throwing being a full-body activity, hip and core strengthening is also encouraged

at this time. Low-level isometric exercises at the forearm and elbow may be appropriate if well tolerated.

The athlete should progress to more direct forearm and elbow strengthening exercises once he is asymptomatic both at rest and with provocative testing. Special emphasis should be placed on exercises that promote both strength and endurance with the forearm flexors and pronators as well as the scapula and rotator cuff. Inclusion of plyometrics are vital as well to establish quick and repetitive movement patterns as required by sport. Plyometrics are especially important in readying the athlete to return to throwing, as they can better mimic the joint kinematics seen during the throwing motion than traditional therapy exercises while also building confidence in the athlete. When prescribing plyometric exercise, dose is extremely important secondary to the higher levels of stress involved. It is the author's opinion that bilateral exercises should be introduced first, progressing to unilateral exercises with an emphasis on movements that mimic the throwing motion.

At this point, after completion of a comprehensive plyometric program, an interval throwing program can begin. The clinician should select a program that best matches the patient; if the patient has had VEO before, a more conservative program should be implemented. It is also during this time that proper throwing mechanics should be reviewed with the athlete; the best course of treatment and rehabilitation can be undone by improper mechanics, so this vital last step must be taken before the athlete can be returned to full competition. Once the athlete has completed an interval throwing program without any issues, he should be released to full competition.

REFERENCES

1. Shanley E, Thigpen C. Throwing injuries in the adolescent athlete. *International J Sports Medicine.* 2013;8(5):630-640.
2. Cain EL Jr, Dugas JR, Wolf RS, Andrews JR. Elbow injuries in throwing athletes: a current concepts review. *Am J Sports Med.* 2003;31(4):621-635.
3. Park JY, Lee JH. Rehabilitation: part III. Throwing athletes. In: Park JY, ed. *Sports Injuries to the Shoulder and Elbow.* Springer; 2015:453-477.
4. Morrey B, An K-N. Articular and ligamentous contributions to the stability of the elbow joint. *Am J Sports Med.* 1983;11:315-319.
5. DiGiovine NM. An electromyographic analysis of the upper extremity in pitching. *J Shoulder Elbow Surg.* 1992;1(1):15-25.
6. Redler LH, Watling JP, Ahmad CS. Physical examination of the throwing athlete's elbow. *Am J Orthop.* 2015;44(1):13-18.
7. Ellenbecker TS, Mattalino AJ, Elam EA, Caplinger RA. Medial elbow laxity in professional baseball pitchers: a bilateral comparison using stress radiography. *Am J Sports Med.* 1998;26(3):420-424.
8. Dines JS, Frank JB, Akerman M, Yocum LA. Glenohumeral internal rotation deficits in baseball players with ulnar collateral ligament insufficiency. *Am J Sports Med.* 2009;37(3):566-570.
9. Day JM, Bush H, Nitz AJ, Uhl TL. Scapular muscle performance in individuals with lateral epicondylalgia. *J Orthop Sports Phys Ther.* 2015;45(5):414-424.
10. Morrey BF. *The Elbow and its Disorders.* 2nd ed. W.B. Saunders Company; 1993.

11. Andrews JR, Wilk KE, Satterwhite YE, Tedder JL. Physical examination of the thrower's elbow. *J Orthop Sports Phys Ther.* 1993;17(6):296-304.

12. O'Driscoll SW, Lawton RL, Smith AM. The "moving valgus stress test" for medial collateral ligament tears of the elbow. *Am J Sports Med.* 2005;33(2):231-239.

13. Kraushaar BS, Nirschl RP. Tendinosis of the elbow (tennis elbow). Clinical features and findings of histopathological, immunohistochemical and electron microscopy studies. *J Bone Joint Surgery Am.* 1999;81:259-278.

14. Bortell DT, Pritchett JW. Straight-line graphs for the prediction of growth of the upper extremities. *J Bone Joint Surg Am.* 1993;75(6):885-892.

15. Dotter WE. Little leaguer's shoulder. *Guthrie Clin Bull.* 1953;23:23-68.

16. Heyworth BE, Kramer DE, Martin DJ, Micheli LJ, Kocher MS, Bae DS. Trends in the presentation, management, and outcomes of little league shoulder. *Am J Sports Med.* 2016;44(6):1431-1438.

17. Fleisig GS, Escamilla RF, Andrews JR. Applied biomechanics of baseball pitching. In: Magee DJ, Manske RC, Zachazewski JE, Quillen W, eds. *Athletic and Sports Issues in Musculoskeletal Rehabilitation.* Elsevier; 2011:331-349.

18. Joyce ME, Jelsma RD, Andrews JR. Throwing injuries to the elbow. *Sports Med Arthroscopy Rev.* 1995;3:224-236.

19. Gruchow HW, Pelletier D. An epidemiologic study of tennis elbow. Incidence, recurrence, and effectiveness of prevention strategies. *Am J Sports Med.* 1979;7:234-238.

20. Kurppa K, Viikari-Juntura E, Kuosma E, Huuskonen M, Kivi P. Incidence of tenosynovitis or peritendinitis and epicondylitis in a meat-processing factory. *Scand J Work Environ Health.* 1991;17:32-37.

21. Amin NH, Kumar NS, Schickendantz MS. Medial epicondylitis: evaluation and management. *J Am Acad Orthop Surg.* 2015;23(6):348-355.

22. Labelle H, Guibert R, Joncas J, Newman N, Fallaha M, Rivard CH. Lack of scientific evidence for the treatment of lateral epicondylitis of the elbow. An attempted meta-analysis. *J Bone Joint Surg Br.* 1992;74:646-651.

23. Coombes BK, Bisset L, Vincenzino B. Management of lateral elbow tendinopathy: one size does not fit all. *J Orthop Sports Phys Ther.* 2015;45(11):938-949.

24. Strujis PA, Kerkhoffs GM, Assendelft WJ, Van Dijk CN. Conservative treatment of lateral epicondylitis: brace versus physical therapy or a combination of both-a randomized clinical trial. *Am J Sports Med.* 2004;32(2):462-469.

25. Weber C, Thai V, Neuheuser K, Groover K, Christ O. Efficacy of physical therapy for the treatment of lateral epicondylitis: a meta-analysis. *BMC Musculoskelet Disord.* 2015;16:223.

26. Taylor SA, Hannafin JA. Evaluation and management of elbow tendinopathy. *Sports Health.* 2012;4(5):384-393.

27. Smidt N, Assendelft WJ, Arola H, et al. Effectiveness of physiotherapy for lateral epicondylitis: a systematic review. *Ann Med.* 2003;35:51-62.

28. Mazzocca AD, Spang JT, Arciero RA. Distal biceps rupture. *Orthop Clin N Am.* 2008;39:237-249. doi:10.1016/j.ocl.2008.01.001

29. Sibley PA, Harman TW, Bamberger HB. Triceps tendinopathy. *J Hand Surg.* 2017;40(7):1446-1448. doi:10.1016/j.jhsa.2015.04.004

30. Erickson BJ, Harris JD, Chalmers PN, et al. Ulnar collateral ligament reconstruction: anatomy, indications, techniques, and outcomes. *Sports Health.* 2015;7(6):511-517.

31. Chang ES, Bishop ME, Baker D, West RV. Interval throwing and hitting programs in baseball: biomechanics and rehabilitation. *Am J Orthop.* 2016;45(3):157-162.

32. Reinold MM, Wilk KE, Reed J, Crenshaw K, Andrews JR. Interval sport programs: guidelines for baseball, tennis, and golf. *J Orthop Sports Phys Ther.* 2002;32(6):293-298.

33. Wilk KE, Hooks TR. Rehabilitation of the throwing athlete: where we are in 2014. *Clin Sports Med.* 2015;34:247-261.

34. Wilk KE, Meister K, Andrews JR. Current concepts in the rehabilitation of the overhead throwing athlete. *Am J Sports Med.* 2002;30(1):136-151.

35. Axe M, Hurd W, Snyder-Mackler L. Data-based interval throwing programs for baseball players. *Sports Health.* 2009;1(2):145-153.

36. Axe MJ, Snyder-Mackler L, Konin JG, Strube MJ. Development of a distance-based interval throwing program for little league-aged athletes. *Am J Sports Med.* 1996;24(5):594-602.

37. Axe MJ, Wickham R, Snyder-Mackler L. Data-based interval throwing programs for little league, high school, college, and professional baseball pitchers. *Sports Med Arthrosc Rev.* 2001;9:24-34.

38. Axe MJ, Windley TC, Snyder-Mackler L. Data-based interval throwing programs for baseball position players from age 13 to college level. *J Sport Rehabil.* 2001;10:267-286.

39. Axe MJ, Windley TC, Snyder-Mackler L. Data-based interval throwing programs for collegiate softball players. *J Ath Train.* 2002;37(2):194-203.

40. Slenker NR, Limpisvasti O, Mohr KJ, Aguinaldo AL, Elattrache NS. Biomechanical comparison of the interval throwing program and baseball pitching: upper extremity loads in training and rehabilitation. *Am J Sports Med.* 2014;42(5):1226-1232. doi:10.1177/0363546514526152

41. Dugas JR. Valgus extension overload: diagnosis and treatment. *Clin Sports Med.* 2010;29(4):645-654.

42. Ahmed CS, ElAttrache NS. Valgus extension overload syndrome and stress injury of the olecranon. *Clin Sports Med.* 2004;23(4):665-676.

43. Paterno MV, Prokop TR, Schmitt LC. Physical therapy management of patients with osteochondritis dissecans: a comprehensive review. *Clin Sports Med.* 2014;33(2):353-374.

44. Nissen CW. Osteochondritis dissecans of the elbow. *Clin Sports Med.* 2014;33(2):251-265.

45. Savoie FH. Osteochondritis dissecans of the elbow. *Oper Tech Sports Med.* 2008;16(4):187-193.

46. Takahara M, Mura N, Sasaki J, Harada M, Ogino T. Classification, treatment, and outcome of osteochondrosis dissecans of the humeral capitellum. *J Bone Joint Surg Am.* 2007;89(6):1205-1214.

47. Mihara JA, Bain GI. Non-operative treatment for osteochondritis dissecans of the capitellum. *Am J Sports Med.* 2009;37(2):298-304.

48. Kodde IF, Kaas L, Flipsen M, van den Bekerom MPJ, Eygendaal D. Current concepts in the management of radial head fractures. *World J Orthop.* 2015;18;6(11):954-960.

49. Nauth A, McKee MD, Ristevski B, Hall J, Schemitsch EH. Distal humerus fractures in adults. *J Bone Joint Surg Am.* 2011;93(7):686-700.

50. Ashwood N, Bain GI, Unni R. Management of Mason type-III radial head fractures with a titanium prosthesis, ligament repair, and early mobilization. *J Bone Joint Surg Am.* 2004;86(2):274-280.

51. Rosenblatt Y, Athwal GS, Faber KJ. Current recommendations for the treatment of radial head fractures. *Orthop Clin North Am.* 2008;39(2):173-185.

52. Pollock JW, Faber KJ, Athwal GS. Distal humerus fractures. *Orthop Clin North Am.* 2008;39(2):187-200.

53. Abrams GD, Bellino MJ, Cheung EV. Risk factors for development of heterotopic ossification of the elbow after fracture fixation. *J Shoulder Elbow Surg.* 2012;21(11):1550-1554.

54. Baecher N, Edwards S. Olecranon fractures. *J Hand Surg Am.* 2013;38(3):593-604.

55. Veillette CJH, Steinmann SP. Olecranon fractures. *Orthop Clin North Am.* 2008;39(2):229-236.

56. McKee MD, Jupiter JB, Bamberger HB. Coronal shear fractures of the distal end of the humerus. *J Bone Joint Surg Am.* 1996;78(1):49-54.

57. Trinh TQ, Harris JD, Kolovich GP, Greisser MJ, Schickendantz MS, Jones GL. Operative management of capitellar fractures: a systematic review. *J Shoulder Elbow Surg.* 2012;21(11):1613-1622.

58. Dizdarevic I, Low S, Currie DW, Comstock RD, Hammoud S, Atanda A Jr. Epidemiology of elbow dislocations in high school athletes. *Am J Sports Med.* 2016;44(1):202-208.

59. McGuire DT, Bain GI. Management of dislocations of the elbow in the athlete. *Sports Med Arthrosc Rev.* 2014;22(3):188-193.

60. Mehta JA, Bain GI. Elbow dislocations in adults and children. *Clin Sports Med.* 2004;23(4):609-627.

61. O'Brien MJ, Savoie FH III. Treatment and rehabilitation of elbow dislocations. In: Brotzman SB, Manske RC, eds. *Clinical Orthopaedic Rehabilitation: An Evidence-Based Approach.* 3rd ed. Elsevier Mosby; 2011:63-65.

62. Josefsson PO, Johnell O, Gentz CF. Long-term sequelae of simple dislocation of the elbow. *J Bone Joint Surg Am.* 1984;66(6):927-930.

7

Dysfunction, Evaluation, and Treatment of the Wrist and Hand

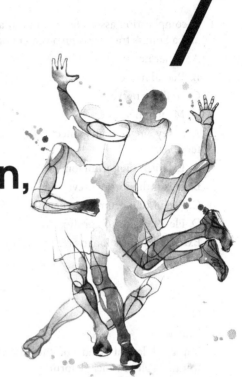

Kevin J. Lawrence, PT, MS, DHS, OCS

KEY TERMS

Bennet's fracture: Fracture of the base of the first metacarpal bone, which extends into the carpometacarpal (CMC) joint. Intra-articular fracture of the thumb—often accompanied by some degree of subluxation.

Boxer's fracture: Fracture of the metacarpal of the hand.

Carpal tunnel: The tunnel on the flexor side wrist under the flexor retinaculum that contains the median nerve, tendons of the flexor digitorum superficialis, flexor digitorum profundus, and the synovial sheaths around each tendon.

Extensor compartment at wrist: Tendons at the wrist on the extensor side cross the wrist in one of 6 compartments

Flexor compartment at wrist: Tendons at the wrist on the flexor side cross the wrist in 1 of 2 compartments.

Lunotriquetral dissociation: Instability between lunate and triquetrum.

Scapholunate dissociation: Instability between scaphoid and lunate.

Tenosynovitis: Inflammation of synovial lining around tendons in the wrist and hand.

Tunnel of Guyon: The tunnel between the pisiform and hook of hamate that contains the ulnar nerve, artery, and vein.

CHAPTER QUESTIONS

1. A fracture to the distal radius where the distal fragment displaced dorsally is known as a:
   A. Smith's fracture
   B. Colles fracture
   C. Barton's fracture
   D. Smith avulsion fracture

2. The poorest outcomes for flexor tendon injuries following repair occur in flexor tendon:
   A. Zone 1
   B. Zone 2
   C. Zone 3
   D. Zone 4

3. Control of peripheral blood supply is controlled by:
   A. Autoimmune nervous system
   B. Central nervous system
   C. Passive nervous system
   D. Collateral nervous system

Wallmann HW, Donatelli R, eds. *Foundations of Orthopedic Physical Therapy* (pp 169-185).
© 2024 Taylor & Francis Group.

4. A complication associated with both a Colles fracture and a Smith's fracture is involvement of the:
   A. Ulnar nerve
   B. Radial nerve
   C. Axillary nerve
   D. Median nerve

5. A jersey finger injury affects which of the following tendons:
   A. Extensor digitorum longus
   B. Flexor digitorum brevis
   C. Flexor digitorum superficialis
   D. Flexor digitorum profundus

6. Extensor pollicis longus tendon is located in extensor compartment:
   A. One
   B. Two
   C. Three
   D. Four

7. Ruptured lateral bands of the extensor mechanism would result in which deformity?
   A. Mallet finger
   B. Jersey finger
   C. Ulnar drift
   D. Volar displacement

8. Volar plates can be found at the:
   A. Proximal interphalangeal (PIP) joints
   B. Distal interphalangeal (DIP) joints
   C. PIP and DIP joints
   D. Metacarpophalangeal (MCP), PIP, and DIP joints

9. Scapholunate dissociation results in a gaping between the scaphoid and the lunate. When this occurs the scaphoid tips _____ and the lunate tips _____.
   A. Medially, laterally
   B. Palmarly, dorsally
   C. Anteriorly, anteriorly
   D. Dorsally, palmarly

10. Kienbock's disease is a:
    A. Vascular condition
    B. Fracture of the pisiform
    C. Autoimmune condition
    D. Fracture of the lunate

11. Watson's test is used to determine?
    A. Diminished vascular supply
    B. Fracture of the lunate
    C. Presence of dissociation of the lunate with the triquetrum
    D. Presence of dissociation of the lunate and the scaphoid

12. The triangular fibrocartilage complex (TFCC) is located between:
    A. Ulna and radius
    B. Ulna and trapezoid
    C. Ulna and triquetrum
    D. Radius and triquetrum

13. Which upper extremity nerve passes through the triangular interval?
    A. Radial
    B. Median
    C. Ulnar
    D. Intraosseous

14. A Rolando fracture is a fracture of:
    A. Distal first metacarpal
    B. Trapezium
    C. Proximal base of first metacarpal
    D. Trapezoid

15. The tunnel of Guyon passes between:
    A. The pisiform and lunate
    B. The hook of the hamate and trapezoid
    C. The pisiform and hook of the hamate
    D. The trapezoid and triquetrum

16. Injury to the anterior interosseous nerve could result in weakness of:
    A. Flexor pollicis brevis and flexor pollicis longus
    B. Flexor carpi radialis and flexor pollicis longus
    C. Flexor pollicis brevis and abductor pollicis
    D. Flexor digitorum profundus to fingers 2 and 3 and flexor pollicis longus

17. Which of the following is not true concerning the posterior interosseous nerve?
    A. Innervates extensor pollicis longus
    B. Provides sensation to the posterior forearm
    C. Innervates extensor indicis
    D. Innervates extensor pollicis brevis

18. Significant angle of the bone associated with a fracture of the shaft of a metacarpal (boxer's fracture) can result in muscle weakness of:
    A. Dorsal interossei
    B. Palmar interossei
    C. Lumbrical muscles
    D. All of the above

19. de Quervain's tenosynovitis involves a tenosynovitis of extensor compartment:
    A. One
    B. Two
    C. Three
    D. Six

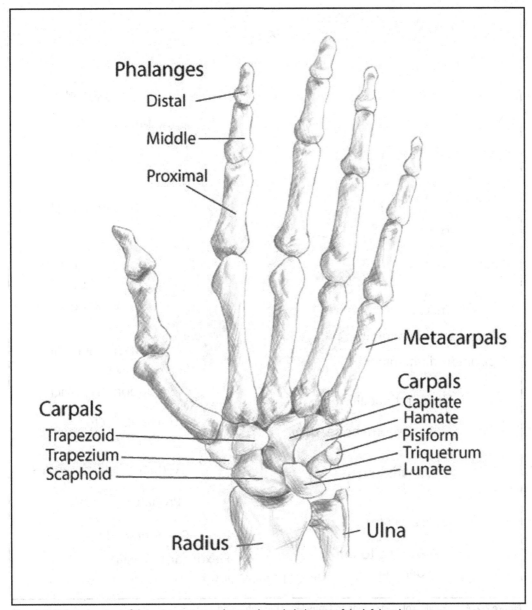

Figure 7-1. Anterior view of the wrist, metacarpals, carpals, and phalanges of the left hand.

20. Thickening of the palmar aponeurosis of the hand is known as _____?
    A. Dupuytren's contracture
    B. Palmar contracture
    C. Palmar neuroma
    D. Supinator contracture

ANATOMY OF THE WRIST JOINT COMPLEX

The wrist joint is made up of 2 rows of bones. From radial to ulnar, the proximal row contains the scaphoid, lunate, and triquetrum. The distal row contains the trapezium, trapezoid, capitate, and hamate (Figure 7-1). Many will include the pisiform in the proximal row, but the pisiform is a sesamoid bone within the tendon of the flexor carpi ulnaris. The pisiform will glide on the trapezium with all wrist motions.[2] There should be minimal motion between carpal bones within the same row. Motion at the wrist occurs at the distal radius and the proximal row of carpals and with the proximal row of carpals and the distal row of carpals.

There are 5 metacarpal bones that are numbered from the radial to the ulnar side.[1] These bones are concave with the concavity on the palmar side. Digits 2 to 5 have 3 phalanx each, whereas the thumb has 2.[1] The tendon for the flexor digitorum superficialis inserts into the base of the middle phalanx. The flexor digitorum inserts into the base of the distal phalanx (Figure 7-2).

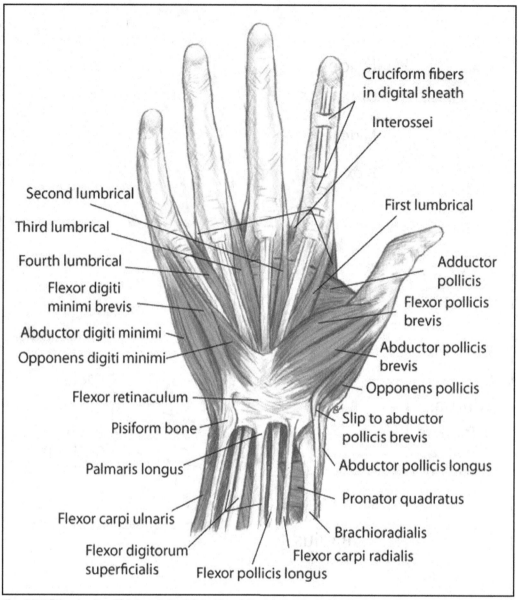

Figure 7-2. Anterior view of the tendons and muscles of the right hand.

Cruciform fibers in digital sheath

Interossei

Second lumbrical

First lumbrical

Third lumbrical

Fourth lumbrical

Adductor pollicis

Flexor digiti minimi brevis

Flexor pollicis brevis

Abductor digiti minimi

Abductor pollicis brevis

Opponens digiti minimi

Opponens pollicis

Flexor retinaculum

Slip to abductor pollicis brevis

Pisiform bone

Palmaris longus

Abductor pollicis longus

Pronator quadratus

Flexor carpi ulnaris

Brachioradialis

Flexor digitorum superficialis

Flexor carpi radialis

Flexor pollicis longus

Normal Biomechanics of the Wrist and Hand

The distal radius articular surface is concave, and the proximal row of the carpals is convex. With wrist flexion, the carpals will anteriorly roll and posteriorly glide. With wrist extension, the carpals will posteriorly roll and anteriorly glide. With radial deviation, the carpals will roll to the radial side and glide toward the ulnar side. With ulnar deviation, the carpals will roll toward the ulnar side and glide toward the radial side.[2] These arthrokinematics are important to understand as the clinician will reproduce the joint glides when producing joint mobilizations.[1]

The distal row of carpals moves on the proximal row of carpals. The trapezium and trapezoid are concave on convex, whereas the capitate and lunate are convex on concave. This mix of joint surfaces will result in slight gliding and rotation motions with all wrist motions.[2] The CMC joints to the carpals 2 and 3 are fixed with little or no motion present. Metacarpals 4 and 5 have anterior and posterior glides present. This motion will allow cupping of the hand.[2]

The MCP, PIP, and DIP joints are all concave on convex. The PIP and DIP joints will roll dorsally and glide palmarly with flexion. For extension, the joint surfaces will roll toward the palmar side and glide toward the dorsal side. The same mechanics occur at the MCP, but additionally, the MCP joints have medial and lateral deviation. These movements are controlled by the dorsal interossei for abduction and the palmar interossei for adduction.[2]

The mechanics are unique at the thumb as the thumb does not move in the same plane as the other fingers. The shape of the CMC joints is saddle shaped, resulting in 2 degrees of freedom. The CMC joint has an ability to flex and extend (concave on convex) and abduct and adduct (convex on concave). With thumb flexion, the first metacarpal rolls medially and glides medially toward the palm. With thumb abduction, the first metacarpal bone rolls anteriorly away from the palm and glides posteriorly.[2]

TRAUMATIC INJURIES TO THE WRIST

Traumatic injuries of the wrist and hand are frequent. Karabay reports that wrist and hand injuries are estimated to be 6 % to 28% of all injuries and 28% of all musculoskeletal injuries.[1] Traumatic injuries in this section will include fractures, ligament injuries, instabilities, and skin lacerations.[3]

Colles Fracture

A Colles fracture is a fracture of the distal radius. The mechanism of injury is generally a fall on an outstretched hand with the forearm in pronation and the wrist extended.[5] The carpal bones are pushed up against the dorsal lip of the radius fracturing the radius just proximal to the distal end. This fracture can often result in a deformity called a *dinner fork deformity*.[3] When this occurs, the distal fragment of bone will displace dorsally. At times, some of the distal bone is crushed making realignment difficult for the surgeon. An open reduction internal fixation (ORIF) may then be required to get satisfactory realignment.

A Colles fracture will generally take 6 weeks or more of immobilization depending on the patient. Longer if an ORIF was necessary, or other comorbidity factors such as advanced age, osteoporosis, or if the patient smokes. Complicating factors with any ORIF can include infection and nonunion.[5]

Assessing the patient must include range of motion (ROM), strength, and sensation. When the ROM is limited, active exercise and joint mobilization techniques can help restore ROM. If the patient is acute, begin with very gentle active exercise and low-grade mobilizations. As long as the bone is well healed and the pain is subsided, higher-grade mobilizations and resistive exercise can be introduced.[5,6]

Sensation is important to assess as the median nerve may have been involved due to changes in its course just above the carpal tunnel or swelling within the carpal tunnel. A thorough median nerve sensory scan and motor scan should be employed. Diminished median nerve function can have a major effect of loss of sensation needed for fine motor control when handling small objects. This is particularly true of the thumb, which may affect the strength of thumb flexion and abduction.[3]

Assessing sensation following any nerve or nerve root involvement can be assessed by first determining if the patient has symmetrical sensation on the right and on the left. Sensation is assessed by comparing the 2 sides using a small, light, stroking touch.[6] Sensation can be further assessed utilizing 2-point discrimination[6] and using Semmes-Weinstein monofilaments.[7] Two-point discrimination is assessed using 2 points at a measured distance apart. The patient will be asked to determine if they were touched with 1 point or 2 points. Normal values range from 2 to 10 mm depending on the region of the body. Most normal patients can determine 2 mm on the fingertips.

The Semmes-Weinstein monofilaments are available in a kit. The monofilaments in the hand kit are color coded. The examiner will touch the patient with the monofilament until the filament flexes into a C shape. If the patient can determine the touch of the green monofilament, the patient will be described as having normal sensation. If they cannot feel the green but can feel the blue, they are said to have diminished sensation. If they can feel the purple, then they have diminished protective sensation. If they cannot feel the red, they have lost protective sensation.[4] The Semmes-Weinstein monofilament test can be used to assess the return of sensation.

Smith's Fracture

A Smith's fracture is similar to a Colles fracture in that both involve the distal radius.[5] The main difference is in the mechanism of the injury. With a Smith's fracture, the patient will fall backward landing on their wrist with the forearm supinated and the wrist flexed. This can result in the distal fragment of bone displacing toward the palmar side.[5] Significant displacement can result in the need for an ORIF and 6 or more weeks of immobilization. Assessment of ROM, strength, and sensation should be employed. Median nerve involvement is common. Interventions will follow the same guideline as a Colles fracture.

Barton's Fracture

A Barton's fracture is a fracture of the distal radius, but in this case, the fracture site is through the distal articular surface of the radius.[8,9] The mechanism of injury is a fall on an outstretched hand with the volar lip of the distal radius fracturing and displacing to the palmar side. Significant displacement will require ORIF. Complicating factors can include early osteoarthritic changes in the radiocarpal joint due to the intra-articular nature of the fracture. Median nerve involvement is common.[9]

Galeazzi Fracture

A Galeazzi fracture is a fracture of the distal one-third of the radius with dislocation of the distal radioulnar joint.[10] The mechanism of injury is generally direct trauma at the wrist or a fall on an outstretched hand. Disruption of the distal radioulnar joint can lead to significant instability. Often the radius will require ORIF, and the distal radioulnar joint will require stabilization. Often supination as well as pronation will be limited. Once full bone healing has occurred, it will be important to mobilize both the distal and proximal radioulnar joints. Other than the usual risk of infection and nonunion, it is important to look for any signs of compartment syndrome or complex regional pain syndrome (CRPS).

Essex-Lopresti Fracture

An Essex-Lopresti fracture is a fracture of the radial head, dislocation of the distal radioulnar joint, and disruption of the interosseous membrane.[11] Depending on the severity of the radial head fracture, the head may be immobilized, surgically repaired, removed, or replaced with a prosthetic radial head. The distal radioulnar joint may require stabilization as well as the interosseous membrane. This injury is generally caused by a fall from a height, and 6 to 8 weeks of immobilization may be required.

Injury to the interosseous membrane can involve instability of the radius and ulna and a risk of injury to either or both the anterior and posterior interosseous nerves.[11] Injury to the anterior interosseous nerve could affect innervation of the flexor pollicis longus, flexor digitorum profundus to fingers 2 and 3, and pronator quadratus. Injury to the anterior interosseous nerve could lead to weakness of thumb flexion, especially affecting a strong tip-to-tip pinch, weakness, or inability to make a full fist (especially to fingers 2 and 3), and weakness of pronation.

Injury to the posterior interosseous nerve could affect innervation to extensor pollicis longus, extensor pollicis brevis, abductor pollicis longus, and extensor indicis. Injury to the posterior interosseous nerve would have the largest effect on positioning the thumb into abduction and extension.[12] Assessing both of these neve injuries requires careful assessment of motor function of each of the muscles that could be affected. Neither of these 2 nerves has a sensory component, so loss of sensation should not be expected.

Distal Ulnar Fracture

Distal ulnar fractures are rare.[12] The distal ulna can fracture with a fall on an outstretched hand and the individual landing in ulnar deviation. In most cases the TFCC will cushion the fall and spare the ulna. The ulna does not directly articulate with any carpal bone but indirectly through the TFCC with the triquetrum.[12] The distal ulna can fracture through the ulna styloid or just proximal to the styloid. Complications of this fracture include a fracture of the triquetrum and or a tear of the TFCC.[12]

Scaphoid Fracture

Scaphoid fractures are the most common carpal fracture. Scaphoid fractures most commonly occur due to a fall on an outstretched hand.[13] The fracture can occur at several places on the scaphoid. The fracture can occur at the proximal tip or the distal tip, but the fracture most commonly occurs through the waist of the scaphoid. This is the region of the scaphoid centrally where the bone is most narrow. Following a wrist fracture of the scaphoid, the fracture may be difficult to visualize on a radiograph. The fracture may not show up well for 7 to 10 days. A magnetic resonance imaging scan or bone scan may be required to determine the presence of a fracture. Nonunion of this fracture is common, especially if no fracture was initially diagnosed. Often these patients are referred to therapy with a diagnosis of wrist sprain. A scaphoid fracture should be suspected with any patient who has had a fall on an outstretched hand, has pain on the radial side of the wrist, and has tenderness and swelling in the anatomical snuff box. Using a tuning fork to vibrate the scaphoid within the anatomical snuff box may give an additional clue that a fracture may be present.[14] Tenosynovitis of compartments 1, 2, and 3 (compartments are discussed later) must be ruled out. If the patient's pain level is not improving over time, the patient should be referred for additional medical imaging.

The proximal end of the bone can become avascular and experience necrosis. This is because the blood supply enters the bone distally and runs proximally within the bone.[16] Excessive movement at the fracture site can cut off the vascular supply to the proximal end of the bone. Necrosis of the proximal end of the bone would lead to severe degeneration of the scaphoid, where it articulates with the distal radius. This would result in severe pain at the proximal radiocarpal joint, especially during upper extremity weight bearing.

If a scaphoid fracture has been found and nonunion is suspected, an ORIF with a compression screw may be used to help assure a reestablishment of the blood supply.[16,17] The wrist will be immobilized for approximately 6 weeks. On examination, this patient will often be found to have limited ROM and pain, especially with wrist extension and radial deviation. Once healing has occurred, therapy can begin with gentle exercise and low-grade joint mobilization. Exercise and higher-grade mobilization can then progress according to patient tolerance.

Lunate Fracture

The lunate is the third most commonly fractured carpal bone behind the scaphoid and triquetrum.[17] The most common cause is a fall on an outstretched hand or a direct trauma. When a nonunion occurs, this is known as Kienböck's disease. A lunate fracture often leads to avascular necrosis. Avascular necrosis of the lunate will result in degenerative changes between the lunate and the distal radius. Individuals with a lunate fracture may not always remember a mechanism of injury such as a fall. They will often report that their wrist slowly began becoming more painful, swollen, and stiff. They will present with limited ROM, especially in extension; weakness in grip strength; and tenderness over the lunate.

In the early stages of lunate degeneration, the radiograph may be inconclusive. Later, the lunate will appear whiter than the surrounding bones as the bone becomes sclerotic. Next, the bone may begin to collapse and fragment. Treatment options may begin with an immobilization splint with the wrist in neutral and instruction to avoid weight bearing through the wrist. Surgical options may include fusion of the radiocarpal joint, a revascularization procedure when vascularized bone is grafted to the lunate, or removal of the proximal rows of carpals.

Rehabilitation would focus on returning mobility, strength, and ROM to the radiocarpal joint. Permanent loss of ROM and strength should be expected following removal of the proximal row of carpals as approximately 50% of the wrist ROM occurs at the radiocarpal joint and 50% at the midcarpal joint.[17]

Triquetrum Fracture

Triquetrum fractures are the second most common carpal fracture behind the scaphoid. The triquetrum most commonly fractures from a fall where the individual lands on a flexed wrist.[17] An avulsion fracture occurs on the dorsal aspect of the bone. This type of fracture can involve ligament disruption that can result in wrist instability. Often this fracture will require surgical stabilization. Smaller chip fractures may be at first nonsymptomatic and heal without intervention. Triquetrum body fractures can result from a direct blow to the bone. They are generally nondisplaced and should be immobilized for 4 to 6 weeks.[14,15]

Pisiform Fracture and Hook of the Hamate Fracture

The most common mechanism for a pisiform fracture or hook of the hamate fracture is due to repeated vibration.[17] This might occur with use of a jack hammer or with the vibration that occurs with excessive hitting of a baseball. The pisiform is a sesamoid bone contained within the flexor carpi ulnaris. The pisiform bone articulates with the triquetrum and can affect the strength of wrist flexion and ulnar deviation. There may be degenerative changes of the articulation between the pisiform and triquetrum resulting in osteoarthritic pain and diminished grip strength. The strength of the abductor digiti minimi may be affected as it originates on the pisiform.[16,17]

Fracture of the hook of the hamate can result in loss of strength of the flexor digiti mini and the opponens digiti minimi, both of which attach to the hook of the hamate. Both the pisiform and hook of the hamate form the borders of the tunnel of Guyon (ulnar tunnel).[1] Displacement or malformation of either bone can result in compression of the ulnar nerve or compression of the ulnar artery, both of which pass through the tunnel of Guyon. Compression of the ulnar nerve can cause decreased sensation of the ulnar side of the hand both anteriorly and posteriorly and weakness of all muscles of the hypothenar eminence, all palmar and dorsal interossei, lumbricals 3 and 4, and the adductor pollicis.[18] Weakness of ulnar nerve innervated muscles to the intrinsic of the hand can result in diminished strength of grip, diminished pad-to-pad pinch, and difficulty with opening the fingers, especially to fingers 4 and 5.[18] A more severe problem with the ulnar nerve intrinsic muscles of the hand can lead to a Bishop's hand deformity. In this situation, the patient would not be able to open fingers 4 and 5 and have no power with a pad-to-pad pinch.

Fracture of the Trapezium

Fractures of the trapezium are often associated with fractures to the first metacarpal or distal radius.[17] Fractures of the trapezium will present with tenderness in the anatomical snuff box. Most will heal following 4 weeks of immobilization. Some of these fractures will be intra-articular with the base of the first metacarpal and may lead to significant degenerative change to the joint over time. Grip strength and pinch strength may be significantly diminished.[17]

Fracture of the Trapezoid

Trapezoid fractures are the least common of carpal fractures. The mechanism is generally a fall on the distal second metacarpal resulting in compression of the trapezoid. Nondisplaced fractures will require 4 to 6 weeks of immobilization. Displaced fractures may require ORIF.[17]

Fracture of the Capitate

Isolated fractures of the capitate are rare. Most capitate fractures will heal with immobilization. At times, a fragment can be separated and result in avascular necrosis of that portion of the bone. Capitate fractures are more commonly associated with scaphoid and lunate fractures and dislocations.[17]

Fracture of the Body of the Hamate

Fractures of the body of the hamate are rare and most commonly associated with fractures to the base of the fourth and fifth metacarpals. Nondisplaced fractures will heal with 4 to 5 weeks of immobilization. Displaced fractures will require ORIF.[17]

Triangular Fibrocartilage Complex Injuries

The TFCC is a structure located between the distal ulna and triquetrum. The TFCC is made up of ligament and fibrocartilage. Injuries to the TFCC can occur from several different mechanisms of injury. Most commonly they can occur from a fall on an outstretched hand when the wrist is in end-range ulnar deviation or with repetitive weight bearing in ulnar deviation. TFCC injuries can also occur from twisting of the forearm or wrist into extremes of ROM.[19] The injury can involve tearing of the ligamentous portion from either its attachment to the ulna or radius. The ulnar attachment is better vascularized and is therefore more likely to heal. The radial attachment is less vascularized and is less likely to heal without surgical intervention. The fibrocartilaginous component is in the center of the TFCC. The fibrocartilage can degenerate with repetitive loading. Another cause of this injury is with distal radioulnar joint dislocation as the ligamentous portion is a key support of this joint.[12]

Signs and symptoms of this injury can include pain and swelling, especially on the ulnar side of the wrist, and diminished grip strength. The patient will report tenderness with palpation over the TFCC, pain with ulnar deviation, and may have pain with end-range supination or pronation. There may also be palpable crepitus with supination, pronation, or ulnar deviation and with compression. Often rest from function, especially repeated loading, will help heal the problem. The patient may benefit from a resting splint designed to hold the distal radioulnar joint in neutral.[19]

The piano key sign can be used to test the stability of the TFCC and the distal radioulnar joint. The patient holds their forearm in pronation and the examiner presses the ulna styloid. If the distal ulna moves excessively compared to the uninvolved side and the patient reports pain, then the test is considered to be positive for a tear of the TFCC and instability of the distal radioulnar joint.[20]

Ulnar Variance

The radial side of the distal ulna and the ulnar side of the distal radius should be in alignment. Asymmetry of this alignment is referred to as *ulnar variance*.[21] A positive ulnar variance is when the ulna is longer than the radius, and a negative ulnar variance is when the ulna is shorter than the radius. Ulnar variance can only be corrected surgically. A difference of 2 to 3 mm has been associated with changes in compressive forces between the radius, ulna and proximal row of carpals, and TFCC. Ulnar variance is best diagnosed with a radiograph. Negative ulnar variance has been associated with Kienböck's disease. A positive ulnar variance has been associated with degenerative changes in the TFCC and sclerotic changes in the triquetrum leading to degeneration of the articular cartilage and inflammation of the joint capsule.[21]

Metacarpal Fracture (Boxer's Fracture)

Metacarpal fractures can occur most commonly from striking a hard object with a closed fist or a crush injury. Injury from striking an object with a closed fist is known as a *boxer's fracture*. The fracture can be simple, requiring only a period of approximately 4 weeks of immobilization, or complex, requiring an ORIF and much longer immobilization. Most of these fractures are in the shaft of the bone. The more complex fractures can displace or spiral or have crushing of the bone, resulting in significant angulation. If the bone angulates significantly and is not properly fixated, there can be permanent shortening of the dorsal and palmar interossei and lumbricals, resulting in weakness of grip strength and difficulty opening the fingers fully.[22]

INJURIES INVOLVING THE THUMB

Ulnar Collateral Ligament of Thumb (Skier's Thumb, Gamekeeper's Thumb)

This injury to the ulnar collateral ligament (UCL) of the MCP joint of the thumb most commonly occurs with hyperextension and radial deviation of the MCP joint of the thumb.[23] Skiers who land on an outstretched hand while holding a ski pole force the MCP joint of the thumb into excessive extension and radial deviation, tearing the ligament or avulsing a fragment of bone. Another mechanism of injury can be landing on any object carried in the hand, such as a football, and the hand is out forward, but the thumb is held back by the object causing excessive abduction. The injury can involve tearing of the ligament or avulsion of the ligament from the bone. The patient will report pain with palpation over the ulnar side of the joint. If a valgus force is applied to the joint, excessive mobility will be found.

A complication of the UCL of the thumb is a Stener lesion.[23] This occurs when the ligament is displaced above the adductor pollicis aponeurosis. When this occurs, the ligament is displaced and will not heal without an ORIF. The patient will require immobilization in a thumb spica splint for up to 6 weeks.[24] Gentle ROM exercises and gentle joint mobilization can begin following removal of the splint. Caution should be used to not move the thumb into radial deviation. The splint can be worn at night to further protect the thumb for several more weeks. Strengthening and mobility exercises should progress to patient tolerance.

Radial Collateral Ligament Injuries

Radial collateral ligament injuries of the MCP joint of the thumb are much less frequent than UCL injuries. The thumb is forced into sudden adduction tensioning the radial side ligament. This injury can result in a ligament tear or an avulsion. The thumb will be immobilized in a spica splint or cast for a minimum of 4 weeks.[25]

Rolando's Fracture

A Rolando's fracture is similar to the Bennett's fracture with the same mechanism of injury except there are bone fragments on both the ulnar and radial side of the base of the first metacarpal. If there is separation of the fragments, then both sides require ORIF. Rolando's fracture will often have poor outcomes due to greater damage to articular cartilage and greater risk of CMC joint instability.[26]

Volar Plate Avulsion

Volar plates are palmar side ligaments at the MCP and interphalangeal (IP) joints of the fingers. These ligaments are covered with articular cartilage to encourage sliding of the flexor digitorum superficialis and flexor digitorum profundus tendons and their synovial sheaths across the MCP and IP joints. An injury to the volar plate is generally caused by forced hyperextension of the joints from either a fall or having a finger forcibly pulled into hyperextension. The volar plate can either rupture or avulse from the bone. Generally, the finger can be splinted and immobilized in some flexion to approximate the ends of the ligament. Healing will often occur in 3 to 4 weeks. At that time, ROM and exercise can be introduced.[27]

Collateral Ligament Injury to the Interphalangeal Joints

Collateral ligament injury to the PIP and DIP joints are most often caused by the individual having their finger held and either an excessive valgus or varus force applied across the joint.[28] Tension across the ligament can result in either a rupture of the ligament or an avulsion. If the joint has dislocated, the joint may be reduced with a traction force and the finger immobilized or taped to an adjacent finger (buddy taping) to limit ROM. If there is any possibility that the finger is fractured, then this procedure should be avoided until x-rays can rule out a fracture. Otherwise, the fracture is at risk of becoming more involved such as displacement of fragments that may now require ORIF.

Carpal Instability

Individuals with carpal instability will often report clicking or popping associated with pain and a feeling that they cannot support weight through the wrist. Carpal instability can be the result of trauma to the wrist, such as a fall, leading to damage to supporting ligaments or from hypermobility that is not well controlled by muscle. Individuals who are hypermobile at the wrist are not necessarily unstable. Carpal instability can present in several patterns. There can be instability of carpal bones within a row, or there can be instability of carpals between rows. Normally, there should be motion within a row of carpals. Flexion/extension and radial/ulnar deviation will occur between the proximal and distal rows.[2]

Scapholunate Dissociation

The instability is generally caused by a load that has been applied to the distal capitate, which is force between the scaphoid and lunate tearing the scapholunate ligament. This will result in a spreading of the 2 bones and an instability. Another mechanism is a result of a twisting injury to the wrist, in which the wrist is loaded in hyperextension and ulnar deviation. This motion can result in disruption of the ligaments that stabilize the scaphoid and lunate.[2] Initially, alignment of the bone may not be altered, but over time a shifting may occur. The tendency is for the scaphoid to collapse into flexion, ulnar deviation, and pronation, while the lunate collapses into extension, radial deviation, and supination. This dissociation often leads to degeneration, especially of the scaphoid.

Clinical examination of this patient may reveal a sharp pain with palpation directly over the lunate. The scaphoid shift test (Watson's test) can be performed to determine instability of the scaphoid.[17] The examiner compresses the scaphoid tubercle on the palmar side of the wrist, while the wrist is passively moved from neutral to radial deviation. With a positive test the examiner will feel the scaphoid shift and pain is often reported by the patient. If the test is repeated without pressure over the scaphoid tubercle, an audible click may be heard. Radiographs may reveal excessive space between the scaphoid and lunate, especially if the patient is asked to make a tight fist during the radiograph. ORIF may be required depending on the level of instability. This procedure may include use of insertion of K-wires, repair of the scapholunate ligaments, bone graft, and tendon realignment of the flexor carpi radialis to support the position of the scaphoid.[17]

Lunotriquetral Dissociation

This instability is generally the result of a fall backward on an outstretched hand with the arm externally rotated, the forearm supinated, and the wrist extended and radially deviated.[17] The result is a tear of the lunotriquetral ligament. The TFCC may also be torn as well as the UCL of the wrist. The patient will complain of painful crepitus with ulnar deviation; point tenderness over the dorsal aspect of the joint; and a feeling of giving way with full supination, ulnar deviation, and extension. Derby's maneuver can assist with the diagnosis. The examiner compresses over the pisiform, thus pushing the triquetrum dorsally. This will help to stabilize the triquetrum and the patient will report a feeling of improved stability.

Initially, treatment may begin with immobilization in a neutral resting splint followed by isometric exercise. If this conservative approach fails, the ORIF with reconstruction of the lunotriquetral ligament or lunotriquetral fusion may be necessary. This procedure may require six weeks of immobilization before exercise can begin.[17]

Dissociation of the Proximal and Distal Row

This injury generally occurs with axial loading of the wrist. The proximal row can shift to either a more dorsal or palmar position. The palmar shift is more common. The wrist can no longer tolerate weight bearing without collapsing, and the wrist will exhibit a clunk with weight bearing as the proximal row shifts. Initially, the treatment may consist of immobilization in a splint and anti-inflammatory medication. An ORIF to reconstruct the ligaments or carpal fusion may be required.[17]

NERVE INJURIES AND ENTRAPMENTS

Whenever there is paresthesia or anesthesia affecting the hand, several factors must be considered. A careful sensory and motor examination must be performed to determine which peripheral nerve, nerve root, or portion of the brachial plexus may be involved and the site of the injury or entrapment. Consideration must be given to the possibility of a nerve root entrapment in the cervical spine; thoracic outlet syndrome; entrapment under the pectoralis minor; or a peripheral nerve entrapment of the medial, ulnar, or radial nerves. Cervical spine entrapments, thoracic outlet syndrome, and entrapment under the pectoralis minor are issues beyond the scope of this chapter, but peripheral nerve entrapments will be discussed. When the sensory and motor patterns are not clear, upper limb tension testing may be helpful to determine the specific peripheral nerve involved.

Median Nerve

Carpal Tunnel Syndrome

Carpal tunnel syndrome (CTS) is an entrapment of the median nerve within the carpal tunnel. Traveling within the carpal tunnel are the tendons of the flexor digitorum superficialis, flexor digitorum profundus, and the flexor pollicis longus. All of these tendons are surrounded by synovial sheaths. Any inflammation of the sheaths will result in compression on the median nerve.

Most often CTS is considered an overuse injury but can be the result of trauma. Swelling of the synovial sheaths within the carpal tunnel or swelling of the wrist joint capsule will place pressure on the median nerve. CTS would affect sensation of the finger pads of the first, second, third, and the radial side of the fourth fingers.[29] Muscles that could be found to be weak are the abductor pollicis brevis, flexor pollicis brevis, opponens pollicis, and the first 2 lumbricals. The patient will most commonly complain of pain in the medial nerve distribution, paresthesia, and weakness. Whenever muscle weakness is involved, the patient may demonstrate an ape-thumb deformity. The patient will hold their hand with the thumb in the plane of the hand and have difficulty abducting their thumb to grasp objects. They will often complain of not being able to feel small objects and often drop them. Tip-to-tip and pad-to-pad pinches will be difficult.

CTS is most likely to occur from a trauma such as a fall on an outstretched hand or due to overuse, especially when the wrist is being held in extremes of flexion or extension. Tapping over the carpal tunnel with a fingertip may produce a paresthesia in the median nerve distribution (Tinel's sign).[29] Taking the wrist and holding it in end-range flexion (Phalen's test) and end-range extension (reverse Phalen's test) may also reproduce the paresthesia and/or pain.[29] A median nerve upper limb tension test to assess the nerve can be helpful if the pattern is not clear.[30] Electromyography and nerve conduction studies may be performed to further assess the level of damage to the median nerve.[31]

Treatment of CTS is often done using a resting splint that allows the fingers to move freely. The splint should be placed at 0 degrees and the distal end should not go past the distal palmar crease. A surgical release of the carpal tunnel is often performed when conservative treatment is not successful. A small incision is made at the wrist to release the flexor retinaculum.[32]

Entrapment of the Median Nerve Between the Two Heads of the Pronator Teres

Entrapment of the median nerve at this location must be ruled out.[33] The sensory pattern will look almost identical as that found with CTS, but the patient will also be found to have weakness of the flexor pollicis longus and flexor digitorum profundus to the second and third fingers. The patient may also experience a double crush injury to the median nerve, where there is entrapment at both the carpal tunnel and between the 2 heads of the pronator teres. A double crush injury will require an electromyography and nerve conduction velocity test to accurately diagnose this condition.

Ulnar Nerve

Tunnel of Guyon

The ulnar nerve can become entrapped within the tunnel of Guyon at the wrist (ulnar tunnel). This is an opening between the pisiform on the medial side, hook of the hamate on the lateral side, and palmar carpal ligament.[1,33] Traveling through the tunnel of Guyon is the ulnar nerve and artery. Trauma to this region, especially to the pisiform or hamate, or swelling within the tunnel can affect the ulnar nerve and artery. Narrowing here could result in paresthesia and or pain on the ulnar side of the hand anteriorly and posteriorly and in the fifth and the ulnar side of the fourth finger. Vascular supply could also affect both the superficial and deep vascular arches leading to diminished blood supply to the intrinsic muscles of the hand. Muscle weakness could be found in all the hypothenar muscles, all dorsal and palmar interossei, lumbricals to the fourth and fifth fingers, and adductor pollicis.

Weakness to the ulnar nerve innervated intrinsic muscles can result in diminished grip and pinch, especially affecting the pinch involving the thumb with the second and or third finger. This would greatly affect the pad-to-pad pinch and key grips. A severe weakness could result in a Bishop's hand deformity, which results in flexion of the fourth and fifth fingers as well as an inability to extend those 2 fingers. Ability to extend the second and third finger would be possible but weak. The individual would only have the first 2 lumbricals going into the extensor mechanism but none of the palmar or dorsal interossei.[2]

Ulnar Nerve Entrapment at the Cubital Tunnel

The ulnar nerve can become entrapped at the cubital tunnel. The cubital tunnel is a passage behind the elbow between the medial epicondyle and the olecranon process.[33] The ulnar nerve is superficial at this point. The roof of the cubital tunnel is covered with fibrous connective tissue. Injury to the ulnar nerve can be the result of fracture of the medial epicondyle or olecranon process or from overuse of elbow flexion repeatedly tensioning the nerve. Chronic medial epicondylitis or an injury to the medial collateral ligament of the elbow is often associated with ulnar nerve involvement and Little League elbow in adolescents. The nerve can become tensioned with repetitive throwing.

When the ulnar nerve is significantly affected at the cubital tunnel, an ulnar nerve transposition can be surgically performed. The nerve will be removed from the cubital tunnel and transferred to cross anterior to the elbow joint.[34]

The sensory pattern is the same as at the tunnel of Guyon, but the motor pattern would also include weakness of the flexor carpi ulnaris and flexor digitorum profundus to fingers 4 and 5. Performing a Tinel's sign can be helpful for diagnosis of this syndrome.[33] If the therapist is not sure that it is the ulnar nerve, an ulnar nerve upper limb tension test may help.

Radial Nerve

Triangular Interval

The radial nerve travels through the triangular interval. This triangle is a small space between the teres major superiorly, the long head of the triceps and humerus laterally, and the short head of the triceps medially.[1,35] The radial nerve and the deep brachial artery pass through this space. Hypertrophy of any of these 3 muscles could entrap the radial nerve or diminish blood flow to the triceps. This could result in weakness of the triceps complex, the brachioradialis, or any of the posterior muscles of the forearm. Sensations could be diminished in the posterior upper arm, posterior forearm, and posterior hand on the radial side.

Midhumeral shaft fractures can result in an injury to the radial nerve. The radial nerve lies posterior on the humeral shaft in the radial groove between the long head of the triceps and the short head of the triceps.[35] A fracture at this location can damage or even sever the radial nerve. Sensory to the dorsal surface of the forearm and radial side of the dorsum of the hand would be affected. Innervation of the brachioradialis and all the muscles of the posterior forearm would be affected. This could result in paresis or paralysis of the ability to extend the wrist, thumb, and fingers. The result would be a drop wrist deformity. Putting the wrist in constant flexion would greatly diminish grip strength by putting all the finger and thumb extrinsic flexor muscles in a position of active insufficiency.

The Radial Nerve at the Elbow

The radial nerve at the elbow crosses the elbow joint on the palmar side and then dives deep between the 2 heads of the supinator.[33] The sensory branch of the radial nerve to the dorsum of the forearm and hand branches off above the elbow joint and would not be affected. Hypertrophy of the supinator muscle could entrap the deep motor branch of the radial nerve (posterior interosseous nerve). This would affect the innervation of the deep compartment of the extensors, extensor pollicis longus, extensor pollicis brevis, abductor pollicis longus, and extensor indicis. Because there is no sensory component, clinical diagnosis may be difficult. A simple clinical test is to ask the patient to place their hand palm down on a tabletop.[4] Then, ask them to lift their thumb straight off the table. If this motion is weak but all other motions of finger extension and wrist extension are strong, then the deep motor branch of the radial nerve should be suspected.

Loss of sensation to the radial side of the dorsum of the hand but no sign of muscle weakness is often simple in nature. The patient may be wearing a watch band or other band or brace too tightly and be compressing the sensory branches of the radial nerve at the wrist. Simply loosen the band or brace, and the symptoms should resolve.

Complex Regional Pain Syndrome

CRPS has been known by several different names over time including *shoulder hand syndrome*, *causalgia*, and *reflex sympathetic dystrophy (RSD)*. CRPS can affect either the upper extremity or the lower extremity. In the upper extremity, any of the joints can become affected, but the hand is generally the most affected.[36] CRPS often follows a trauma to the upper extremity. Signs and symptoms of CRPS include severe pain, burning sensations, joint stiffness, and edema. Over time, decreased bone density may become evident.

In the early stages of CRPS, pain is severe with joint stiffness and pitting edema. The skin will be cold and clammy. Later, the pain will become more severe; the edema may become firm and the skin hot and dry. In the third stage, the pain may begin to decrease, and the skin is cool and dry. At this point, the joints may have become severely stiff and nonfunctional.[36]

Treatment of CRPS must prioritize pain control. This may be accomplished with electrical modalities and gentle rocking rhythmic exercise and low-grade joint mobilizations. Frequent active exercise is essential for self-treatment and must be done by the patient frequently. Edema control can be accomplished with compression garments or pneumatic pumps. A wrist continuous passive motion can be used to promote motion. Joint mobilization to all joints involved should be performed progressively but to patient tolerance. Without the proper treatment, the patient may be left with a completely nonfunctional hand.[36]

Peripheral Neuropathy

Peripheral neuropathy is a condition affecting the peripheral nervous system.[37] This condition is most commonly seen in people with diabetes and people with alcohol use disorder. Peripheral neuropathy will affect sensory and motor function of peripheral nerves. This effect is caused by diminished blood flow affecting swan cells and axons of the peripheral nerves. The peripheral nerves are affected from distal to proximal as the condition progresses, regardless of the specific peripheral nerves in the region. Therefore, the condition initially affects hands and feet.

The first signs of peripheral neuropathy are diminished sensation initially in the fingertips and progression proximally.[38] The sensory loss pattern is known as an opera glove sensory loss as the pattern can progress up into the forearm. Sensory changes can include paresthesia, hyperesthesia, hypoesthesia, and anesthesia. Joint proprioception is diminished as well. These sensory changes can have a negative effect on a patient's ability to handle small objects and do activities that require fine motor coordination. Often the patients will report that they frequently drop small objects.

Innervation of the most peripheral muscle is affected next. The first muscles in the upper extremities will be the intrinsic muscles of the hand. The patient may develop weakness of pinch and grips and difficulty opening their hand. When the condition becomes severe the patient can develop a claw hand deformity. The thumb will drop dorsally into the plane of the hand due to atrophy of the thenar eminence muscles. The hand will appear exceptionally bony due to loss of the intrinsic muscles. When the patient attempts to open the hand, they will have MCP joint hyperextension and IP flexion due to the loss of the palmar and dorsal interossei and lumbricals.[39]

The autonomic nervous system can also be affected. This can involve control of the distal vascular supply and sweat glands. Loss of peripheral vascular supply can lead to diminished response to temperature changes, hot or cold intolerance, and risk of burns or frostbite. Diminished sweat gland function can lead to anhidrosis, causing exceptionally dry skin and risk of skin breakdown and infection.[37]

ARTHRITIS

Arthritic changes can be classified into several different categories including osteoarthritis, rheumatoid arthritis, and those associated with gout and psoriasis. Each of these conditions are associated with inflammation and degenerative changes of the joints of the wrist and hand.

Osteoarthritis

Osteoarthritis is often known as *wear-and-tear arthritis*. This occurs when joints are overused in daily activities.[40] The wearing of articular cartilage does not result in the pain associated with osteoarthritis as articular cartilage is not innervated. Pain will initially come from inflammation of the joint capsule, which is highly innervated. Eventually pain may come from the subchondral bone if the articular cartilage is completely worn away. Many joints in the wrist and hand region commonly experience osteoarthritis including the carpal articulations; CMC joints, especially at the base of the thumb; MCP joints; and IP joints. When these joints are significantly affected then arthroplasty can be performed.

Rheumatoid Arthritis

Rheumatoid arthritis is an autoimmune disease that is systemic in nature. It is of an inflammatory nature and will affect multiple joints.[40,41] Synovial membranes will become inflamed resulting in pain, stiffness, and weakness. The patient may also report depression, low-grade fever, and weight loss. Rheumatoid arthritis is best known to affect synovial joints and synovial linings of sheaths and bursae, but it can also have an effect on lungs, the vascular system, and the neurological system. Rheumatoid arthritis can result in degenerative changes in the synovial linings, articular cartilage, and adjacent ligaments and tendons all of which can result in significant deformity and loss of function.

A common deformity affecting the wrist and hand is a zigzag deformity in which the wrist tends to go into radial deviation while the MCP joints go into ulnar deviation. The ulnar deviation of the MCP joints, also known as *ulnar drift*, can become so severe that the joints may disarticulate. The carpal bones can also dislocate in a volar direction. A Boutonniere deformity occurs when the lateral bands of the extensor mechanism migrate to the palmar side of the fingers at the PIP joints. The central slip ruptures and can no longer extend the PIP joints resulting in PIP flexion and DIP hyperextension. A swan neck deformity is due to failure of the volar plates at the PIP joints. The volar plates can no longer resist hyperextension at the joints and the PIP joints go into hyperextension while the DIP joints go into flexion. Mallet finger can also occur due to rupture of the lateral bands at the DIP joints resulting in an inability to extend the DIP joints.[41]

Many of these deformities should be splinted especially when the inflammatory process is acute to help diminish the deformity. These splints are designed to be static resting splints to support the joints in a stable, functional position.[24]

Many of these deformities can be minimized due to the use of new medications that affect the autoimmune system. Unfortunately, not all patients can take these medications, especially if the patient has an infection or is prone to infection.[41] The medication will diminish the effectiveness of a patient's ability to fight the infection as the medication inhibits their autoimmune system.

Tendon Injuries, Tenosynovitis, Avulsions, and Lacerations

Extensor Tendon Tenosynovitis

The extensor tendons cross the wrist in 6 separate compartments, each with its own synovial sheath.[1] When any of the wrist extensor compartments are involved it is known as *tenosynovitis*. Tenosynovitis is generally caused by either overuse or a direct blow to the tendon sheaths. Involvement of the radial side compartments are most common and ulnar side compartments are progressively less common from radial to ulnar.

Extensor compartment 1 includes involvement of extensor pollicis brevis and abductor pollicis longus. The 2 tendons are within 1 synovial sheath. This condition is known as *de Quervain's tenosynovitis* and can be caused by either a direct blow or overuse of thumb extension. This condition, like all tenosynovitis conditions, is generally simple to diagnose but may be difficult to treat. The first examination procedure is palpation of the tendons at the wrist, the second is to put the tendons on a stretch, and the third is to do a resisted isometric contraction of the muscles involved. For all 3 tests, a positive finding is pain. A good way to apply a stretch to the tendons is to have the patient place their thumb into the palm of the hand, hold it down with the other fingers and ulnarly deviate the wrist. This is known as *Finkelstein's test*.[42]

Extensor compartment 2 involves the extensor carpi radialis longus and extensor carpi radialis brevis in one synovial sheath.[1] Involvement of compartment 2 would result from a direct blow or repetitive overuse of wrist extension. Diagnosis of this condition would again be best determined with palpation, resisted isometric contraction, and putting the wrist into full flexion. A positive test is pain resulting from each test.[42]

Extensor compartment 3 is the extensor pollicis longus.[1] This generally occurs from a direct blow or overuse as the tendon rubs on the dorsal radial tubercle (Lister's tubercle). This condition can be diagnosed with palpation of the tendon at the wrist at or just distal to the dorsal radial tubercle, resisted thumb extension, or flexing the thumb to end range.[42]

Extensor compartment 4 has 5 tendons. The 4 tendons of extensor digitorum and the tendon of extensor indicis are all within 1 sheath.[1] When doing a resisted isometric or putting these tendons on a stretch, care must be taken to only contract these muscles or only stretch these muscles, but to not involve contraction of the wrist extensors or stretching of the wrist into flexion. Doing this can give a false positive.[42]

Extensor compartment 5 contains the extensor digiti minimi tendon. It can be best palpated just to the radial side of the ulnar styloid or slightly distal to it.[43] Overuse of this compartment would be quite rare, but a direct blow should be considered.[42]

Extensor compartment 6 is the extensor carpi ulnaris.[1] This compartment will be found just to the ulnar side or just distal to the ulna styloid.[43] Wrist extension and or ulnar deviation should be resisted. Stretching into flexion and or radial deviation should be used to produce the stretch. Generally, only one compartment will be involved at a time. The exception to that rule is if the patient has rheumatoid arthritis, then any or all of the extensor compartments may be involved. Occasionally patients with rheumatoid arthritis may experience rupture of any of the extensor compartment tendons and would require surgical repair.

All of the extensor compartment tenosynovitis conditions can be successfully treated similarly. The first approach should be rest from function. This is generally best achieved by making a resting splint to immobilize the tendons in question. Compartment 1 is best splinted with a thumb spica splint with a gutter support on the radial side of the forearm.[24] This will immobilize both the thumb and the wrist. The forearm component should extend approximately two-thirds up the forearm in order to assure immobilization of the wrist. Three-point fixation of the thumb is best achieved with a cylinder shape around the thumb and a strap at the wrist and more proximal on the forearm. The thumb should be positioned in partial abduction.

The splint for compartments 2 and 6 is a resting splint that will place the wrist in neutral but allow active mobility of the thumb and fingers. The splint should not go past the distal palmar crease or motion may be blocked.[24]

The splint for compartment 3 will be very similar to compartment 1.[24] The difference would be that the splint should cover more of the dorsal surface of the wrist. Compartments 4 and 5 would require a splint that would immobilize both the wrist and all 4 ulnar side digits.[24] This splint would extend all the way to the distal end of the digits and immobilize both the wrist and the fingers. The MCP joints should be immobilized in flexion, but the IP joints should be immobilized in extension. This puts these joints closer to their closed-pack position helping to assure that the collateral ligaments will maintain some tension on them and not become overly shortened.

Initially the splints can be removed several times per day for gentle ROM exercise to maintain joint mobility and tendon gliding. Modalities can be utilized for pain control. Once the pain has subsided, then exercise can be done more frequently, slowly adding resistance and finally stretching to end range.

Jersey Finger

Jersey finger can be either an avulsion of the flexor digitorum profundus tendon from the base of the distal phalanx or a rupture of the distal tendon.[44] This injury is most common in football when one individual tackles another by the shirt collar from behind with one fingertip and drops to the ground hanging their entire body weight by the one finger tip.

This injury most commonly involves the middle finger. The bone fragment with an avulsion will require ORIF and immobilization. If the tendon is torn, it will require repair. If this injury is not repaired, there is a risk of retraction of the flexor digitorum profundus tendon proximally. The longer the period of time between injury and repair, the more difficult the repair becomes if retraction of the tendon occurs.

These patients will need to be immobilized in a splint for a minimum of 6 weeks.[24] Depending on the quality of the repair, they may not be allowed to put tension on the tendon for up to 12 weeks. They may then be placed in a dynamic splint where the fingers are pulled passively into flexion by rubber bands or springs and the patient is permitted to extend approximately 50% of the range. This assures that further tension will not be applied to the newly repaired tendon. Exercises must progress gently and slowly progress to resistive exercise.

Mallet Finger

A mallet finger is an injury to the extensor mechanism of the finger at the DIP joint.[45] The mechanism of injury is most often when the individual is hit on the distal end of the finger and the joint is suddenly forced into flexion. This injury commonly occurs in athletics when attempting to catch a ball. A common name for this injury is *baseball finger*. As a result of this trauma, either the lateral bands will rupture, or the lateral bands will avulse for the dorsal side base of the distal phalanx. If there is significant displacement of bone, the fragment of bone following an avulsion may require an ORIF. If the bone fragments remain approximated, then splinting the DIP joint in full extension may be adequate to allow healing to occur.[24]

The patient will generally hold the DIP joint in flexion. This injury can be assessed by the examiner stabilizing the middle phalanx and asking the patient to extend the DIP joint. If the patient cannot extend the DIP joint, then the lateral bands are most likely torn.[45]

Tendon Laceration Injuries

Tendon laceration injuries generally occur with a slicing injury with a sharp object such as a knife, glass, or sheet metal. These injuries are classified as either a flexor tendon injury or an extensor tendon injury. They are further divided into zones of injury. Each zone has specific anatomy that may have been injured. Complete tendon laceration injuries must be surgically repaired. The therapist must understand exactly which tissues were injured and whether they were surgically repaired. Different tissues will heal at different rates and must be protected from tensile forces.

All long tendons tend to have a poor blood supply, with the blood supply coming from the muscle on one end and the bone on the other.[46] Further nutrition is provided by the synovial fluid within the tendon sheaths and a small connective tissue that contains a small artery for the middle and distal phalanx called the *vincula*. The vincula gives additional blood supply to both the flexor digitorum superficialis and profundus tendons in zone 2. Despite nutrition coming from multiple sources, a typical repaired tendon laceration will take 6 weeks or longer to heal.

Flexor Tendons Zone One

This zone of injury is at the distal end of a finger just proximal to or at the DIP joint.[47] In this zone, the key structure involved is the tendon of flexor digitorum profundus. Following repair, the tendon will then need to be protected in a splint for approximately 6 weeks. After that time, gentle ROM exercise may begin with care taken to not go to end-range extension for several more weeks.

Flexor Tendons Zone Two

Zone 2 is from just proximal to the MCP joints to just proximal to the DIP joints.[47] Zone 2 contains the flexor digitorum profundus and superficialis tendons and tendon sheaths. Laceration injuries in this region will often have the poorest outcomes. Here, the tendons have the least blood supply and are most likely to scar together as one. The tendon is at risk for rerupture, or the 2 tendons and sheath will scar together risking losing significant function of both flexion and extension activities.

A special dynamic splint must be fabricated to properly protect repaired tendons in this zone. This splint is generally dorsal based with the wrist positioned in flexion.[24] The splint will be designed to block extension of the MCP joints at 90 degrees and the PIP and DIP joints at 0 degrees. The dynamic portion of the splint is often either springs or rubber bands fixed to the distal end of the fingers. The surgeon may either sew a small button into the patient's fingernail or the therapist may glue a hook to the fingernail. The fingers will then be passively pulled into flexion, and the patient is allowed to actively move into extension with the PIP and DIP joints at 0 degrees. The springs or rubber bands fixed to the distal end of the fingers passively pull the fingers into flexion and the patient is allowed to actively move into extension. The splint will keep tension off the flexor tendons but allow for movement helping to prevent scarring between the flexor tendons. Since the development of this type of splint, flexor tendon injuries in zone 2 have greatly improved outcomes. The splint will be maintained for a minimum of 6 weeks before active exercise will be permitted. No stretching of the fingers into full extension and with wrist extension will be allowed for at least 12 weeks.

Flexor Tendons Zone Three

Zone 3 is from the distal row of carpals to just proximal to the MCP joints.[47] This region contains many structures. From superficial to deep, there is the skin, palmar aponeurosis, superficial vascular arch, flexor digitorum superficialis, deep vascular arch, flexor digitorum profundus and lumbricals, and branches of the median and ulnar nerves. Normally, the interossei are protected by the metacarpals unless the bone is also fractured. The muscles of the thenar and hypothenar eminence may also be affected. All of these structures must be individually repaired by the surgeon.

Once the vascular arches are repaired, blood supply will be restored. Blood supply to the hand can be verified by the therapist once healing of the tendons has occurred by utilizing a clinical test called the Allen's test of the wrist.[4] The therapist will ask the patient to pump their fingers for approximately 1 minute. The patient will continue to pump their fingers as the therapist occludes both the median and ulnar arteries at the wrist until pallor is observed in the hand. The therapist will then release one artery while maintaining pressure on the other. The therapist should observe the blood returning to the hand first on the side released and then across to the opposite side of the hand. The test should then be repeated with a reversal of the release of the opposite artery. In both scenarios, the blood supply to the hand should return within several seconds, letting the therapist know that the vascular arches are operating adequately.

Flexor Tendons Zone Four

The tendons in zone 4 are at the wrist in the region of the carpal tunnel and the tunnel of Guyon.[47] The structures that are injured in this region can be quite variable depending on the depth of the laceration. This injury can be the result of a laceration accident with a sharp object or an attempted suicide. The most likely structures to be injured would include the tendons of the palmaris longus, flexor carpi radialis, and flexor carpi ulnaris. The ulnar artery and nerve could be injured as the tunnel of Guyon is not as deep as the structures within the carpal tunnel. Most of the time the tendons and the median nerve in the carpal tunnel would be protected by the flexor retinaculum and the arching shape of the carpal bones.

Flexor Tendons Zone Five

Zone 5 includes all of the tendons, nerves, and muscle bellies within the anterior forearm.[47] Injury here would be dependent on depth and level of injury.[1]

Extensor Tendon Injuries

The zones of these injuries are classified slightly differently but again are related to the anatomy and the structures injured. All of these structures must be surgically repaired in order to assure full return of function.[48]

Zone One

This injury involves the insertion of the lateral bands into the base of the distal phalanx. This injury would make it impossible for the patient to extend the DIP joint actively.[48]

Zone Two

This injury would involve the lateral bands before they join together just proximal to the DIP joint. This injury would make it impossible for the patient to extend the DIP joint actively.[48]

Zone Three

This injury would involve the lateral bands and central slip at the PIP joint. The patient would lose the ability to extend the PIP and DIP joints.[48]

Zone Four

This injury would affect both the central slip and lateral bands just proximal to the PIP joint. This patient would lose the ability to extend the PIP and DIP joints.[48]

Zone Five

This is an injury through the extensor hood at the MCP joint. This patient would lose the ability to extend the MCP, PIP, and DIP joints.[48]

Zone Six

Zone 6 is on the dorsum of the hand across the metacarpal shafts. The injury would lacerate the tendons of the extensor digitorum. This patient would lose the ability to extend the MCP, PIP, and DIP joints.[48]

Zone Seven

Zone 7 is across the dorsal surface of the carpal bones. Tendons in this region are grouped together in extensor compartments within synovial sheaths. Injury to compartment 1 would involve extensor pollicis brevis and abductor pollicis longus and its sheath. Compartment 2 would involve extensor carpi radialis longus and extensor carpi radialis brevis and its sheath. Compartment 3 would involve extensor pollicis longus and its sheath. Compartment 4 would involve all 4 tendons of the extensor digitorum and extensor indicis and its sheath. Compartment 5 would involve the extensor digiti minimi and its sheath. Compartment 6 would involve the extensor carpi ulnaris and its sheath. Sensory branches of the radial nerve supply the radial side dorsum of the hand and could also be involved.[48]

INJURIES TO SKIN

Injuries to the skin are very common with hand injuries. Careful examination and debridement are necessary to prevent infection.[49] The therapist should first inspect the color of the wound. Pink or red is a sign of granulation and return of blood flow and is a sign of proper healing. Yellow or green is a sign of infection indicating that this tissue needs to be debrided. The therapist should also be alert of any foul smell from the wound. Brown or black is a sign of necrosis also indicating debridement. If the wound is narrow and free from infection the wound can be closed with sutures. If the wound is wide or has shown signs of infection, then the wound will be left open to drain and only be closed when all signs of infection have resolved. If the wound is wide, then the wound will be left open to granulate. The wound will then close by filling in from the outside in.

A wound can occur when the skin is stripped off, most commonly from the dorsum of the hand.[50] This injury is known as a *degloving* or *denuding* and occurs when an individual gets their hand caught between 2 structures such as rollers. This injury generally requires a skin graft. A partial-thickness skin graft can be harvested from any broad region of the body.[50] Some surgeons prefer a full-thickness skin graft. This can be achieved by creating a pocket of skin into the abdomen of the patient and placing the hand under the skin.[50] This skin, while still attached to the abdomen, will have a good blood supply. Once the skin has adhered to the dorsum of the hand and blood supply is viable from the hand to the grafted skin, the skin can then be released from the abdomen. This healing can take up to 6 weeks. A partial-thickness graft can then be applied to the abdominal site. Smaller flaps can be used for smaller areas such as fingertips.[51]

Burns of the Hand

Burns involving the hand can result in significant and lifelong deformity if not treated properly. Burns can occur due to hot water, direct flame, or touching a hot object. Burns of the hand can result in dysfunction due to loss of sensation from damage of the sensory nerves or loss of mobility due to excessive scarring.[52] Scarring from burns can often adhere to the underlying tissue. Hypertrophic scarring and scar contracture may occur. Edema may also be excessive. A circumferential burn can be especially problematic if there is excessive scarring, which risks compromise of blood circulation. An escharotomy may be necessary to restore circulation.[53] The patient should then be positioned in a protective splint while healing occurs.[53] Skin grafting may then be performed to close the wound. Once healing is determined to be adequate, scar massage, mobilization, and strengthening exercise may begin. Often, the patient will be placed in a custom-fitted compression garment to help minimize further scar formation.

REFERENCES

1. Drake RL, Vogl AW, Mitchell AWM. *Gray's Anatomy for Students.* 2nd ed. Churchill Livingston, Elsevier; 2015.
2. Neumann DA. *Kinesiology of the Musculoskeletal System: Foundations for Rehabilitation.* 3rd ed. Elsevier; 2017.
3. Karabay N. US findings in traumatic wrist and hand injuries. *Diagn Interv Radiol.* 2013;19:320-325.
4. Khader BA, Towler MR. Common treatments and procedures used for distal radius and scaphoid: a review. *Mater Sci Eng C Mater Biol Appl.* 2017;74:422-433.
5. Jenkins NH. The unstable Colles fracture. *J Hand Surg.* 1989;14:149-154.
6. Kenney RJ, Hammert WC. Physical examination of the hand. *J Hand Surg.* 2014;11:2325-2334.
7. Campbell DA, Wilkinson TC. Wrist fractures. *Ortho Trauma.* 2011;25:324-335.
8. Medoff RJ. Distal radial fractures In: Skirven TM, Osterman AL, Fedorczyk JM, Amadio PC. *Rehabilitation of the Hand and Upper Extremity.* 6th ed. Elsevier; 2011.
9. Mehara AK, Rostogi S, Bhan S, Dave PK. Classification and treatment of volar Barton's fractures. *Injury.* 1993;24:55-59.
10. Giannoulis FS, Sotereanos DG. Galeazzi fractures and dislocations. *Hand Clinics.* 2007;23:153-163.
11. Dodds SD, Yeh PC, Slade JF. Essex-Lopresti injuries. *Hand Clinics.* 2008;24:436-438.
12. Daneshvar P, Chan R, MacDermind J, Grewal R. The effects of ulnar styloid fracture on patients sustain distal radial fracture. *J Hand Surg.* 2014;39:1015-1920.
13. Fowler JR, Hughes TB. Scaphoid fractures. *Clin Sports Med.* 2015;34(1):37-50.
14. Charles D, Elkins A, Kneeburg A, Nikkila K. A comparison of diagnostic imaging and vibrating tuning forks in the detection of fractures. *Int J health Sciences Research.* 2017;7(8):473-478.
15. Karamura K, Chang KE. Treatment of scaphoid fractures and nonunion. *J Hand Surg.* 2008;33:988-997.
16. Suh N, Ek ET, Wolfe SW. Carpal fractures. *J Hand Surg.* 2014;39:785-791.
17. Dell PC, Dell RB, Griggs R. Management of carpal fractures and dislocations. In: Skirven TM, Osterman AL, Fedorczyk JM, Amadio PC. *Rehabilitation of the Hand and Upper Extremity.* 6th ed. Elsevier; 2011.
18. Earp BE, Floyd WE, Louis D, Koris M, Protomastro P. Ulnar nerve entrapment at the wrist. *J Am Acad Ortho Surg.* 2014;22:699-706.
19. Doarn MC, Wysocki RW. Acute TFCC injury. *Op Tech Sports Med.* 2016;24:123-125.
20. Rhee PC, Sauve PS, Lindau T, Shin AY. Examination of the wrist: ulnar side wrist pain due to ligament injury. *J Hand Surg.* 2014;39:1859-1862.
21. Taras JS, D'Addesi LL. Diagnostic imaging of the upper extremity. In: Skirven TM, Osterman AL, Fedorczyk JM, Amadio PC. *Rehabilitation of the Hand and Upper Extremity.* 6th ed. Elsevier; 2011.
22. McNamer TB, Howell JW, Chang E. Management of metacarpal fractures. *J Hand Ther.* 2003;69:143-151.
23. Mahagan M, Rhemrev SJ. Rupture of the ulnar collateral ligament of the thumb: a review. *Inter J Emerg Med.* 213;6:31-37.
24. Jacobs MAS, Austin NM. *Splinting the Hand and Upper Extremity.* Lippincott, Williams & Wilkins; 2003.
25. Edelstein DM, Kardashian J, Lee SK. Radial collateral injuries of the thumb. *Am Soc Surg Hand.* 2008;33:760-770.
26. Carlsen BT, Moran SL. Thumb trauma: Bennett's fracture, Rolando's fracture and ulnar collateral ligament injuries. *Am Soc Surg Hand.* 2009;34:945-962.
27. Pruez RB, Friedrich JB. Finger joint injuries. *Clin Sports Med.* 2015;34:99-116.
28. Roh YK, Koh YD, Go JY, Noh JH, Gong HS, Beak GH. Factors influencing functional outcome of proximal interphalangeal joint collateral ligament injury when treated with buddy strapping and exercise. *J Hand Ther.* 2018;31(3):295-300.
29. Burton C, Chesterton LS, Davenport G. Diagnosing and treating carpal tunnel syndrome in primary care. *Br J Gen Pract.* 2014;64(622):262-263.
30. Elvey RL. Physical examination of the peripheral nervous system in disorders of pain and dysfunction. *J Hand Ther.* 1997;10:122-129.
31. Nelson C. Electrical evaluation of nerve and muscle excitability. In: Gersh MR. *Electrotherapy in Rehabilitation.* FA Davis; 1992.
32. Bickel KD. Carpal tunnel syndrome. *J Hand Surg.* 2010;35:147-153.
33. Miller TT, Renus WR. Nerve entrapments of the elbow, forearm and wrist. *Am J Roentgenology.* 2010;195:585-594.
34. Catalano LW, Barron OA. Anterior subcutaneous transposition of the ulnar nerve. *Hand Clinics.* 2007;23:339-344.
35. Pidhorz L. Acute and chronic humeral shaft fractures in adults. *Ortho Trauma Surg Res.* 2015;101:541-549.

36. Zyluk A, Puchalski P. Complex regional pain syndrome of the upper limb: a review. *Neuro Pol.* 2014;148:200-208.

37. Gries F, Cameron N, Low P, Ziegler D. *Textbook of Diabetic Neuropathy.* Thieme; 2003.

38. Hanewinckel R, Ikram MA, Van Doorn PA. Peripheral neuropathy. *Handbook Clin Neuro.* 2016;138:263-282.

39. Seu M, Pasqualetto M. Hand therapy for dysfunction of intrinsic muscles. *Hand Clinics.* 2012;28:87-100.

40. Lawrence KJ. The aging wrist and hand. In: Kauffman TL, Scott R, Barr JO, Moran ML. *A Comprehensive Guide to Geriatric Rehabilitation.* Churchill Livingston Elsevier; 2014.

41. Gabay O, Gabay C. Hand osteoarthritis: new insights. *Joint Bone Spine.* 2013;80(2):130-134

42. Rosenthal EA, Elhassan BT. The extensor tendons: evaluation and surgical management. In: Skirven TM, Osterman AL, Fedorczyk JM, Amadio PC. *Rehabilitation of the Hand and Upper Extremity.* 6th ed. Elsevier; 2011.

43. Biel A. *Trail Guide to the Body: How to Locate Muscles, Bone and More.* 5th ed. Books of Discovery;. 2016.

44. Tempelaere C, Brun M, Daursounian J, Feron JM. Traumatic avulsion of flexor digitorum profundus tendon. Jersey finger, a 29 cases report. *Hand Surg Rehab.* 2017;36(5):368-372.

45. Patel D, Dean C, Baker RJ. The hand in sports: an update on the clinical anatomy and physical examination. *Prim Care Clin Office Pract.* 2005;32:71-89.

46. Fenwick SA, Hazleman BL, Riley GP. The vasculature and its role in tendon healing. *Arthritis Res.* 2002;4;252-260.

47. Lutsku KF, Giang EL, Matzon JL. Flexor tendon injuries: repair and rehabilitation. *Ortho Clinics North Am.* 2015;46:67-76.

48. Owen JM, Watts AC. (iii) Extensor tendon injuries. *Ortho Trauma.* 2014;28(4):214-218. doi:10.1016/j.mporth.2014.07.005

49. Kamolz LP, Wild T. Wound bed preparation: the impact of debridement and wound cleaning. *Wound Med.* 2013;1:44-50.

50. Sabapathy SR, Ventakatramani H, Paya PM. The use of pedicled abdominal flaps for coverage of acute bilateral circumferential degloving injuries of the hand. *Trauma Case Rep.* 2015;1(3-4):25-31.

51. Rehim SA, Chung KC. Local flaps of the hand. *Hand Clin.* 2014;30(2):137-151.

52. Soni A, Pham TM, Ko JH. Acute management of hand burns. *Hand Clin.* 2017;33:229-236.

53. Tufarro PA, Bondoc SL. Therapist management of the burned hand. In: Skirven TM, Osterman AL, Fedorczyk JM, Amadio PC. *Rehabilitation of the Hand and Upper Extremity.* 6th ed. Elsevier; 2011.

PART III

Lower Extremity

8

Lower Quarter Systems Review, Postural Assessment, and Referred Pain Patterns

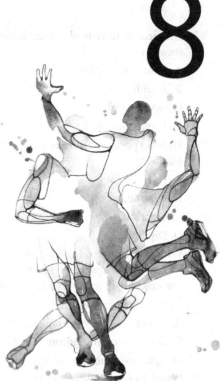

Kristi M. Angelopoulou, PT, DPT, OCS, MCMT, Cert.MSKUS
and William R. VanWye, PT, DPT, PhD

KEY TERMS

Clinical decision-making process for referral: The process outlined by the American Physical Therapy Association's *Guide to Physical Therapist Practice* that indicates the responsibility of a practicing physical therapist to screen patients for medical conditions that require a referral to another practitioner.

Lower extremity functional screen: Application of loaded or weightbearing forces in functional patterns to assess the gross musculoskeletal integrity of a patient's lower extremities.

Lower quarter systems review: A hands-on brief scan examination focusing on the 5 systems deemed most related to physical therapist practice: (1) communication, (2) cardiovascular/pulmonary, (3) integumentary, (4) musculoskeletal, and (5) neuromuscular.

Postural scan: The process of visual inspection of a patient from the 3 cardinal planes, with comparison to a reference point, to detect skeletal malalignments or adaptive compensation patterns, which may assist the clinician in identifying the biomechanical or underlying structural causes of a patient's chief complaint.

Referred pain: Pain that is generated by a nociceptive stimulus within a somatic or visceral structure, which refers pain to regions outside of that structure, and is perceived by the patient in regions that share the same innervation source.

CHAPTER QUESTIONS

1. What is the primary purpose of performing a lower quarter screening examination?

   A. To determine if the symptoms are systemic or musculoskeletal in origin

   B. To determine the exact location of the patients' complaints

   C. To make a medical diagnosis of the patients' condition

   D. To cover yourself from legal claims and protect your license

2. True or False—Abnormal posture has been found to be a predictor of pain and dysfunction.

Wallmann HW, Donatelli R, eds. *Foundations of Orthopedic Physical Therapy* (pp 189-209).
© 2024 Taylor & Francis Group.

3. An ideal posture is identified through which objective measure?

   A. Visual inspection

   B. Plumb line

   C. Goniometry

   D. Dynamometry

4. Hyperkyphotic posture is a risk factor to which of the following?

   A. Falls

   B. Dizziness

   C. Fracture

   D. Diplopia

5. Which of the following is a clinical sign that is frequently observed in a patient with low back pain (LBP) that is associated with an intervertebral disk lesion?

   A. Forward head posture

   B. Upper crossed syndrome (UCS)

   C. Lower crossed syndrome (LCS)

   D. Gravity-induced trunk list

6. Which of the following is a frontal plane deviation seen as associated with a postural screen?

   A. Genu valgum

   B. Anterior pelvic tilt

   C. Hyperkyphosis

   D. Genu recurvatum

7. Which of the following measures should be assessed to screen for underlying cardiovascular conditions?

   A. Resting heart rate (HR)

   B. Respiratory rate (RR)

   C. Blood pressure (BP)

   D. All of the above

8. When screening a patient with a known history of heart failure, a daily weight change of more than _____ pound/s is considered abnormal.

   A. 1

   B. 3

   C. 5

   D. 7

9. Which of the following subset of patients should receive a gait screen as a part of the initial evaluation process?

   A. Patient with a referral for a lower extremity disorder

   B. Patient with a referral for a balance disorder

   C. Patient with a referral for an upper extremity disorder

   D. All patients should receive a gait screen

10. Performing a functional squat can be best used to screen which level of motor nerve innervation?

    A. T12-L1

    B. L1-L2

    C. L2-L4

    D. S2-S4

11. When performing a functional squat, the therapist can use which parameters to positively differentiate a neuromusculoskeletal pathology from a musculoskeletal pathology?

    A. Pain without the presence of weakness

    B. Weakness without the presence of pain

    C. Capsular stiffness without loss of range of motion (ROM)

    D. Loss of ROM without capsular stiffness

12. If a patient is unable to independently and safely perform a functional squat, what alternative activity should be assessed?

    A. Sit to stand from a chair

    B. Single leg stance

    C. Single leg lunge

    D. Step up

13. Which of the following tests is used to differentiate balance impairment between the visual, proprioceptive and vestibular systems?

    A. Tinetti

    B. Berg Balance

    C. Modified Romberg

    D. Timed Up and Go

14. A patient is having difficulty lifting their foot to clear the foot and ankle during swing phase of gait. Weakness in which of the following lower extremity myotomes could contribute to this neurological weakness pattern?

    A. L2-L3

    B. L3-L4

    C. L4-L5

    D. L5-S1

15. While performing a deep tendon reflex (DTR) screen on a patient at the level of S1-S2, you score it as a 4+ with clonus. What do these findings indicate?

    A. Upper motor neuron disorder

    B. Lower motor neuron disorder

    C. Ataxia disorder

    D. Lower limb neural tension

16. A 68-year-old male patient is referred to your clinic for LBP. While performing an abdominal screening, you observe a pulse present in the abdomen. Upon auscultation of the pulse, there is presence of a bruit. Which of the following clinical decisions should be made at this time?

    A. This is a normal finding. Treat the patient.

    B. This is a normal finding; however, you would like the patient to follow up with their primary medical provider.

    C. This is an abnormal finding; suggest that the patient mention it to their primary care provider on their next visit.

    D. This is an abnormal finding, and the patient should be referred for immediate medical attention.

17. Pain which is referred from an internal body organ such as the spleen or the heart is known as _____.

    A. Radiculopathy

    B. Myofascial

    C. Myogenic

    D. Viscerogenic

18. Which of the following patient descriptions of pain should be considered a red flag finding in the screening process?

    A. Radiating, numbness

    B. Poorly localized and diffuse

    C. Sharp, pinpoint

    D. Aching, tightness

19. Which of the following terms indicates a constellation of signs and symptoms including diminished reflexes, dermatomal numbness, myotomal weakness and pain?

    A. Referred pain

    B. Radiating pain

    C. Radiculopathy

    D. Radicular pain

20. Which of the following statements reflects current best practices of lumbar spine evaluation and treatment?

    A. Treat the patient based upon the findings of the MRI

    B. Treat the patient based upon the pathoanatomical diagnosis

    C. Treat the patient based upon the examination findings and response to movement

    D. Treat the patient based upon the pain and referred pain patterns into the lower extremities

LOWER QUARTER SYSTEMS REVIEW

Examination of the lower quarter begins with a screening process to determine whether the patient's pain is coming from a potentially serious or life-threatening disorder (see Chapter 2), systemic origin, or from a

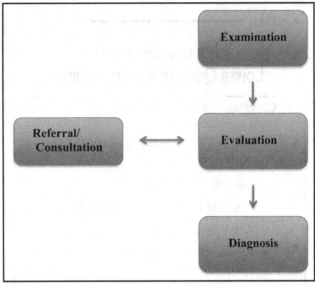

Figure 8-1. Patient/client management and clinical decision-making process for referral. (Adapted from American Physical Therapy Association. *Guide to Physical Therapist Practice*. Accessed November 23, 2021. http://guidetoptpractice.apta.org/)

musculoskeletal condition. The screening examination allows the physical therapist to narrow the search for the underlying source of symptoms, identify red flag findings that would warrant a referral to another medical provider, and determine body regions or systems that may require a more detailed examination. The clinical decision-making process, outlined by the American Physical Therapy Association's *Guide to Physical Therapist Practice*, indicates that the physical therapist must decide when a referral to another provider is necessary as a part of the differential diagnosis process (Figure 8-1).[1] For an overview of the sequence of a complete lower quarter systems review, see Table 8-1.

Observation

Patient position: Variable

Observation begins as soon as you greet the patient and continues throughout the examination and treatment. Also, observe for possible cognitive impairment throughout the examination and if a more detailed examination is required (eg, Mini-Mental State Examination).

Examination of the integumentary system includes observation of the skin, including hair and nails. Observe skin contour, color, and condition, as well as noting any rashes, ulcers, scars, or swelling. Also, a useful screen for skin cancer is the ABCDEF method.[2] The addition of F helps improve the sensitivity of the screening tool as F stands for "funny looking", which accounts for the "ugly duckling sign" (ie, a spot unlike the others). Any abnormal finding should be brought to the patient's attention along with follow-up questioning to determine whether the change is new, if the patient's physician is aware of the change, and if it is worsening.[3]

Table 8-1

INTEGRATION OF THE LOWER QUARTER SYSTEMS REVIEW

- Observation, including posture and gross symmetry
- Cardiovascular and pulmonary screen
- Gross functional screen, including gait and balance
- Gross ROM of trunk and lower extremities
    - Active range of motion (AROM)
    - Passive range of motion (PROM) including overpressures
- Neurological*—trunk and lower extremities
    - Dermatomes
    - Myotomes
    - Reflexes
    - Lower limb tension testing
- Palpation
- Abdominal screening*
- Tests and measures*

* Not part of the system review but included to show its position in the sequence.

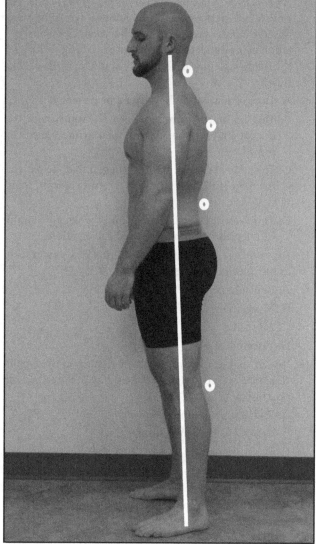

Figure 8-2. Postural observation: lateral view.

- A—Asymmetry
- B—Borders
- C—Color
- D—Diameter
- E—Evolving
- F—Funny looking

Postural Assessment of the Upper and Lower Quarters

A postural scan, in the context of an upper quarter or lower quarter screening examination, can assist in identifying gross postural abnormalities or skeletal malalignment, which could be contributing to a neuromusculoskeletal, biomechanical, or systemic pathology. While abnormal posture alone has not been found to be a predictor of pain or dysfunction, a significantly higher incidence of pain has been found in participants with more severe postural abnormalities. Skeletal malalignment can alter joint load distribution and, therefore, joint contact pressure distribution of adjacent

or distant joints.[4] A screening examination for skeletal alignment of the lower quarter may assist the clinician in identifying skeletal malalignments that are associated with a musculoskeletal complaint.[5] Abnormal findings during the postural screen may direct the clinician toward further investigation of signs or symptoms correlating with the patient history or other positive tests and measures.

Postural assessment should be performed through gross inspection of the patient from lateral, anterior, and posterior views (Figures 8-2 through 8-4). If practical, the patient should disrobe as appropriate for adequate visualization of landmarks. The physical therapist should observe for symmetry of major bony landmarks, soft tissue folds, muscle size, as well as for compensatory patterns of standing including sway, shifting of the trunk, and weightbearing/weight acceptance through the lower extremities. For a checklist of the postural scan, see Table 8-2.

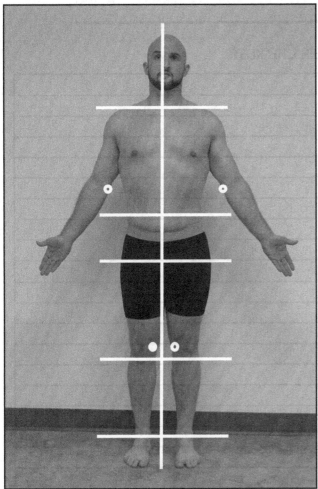

Figure 8-3. Postural observation: anterior view.

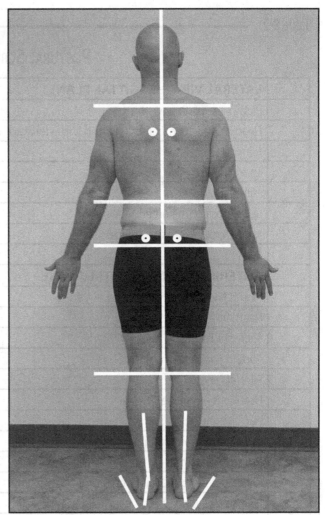

Figure 8-4. Postural observation: posterior view.

Observation by Plane

Lateral View

An ideal static erect posture can be identified through a plumb line in the lateral view, which is a line that falls through the ear lobe, the tip of the shoulder, the center of the hip and knee joints, and just anterior to the lateral malleolus. From the lateral view (see Figure 8-2), the clinician can observe the spinal curvatures including the cervical and lumbar lordosis, as well as the thoracic kyphosis. Lumbar lordosis is unique to the human spine and is necessary to facilitate upright posture and balance; however, decreased lumbar lordosis and increased thoracic kyphosis are hallmarks of an aging human spinal column.[6] Malalignments within the sagittal plane result in increased energy expenditure and induce a variety of compensatory measures, which over time can induce a number of degenerative conditions.[6]

Forward head posture can be identified as the head falling anterior to the sagittal plane plumb line. An excessive kyphosis, as observed from the lateral view can originate as postural or structural. A postural increase in the thoracic kyphosis is one that can be self-corrected, in the sense that

there have not been vertebral or structural changes associated with the spinal curve and may imply a muscular imbalance or specific postural weaknesses. Vladimir Janda was the first to recognize UCS as a specific pattern of muscle imbalance and postural abnormality in the upper quarter. In UCS, tightness of the upper trapezius and levator scapula crosses with tightness of the pectoralis major and minor. Weakness of the deep cervical flexors crosses with weakness of the middle and lower trapezius.[7] According to Janda, this pattern of imbalance creates joint dysfunction, particularly at the atlanto-occipital joint, C4-C5 segment, cervicothoracic joint, glenohumeral joint, and T4-T5 segment. The specific postural changes seen in UCS include forward head posture, increased cervical lordosis and thoracic kyphosis, elevated and protracted shoulders and rotation or abduction, and winging of the scapulae.[7]

In the older adult, hyperkyphosis is often equated with osteoporosis because vertebral fractures are assumed to be a major causative factor.[8] When screening an older patient with hyperkyphosis, particular attention should be directed toward their medical history, history of osteoporosis, and

Table 8-2

POSTURAL SCREEN CHECKLIST

	LATERAL VIEW—SAGITTAL PLANE
	Plumb line of gravity
	Head position compared to plumb line—forward head posture
	Cervical lordosis
	Thoracic kyphosis
	Lumbar lordosis
	Pelvic position/tilt anterior/posterior
	Knees hyperflexed or extended
	Sway
	ANTERIOR VIEW—FRONTAL PLANE
	Plumb line of gravity bisecting the torso
	Head tilt
	Shoulder height
	Carrying angle of the elbow
	Ribs left and right
	Umbilicus—midline
	Iliac crest height
	Greater trochanter height
	Hip-to-knee angle—Q-angle (observational)
	Knee angles—genu valgum/varum
	Patellar position
	Foot—pes cavus, pes planus
	Toe deformities
	Callous patterns of the foot (seated or supine)

(continued)

potential risk for vertebral fractures. It has recently been suggested that hyperkyphotic posture itself may be a risk factor for future fractures, independent of low bone mineral density or fracture history.[8] Older patients with hyperkyphotic postures are more likely to have self-reported difficulty in bending, walking, and/or climbing; worse measured hand grip strength; and have been found to have higher mortality rates.[9,10]

From the lateral view, the clinician can also view pelvic tilt abnormalities (anterior or posterior), genu recurvatum, or flexion contractures of the knee and sway. A patient with an excessive lumbar lordosis may present with an anterior pelvic tilt that may correlate to adaptive shortening of the hip flexor and lumbar extensor musculature and weakness of the abdominals and gluteus maximus and medius, a pattern referred to as *LCS*. This pattern of muscle imbalance

creates joint dysfunction, particularly at the L4-L5 and L5-S1 segments, sacroiliac joint, and hip joint.[11] Specific postural changes seen in LCS include anterior pelvic tilt, increased lumbar lordosis, lateral lumbar shift, lateral leg rotation, and knee hyperextension.[7] A loss of the lumbar lordosis presenting as a flattened curvature of the lower back may be present and may accompany a posteriorly tilted pelvis.

Anterior View

From the anterior view (see Figure 8-3), a frontal plane analysis can be performed by the clinician. A vertical line bisecting the torso into left and right halves can be composed through the midline of the sternum, the umbilicus, and the pubic symphysis. Key observational points from this plane include head tilt, shoulder height, ribs and umbilicus, iliac crest height, greater trochanter height, and

Table 8-2 (continued) ─────────────────────────────

POSTURAL SCREEN CHECKLIST

	POSTERIOR VIEW—FRONTAL/TRANSVERSE PLANES
	Plumb line of gravity C1 to sacrum
	Head tilt
	Shoulder height
	Scapular position symmetry
	Distance from midline
	Inferior angle (rotation or tipping)
	Medial border winging (transverse plane)
	Lateral deviation of the spine from midline
	Trunk list
	Scoliosis
	Leg-length discrepancy
	Iliac crest height—pelvic obliquity
	Posterior superior iliac spine (PSIS) levels
	Gluteal line symmetry
	Popliteal folds bilateral
	Rearfoot calcaneal angle
	Angulation of foot in standing (transverse plane)

tibial plateau height. Additional frontal plane deviations that should be noted include the carrying angle of elbow, genu valgum or genu varum of the knee, and the pronation or supination stance of the foot. The foot should be inspected for arch structure including pes cavus, and pes planus, as well as structural deformities of the toes (eg, hallux valgus, claw toes, hammer toes) and callous patterns of the foot. Identifying a postural abnormality in a patient cannot be directly correlated with pain or pathology; however, identification of a unilateral or segmental deviation such as one iliac crest being significantly more elevated, unilateral genu valgum, or unilateral hyperpronation can lead the clinician to further assessment for deformity, compensatory patterns, or pathology, which may correlate with the patient's chief complaints.

A gross observation of hip-to-knee angle and patellar positioning can be observed anteriorly. A more precise measurement of this, known as the *Q-angle*, is used as an index of the vector for the combined pull of the extensor mechanism of the knee on the patellar tendon and is used as an indicator for patellofemoral joint dysfunction, which can be correlated to anterior knee pain.

Posterior View

A posterior observation of the patient (see Figure 8-4) gives the physical therapist an alternate frontal plane analysis and can be used as a comparison to the anterior view. From a superior to inferior approach, one can observe head tilting. A close observation of the scapular position at rest should be performed. Note the bilateral position of the medial scapular border from midline, the inferior angle, and tilting away from the thorax in either the transverse or frontal plane. The posterior view allows an objective observation of lateral deviation of the spine from midline indicating scoliosis, a structural or functional discrepancy in leg length, or a trunk list. A gravity induced trunk list is a clinical sign that is frequently observed in patients with LBP and has been associated with intervertebral disk lesions.[12] A lateral list can be observed as a shifting of the lower thoracic and/or upper lumbar spine away from a painful spinal stimulus. The amount of trunk list can be observed as the horizontal displacement of T12 away from a central vertical plumb line intersecting S1. Plumb line measurement of a lateral list has been cited as the most useful instrument for measuring a static trunk list due to the advantage of simplicity and the ease of use as a suitable bedside test.[12]

Observation for inequality in leg length can be performed from this view. Inequality in leg length is commonly associated with compensatory gait abnormalities and may lead to degenerative arthritis of the lower extremity and lumbar spine.[13] Patients with leg-length discrepancy can also have angular and torsional deformities as well as soft tissue contractures of the hip or equinus deformity of the ankle[13]; therefore, identification of such a skeletal abnormality is essential for the physical therapist. Pelvic obliquity, an angulation of the pelvis in the frontal plane, can be caused by leg-length discrepancy, contractures about the hips, as a part of a structural scoliosis, or as a combination of 2 or more of these causes.[14] Careful observation and measurement of skeletal malalignments can assist the clinician with identifying an underlying cause of an observed pelvic obliquity angle. The therapist should observe and palpate bilateral iliac crest levels, note for abnormal skin folds, note PSIS levels, gluteal line bilaterally, and observe popliteal folds for symmetry. Furthermore, postural assessment and comparison of pelvic obliquity angle in a seated, rather than standing position, removes the influence of the leg length on pelvis height.

There is preliminary support of a mechanistic link between foot posture and lower extremity pain.[15] Planus foot posture, has been associated with greater risk of knee and widespread lower extremity pain, whereas a pes cavus foot posture has been associated with ankle joint pain.[15] Observation of the rear-foot (calcaneal) angle in weightbearing should be performed from the posterior view along with transverse angulation of the foot stance in relaxed standing. Excessive in-toeing or out-toeing correlates to torsional abnormalities in the hip and/or lower leg.

Cardiovascular and Pulmonary Screen

Patient position: Seated, feet supported

It is essential for all primary care providers, including physical therapists, to screen for underlying cardiovascular conditions. At a minimum, during the initial examination the patient's HR, RR, and BP should be assessed. If a patient has a history of cardiovascular disease, these values should be checked each session. These values should be assessed prior to any physical activity, preferably after sitting quietly for at least 5 minutes, in order to achieve resting values.[16]

Additional considerations:

- During the initial examination, height and weight should be assessed, which also allows for calculation of body mass index.
- Patients with a history of heart failure should monitor their weight daily using the same scale, time of day, and similar clothing as a screening tool to detect the potential onset of acute heart failure. A weight change of more than 3 pounds is considered abnormal.[17]

- Auscultation of heart sounds is indicated for patients with a history of heart failure. The presence of an S3 sound or "gallop" is abnormal and indicates exacerbation of the patient's condition. Urgent referral to the physician is warranted.[17]
- In addition to HR, RR, and BP, patients with known lung disease should have their oxygen saturation (SpO_2) assessed each session. In addition, lung sounds should be assessed during the initial examination and again if the patient presents with increased shortness of breath.
- Postoperative patients should have their temperature assessed.

Gross Functional Screen

Gait

A screening of gait should be performed on all patients, regardless of their presentation or chief complaint. Observation of the patient during gait should occur in all 3 planes: anterior, posterior, and lateral. The physical therapist screens for abnormalities in gross motor control with attention to signs of neuromusculoskeletal involvement such as scissoring, festination, or foot slap. A gross assessment of balance is noted during ambulation as well as with changes in direction. Attention should be drawn to coordination and quality of movement of both upper and lower quadrants. Note the weight distribution through bilateral lower extremities along with stride and step length and the weight shifting during stance phase on each of the lower extremities. Finally, close observation to lower extremity joints can cue the therapist to biomechanical dysfunctions. Safety measures should be applied to all patients with the appropriate amount of guarding, gait belt usage, and/or use of adaptive equipment if required. Further objective outcome measures can be applied to the appropriate population for advanced assessment. See Table 8-3[18] for some suggested tests that should be chosen based on the patient's perceived level of function.

Squatting

A standing squat screening allows the clinician to observe for abnormalities in gross motor function, overall lower extremity strength and coordination, and response to loading the joints of the lower extremity. The patient may hold onto the treatment table or the back of a chair for balance. The patient is asked to squat down, sitting back to avoid excessive stress through the knees. The physical therapist observes the quality and quantity of movement through the lower extremity and provides appropriate guarding for the patient for safety. A patient with a musculoskeletal pathology of the lower extremity may have either pain, weakness, or both with performing this task. A patient with a neuromusculoskeletal pathology may present with weakness alone. The squat can be used as a functional screen for quadriceps weakness (L2-L4 innervation). If the patient is unable to perform a standing squat safely, an alternate method for

Table 8-3
FUNCTIONAL OUTCOME MEASURES FOR GAIT AND BALANCE
• Timed Up and Go Test • 10-Meter Walk Test • 6-Minute Walk Test • Dynamic Gait Index • Berg Balance Scale • Tinetti Balance Scale
Data Source: American Physical Therapy Association. 2023. Accessed March 8, 2023. https://www.apta.org/patient-care

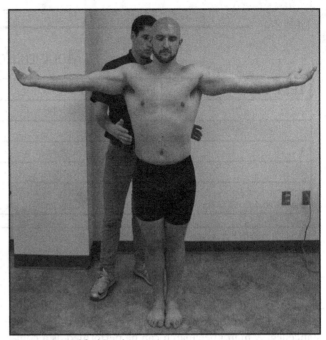

Figure 8-5. Modified Romberg test.

assessing this functional task is sit to stand from a chair. Safety should always be the first priority when performing functional assessments. The Five Times Sit to Stand Test can be used to assess increased disability and morbidity, as well as predict recurrent falls in older populations (aged 65 years and over).[19]

Balance

According to the Centers for Disease Control and Prevention, more than one-third of adults 65 years and older fall each year in the United States, and 20% to 30% of people who fall suffer moderate to severe injuries. Falls among older adults is the number one cause of injuries and death in the United States.[20] Balance disturbance can originate from multiple systems and impairments as well as from external or environmental factors. There are 5 key areas that are the most common factors in falls among the aging adult population[21]:

1. Vision/hearing
2. Balance
3. BP regulation
4. Medications/substances
5. Assaults of older adults

Balance impairment and fall risk assessment is very important for the physical therapist, specifically in the older adult population. Multiple comorbidities and polypharmacy alone are risk factors for falling in older adults. The Modified Romberg Test (Figure 8-5) can be used to differentiate impairments in the visual, proprioceptive, and vestibular systems by systematically eliminating the source of stimuli for each system including visual input, proprioceptive sense of the body in space and proprioceptive sense of the head in space.[22] Table 8-3 lists other common balance tests used in the clinical setting. See Table 8-4 for sequencing of the Romberg test.

Gross Range of Motion of Trunk and Lower Extremities

Active Range of Motion Screen

Patient position: Standing, feet slightly apart

For the purpose of a screen, use visual observation of AROM to note any gross asymmetries or abnormal movement patterns, and if found, more detailed test and measures (eg, goniometry, inclinometry) are indicated for a more objective measurement. Observe and note the quality and quantity of motion and if symptoms are altered (provoked or reduced) with motion. When performing ROM of the lumbar spine, pay particular attention to complaints of pain patterns evoked in the lower extremity with motion of the spine. Begin by assessing trunk motion in all planes including flexion, extension, lateral flexion, and lateral rotation bilaterally. Quadrant positioning (combined movement patterns) may also be performed at this time if indicated. The amount of forward bend that a patient can achieve is a combined osteokinematic pattern of true lumbar spine segmental flexion with closed kinetic chain flexion of the pelvis on the femur. Observe the lumbopelvic rhythm during flexion and extension for quality of motion from the spine on pelvis (segmental flexion) vs the pelvis on femur (hip flexion/extension and anterior and posterior pelvic tilting). Pathology in any of these structures can generate pain or a limitation of forward bending motion. A patient with pain or dysfunction originating in the lumbar spine may demonstrate limited segmental spinal flexion but excessive pelvic on hip motion, whereas a patient with pain or dysfunction of the femoral head or acetabulum may demonstrate limited pelvic on femur flexion, but excessive lumbar segmental flexion.[23]

Table 8-4

MODIFIED ROMBERG TEST

TEST CONDITION	DESCRIPTION	SENSORY INPUTS
1	Eyes open, firm surface	Visual, proprioceptive, vestibular
2	Eyes closed, firm surface	Proprioceptive, vestibular
3	Eyes open, compliant surface	Visual, vestibular
4	Eyes closed, compliant surface	Vestibular only

Adapted from Agrawal Y, Carey JP, Hoffman HJ, Sklare DA, Schubert MC. The modified Romberg balance test: normative data in US adults. *Otol Neurotol Off Publ Am Otol Soc Am Neurotol Soc Eur Acad Otol Neurotol.* 2011;32(8):1309-1311.

AROM screening of the lower extremities can be performed in a number of positions. Performed in the standing position, the patient must be able to overcome gravity of the leg being tested, while at the same time, this position challenges weight shifting, balance, and proprioception on the stance leg. A high knee march can be performed as a combined assessment of hip and knee flexion, while heel and toe raising can be performed at the ankle. In supine, the patient is asked to bring bilateral knees to chest as a gross screen of lumbar, hip, and knee mobility bilaterally.

Passive Range of Motion Including Overpressures

If active motions do not provoke the patient's symptoms, overpressure may be applied to each trunk motion in standing. It is important to note that if a patient reports reproduction of their symptoms with AROM, then proceeding to more provocative testing with overpressure may not be appropriate. Perform PROM of the lower extremities in supine and add overpressure to assess end-feels.

Lower Quarter Neurological Screen

Patient position: Seated, feet relaxed
- Dermatomes[24]: Assess sensation to light touch for levels L1-S2 nerve roots (Figures 8-6 and 8-7)
- Myotomes[24]: Assess motor function of L1-S2 nerve roots (Figure 8-8). Assess bilaterally, grade as either within normal limits (WNL) or diminished. If a deficiency is noted, more detailed tests and measures (eg, manual muscle testing, dynamometry) are indicated.
  - L1-L2 hip flexion
  - L3-L4 knee extension
  - L4-L5 ankle dorsiflexion
  - L5-S1 great toe extension
  - S1-S2 ankle plantarflexion

Heel walking and toe walking tasks are a quick myotomal screen for the L4-L5 and S1-S2 myotomes, respectively (Figure 8-9).

- Reflexes[25]: Evaluate in a seated position. Focus the patient's attention on an alternated muscle contraction (Jendrasik maneuver) by having the patient perform an isometric contraction in another muscle group, it may help prevent a patient's exaggerated or diminished response (Figure 8-10). Position the limb with slight tension on the tendon to be tapped and palpate the tendon to locate the correct point for stimulation. Hold the reflex hammer loosely between the thumb and index finger and briskly tap the tendon with moderate force.
  - Lower motor neuron: Assess DTRs (Figure 8-11)
    - L2-L4 patellar tendon
    - S1-S2 Achilles tendon
  - Scoring DTR (Table 8-5)
  - Upper motor neuron
    - Babinski sign[24] (Figure 8-12) is performed with the patient supine in long-sitting. The lateral aspect of the sole of the foot is stroked with a blunt object, such as the handle of a reflex hammer or a tongue depressor, beginning at the bottom toward the heel and crossing to the base of the great toe. The motion is firm and continuous. A normal response is flexion of the toes. An abnormal response is slight fanning of the lateral 4 toes and dorsiflexion of the great toe. A positive Babinski sign indicates brain injury or cerebral disease. Note: Babinski sign may be present in children until 4 years of age.
    - Clonus[26] test for clonus should be performed if the DTR are hyperactive/very brisk, or there is suspicion for upper motor neuron disease. Briskly apply a dorsiflexion force through the plantar aspect of the patient's foot. An abnormal response is sustained rhythmic oscillating movements of the patient's foot into dorsiflexion and plantarflexion. Clonus is associated with upper motor neuron disease.

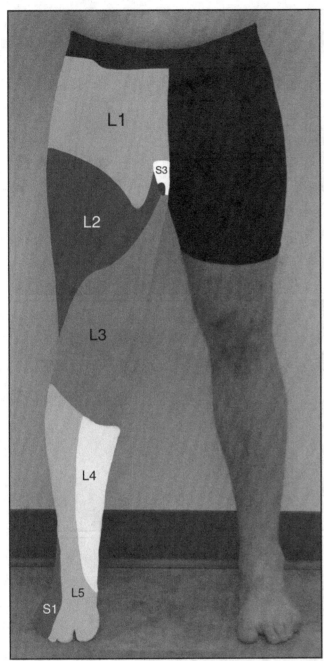

Figure 8-6. Dermatome patterns: anterior view.

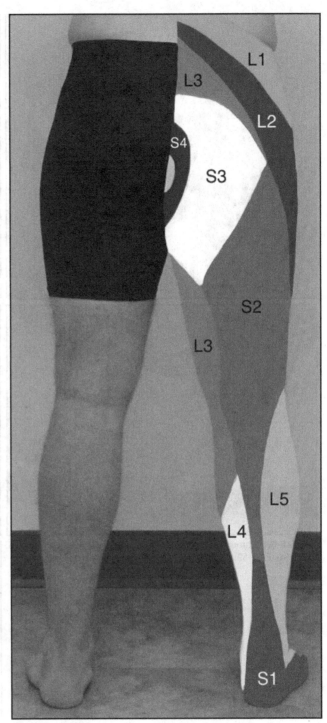

Figure 8-7. Dermatome patterns: posterior view.

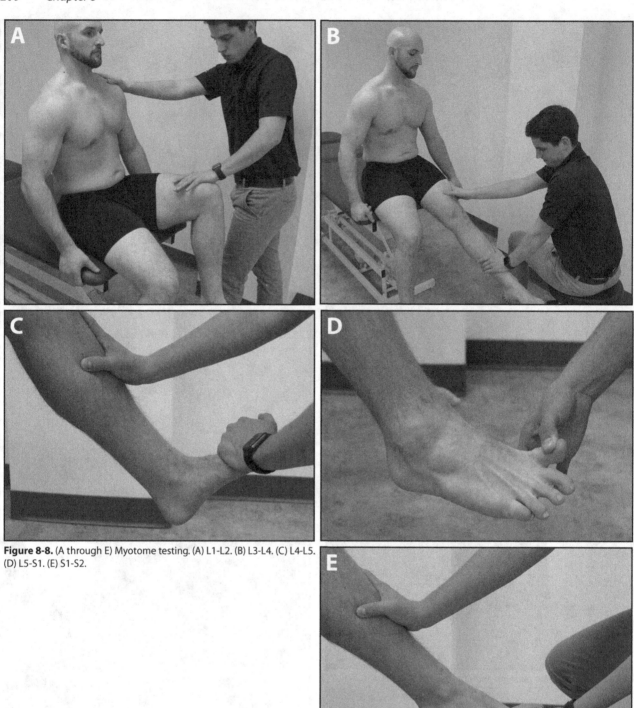

Figure 8-8. (A through E) Myotome testing. (A) L1-L2. (B) L3-L4. (C) L4-L5. (D) L5-S1. (E) S1-S2.

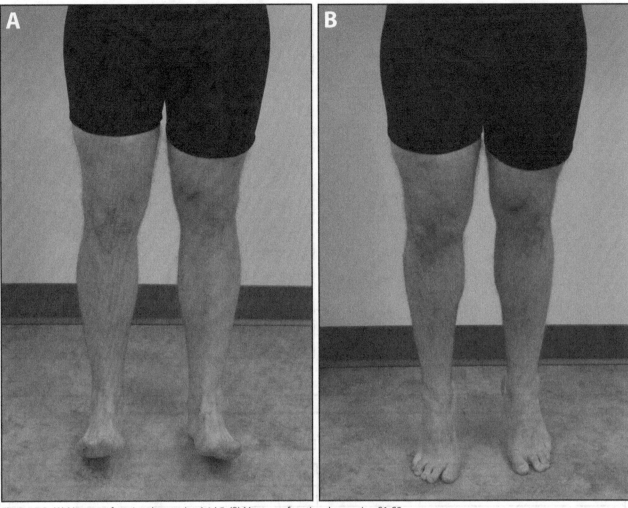

Figure 8-9. (A) Myotome functional screening L4-L5. (B) Myotome functional screening S1-S2.

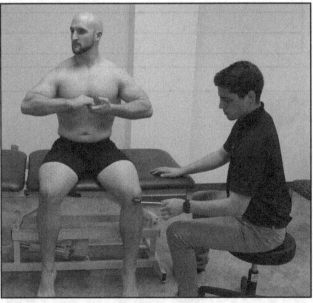

Figure 8-10. Jendrasik maneuver.

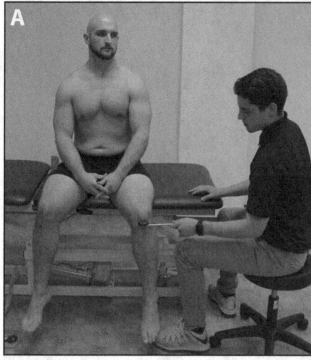
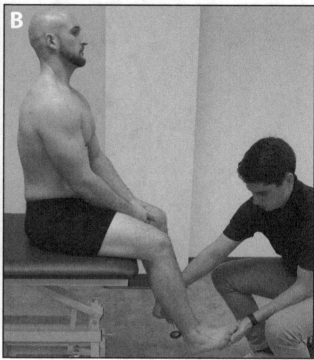

Figure 8-11. (A) DTR patellar tendon L2-L4. (B) DTR Achilles tendon S1-S2.

Table 8-5

SCORING DEEP TENDON REFLEXES

GRADE RESPONSE	DEEP TENDON REFLEX
0	No response/absent
1+	Diminished
2+	Normal
3+	Brisk/slightly hyperactive
4+	Brisk/hyperactive

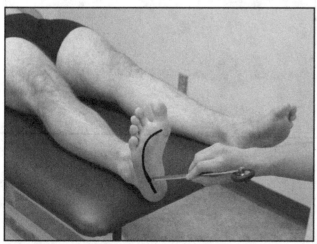

Figure 8-12. Babinski sign.

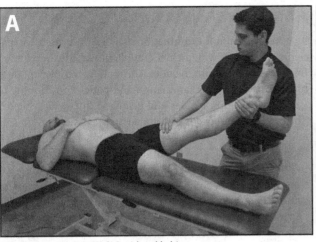 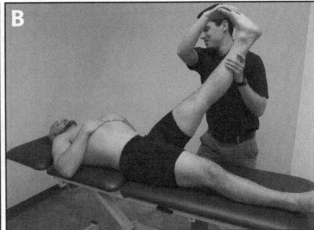

Figure 8-13. (A) SLR. (B) SLR with ankle bias.

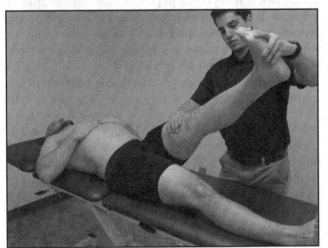

Figure 8-14. SLR with tibial nerve bias.

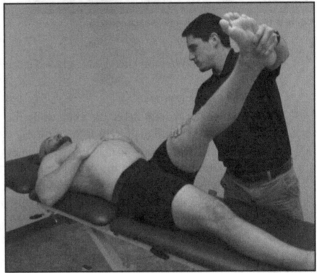

Figure 8-15. SLR with common fibular nerve bias.

- Lower limb tension testing
  - Straight leg raise (SLR; sciatic nerve L4-S2; Figure 8-13A)
    - The patient is supine with no pillow under the head.
    - The leg is placed in slight internal rotation and adduction with extension at the knee and neutral ankle.
    - Examiner passively raises the leg until complaints of pain or tightness in the posterior leg or until tissue resistance is met.
    - Ankle bias may be added to the sequence (Figure 8-13B).
  - SLR (tibial nerve bias; Figure 8-14)
    - The patient is supine with no pillow under the head.
    - The foot is placed into dorsiflexion and eversion.

- The hip is then taken into flexion, internal rotation, and adduction.
    - Examiner passively raises the leg until complaints of pain or tightness in the lower leg and/or foot or until tissue resistance is met.
  - SLR (common fibular nerve bias; Figure 8-15)
    - The patient is supine with no pillow under the head.
    - To stress the deep fibular nerve, the foot is placed into plantarflexion.
    - To stress the superficial fibular nerve, the foot is placed into dorsiflexion.
    - The hip is then taken into flexion, internal rotation, and adduction.
    - Examiner passively raises the leg until complaints of pain or tightness in the lower leg and/or foot or until tissue resistance is met.

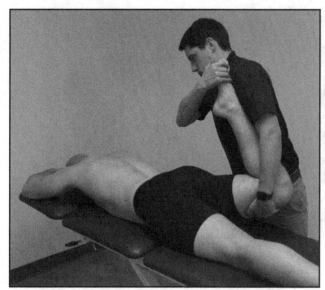

Figure 8-16. Prone knee bend with femoral nerve bias.

- ○ Prone knee bend (femoral nerve L2-L4 bias; Figure 8-16)
  - ▪ The patient is prone.
  - ▪ Examiner passively flexes the knee while the pelvis is stabilized to prevent anterior tilting.
  - ▪ Knee flexion to approximately 100 degrees may be performed, and then hip extension or foot plantarflexion bias may be added until complaints of pain or tightness occur in the femoral nerve distribution or until tissue resistance is met.

Palpation

Patient position: Variable

Various texts recommend performing palpation early in the physical examination sequence. However, from clinical experience, early palpation can cause irritation, possibly altering the results of the remaining physical examination components. Regardless, layer palpation should be performed, which means the examiner works from superficial to deeper tissues. Any change in contour (ie, lump, bump, or lesion) should be brought to the patient's attention. Follow-up questions include determining whether the physician is aware of the lump and if there has been any change to it. Palpate in a systematic fashion in the lower quarter soft tissues and bony structures. Knowledge of lower quarter lymph nodes and arteries is important, and they should be palpated. In general, during palpation ask the patient if there is any discomfort or change in symptoms. The following grading scale can be used to quantify palpation:

- Grade 1 = Tenderness
- Grade 2 = Tenderness with flinch
- Grade 3 = Severe tenderness, withdrawal
- Grade 4 = Hyperalgesia

Abdominal Screening

An abdominal examination may be indicated for patients presenting with a chief complaint of LBP. Preparation for the examination includes the patient emptying their bladder prior to the examination and patient positioning in supine with hands at sides and head and knees supported.[27] The physical therapist is positioned on the patient's right side and in a position to observe the patient's face throughout the examination.[27] The examination should be performed in a systematic manner using the following order: observation, auscultation, and palpation.[28] Observe the abdomen for symmetry, contour, scarring, color changes, or distension. During auscultation, the therapist is listening for the absence of bowel sounds or the presence of bruits over the major arteries such as the abdominal aorta, iliac arteries, and femoral arteries. It is important to perform auscultation prior to palpation in order to avoid altering bowel sounds.[27,28] Lastly, palpation of the 4 abdominal quadrants is completed, beginning with light palpation and progressing to deep, making note of pain and/or any abnormalities.[27]

An individual with an underlying aortic abdominal aneurysm (AAA) may present with a chief complaint of back pain. Absence of a visual or palpable abdominal pulse has a 100% sensitivity for ruling out an AAA of 5 cm or greater in diameter for patients with a waist circumference of less than 100 cm.[29] If a pulse is observed, auscultation should be performed to assess for the presence of a bruit. The presence of a bruit would be indicative of an AAA (95% specificity), and therefore, the patient should be referred for immediate medical attention.[30] Patients with back pain should be screened for an AAA if they are 65 years or more, have known atherosclerotic disease, or have risk factors for atherosclerotic disease such as sedentary lifestyle, obesity, diabetes, dyslipidemia, hypertension, or smoking.

Lower Quarter Referred Pain Patterns

A global review of the prevalence of LBP in the adult general population has shown a lifetime prevalence of approximately 40%.[31] LBP and lower extremity pain symptoms can originate from many potential sources including joints, intervertebral disks, muscles, nerve roots, and organs within the abdominal cavity.[32] Anatomic structures within the lumbar spine and pelvis, additionally have potential to refer pain to other regions of the body, thus challenging the differential diagnosis and the clinical decision-making process associated with the physical therapy evaluation. Intervertebral disks, facet joints, and sacroiliac joints have been observed to refer pain to the lower lumbar spine, PSIS, buttock, trochanteric region, groin, ischial tuberosity, thigh, leg, ankle, and foot.[33] Distinguishing pain due to primary extremity pathology vs lumbar pathology can be challenging. Additionally, there remains a degree of confusion in the medical community regarding the definitions of back pain, referred pain, radicular pain, and radiculopathy.[32]

While it may be useful from a prognosis standpoint to identify the pathoanatomical structure as the pain generator, it is well known that lumbar spine pathological changes observed on imaging is common in asymptomatic individuals, making pathoanatomical findings suspect and less likely to help guide treatment in symptomatic individuals.[34] As musculoskeletal experts, physical therapists can best guide examination and treatment by response to movement and/or loading, which is congruent with the emergence of treatment-based classifications that use physical therapist examination findings to establish and guide the physical therapist treatment plan.

The following section on lower quarter referred pain patterns identifies specific anatomic structures as potential pain generators, along with some common referred pain patterns of the lower extremity.

Radicular Pain

It is important to recognize that radicular pain and referred pain are not synonymous. Furthermore, radicular pain must be differentiated from radiculopathy. That is, radicular pain is limited to a single symptom (ie, pain) that stems from a dorsal root or its ganglion, whereas radiculopathy is a constellation of signs and symptoms including diminished reflexes, dermatomal numbness, myotomal weakness, and can include pain.[35,36] Radiculopathy is not defined by pain, it is defined by objective neurological signs.[35] Sensory change associated with radiculopathy will typically follow a dermatomal pattern, whereas radicular pain and referred pain do not.

Referred Pain

Intervertebral Disk

There are many structures in the lumbar spine that can serve as pain generators, and often times the etiology of lower back and lower quadrant pain is multifactorial. Referred pain results from activation of nociceptive free nerve ending (nociceptors) in somatic or visceral tissue; thus, the physiologic basis for referred pain is convergence of afferent neurons onto common neurons within the central nervous system.[35,37] In the lumbar spine, the somatic structures including muscle, ligament, synovial joints, and intervertebral disks converge on the same neurons as the afferent nerves from the lower extremity; thus, noxious stimulation of any of these spinal structures can be associated with referred pain into the lower extremity.[37] Noxious stimulation of the intervertebral disks of the lower back has been found to cause referred pain patterns to the lower back, the thighs, and into the lower extremities below the level of the knee.[37] Clinically, these findings are important for the physical therapist evaluating a patient who presents with symptoms of LBP or complains of pain radiating into the lower extremity, as not all pain radiating below the knee can be classified as nerve root or radicular.

Facet Joints (Zygapophyseal Joints)

While there are many pain generators for the lower back, the facet joint has been increasingly recognized as a contributing source. The facet joint is the articulating surfaces of the superior and inferior articular processes of adjacent vertebral segments and are classified as synovial joints. Facet joints have been shown capable of causing pain in the neck, upper and mid back, and low back with pain referred to the head or upper extremity, chest wall, and lower extremity.[38] Facet joint mediated pain involves both biomechanical and inflammatory components.[39] It has been estimated that facet joint pathology is a contributory factor in 15% to 52% of patients with chronic LBP.[39] Specific pain referral patterns have been identified associated with the lumbar facet joint, including the lower back and lower extremities; however, investigators have been unable to correlate specific patterns associated with individual spinal levels of the lumbar spine.[39,40]

Muscular (Myofascial)

As discussed in Chapter 6, common terminology to describe muscular pain includes *myofascial pain*, *myofascial trigger points (MTrP)*, or simply *trigger point*. An MTrP has been defined as a palpable discrete nodule located within a taut band of skeletal muscle that produces pain in a predictable referral pattern.[41] The clinical criteria for the diagnosis of myofascial pain has historically relied heavily on the clinical history and careful physical examination of the myofascial tissue.[42] An active MTrP is clinically associated with localized pain at the area of the taut band, and radiating pain in an identified pain pattern associated with the originating muscle's MTrP.

Although MTrP is a common physical finding, it is often an overlooked component of nonarticular musculoskeletal pain because its pathophysiology is currently not fully understood or quantified. Besides the use of palpation, there are currently no accepted criteria (eg, biomarkers, electrodiagnostic testing, imaging) for identifying or quantitatively describing MTrPs.[42] Recently, investigators indicate preliminary findings that ultrasound imaging techniques can be used to distinguish myofascial tissue containing MTrPs from normal myofascial tissue.[43-45]

Viscerogenic

Visceral sources of pain include all internal body organs located in the trunk or abdomen including respiratory, digestive, urogenital, endocrine, spleen, heart, and great vessels.[21] Viscerogenic referred pain is believed to be a result of 3 mechanisms. First, embryologic development is believed to play a role. For example, during human embryonic development the pericardium is formed in the gut, which may help explain why a myocardial infarction can refer pain to the abdomen.[21] Second, there is multisegmental innervation of viscera, resulting in overlap with somatic structures that

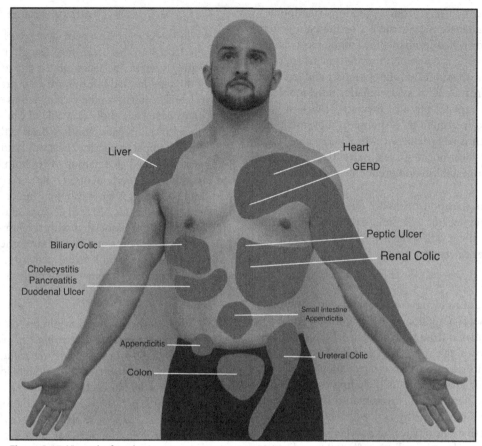

Figure 8-17. Visceral referred pain patterns: anterior view. (GERD = gastroesophageal reflux disease.)

share the same spinal afferent pathway, a concept known as *visceral-organ cross-sensitization*. Last, viscerogenic referred pain can be caused by direct pressure of an inflamed visceral structure on the respiratory diaphragm.[21]

In the early stages of visceral disease, symptoms may present as sensory, motor, and/or trophic changes in the skin, subcutaneous tissues, and/or muscle. The patient may note itching, dysesthesia, skin temperature changes, or dry skin. Additionally, pain and symptoms of a visceral source are usually accompanied by an autonomic nervous system response such as a change in vital signs, unexplained perspiration, or skin pallor and should be considered as red flags in the screening process.[21] There are some characteristics of viscerogenic pain that can occur regardless of which organ or system is involved.[21] These characteristics are identified as pain that is gradual, progressive, and cyclical in pattern, as well as poorly localized and diffuse in location.[21,46] See Figures 8-17 and 8-18[21] for referral patterns of visceral pain.

CONCLUSION

The medical screening process to determine whether the patient's pain is coming from a potentially serious or life-threatening disorder, systemic origin, or from a musculoskeletal condition is a vital component of the physical therapist's examination. The clinical decision-making process to evaluate and treat or refer the patient to another provider is rooted in a screening process that is comprehensive and systematic in nature. In addition to the systems review, a lower quarter functional screen, postural assessment, and gait assessment aid the physical therapist in collecting information to complete the differential diagnosis, prognosis, and appropriate clinical decision making for the patient.

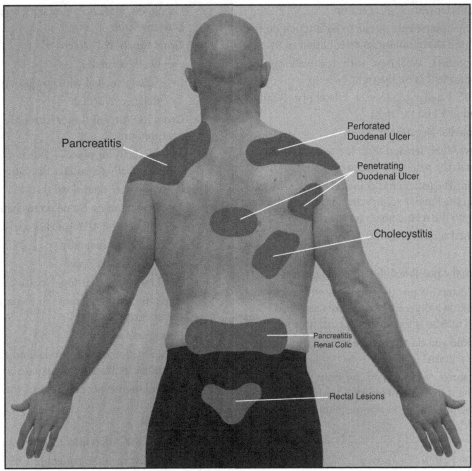

Figure 8-18. Visceral referred pain patterns: posterior view.

CASE STUDIES

Case Study One

- Patient: 41-year-old woman.
- Chief complaint: Acute LBP with radiating pain into the right lower leg of 10 days' duration
- Subjective examination
  - Review of systems: Unremarkable
  - Patient interview: The patient is an active parent of 2 and is employed full time as a teacher. Recreationally, she bikes, jogs, and coaches soccer for her kindergartener's team. History of intermittent LBP since high school. The patient is otherwise healthy and is not taking any medication. Pain is rated 5/10 on Visual Analog Scale. Pain behavior: Symptoms in the right lower leg are made worse with sitting, bending, and prolonged standing and relieved with lying supine.
- Physical examination
  - Observation: Postural assessment reveals a trunk list toward the left

- Cardiovascular and pulmonary screen: Vitals were all WNL for age
- Gross functional screen
  - Gait: The patient ambulates with guarding and limited trunk rotation and decreased arm swing. Decreased weight shifting during stance phase of the right leg.
  - Squat: The patient is able to perform a squat with appropriate amount of guarding; however, she demonstrates antalgic return from flexion.
  - Balance: The patient demonstrates appropriate balance with single leg stance on the left, but is unable to accept all weight on the right secondary to pain in the lower back.
- Gross ROM trunk/lower extremity with overpressure: The patient has decreased lumbar flexion AROM with increased radiating pain into the right lower leg in flexion pattern. Extension ROM was WNL and not painful. The patient has increased LBP and right leg pain with side flexion to the left. The patient is guarded with motions. Lower extremity ROM is limited secondary to guarding and pain, greater on the right than left.

- ○ Lower quarter neurological screen
  - Dermatomes: Paresthesia to light touch on the right in the dermatomal distribution of S1
  - Myotomes: Weakness with toe walking and plantarflexion on the right 4-/5
  - DTR: Patellar tendon 2+ bilaterally; Achilles tendon 1+ on the right
  - Babinski: Negative
  - Lower limb tension test: The test was deferred due to the patient's acute presentation
- ○ Palpation: The patient has pain and turgor with palpation to the lumbar spine extensor musculature as well as into the sciatic notch on the right
- ○ Abdominal screen: Negative
- Discussion
  - ○ What are the possible differential diagnoses?
  - ○ What clusters of positive findings will assist you with making a differential diagnosis and lead your tests and measures for further special testing?
  - ○ How would you classify/define this patients' radiating pain pattern?
  - ○ What features of this screen can assist you with determining if this patient's referred pain is mechanical (musculoskeletal) vs nonmechanical (systemic) in nature?

Case Study Two

- Patient: 67-year-old man
- Chief complaint: 4-month history of lower back pain
- Subjective examination
  - ○ Review of systems: History of smoking, hypercholesterolemia, and coronary heart disease. Medications include Lipitor (atorvastatin) and low-dose aspirin.
  - ○ Patient interview: The patient was referred to physical therapy from his primary care physician for an insidious onset of LBP. Radiographs in the physician's office reveal mild degenerative changes. The patient notes the LBP to be continuous, described as an ache that is vague in the lower back with pain occasionally into the left groin. The patient is unable to identify positions or activities that make the pain better or worse. He has been having a difficult time sleeping at night and is unable to find a comfortable position. He has no history of LBP. Social history: The patient is retired and lives in a single story home with his wife. The patient is relatively inactive with the exception of household chores.
- Physical examination
  - ○ Observation: Flattened lumbar lordosis with excessive kyphosis noted from the lateral view

- ○ Cardiovascular and pulmonary screen: Unremarkable
- ○ Gross functional screen
  - Gait: Normal
  - Squat: Normal with good control
  - Balance: Normal
- ○ Gross ROM trunk/lower extremity with overpressure
  - WNL in all planes—Did not provoke or mechanically reproduce the patient's symptoms
- ○ Lower quarter neurological screen
  - Dermatomes: No detected changes in sensation
  - Myotomes: All segments tested 5/5
  - DTR: 2+ bilaterally
  - Babinski: Negative
  - Lower limb tension: Negative
- ○ Palpation: No tenderness to palpation, normal tissue integrity
- ○ Abdominal screen
  - Palpation over the midabdomen aorta reveals a pulse with a laterally expansive pulsation
  - Follow-up auscultation of the pulse reveals a bruit
- Discussion
  - ○ What is the differential diagnosis in this case?
  - ○ What factors in the patient history and physical examination lead the clinician to the above differential diagnosis?
  - ○ What is the plan of action for this patient (clinical decision-making process)? Why?

References

1. American Physical Therapy Association. *Guide to Physical Therapist Practice*. Accessed November 23, 2021. http://guidetoptpractice.apta.org/

2. Jensen JD, Elewski BE. The ABCDEF rule: combining the "ABCDE rule" and the "ugly duckling sign" in an effort to improve patient self-screening examinations. *J Clin Aesthetic Dermatol.* 2015;8(2):15.

3. Boissonnault WG. *Primary Care for the Physical Therapist: Examination and Triage.* 2nd ed. Elsevier/Saunders; 2011.

4. Riegger-Krugh C, Keysor JJ. Skeletal malalignments of the lower quarter: correlated and compensatory motions and postures. *J Orthop Sports Phys Ther.* 1996;23(2):164-170. doi:10.2519/jospt.1996.23.2.164

5. Gross MT. Lower quarter screening for skeletal malalignment—suggestions for orthotics and shoewear. *J Orthop Sports Phys Ther.* 1995;21(6):389-405. doi:10.2519/jospt.1995.21.6.389

6. Sparrey CJ, Bailey JF, Safaee M, et al. Etiology of lumbar lordosis and its pathophysiology: a review of the evolution of lumbar lordosis, and the mechanics and biology of lumbar degeneration. *Neurosurg Focus.* 2014;36(5):E1. doi:10.3171/2014.1.FOCUS13551

7. Page P, Frank C, Lardner R. *Assessment and Treatment of Muscle Imbalance: The Janda Approach.* Human Kinetics; 2009.

8. Huang M-H, Barrett-Connor E, Greendale GA, Kado DM. Hyperkyphotic posture and risk of future osteoporotic fractures: the Rancho Bernardo study. *J Bone Miner Res.* 2006;21(3):419-423. doi:10.1359/JBMR.051201

9. Kado DM, Huang M-H, Karlamangla AS, Barrett-Connor E, Greendale GA. Hyperkyphotic posture predicts mortality in older community-dwelling men and women: a prospective study. *J Am Geriatr Soc.* 2004;52(10):1662-1667. doi:10.1111/j.1532-5415.2004.52458.x

10. Kado DM, Huang M-H, Barrett-Connor E, Greendale GA. Hyperkyphotic posture and poor physical functional ability in older community-dwelling men and women: The Rancho Bernardo study. *J Gerontol Ser A.* 2005;60(5):633-637. doi:10.1093/gerona/60.5.633

11. Lower Crossed Syndrome. Accessed January 31, 2017. http://www.jandaapproach.com/

12. McLean IP, Gillan MGC, Ross JC, Aspden RM, Porter RW. A comparison of methods for measuring trunk list. A simple plumbline is the best. *Spine.* 1996;21(14):1667-1670. doi:10.1097/00007632-199607150-00011

13. Sabharwal S, Kumar A. Methods for assessing leg length discrepancy. *Clin Orthop.* 2008;466(12):2910-2922. doi:10.1007/s11999-008-0524-9

14. Winter RB, Pinto WC. Pelvic obliquity. Its causes and its treatment. *Spine.* 1986;11(3):225-234.

15. Riskowski JL, Dufour AB, Hagedorn TJ, Hillstrom HJ, Casey VA, Hannan MT. Associations of foot posture and function to lower extremity pain: results from a population-based foot study. *Arthritis Care Res.* 2013;65(11):1804-1812. doi:10.1002/acr.22049

16. American College of Sports Medicine. *ACSM's Guidelines for Exercise Testing and Prescription.* 9th ed. Lippincot Williams & Wilkins; 2013.

17. Hillegass E. *Essentials of Cardiopulmonary Physical Therapy.* 4th ed. Saunders; 2016.

18. Functional Limitation Reporting: Tests and Measures for High-Volume Conditions - PTNow. Accessed February 2, 2017. http://www.ptnow.org/FunctionalLimitationReporting/TestsMeasures/

19. Buatois S, Miljkovic D, Manckoundia P, et al. Five Times Sit to Stand Test is a predictor of recurrent falls in healthy community-living subjects aged 65 and older. *J Am Geriatr Soc.* 2008;56(8):1575-1577. doi:10.1111/j.1532-5415.2008.01777.x

20. Centers for Disease Control and Prevention. Falls are leading cause of injury and death in older Americans: healthcare providers play an important role in falls and prevention. Published January 1, 2016. Accessed November 23, 2021. http://www.cdc.gov/media/releases/2016/p0922-older-adult-falls.html

21. Goodman CC, Kelly Snyder TE. *Differential Diagnosis for Physical Therapists: Screening for Referral.* 5th ed. Saunders; 2012.

22. Agrawal Y, Carey JP, Hoffman HJ, Sklare DA, Schubert MC. The modified Romberg balance test: normative data in US adults. *Otol Neurotol Off Publ Am Otol Soc Am Neurotol Soc Eur Acad Otol Neurotol.* 2011;32(8):1309-1311. doi:10.1097/MAO.0b013e31822e5bee

23. Neumann DA. *Kinesiology of the Musculoskeletal System: Foundations for Rehabilitation.* 2nd ed. Mosby; 2009.

24. Moore KL, Dalley AF II, Agur AMR. *Clinically Oriented Anatomy.* 7th ed. Lippincott Williams & Wilkins; 2014.

25. Jarvis C. *Physical Examination and Health Assessment.* 7th ed. Saunders; 2015.

26. Seidel HM, Stewart RW, Ball JW, Dains JE, Flynn JA, Solomon BS. *Mosby's Guide to Physical Examination.* 7th ed. Mosby; 2010.

27. Jarvis C. *Physical Examination & Health Assessment.* 7th ed. Elsevier; 2016.

28. Goodman CC, Snyder TEK. *Differential Diagnosis for Physical Therapists: Screening for Referral.* 5th ed. Elsevier; 2013.

29. Fink HA, Lederle FA, Roth CS, Bowles CA, Nelson DB, Haas MA. The accuracy of physical examination to detect abdominal aortic aneurysm. *Arch Intern Med.* 2000;160(6):833-836.

30. Lederle FA, Walker JM, Reinke DB. Selective screening for abdominal aortic aneurysms with physical examination and ultrasound. *Arch Intern Med.* 1988;148(8):1753-1756.

31. Manchikanti L, Singh V, Falco FJE, Benyamin RM, Hirsch JA. Epidemiology of low back pain in adults. *Neuromodulation.* 2014;17(suppl 2):3-10. doi:10.1111/ner.12018

32. Allegri M, Montella S, Salici F, et al. Mechanisms of low back pain: a guide for diagnosis and therapy. *F1000Res.* 2016;5. doi:10.12688/f1000research.8105.2

33. Laplante BL, Ketchum JM, Saullo TR, DePalma MJ. Multivariable analysis of the relationship between pain referral patterns and the source of chronic low back pain. *Pain Physician.* 2012;15:171-178.

34. Brinjikji W, Luetmer PH, Comstock B, et al. Systematic literature review of imaging features of spinal degeneration in asymptomatic populations. *AJNR Am J Neuroradiol.* 2015;36(4):811-816. doi:10.3174/ajnr.A4173

35. Bogduk N. On the definitions and physiology of back pain, referred pain, and radicular pain. *Pain.* 2009;147(1):17-19.

36. Murphy DR, Hurwitz EL, Gerrard JK, Clary R. Pain patterns and descriptions in patients with radicular pain: does the pain necessarily follow a specific dermatome? *Chiropr Osteopat.* 2009;17:9. doi:10.1186/1746-1340-17-9

37. O'Neil CW, Kurgansky ME, Derby R, Ryan DP. Disc stimulation and patterns of referred pain. *Spine.* 2002;27(24):2776-2781.

38. Manchikanti L, Boswell MV, Singh V, Pampati V, Damron KS, Beyer CD. Prevalence of facet joint pain in chronic spinal pain of cervical, thoracic, and lumbar regions. *BMC Musculoskelet Disord.* 2004;5:15. doi:10.1186/1471-2474-5-15

39. Binder DS, Nampiaparampil DE. The provocative lumbar facet joint. *Curr Rev Musculoskelet Med.* 2009;2(1):15-24. doi:10.1007/s12178-008-9039-y

40. Datta S, Lee M, Falco FJE, Bryce DA, Hayek SM. Systematic assessment of diagnostic accuracy and therapeutic utility of lumbar facet joint interventions. *Pain Physician.* 2009;12(2):437-460.

41. Simons DG, Travell JG, Simons LS. *Myofascial Pain and Dysfunction: The Trigger Point Manual. Vol. 1 - Upper Half of Body.* 2nd ed. Lippincott William & Wilkins; 1998.

42. Shah JP, Thaker N, Heimur J, Aredo JV, Sikdar S, Gerber LH. Myofascial trigger points then and now: a historical and scientific perspective. *PM R.* 2015;7(7):746-761. doi:10.1016/j.pmrj.2015.01.024

43. Sikdar S, Shah JP, Gebreab T, et al. Novel applications of ultrasound technology to visualize and characterize myofascial trigger points and surrounding soft tissue. *Arch Phys Med Rehabil.* 2009;90(11):1829-1838. doi:10.1016/j.apmr.2009.04.015

44. Sikdar S, Ortiz R, Gebreab T, Gerber LH, Shah JP. Understanding the vascular environment of myofascial trigger points using ultrasonic imaging and computational modeling. *Annu Int Conf IEEE Eng Med Biol Soc.* 2010;2010:5302-5305. doi:10.1109/IEMBS.2010.5626326

45. Turo D, Otto P, Shah JP, et al. Ultrasonic tissue characterization of the upper trapezius muscle in patients with myofascial pain syndrome. *Annu Int Conf IEEE Eng Med Biol Soc.* 2012;2012:4386-4389. doi:10.1109/EMBC.2012.6346938

46. Gebhart GF, Bielefeldt K. Physiology of visceral pain. *Compr Physiol.* 2016;6(4):1609-1633. doi:10.1002/cphy.c150049

Dysfunction, Evaluation, Diagnosis, and Treatment of the Hip Complex
Nonsurgical and Surgical

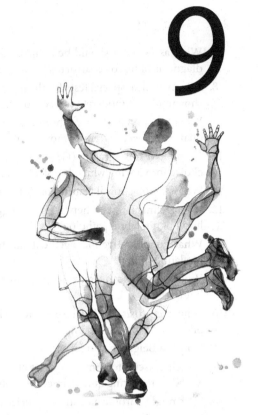

Janette Powell, PT, MHSC, OCS, SCS; Tyler Kent, MD; and Chad Hanson, MD

CHAPTER QUESTIONS

1. Why is the hip musculature a frequent source of pain and dysfunction?
2. How is acetabular labral injury thought to accelerate degenerative change and thereby be implicated in osteoarthritis?
3. Where is pain typically perceived when it is originating from the hip joint?
4. Which hip structures are associated with mechanical symptoms such as locking, clicking, and giving way?
5. Which functional activity is most typically altered with the presentation of hip pain?
6. What is the clinical prediction rule for hip osteoarthritis?

Wallmann HW, Donatelli R, eds. *Foundations of Orthopedic Physical Therapy* (pp 211-239).
© 2024 Taylor & Francis Group.

7. What assessment should be completed to confirm the diagnosis of hip osteoarthritis?

8. Which clinical special tests for the hip region have been shown to have moderate utility scores?

9. What functional tests have been described to assess the quality of lower extremity movement?

10. Computed tomography (CT) is the imaging study of choice for viewing which hip structures?

11. What are the clinical features of FAI syndrome?

12. Which clinical tests, when negative, suggest a low likelihood of hip labral pathology?

13. What nonoperative management can be utilized for a hip labral injury?

14. What surgical strategies are available for hip labral injuries?

15. A hemarthrosis has been associated with which complication following hip injuries?

16. How is a Beighton score interpreted?

17. Which musculotendinous injuries at the hip are seen in activities requiring quick direction changes?

18. Why might chronic hamstring injuries occur?

19. What are the risk factors for the development of myositis ossificans?

20. What are the physical therapy treatment goals for extracapsular hip injuries?

INTRODUCTION

The hip complex is an important region in the human body. It is the critical link between the lower extremity and the trunk, the pivot on which the body moves.[2] This superbly organized array of tissues both absorbs and transmits enormous forces repeatedly, while also allowing a large arc of motion. It bears the body's weight and the force of the strong musculature of the pelvis and thigh. It is also one of the most flexible joints of the body. It enables walking, running, jumping, and squatting. As such, the hip complex presents as a fascinating dichotomy of stability and mobility.[3]

The hip complex has a number of features that facilitate its stability functions: articular surfaces that are nearly congruent during weightbearing; a deep concave joint surface reinforced and deepened by the labrum that forms a bony ring around the femoral head; bony trabeculae reinforce the femur and pelvis in the direction of weightbearing; and a large muscle mass acting through well-placed, bony lever arms. The features of the hip complex that enhance mobility include the large articular surface area, a lack of barriers to motion from adjacent structures, and extensive capsular redundancy.

Hip region pain is a common cause of activity and self-care limitations. Additionally, hip pain frequently affects gait. Numerous factors can contribute to hip dysfunction, pain, and injury. The hip relies on precise bony alignment and is dramatically influenced by alterations in muscle tension and ligamentous support. The hip joint transmits large forces repetitively throughout life, and therefore, it is subjected to enormous wear and tear over time, which is typically related to a person's occupational demands and recreational pursuits.[3] The likelihood of an individual sustaining an injury to the hip joint can be increased by the demands of the sport, acrobatics, or employment that require repetitive hip flexion, adduction, and rotation and by occupational demands such as heavy lifting and stair climbing.[4-8] Normal functioning of the hip region is based upon the complex interplay of the tissues in the lower quarter. Because of its pivotal location, the tissues of the hip joint complex are susceptible to strain due to a variety of extrinsic causes.[3]

Hip disorders have long been recognized in the pediatric population (Perthes disease, slipped capital femoral epiphysis) and in older people (osteoarthritis).[3,9] With imaging and surgical advances, it has been noted that the incidence of hip labral and acetabular rim pathology is high, and that anatomical variants such as FAI syndrome or developmental dysplasia of the hip are a common underlying cause of hip and/or groin pain. In addition, subtle malalignments of the lower extremity, such as leg-length asymmetries or torsional deformities, can adversely affect the hip.[7,9-13] Contact injuries such as hip pointers, hematoma, traumatic dislocations, and fractures are noted in both contact sports and in speed-related activities. Stress fractures and repetitive strain injuries such as bursitis and tendonitis are noted with variable incidence in endurance sports and military activities. Reduced bone mass (osteopenia) in the femoral neck area is common and can predispose to fractures.[3,14]

The hip complex is a transition zone and is influenced by the regions above and below: the lumbar spine, knee and lower leg, and ankle and foot. This chapter reviews the hip complex in isolation, but keep in mind its important functional role within the kinetic chain of the lower extremity. It is rare for a joint to truly function in isolation without influence from surrounding regions.

ANATOMY AND BIOMECHANICS

The anatomic and biomechanical principles provided in this chapter are meant to provide an overview and are in no way exhaustive. We recommend that the student unfamiliar with basic anatomy refer to a text dedicated to such. Our intent is that this material will provide a background to allow discussion of clinically relevant evaluation and treatment of the hip.

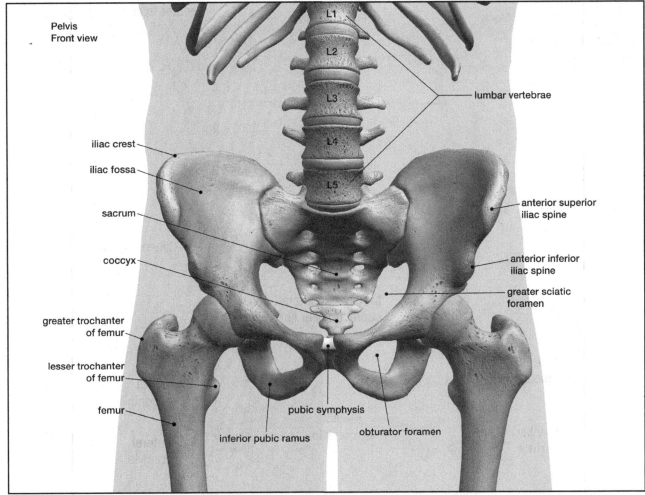

Figure 9-1. Components of the pelvic bone. (Hank Grebe/Shutterstock.com)

OSTEOLOGY

What is known as the *hip* in colloquial terms is actually made of up the pelvis and proximal femur. It is referred to as a *ball and socket joint* due to the intimate interdigitation of the 2 bones.[15] The arrangement of this joint allows for tremendous freedom of movement, but also makes it prone to injury. The osseous relationship of the pelvis and femur, along with other nearby bony landmarks and structures must be understood to fully appreciate the function of the hip.

The pelvic component of the hip joint is called the *acetabulum* and is composed of 3 bones: the ilium, ischium, and pubis (Figure 9-1). These bones fuse in adolescence and the hemipelvis is one continuous bone in adults. Each hemipelvis is joined anteriorly at the pubic symphysis and posteriorly with the sacrum. The sacroiliac joints unite the lower extremities with the axial skeleton. The pelvis serves as the origin for many of the soft tissues that cross the hip joint and provide motion and stability. It is important to keep in mind the close relationship between the hip joint and the pelvic and abdominal viscera when considering hip pathology.

The proximal femur has several distinct regions to consider in regard to the hip joint: the head, neck, intertrochanteric area, and diaphysis (Figure 9-2). The femoral head is entirely covered with articular cartilage and serves as the pivot of the lower extremity. Its blood supply is tenuous in adults, which makes it prone to poor healing in pathologic states.[16] The femoral neck connects the head to the shaft and provides a mechanical advantage for motion. Part of the neck lies inside the hip joint capsule, while part is extracapsular. This becomes important when considering fractures and pathology of the femoral neck. The intertrochanteric region is composed of the greater and lesser trochanter and serves as the insertion site for many of the muscles that provide motion to the hip. The greater trochanter is the palpable, most lateral portion of the hip. The diaphysis, or shaft, of the femur provides stability for the lower extremity, an anchor for the soft tissues that control motion about the hip and knee, and serves as a reservoir for bone marrow.[15]

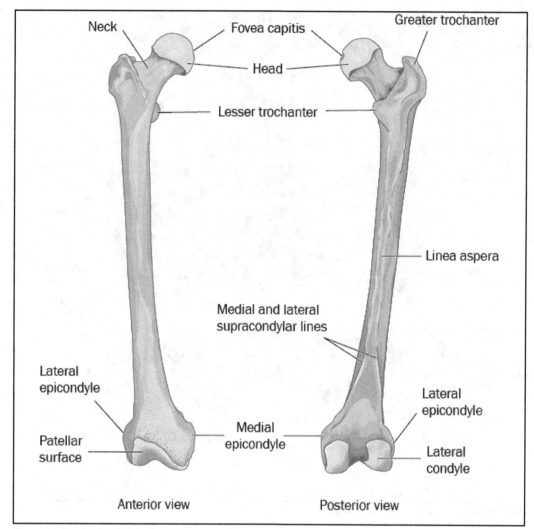

Figure 9-2. Proximal end of the femur. Anterior and posterior view. (Blamb/Shutterstock.com)

MYOLOGY

When studying the muscles of the hip, it is often most pragmatic to consider them in distinct groups based on the movement they produce (Table 9-1). Studying the origin and insertion of individual muscles helps reveal the action of that particular muscle and can be of great value to the student in visualizing movement in its simplest form. However, it is also important to remember that although individual muscles typically produce only one primary motion, muscle groups often work in concert to synthesize the vast arcade of motion capable at the hip. Furthermore, due to the high demand placed on these muscles, they are a frequent source of pain and dysfunction.

NEUROVASCULAR ANATOMY

The nerves of the hip and lower extremity originate from the lumbosacral plexus (Figure 9-3). Nerves exiting posteriorly to innervate the abductors, extensors, and external rotators include the superior and inferior gluteal nerves (named for their relation to the piriformis), as well as the named nerves to the individual external rotators. These exit the pelvis through the greater sciatic foramen, which is formed by the ilium and sacrospinous ligament. The sciatic nerve also follows this trajectory, and although not responsible for motion or sensation at the hip, it is important to consider due to its intimate association with the hip and the possibility for pathology that can be confused as hip pain. Nerves exiting

Table 9-1

MUSCULATURE ABOUT THE HIP COMPLEX

FLEXORS	EXTENDERS	ABDUCTORS	ADDUCTORS	EXTERNAL ROTATORS	INTERNAL ROTATORS**
• Psoas • Iliac • Sartorius • Pectineus	• Gluteus maximus • Gluteus medius	• Gluteus maximus (anterior fibers) • Gluteus medius • Gluteus minimus • Tensor fascia lata • Iliotibial band*	• Adductor magnus • Adductor longus • Adductor brevis • Gracilis	• Piriformis • Superior and inferior gemelli • Obturator internus • Obturator externus • Quadratus femoris	• Gluteus medius • Gluteus minimus • Tensor fascia lata • Pectineus • Adductor magnus (posterior head), longus, and brevis • Iliopsoas

* The tensor fascia lata and gluteus maximus insert onto the iliotibial band. While the iliotibial band is not a muscle, it plays an important role in abduction, extension, and stabilization during stance and gait.

** While there are no true internal rotators of the hip, several muscles have secondary function that allow them to aid in internal rotation.[17]

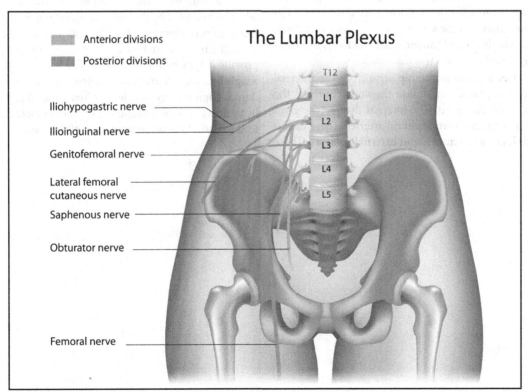

The Lumbar Plexus

Anterior divisions
Posterior divisions

T12
L1
L2
L3
L4
L5

Iliohypogastric nerve
Ilioinguinal nerve
Genitofemoral nerve
Lateral femoral cutaneous nerve
Saphenous nerve
Obturator nerve
Femoral nerve

Figure 9-3. Branches of the lumbosacral plexus. (Alila Medical Media/Shutterstock.com)

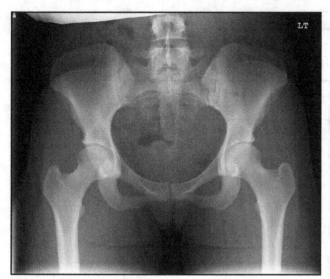

Figure 9-4. Normal pelvis radiograph.

anteriorly to innervate the flexors and adductors include the femoral and obturator. The femoral nerve passes inferior to the inguinal ligament and superior to the superior pubic ramus to enter the femoral triangle (an anatomic area defined by the knee extensors and hip adductors) and innervates the iliacus and secondary hip flexors. The primary hip flexor, or psoas major, is innervated directly from spinal nerve roots. The obturator nerve passes through the obturator foramen to innervate the adductors. These nerves also innervate the hip joint and capsule to allow for proprioception and nociception. Various cutaneous (or sensory) nerves also arise from the lumbosacral plexus and similarly exit anteriorly or posteriorly to arrive at their respective dermatomes.

The arteries integral to the hip arise from the internal and external iliac arteries and follow the same course as the nerves previously discussed. The internal iliac artery gives rise to the superior and inferior gluteal arteries. These vascularize the abductors, extensors, and external rotators. These

branches also contribute to the vascularization of the joint and capsule via an arterial plexus that forms from contributions from the major arteries of the hip. As the external iliac artery passes under the inguinal ligament, it becomes known as the *femoral artery*. Its first branch is the profunda femoris artery, which gives off the medial and lateral circumflex arteries. These are important in supplying blood to the femoral head and neck and are often implicated in cases of avascular necrosis (AVN) of the head. The profunda femoris also gives off the perforating arteries, which ascend to join the anastomosis, that supplies the hip joint. The obturator artery branches off the internal iliac artery and descends through the obturator foramen to supply the muscles of the medial compartment. It also gives off branches, which join the anastomosis to supply the femoral head. The veins and lymphatics follow the course of the arteries and nerves. There are deep and superficial veins, with the deep veins usually having the same name as the artery to which they are adjacent. The superficial veins return blood from the lower extremity and have an independent nomenclature (eg, sural, saphenous).

ARTICULAR ANATOMY

The acetabulum is the major weightbearing portion of the hip. Although it is shaped like a cup, only a portion of the surface actually bears weight. This portion is lunate, or horseshoe shaped, and runs anterior to posterior and superior to inferior.[15] There is an acetabular notch inferiorly, which is bounded by the transverse acetabular ligament. This ligament provides stability and continuity to the hip (Figure 9-4). The bone is thickest in the posterosuperior position to provide a buttressing reinforcement.[18] The majority of the weightbearing occurs in the anterosuperior portion of the dome. High energy accidents often cause damage to these bony areas. Trauma, dysplasia, or altered biomechanics can lead to pathology or degeneration of the joint.

The articulating joint surface is covered with hyaline cartilage, with the femoral head being completely covered. The thickest portion of acetabular cartilage is in the antero-superior portion where the highest loads are seen. The purpose of articular cartilage is to absorb shock and dissipate force. It essentially acts as a load sharing sponge to minimize force over any single area. Synovial fluid bathes the cells of the articular surface to help lubricate the joint, prevent friction, and provide nutrition. Blood supply is limited, so nutrition by diffusion, provided via the synovial fluid, is essential.

The ligamentum teres is a pyramidal-shaped structure that originates from the acetabular fossa inserting into the femoral head and is surrounded by a synovial lining that is intimately attached to the posterior branch of the obturator artery and a sensory nerve supply.[19] Ligamentum teres appears to have a role in stabilization, supplementing the work of the capsular ligaments in addition to functioning as a sling around the femoral head.[20] This ligament and its associated structures may also serve a proprioceptive role and be a source of intra-articular hip pain.[20,21] It has been postulated that ligamentum teres functions to distribute synovial fluid within the hip joint via a "windshield wiper" effect.[20,22]

The acetabular labrum is a fibrocartilaginous structure that circumferentially attaches to the outermost edge of the acetabulum. It is wedge shaped, with the base at the attachment and the apex toward the femur. There are 3 histologic zones in the labrum, with fibers being oriented based on the relative strain placed upon them.[23,24] The labrum has no intrinsic vascularity, but rather receives contributions from the anastomosis that feeds the capsule and synovium. Furthermore, only the outermost (or capsular) portion of the labrum has any substantial blood supply, but even this is tenuous.[11,24] This has implications for healing that will be discussed later. The labrum has been shown to contain various types of nerves and nervous organs.[24-26] This implies that the labrum takes part in nociception and proprioception. The labrum increases the acetabular surface area and deepens the volume by approximately 25% and 30%, respectively.[27,28] The labrum creates a seal around the femoral head inside the acetabulum. This seal creates a suction effect, a negative intra-articular hydrostatic pressure that prevents distraction/dislocation of the femoral head. A recent biomechanical study demonstrated that 43% less force was required to distract the femoral head by 3 mm after the labral seal was vented, and that 60% less force was required after a labral tear.[29] The labrum also helps contain joint fluid and acts as a seal to prevent the escape of synovial fluid. This allows pressurization of the joint fluid, which helps distribute joint forces and protect cartilage. This pressurization also keeps the cartilage from deforming under pressure, which allows for the preservation of the spherical shape of the head and further dissipates force.[30] When the labrum is injured, the suction seal is broken and synovial fluid escapes. This prevents all its protective functions and also causes altered joint geometry. These changes allow for uneven wear and tear on the joint surface, which accelerates degenerative changes and has been implicated in osteoarthritis.[30] Thus, any injury to the labrum can have drastic consequences. The distal portion of the labrum becomes continuous with the transverse acetabular ligament and the joint capsule, which provides further stability to the joint.

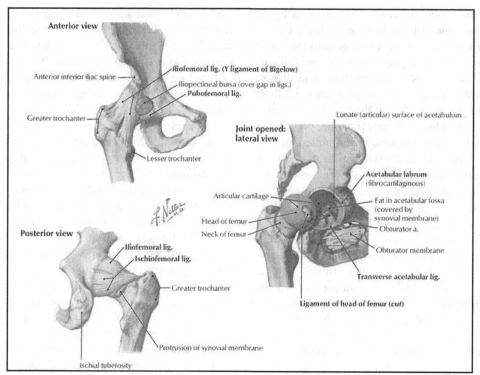

Figure 9-5. Hip joint and its ligaments.[31] (Reproduced with permission from Hansen JT. *Netter's Clinical Anatomy.* 2nd ed. Saunders; 2010.)

The hip joint capsule is a thick fibrous structure that provides stability to the hip and helps prevent dislocation (Figure 9-5).[31] There is a superficial and a deep layer to the capsule. The deep layer contains circumferential fibers and is lined by the synovium, which, as mentioned, produces the synovial fluid.[15] This layer also contains the pubofemoral ligament, which is important in limiting extremes of flexion and extension.[32] The superficial layer is primarily composed of the ischiofemoral and iliofemoral ligaments. The ischiofemoral ligament restricts internal rotation and adduction when the hip is flexed.[32] The iliofemoral ligament, or Y ligament of Bigelow, is the strongest of the 3 and 1 of the strongest ligaments in the body and acts to restrict hip extension.[32] These ligaments and the capsule are pivotal in providing strength and support to the hip, as well as a favorable cellular and mechanical environment for the joint surface.

SURFACE ANATOMY

Despite technological advances, physical examination is still the greatest tool available for deciphering patients' complaints. Therefore, an understanding of how internal anatomy can be visualized by external inspection is indispensable.

There are several bony and soft tissue prominences that provide great detail to the overall examination. The greater trochanter is the lateral-most prominence seen on the leg. The anterior superior iliac spine (ASIS) is the most anterosuperior bony prominence that is readily visible and palpable, even in patients who are obese. The pubic tubercle is only several centimeters from the midline and is just superior to the external genitalia. The inguinal ligament is oriented roughly 45 degrees medioinferiorly from the ASIS and attaches to the pubic tubercle. The femoral artery is approximately halfway between the ASIS and the pubic tubercle and inferior to the inguinal ligament. The posterior superior iliac spine often forms dimples on the back at the level of the iliac crests. The sacroiliac joints can be palpated medial and inferiorly to the posterior superior iliac spine. Keeping these relationships in mind can provide invaluable information to the practitioner.

Another important concept to keep in mind is that patients will often complain of hip pain, and this can refer to anywhere in the gluteal, pelvic, or trochanteric regions. It is essential to differentiate specifically where the pain is located as it can tell you much regarding the nature of their pain. For example, anterior pain located in the groin is often associated with the hip joint, whereas posterior pain is often associated with sacroiliac or lumbosacral pain. These are very different entities that may both be described as hip pain.

The final consideration in regard to surface anatomy is the modesty of the patient; it is essential to protect at all times. Physical evaluations often necessitate that a patient be in a state of undress. This can be intimidating, awkward, or embarrassing to the patient. Be aware of things like patient positioning, positioning of practitioners or students, proper gowning, hand placement during palpation and examination maneuvers, language (eg, "elevate" or "relax" instead of "spread" or "open" when referring to the leg), and overall conduct to provide a comfortable environment for the patient and to protect oneself from litigious claims. It is often prudent to have a chaperone present during this examination.

Biomechanics

An understanding of hip biomechanics allows for appreciation of healthy hip function as well as clinical assessment of hip pathology. Due to the congruency of the hip joint, all motion is rotational. The rotational motion of the hip can be described as occurring in 3 planes: coronal, sagittal, and axial. This allows for 6 basic movements about the hip: abduction/adduction, flexion/extension, and internal/external rotation. The limits of motion are defined by the bony confines that occur at the extremes of motion. While individuals may vary slightly, averages are as follows: abduction 45 degrees, adduction 25 degrees, flexion 120 degrees, extension 10 degrees, internal rotation 15 degrees, and external rotation 35 degrees.[33] Combinations of these movements allow for the wide variety of functions for which the hip and lower extremity are capable.

The center of rotation (COR) for the hip occurs at roughly the center of the femoral head. The greater the distance from the COR, the less force is required to displace it. This is the basic principle behind a lever. A moment, or torque, is the force times the distance from the COR and is essentially a description of the required force applied through a lever arm to cause rotation about the COR. These principles are applied to describe the forces necessary to balance the joint reactive forces at the hip. The weight of the body directs a force toward the floor with the distal end of the moment arm being the center of the pubic symphysis during 2-legged stance. The opposite moment is created by the hip abductors acting on the greater trochanter. Thus, any traumatic, degenerative, or surgical event that changes femoral offset will change the length of the moment arms and can have drastic implications for the forces required for stance, gait, and other complex motions at the hip.[33,34]

When considering movement at the hip and the forces required to maintain balance, one can think of motion in 1 of 2 ways: Either the foot is planted and the body moves in relation to the lower extremity, or the foot is free and the lower extremity moves in relation to the body. Consider the following simplified example to see how this helps understand the forces at play during single-leg stance (which occurs 60% of the time during gait). With the foot planted and no other forces working at the hip, the weight of the body would cause adduction of the lower extremity. Therefore, to prevent tipping over and to maintain an upright posture, the abductors must exert an equal (and opposite) abduction force. The same is true in the sagittal plane with forward flexion of the body and concomitant firing of the extensors.

An understanding of the basic forces required to produce locomotion enables the practitioner to begin to analyze gait disturbances and pathological movement at the hip. Two classic examples are the Trendelenburg stance and gait. Both of these pathologic signs involve weakened abductor muscles, typically the gluteus medius and/or minimus. When attempting to stand on one leg with weakened abductors, the nonstance side of the pelvis will droop toward the floor due to an inability of the stance-side abductors to maintain upright posture. The side that drops occurs because of weakness or a torn abductor on the weightbearing side. During gait, the patient lurches toward the affected side in order to prevent the swinging leg from striking the ground.[35]

Assessment

The purpose of assessment is to understand the patient's problems, from the patient's perspective as well as the clinician's, and the physical basis for the symptoms that have caused the patient to complain. As James Cyriax stated, "Diagnosis is only a matter of applying one's anatomy."[36] A clinical assessment requires a thorough systematic examination of the patient. The clinical diagnosis depends on a knowledge of functional anatomy, an accurate patient history, diligent observation, and a thorough examination. The differential diagnosis process involves the use of clinical signs and symptoms, a knowledge of pathology and mechanisms of injury and/or dysfunction, physical examination involving provocative and palpation (motion) tests, and laboratory and diagnostic imaging techniques when appropriate. A systematic evaluation enables the clinician to collate and develop a clinical picture of the integrity and function of the hip's osseous, intra-articular, extra-articular, musculotendinous, and neurovascular structures.[36,37]

Table 9-2

HIP PAIN PATTERN AND BEHAVIOR[37,41]

TYPE OF PAIN	POSSIBLE CAUSES
Dull, deep, aching	Osteoarthritis, Paget disease
Sharp, intense, sudden, associated with weightbearing	Fracture
Tingling that radiates	Radiculopathy, spinal stenosis, meralgia paresthetica
Increased pain while sitting with the affected leg crossed or laying on one side	Trochanteric bursitis
Pain at sitting, legs not crossed	Ischiogluteal bursitis
Pain after standing, walking	Hip arthrosis
Pain on attempted weightbearing	Occult fracture, severe arthrosis
Unremitting, long duration	Paget disease, metastatic carcinoma, severe arthrosis (occasionally)

Table 9-3

HIP PAIN LOCATION[9,37,41]

LOCATION OF PAIN	POSSIBLE CAUSES
Anterior hip, groin pain (+/- radiation to medial thigh and/or medial knee)	Osteoarthritis, AVN, labral tear, FAI, hernia, neck of femur fracture
Medial thigh	Adductor strain, inguinal disruption
Buttock pain	Lumbar spine, sacroiliac strain/dysfunction, posterior labral tears, piriformis syndrome, hamstring strain, ischial bursitis
Lateral thigh	Lumbar spine, trochanteric bursitis, meralgia paresthesia

A full history of hip region pain typically involves obtaining information from the patient regarding their age, general health, and past medical history (including childhood conditions of the hip). Note that different conditions occur in different age groups and may be related to current symptoms (eg, infantile dysplasia, slipped capital femoral epiphysis, Legg-Calvé-Perthes, osteopenic fractures, osteoarthritis).[37] When exploring hip pain pattern and behavior, note that pain originating from the hip joint is often perceived in the inguinal area and can radiate to the medial knee.[9] Additionally, note that the presence of mechanical symptoms, such as locking, clicking, and giving way have been associated with labral or ligamentum teres pathology.[9,38-40] Keep in mind the possibility of, and/or influence of, neurological and low back symptoms. Tables 9-2 through 9-4 review diagnostic clues related to hip pain presentation and behavior.

It can be useful to obtain or calculate the body mass index (BMI) of the individual presenting with hip pain as a

BMI greater than 25 has been associated by some with an increase severity of osteoarthritis and tendinopathy symptoms.[9,49-52] Conversely, keep in mind that the strength of the relationship between BMI and hip osteoarthritis has been questioned.[53] The mechanism of injury, in addition to the current and previous daily and athletic activities, provides insight into which structures of the hip region have been optimally conditioned and/or abnormally loaded. Be attentive to the posture, frequency, duration, and intensity of hip region loading. It can be clinically valuable to review any prior treatments, in light of any prior benefit or adverse effect.

Self-reporting questionnaires are valuable tools to assess and monitor hip function. Self-reported measures are a feasible and cost-effective means of obtaining standardized data from large numbers of individuals.[54] With the current emphasis on patient-centered care,[55] Guccione et al[56] proposed that self-reported measures are most consistent with the tenets of evidence-based practice in that an individual's judgment about their level of function (ie, patient's values)

Table 9-4

INITIAL HYPOTHESES BASED ON HISTORY FINDINGS[38]

HISTORY	POSSIBLE CAUSES
Lateral thigh pain, exacerbated during sit to stand.	Greater trochanteric bursitis[42] Muscle strain[43]
Age > 60 years. Pain and stiffness are in the hip with possible radiation into the groin.	Osteoarthritis[44]
Clicking or catching in the hip joint. Pain is exacerbated at end-range flexion or extension.	Labral tear[39,40,45]
Reports of a repetitive or an overuse injury.	Muscle sprain/strain[43]
Deep aching throb in the hip or groin; possible history of prolonged steroid use.	AVN[45,46]
Sharp pain in groin (often misdiagnosed by multiple providers).	FAI (anterior)[47]
Pain in the gluteal region with occasional radiation into the posterior thigh and calf.	Piriformis syndrome[48] Hamstring strain[43,45] Ischial bursitis[43]

are conjoined to best clinical practice.[57] There is a variety of outcome assessment tools for hip pain and dysfunction, and we briefly review the more commonly utilized hip outcome scores here.

The Harris Hip Scale (HHS) was developed for the assessment of the results of hip surgery and is intended to evaluate various hip disabilities and methods of treatment in an adult population. The original version was published 1969.[58] The HHS is widely used throughout the world for evaluating outcome after total hip replacement (THR) and femoral neck fractures.[59] The Modified HHS is a modification of the HHS and is intended to evaluate hip pain and function in hip arthroscopy patients.[60] The Hip Disability and Osteoarthritis Outcome Score is a disease-specific questionnaire that is intended to be used in an adult population with hip disability with or without osteoarthritis.[59] The Oxford Hip Score was designed to assess outcomes after THR and has also been validated and used in revision hip replacement. It has been reported to be a useful predictor of early revision after THR. Due to its brevity, the Oxford Hip Score questionnaire yields a high response rate and is therefore preferred for larger studies used in several countries in large registry studies.[59] The Lower Extremity Function Scale was developed to evaluate clinically important and patient-relevant changes in health status as influenced by the lower extremity (hip, knee, foot, and ankle). The Lower Extremity Function Scale has test-retest reliability and cross-sectional construct validity in addition to discriminatory validity.[3,9,37,57,61-63]

For the active individual presenting with hip pain consider the iHOT scales.[64,65] The iHOT-33 subscales include symptoms and functional limitations; sports and recreational physical activities; job-related concerns; and social, emotional, and lifestyle concerns. A shorter version, the iHOT-12, has been introduced for clinical use.[64,66] The iHOT tools have been introduced to limit the ceiling effect observed in the younger active patient and both versions have been rigorously validated and shown to be responsive to change.[67]

A thorough clinical examination of the hip region typically involves observation, both stationary and dynamic, maybe even nonweightbearing in addition to weightbearing. If the hip is injured or exhibits pathology, the lesion is often perceptible during walking; therefore, observation of gait is critical.[3,9,37,68] Observe the gait for symmetry in alignment, in distances, in motion, and in timing, and be very attentive for deviations from normal in addition to deviations from the contralateral side. An antalgic gait is often present, but dependent on the severity of symptoms. Typically, the stance phase is shortened, and hip flexion appears accentuated as hip extension is avoided during stance. Varying degrees of abductor lurch may be present as the patient attempts to place the center of gravity over the hip, reducing the forces on the joint.[68]

Observe pelvic alignment and control in both dynamic activities such as gait, step up and down, squat, forward bend, and lunge, and in static postures such as stand and single leg stance. As the hip has a critical role in transferring forces between the trunk and the lower extremity, it is of great value to observe the individual's ability to stabilize both the pelvis and the lower extremity alignment during functional activities. An inability to control the pelvis can often be seen in a Trendelenburg gait or a Trendelenburg stance. An inability to control the whole leg rotation can often be seen in a squat,

Table 9-5 ━━━━━━━━━━━━

CLINICAL PREDICTION RULE FOR HIP OSTEOARTHRITIS*[69]

- Limited active hip flexion with lateral hip pain
- Active hip extension causes pain
- Limited passive hip medial rotation (25 degrees or less)
- Squatting limited and painful
- Scour test with adduction causes lateral hip or groin pain

* 4 out of 5 variables must be positive.

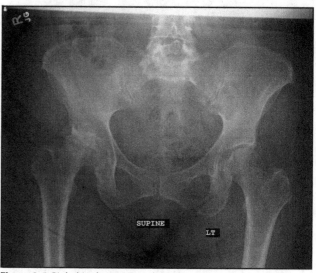

Figure 9-6. Right hip degenerative joint disease.

step down, lunge, or sit-to-stand transfer activities. Both these deviations have consequences for a number of hip pain presentations (including, but not limited to, trochanteric bursitis, iliotibial band syndrome, piriformis syndrome, FAI, labral tears, and osteoarthritis).[68]

Byrd[68] has described a common characteristic sign of patients presenting with hip joint disorders. The patient will cup their hand above the greater trochanter with the thumb posterior and the fingers gripping deep into the anterior groin when describing deep interior hip pain. The hand forms a C and thus this has been termed the *C-sign*. Byrd notes that due to the position of the hand, this sign can be misinterpreted as indicating lateral pathology such as the iliotibial band or trochanteric bursitis, but he notes that the patient is describing deep interior hip pain.[68]

Hip motion is necessary for more activities than just ambulation. In fact, greater hip mobility is required for activities of daily living than is required for gait; activities such as shoe tying, sitting, getting up from a chair, and picking up things from the floor all require a greater range of hip motion.[37] Mobility tests typically include active and passive motion and may include tests of passive accessory joint motion. Passive accessory joint motion at the hip often includes long axis traction, compression, and lateral distraction. Magee[37] explains how small differences of joint motion may be difficult to detect because of the large muscle bulk in the area. It can be valuable to assess sustained or repeated postures, if necessary, in addition to combined movements.[37] There can be a large spectrum of motion variability among individuals, so it is valuable to compare mobility tests between the left and right hip.

Sutlive et al[69] have developed a clinical prediction rule (Table 9-5) for hip osteoarthritis involving active and passive movement, whereby if 4 of the 5 variables are positive, there is a high probability of hip osteoarthritis. Diagnostic imaging should then be ordered to confirm the diagnosis (Figure 9-6).

Cleland et al[70] note that assessing hip motion has consistently been shown to be highly reliable, and when limited in 3 planes, it is useful in identifying hip osteoarthritis (positive likelihood ratio [+LR] = 4.5 to 4.7). Cleland et al[70] additionally explain how lateral hip pain during passive abduction is strongly suggestive of lateral tendon pathologic disorders (+LR = 8.3), whereas groin pain during active hip abduction or adduction is moderately suggestive of osteoarthritis (+LR = 5.7). Limited hip abduction in infants has been long associated with identifying hip dysplasia or instability.

Manual muscle tests around the hip region are also compared left and right and provide valuable insight into strength, and because some of the hip musculature also crosses the knee joint, these tests typically involve manual muscle tests at the knee. Cleland et al[70] explain how evaluation of hip muscle strength has been shown to be FAI syndrome reliable, but it is less helpful in identifying lateral tendon pathologic conditions than simply reports of pain during resisted tests, especially of the gluteus minimus and medius muscles (+LR = 3.27). Similarly, a report of posterior pain with a squat is also useful in identifying hip osteoarthritis (+LR = 6.1).[70] It has been reported that hip flexors and hip extensors are almost equal in strength[71] and that the adductors are 2.5 times as strong as the abductors.[72] These ratios may vary depending on whether the movement is tested isometrically or isokinetically.

When assessing the hip region via palpation explore all 4 quadrants of the area: anterior, posterior, medial, and lateral. During palpation of the hip region, the examiner should note any tenderness, temperature, muscle spasm, or other signs and symptoms that may indicate the source of pathology. Intra-articular pain in the hip is rarely palpable.[73]

There are a vast number of clinical tests for hip pain. This chapter focuses on common clinical (special) tests for hip pain. Only those tests that the examiner believes are necessary should be performed when assessing the hip. Most tests are done primarily to confirm a diagnosis or to determine pathology and should not be used as standalone tests when considering a diagnosis. As with all special tests, if the test is positive, it is highly suggestive that the problem exists, but if it is negative, it does not necessarily rule out the problem. Therefore, special tests should not be taken in isolation but should be used to support the history, observation, and clinical examination.[37]

HIP SCOUR/QUADRANT TEST

The patient is supine; the examiner flexes the patient's knee and provides an axial/compressive load through the femur (Figure 9-7). The examiner performs a sweeping compression and rotation (scour) motion from external rotation to internal rotation. The hip quadrant has been described to differ from the hip scour, whereby the quadrant test does not compress the acetabular rim during the arc of movement from abduction to adduction. A positive test is pain or apprehension during the examination. These tests have been considered a test for hip labrum, capsulitis, osteoarthritis, and FAI syndrome. This test has been categorized with a minimal (quadrant) to moderate (scour) utility score by Hegedus and Cook.[74]

TRENDELENBURG'S SIGN

The patient stands and the examiner instructs the patient to stand on one leg. The examiner observes for a drop in the contralateral pelvis once the leg is lifted. Confirmation of abnormal pelvic drop can be additionally observed during gait (Trendelenburg gait; Figure 9-8). A positive test is an asymmetric drop of one hip compared to the other during single leg stance. This test is for a tear and/or weakness of the gluteus medius muscle. This test has been categorized with a moderate utility score by Hegedus and Cook.[74] Cleland et al[70] explain that although less reliable than strength tests, the Trendelenburg test is also moderately useful in identifying both lateral tendon pathologic conditions and gluteus medius tears.

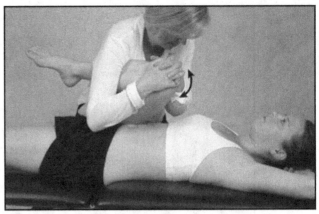

Figure 9-7. Hip scour test.[37] (Reproduced with permission from Magee DJ. Hip. In: *Orthopedic Physical Assessment*. 6th ed. Elsevier; 2014:689-764.)

OBER'S TEST

The patient is side-lying with the symptomatic leg upward and the asymptomatic leg on the plinth (Figure 9-9). The examiner positions the knee of the symptomatic leg into flex and stabilizes the pelvis at the iliac crest. The examiner then glides the hip of the symptomatic leg into extension and slight abduction. A positive test is a failure of the knee to drop toward the plinth, indicative of tightness of the structures. A comparison of both sides is warranted. This test is for iliotibial band restriction. This test has been categorized with an unknown utility score by Hegedus and Cook; they note this extremely common technique has not been assessed for diagnostic value.[74]

THOMAS TEST

The patient sits at the edge of the plinth or table. The patient then lies back pulling both knees to their chest. One knee (asymptomatic side) is held to the chest and the other is lowered into extension of the hip while the knee is allowed to extend. The patient is instructed to pull their pelvis into posterior ration. The angle of the hip and knee on the symptomatic side is noted. A comparison of both sides is warranted. A positive test is significant tightness on the hip flexors of the extended leg. This test is for anterior or lateral capsular restriction or hip flexor tightness. This test has been categorized with a minimal utility score by Hegedus and Cook.[74] They note there are multiple suggested iterations of the test, none of which have been substantiated.

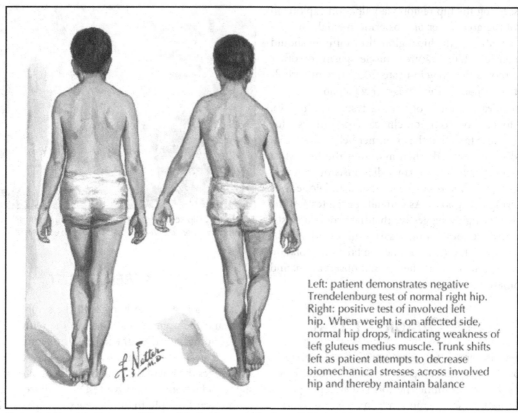

Left: patient demonstrates negative Trendelenburg test of normal right hip. Right: positive test of involved left hip. When weight is on affected side, normal hip drops, indicating weakness of left gluteus medius muscle. Trunk shifts left as patient attempts to decrease biomechanical stresses across involved hip and thereby maintain balance

Figure 9-8. Trendelenburg test.[70] (Reproduced with permission from Cleland JA, Koppenhaver S, Su J. *Netter's Orthopaedic Clinical Examination.* Elsevier; 2016.)

DIAL TEST/LOG ROLL TEST OF THE HIP

The patient lies supine with the hips in neutral (ie, no rotation; Figure 9-10). The examiner internally rotates the limb and then releases it, allowing the leg to go into lateral rotation. If the patient's leg passively rotates greater than 45 degrees from vertical in the axial plane, and if on testing, there is no mechanical end point, the test is positive for hip instability. Both limbs are compared starting with the unaffected side.[37] This test is very similar to the Log Roll Test where the examiner passively, medially, and laterally rotates the femur to end range comparing both hips. For the Log Roll Test, if a click is present, it may indicate a labral tear. The maneuver also shows hip rotational mobility, and if restricted or painful, indicates hip pathology.[37] There is no research on the diagnostic value of either of these clinical tests.

FLEXION ABDUCTION EXTERNAL ROTATION TEST (PATRICK'S TEST)

The patient is positioned supine, and the painful side leg is placed in a "figure four" position with the ankle just above the knee on the other leg (Figure 9-11). The examiner provides a gentle downward pressure on both the knee of the painful side and the ASIS of the nonpainful side. A comparison of both sides is warranted. A positive test is pain near the anterior or lateral capsule of the hip. This test is for anterior or lateral capsular restriction or hip flexor tightness.[37] This test has been categorized with a moderate utility score by Hegedus and Cook.[74] This test is also a test for sacroiliac pain as pain posteriorly is associated with sacroiliac dysfunction. Mitchel et al[75] found high sensitivity noting its value as a sacroiliac joint screen.

ANTERIOR IMPINGEMENT TEST

The patient lies supine with the hip flexed to 90 degrees. The examiner then internally rotates and adducts the hip, which leads to impingement of femoral neck against the acetabular rim. Forced internal rotation in a flexed hip can lead to a labral lesion, chondral lesion, or both. Pain is a positive sign. The hip is similarly tested in different degrees of flexion (45 degrees to 120 degrees) with pain typically increasing with increased flexion. This test is a test for hip dysplasia (eg, acetabular retroversion), slipped capital femoral epiphysis, and FAI syndrome.[37] In a meta-analysis study, the sensitivity of this clinical test has been described as excellent, but the specificity has been conversely described as poor.[76]

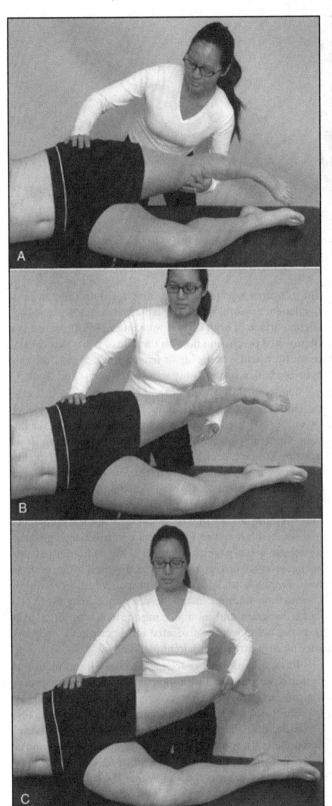

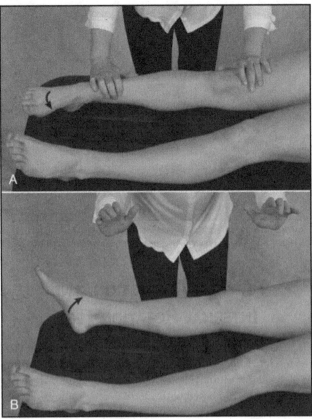

Figure 9-10. Dial test of the hip. (A) The examiner medially rotates the hip. (B) The examiner releases the medial rotation and watches the hip roll into lateral rotation.[37] (Reproduced with permission from Magee DJ. Hip. In: *Orthopedic Physical Assessment*. 6th ed. Elsevier; 2014:689-764.)

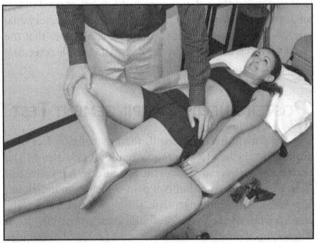

Figure 9-11. Flexion, abduction, and external rotation (FABER; Patrick's) test.[70] (Reproduced with permission from Cleland JA, Koppenhaver S, Su J. *Netter's Orthopaedic Clinical Examination*. Elsevier; 2016.)

Figure 9-9. Ober's test. (A) Knee straight. (B) The hip is passively extended by the examiner to ensure that the tensor fasciae latae runs over the greater trochanter. A positive test is indicated when the leg remains abducted while the patient's muscles are relaxed. (C) Test done with the knee flexed.[37] (Reproduced with permission from Magee DJ. Hip. In: *Orthopedic Physical Assessment*. 6th ed. Elsevier; 2014:689-764.)

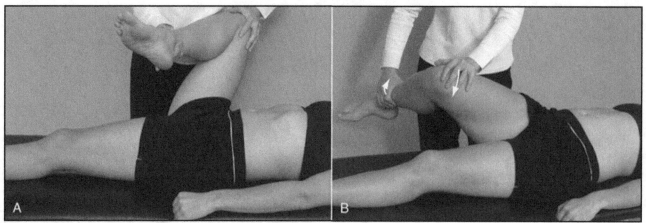

Figure 9-12. Flexion, adduction, and internal rotation (FADDIR) test. (A) Starting position. (B) End position.[37] (Reproduced with permission from Magee DJ. Hip. In: *Orthopedic Physical Assessment*. 6th ed. Elsevier; 2014:689-764.)

FLEXION, ADDUCTION, AND INTERNAL ROTATION TEST

The patient is in a supine position and the examiner takes the hip into full flexion, external rotation, and full abduction as a starting position (Figure 9-12). The examiner then extends the hip combined with internal rotation and adduction. A positive test is indicated by the production of pain, the reproduction of the patient's symptoms with or without a click, or apprehension. The test places the greatest strain on the anterolateral labrum, and the examiner should be careful to equate any findings with the patient's symptoms. This test, also called the *anterior apprehension test*, is used to test for anterior-superior impingement syndrome, anterior labial tear, and iliopsoas tendinitis.[37] Reiman et al[76] note that the FADDIR test is supported by the data as a valuable screening test for FAI syndrome/labral tear pathology.

POSTEROINFERIOR IMPINGEMENT TEST

The patient lies supine with the legs hanging free over the edge of the bed to ensure maximum hip extension. The examiner then laterally rotates the hip quickly. A positive test is deep-seated groin or buttock pain, which is an indication of posteroinferior impingement. This tests for global acetabular overcoverage (eg, coxa profunda, coxa protrusio), global femoral neck offset abnormalities, and posterior acetabular cartilage damage. The test can also be positive in people who place the hip in extremes of range of motion (ROM; eg, ballet dancers, martial artists, hockey goal tenders, mountain climbers, yoga practitioners, long striding runners).[37] There has been minimal research into the clinical utility of this test.

PATELLAR-PUBIC PERCUSSION TEST

The patient is positioned supine and the examiner places a stethoscope over the pubic symphysis of the patient.

The examiner taps (or uses a tuning fork) on the patella of the patient's painful side and qualitatively reports the sound. A comparison of both sides is warranted. A positive test is a diminished percussion note on the side of pain. This clinical test is for fracture of the hip or femur. This test has been categorized with a strong utility score by Hegedus and Cook.[74]

Differential diagnosis of the hip joint poses a diagnostic clinical challenge. Currently, there is limited evidence in support of the diagnostic utility of special tests for hip pain. Generally, special tests of the hip have not been demonstrated to be especially helpful in identifying specific hip pathologic conditions. Owing to the low quality and biased sampling of patients with high probability of disease, hip physical examination tests do not appear to currently provide the clinician any significant value in altering probability of disease with their use. Further studies involving high quality designs across a wider spectrum of hip pathology patients are necessary to discern the confirmed clinical utility of these tests. Emphasis to date has been on patient history, clinical examination findings, magnetic resonance imaging (MRI) and arthrogram, and anesthetic intra-articular injection pain response are currently advocated for determining the presence of intra-articular hip joint pathology.[70,74,76-78]

Physical performance tests add to the clinical picture of dysfunction associated with hip pain. In addition to observing the gait pattern, which is often altered with hip pain, it is useful to observe single leg stance, balance activities (eg, Y balance test,[79,80] star balance test[81,82]), squatting (bilateral and unilateral), and ascending and descending stairs (one or more at a time). There is also value in observing the individual's ability to cross the legs so that the ankle of one foot rests on the knee of the opposite leg (figure 4 sitting). The examiner should be attentive to motions that are painful and/or limited in addition to the individual's capacity to control and stabilize both the core and pelvis in addition to the lower extremity. This might include a crunch or resisted sit up. The assessor should also observe what happens to the motion control around the hip region during repetitive tasks. If relevant to the functional activities of the individual, additionally observe agility tasks: running straight ahead, take off and deceleration, pivoting and twisting, single leg hopping (single, triple, time, distance, and crossover) in addition to jumping (tuck jump, vertical drop down) and landing (controlling the impact with optimal form).[14,37,83]

There are functional tests described in the literature that are used to assess the overall quality of lower extremity movement: the Functional Movement Screen[84-86] and the Vail Sport Test.[87,88] Both these functional screens purport to assess the qualitative ability to control the lower extremity during a variety of tasks; the Functional Movement Screen assesses 7 movement patterns (deep squat, hurdle step, inline lunge, shoulder mobility, active straight leg raise, trunk stability push-up, and rotary stability) and the Vail Sport Test involves dynamic and plyometric activities in multiplanar movements (single leg squat, lateral bounding, diagonal bounding, and forward box lunge).

Hegedus et al[89] note how physical performance tests are used by coaches, strength and conditioning experts, and health care professionals to estimate function, gauge progress after surgery or injury, predict which athletes are at a greater risk for injury, and make a return-to-play decision. Their research urges caution in making any firm clinical conclusions based on the results of functional lower extremity tests while additionally noting that the hip region is understudied in relation to physical performance tests. They highlight how the current body of knowledge should leave the clinician-scientist skeptical about the use of these tests for preseason screening, as predictors of injury, and as outcome measures after injury or surgery. There is both an opportunity and an urgent need for further research on these tests.[89]

Do not overlook clearing screens for the lumbar and knee regions when considering their influence on the presentation of hip region pain or dysfunction. Pain in the hip can be referred to or from the sacroiliac joints or the lumbar spine, it is imperative—unless there is evidence of direct trauma to the hip—that these joints be examined along with the hip.[3,9,37]

A comprehensive assessment of the hip complex typically involves imaging. Options include the following:

- Ultrasound
- Radiographs
- CT
- MRI
- Bone scintigraphy
- Bone scans

Ultrasound uses sound waves to determine density and distance, and thus does not expose patients to radiation. Sound waves are best propagated through fluid, are poorly propagated through dense tissues such as bone, and are not propagated through air. Thus, the ideal use of ultrasound is to evaluate fluid-filled structures such as an inflamed bursa, a joint with an effusion, or an abscess. They are also helpful in delineating tissue planes and are often used to facilitate targeted injections. They can assess blood flow and are a useful tool in the diagnosis of lower extremity deep vein thrombosis. In comparison to other imaging studies, they are inexpensive and highly portable. Furthermore, they offer results in real time and can be used in the clinic. However, they are operator and patient body habitus dependent, and offer poor resolution. In general, ultrasound is safe and widely used in clinical settings.[90,91]

Radiography, or x-ray, uses ionizing radiation to produce a projectional image. In other words, the image seen contains all imaged objects "stacked on top of one another," making it impossible to determine the 3-dimensional (3D) relationship of objects within the image. Another way of saying this is that an x-ray is a 2-dimensional (2D) image of a 3D object. Radiation passes freely through air and appears black, whereas dense tissues such as bone absorb radiation and appear white. X-ray is therefore extremely useful for evaluating bony structures. It is also helpful to look for gas trapped within tissues, such as in an abscess, a puncture wound, or evaluating for an open fracture. Contrast can be added (typically into joints) to obtain a better view of the joint. For musculoskeletal purposes, it does poorly at evaluating soft tissues. It can be moderately useful to appreciate a joint effusion. In comparison to CT scans, they are inexpensive and incur much less radiation exposure. Weaknesses include ionizing radiation and inability to appreciate objects in 3 dimensions. Overall, x-ray is often the first imaging modality employed by most orthopedists.

CT scans use ionizing radiation to create a tomographic image. The scanner assesses the radiation in 360 degrees and uses thin slices to create tens or even hundreds of 2D images. When these slices are viewed in sequence, the 3D structure of the imaged object is able to be appreciated. Coronal, sagittal, and axial slices are obtained from a single scan. Also, 3D reconstructions can be performed. CT gives astounding resolution and is best suited for viewing bony structures. Soft tissues can also be appreciated. Contrast is often used for vascular studies or for arthrograms. Scans can be obtained in seconds, even of large areas or in patients who are morbidly obese. CT is also used to guide injections for difficult or deep joints such as the hip. In comparison to x-ray or ultrasound, CT is significantly more expensive and exposes the patient to much higher doses of radiation. In the end, there is no imaging modality that gives better resolution of bony structures. It is the study of choice for evaluating complex fractures or bony anatomic abnormalities about the hip.[90,92-94]

MRI creates a powerful magnetic field that causes atomic distortion. This slight distortion is what produces the images, and thus provides a level of detail that is unmatched by any other imaging modality. Similar to CT, 2D slices are used to appreciate 3D structures. 3D reconstructions are not possible. MRI does not use radiation but cannot be used in patients with any metallic object in their body that is not MRI compatible (most modern medical implants are MRI-safe). MRI is expensive, time-consuming (studies often take up to 1 hour), and the machine itself forces patients to be fully enclosed in a confined space. The ideal use of MRI is evaluation of soft tissues. When contrast is added, the level of detail increases.[90,92,94]

Other imaging modalities less frequently used include bone scintigraphy (or bone scan) and bone density. Bone scans use a radioactive medication that isolates osteoblast activity. X-ray is used to identify locations of increased uptake of the tracer. These "hot spots" can be used to identify occult fractures, bony cancers or metastases, inflammation, or infection.[90] Bone density scans, or dual-energy x-ray absorptiometry, use low-dose radiography to determine the density of a given bone (usually lumbar vertebrae). This density is then compared to a standard. This is helpful to diagnose osteoporosis and assess fracture risk.[95]

Another consideration when ordering imaging is the amount of radiation the patient will receive. Although x-rays and CT scans are ordered routinely, the risks of radiation are not negligible. Radiation exposure from imaging has been well studied and can be quantified. Amounts of radiation exposure are measured in the SI unit called the *Gray (G)*, or more commonly, *miliGray (mGy)*. A Gray is the amount of radiation present from one joule of energy absorbed per one kilogram of tissue. The Sievert (SV) is an attempt to quantify the effective dose of radiation on biological tissue depending on its weight and density. The unit is still J/kg, but is multiplied by the relative density of the tissue being imaged with most tissues having a value near 1.[96] Thus, the Sievert is roughly equivalent to the Gray. Applying these concepts to risk stratification is useful. For example, a single dose of approximately 4 SV is thought to be lethal.[97] Furthermore, according to the Food and Drug Administration, a CT examination with 10 mSv may increase the risk of acquiring a fatal cancer by 2 chance in 2000.[93] Each dose is cumulative, so every study increases that risk. With that in mind, consider the dosage of some standard imaging of the pelvis. X-ray of the pelvis is 1.3 mGy,[98] or roughly 1.0 mSv.[99] CT pelvis without contrast is 17 mGy, and that of the thigh is 13 mGy.[100] Again, these doses and their associated risks are small, but it is important to mitigate and minimize them by any means necessary.

DIAGNOSIS AND MANAGEMENT OF HIP COMPLEX DYSFUNCTION: DISORDERS AND PATHOLOGY

Diagnosis of Labral Injuries and Femoral Acetabular Impingement Syndrome

Diagnosing labral injuries can be difficult. Symptoms are nonspecific, and various pathology can present the same way. A recent meta-analysis[76] and systematic review[101] looked at the various physical examination maneuvers described in the literature to aid in diagnosing hip pathology. The authors concluded that no single maneuver has the sensitivity or specificity to make an accurate diagnosis for hip pathology. Does this mean that the physical examination is obsolete or unnecessary? Of course not. What it means is that when evaluating a patient, the practitioner must use all available information provided by the history and physical examination and rely on a series of maneuvers and tests in order to develop an accurate differential diagnosis. One must take caution to not be fooled into thinking that assessments are like if/then equations; No 2 patients are alike, and the same pathological process can present in myriad ways. However, there are certain characteristics that allow for the formation of a differential diagnosis.

Patients with labral pathology often complain of anterior inguinal or groin pain. It can occasionally present with mechanical symptoms such as limping, catching, clicking, or locking.[101,102] Labral cysts can also present with pain and/or mechanical symptoms.[103] Night pain is uncommon. Onset of pain is usually gradual, which reflects the idea that most labral pathology is due to repetitive microtrauma rather than acute traumatic events. It is important to distinguish the source of pain to rule out other pathology (eg, pubic symphysis, greater trochanter, sacroiliac joints). Patients will often describe their pain as aching or gnawing at baseline, whereas sharp pain is associated with extremes of motion or particular movements related to sport or profession. Pain typically does not radiate, although if it does, it tends to radiate laterally.

Individual tests can be a helpful snapshot of the overall picture of pathology. The FADDIR test has been shown to be particularly helpful in the diagnosis of labral pathology because when absent, labral pathology is not likely.[87] However, a positive FADDIR test does not necessarily rule it in. Other tests include the scour/quadrant, FABER, and FADDIR plus axial compression. The authors of a recent systematic review concluded that if these tests are negative, there is a low likelihood of labral pathology.[101] Furthermore, a recent biomechanical study showed that flexion, adduction, and internal rotation placed the greatest amount of strain in the anterolateral labrum, when compared to various other hip positions. Abduction and external rotation also placed significant strain on the anterolateral labrum.[39] This provides an explanation as to why certain examination maneuvers are more likely to reveal pathology.

Beyond history and physical examination, radiography or invasive procedures are typically required to make an accurate diagnosis. X-ray is inexpensive and allows for inspection of the bony morphology around the hip. It is usually the first form of imaging obtained and can rule out any gross or potentially mechanical abnormalities. CT scan is not routinely used when suspicious of labral or soft tissue irregularity around the hip due to the superiority of MRI at visualizing soft tissues and fluid. Magnetic resonance arthrography with the addition of contrast can be extremely sensitive for detecting labral pathology and is the imaging gold standard.[90] However, labral tears can occasionally be missed on imaging

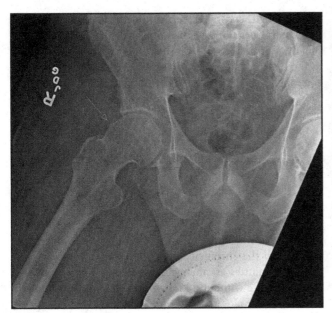

Figure 9-13. A cam lesion.

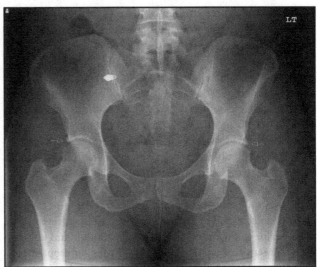

Figure 9-14. Bilateral pincer lesions.

because the images are static and the 2 ends of the tear may fit together like puzzle pieces when not under stress. If imaging is negative, but there is still high suspicion for labral pathology, more invasive procedures may be required.

One option involves fluoroscopic-guided injection of local anesthetic (and potentially an anti-inflammatory medication) into the joint. If this alleviates pain, then the diagnosis becomes much clearer. One group described a method of determining labral tears using this principle. The authors subjected athletes with suspected labral injuries to a battery of active maneuvers (eg, single leg squats, box jumps) and scored their performance and degree of symptoms. They then injected lidocaine into the hip joint and repeated the test. One hundred percent of the athletes who had an improved score on the test were shown to have a labral tear at the time of surgery.[7]

The final option for diagnosis is arthroscopy, and this is the current gold standard. The only sure way to determine labral pathology is to visualize and probe it. Obviously, this is a technique of last resort and should not be the routine manner in which injuries are diagnosed.

Another cause of labral pathology is FAI syndrome. FAI syndrome is a common source of hip pain. Although hip impingement has been a known entity for a long time, FAI syndrome has only recently been described.[104,105] Pain occurs when soft tissues, namely the labrum, are impinged between the femur and acetabulum during extremes of motion, or with pathologic morphologies. As bony contact occurs, the soft tissues between them break down over time. This eventually leads to symptomatic dysfunction.

FAI syndrome has recently been defined as a triad of symptoms, clinical signs, and imaging findings.[106] Without all 3 elements, the diagnosis of FAI syndrome is less likely. The principal complaint from patients with FAI syndrome

is pain, specifically, anterior groin pain. This is similar to those with labral pathology and reflects the close interrelationship between the 2 entities. Typically, pain is reproduced with extremes of motion, or certain positions (ie, sitting with the hips adducted and flexed). The pain experienced can be varied because impingement can occur anywhere along the acetabular rim. Mechanical symptoms can be present but are less likely. When a patient presents with hip and/or groin pain, FAI syndrome should be in the differential diagnosis.

Clinical examination for FAI syndrome is similar to that of labral tears. Again, there is no single sign that can rule it in or out, but rather a multitude of maneuvers should be performed. FADDIR test is often positive, as has been previously shown for labral tears. Another sign is a limited arc of motion when compared to the other side. Furthermore, patients may guard the injured side when walking, so gait disturbance may be present. This can also lead to muscle weakness or pain in other areas due to overcompensation. Therefore, other tests should include observation of gait, single leg stance, double and (if possible) single leg squats. Limp, pain, or inability to perform these maneuvers can give clues as to what is happening locally and globally.

Imaging studies are often required to make a definitive diagnosis. Before discussing imaging techniques and measurements, several morphologic descriptions must be made. A cam lesion is the loss of sphericity of the femoral head with a noticeable bony hypertrophy in the basicervical region (Figure 9-13). A pincer lesion is a bony overgrowth on the rim of the acetabulum (Figure 9-14).[92] This creates overcoverage of the femoral head and leads to increased impingement. An individual may have one or both of these lesions. One can easily imagine increased contact between the femur and acetabulum during movement secondary to these overgrowths. The term *head-neck offset* is defined as the distance between the outer circumferential edge of the femoral neck compared to that of the femoral head. This is best envisioned by imagining looking "down the barrel" of the femoral neck.

Doing so would present the neck as a 2D circle and would allow for measurement of the diameter. Now, imagine the femoral head interposed over the neck with the center of the neck and center the head perfectly aligned. The head would also be appreciated as a 2D circle and a measurement of its diameter could also be made. The distance between the circumferential lines of the neck and head is the offset distance or ratio. A shortened offset, or a larger neck diameter, has been implicated with higher incidence of impingement.[47,107] Also, if the center of the neck is literally offset from the center of the head, this could also lead to increased impingement. Acetabular version is the final element to consider. Version is the natural angle of the acetabulum in relation to the pelvis. It is determined by the angle between a line drawn from the anterior to posterior rim of the acetabulum and another drawn anterior to posterior in line with the anteroposterior axis. It does not project directly laterally, but rather is angled anteriorly approximately 15 to 20 degrees and inferiorly due to sacral tilt.[108] Increased acetabular retroversion (or more lateral projection) is associated with increased impingement, especially during hip flexion.[108,109] With these concepts in mind, we can now discuss imaging modalities and measurements.

Plain film radiography is the best place to start. They are inexpensive and easy to obtain. An anteroposterior view of the hips and a lateral femoral neck view should be obtained. Initial inspection includes overall bony morphology, evaluation of the joint space, identification of cam and pincer lesions, some degree of acetabular version, and head-neck offset. The crossover sign can be appreciated on plain films and gives an idea of the presence of acetabular retroversion. Normally, the anterior rim is more medial than the posterior rim. In retroversion, the proximal portion of the anterior rim is lateral to the posterior rim and then "crosses over" to become more medial inferiorly.[108,110,111] More advanced imaging is required to determine the degree of retroversion.

Several more concrete measurements can be made from plain films to help define or predict the level of impingement and degree of FAI syndrome. The first is called the alpha angle. It is measured by creating a perfect circle overlying the articular sphericity of the femoral head. A radial line is drawn at the first instance of loss or incongruence of sphericity. The alpha angle is the angle at which this line intersects with a line drawn from the center of the head down the axis of the neck. This is used to evaluate cam lesions. The larger the angle, the less spherical the head and the greater the cam lesion. Angles greater than 55 degrees are associated with impingement.[108,112]

Another measurement is the head-neck offset as described earlier. A decreased offset has been implicated in cam lesions and impingement. One group found that symptomatic patients had an average offset of 7.2 mm, whereas healthy control participants had an offset of 11.6 mm.[113]

A final measurement is called the center edge angle.[114] First, draw a horizontal line connecting bilateral lesser trochanters or inferior pubic rami on an anteroposterior

radiograph. Then draw a vertical line through the center of the femoral head and perpendicular to the horizontal line. Finally, a line is drawn from the center of the femoral head to the most lateral projection of the acetabulum. The center edge angle is the angle between this line and the vertical line. This is used to evaluate acetabular overcoverage, or pincer lesion. Angles greater than 40 degrees have been implicated in impingement.[115]

Management of Labral Injuries and Femoral Acetabular Impingement Syndrome

When considering treatment options, it is important to establish the chronicity and nature of the injury. Acute, traumatic injuries are managed differently than chronic injuries or those without a known inciting event. Atraumatic or chronic pathology should initially be managed nonoperatively.[116,117] Because the labrum has some vascularity, there is potential for healing. This is why nonoperative management should be attempted initially. That may mean cessation of athletic competition, alteration of work responsibilities (ie, light duty), or a trial of limited weightbearing. This should be tailored to the patient's activity level, needs, and severity of symptoms. One may also consider short-term use of nonsteroidal anti-inflammatory drugs (NSAIDs) to alleviate pain and inflammation. Another approach is to implement a course of physical therapy aimed at strengthening not only the muscles of the pelvic girdle, but also the core, low back, quadriceps, and hamstrings.[118] It is important to remember to not treat the hip in isolation,[119] and that hip pain is often caused or referred by areas above or below. It is essential to consider the needs and desires of your patient to ensure that conservative treatment plans are realistic (eg, asking a day laborer to stop working for several weeks may not be possible).

Physical therapy treatment goals for labral injuries and FAI syndrome are likely to include optimizing mobility and motion of the hip joint. The articular cartilage and surrounding structures obtain oxygen and nutrients from the synovial joint fluid. When a joint is loaded, the pressure squeezes fluid including waste products out of the cartilage, and when the pressure is relieved, the fluid seeps back in together with oxygen and nutrients. Thus, the health of cartilage depends on it being used. Treatment activities with this goal in mind might include joint mobilizations and/or manipulations, mobility exercises, stretches, and gentle cyclic repetitive activities. Physical therapy treatment will also be aimed at addressing muscle imbalances, weaknesses, or instabilities found on assessment. The hip abductors and hip extensors are often noted to be weak in addition to a lack of core/pelvic girdle control. Be mindful that it has been proposed the acetabulum collapses onto the femoral head when the pelvis is inadequately controlled by the core musculature.[120]

If conservative treatment fails, or in cases of acute injuries, surgery is often required. Although open surgery was initially described for labral repair, advances in arthroscopic visualization and instrumentation have made arthroscopy the gold standard. Basic principles and goals are aimed at restoring natural morphology and preventing further injury or degeneration. Pincer lesion removal, or "rim trimming," helps correct acetabular overcoverage, and shaving of cam lesions restores femoral sphericity. These corrections help reduce further impingement. Shaving of frayed cartilage fibers removes exposed nerve endings and helps reduce pain. Repair of the labrum can restore its natural function. When repair is not possible, loose edges are removed through debridement to prevent mechanical symptoms. The joint space is evaluated, and loose bodies are removed to prevent pain or mechanical symptoms. In cases of severe articular cartilage damage, procedures such as microfracture or osteochondral autograft transfers can be performed to help stimulate new cartilage growth. The goal of all surgery is to correct deformity or degeneration and preserve function.

Although surgery should not be taken lightly, it often provides significant relief. One study performed on National Hockey League players showed excellent outcomes and high patient satisfaction after arthroscopic intervention for FAI syndrome. It also showed that the longer a patient waited to have surgery after symptom onset, the longer it took for them to return to sport.[7] The authors also showed that arthroscopic repair allowed athletes to return to sport faster than open repair.[7] A large body of evidence is accumulating that shows that arthroscopic surgery for labral injuries and FAI syndrome is safe and effective.

Diagnosis of Osteoarthritis

Primary osteoarthritis of the hip is one of the most common causes of hip pain in older adults and will very likely be encountered in a clinical setting. There are many proposed causes of hip arthritis (eg, genetics, wear and tear, endocrinopathies, cell-signaling), but most cases are thought to be multifactorial. Patients will often complain of deep, aching pain in the groin, and often present with a C-sign. The C-sign is made when the patient places their index finger toward the groin with their thumb toward their buttock in an attempt to demonstrate where they feel their pain. Patients may also complain of vague anterior or medial thigh pain.

Important factors to consider in the patient's history and examination are age, function-limiting pain, ROM limitation, and a radiographic evaluation.[121] Age can have an effect on the diagnosis and prognosis of hip arthritis; treatments may differ based on age, and the younger the patient the more significant the disease burden. When evaluating function, one should consider the ability to perform daily activities, hobbies, or other necessary functions. The presence of night pain should also be determined. A thorough examination should be performed to determine ROM. The patient should also be asked about their ROM and how it affects their daily life. Radiographs of the hip will show the classic findings of decreased joint space, subchondral sclerosis,

osteophyte formation, and subchondral cysts, and can be graded based on severity.[122] All of these evaluations are performed with the goal of defining the patient's disease burden and how it affects their life; this gives the practitioner the ability to formulate effective interventions.

Secondary arthritis of the hip is that which arises due to a known entity, such as trauma or hip dysplasia. In addition to the previously mentioned factors that affect symptoms and function, these cases require a thorough understanding of the predisposing entity to help guide treatment. In the case of hip dysplasia, for example, a thorough radiographic evaluation is necessary to understand the degree of dysplasia because some cases require extreme interventions such as periacetabular osteotomies to reshape the pelvis and restore bony congruity and function.

Management of Osteoarthritis

It is helpful to discuss goals of treatment with each patient; some patients desire to be pain free and have near normal function, whereas others simply want to return to daily activities and are willing to accommodate some dysfunction. Understanding a patient's goals and expectations can help guide treatment. In regard to conservative strategies, there is strong evidence to support NSAIDs, physical therapy, and steroid injections. These modalities have been proven to improve function and reduce pain in the short term.[123] A common misconception is that physical therapy and activity will worsen symptoms because osteoarthritis is often thought of as wear and tear. Physical activity has been shown time and again to offer improvement in function and relief of pain. Injections can also be helpful to alleviate inflammation in the short term, which may provide enough relief to start physical therapy.

When conservative treatments fail, hip arthroplasty is the most reliable surgical intervention. This surgery has consistently been rated as having a very high patient satisfaction.[124] Referral to an orthopedic surgeon should be considered if conservative measures fail to provide relief and if a patient is interested in undergoing surgical management.

Diagnosis of Chondral Injuries

Traumatic hip dislocation (THD) is a relatively rare injury. Dislocation of the hip is a true orthopedic emergency, requiring prompt reduction to reduce the risk of AVN of the femoral head. The hip joint is inherently very stable, with a high degree of bony conformity and stout surrounding capsular and ligamentous structures. A considerable amount of force, acting across the joint, is required to dislocate the joint. Traumatic dislocation of the hip joint is therefore the result of high-energy trauma, typically occurring in young adults.[125,126] Posterior dislocations of the hip represent 85% to 90% of all THDs.[126] A simple dislocation is one without a fracture. Complex fracture dislocations involve an associated fracture of the acetabulum and femoral head or neck. The reported rate of arthrosis after hip dislocation is 24% for simple dislocations and 88% for those associated with acetabular fractures.[127] Timely reduction is essential to the survival of the femoral head. Osteonecrosis has been reported to occur in 10% to 34% of hip dislocations[127] and depends on the severity of the injury and time between dislocation and reduction. Up to 58% of the patients may have subsequent hip osteonecrosis if the hip was reduced more than 6 hours after dislocation.[128]

A study of hip arthroscopy following posterior hip dislocations found intra-articular damage was demonstrated in every case. In the review of these 17 posterior hip dislocations, 14 had anterior labral tears, 6 had posterior labral tears, 16 had acetabular chondral damage, all had femoral chondral damage, and 14 had intra-articular fragments.[125] Obakponovwe et al[126] explain how in addition to the obvious joint disruption and soft tissue injury to the hip, associated fractures of the femur, acetabulum, and chondral disruptions of the femoral head are also common. These associated injuries not only compromise joint integrity but also inhibit joint recovery, leading to chronic morbidity of the affected joint.[126]

Subluxation of the hip joint is less clearly understood. Moorman et al[127] presented a study of 8 posterior hip subluxations in American football players and reported this injury likely occurs more commonly than is recognized as many hip sprains may actually represent traumatic hip subluxations.[127,129,130] The transient nature of the subluxation episode, the subtlety of the physical findings, and the difficulty of identifying small acetabular lip fractures on standard anteroposterior pelvic radiographs combine to make diagnosis a challenge. Despite the lower-energy trauma, osteonecrosis developed in 2 of the 8 patients in their small series.[127]

Although the cause of osteonecrosis following hip subluxation is not completely understood, Moorman et al[127] propose that intracapsular tamponade further reduces blood flow in patients in whom the extraosseous blood supply to the femoral head has been disrupted as the result of the hip subluxation. It has been suggested that increased pressure in the joint cavity may be sufficiently high to obstruct the blood flow to the femoral head and that aspiration of an intra-articular hematoma produces an increase in blood flow to the femoral head by relieving tamponade.[131-134] It is unclear why some have complete disruption of the capsule with hip subluxation and therefore decompression of the hematoma, while others do not. Additionally, Moorman et al[127] suggested that the intra-articular hematoma resulted in enzymatic degradation of the articular cartilage, whereby in addition to osteonecrosis, posttraumatic chondrolysis occurred as extensive joint-space narrowing was noted over a 3-month period without evidence of subchondral collapse.

Moorman et al[127] proposed that the radiographic workup of a patient who has a suspected hip subluxation should include radiographs (oblique views) to evaluate for posterior acetabular lip fracture. They noted how MRI in the acute period provides an evaluation of the iliofemoral ligament as well as the presence/size of a hemarthrosis. Magnetic resonance angiography would provide additional assessment of the circumflex vessels. The timing of MRI for the prediction of osteonecrosis has been somewhat controversial. A study by Poggi et al[135] demonstrated that MRI is not useful for the detection of osteonecrosis until 4 to 6 weeks following a THD. If the scan shows a normal marrow signal at 4 to 6 weeks, then the patient is at low risk for the development of osteonecrosis and no further imaging is necessary. If the MRI scan is abnormal, a repeat scan should be done at 3 months. If the initial marrow changes persist or worsen, the diagnosis of osteonecrosis can be made with confidence.

Injury and changes to the chondral surfaces of the hip are also seen in conjunction with other hip pathologies. It is reported that the presence of FAI syndrome, decreased acetabular anteversion, labral pathology, and developmental dysplasia of the hip will lead to an increased risk of chondropathy and ultimately osteoarthritis of the hip. In patients with significant labral pathology, chondral loss is often up to 70% of the full thickness. It is also proposed that the presence of longstanding synovitis may also affect the nutrition of chondral surfaces, possibly exacerbating chondral damage.[9] The clinical diagnosis of chondropathy may be confirmed with plain radiographs, although early chondral changes will not be visible. MRI may identify earlier chondral lesions, although the extent of chondropathy is often only evident on hip arthroscopy.[9]

Management of Chondral Injuries

Once a hip chondral injury has been confirmed, it is possible that hip aspiration and partial weightbearing may be appropriate management strategies to minimize the extent of the injury, and diminish the likelihood that this injury would progress to osteonecrosis.[127] Relative rest and/or anti-inflammatory strategies will also likely be of benefit in the early management of these injuries.

Physical therapy treatment goals for chondral injuries will be focused on 3 facets of treatment: (1) unload and protection of any healing and/or vulnerable structures, (2) optimizing mobility and motion of the hip joint, and (3) addressing any muscle imbalances, weaknesses, or instabilities found on the assessment. This will restore normal dynamic and neuromotor control around the hip joint in addition to addressing remote factors that may be altering the dynamics and function of the entire kinetic chain.[9]

Diagnosis of Capsular Injuries (Laxity Ehlers-Danlos Syndrome, Adhesions, Synovitis)

Ehlers-Danlos syndrome (EDS) is one of many heritable connective tissue disorders causing generalized joint hypermobility. EDS is characterized by major criteria of a Beighton score of 5 of 9 or greater[136,137] and skin hyperextensibility and

Table 9-6

BEIGHTON SCREEN FOR HYPERMOBILITY[136,137]

JOINT	FINDING
Left little (fifth) finger	Passive dorsiflexion beyond 90 degrees
Right little (fifth) finger	Passive dorsiflexion beyond 90 degrees
Left thumb	Passive dorsiflexion to the flexor aspect of the forearm
Right thumb	Passive dorsiflexion to the flexor aspect of the forearm
Left elbow	Hyperextends beyond 10 degrees
Right elbow	Hyperextends beyond 10 degrees
Left knee	Hyperextends beyond 10 degrees
Right knee	Hyperextends beyond 10 degrees
Forward flexion of trunk with knees fully extended	Palms and hands can rest flat on the floor

minor criteria including recurring joint dislocations and chronic joint pain. The Beighton screen for hypermobility is outlined in Table 9-6. The primary orthopedic feature of EDS is capsuloligamentous laxity.[138-140] Additionally, flexible acrobats and athletes such as contortion artists, dancers, cheerleaders, and gymnasts with hip pain are a challenging population because of the extreme ROM requirements for their sports and compensatory soft tissue laxity. As a result, they are able to place their hips in impinging positions even in the setting of normal osseous anatomy and often have combinations of impingement and instability. These hips are complex, and decision making regarding biomechanical abnormalities can be challenging.[141]

Synovitis is often seen in active individuals with other intra-articular hip problems—FAI syndrome, labral tears, ligamentum teres tears, or chondropathy. Synovitis has been found coexisting in 70% of athletes with hip joint pathology and therefore is rarely seen as a primary entity.[142] Synovitis can cause considerable pain in the hip joint, with night pain and resting pain being common presentations.

Kemp explains how there are considerable alterations in muscle activation around the hip in the presence of hip pain.[9] Kemp further highlights the implications of synovial dysfunction on cytokine production, nutrition, and hydration of articular cartilage in a joint that may already show signs of chondropathy, outlining how inflammation of the synovial structures may accelerate the deterioration of chondral tissue and thereby have long-term consequences for the health of the hip joint.[9]

Synovitis may contribute to stiffness and motion limitations in the hip joint. Both capsular contractions and intra-articular adhesions will result in a lack of active and accessory motion within the hip joint. The diagnosis of capsular laxity (hypermobility), inflammation (synovitis), and contracture (adhesions) is typically made via clinical assessment utilizing generalized ROM (passive and active), accessory joint mobility (joint glides), and Beighton's score.

Management of Capsular Injuries

It is possible that arthroscopy may have a role in the management of painful capsular hypermobility. Larson et al[143] completed a retrospective study of 16 hips with confirmed EDS-hypermobility type that underwent hip arthroscopy for continued pain and capsular laxity. All patients had complaints of "giving way" and pain, an easily distractible hip with manual traction under fluoroscopy, and a patulous capsule at the time of surgery. Meticulous capsular plication, arthroscopic correction of FAI syndrome when present, and labral preservation led to dramatic improvements in functional outcomes and subjective stability without iatrogenic dislocations over a follow-up period averaging 44 months (range, 12 to 99 months).[143]

Physical therapy treatment goals for capsular injuries should be focused on controlling motion with optimal core and lower extremity alignment in the hypermobile population via stabilization-focused rehabilitation strategies. Conversely, treatment focused on optimizing motion in the stiff and/or inflamed hip joint may involve manual treatment techniques and active and passive therapeutic strategies such as joint mobilizations, traction, passive motion, mobility exercises, low resistance cycling, and deep water running. Mobility activities including joint mobilizations, low-load repetitive motion activities (eg, cycling with minimal resistance) often facilitate joint lubrication and nutrition in addition to joint motion. Prolonged stretches are also beneficial for increasing the length of any concurrently shortened connective tissue structures. To ensure optimal function, it is important that the clinician address any muscle imbalances, weaknesses, or instabilities in both these diagnostic groups found on their assessment; again, the aim is to restore normal dynamic and neuromotor control around the hip joint while considering remote factors that may be altering the dynamics and function of the entire kinetic chain.[9]

Diagnosis of Extra-Articular Injuries

Musculotendinous strains of the lower extremity are among the most common injuries in sports. Injury typically occurs during an eccentric load and is typically located at the musculotendinous junction. Muscles at the highest injury risk are "two-joint" muscles, such as the hamstring muscles. Muscle strains can range from minimal tissue disruption with a low-grade inflammatory response to complete disruption of the musculotendinous unit (ruptures) with grossly visible and palpable damage and complete loss of function of the unit.[14]

Gluteus medius strains and tendinitis have been noted to be frequent causes of hip pain. Lloyd-Smith et al[144] report gluteus medius injuries accounted for 18% of total hip and pelvis injuries. Gluteus medius insertion tendonitis can be challenging to differentiate from trochanteric bursitis as both are tender in the region of the greater trochanter and both can be painful with resisted hip abduction. Mechanism of injury is thought to be related to the seesaw tilt action of the pelvis (Trendelenburg) when running. Uneven terrain and/or leg-length discrepancies (greater than 2.5 cm) exacerbate this action and concurrently increase the stress involved with dynamic pelvic stabilization.[144]

Adductor strains are frequently seen in activities requiring quick direction changes such as hockey, soccer, football, high jump, and skiing. These injuries typically occur at the muscle-tendon junction with less severe injuries commonly occurring in the muscle belly. Adductor longus is the most frequently involved. It has been described that the typical mechanism of injury involves a sudden eccentric load via forced external rotation of an adducted leg. The clinical presentation typically includes pain with passive abduction, resisted adduction, and tenderness along the border of the pubic ramus.[14]

Hamstrings injuries have been described as the most frequently strained muscle in the body and are often seen in running, sprinting, soccer, football, and rugby. Recurrence is common with hamstring strains. Most of the hamstring activity is eccentric to decelerate walking or running activities. There has been some support for the theory that an imbalance in strength of the hamstrings bilaterally or in comparison with the quadriceps predisposes an individual to hamstring injury.[145] There has also been some support for a relationship between hamstring flexibility and hamstring injury.[145,146] Most injuries to the hamstrings are mild to moderate strains, but occasionally the tendon is avulsed from the tendon-bone interface. The patient may report to have heard or felt a pop during activity, accompanied by immediate pain. Physical examination reveals tenderness, limited passive straight leg raise, and limited strength. There may be a notable defect in the muscle. Imaging can be useful to determine the severity of the injury. Chronic hamstring injuries have been noted to occur due to insufficient rehabilitation or inappropriate progression of activities.[147,148]

Contusions occur when a direct blow produces significant bruising in and around a muscle (often in the proximity of a bony prominence such as the iliac crest or greater trochanter). This type of injury is associated with localized pain and swelling, decreased motion, and occasionally a palpable mass or hematoma.[149] Hip pointer is a nonspecific term and generally refers to contusion of the iliac crest over the tensor fascia lata muscle belly with an associated hematoma, but it may include tearing of the external oblique muscle from the iliac crest, periostitis of the iliac crest, and trochanteric contusions. Contusions of the anterolateral thigh are quite common. The region of the contusion is exquisitely tender to palpation, swelling is present and motion of the surrounding structures will be limited.[14]

Myositis ossificans is the development of heterotopic bone in soft tissue adjacent to bone and associated with trauma, surgery, or disease. It is a frequent complication of a muscular contusion.[14] Contusions are usually viewed as minor injuries and thus are not treated with much concern, although appropriate management of this initial injury can prevent or lessen the development of myositis ossificans. The symptoms include a palpable, painful mass associated with progressive loss of motion in the involved muscle and its associated region. There are several risk factors: continued activity or premature return to activity after injury, early massage to the injured area, heat application to the area, rapid progression in rehabilitation, passive forceful stretching, re-injury of the same area, and an innate predisposition to ectopic bone formation. Symptoms and findings may be confused with a femoral stress fracture or neoplasm. Clinical findings may also include the persistence of warmth to palpation at the site of injury, or the palpation of increasing induration in the hematoma. Radiographic signs of this injury are typically present by weeks 3 to 6. The initial appearance is that of fluffy calcification with indistinct margins in the soft tissue adjacent to the bony margins. As the lesion matures, it enlarges, margins become more distinct, and it may coalesce with the neighboring bone.[14]

Three major bursae around the hip are susceptible to bursitis: iliopsoas (iliopectineal), greater trochanteric, and the ischial bursa. Bursitis is an inflammation of the bursal sac and this typically occurs from either trauma (direct blows and contusions) or from excessive friction and shear forces. There is tenderness to palpation of the bursal region, and motion may be limited should any structures contact/compress the irritated bursal sacs. Gait may be disturbed and typically the symptoms progress with increased activity (continued friction to the inflamed bursal tissues).[150]

A snapping hip syndrome has been described as having a variety of intra-articular causes (synovial chondromatosis, loose bodies, osteocartilaginous exostosis, and subluxation of the hip)[151] and extra-articular causes. The most common extra-articular cause is snapping of the iliotibial band over the great trochanter (which can also result in trochanteric bursitis). Snapping can also arise from the iliopsoas tendon fractioning over the iliopectineal eminence, the iliofemoral ligaments over the femoral head, and the long head of biceps femoris over the ischial tuberosity.[152-154] The snapping hip is common and most complaints concern the sound or sensation rather than pain. This condition is generally present with specific flexion maneuvers of the hip. Should pain be present, evaluation for contributing factors should be completed and treatment directed toward these factors—muscle tightness, muscle imbalance, poor training techniques and/or biomechanics of movement.[14]

Osteitis pubis is an inflammatory condition involving the pubic symphysis. The pain is insidious and may radiate into the groin or medial thigh. The characteristic finding is pain over the pubic symphysis. Early on, mild radiographic changes may be apparent, such as mild widening of the pubic symphysis, erosion along the cortical margins, and sclerotic reactive bone in the metaphyseal regions around the symphysis. In the chronic form, this area can appear moth-eaten on x-ray film. The precise cause of this problem is unknown, although it has been thought to be a traction injury at the origin of muscles from the pubic symphysis, where the adductor longus and brevis and gracilis musculature originate. This may also be an overuse or bone stress reaction injury.[155-157] It is found in athletes whose sports involve kicking and rapid accelerations, decelerations, and abrupt directional changes. Athletes most commonly present with a complaint of anterior and/or medial groin pain, but also can present with lower abdominal, adductor, inguinal, perineal, and/or scrotal pain. Symptoms can be severe and can limit activity participation until treatment is instituted. Imaging is useful for ruling out other etiologies of groin pain, identifying concomitant pathology, and confirming the diagnosis itself.[157]

Another condition that causes anterior pubic or groin pain is called core muscle injury,[158,159] or commonly known as *athletic pubalgia* or *sports hernia*. This condition results from fraying or tearing of the abdominal musculature from the pubic bone and is not associated with herniation of abdominal contents. This condition is common in sports that require repetitive pivoting and cutting. Patients may complain of pain during activity, with cessation of symptoms during inactivity.[160] Diagnosis can be made with pain during a resisted sit-up or with palpation of the superior pubic bones. Management begins with conservative measures and steroid injections, but this condition often requires surgical intervention.

Less commonly, conditions affecting the pelvic floor may also result in hip pain. While possible in men, this condition affects women much more frequently.[161] Conditions that can lead to pelvic floor incompetence include pelvic trauma and/or fractures, surgery, congenital deformity, hormonal imbalance, or from connective tissue disease. The most common symptoms are urinary incontinence and dyspareunia. If pain radiates, it is often described as being localized to the buttock or posterior thigh. Management usually consists of pelvic floor exercises.[162]

Management of Extra-Articular Injuries

The initial treatment of an acute extra-articular injury typically involves rest, ice, compression, and elevation. Comprehensive treatment likely includes stretching to improve motion, strengthening exercises, support bandaging and/or taping, and medication. Medication options include analgesics, NSAIDs, and occasionally steroids. Surgical intervention is rare but can be beneficial when there is significant tissue disruption or chronic tissue irritation that has minimally responded to conservative care. Prevention is a key component in managing muscle strains. Optimizing muscle strength, length, and warmup strategies, in addition to minimizing fatigue have been described to minimize muscular, tendon, and bone reaction injuries.[14]

Early treatment of myositis ossificans consists of rest, and even immobilization, anti-inflammatory agents accompanied by frequent reevaluation. Initiation and progression of activity and rehabilitation should be slow and cautious. Activity progresses when the bone mass shows signs of stabilizing or maturing. Surgery is indicated only to reduce the mass effect of the ectopic bone and should never be done until a bone scan shows quiescence of activity, generally 9 to 12 months after injury, as early surgery usually results in recurrence. Prevention of myositis ossificans is the best treatment. Clinicians, patients, and coaches should understand the seriousness of this injury and recognize the need for careful and considerate progressive activity and rehabilitation.[14]

Physical therapy treatment goals for extracapsular injuries should be focused on optimizing tissue healing and addressing any muscle imbalances, weaknesses, or instabilities found on their assessment as these likely had a role in contributing to the inflammation of the specific structure that has presented as hip pain. Often a tight/restrictive connective tissue presents with a concurrent weakness (tight hip flexor can accompany a weak hip adductor and/or extensor, tight iliopsoas and/or iliotibial band, weak gluteals). Physical therapy can also use manual treatment techniques to optimize motion (joint and soft tissue mobilizations/manipulations) and anti-inflammatory strategies (electrotherapeutic and mechanotherapeutic).[163]

Diagnosis of Systemic Problems About the Hip

As with other joints, it is critical to remember the many systemic diagnoses that could manifest as primary hip pain. This could include tumors, nerve impingement (eg, meralgia paresthetica—compression/injury to the lateral femoral cutaneous nerve), complex regional pain syndrome, rheumatoid arthritis, and metabolic disturbances. With a confusing or complex presentation, one might entertain these less common diagnoses and order appropriate workup and testing (eg, blood testing, electromyography/nerve conduction velocity, neurologic, rheumatologic consultation).

CONCLUSION

This chapter should serve as a good starting point for the clinician evaluating individuals with pain in and around the hip. Using sound principles of obtaining a thorough history, performing a directed physical examination, and utilizing appropriate diagnostic studies will allow the clinician to accurately and predictably understand and treat those with pain around the hip complex.

REFERENCES

1. Griffin DR, Dickenson EJ, O'Donnell J, et al. The Warwick Agreement on femoroacetabular impingement syndrome (FAI syndrome): an international consensus statement. *Br J Sports Med.* 2016;50(19):1169-1176.

2. Radin EL. Biomechanics of the human hip. *Clin Orthop.* 1980;152:28-34.

3. Beattie P. The hip. In: *Orthopedic and Sports Physical Therapy.* Mosby; 1997:459-508.

4. Stähelin L, Stähelin T, Jolles BM, Herzog RF. Arthroscopic offset restoration in femoroacetabular cam impingement: accuracy and early clinical outcome. *Arthroscopy.* 2008;24(1):51-57.e1.

5. Crawford MJ, Dy CJ, Alexander JW, et al. The 2007 Frank Stinchfield Award. The biomechanics of the hip labrum and the stability of the hip. *Clin Orthop.* 2007;(465):16-22.

6. Teichtahl AJ, Smith S, Wang Y, et al. Occupational risk factors for hip osteoarthritis are associated with early hip structural abnormalities: a 3.0 T magnetic resonance imaging study of community-based adults. *Arthritis Res Ther.* 2015;17(1):19.

7. Philippon MJ, Weiss DR, Kuppersmith DA, Briggs KK, Hay CJ. Arthroscopic labral repair and treatment of femoroacetabular impingement in professional hockey players. *Am J Sports Med.* 2010;38(1):99-104.

8. Nepple JJ, Riggs CN, Ross JR, Clohisy JC. Clinical presentation and disease characteristics of femoroacetabular impingement are sex-dependent. *J Bone Joint Surg Am.* 2014;96(20):1683-1689.

9. Kemp J, Crossley K, Schache A, Pritchard M. Hip-related pain. In: Brukner P, Khan K, eds, *Clinical Sports Medicine.* 4th ed. McGraw-Hill; 2012:510-544.

10. Tanzer M, Noiseux N. Osseous abnormalities and early osteoarthritis: the role of hip impingement. *Clin Orthop Relat Res.* 2004;(429):170-177.

11. McCarthy J, Noble P, Aluisio FV, Schuck M, Wright J, Lee J. Anatomy, pathologic features, and treatment of acetabular labral tears. *Clin Orthop Relat Res.* 2003;(406):38-47.

12. Ito K, Minka MA Jr, Leunig M, Werlen S, Ganz R. Femoroacetabular impingement and the cam-effect: a MRI-based quantitative anatomical study of the femoral head-neck offset. *J Bone Joint Surg Br.* 2001;83(2):171-176.

13. Nepple JJ, Carlisle JC, Nunley RM, Clohisy JC. Clinical and radiographic predictors of intra-articular hip disease in arthroscopy. *Am J Sports Med.* 2011;39(2):296-303.

14. Sanders B, Nemeth W. Hip and thigh injuries. In: Zachazewski JE, Magee DJ, Quillen WS, eds, *Athletic Injuries and Rehabilitation.* WB Saunders Company; 1996:599-622.

15. Vogl W, Mitchell AWM, Drack RL. *Gray's Anatomy for Students.* 3rd ed. Churchill Livingstone; 2015.

16. Dewar DC, Lazaro LE, Klinger CE, et al. The relative contribution of the medial and lateral femoral circumflex arteries to the vascularity of the head and neck of the femur: a quantitative MRI-based assessment. *Bone Joint J.* 2016;98-B(12):1582-1588.

17. Neumann DA. Kinesiology of the hip: a focus on muscular actions. *J Orthop Sports Phys Ther.* 2010;40(2):82-94.

18. Field RE, Rajakulendran K. The labro-acetabular complex. *J Bone Joint Surg Am.* 2011;93(suppl 2):22-27.

19. de Sa D, Phillips M, Philippon MJ, Letkemann S, Simunovic N, Ayeni OR. Ligamentum teres injuries of the hip: a systematic review examining surgical indications, treatment options, and outcomes. *Arthroscopy.* 2014;30(12):1634-1641.

20. O'Donnell JM, Devitt BM, Arora M. The role of the ligamentum teres in the adult hip: redundant or relevant? A review. *J Hip Preserv Surg.* 2018;5(1):15-22.

21. Moraes MRB, Cavalcante MLC, Leite JAD, et al. The characteristics of the mechanoreceptors of the hip with arthrosis. *J Orthop Surg Res.* 2011;6:58.

22. Phillips A, Bartlett G, Norton M, Fern D. Ligamentum teres: vital or vestigial? *Orthopaedic Proceedings.* 2018;94-B(suppl XLII).

23. Petersen W, Petersen F, Tillmann B. Structure and vascularization of the acetabular labrum with regard to the pathogenesis and healing of labral lesions. *Arch Orthop Trauma Surg.* 2003;123(6):283-288.

24. Safran M. The acetabular labrum: anatomic and functional characteristics and rationale for surgical intervention. *J Am Acad Orthop Surg.* 2010;18(6):338-345.

25. Hosokawa O. Histological study on the type and distribution of the sensory nerve endings in human hip joint capsule and ligament. *Nippon Seikeigeka Gakkai Zasshi.* 1964;38:887-901.

26. Kim Y, Azuma H. The nerve-endings of the acetabular labrum. *Clin Orthop Relat Res.* 1995;(320):176-181.

27. Tan V, Seldes RM, Katz MA, Freedhand AM, Klimkiewicz JJ, Fitzgerald RH Jr. Contribution of acetabular labrum to articulating surface area and femoral head coverage in adult hip joints: an anatomic study in cadavera. *Am J Orthop.* 2001;30(11):809-812.

28. Buckwalter JA, Einhorn TA, Simon SR. *Orthopaedic Basic Science: Biology and Biomechanics of the Musculoskeletal System.* American Academy of Orthopaedic Surgeons; 2000:782-788.

29. Crawford MJ, Dy CJ, Alexander JW, et al. The biomechanics of the hip labrum and the stability of the hip. *Clin Orthop Relat Res.* 2007;(465):16-22.

30. Ferguson SJ, Bryant JT, Ganz R, Ito K. An in vitro investigation of the acetabular labral seal in hip joint mechanics. *J Biomech.* 2003;36(2):171-178.

31. Hansen JT. *Netter's Clinical Anatomy.* 3rd ed. Saunders; 2014.

32. Hewitt JD, Glisson RR, Guilak F, Vail TP. The mechanical properties of the human hip capsule ligaments. *J Arthroplasty.* 2002;17(1):82-89.

33. Bowman KF, Fox J, Sekiya JK. A clinically relevant review of hip biomechanics. *Arthroscopy.* 2010;26(8):1118-1129.

34. Krebs DE, Robbins CE, Lavine L, Mann RW. Hip biomechanics during gait. *J Orthop Sports Phys Ther.* 1998;28(1):51-59.

35. Hardcastle P, Nade S. The significance of the Trendelenburg test. *J Bone Joint Surg Br.* 1985;67(5):741-746.

36. Cyriax J. *Textbook of Orthopaedic Medicine. Volume 1: Diagnosis of Soft Tissue Lesions.* Baillière Tindall; 1982.

37. Magee DJ. *Orthopedic Physical Assessment.* 6th ed. Elsevier Saunders; 2014.

38. Cleland JA, Koppenhaver S, Su J. *Netter's Orthopaedic Clinical Examination: An Evidence-Based Approach.* 3rd ed. Elsevier; 2016.

39. Safran MR, Giordano G, Lindsey DP, et al. Strains across the acetabular labrum during hip motion: a cadaveric model. *Am J Sports Med.* 2011;39(suppl 1):92S-102S.

40. Narvani AA, Tsiridis E, Kendall S, Chaudhuri R, Thomas P. A preliminary report on prevalence of acetabular labrum tears in sports patients with groin pain. *Knee Surg Sports Traumatol Arthrosc.* 2003;11(6):403-408.

41. Schon L, Zuckerman JD. Hip pain in the elderly: evaluation and diagnosis. *Geriatrics.* 1988;43(1):48-62.

42. Hertling D, Kessler RM. *Management of Common Musculoskeletal Disorders: Physical Therapy Principles and Methods.* 3rd ed. Lippincott; 1996.

43. Pecina MM, Bojanic I. *Overuse Injuries of the Musculoskeletal System.* CRC Press; 1993.

44. Altman R, Alarcón G, Appelrouth D, et al. The American College of Rheumatology criteria for the classification and reporting of osteoarthritis of the hip. *Arthritis Rheum.* 1991;34(5):505-514.

45. Hartley A. *Practical Joint Assessment Lower Quadrant: A Sports Medicine Manual.* Mosby; 1995.

46. Plante M, Wallace R, Busconi BD. Clinical diagnosis of hip pain. *Clin Sports Med.* 2011;30(2):225-238.

47. Clohisy JC, Knaus ER, Hunt DM, Lesher JM, Harris-Hayes M, Prather H. Clinical presentation of patients with symptomatic anterior hip impingement. *Clin Orthop Relat Res.* 2009;467(3):638-644.

48. Fishman LM, Dombi GW, Michaelsen C, et al. Piriformis syndrome: diagnosis, treatment, and outcome—a 10-year study. *Arch Phys Med Rehabil.* 2002;83(3):295-301.

49. Andersen RE, Crespo CJ, Bartlett SJ, Bathon JM, Fontaine KR. Relationship between body weight gain and significant knee, hip, and back pain in older Americans. *Obes Res.* 2003;11(10):1159-1162.

50. Gaida JE, Ashe MC, Bass SL, Cook JL. Is adiposity an under-recognized risk factor for tendinopathy? A systematic review. *Arthritis Rheum.* 2009;61(6):840-849.

51. Gaida JE, Cook JL, Bass SL. Adiposity and tendinopathy. *Disabil Rehabil.* 2008;30(20-22):1555-1562.

52. Franceschi F, Papalia R, Paciotti M, et al. Obesity as a risk factor for tendinopathy: a systematic review. *Int J Endocrinol.* 2014;2014:670262.

53. Reijman M, Pols HAP, Bergink AP, et al. Body mass index associated with onset and progression of osteoarthritis of the knee but not of the hip: the Rotterdam study. *Ann Rheum Dis.* 2007;66(2):158-162.

54. Myers AM, Holliday PJ, Harvey KA, Hutchinson KS. Functional performance measures: are they superior to self-assessments? *J Gerontol.* 1993;48(5):M196-M206.

55. Woolf SH, Chan ECY, Harris R, et al. Promoting informed choice: transforming health care to dispense knowledge for decision making. *Ann Intern Med.* 2005;143(4):293-300.

56. Guccione AA, Mielenz TJ, Devellis RF, et al. Development and testing of a self-report instrument to measure actions: outpatient physical therapy improvement in movement assessment log (OPTIMAL). *Phys Ther.* 2005;85(6):515-530.

57. Pua Y-H, Cowan SM, Wrigley TV, Bennell KL. The Lower Extremity Functional Scale could be an alternative to the Western Ontario and McMaster Universities Osteoarthritis Index physical function scale. *J Clin Epidemiol.* 2009;62(10):1103-1111.

58. Harris WH. Traumatic arthritis of the hip after dislocation and acetabular fractures: treatment by mold arthroplasty. An end-result study using a new method of result evaluation. *J Bone Joint Surg Am.* 1969;51(4):737-755.

59. Nilsdotter A, Bremander A. Measures of hip function and symptoms: Harris Hip Score (HHS), Hip Disability and Osteoarthritis Outcome Score (HOOS), Oxford Hip Score (OHS), Lequesne Index of Severity for Osteoarthritis of the Hip (LISOH), and American Academy of Orthopedic Surgeons (AAOS) Hip and Knee Questionnaire. *Arthritis Care Res.* 2011;63(S11):S200-S207.

60. Tijssen M, van Cingel R, van Melick N, de Visser E. Patient-reported outcome questionnaires for hip arthroscopy: a systematic review of the psychometric evidence. *BMC Musculoskelet Disord.* 2011;12:117.

61. Mehta SP, Fulton A, Quach C, Thistle M, Toledo C, Evans NA. Measurement properties of the Lower Extremity Functional Scale: a systematic review. *J Orthop Sports Phys Ther.* 2016;46(3):200-216.

62. Binkley JM, Stratford PW, Lott SA, Riddle DL. The Lower Extremity Functional Scale (LEFS): scale development, measurement properties, and clinical application. North American Orthopaedic Rehabilitation Research Network. *Phys Ther.* 1999;79(4):371-383.

63. Cleland J. *Orthopaedic Clinical Examination: An Evidence-Based Approach for Physical Therapists.* Saunders Elsevier; 2007.

64. Harris-Hayes M, McDonough CM, Leunig M, Lee CB, Callaghan JJ, Roos EM. Clinical outcomes assessment in clinical trials to assess treatment of femoroacetabular impingement: use of patient-reported outcome measures. *J Am Acad Orthop Surg.* 2013;21(suppl 1):S39-S46.

65. Dwyer MK, Green M, McCarthy JC. Assessing outcomes following arthroscopic labral debridement—what can the IHOT-33 reveal? *J Hip Preserv Surg.* 2015;2(2):152-157.

66. Harris-Hayes M, McDonough CM, Leunig M, Lee CB, Callaghan JJ, Roos EM. Clinical outcomes assessment in clinical trials to assess treatment of femoroacetabular impingement: use of patient-reported outcome measures. *J Am Acad Orthop Surg.* 2013;21(suppl 1):S39-S46.

67. Nwachukwu BU, Chang B, Beck EC, et al. How should we define clinically significant outcome improvement on the iHOT-12? *HSS J.* 2019;15(2):103-108.

68. Byrd JWT. Evaluation of the hip: history and physical examination. *N Am J Sports Phys Ther.* 2007;2(4):231-240.

69. Sutlive TG, Lopez HP, Schnitker DE, et al. Development of a clinical prediction rule for diagnosing hip osteoarthritis in individuals with unilateral hip pain. *J Orthop Sports Phys Ther.* 2008;38(9):542-550.

70. Cleland JA, Koppenhaver S, Su J. *Netter's Orthopaedic Clinical Examination: An Evidence-Based Approach.* 3rd ed. Elsevier; 2016.

71. Tis LL, Perrin DH, Snead DB, Weltman A. Isokinetic strength of the trunk and hip in female runners. *Isokinetics and Exercise Science.* 1991;1(1):22-25.

72. Donatelli R, Catlin PA, Backer GS, Drane DL, Slater SM. Isokinetic hip abductor to adductor torque ratio in normals. *Isokinetics and Exercise Science.* 1991;1(2):103-111.

73. Kelly BT, Williams RJ III, Philippon MJ. Hip arthroscopy: current indications, treatment options, and managment issues. *Am J Sports Med.* 2003;31(6):1020-1037.

74. Hegedus EJ, Cook C. *Orthopedic Physical Examination Tests: An Evidence-Based Approach.* 2nd ed. Pearson; 2013.

75. Mitchell B, McCrory P, Brukner P, O'Donnell J, Colson E, Howells R. Hip joint pathology: clinical presentation and correlation between magnetic resonance arthrography, ultrasound, and arthroscopic findings in 25 consecutive cases. *Clin J Sport Med.* 2003;13(3):152-156.

76. Reiman MP, Goode AP, Cook CE, Hölmich P, Thorborg K. Diagnostic accuracy of clinical tests for the diagnosis of hip femoroacetabular impingement/labral tear: a systematic review with meta-analysis. *Br J Sports Med.* 2015;49(12):811.

77. Reiman MP, Goode AP, Hegedus EJ, Cook CE, Wright AA. Diagnostic accuracy of clinical tests of the hip: a systematic review with meta-analysis. *Br J Sports Med.* 2013;47(14):893-902.

78. Reiman MP, Thorborg K. Clinical examination and physical assessment of hip joint-related pain in athletes. *Int J Sports Phys Ther.* 2014;9(6):737-755.

79. Robertson K, Burnham J, Yonz C, Akash P, Ireland ML, Noehren B. The relationship between hip strength and the Y balance test. (Report). *Medicine and Science in Sports and Exercise.* 2014;46(5):693.

80. Overmoyer GV, Reiser RF. Relationships between lower-extremity flexibility, asymmetries, and the Y balance test. *J Strength Cond Res.* 2015;29(5):1240-1247.

81. Stiffler MR, Sanfilippo JL, Brooks MA, Heiderscheit BC. Star Excursion Balance Test performance varies by sport in healthy division I collegiate athletes. *J Orthop Sports Phys Ther.* 2015;45(10):772-780. doi:10.2519/jospt.2015.5777. PMID:26304643.

82. Overmoyer GV, Reiser RF. Relationships between asymmetries in functional movements and the star excursion balance test. *J Strength Cond Res.* 2013;27(7):2013-2024.

83. Brukner P, Khan K. *Brukner & Khan's Clinical Sports Medicine.* 4th ed. McGraw-Hill; 2012.

84. Bushman TT, Grier TL, Canham-Chervak M, Anderson MK, North WJ, Jones BH. The Functional Movement Screen and injury risk. *Am J Sports Med.* 2016;44(2):297-304.

85. Cook G, Burton L, Hoogenboom B. Pre-participation screening: the use of fundamental movements as an assessment of function-part 1. *N Am J Sports Phys Ther.* 2006;1(2):62-72.

86. Cook G, Burton L, Hoogenboom B. Pre-participation screening: the use of fundamental movements as an assessment of function-part 2. *N Am J Sports Phys Ther.* 2006;1(3):132-139.

87. Garrison JC, Shanley E, Thigpen C, Geary R, Osler M, DelGiorno J. The reliability of the vail sport test as a measure of physical performance following anterior cruciate ligament reconstruction. *Int J Sports Phys Ther.* 2012;7(1):20-30.

88. Kokmeyer D, Wahoff M, Mymern M. Suggestions from the field for return-to-sport rehabilitation following anterior cruciate ligament reconstruction: alpine skiing. *J Orthop Sports Phys Ther.* 2012;42(4):313-325.

89. Hegedus EJ, McDonough SM, Bleakley C, Baxter D, Cook CE. Clinician-friendly lower extremity physical performance tests in athletes: a systematic review of measurement properties and correlation with injury. Part 2—the tests for the hip, thigh, foot and ankle including the star excursion balance test. *Br J Sports Med.* 2015;49(10):649-656.

90. Expert Panel on Musculoskeletal Imaging; Mintz DN, Roberts CC, Bencardino JT, et al. ACR appropriateness criteria chronic hip pain. *J Am Coll Radiol.* 2017;14(5S):S90-S102.

91. Jacobson JA, van Holsbeeck MT. Musculoskeletal ultrasonography. *Orthopedic Clinics of North America.* 1998;29(1):135-167.

92. Suarez J, Ely EE, Mutnal AB, et al. Comprehensive approach to the evaluation of groin pain. *J Am Acad Orthop Surg.* 2013;21(9):558-570.

93. US Food & Drug Administration. What are the radiation risks from CT? December 5, 2017. Accessed November 29, 2021. https://www.fda.gov/radiation-emitting-products/medical-x-ray-imaging/what-are-radiation-risks-ct

94. Armfield DR, Towers JD, Robertson DD. Clinical evaluation of the hip: radiologic evaluation. *Operative Techniques in Orthopaedics.* 2005;15(3):182-190.

95. Forstein DA, Bernadini C, Cole RE, Harris ST, Singer A. Before the breaking point: reducing the risk of osteoporotic fracture. *J Am Osteopath Assoc.* 2013;113(2 Suppl 1):S5-S24.

96. Amis ES, Butler P F, Applegate KE, et al. American College of Radiology white paper on radiation dose in medicine. *J Am Coll Radiol.* 2007;4(5):272-284.

97. Commission, U.S.N.R., Lethal Dose. Updated March 9, 2021. Accessed April 24, 2023. https://www.nrc.gov/reading-rm/basic-ref/glossary/lethal-dose-ld.html

98. Ofori K, Gordon SW, Akrobortu E, Ampene AA, Darko EO. Estimation of adult patient doses for selected x-ray diagnostic examinations. *Journal of Radiation Research and Applied Sciences.* 2014;7(4):459-462.

99. Jordan DW, Becker M, Brady S, et al. ACR Appropriateness Criteria Radiation Dose Assessment Introduction. 2017. Revised February 2020. Accessed April 24, 2023. https://www.acr.org/-/media/ACR/Files/Appropriateness-Criteria/RadiationDoseAssessmentIntro.pdf

100. National Radiology Data Registry: American College of Radiology. Radiology, A.C.o., National Radiology Data Registry Semiannual Report - Adult. 2016.

101. Leibold MR, Huijbregts PA, Jensen R. Concurrent criterion-related validity of physical examination tests for hip labral lesions: a systematic review. *J Man Manip Ther.* 2008;16(2):E24-E41.

102. Keeney JA, Peelle MW, Jackson J, Rubin D, Maloney WJ, Clohisy JC. Magnetic resonance arthrography versus arthroscopy in the evaluation of articular hip pathology. *Clin Orthop Relat Res.* 2004;(429):163-169.

103. Stubbs AJ, Atilla HA. The hip restoration algorithm. *Muscles Ligaments Tendons J.* 2016;6(3):300-308.

104. Ganz R, Gill TJ, Gautier E, Ganz K, Krügel N, Berlemann U. Surgical dislocation of the adult hip: a technique with full access to the femoral head and acetabulum without the risk of avascular necrosis. *J Bone Joint Surg Br.* 2001;83(8):1119-1124.

105. Ganz R, Parvizi J, Beck M, Leunig M, Nötzli H, Siebenrock KA. Femoroacetabular impingement—a cause for osteoarthritis of the hip. *Clin Orthop Relat Res.* 2003;(417):112-120.

106. Griffin DR, Dickenson EJ, O'Donnell J, et al. The Warwick Agreement on femoroacetabular impingement syndrome (FAI syndrome): an international consensus statement. *Br J Sports Med.* 2016;50(19):1169-1176.

107. Eijer H, Leunig M, Mahomed MN, Ganz R. Cross table lateral radiographs for screening of anterior femoral head-neck offset in patients with femoro-acetabular impingement. *Hip Int.* 2001;11(1):37-41.

108. Audenaert EA, Peeters I, Vigneron L, Baelde N, Pattyn C. Hip morphological characteristics and range of internal rotation in femoroacetabular impingement. *Am J Sports Med.* 2012;40(6):1329-1336.

109. Reynolds D, Lucas J, Klaue K. Retroversion of the acetabulum. A cause of hip pain. *J Bone Joint Surg Br.* 1999;81(2):281-288.

110. Byrd JWT. Femoroacetabular impingement in athletes. *Am J Sports Med.* 2014;42(3):737-751.

111. Zaltz I, Kelly BT, Hetsroni I, Bedi A. The crossover sign overestimates acetabular retroversion. *Clin Orthop Relat Res.* 2013;471(8):2463-2470.

112. Nötzli H, Wyss TF, Stoecklin CH, Schmid MR, Treiber K, Hodler J. The contour of the femoral head-neck junction as a predictor for the risk of anterior impingement. *J Bone Joint Surg Br.* 2002;84(4):556-560.

113. Eijer H, Leunig M, Mahomed MN, Ganz R. Cross table lateral radiographs for screening of anterior femoral head-neck offset in patients with femoro-acetabular impingement. *Hip Int.* 2001;11(1):37-41.

114. Anderson LA, Gililland J, Pelt C, Linford S, Stoddard GJ, Peters CL. Center edge angle measurement for hip preservation surgery: technique and caveats. *Orthopedics.* 2011;34(2):86.

115. Jaberi FM, Parvizi J. Hip pain in young adults: femoroacetabular impingement. *J Arthroplasty.* 2007;22(7):37.e1-42.e1.

116. Ward D, Parvizi J. Management of hip pain in young adults. *Orthop Clin North Am.* 2016;47(3):485-496.

117. Boykin RE, Anz AW, Bushnell BD, Kocher MS, Stubbs AJ, Philippon MJ. Hip instability. *J Am Acad Orthop Surg.* 2011;19(6):340-349.

118. Machotka Z, Kumar S, Perraton LG. A systematic review of the literature on the effectiveness of exercise therapy for groin pain in athletes. *Sports Med Arthrosc Rehabil Ther Technol.* 2009;1(1):5.

119. Kibler W, Press J, Sciascia A. The role of core stability in athletic function. *Sports Med.* 2006;36(3):189-198.

120. Casartelli NC, Maffiuletti NA, Bizzini M, Kelly BT, Naal FD, Leunig M. The management of symptomatic femoroacetabular impingement: what is the rationale for non-surgical treatment? *Br J Sports Med.* 2016;50(9):511-512.

121. Quinn RH, Murray J, Pezold R, Hall Q. Management of osteoarthritis of the hip. *J Am Acad Orthop Surg.* 2018;26(20):e434-e436.

122. Symposium on Population Studies in Relation to Chronic Rheumatic Diseases Symposium on Population Studies in Relation to Chronic Rheumatic Diseases; Kellegren JH, Jeffrey MR, Ball J. The epidemiology of chronic rheumatism; a symposium organized by the Council for International Organizations of Medical Sciences. Blackwell;1963.

123. The American Academy of Orthopaedic Surgeons. Management of osteoarthritis of the hip: evidence-based clinical practice guideline. Published March 13, 2017. Accessed February 20, 2023. https://www.aaos.org/oahcpg

124. Okafor L, Chen AF. Patient satisfaction and total hip arthroplasty: a review. *Arthroplasty*. 2019;1(1):6.

125. Ilizaliturri VM, Gonzalez-Gutierrez B, Gonzalez-Ugalde H, Camacho-Galindo J. Hip arthroscopy after traumatic hip dislocation. *Am J Sports Med*. 2011;39(1_suppl):50S-57S.

126. Obakponovwe O, Morell D, Ahmad M, Nunn T, Giannoudis PV. Traumatic hip dislocation. *Orthop Trauma*. 2011;25(3):214-222.

127. Moorman CT, Warren RF, Hershman EB, et al. Traumatic posterior hip subluxation in American football. *J Bone Joint Surg Am*. 2003;85(7):1190-1196.

128. Hougaard K, Thomsen PB. Coxarthrosis following traumatic posterior dislocation of the hip. *J Bone Joint Surg Am*. 1987;69(5):679-683.

129. Cooper DE, Warren RF, Barnes R. Traumatic subluxation of the hip resulting in aseptic necrosis and chondrolysis in a professional football player. *Am J Sports Med*. 1991;19(3):322-324.

130. Weiker GG, Munnings F. How I manage hip and pelvis injuries in adolescents. *Phys Sportsmed*. 1993;21(12):72-82.

131. Soto-Hall R, Johnson LH, Johnson RA. Variation in the intra-articular pressure of the hip joint in injury and disease. A probable factor in avascular necrosis. *J Bone Joint Surg Am*. 1964;46:509-516.

132. Crawfurd EJP, Emery RJ, Hansell DM, Phelan M, Andrews BG. Capsular distension and intracapsular pressure in subcapital fractures of the femur. *J Bone Joint Surg Br*. 1988;70(2):195-198.

133. Holmberg S, Dalen N. Intracapsular pressure and caput circulation in nondisplaced femoral neck fractures. *Clin Orthop Relat Res*. 1987;(219):124-126.

134. Harper WM, Barnes MR, Gregg PJ. Femoral head blood flow in femoral neck fractures. An analysis using intra-osseous pressure measurement. *J Bone Joint Surg Br*. 1991;73(1):73-75.

135. Poggi JJ, Callaghan JJ, Spritzer CE, Roark T, Goldner RD. Changes on magnetic-resonance images after traumatic hip dislocation. *Clin Orthop Relat Res*. 1995;(319):249-259.

136. Beighton P, Solomon L, Soskolne CL. Articular mobility in an African population. *Ann Rheum Dis*. 1973;32(5):413-418.

137. Smits-Engelsman B, Klerks M, Kirby A. Beighton score: a valid measure for generalized hypermobility in children. *J Pediatr*. 2011;158(1):130.e4-134.e4.

138. Castori M. Ehlers-Danlos syndrome, hypermobility type: an underdiagnosed hereditary connective tissue disorder with mucocutaneous, articular, and systemic manifestations. *ISRN Dermatol*. 2012;2012:751768.

139. Sobey G. Ehlers-Danlos syndrome—a commonly misunderstood group of conditions. *Clin Med*. 2014;14(4):432-436.

140. Castori M. Joint hypermobility syndrome (a.k.a. Ehlers-Danlos syndrome, hypermobility type): an updated critique. *Giornale Italiano Di Dermatologia E Venereologia*. 2013;148(1):13-36.

141. Weber AE, Bedi A, Tibor LM, Zaltz I, Larson CM. The hyperflexible hip: managing hip pain in the dancer and gymnast. *Sports Health*. 2015;7(4):346-358.

142. Singh PJ, O'Donnell JM. The outcome of hip arthroscopy in Australian football league players: a review of 27 hips. *Arthroscopy*. 2010;26(6):743-749.

143. Larson CM, Stone RM, Grossi EF, Giveans MR, Cornelsen GD. Ehlers-Danlos syndrome: arthroscopic management for extreme soft-tissue hip instability. *Arthroscopy*. 2015;31(12):2287-2294.

144. Lloyd-Smith R, Clement DB, McKenzie DC, Taunton JE. A survey of overuse and traumatic hip and pelvic injuries in athletes. *Phys Sportsmed*. 1985;13(10):131-141.

145. Heiser TM, Weber J, Sullivan G, Clare P, Jacobs RR. Prophylaxis and management of hamstring muscle injuries in intercollegiate football players. *Am J Sports Med*. 1984;12(5):368-370.

146. Liemohn W. Factors related to hamstring strains. *J Sports Med Phys Fitness*. 1978;18(1):71-76.

147. Agre JC. Hamstring injuries. Proposed aetiological factors, prevention, and treatment. *Sports Med*. 1985;2(1):21-33.

148. Ekstrand J, Gillquist J, Möller M, Oberg B, Liljedahl SO. Incidence of soccer injuries and their relation to training and team success. *Am J Sports Med*. 1983;11(2):63-67.

149. Ryan JB, Wheeler JH, Hopkinson WJ, Arciero RA, Kolakowski KR. Quadriceps contusions. West Point update. *Am J Sports Med*. 1991;19(3):299-304.

150. Fearon AM, Scarvell JM, Neeman T, Cook JL, Cormick W, Smith PN. Greater trochanteric pain syndrome: defining the clinical syndrome. *Br J Sports Med*. 2013;47(10):649-653.

151. Micheli LJ. Overuse injuries in children's sports: the growth factor. *Orthop Clin North Am*. 1983;14(2):337-360.

152. Schaberg JE, Harper MC, Allen WC. The snapping hip syndrome. *Am J Sports Med*. 1984;12(5):361-365.

153. Chang K-S, Cheng Y-H, Wu C-H, Özçakar L. Dynamic ultrasound imaging for the iliotibial band/snapping hip syndrome. *Am J Phys Med Rehabil*. 2015;94(6):e55-e56.

154. Cheatham S, Cain M, Ernst MP. Snapping hip syndrome: a review for the strength and conditioning professional. *Strength Cond J*. 2015;37(5):97-104.

155. Hiti CJ, Stevens KJ, Jamati MK, Garza D, Matheson GO. Athletic osteitis pubis. *Sports Med*. 2011;41(5):361-376.

156. Vitanzo PC, McShane JM. Osteitis pubis: solving a perplexing problem. *Phys Sportsmed*. 2001;29(7):33-48.

157. Beatty T. Osteitis pubis in athletes. *Curr Sports Med Rep*. 2012;11(2):96-98.

158. Poor AE, Roedl JB, Zoga AC, Meyers WC. Core muscle injuries in athletes. *Curr Sports Med Rep*. 2018;17(2):54-58.

159. Scillia AJ, Pierce TP, Simone E, Novak RC, Emblom BA. Mini-open incision sports hernia repair: a surgical technique for core muscle injury. *Arthrosc Tech*. 2017;6(4):e1281-e1284.

160. Lynch TS, Bedi A, Larson CM. Athletic hip injuries. *J Am Acad Orthop Surg*. 2017;25(4):269-279.

161. Rebullido TR, Stracciolini A. Pelvic floor dysfunction in female athletes: is relative energy deficiency in sport a risk factor? *Curr Sports Med Rep*. 2019;18(7):255-257.

162. Teitz CC, Hu SS, Arendt EA. The female athlete: evaluation and treatment of sports-related problems. *J Am Acad Orthop Surg*. 1997;5(2):87-96.

163. Warden SJ, Thompson WR. Become one with the force: optimising mechanotherapy through an understanding of mechanobiology. *Br J Sports Med*. 2017;51(13):989-990.

10

Dysfunction, Evaluation, Diagnosis, and Treatment of the Knee

Nonsurgical and Surgical

Beth Stone Norris, PhD, PT, OCS, E-RYT 500

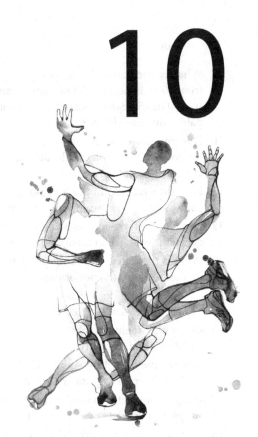

Wallmann HW, Donatelli R, eds. *Foundations of Orthopedic Physical Therapy* (pp 241-307).
© 2024 Taylor & Francis Group.

KEY TERMS

Dynamic knee valgus: Excessive movement of the lower extremity into femoral internal rotation and adduction, knee abduction, tibial external rotation, and foot pronation during the deceleration phases of double or single leg functional tasks.

Kinesiopathologic perspective: Conducting assessment and intervention from the concept that abnormal movement contributes to pathologic conditions.[1]

Neuromuscular control: The integration of muscle strength, balance, coordination, and proprioception during the performance of motor tasks that allows movement execution to occur with optimal dynamic alignment, joint stability, and reactive muscle firing patterns.[2,3]

Patellar tilt: The anteroposterior orientation of the patella in a manner that one border of the patella is more posterior, and the opposite border position is more anterior.

Pathokinesiologic perspective: Conducting assessment and intervention from the concept that abnormal movement is the result of pathologic conditions.[1]

Regional interdependence: "The identification of other factors or regions that may contribute to the patient's complaints."[4]

CHAPTER QUESTIONS

1. Describe the osseous components of the tibiofemoral joint and the patellofemoral joint (PFJ).
2. In what directions do the tibial condyles glide during open kinetic chain (OKC) knee flexion and knee extension?
3. In what directions do the femoral condyles glide during closed kinetic chain (CKC) knee flexion and knee extension?
4. How does the contact surface of the patella change as knee flexion proceeds from 0 to 135 degrees?
5. What structures provide static resistance to excessive anterior translation of the tibia?
6. What structures provide static resistance to excessive posterior translation of the tibia?
7. What tissues provide the restraint to lateral patella displacement?
8. Describe common alterations of static knee alignment in the sagittal and frontal planes.

9. What is the rationale for performing OKC exercise from 90 to 45 degrees of knee flexion and CKC exercise from 0 to 45 degrees of knee flexion for patellofemoral pain syndrome (PFPS)?

10. Dynamic lower extremity valgus is characterized by excessive movements of the hip and knee in which directions?

11. How do weakness of the hip abductors and extensors contribute to dynamic lower extremity valgus?

12. Describe criteria for assessment of trunk and lower quarter postural alignment during functional tasks.

13. What is the criteria for limb symmetry index (LSI) on hop tests of physical performance?

14. Identify self-report outcome measures (SROM) that can be used to assess perceived knee function.

15. Define the staging of rehabilitation in consideration of irritability and disability.

16. Identify methods to assess psychological factors that may affect recovery from knee pain.

17. What are the neuromuscular risk factors for sustaining an anterior cruciate ligament (ACL) injury?

18. How do quadriceps strengthening interventions differ between the rehabilitation of muscle performance impairments related to PFPS and post–anterior cruciate ligament reconstruction (ACLR)?

19. How do range of motion (ROM) interventions differ during rehabilitation following partial meniscectomy and meniscal repair?

20. How are ROM interventions and muscle performance interventions implemented to protect a meniscal repair?

INTRODUCTION

Musculoskeletal knee pain encompasses many medical diagnoses and constitutes a high percentage of patients seeking rehabilitative care. Knee pain can develop insidiously in conditions such as osteoarthritis and patellofemoral pain, can be the result of contact or noncontact injury in conditions such as ligament and meniscal tears, or can occur subsequent to trauma in conditions such as posttraumatic arthritis or articular cartilage lesions. Effective management of knee disorders involves understanding the effect of impairments of knee structures on function and establishing the skills to evaluate and implement treatment from both a pathokinesiologic or kinesiopathologic perspective. This chapter begins with an overview of anatomy and biomechanics of the knee, provides a comprehensive clinical examination of the knee, discusses knee rehabilitation from a stage-based impairment model, and presents current concepts in the conservative and postsurgical management of common knee disorders utilizing a classification-based physical therapy diagnosis.

ANATOMICAL AND BIOMECHANICAL CONSIDERATIONS OF THE KNEE

Articulations

The knee is composed of the tibiofemoral joint and PFJ. The tibiofemoral joint is a diarthrodial joint that consists of the articulation between the convex medial and lateral femoral condyles and the shallow, relatively flat medial and lateral plateaus of the tibia condyles. The intercondylar eminence between the tibial plateaus divides this articulation into medial and lateral compartments. Disparity in the shape of the tibiofemoral articulating surfaces contributes to the triplane motion and to the reliance on connective tissues to provide joint stability.[5] The femoral and tibial condyles are lined with hyaline cartilage that is 2 to 4 mm in thickness.[6] Between the femoral and tibial condyles are 2 menisci—fibrocartilage disks that are concave superiorly to enhance the congruence of the tibiofemoral articulation. Additional functions of the menisci are to increase the contact area between the joint surfaces, which assists in load dispersion, and to guide knee motion.[5] Both menisci are semicircular in shape, have anterior and posterior horns that attach to the intercondylar area of the tibia, and are attached to the periphery of the tibia via coronary ligaments. The medial meniscus is larger, more C-shaped, and attached to the joint capsule and medial collateral ligament (MCL), making it less mobile than the lateral meniscus.[7] While the lateral meniscus attaches to the popliteus, it has a less firm attachment to the lateral joint capsule and no attachment to the lateral collateral ligament (LCL), factors that contribute to its mobility. The tibiofemoral joint is surrounded by a joint capsule that consists of an inner synovial layer and outer fibrous layer.

The PFJ consists of the posterior surface of the patella and the intercondylar groove (the trochlea) of the femur. The posterior articular surface of the patella is lined with thick articular cartilage (up to 7 mm in depth) and contains a vertical ridge that divides the surface into a lateral and medial facet.[8] The lateral facet is larger and the medial facet contains the odd facet. Patella orientation is with the base (top) superior and the apex (inferior aspect) inferior. The patella is contained within the quadriceps tendon, superiorly, and the patella tendon, inferiorly, which increases the internal moment arm of the quadriceps.

The superior tibiofibular joint is located lateral and inferior to the knee and consists of the head of the fibula and the posterior aspect of the lateral condyle of the tibia. While this joint is not considered an articulating component of the knee, the head of the fibula is an attachment point for the biceps femoris and LCL.[5,9]

Mobility

The primary motions at the knee occur in the sagittal plane as flexion and extension. These motions are produced by movement at both the tibiofemoral joint and PFJ. Tibiofemoral joint arthrokinematics consist of rolling and gliding accessory motions between the convex femoral condyles and concave tibial plateaus and are described in reference to OKC motion and CKC motion. During OKC knee extension, the concave tibia rolls and glides anteriorly on the femoral condyles.[5] During CKC knee extension, the convex femoral condyles roll anterior and glide posterior on the tibia.[5] The opposite occurs with knee flexion; during OKC knee flexion, the concave tibia rolls and glides posteriorly, and during CKC knee flexion, the convex femoral condyles roll posteriorly and glide anteriorly.

Secondary motion occurs at the tibiofemoral joint in the transverse plane as medial and lateral rotation, and, to a lesser extent, in the frontal plane as abduction and adduction. Secondary motion is a result of the shape and congruence differences between the medial and lateral compartments of the tibiofemoral joint. In OKC knee motion, the tibia externally rotates on the femur during extension and internally rotates during flexion. In CKC knee motion, the femur internally rotates on the tibia during knee extension, resulting in relative external rotation at the tibiofemoral joint, and externally rotates on the tibia during knee flexion, resulting in relative internal rotation at the tibiofemoral joint. The amount of external and internal rotation is greatest when the knee is flexed to 90 degrees and is restricted when the knee is in full extension. The "screw-home" mechanism refers to external rotation of the tibiofemoral joint that occurs during terminal range of knee extension.[5]

Mobility of the PFJ consists of the patella translating superiorly in the trochlea during extension and inferiorly during flexion, totaling 5 to 7 cm of mobility.[8] The intercondylar groove of the femur helps to stabilize the patella during knee motion, but allows the patella to glide in a C shape (laterally to medially then laterally) as the patella translates inferiorly during flexion and reverse C shape as the patella translates superiorly during knee extension (Figure 10-1).[8] Full knee extension to 5 degrees flexion is the open-packed position of the PFJ. In the open-packed position, the patella rests proximal to the trochlea and passive mobility of the patella can be performed superiorly, inferiorly, medially, and laterally. At approximately 20 degrees of knee flexion, the inferior pole of the patella contacts the patella. As knee flexion continues, the contact area of the patella moves proximally to the superior pole at 90 degrees of flexion and toward the lateral facet and odd facet at approximately 135 degrees of knee flexion.[8]

Stability

In addition to stability provided by the joint capsule and menisci, reinforcement to the tibiofemoral joint is provided by ligaments as static stabilizers and muscles as

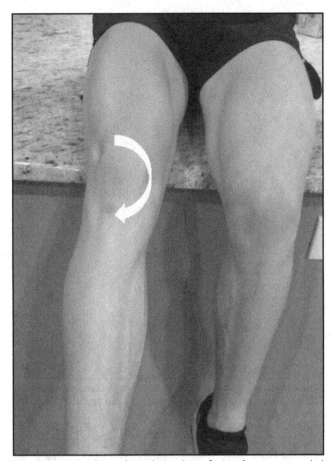

Figure 10-1. Patella tracking during knee flexion from an extended position.

dynamic stabilizers. The 4 major ligaments in the knee are the MCL, LCL, ACL, and posterior cruciate ligament (PCL). Excessive anterior and posterior displacement of the tibia is primarily resisted by the ACL and PCL, respectively. The ACL provides greatest resistance to anterior translation of the tibia in all angles of knee flexion, with highest resistance provided when the knee is in 20 to 30 degrees of flexion.[10] The ACL consists of 2 fiber bundles: the anteromedial bundle, which is taut from 20 to 90 degrees of flexion, and the posterolateral bundle, which is taut in extension.[10] The PCL consists of a posteromedial bundle and an anterolateral bundle, which have been shown to remain taut throughout most of flexion and extension.[5] It provides greatest resistance to posterior translation of the tibia when the knee is flexed to 90 degrees or greater. Excessive anterior displacement of the tibia is reinforced dynamically by the hamstrings, iliotibial band (ITB), and posterior capsule, whereas excessive posterior displacement of the tibia is reinforced dynamically by the quadriceps muscles, the popliteus, and the posterolateral capsule. In addition to resisting excessive sagittal plane translation of the tibia, the ACL and PCL also serve as secondary restraints to excessive frontal plane motion (tibial abduction and adduction) when the knee is in or near full extension. The primary stabilizer against excessive tibiofemoral internal

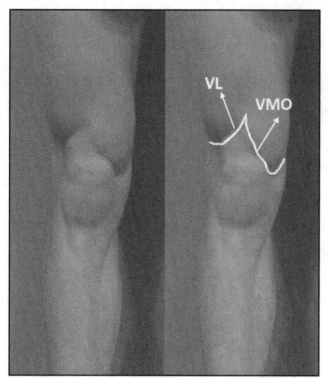

Figure 10-2. Synergistic relationship between VMO and vastus lateralis (VL) that promotes concurrent dynamic medial and lateral stability of the patella.

rotation is the ACL with secondary restraint coming from the posteromedial capsule, while the primary stabilizers for tibiofemoral external rotation are the posterolateral capsule and MCL.[10,11]

The primary stabilizers against excessive lateral displacement of the tibia (abduction or valgus) and medial displacement of the tibia (adduction or varus) are the MCL and LCL, respectively. The MCL and LCL provide the greatest resistance to frontal plane translation of the tibia when the knee is in slight flexion.[12] Medial stability (ie, resistance to excessive lateral tibial displacement or tibial abduction) of the knee is reinforced by the semimembranosus tendon, pes anserine, medial head of the gastrocnemius muscle, and the posteromedial capsular structures (knee capsule reinforced by posterior oblique ligament and oblique popliteal ligament).[13] Lateral stability (ie, resistance to excessive medial tibial displacement or tibial adduction) of the knee is reinforced by the popliteus tendon, biceps femoris tendon, ITB, and posterolateral capsular structures (knee capsule and arcuate ligament).[14,15] In addition to resisting excessive frontal plane movement of the tibia, the MCL and LCL also provide resistance to extreme external rotation of the tibia.[16,17]

Static stability of the PFJ is provided by the trochlea, retinaculum, and ligaments.[8] The shape of the trochlea combined with the lateral femoral condyle projecting anteriorly more than the medial femoral condyle prevents excessive lateral movement of the patella at angles greater than 20 to 30 degrees of knee flexion. From 20 to 0 degrees of knee flexion,

the patella rests above the trochlea and is dependent upon stability provided by soft tissues, such as the patella retinaculum. Medial ligament stabilizers of the patella include the medial patellofemoral ligament (MPFL), the medial patellomeniscal, and medial patellotibial ligament, of which the MPFL is the primary static restraint to lateral patella displacement.[18] The MPFL is a continuation of the retinaculum of the vastus medialis oblique (VMO) and runs from the medial epicondyle to the adductor tubercle. The lateral static stabilizers include the lateral retinaculum, ITB, and joint capsule. The lateral retinaculum consists of a superficial layer, which contains fibers from the vastus lateralis and ITB, and a deep layer, which contains the lateral patellofemoral ligament and lateral patellotibial ligament. The lateral patellofemoral ligament attaches to the femur indirectly via attachments to the ITB. Given the connections of the lateral retinaculum to the ITB and the lateral retinaculum to the patella, tightness of the ITB can exert a lateral force on the patella and affect the stability of the patella.[19] When functioning optimally, dynamic stability is provided by the quadriceps muscle and extensor mechanism. In particular, the fiber orientation of the VMO and the vastus lateralis provides a synergistic relationship, promoting concurrent dynamic medial and lateral stability of the patella in the trochlea (Figure 10-2). Laxity in the static medial stabilizers, insufficiency in the VMO, or tightness in the lateral retinaculum can contribute to altered alignment of the patella in a position of lateral tilt. Lateral patella tilt of more than 11 degrees has been found to occur in 93% of individuals with objective patella instability.[20]

Muscle Considerations at the Knee

Muscles acting on the knee are best considered by location (anterior, posterior, medial, or lateral) in their contributions to dynamic stability, as previously mentioned, and to knee motion production via concentric or eccentric contraction, or limitation via flexibility deficits. Anteriorly, the quadriceps consist of the rectus femoris, vastus lateralis, vastus medialis, and vastus intermedius. Together these muscles extend the knee (acting concentrically), control knee flexion (acting eccentrically), and can contribute to impairment of knee flexion mobility when quadriceps muscle extensibility deficits exist. As a 2-joint muscle, the rectus femoris can limit knee flexion through passive insufficiency as the muscle is simultaneously lengthened across both the hip and knee. The orientation of the distal portion of the vastus medialis, the VMO, contributes to control of patella tracking against dominance of lateral structures. The vastus lateralis is one of the lateral structures that can contribute to lateral tracking of the patella through knee ROM and potential lateral instability. Quadriceps strength has a strong association with knee function related to PFPS, knee osteoarthritis, and after ACLR.[21-24]

Posteriorly located muscles at the knee are the hamstrings (semimembranosus, semitendinosus, and the biceps femoris), popliteus, and gastrocnemius (medial and lateral heads). Together, the hamstrings, popliteus, and

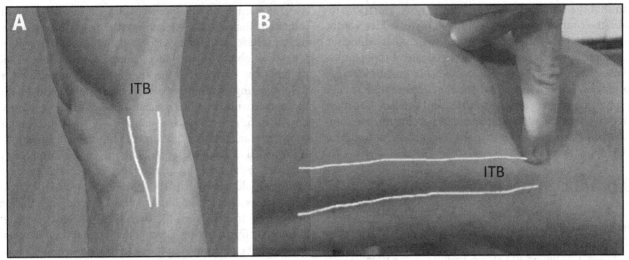

Figure 10-3. ITB with the knee (A) extended and (B) flexed.

gastrocnemius provide dynamic stability to the posterior capsule, with the biceps femoris, popliteus, and lateral head of the gastrocnemius providing posterolateral reinforcement and the semimembranous, semitendinous, and medial head of the gastrocnemius providing posteromedial reinforcement. Acting on the knee, these muscles perform knee flexion and tibial internal rotation (semimembranosus, semitendinosus, and popliteus) and tibial external rotation (biceps femoris). As 2-joint muscles (with the exception of the short head of the biceps femoris), the hamstrings produce hip extension and can become overused when weakness or activation deficits of the gluteus maximus exist. The hamstrings can limit knee extension mobility through passive insufficiency as the muscle is simultaneously lengthened across both the hip and knee. In addition to hip extension, the hamstrings assist with hip internal rotation (semitendinosus and semimembranosus) and external rotation (biceps femoris). Hamstring activation is an important component of knee stability after ACL injury and reconstruction, with deficits in the hamstring/quadriceps ratio being a key component in the risk of primary ACL injury.[21]

Medially, the tendons of the sartorius, gracilis, and semitendinosus attach to the tibia as the pes anserine. Together, this group provide dynamic stability to the medial aspect of the knee, resisting tibial abduction and external rotation. Acting on the knee, these muscles contribute to knee flexion and internal rotation. Laterally, the biceps femoris provides dynamic stability by resisting excessive tibial adduction in addition to providing support to the posterolateral capsule. The ITB is a dense fibrous band of connective tissue that originates proximally from the fascia of the tensor fascia lata (TFL) and the gluteus maximus and medius muscles. It extends down the lateral aspect of the thigh, crossing the lateral femoral epicondyle to attach on the anterior lateral tibia at Gerdy's tubercle (Figure 10-3). Via this lateral attachment to the tibia, the ITB provides a secondary restraint to anterolateral stability at the knee.[25] Acting on the hip, the TFL-ITB

flexes, abducts, and internally rotates the femur. Weakness of the synergistic hip flexors (iliopsoas and rectus femoris) and abductors (gluteus medius) may lead to overdominance and shortness of the TFL-ITB, which can contribute to femoral internal rotation, genu valgus, and lateral tracking of the patella.

Muscle Considerations at the Hip

Although located proximally to the knee, the hip muscles can exert regional interdependence on knee function through their control on the orientation of the femur in the frontal, sagittal, and transverse planes during weightbearing tasks. Deficits in hip muscle strength can lead to excessive motion of the femur in any or all planes, effecting dynamic lower extremity alignment, asymmetrical forces at the knee, and loading of the knee joints.[26-30] In particular, hip abductor and extensor weakness can lead to excessive hip adduction and internal rotation during weightbearing tasks, resulting in dynamic lower extremity valgus and increased loading of the tibiofemoral joints.[26] Excessive hip adduction and internal rotation is controlled by optimal function of the hip abductors, external rotators, and extensors. While many muscles perform or contribute to hip abduction, external rotation, and extension, the gluteus medius and maximus have been the primary muscles of consideration in research investigating the association of hip strength to knee dysfunction[27,31-35] and research investigating the effectiveness of hip strengthening in knee rehabilitation.[36-38] The primary action of the gluteus medius is hip abduction, whereas the posterior fibers contribute to external rotation.[39] The gluteus maximus produces hip extension and is the largest of the hip external rotator muscles. When functioning in weightbearing, the gluteus medius provides frontal plane stability of the pelvis and controls against a hip adduction moment.[39] Weakness of the gluteus medius may result in contralateral pelvic drop or excessive femoral adduction.[40] Contralateral pelvic drop can shift the center of mass of the head, neck, and trunk toward the contralateral side resulting in increased load at the medial tibiofemoral joint.[41,42] Excessive femoral adduction can contribute to excess loading of the lateral tibiofemoral joint. Weakness of the gluteus maximus or medius can lead to excessive femoral internal rotation, which may change the orientation between the trochlea and patella.[43] Together, excessive femoral adduction and internal rotation are components of dynamic lower extremity valgus, a risk factor for ACL injury and PFPS.[26,28,44]

Biomechanical Factors

A primary consideration during knee rehabilitation is the minimization of factors that contribute to excess loading of soft tissues and increased joint stress. Of particular importance is reducing PFJ stress, loading of the tibiofemoral articular cartilage, and loading of the injured or postsurgical ACL and PCL. Joint stress is a product of force applied over a contact area.[8] When a force is applied over a small contact area, joint stress increases. Knowledge of the contact area of the patella in relation to the trochlea and of the forces produced by the external moment arm at differing angles of sagittal plane knee motion assists the clinician in selecting the ROM to perform quadriceps strengthening exercises.

The contact area of the patella increases from 20 to 90 degrees of flexion as the contact area of the patella on the trochlea moves from the inferior pole to the superior pole during this range.[8,23,45] During OKC motion with an external load applied at the ankle (using variable resistance), the external flexion moment arm is greatest at 0 degrees of knee extension and decreases as the knee flexes.[40] Thus, as the knee extends from 90 to 0 degrees, a greater amount of quadriceps force is needed to overcome the external flexion moment arm and the patellofemoral joint reaction (PFJR) force increases. Together, during OKC knee extension the contact area of the patella decreases while the PFJR force increases, resulting in greater PFJ stress as the knee nears full extension. The opposite occurs during CKC knee motion when the external flexion moment arm increases as the knee flexes contributing to an increase in PFJR force.[40] From 0 to 45 degrees CKC knee flexion, PFJ stress increases linearly with a more rapid increase occurring from 45 to 100 degrees.[45]

When prescribing quadriceps strengthening exercises for a patient with patellofemoral pain, the 90- to 45-degree range of extension is recommended for OKC exercise using variable resistance loading, and the 0- to 45-degree range is recommended for CKC exercise.[8,45] When constant loading is applied, as through a knee extension machine with cable system, the PFJ stress remains constant from 0 to 90 degrees, at a level between the stress produced with variable resistance OKC and CKC quadriceps strengthening.[45] Consideration should also be given to loading of the PFJ during weightbearing activities. Walking generates loading of the PFJ that is 1 to 3 times body weight, whereas, running increases the loading to 5.6 times body weight.[8,23]

Knowledge of the biomechanics of the tibiofemoral joint contributes to the selection of the range in which mobility exercises should be performed after articular cartilage repair. Weightbearing produces compressive loading of the tibiofemoral joint, and as the knee moves through ROM in weightbearing, different aspects of the femoral condyles are in contact with the tibial plateaus. For example, when the knee is in full extension, the anterior aspects of the femoral condyles contact the middle aspect of the tibial plateaus.[46-48] If the articular cartilage lesion is on the anterior aspect of a femoral condyle, exercise in the range of terminal knee extension would be avoided. The posterior aspect of the femoral condyles contact the tibial plateaus during knee flexion between 90 to 120 degrees.[49] Thus, if the articular cartilage lesion is on the posterior aspect of the femoral condyle, exercise would be performed in the 0- to 80-degree range.[49]

During postsurgical rehabilitation of the ACL and PCL, prescribing exercises that limit anterior or posterior tibial translation is of importance to minimize loading of the ACL and PCL, respectively.[50,51] This is accomplished by considering the effect of quadriceps and hamstring force production on tibial translation, the placement of external resistance, the knee angle in which exercise is performed, and the mode of exercise (OKC or CKC). Contracting the quadriceps creates an anterior force on the tibia, especially in the 30- to 10-degree range, and contracting the hamstrings creates a posterior force on the tibia throughout the full range of knee motion.[51] When using constant resistance, such as an ankle weight, placement of the external resistance proximal to the knee on the lower leg will decrease ACL loading as compared to a more distal placement.[52] To minimize ACL loading, OKC knee extension should be performed at higher angles, 100 to 50 degrees to avoid greater anterior shear forces on the tibia.[51,53] OKC-resisted knee flexion creates no loading to the ACL; however, PCL loading occurs throughout the full range of knee flexion motion, which is why OKC knee flexion is contraindicated in the early stage of postsurgical PCL rehabilitation.[54] CKC knee exercise involving double leg squat (DLS) from 0 to 90 degrees is found to have minimal loading of the ACL, which is thought to be due to the high amount of hamstring force being generated.[51] Hamstring activity is further increased by incorporating trunk inclination when performing CKC squat.[51] Due to the high amount of hamstring activity and posterior tibial translation, use of a CKC squat exercise is delayed in the early stages of postsurgical PCL rehabilitation or is performed in the 0- to 45-degree range where posterior tibial shear is less.[54]

Static Lower Quarter Postural Alignment Considerations

Deviations in postural alignment in the lower extremity may create alterations in stress applied to connective tissue structures at the knee, which may contribute to knee pain and movement dysfunction. Given that the knee is a linking joint between the ankle and foot distally and the hip and pelvis proximally, examination for postural malalignment should include regions above and below the knee. Examination of lower extremity posture should be conducted in consideration of what constitutes "optimal" alignment. When deviations from optimal alignment are observed, the distinction between structural and acquired or dynamic postural malalignment should be determined. When the observed posture can be modified by the clinician or patient, the postural malalignment is considered acquired, whereas postural deviations that are not modifiable are considered as a structural malalignment.[55] In cases of acquired postural malalignment, the effect of posture modification on current knee related symptoms is assessed and modifications that result in symptom reduction can be considered as potential treatment interventions. There is also the possibility that lower extremity postural malalignment may not be associated with the current condition but could lead to future dysfunction, and, thus, should be considered as a potential risk factor necessitating appropriately directed interventions that are preventive in nature. The presence of pelvic, hip, knee, ankle, and foot malalignment may also lead the examiner to conduct tests of muscle length and strength.

Optimal alignment of the lower extremity in the sagittal plane occurs when the anterior superior iliac spine (ASIS) and pubic symphysis are in line vertically, and the line of gravity passes slightly posterior to the hip joint, anterior to the knee joint, and anterior to the lateral malleolus. The hip and knee should be in 0 degrees of knee extension and the ankle in 0 degrees of dorsiflexion. Optimal alignment of the lower extremity in the frontal plane occurs when symmetry exists between the right and left halves of the body, the right and left ASIS, posterior superior iliac spine, patella, popliteal spaces, and medial malleoli are level horizontally. In adults, the femur, which inclines medially, and the tibia are oriented vertically to the longitudinal axis of the lower extremity. This results in 170 to 175 degrees of physiological valgus at the knee. Frontal plane orientation of the foot consists of the calcanei oriented in slight valgus relative to the longitudinal axis of the lower extremity. Optimal alignment of the lower extremity in the horizontal plane is neutral rotation of the femur and tibia and there is equal visibility of the lateral and medial toes.

Alternations in postural alignment in the sagittal plane are identified by examining standing posture from the right and left sides. Specific to the knee, the clinician should observe for deviation of the knee alignment into knee hyperextension or knee flexion. Knee hyperextension, genu recurvatum, moves the line of gravity anterior to the knee joint, reducing demands on the quadriceps to maintain postural stability. Genu recurvatum posture reflects posterior displacement of the lower leg and usually occurs with posterior tilt of the pelvis, inferior positioning of the patella, and ankle plantarflexion. Over time, this malalignment can increase the loading of the anterior aspect of the tibiofemoral joint, create strain on the PCL, and can contribute to shortening of the patella tendon, the hip extensors, and ankle plantarflexors.[55] A posture of knee flexion moves the line of gravity posterior to the knee joint, increasing quadriceps demands to maintain static postural stability. This posture malalignment is associated with anterior pelvic tilt and ankle dorsiflexion, which over time may contribute to shortening of the hip flexors and ankle dorsiflexors.

Alterations in postural alignment in the frontal plane are identified by examining standing posture from the front and back views. Lateral pelvic tilt is observed through iliac crest height symmetry and may provide an indirect indication of leg length discrepancy (LLD) when observed in double leg stance or pelvic stability impairment when observed in single leg stance. LLDs have been associated with knee osteoarthritis; however, it is unclear if the association is with the shorter or longer leg.[56-59] Harvey et al[58] found that an LLD of 1.0 cm or more measured with radiography to be significantly associated with radiographic and symptomatic knee osteoarthritis at baseline and predicted symptomatic knee osteoarthritis in a 30-month follow-up. Leg length can be measured directly in standing and in supine with a flexible tape measure using the distance from the ASIS to the medial malleolus.[60,61] Genu valgus and varus is assessed according to the position of the knees and distal tibia relative to midline with genu valgus reflected by knee adduction toward midline and tibia abduction and genu varum reflected by knee abduction from midline and tibia adduction. Knee ligament laxity may occur in consequence of genu valgus (laxity of MCL) or varum (laxity of LCL), which could be examined using valgus or varus ligament stability tests. Calcaneal varus (distal calcaneus positioned toward midline) or excessive calcaneal valgus (distal calcaneus positioned away from midline) suggests potential supination or pronation malalignment, respectively, which is discussed in the next paragraph.

Anterior and posterior views of postural inspection conducted with the patient standing best provide identification of alterations in postural alignment in the transverse plan. Femoral rotation may be suspected if the patella is facing inward (internal rotation) or outward (external femoral rotation). External tibia torsion may be suspected if toeing out is present with the patella facing forward. Foot pronation/supination, which consists of triplane motion, may be suspected by viewing the calcaneus for valgus (pronation) or varus (supination) alignment and by observing the medial longitudinal arch for lowering (pronation) or elevating (supination) in height. When transverse plane postural malalignment is suspected, the magnitude of the malalignment can be further examined with clinical tests such as Craig's test to measure femoral anteversion or retroversion, the foot posture index, medial longitudinal arch angle, or rearfoot angle to assess foot pronation/supination, and the thigh-foot angle to assess tibial torsion.

Static alignment of the patella can be measured via the quadriceps angle (Q-angle) and the Insall-Salvati ratio.[62-64] The Q-angle is the angle formed by the bisection of a line from the ASIS to the midpoint of the patella and a line from

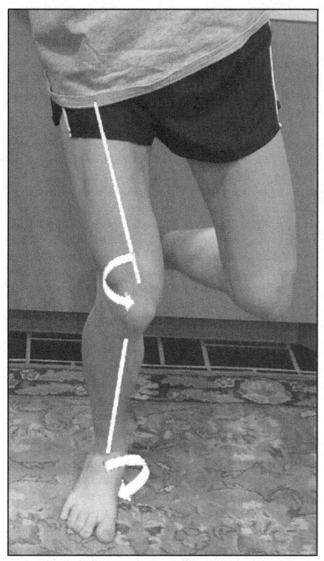

Figure 10-4. Dynamic knee valgus.

height of the patella. A ratio of less than 0.80 reflects patella baja and a ratio of greater than 1.2 reflects patella alta.[8] The alignment of the patella should also be such that the superior, inferior, medial, and lateral borders of the patella are equidistant from the femur. An anterior or posterior deviation of the patella creates a malalignment referred to as a *tilt*. For example, when the lateral border of the patella is more posterior or closer to the femur than the medial border, the medial border would be palpated to be higher than the lateral border creating a lateral tilt of the surface of the patella. Similarly, an inferior tilt occurs when the surface of the patella is tilted inferiorly and the inferior border is closer to the femur. Patella rotation occurs when the inferior pole of the patella is oriented medially (medial rotation) or laterally (lateral rotation) instead of directly inferior to the superior pole.

Dynamic Lower Quarter Alignment and Neuromuscular Control

While static postural alignment may provide insight to potential muscle imbalances and altered tissue stress in the lower quarter, examination of dynamic alignment during functional tasks provides insight to neuromuscular control of the lower quarter and trunk. Impairments of neuromuscular control of the lower quarter are frequently identified in individuals with knee pain and dysfunction and have been identified as potential risk factors for future ligament injury or re-injury.[29,44,67-70] Neuromuscular control is a multifactorial construct that integrates muscle strength, balance, coordination, and proprioception during the performance of functional motor tasks. Alternations in neuromuscular control can be identified through the assessment of dynamic movement patterns during functional task performance. The most implicated abnormal movement pattern is dynamic knee valgus in which the femur internally rotates and adducts, the knee abducts, the tibia externally rotates, and the foot pronates excessively during deceleration phases of double or single leg functional tasks (Figure 10-4).[26,29,71] Research has found that high knee abduction moments (KAM) generated through dynamic valgus movement patterns predict risk of future ACL injury and PFPS.[29,44,72] Furthermore, women tend to have a higher KAM than men, and high KAM during a drop-vertical jump task is one of the predominant clinical measures to predict risk of future ACL injury in female athletes.[29,73,74]

Three-dimensional (3D) motion analysis is the gold standard for quantifying multiplane alignment deviations that constitute dynamic knee valgus; however, this measurement method lacks clinical applicability. Alternative clinical measurement methods for dynamic knee valgus include 2-dimensional (2D) motion analysis and visual assessment of lower extremity movement patterns during the performance of functional tasks.[75-82] 2D motion analysis provides quantitative angular measurement of lateral pelvic tilt and the frontal

the midpoint of the patella to the tibial tuberosity. Women tend to have a larger Q-angle than men (15 to 17 degrees for women; 10 to 13 degrees for men).[8] A Q-angle that exceeds 15 to 20 degrees may create excessive lateral forces on the patella with subsequent changes to patella contact area and stability.[65] Because the Q-angle is intended to reflect the effects of contraction of the quadriceps on the tracking of the patella, the validity of a static measure to assess dynamic function is questionable.[66] In the sagittal plane, the patella rests just above the tibiofemoral joint line. A lower positioned patella is considered patella baja, which could occur due to a shortened patella tendon. A higher positioned patella is considered patella alta, which could occur due to quadriceps tightness. Patella alta is a factor that may contribute to patella instability due to the lack of soft tissue restraints around the patella in this position. The Insall-Salvati ratio provides a quantification of the sagittal plane position of the patella by dividing the patella tendon length by the plane projection angle of the knee. There are 2 methods to measure the frontal plane projection angle at the knee. One method measures the angle formed by a line bisecting the thigh and a second line bisecting the lower leg. The second method measures the angle formed from a line bisecting the lower leg and a vertical reference line.[82,83] Other methods to quantify dynamic knee valgus during 2D motion analysis of functional tasks performance include the knee foot separation ratio and the knee separation distance.[71] Visual assessment involves rating the magnitude of or presence of errors in trunk and lower extremity postural alignment during the performance of physical and functional tasks.[80,81,83,84] Visual assessment rating methods have ranged from "yes"/"no" ratings where "yes" is the presence of the postural malalignment and "no" is the absence of the malalignment[79,83] to assignment of 0, 1, or 2 points[80,85] where 0 points reflects absence of the postural malalignment or good movement strategy and 1 to 2 points reflect presence of the postural malalignment or poor movement strategy. Visual assessments of movement quality can be performed for an individual functional task or a sum score over multiple functional tasks.

In addition to frontal plane dynamic alignment, alternations in sagittal plane dynamic alignment of the trunk and lower quarter are of concern in regard to knee dysfunction. For athletes with knee dysfunction, examination of sagittal plane trunk, hip, and knee positioning during the landing phase of jumping tasks provides insight to risk of knee injury.[26,72,86] Landing from a jump with the trunk upright has been found to lead to decreased knee flexion angles, increased force of landing, and greater quadriceps activity, which leads to anterior tibial shear and ACL loading.[86,87] When exploring gender differences in landing strategies, men demonstrated increased hip flexion at initial contact than women and women had a tendency to underutilize the hip as compared to the knee.[88] These finding have led to incorporation of neuromuscular training of the trunk and hip to improve landing mechanics and reduce loading at the knee.[21,26,72]

Functional tasks for the assessment of abnormal lower quarter movement patterns include DLS, single leg minisquat (SLS), front step down, lateral step down (LSD), drop vertical jump (DVJ), forward lunge, and single leg hop (SLH) for distance (Table 10-1). Nae et al[81] established a battery of 4 functional tasks (SLS, stair descent, forward lunge, and SLH) to have good content validity (Cronbach alpha = 0.70 to 0.90) and substantial interrater reliability (kappa = 0.664 to 0.863) when assessing movement patterns in individuals following ACL injury. Visual assessment of the tasks was performed using postural orientation errors targeting the foot, knee, pelvis/hip, and trunk. A recent systematic review and meta-analysis found the visual observation of knee valgus using the alignment of the medial patella over the foot to support intrarater and interrater reliability and to be valid against 2D and 3D motion analysis.[80] A summary of criteria for visual assessment of the trunk and lower quarter postural alignment during functional tasks is presented in Table 10-2.

Alterations in postural alignment during static and dynamic weightbearing positions may suggest the presence of muscle imbalances and uneven load distribution at the knee joints, which would direct the clinician to consider the use of muscle strength, muscle length, and/or ligamentous stability tests during the examination process. For example, genu varum knee alignment may increase stress at the medial compartment of the tibiofemoral joint, contribute to greater knee adduction moment during walking, and create strain of the LCL.[89-91] The integrity of the LCL could be examined with a varus stress test. Hip malalignment involving excessive femoral adduction and internal rotation may have associated weakness of the hip abductors and external rotators, and shortness of the hip internal rotators, specifically the ITB-TFL. If this malalignment was observed, further clinical tests could include hip abductor and external rotation isometric strength testing and muscle length test for the ITB-TFL. Dynamic posture alignment of the lower quarter could also be impaired secondary to deficits of balance and proprioception, necessitating conducting clinical measurements of these aspects of neuromuscular control.[21,72]

Physical Performance Tests

Physical performance tests (PPT) are often used to establish functional ability of individuals with knee dysfunction. Depending upon the irritability of the condition, these tests can be conducted during the examination process to assess baseline activity limitations and participation restrictions, as a component of screening for risk of injury, during the rehabilitation process to determine criterion for progression within rehabilitation phases, and at discharge as a criterion of readiness for return to activity and sport. Clinic-based PPT are simple to administer, do not require laboratory-based motion analysis systems, and are portable to multiple settings. A systematic review of clinician-friendly PPT found that the most common PPT used assessed the function of athletes with knee dysfunction to include one leg hop for distance (single and triple hop), 6-meter timed hop, crossover hop for distance, one leg triple hop for distance, and single leg vertical jump (Table 10-3).[92] Of these tests, the one leg single hop for distance is the most commonly used and is the only hop test found to be responsive to change after rehabilitation for ACL injury. Despite the frequent use of hop tests, there is little evidence supporting their reliability, validity, responsiveness, and measurement error.[92] Hop tests are interpreted through calculation of LSI based on the ratio of the involved lower extremity performance divided by the uninvolved lower extremity performance. LSI criteria on hop tests for return to sport is 90% or greater.[93,94]

Table 10-1

FUNCTIONAL TASKS USED FOR ASSESSMENT OF DYNAMIC MOVEMENT CONTROL

FUNCTIONAL TASK	DESCRIPTION	FIGURE
DLS	Position: Standing, feet hip width apart. Movement: Bend both knees to perform a partial squat as far as possible without lifting the heels or loss of balance.	
Forward step down	Position: Standing on a 20-cm box, arms folded across chest or hands on hips. Movement: Forward step down is performed until the heel touches the floor, then return to the starting position. Patient performs 5 to 10 repetitions.	
LSD	Position: Standing on a 15-cm box, arms folded across chest or hands on hips. Movement: LSD is performed until the heel touches the floor, then return to the starting position. Patient performs 5 to 10 repetitions.	

(continued)

Table 10-1 (continued)

FUNCTIONAL TASKS USED FOR ASSESSMENT OF DYNAMIC MOVEMENT CONTROL

FUNCTIONAL TASK	DESCRIPTION	FIGURE
SLS	Position: Standing on the floor on one lower extremity. Movement: Bend the knee of the supporting lower extremity as far as possible without lifting the stance heel or loss of balance.	
Forward lunge	Position: Standing feet together. Movement: Step forward with one lower extremity, place the foot on the ground, bend both knees to approximately 90 degrees, push back to starting position.	
SLH for distance	Position: Standing on one lower extremity Movement: Hop as far forward as possible and land on the same lower extremity, maintaining the landing for a minimum of 2 seconds.	

Table 10-2

CRITERIA FOR TRUNK AND LOWER QUARTER POSTURAL ALIGNMENT DURING FUNCTIONAL TASKS OF DYNAMIC MOVEMENT CONTROL

LOWER EXTREMITY MALALIGNMENT	VISUAL OBSERVATION DESCRIPTION	MEASUREMENT PROPERTIES
Foot pronation	• Lowering of medial longitudinal arch	• Interrater reliability: k=0.517[95]; task: SLS
Knee valgus/varus	• Midpoint of patella is medial to second toe	• Interrater reliability: k=0.592 to 0.808[95]; tasks: SLS, stair descent, forward lunge, SLH • Interrater reliability: k=0.54 to 0.92; task: DVJ[96]
Pelvic deviation	• Lateral pelvic tilt: Lowering of one side of the pelvis • Pelvic rotation: Forward or backward movement of one side of the pelvis	• Interrater reliability: k=0.429 to 0.768[95]; tasks: SLS, stair descent, forward lunge, SLH
Trunk deviation	• Lateral tilt of the trunk • Rotation of the trunk	• Interrater reliability: k=0.524 to 0.875[95]; tasks: SLS, stair descent, SLH

Although hop tests performed preoperatively have not been found to predict self-reported knee function that is within normal values, hop tests performed 6 months post-ACLR were able to predict self-reported knee function below and above normal values.[100] Specifically, at 6 months post-ACLR, patients with self-reported knee function within normal ranges on the International Knee Documentation Committee (IKDC) 2000 outcome measure were 4 times more likely to have a crossover hop LSI greater than 95% as compared to those with knee function on the IKDC 2000 below normal values. In addition, patients 6 months post-ACLR with self-reported knee function below normal values were 5 times more likely to have a 6-m hop LSI lower than 88% as compared to those with normal self-reported knee function.[92]

For individuals with knee osteoarthritis, the recommended core set of PPT by the Osteoarthritis Research Society International is the 30-second chair stand test, 40-m fast-paced walk test, stair climb test, timed up and go test, and 6-minute walk test.[101] For clinical practice and research, the minimum core set of PPT outcome measures for knee osteoarthritis is the 30-second chair stand test, 40-m fast-paced walk test, and stair climb test.[101] The reliability, standard error of measurement (SEM), SEM% (SEM/mean x 100), and minimal detectable change (MDC) for these tests are provided in Table 10-4.

Table 10-3

PHYSICAL PERFORMANCE TESTS FOR ASSESSMENT OF FUNCTIONAL ABILITY IN INDIVIDUALS WITH KNEE DYSFUNCTION

TEST	DESCRIPTION	CRITERIA	STANDARD ERROR OF MEASUREMENT[98]
SLH	Position: Standing on one lower extremity (take-off lower extremity). Movement: The patient performs a maximum hop forward, landing on the take-off lower extremity.	• Stick the landing • Distance hopped from the toe of the take-off lower extremity to the toe of the landing lower extremity • LSI = (distance hopped involved lower extremity/ distance hopped uninvolved lower extremity)*100 • ≥90% LSI[97]	4.56 to 7.93 cm
Triple single leg	Position: Standing on one lower extremity (take-off lower extremity). Movement: The patient performs a series of 3 maximum hops forward, landing on the take-off lower extremity.	• Stick the landing • Distance hopped from the toe of the take-off lower extremity to the toe of the landing lower extremity • LSI = (distance hopped involved lower extremity/ distance hopped uninvolved lower extremity)*100 • ≥90% LSI[97]	15.44 to 23.18 cm
Triple single leg crossover hop	Position: Standing on one lower extremity (take-off lower extremity) to the side of a line on the floor that extends forward in the direction of the hop. Movement: The patient performs a series of 3 hops with each hop crossing over the midline, landing on the opposite side on the take-off lower extremity.	• Stick the landing • Distance hopped from the toe of the take-off lower extremity to the toe of the landing lower extremity • LSI = (distance hopped involved lower extremity/ distance hopped uninvolved lower extremity)*100 • ≥90% LSI[97]	15.95 to 21.16 cm
Single leg timed	Position: standing on one lower extremity (take-off lower extremity) to the side of a line on the floor that extends forward 6 meters (m) in the direction of the hop. Movement: The patient performs a series of hops forward as fast as possible for 6 m, landing on the take-off lower extremity.	• Stick the landing • Time to complete the 6-m distance • LSI = (time hopped involved lower extremity/ time hopped uninvolved lower extremity)*100 • ≥90% LSI[97]	0.08 to 0.21 seconds

Table 10-4 ━━

MEASUREMENT PROPERTIES OF PHYSICAL PERFORMANCE-BASED TESTS FOR INDIVIDUALS WITH KNEE OSTEOARTHRITIS[99]

TEST	INTRARATER RELIABILITY (ICC)	INTERRATER RELIABILITY (ICC)	STANDARD ERROR OF MEASUREMENT (BASED ON INTRARATER RELIABILITY)	STANDARD ERROR OF MEASUREMENT% (BASED ON INTRARATER RELIABILITY)	MDC
30-s chair stand test (number completed)	0.85	0.86	0.9	7.3	2.0
40-m fast-paced walk (m/s)	0.92	0.96	0.007	4.1	0.19
11-step stair climb test (seconds)	0.78	1.00	0.99	8.1	2.33
Timed Up and Go (seconds)	0.78	0.81	0.5	6.3	1.21
6-Minute Walk test (m)	0.94	0.93	18.12	3.3	50.23

ICC=intraclass correlation coefficient; m/s=meters/second; s=seconds.

DIAGNOSIS

The physical therapy examination of an individual with knee pain and dysfunction combines subjective and objective examination findings to provide an impairment-based classification diagnosis that guides the rehabilitation approach. The physical therapy diagnosis classification identifies primary musculoskeletal functional impairments that are often related to impairments of body structures, such as ACL tear, which provides an association to a pathoanatomic-based medical diagnosis. The diagnosis process includes medical screening to differentially diagnosis knee symptomology, which may be related to serious medical pathologies or psychosocial factors, red and yellow flags, respectively. Lastly, the physical therapy diagnosis classification process includes the assimilation of information related to the tissue irritability and the level of disability associated with knee symptomology to provide a staging of the condition that guides the selection and delivery of rehabilitation interventions for the attainment of optimal outcomes.

MUSCULOSKELETAL EXAMINATION OF THE KNEE

This section focuses on the subjective and objective examination components of a region-specific knee examination assuming that the clinician has, through the process of medical screening, determined the appropriateness for physical therapy, and through a lower quarter scan examination, determined the current symptomology to be related to the knee and confirmed the absence of neurological system involvement or referred pain from an adjacent region.

Subjective Examination

The subjective examination consists of focused inquiry to establish the history of the condition and mechanism of injury. Inquiring about symptom onset or mechanism of injury assists the clinician in discerning traumatic vs nontraumatic causes of knee pain and will assist in selecting clinical tests and measures for the objective examination. The term *traumatic knee pain* is defined as pain caused by an accident or sport injury.[102] Knee pain of traumatic origin may necessitate implementing screening processes for potential fractures, such as the Ottawa Knee Rules, and inclusion of ligamentous/soft tissue stress tests to determine the integrity of anatomical structures. Traumatic knee pain can be the result of contact or noncontact forces, of which noncontact traumatic injuries most commonly involve the ACL. Further questioning about the direction of forces sustained to the proximal tibia and the position of the knee when the injury occurred can assist in differentiating tissues that may be implicated. For example, anteriorly directed forces with the knee in full extension may suggest an ACL sprain, whereas posteriorly directed forces with the knee flexed may suggest a PCL sprain. A valgus or medially directed force may disrupt the MCL, and a varus or laterally directed force may disrupt the LCL. Twisting forces that involve rotation over a planted foot may result in additional injuries to the meniscus, ligaments, or both. Musculoskeletal knee pain of nontraumatic origin is usually described as insidious onset and related to degenerative conditions, such as osteoarthritis, or overuse/overload, such as PFPS.

A key component of the subjective examination is gathering information that will contribute to the staging of the condition. Subjective examination information used in the staging process includes assessment of the severity and irritability of presenting symptoms, symptom effect on function and disability, and psychosocial status.

Subjective assessment of the severity of a patient's knee symptomology includes use of a pain rating scale and information gathered from patient-reported outcome measures. The Numeric Pain Rating Scale (NPRS) and the Visual Analog Scale (VAS) are valid and reliable instruments commonly used to assess pain severity.[103,104] The NPRS is an 11-point scale ranging from 0 (no pain) to 10 (worst imaginable pain).[105] The VAS consists of a 100-mm horizontal line that represents a continuum from no pain on one end to extreme pain on the other end. In individuals with PFPS, the minimal clinically important difference (MCID) of the NPRS is 1.2 points.[106] The MCID for individuals with chronic musculoskeletal pain is reported to be 2 points for the NPRS[107] and 1.4 cm for the VAS.[108] While both instruments can be used to assess pain at a single point in time, the NPRS is often used to obtain multiple pain ratings over the last 24 hours (current, worse, and best level of pain) and the average of the 3 ratings is used to provide a measure of pain intensity.[109] The Four-Item Pain Intensity Measure (P4) involves obtaining 4 ratings of pain using the NPRS over the past 2 days.[110] The patient is asked to provide their average pain in the morning, afternoon, evening, and with activity using the NPRS resulting in a score range of 0 (no pain) to 40 (worst pain). The P4 questionnaire has established reliability and validity, with a MCID of 9.1 points.[110]

Identifying movements, positions, and activities that provoke or increase knee symptoms assists with establishing the concordant sign and can serve as a reassessment measure to determine treatment effectiveness. The irritability of the condition is assessed through gauging the tissue's ability to handle stress.[111,112] This can be done by determining how quickly symptoms develop when performing the provoking movement and the time frame required for symptoms to abate after activity cessation. High irritability is considered to be easily aggravated with activity to a moderate to high level of severity and slow to abate after activity cessation. In contrast, low irritability is considered to be not easily aggravated, has a low severity level, and is quick to abate after activity cessation.

SROM assist in the staging process through identifying the presence and extent of functional limitations and participation restrictions to determine the level of disability related to the knee condition. SROM can be divided into those that are region specific to the knee or lower extremity and those that are specific to the health condition (Table 10-5). Assessment of psychological distress provides an avenue to examine personal factors that may present as a barrier or facilitator to recovery. There are multiple constructs of psychological distress, referred to as *yellow flags*, including fear-avoidance beliefs, pain catastrophizing, kinesiophobia, depression, and anxiety. In regard to musculoskeletal knee dysfunction, psychological distress has been investigated primarily in individuals recovering from ACL injury, ACLR, and PFPS.[113-116] Several questionnaires can be used to assess the effect of psychosocial factors on recovery from knee pain (Table 10-6). While these questionnaires provide an assessment of individual dimensions of psychological status, the Optimal Screening for Prediction of Referral and Outcome Yellow Flag (OSPRO-YF) is a 17-item multidimensional assessment tool developed in support by the Orthopaedic Section of the American Physical Therapy Association.[117] The OSPRO-YF was designed for use by physical therapists treating musculoskeletal conditions to provide an estimate of individual psychological questionnaire scores and to identify yellow flags. A development study found the 17-item OSPRO-YF tool to have 85% accuracy when compared to individual questionnaire scores and 2 shorter instruments, 10- and 7-item tools, to have 81% and 75% accuracy, respectfully.[130] The OSPRO-YF is undergoing longitudinal validation, and no additional psychometrics have been reported.[117,131]

Objective Examination

The objective knee examination consists of physical impairment tests and measures administered in standing, seated, supine, and prone positions. Components of the objective examination include observation, motion testing, muscle performance testing, and special tests. Each component of the knee examination is presented in this section, followed by a summary of examination procedures by position in Table 10-7.

Table 10-5

SELF-REPORT OUTCOME MEASURES RELATED TO KNEE DYSFUNCTION

PATIENT-REPORTED OUTCOME MEASURES	DESCRIPTION	PROPERTIES
Anterior Knee Pain Scale (AKPS)	Consists of 13 items. The patient is asked to rate the level of disability in performing related to their anterior knee pain. Scores range from 0 (unable to perform) to 100 (no disability).	MDC = 13 points[118] (population = anterior knee pain)
Patient Specific Functional Scale (PSFS)	The patient is asked to identify up to x activities that they have difficulty or are unable to perform due to current symptoms. Difficulty in performance is rated from 0 (unable to perform) to 10 (able to perform at the prior level).	MDC = 1.5 points[119] (population = knee dysfunction)
Lower Extremity Functional Scale	Consists of 21 activities the patient rates their level of disability in performing as related to their lower limb problem. Difficulty in performance is rated from 0 (extreme difficulty) to 4 (no difficulty). High scores reflect less disability.	MDC = 8 points[118] (population = anterior knee pain)
Knee Outcome Survey-Activity of Daily Living (KOS-ADL)	Consists of 14 activities of daily living the patient rates their symptoms (6 items) and functional limitations (8 items) using a 6-point Likert scale. Scores range from 0 to 100, where 100 is no symptoms or limitations.	MCID = 7 points (population = PFPS)[120]
Knee Injury and Osteoarthritis Outcome Score (KOOS)	Consists of 42 items that represent 5 domains (pain, other symptoms, function in daily living, function in sport and recreation, knee-related quality of life) using a 5-point Likert scale. Scores range from 0 (extreme problems) to 100 (no problems).	MDC[121]: Pain = 13.4; symptoms = 15.5; Activities of daily living = 15.4; sport/ recreation = 19.6; quality of life = 21.1 (population = knee osteoarthritis)
IKDC	Consists of 18 items that assess knee symptoms, sports activity, and knee function. Scores range from 0 to 100 (100 = no limitation and no symptoms).	MCID[122] = 6.3 (at 6 months), 16.7 (at 12 months); population = articular cartilage repair MCID[123] = 11.5; population = varying knee conditions MDC[124] = 8.8; population = knee meniscus pathology
Western Ontario and McMaster Universities Arthritis Index	Consists of 24 items divided into 3 subscales: (1) pain (5 items); (2) stiffness (2 items); and (3) physical function (17 items). Items are scored on a 0 to 4 scale (0 = none, 4 = extreme). Targeted population is individuals with hip and knee osteoarthritis.	MDIC[125] = 17% to 22% change from baseline score; population = patients with lower extremity osteoarthritis

(continued)

Table 10-5 (continued) ──────────────────────────────────

SELF-REPORT OUTCOME MEASURES RELATED TO KNEE DYSFUNCTION

PATIENT-REPORTED OUTCOME MEASURES	DESCRIPTION	PROPERTIES
Lysholm Score	Consists of 8 items that assess knee symptoms related to instability. Score range is 0 to 100 (100 = no symptoms or disability).	MDC[126] = 8.9 (population = ACL injury)
Tegner Activity Score	From a range of 11 levels (Level 0 = sick leave or disability because of the knee problem; level 10 = competitive sports, national elite), the patient rates the highest level of activity they participated in before the knee injury/condition and the highest level of activity they are able to currently participate in.	MDC[126] = 1 (population = ACL injury)

Table 10-6 ──────────────────────────────────

SELF-REPORT QUESTIONNAIRES TO ASSESS PSYCHOLOGICAL FACTORS ON RECOVERY FROM KNEE DYSFUNCTION

QUESTIONNAIRE	DESCRIPTION
Tampa Scale for Kinesiophobia-11[127]	Consists of 11 items. The patient rates their fear of movement and re-injury using a 4-point Likert scale (0 to 4 points). Scores range from 11 to 44, where higher scores reflect greater kinesiophobia.
Fear-Avoidance Belief Questionnaire (FABQ)[128]	Consists of 2 subscales and 16 items that are scored on a 7-point Likert scale (completely disagree = 0; to completely agree = 6). Physical activity subscale contains 5 items and the work subscale contains 11 items. Higher scores represent greater fear-avoidance beliefs.
Pain Catastrophizing Scale[129]	Consists of a 13-item questionnaire in which each item is rated based on the degree to which the person has the feelings or thoughts when they are experiencing pain. A 0-to-4 Likert scale is used where 0 = not at all and 4 = all the time. Scores range from 0 to 52, with a score of 30 representing a high level of pain catastrophizing.

Observation

Observation consists of assessment of appearance, postural alignment, gait, and dynamic movements. Depending upon the severity of the presenting symptoms and weight-bearing status, observation is best performed with the patient in standing. The appearance of the lower extremity is assessed using visual identification of deformity or swelling in the knee region and atrophy of the thigh and calf muscles. Any appearance impairments are compared bilaterally for the presence of asymmetry. When present, the type of swelling, effusion, or edema can be assessed with special tests (eg, milking, sweeping, stroke tests), and the magnitude of swelling or atrophy can be measured in the supine position.

Static posture assessment for lower quarter postural malalignment is performed in standing by viewing the patient from the anterior, posterior, and lateral aspects as described previously in this chapter. If postural malalignment is observed, the therapist should manually attempt to correct the deviation or provide visual or verbal cues to guide the patient in postural correction to determine if the deviation is acquired and, if so, the effects of the correction on presenting symptoms. The presence of postural malalignments may suggest use for specific tests of muscle length and strength described in a corresponding section of this chapter.

Table 10-7

ORGANIZATION OF KNEE EXAMINATION BY POSITION

POSITION	CLINICAL TEST/MEASURE
Standing	• Observation • Static posture alignment: Visual inspection, Q-angle, leg length • Gait • Dynamic posture alignment/movement control • Static balance: DLS, SLS • Dynamic balance: Star Excursion Balance Test • Physical performance hop tests • Meniscus special tests: Thesslay's test
Seated	• Proprioception • Resisted movement testing: Knee extension, knee flexion • Patellofemoral special tests: Passive and active patella tracking • Meniscus special tests: Joint line tenderness • Palpation: See Table 10-8
Supine	• Knee ROM • Accessory motion testing: Tibiofemoral joint, PFJ • Resisted movement testing: Hip flexion • Muscle length: Hamstring 90/90, Thomas test, gastrocnemius, soleus • Patellofemoral special tests: Patella glides, patella apprehension, patella tilt and alignment tests • Ligament instability special tests: Anterior drawer, Lachman's, pivot-shift test, sag test, posterior drawer, valgus stress test, varus stress test, rotatory instability tests • Meniscus special tests: McMurrary's • Palpation: See Table 10-8
Side-lying	• Muscle length: Ober's • Resisted movement testing: Knee flexion, hip abduction, hip adduction
Prone	• Muscle length: Ely's, gastrocnemius, soleus • Resisted movement testing: hip extension, hip internal and external rotation • Palpation: See Table 10-8

A qualitative gait assessment is performed by watching the patient walk to observe for altered gait patterns related to knee pain, hip or thigh muscle weakness, motion impairments at the knee, or abnormal foot mechanics. The gait assessment should be conducted with the patient wearing shoes as well as bare foot to allow for observation of foot mechanics. Preferred gait speed is instructed during the assessment; however, use of fast gait speed or running may be indicated to identify gait alterations related to knee symptoms and impairments. Common gait abnormalities associated with knee pain include quadriceps avoidance gait pattern, decreased knee flexion during loading response, maintenance of knee flexion during stance, and knee hyperextension. Quadriceps avoidance gait can result secondary to quadriceps weakness or inhibition of the quadriceps by pain or swelling and is characterized by keeping the knee extended during loading response to avoid activation of the quadriceps. Similarly, a gait pattern of decreased knee flexion during loading response may be acquired to minimize compressive loading of the PFJ.[132] Maintenance of knee flexion during the stance phase of gait may reflect a limitation of knee extension ROM. Knee hyperextension may result due to insufficiency of the posterior and posterolateral structures of the knee.

Dynamic movement assessment allows identification of abnormal lower quarter movement patterns that may reflect postural malalignment observed in standing or may occur in absence of identification of standing postural impairments. Table 10-1 outlines bilateral and unilateral functional tasks commonly used for dynamic movement assessment. Both bilateral and unilateral functional tasks consist of the patient performing weightbearing knee flexion to 45 to 60 degrees, while the examiner observes for movement quality at the trunk, pelvis, hips, knees, and feet as described in Table 10-2. The irritability and disability level of the patient may necessitate deferral of dynamic movement assessment in whole to a later stage of rehabilitation or in part by performing bilateral functional task assessment and deferring unilateral tests.

Motion Testing

Motion testing of the knee consists of tibiofemoral active and passive mobility, dynamic patella tracking, and passive patella mobility. Because mobility limitations of the proximal and distal joints could affect knee function, examination of hip, ankle, and foot ROM should also be conducted either through a functional squat to screen the lower quarter joints or through individual joint motion testing. Knee ROM is most commonly assessed with the universal goniometer. Measurement properties of goniometric knee active range of motion (AROM) have been reported as good intrarater reliability for the universal goniometer (flexion ICC = 0.95; extension ICC = 0.87) and SEM of 3.4 degrees for knee flexion and 1.62 degrees for knee extension.[133] More recently, smartphone applications have been developed that allow for joint ROM measurements. When investigating the i-Goni application (June Software Inc., v.1.1, San Francisco, CA) for measurement of knee AROM, Mehta et al[133] reported the i-Goni application to have good concurrent validity with the universal goniometer, intrarater reliability of i-Goni knee flexion and extension to be 0.97 and 0.94, respectively, and i-Goni MDC values of 6.3 degrees for knee flexion and 2.7 degrees for knee extension. Other research has also found high concurrent validity for smartphone knee measurements when compared to the universal goniometer.[134,135]

Tibiofemoral active mobility involves the physiologic motions of flexion, extension, tibia internal rotation, and tibia external rotation. During active mobility testing, movement quantity, pain response during movement, dynamic tracking of the patella, and alignment changes of the patella are assessed. Normal AROM at the knee is 135 to 140 degrees of flexion and 10 to 15 degrees of extension.[136] For the secondary motions of tibial internal and external rotation, normal values are 20 to 25 degrees internal rotation (with knee flexed) and 30 to 35 degrees external rotation (with knee flexed). When knee extension AROM is less than passive range of motion (PROM), a quadriceps lag exists suggesting muscle performance deficits of the knee extensors.

PROM allows for the assessment of end-feel with normal end-feel being tissue approximation for knee flexion and tissue stretch for knee extension and tibial rotation. The relationship of PROM limitation and pain can contribute to irritability assessment. Pain before PROM limitation would suggest high irritability, PROM limitation coinciding with pain occurrence would suggest moderate irritability and pain with overpressure would suggest low irritability. When PROM is limited, testing of passive accessory mobility and muscle length can be performed to determine if the motion restriction is due to deficits of joint glide or muscle flexibility, respectively.

Passive accessory mobility testing at the knee is performed at the tibiofemoral joint and PFJ. Tibiofemoral joint accessory motion testing consists of anterior tibial glides for knee extension and posterior tibial glides for knee flexion. PFJ passive accessory motion testing consists of superior patella glide for knee extension and inferior patella glide for knee flexion. Passive medial and lateral patella glides are conducted to examine the integrity of the lateral and medial soft tissue restrains, respectively. When performed with the knee in full extension, medial and lateral glides examine soft tissue restraints, whereas positioning the knee in 30 degrees of flexion, the trochlea provides additional resistance to mobility. Approximately 8 to 20 mm of mediolateral patella glide has been reported as normal motion.[137] Decreased glide in the medial direction would suggest tightness of the lateral tissues, while decreased glide in the lateral direction would suggest tightness of the medial tissues. Conversely, increased medial or lateral mobility would be suggestive of hypermobility. Another method of assessing mediolateral patella mobility is describe by Kolowich et al,[138] which involves dividing the patella into 4 longitudinal quadrants, placing the knee in 20 to 30 degrees of flexion, and passively moving the patella medially and laterally. A medial glide of less than 1 quadrant suggests hypomobility of the lateral soft tissues, whereas a medial or lateral glide of 3 quadrants or greater suggests hypermobility of the patella. When patella instability is suspected, patient apprehension may accompany the passive mobility testing as describe by the Fairbank's sign (Appendix). Hypermobility in either the tibiofemoral joint or PFJ may also be related to general ligamentous laxity, which could be assessed using the Beighton and Horan Joint Mobility Index in which a score of 5 or greater out of 9 is indicative of generalized joint laxity.[139]

Muscle Performance Testing

Muscle performance deficits of the hip and thigh muscles are common impairments associated with knee disorders such as patellofemoral pain, ACL injury, and knee osteoarthritis.[27,31-33] Additional research has found that impaired hip abductor and external rotation strength assessed preseason predicts future noncontact ACL injuries,[28] decreased hamstring and quadriceps strength are risk factors for the development of patellofemoral pain,[140] and deficits in hip abduction strength[27] and knee extensor strength[141,142] are risk factors for the development of symptomatic knee osteoarthritis. Given these findings, assessment of knee and hip strength should be included in the knee examination.

Muscle performance testing of the hip and knee muscles can be performed through manual muscle testing, handheld dynamometry (HHD), isokinetic testing, and as a component of functional tasks and PPTs. During the lower quarter scan examination or in the earlier stages of rehabilitation when significant weakness exists, manual muscle testing is appropriate to identify muscle performance deficits in order to direct treatment. Similarly, an active lag test can assist in identifying the presence of quadriceps muscle performance deficit without the use of manual resistance, which may be contraindicated in the postsurgical knee. A positive active lag test occurs when a patient cannot actively extend the knee equal to motion attained during passive extension testing when the patient is positioned in a semi-recumbent position. A supine straight leg raise (SLR) can also be used to determine an active lag, or quadriceps lag, with a positive test being the inability to actively maintain the knee in an extended position during the SLR in the presence of full knee extension PROM.[143] A small, initial arc of an SLR should be used to prevent potential active insufficiency when the rectus femoris is shortened over both the hip and knee at higher angles of the SLR. HHD is appropriate when more precise quantification of hip/knee strength is needed, such as determination of limb symmetry in the later stages of rehabilitation or for screening of risk of knee injury. A limitation of HHD for the lower quarter muscles is the ability of the tester to generate forces at or above the level the patient could produce. Thus, use of belt-stabilization methods has been recommended when performing HHD of the hip and knee muscles.[144,145] Moderate to high interrater reliability (ICC ≥ 0.40) of belt-stabilized HHD have been reported hip abduction (ICC = 0.81 to 0.87), hip adduction (ICC = 0.88 to 0.90), hip external rotation (ICC = 0.80 to 0.90), hip internal rotation (ICC = 0.70 to 0.80), hip flexion (ICC = 0.90 to 0.96), hip extension (ICC = 0.91 to 0.94), knee extension (ICC = 0.91 to 0.93), and knee flexion (ICC = 0.62 to 0.66).[146] When belt-stabilized HHD was compared to isokinetic dynamometry, moderate to high correlation was found (Pearson correlation coefficient [r] = 0.52 to 0.90)[146-148]; however, absolute agreement between the 2 devices was not supported in the study by Martins et al.[146] Isokinetic concentric and eccentric testing provides another modality to assess knee strength by quantifying quadriceps/hamstring ratio and limb symmetry between the injured and uninjured lower extremity. Results from isokinetic testing is most commonly used to determine treatment progression and return-to-activity readiness.

Lower extremity strength can also be assessed with functional tasks such as sit to stand performed repeatedly over a determined number of repetitions (5 times or 10 times chair stand test) or duration (30-second chair stand test). The 30-second chair stand test is included in the Osteoarthritis Research Society International recommended PPTs as a measure of lower extremity strength in individuals with knee or hip osteoarthritis or following joint replacement.[101] Acceptable intrarater and interrater reliability have been reported for the 30-second chair stand test.[149,150] Normative data for healthy adults aged 60 to 94 years are provided by Rikli and Jones.[151]

Muscle Length Tests

Knee disorders such as PFPS and knee osteoarthritis often have associated ROM limitations associated with muscle length impairments.[152-154] Given the interrelationship of muscles between the hip-knee and the knee-ankle, muscle length tests should include flexibility assessment of the hip flexors, knee extensors, knee flexors, and ankle plantarflexors. Flexibility tests of muscle length are outlined in Table 10-8. Hip flexor flexibility assessment includes the Thomas test (assessment of iliopsoas, rectus femoris, TFL, and sartorius length) and Ely's test (assessment of rectus femoris length). Hamstring flexibility assessment can be performed by measuring popliteal angle during the 90/90 knee extension test or passive SLR test. ITB and TFL flexibility is assessed with the Ober's test or modified Ober's test. Flexibility of the ankle plantarflexors involves muscle length assessment of gastrocnemius and soleus in nonweightbearing and in weightbearing.

Balance and Proprioception

Knee dysfunction or injury can disrupt the mechanoreceptors in the joint capsule, ligaments, muscles, and tendons, creating sensorimotor deficits that result in impairments in proprioception and balance. Proprioceptive testing is most commonly conducted by using joint position sense or threshold to detect passive movement.[155] Research has found deficits in joint position sense and threshold to detect passive movement in individuals with knee osteoarthritis and ACL injury.[156-158] An association of reduced proprioception deficits and medial meniscal abnormalities has also been reported.[159] Joint position sense involves the clinician passively positioning the knee at a target angle without allowing the patient to visually observe the position, maintaining the position for 10 seconds, then returning the lower extremity to the resting position. The patient is then asked to actively reproduce the joint angle position. The difference between the active angle position and passive positioning by the clinician determines angular displacement for joint positioning. Active angle position reproduction assesses the ability of the muscle and joint capsule receptors. Kinesthesia can be examined by the clinician passively moving the knee at a slow angular velocity without visual awareness of the patient. The patient is instructed to indicate when perception of movement occurs. The time to detection of movement perception or the degree of angular displacement before detection of movement perception is assessed.

Table 10-8

FLEXIBILITY TESTS OF MUSCLE LENGTH AT THE HIP, KNEE, AND ANKLE

CLINICAL TEST	DESCRIPTION	FIGURE
Thomas test	Position: Supine with the patient holding both knees toward the chest. The buttocks are near the end of the table. Movement: Clinician palpates the lumbar lordosis with one hand while the patient lowers one lower extremity toward the table with the leg relaxed until the thigh reaches the table or an increase in lumbar lordosis occurs. Positive findings: Limited hip extension (the thigh does not reach the table) with (1) knee flexion > 45 degrees indicates tightness of iliopsoas; (2) knee flexion < 45 degrees indicates rectus femoris tightness; and (3) occurrence of hip abduction indicates tightness of the ITB.	
Ely's test	Position: Prone. Movement: Clinician palpates the lumbar spine while passively flexing the knee of the lower extremity to be tested until the heel touches the buttocks or the lumbar spine moves into lordosis. Positive findings: The heel does not touch the buttocks (measured as knee flexion angle) while maintaining lumbar lordosis without the hip rising off of the table.	
Ober's test	Position: Side-lying with the bottom lower extremity flexed at the hip and knee for stability. Movement: The top lower extremity is passively abducted and slightly extended while stabilizing the pelvis. The lower extremity is allowed to adduct with the force of gravity toward the table. Positive findings: The thigh remains elevated past the horizontal.	

Balance involves the maintenance of postural control during static and dynamic conditions. During static balance assessment, the ability to maintain postural control within the base of support with minimal body or segment movement is examined.[160] In contrast, during dynamic balance assessment, the ability to maintain postural control within the base of support is examined while performing body or segment movement.[160] Postural control can be quantified during static and dynamic tasks with force platform systems that calculate center of pressure movements. Research using instrumented force plate systems has found deficits in single leg balance in individuals with ACL injury,[161-163] patellofemoral pain,[164] and knee osteoarthritis.[165] Cost, time, and clinician experience present as limitations with the use of instrumented systems to assess balance in the clinical setting. Alternative methods to assess balance that are more applicable to the clinic include the measurement of time that balance is maintained, time to complete a balance task, or distance of body or segment movement. Static balance can be assessed with double or single leg standing with variations in vision or support surface. Single leg stance time has been found to be significantly less for individuals with knee osteoarthritis (mean = 41.7 ± 33.2 seconds) as compared to healthy controls (mean = 66.1 ± 30.7 seconds).[166] Individuals post-ACLR were found to have significantly greater total errors during static balance assessed with the Balance Error Scoring System (BESS) as compared to healthy controls and significantly greater errors during single leg balance on foam with eyes closed.[167]

The Star Excursion Balance Test (SEBT) is a dynamic balance test that measures the distance reach by one lower extremity while performing a single-limb squat on the opposite lower extremity. Reaches are performed in 8 directions along lines placed on the floor, oriented 45 degrees from one another to form a star-shaped grid. Reach direction is named in reference to the stance lower extremity placed in the center of the grid. The maximum distance an individual can reach in a direction while maintaining single-limb stance control is measured and normalized by dividing the distance reach by the lower extremity limb length. The SEBT identified balance deficits in individuals with ACL deficiency,[168,169] individuals with ACLR at the time of return to sport,[170] and individuals with PFPS[171] when compared to healthy controls. A modification of the SEBT is the Y Balance Test which consists of the anterior, posteromedial, and posterolateral directions. The sum of the reach distances in the 3 directions divided by 3 times lower extremity limb length provides a composite score. Both the SEBT and the Y Balance Test have been found to be a reliable and valid measures to predict risk of lower extremity injury in active individuals.[160,172-174] Composite Y Balance Tests scores below 94% of limb length have been found to predict lower extremity injury in female basketball players and a side-to-side difference

in the anterior reach distance was associated with increased risk of lower extremity injury in male and female basketball players.[175] The MDC for composite Y Balance Test scores of healthy, young adults (aged 18 to 30 years) is reported to be 7.2% for the right lower extremity and 6.2% for the left lower extremity when testing is performed by the same tester.[174] For healthy adolescents (aged 12 to 14 years), the intrarater MDC of composite Y Balance Test scores are 2.3% and 2.6% for the right and left lower extremities, respectively.[176]

Palpation

The palpation component of the examination is conducted to identify anatomical structures that may be contributing to knee symptomology. The process of palpation may create sensitivity in uninvolved structures; thus, palpation is usually performed at the end of the objective examination. By organizing the objective examination in this manner, the clinician should have an idea of which structures to palpate that will eliminate the need to palpate all accessible structures in the knee region. Palpation should be performed on the uninvolved knee first in the case of unilateral pain or on the side of less pain in the case of bilateral involvement. As palpation is performed, the clinician assesses patient response to tenderness or pain as well as assesses for changes in temperature and presence of edema. Because positioning improves accessibility of certain knee structures, the palpation examination is best performed by position as outlined in Table 10-9 instead of structure type (patellofemoral vs tibiofemoral structures, osseous vs soft tissue structures) or location (anterior, posterior, lateral, or medial). Assessment of palpation findings can use a dichotomous rating in which a rating of positive indicates tenderness or warmth with palpation and a rating of negative indicates absence of tenderness or warmth with palpation.

Special Tests

Special tests of the knee can be divided into categories related to the PFJ, knee ligament sprain, and meniscal tears (Appendix). Information gathered thus far during the subjective and objective examination should guide the clinician toward special tests indicated to further assess the condition. Diagnosis accuracy of clinical test findings associated with PFPS, ACL tears and meniscal tears can be found in Tables 10-10, 10-11, and 10-12, respectively.

Physical Performance Tests

PPTs provide a quantitative assessment of function through measurement of time, distance, or repetitions. If the irritability of the condition is low, these tests may be included in the initial examination. More commonly, PPT are used as criterion for progression between rehabilitation phases or at discharge for outcome assessment and return-to-activity readiness. Common PPTs are provided in Table 10-3.

Table 10-9

SELECTED TISSUES FOR PALPATION RELATED TO KNEE DYSFUNCTION

SUPINE	SEATED	PRONE
• Superior and inferior pole patella • Medial and lateral retinaculum • Medial and lateral facets • Adductor tubercle • Tibial tuberosity • MCL • Patella tendon • Quadriceps tendon • VMO • Rectus femoris • ITB	• Medial and lateral joint line • Medial and lateral femoral condyles • Medial and lateral femoral epicondyles • Medial and lateral tibial condyles • LCL • Fibula head	• Biceps femoris • Semimembranous • Semitendinous • Popliteal fossa

Table 10-10

SUMMARY OF SYSTEMATIC REVIEWS WITH META-ANALYSES OF DIAGNOSTIC ACCURACY OF CLINICAL TESTS FOR MENISCAL TEARS

TEST	STUDY	SENSITIVITY (95% CI)	SPECIFICITY (95% CI)	+LR (95% CI)	−LR (95% CI)
McMurray's test	Smith et al[181]	0.61 (0.45 to 0.74)	0.84 (0.69 to 0.92)	3.2	0.52
	Meserve et al[182]	55 (50, 60)	77 (62, 87)	2.4	0.58
	Hegedus et al[183]	70.5 (67.4, 73.4)	71.1 (69.3, 72.9)		
Joint line tenderness	Smith et al[181]	0.83 (0.73 to 0.90)	0.83 (0.63 to 0.94)	4.0	0.23
	Meserve et al[182]	76 (73, 80)	77 (64, 87)	3.3	0.31
	Hegedus et al[183]	63.3 (60.9, 65.7)	77.4 (75.6, 79.1)		
Thesslay's test at 20 degrees	Smith et al[181]	0.75 (0.53 to 0.89)	0.87 (0.65 to 0.98)	5.6	0.28
Apley's test	Meserve et al[182]	22 (17, 28)	88 (72, 96)	—	—
	Hegedus et al[183]	60.7 (55.7, 65.5)	70.2 (68, 72.4)	—	—

CI = confidence interval; LR = likelihood ratio.

Table 10-11

SUMMARY OF SYSTEMATIC REVIEWS WITH META-ANALYSES OF DIAGNOSTIC ACCURACY OF CLINICAL TESTS FOR ANTERIOR CRUCIATE LIGAMENT TEARS

TEST	STUDY	SENSITIVITY (95% CI)	SPECIFICITY (95% CI)	+LR (95% CI)	-LR (95% CI)
Lachman	Leblanc et al[184]	89% (76%, 98%)	—	—	—
	van Eck et al[185]	81%	81%	4.5	0.22
	Benjaminse et al[186]	85% (83%, 87%)	94% (92%, 95%)	10.2	0.20
Pivot shift	Leblanc et al[184]	79% (63%, 91%)	—	—	—
	van Eck et al[185]	28%	81%	5.35	0.84
	Benjaminse et al[186]	24% (21%, 27%)	98% (96%, 99%)	8.5	0.90
Anterior drawer	van Eck et al[185]	38%	81%	4.52	0.67
	Benjaminse et al[186]	55% (52%, 58%)	92% (90%, 94%)	7.3	0.50
Lever sign	Abruscato et al[187]	77% (56%, 90%)	90% (77%, 96%)	6.60 (2.48, 17.59)	0.22 (0.09, 0.57)

CI = confidence interval.

Table 10-12

SUMMARY OF SYSTEMATIC REVIEWS WITH META-ANALYSES AND INDIVIDUAL STUDIES OF DIAGNOSTIC ACCURACY OF CLINICAL TESTS FOR PATELLOFEMORAL PAIN SYNDROME

TEST	STUDY	INTERRATER RELIABILITY (KAPPA)	SENSITIVITY (95% CI)	SPECIFICITY (95% CI)	+LR (95% CI)	-LR (95% CI)
Systematic Review With Meta-Analysis						
Patella apprehension	Nunes et al[188]	—	15% (9%, 24%)	89% (77%, 95%)	1.3 (0.6, 3.3)	1.0 (0.8, 1.1)
Individual Studies						
Manual compression	Cook et al[189]	—	68%	54%	1.5 (0.99, 2.3)	0.6 (0.3, 1.0)
Resisted isometric quadriceps	Cook et al[189]	—	39%	82%	2.2 (0.99, 5.2)	0.75 (0.6, 1.1)
Palpation	Cook et al[189]	—	47%	68%	1.5 (0.85, 2.8)	0.8 (0.6, 1.1)
Patella tilt	Haim et al[190]	—	43% (31%, 55%)	92% (75%, 98%)	5.4 (1.4, 20.8)	0.6 (0.5, 0.8)
Patella M/L glide	Sweitzer et al[191]	0.59 (0.42, 0.72)	54% (47%, 59%)	69% (52%, 83%)	1.8 (0.9, 3.6)	0.7 (0.5, 1.0)

CI = confidence interval; M/L = medial/lateral; — = not reported.

CLASSIFICATION OF KNEE DYSFUNCTION

Through the evaluation of subjective and objective examination findings, key impairment patterns are identified and the stage of the condition is determined. This process provides a physical therapy classification-based diagnosis that guides the selection and delivery of interventions to minimize impairments of body function, activity limitations, and participation restrictions.[111,177,178] The *International Classification of Functioning, Disability and Health* model provides a framework to classify examination findings to determine the key impairment patterns.[179] While traditional staging methods have utilized timelines defined as acute, subacute, and chronic, associated with symptom duration and tissue healing, use of subjective information related to irritability and disability, clinical tests, and measures are suggested as criteria to guide the selection of intervention and progression of the rehabilitative process. Information related to tissue irritability and level of disability determined from SROM gauge the irritability of the condition.[21,111,177] A rehabilitative staging model has been proposed by Sahrmann[55] and consists of 3 stages. The stages are identified according to level of irritability and to the amount of protection needed to minimize stress to the healing tissues and to prevent re-injury.[55,180] In stage 1 (maximum protection phase), the irritability level is high (pain ≥ 7/10), SROM suggest high disability, and the emphasis of intervention procedures is to provide high protection (maximum protection phase). In stage 2 (moderate protection phase), the irritability level is moderate (pain 4 to 6/10), SROM suggest moderate disability, and the emphasis of the intervention procedures is to provide moderate protection (moderate protection phase). In stage 3, the irritability is low (pain ≤ 3/10), SROM suggest a low level of disability, and intervention procedures are selected based on the need for low protection (minimum protection phase).

GENERAL INTERVENTIONS FOR KNEE REHABILITATION

This section provides general guidelines for impairment-based interventions during knee rehabilitation.

Stage One: Maximum Protection Phase

The primary goals for rehabilitation during stage 1 are to minimize pain, control swelling, maintain joint and soft tissue mobility, and prevent ROM loss. Modalities (eg, transcutaneous electrical stimulation, interferential current) and physical agents (eg, cold, heat) are commonly employed during stage 1 to address pain and swelling. Early mobilization while protecting injured tissues is a component of stage 1 rehabilitation of knee dysfunction for the goal of restoration of or prevention of knee ROM impairments.[111,177] While continuous passive motion is recommended in the 2017 Knee Ligament Clinical Practice Guideline as an intervention for the management of pain in the immediate postoperative period of post-ACLR,[111] Continuous passive motion following total knee arthroplasty[192] was not found to have clinically important effects on pain or ROM. Gentle grade I or II mobilizations to the tibiofemoral joint can also be used for pain control. Soft tissue massage can be used to mobilize fluid and to prevent adhesion formation in soft tissues.

PROM exercises can be used to prevent mobility deficits and to maintain ROM. If active muscle contraction is allowed, AROM or active assisted ROM will assist in minimizing muscle atrophy, mobilizing fluid, and stimulating joint receptors.[193] Joint position reproduction can be performed in nonweightbearing positions to provide proprioception training through pain-free angles of motion. Muscle setting involving low intensity contraction can be used to improve local circulation.

Muscle performance exercises can be initiated beginning with isometric contractions of the quadriceps and hamstrings as appropriate to protect the injured or repaired tissues. Muscle setting can be progressed to include multiangle isometrics as ROM ability and restrictions allow. Emphasis on the lowering phase of an SLR exercise may assist in recruiting quadriceps activation and control. Pain and swelling inhibits neural activation and subsequent motor output of the quadriceps; therefore, the ability to make voluntary quadriceps contractions may be diminished even in the absence of muscle injury, a condition known as *autogenic muscle inhibition*.[194-197] The use of neuromuscular electrical stimulation (NMES) can be effective in improving quadriceps function in individuals with knee osteoarthritis and following knee replacement and ligament reconstruction, as well as preventing the development of inhibition associated quadriceps weakness.[196,198-200]

If weightbearing is allowed, balance interventions can be introduced in double leg stance with progressions to incorporate variations in vision, support surface, and use of tandem stance. Use of cocontraction of the quadriceps and hamstrings during weightbearing balance activities will promote stability of the knee. Pending weightbearing status, protected ambulation can be instructed with an assistive device, if appropriate, to minimize joint and tissue stress. Emphasis is placed on utilizing a normal gait pattern with heel strike, full knee extension during stance, and knee flexion in the swing phase.

Patient education in avoidance of activities that load the knee joints and use of controlled rest from repetitive or high intensity activities is important for self-management of pain. In addition, patient education including instruction in safe movement patterns to optimize dynamic postural control of the lower extremity can assist in managing pain and reducing joint load. Due to regional interdependence, flexibility and resistance exercises directed to muscles proximal and distal to the knee may also be indicated targeting the hip adductors, hip extensors, ITB, iliopsoas, gastrocnemius, and soleus. These exercises should be monitored to ensure they do not disrupt healing of knee-related structures or increase pain at the knee. Box 10-1 provides examples of knee-related therapeutic interventions appropriate for stage 1 rehabilitation.

Stage Two: Moderate Protection Phase

The primary goals for rehabilitation during stage 2 are to manage pain and inflammation, restore knee ROM, improve knee and hip muscle performance, minimize balance deficits, and develop neuromuscular control. If pain is still present and inflammation remains, modalities and physical agents will continue to be appropriate in management impairments of pain and inflammation. ROM exercises remain important to restore full knee extension and flexion. Given that small amounts of knee extension deficits result in significant gait impairments and may lead to postoperative complications of arthrofibrosis, low-load positional stretching techniques may be used to restore knee extension such as prone hangs and heel props with limb loading, progressing to loadings with the application of an external weight such as a cuff weight. When tests of tibiofemoral or patellofemoral accessory mobility are found to be hypomobile, joint mobilization interventions can be employed using an anterior tibial glide and superior mobilization of the patella to address knee extension impairment and a posterior tibial glide and inferior patella mobilization to address knee flexion impairment. Joint mobilization techniques would involve use of grades III and IV (Maitland) to address mobility deficits. Similarly, impairments of muscle length may be contributing to knee mobility deficits, in which hamstring stretching would address knee extension flexibility impairments and quadriceps stretching would address knee flexion flexibility impairments.

Muscle performance interventions can be progressed with sitting knee dynamic extension through a protected range in consideration of biomechanical factors to minimize loading of the PFJ, articular cartilage and injured or repaired ligaments, and prone knee flexion. CKC exercise can be used to promote muscle performance through DLS through the 0- to 45-degree range, partial lunges, and calf raises. Hip extensor and abductor strengthening should also be instituted to assist with minimization of hip adduction and internal rotation during dynamic movements.[201-203] Trunk stabilization interventions targeting muscle performance and motor control are also indicated given the findings of poor trunk control in individuals with PFPS and ACL injury.[204] Static balance training can progress from double leg stance to single leg stance with vision and surface variations. Due to research findings of strength and balance deficits in the uninvolved lower extremity following ACL injury, rehabilitation interventions should also address muscle performance, balance, and dynamic movement control of the uninvolved side.[21]

Attainment of normal gait pattern with quadriceps control is a prerequisite to ambulation without an assistive device or progression of ambulation interventions. Ambulation progression includes directional ambulation in forward, backward, and side directions; ambulation on surface variations; and ambulation around obstacles. Functional mobility interventions involve use of available ROM during functional activities such as placing one foot on/off steps of progressive height to incorporate knee flexion, squatting to pick up objects from the floor, and sit-to-stand transitions.[205,206]

Utilization of optimal movement patterns during CKC exercises and functional mobility tasks is a key component of improving neuromuscular control. This can be accomplished by incorporating motor learning principles during CKC exercises and functional task activities such as verbal, tactile, and visual feedback for knee-over-toe positioning and use of hip flexion with trunk inclination to activate posterior chain muscles during double leg partial squats, partial lunges, functional squat tasks, and sit-to-stand-to-sit transitions.[207-210] Incorporating holding of knee flexion in DLS and partial lunges will promote joint stability. Box 10-2 provides examples of therapeutic interventions appropriate for stage 2 rehabilitation.

Stage Three: Minimum Protection Phase/Return to Function

The primary goals for rehabilitation during stage 3 are to restore full extensibility of soft tissue structures, attain neuromuscular control during dynamic movements, restore strength and endurance in knee and hip musculature, achieve limb symmetry in strength and PPTs, and return to functional or sport activities. Stretching of periarticular soft tissues through high-grade joint mobilizations and of muscles through flexibility exercises is indicated if end-range motion restrictions persist or as mobility maintenance when full ROM has been achieved in prior stages.

Knee rehabilitation and injury prevention programs are most effective when multiple components of neuromuscular control are included instead of focus on a single intervention type in isolation.[210,211] The recommended component interventions for retraining of neuromuscular control include balance, strength, proximal control, and plyometrics.[211] Balance, strength, and proximal control (hip and trunk muscle performance) were introduced or progressed in stage 1 and 2 guidelines thus far. In stage 3, hip, knee, and calf strengthening is progressed through increasing dosage intensity using variations in loading, repetitions, and sets to address muscular endurance as well as strength.[193] Unilateral CKC exercises, such as SLS and step down, are used to target both eccentric and concentric components of muscle performance. During the performance of these unilateral CKC exercises, the clinician should provide verbal and visual cues regarding use of optimum movement strategies as discussed previously. Balance training is progressed to include perturbation training during single leg balance tasks to enhance knee stability through

Box 10-1. Example Interventions for Stage One Knee Rehabilitation

INTERVENTION	FIGURE
Mobility	
Active assisted range of motion (AAROM) heel slides	
AAROM wall slides	
AAROM seated flexion	

(continued)

Box 10-1 (continued). Example Interventions for Stage One Knee Rehabilitation

INTERVENTION	FIGURE
Patella mobilizations	
Calf stretching nonweightbearing	
Knee Muscle Performance	
Quadriceps muscle sets	
Hamstring muscle sets	

(continued)

Box 10-1 (continued). Example Interventions for Stage One Knee Rehabilitation

INTERVENTION	FIGURE
Multiangle isometrics	
SLR	
Straight leg lowering	

(continued)

Box 10-1 (continued). Example Interventions for Stage One Knee Rehabilitation

INTERVENTION	FIGURE
CKC terminal knee extension	
CKC mini squats 0 to 30 degrees	
Hip Muscle Performance	
Four-way SLR: A. Adduction B. Flexion C. Extension D. Abduction	

(continued)

Box 10-1 (continued). Example Interventions for Stage One Knee Rehabilitation

INTERVENTION	FIGURE
Trunk Muscle Performance	
Prone plank	
Side plank	
Neuromuscular Training	
Double leg stance with perturbation	

(continued)

Box 10-1 (continued). Example Interventions for Stage One Knee Rehabilitation

INTERVENTION	FIGURE
Tandem stance progression from stride stance to heel-toe stance	
Single leg stance	

establishing open loop feedback for motor control.[212-214] Dynamic balance training is accomplished through agility and coordination training such as braiding, front and back crossover steps during forward and backward walking, respectively; shuttle walking; and multiple changes in direction during walking upon command using a random practice schedule.[212,214] As for the individual with activity limitations related to running, gait training should include assessment of and instruction in running mechanics and technique. Agility and coordination activities can be progressed from walking to running as the knee joints attain the ability to attenuate higher loading incurred during running.

Once full knee ROM is attained, pain and effusion are resolved and quadriceps strength is 80% of the uninvolved side, plyometric exercises can be instituted if appropriate for the functional activities and participations the individual desires to resume.[215] Plyometric exercises are more commonly used for rehabilitation of knee ligament instability. During plyometric exercise, emphasis is placed on landing strategy during bilateral progressing to unilateral jump tasks. Examples include vertical jump, DVJ, and hopping. Box 10-3 provides examples of therapeutic interventions appropriate for stage 3 rehabilitation.

Box 10-2. Example Interventions for Stage Two Knee Rehabilitation

INTERVENTION	FIGURE
Mobility	
Tibiofemoral joint mobilizations A. Flexion progression in prone B. Flexion progression in supine C. Extension in prone	
Prone hang for knee extension	
Heel prop for knee extension	
Knee flexion overpressure	

(continued)

Box 10-2 (continued). Example Interventions for Stage Two Knee Rehabilitation

INTERVENTION	FIGURE
Hamstring stretching	
Quadriceps stretching	
Gastrocsoleus weightbearing stretching	

(continued)

Box 10-2 (continued). Example Interventions for Stage Two Knee Rehabilitation

INTERVENTION	FIGURE
Knee Muscle Performance	
OKC knee extension 90 to 45 degrees	
OKC hamstring curl A. Prone B. Standing maintaining hip-knee alignment to isolate hamstrings	

(continued)

Box 10-2 (continued). Example Interventions for Stage Two Knee Rehabilitation

INTERVENTION	FIGURE
CKC SLS (0 to 45 degrees) A. TRX (Fitness Anywhere LLC) unloading assistance B. Body weight resistance with alignment of knee over medial toes	
CKC partial forward lunges A. Sagittal plane forward lunge with trunk, hip, and knee alignment B. Sagittal plane forward lunge with TRX to engage posterior chain muscles	
Hip Muscle Performance	
Bridging with alignment of trunk-hip-knee for trunk stability and alignment of knee over or slightly behind the heel to promote gluteal muscle activation A. Double leg bridge B. Single leg bridge	

(continued)

Box 10-2 (continued). Example Interventions for Stage Two Knee Rehabilitation

INTERVENTION	FIGURE
Four-way SLR weightbearing on involved lower extremity A. Abduction B. Extension C. Flexion D. Adduction	
Trunk Muscle Performance	
TRX suspension training A. Plank B. Plank tucks	

(continued)

Box 10-2 (continued). Example Interventions for Stage Two Knee Rehabilitation

INTERVENTION	FIGURE
Neuromuscular Training	
Double leg stance progressions A. Addition of surface instability B. Addition of perturbations with surface instability C. Tandem stance on unstable surface	
Single leg stance progressions A. Contralateral weight destabilization B. Ipsilateral weight destabilization C. Overhead weight destabilization D. Unstable surface	
Y-balance A. Anterior B. Posteromedial C. Posterolateral	
DLS and hold	

Box 10-3. Example Interventions for Stage Three Knee Rehabilitation

INTERVENTION	FIGURE
Knee Muscle Performance	
OKC knee extension 90 to 0 degrees	
CKC step down A. Front B. Lateral	
Hip Muscle Performance	
Bridge progression	
Single leg deadlift	

(continued)

Box 10-3 (continued). Example Interventions for Stage Three Knee Rehabilitation

INTERVENTION	FIGURE
Trunk Muscle Performance	
Kneeling stability	
Frontal plane trunk lifts	

(continued)

Box 10-3 (continued). Example Interventions for Stage Three Knee Rehabilitation

INTERVENTION	FIGURE
Neuromuscular Training: Running Program	
Perturbation training	
Double leg vertical jumps	
Single leg vertical jump	
Forward hopping— Double leg progressing to SLH	

(continued)

Box 10-3 (continued). Example Interventions for Stage Three Knee Rehabilitation

INTERVENTION	FIGURE
Lateral hopping A. Double leg lateral hops B. Single leg lateral hops C. Side-to-side lateral hops with TRX	
DVJ	
Agility drills A. Grapevine B. Shuttle run C. Ladder drills	

An Overview of Common Knee-Related Physical Therapy Classification-Based Diagnoses and Associated Health Conditions

Knee Pain Impairment

Anterior knee pain is a leading cause for patients to seek physical therapy and comprises many subcategories, of which the health condition or pathoanatomical diagnosis of PFPS is the most common. The onset of PFPS is usually insidious and the associated pain is often persistent.[65] Both intrinsic and extrinsic contributing and prognostic factors have been identified. No one factor has been consistently identified as a risk to the development of PFPS or as a barrier to symptom resolution, thus, necessitating the clinician to consider PFPS from a multifactorial and individualistic perspective. The lack of specific imaging studies to confirm PFPS has led to the reliance on the clinical examination process. However, research regarding clinical tests for PFPS does not support the diagnostic use of individual tests but the use of clusters of subjective and objective examination findings that have been found to yield higher diagnostic accuracy in the diagnosis of PFPS.[216-218] In an initial derivation diagnostic study, Décary et al[217] identified 2 clusters of examination tests with 93% and 96% specificity for differentially diagnosing individuals with PFPS. Components of the first cluster were less than 40 years old, isolated anterior knee pain, and medial patellar facet tenderness (specificity 93%, +LR 8.70). The second cluster included age 40 to 58 years, isolated anterior or diffuse knee pain, mild to moderate difficulty descending stairs, medial patellar facet tenderness, and full passive knee extension (specificity 96%, +LR 14.28).[217]

Although PFPS is characterized by both intrinsic and extrinsic factors, it is the repetitive accumulation of stress to the joint through combinations of these factors that disrupts the homeostasis at the PFJ leading to symptom development.[219] This explains why individuals with patella or lower extremity malalignment may be asymptomatic until tissue loading exceeds tissue tolerance. An intervention program directed toward minimization of malalignment and associated movement impairments would not be effective for these individuals. Instead, a more effective rehabilitation strategy for these individuals would employ interventions targeting minimization of factors contributing to tissue overload, such as training parameters, in the early stages of rehabilitation followed by interventions that increase tissue tolerance to the loads the individual is required to function under in the later stages of rehabilitation.[23,178,220]

Intrinsic factors associated with PFPS can be classified at the personal level and as impairments of body structure and function. At the personal level, physical factors associated with PFPS include female sex, young age, and athletes or individuals who perform repetitive loading of the knee in a flexed position.[68,221,222] Recent findings also suggest that psychosocial, nonphysical personal factors may present as barriers to recovery from PFPS.[68,115,116] Psychosocial factors include pain catastrophizing, fear of movement, anxiety, and depression. Intrinsic factors that may present as impairments include lower quarter malalignment during weightbearing, muscle imbalance at the local and regional levels, and soft tissue dysfuction.[65,68] Dynamic valgus malalignment is frequently observed in individuals with PFPS and is characterized by varying combinations of contralateral pelvic drop, hip adduction, femoral internal rotation, knee valgus, tibial internal rotation, and foot pronation.[223] Ways in which dynamic valgus malalignment can contribute to PFPS center around altered hip and knee kinematics that increase laterally directed forces at the PFJ. Laterally directed forces at the PFJ can lead to lateralization of the patella and decreased patellofemoral contact area, which increases patellofemoral stress during weightbearing loading conditions.[223,224] Specifically, the components of dynamic valgus that have been found to increase lateral forces at the PFJ are femoral internal rotation and increased knee abduction moment.[225]

Muscle imbalances at the hip and knee have been found in individuals with PFPS (as compared to healthy controls) and are thought to contribute to dynamic valgus. These imbalances include weakness or activation dysfunction of hip extensors, external rotators and abductors, and knee extensors.[28,65,69,224] While evidence of hip and knee muscle weakness exists in individuals with PFPS, it is unclear if this weakness is causative or subsequent from the condition.[23,226]

Soft tissue dysfunction related to PFPS includes tightness of the quadriceps, hamstrings, gastrocnemius, lateral retinaculum, and ITB. Proposed mechanisms for the contribution of quadriceps and hamstring tightness to PFPS relate to increased PFJ stress created by compression of the patella against the trochlea secondary to quadriceps tightness and increased PFJR forces resulting from increased quadriceps force demands to overcome the knee flexion moment created by hamstring tightness. Soft tissue tightness of the lateral retinaculum and ITB may contribute to PFPS by increasing the lateral vector acting on the patella, which over time creates lateralization of the patella and subsequent alterations in patellofemoral contact area and stress as described previously.[227,228] Tightness of the ITB-TFL may also contribute to PFPS by causing ipsilateral hip internal rotation under a stable patella, which creates a relative lateralization of the patella.[43] Gastrocnemius tightness is proposed to have an indirect effect by altering foot mechanics toward excessive pronation and the resulting dynamic valgus malalignment.[229,230]

Extrinsic contributors include factors associated with training errors such as wearing shoes that are worn or fit improperly, performing weightbearing activities on hard or irregular surfaces, and changes in type and dosage of training or work activities. Activities that increase PFPS include sustained positions of knee flexion (eg, sitting), movements involving deep knee flexion (eg, squatting), and high loading

HEALTH CONDITION		
PATELLOFEMORAL PAIN SYNDROME	• Anterior knee pain in the retropatella or peripatella area that is aggravated by activity that loads the patellofemoral joint.	
BODY STRUCTURE/FUNCTION (IMPAIRMENTS)	**ACTIVITY**	**PARTICIPATION**
• Malalignment- dynamic valgus • Hip muscle weakness-extensors, external rotators, abductors • Knee muscle weakness-quadriceps • Soft tissue dysfunction-lateral retinaculum, ITB • Flexibility deficits-hamstring, quadriceps, gastrocnemius tightness	• Sustained sitting • Squatting • Descending or ascending stairs • Running • Jumping	• Work/employment • Leisure/athletic • Social/community
CONTEXTUAL FACTORS		
PERSONAL	**ENVIRONMENTAL**	
• Gender – female • Age – adolescents, young adults • Psychosocial –fear of movement, pain catastrophizing, depression, anxiety	• Training surface • Work surface • Shoewear • Abrupt changes in training parameters	

Figure 10-5. Common impairments, activity limitations, and participation restrictions associated with PFPS.

tasks (eg, stair ambulation, running, jumping). These provoking activities may contribute to participation restrictions in work, leisure, or athletic events and social or community activities. Figure 10-5 summarizes the common impairments, activity limitations, and participation restrictions associated with PFPS including contextual factors.

Treatment of PFPS is multifaceted and encompasses pain management, modification of extrinsic contributing factors such as shoewear and training practices, education to address psychosocial issues associated with fear avoidance of activities, improving soft tissue extensibility of muscles and peripatella connective tissues, improving strength at the hip and knee, restoring neuromuscular control and the trunk and lower extremity, and improving tissue tolerance to sport and activity with an emphasis on trunk and lower extremity mechanics and dynamic alignment during functional tasks.[36,116,231-233] Table 10-13 provides examples of interventions related to rehabilitation of knee pain impairment related to PFPS. Recent research has highlighted the importance of including proximal strengthening as an intervention for individuals with PFPS. When compared to knee strengthening alone, hip and knee strengthening is more effective in pain reduction and improved function.[36,178,220,233,234] Conflicting findings have been reported regarding the use of patella taping for the management of long-term pain in PFPS with an earlier systematic review and meta-analysis concluding that medially directed tape produced a clinically meaningful reduction in pain when compared to sham tape or no tape,[235] whereas a more recent meta-analysis[236] found no statistical or clinically meaningful difference in pain between patella taping interventions and nontaping.

Due to the multiple factors that can contribute to PFPS, classifying individuals in subgroups to direct treatment has been proposed. Selhorst et al[154] have presented an algorithm for the treatment of PFPS that divides treatment into 4 impairment-based subgroups dependent upon examination findings. The 4 PFPS subgroups are (1) fear avoidance, (2) flexibility, (3) functional malalignment, and (4) strengthening/functional progression. Placement into a subgroup involves a stepwise process of evaluating examination findings that proceeds from interpretation of (1) FABQ scores; (2) muscle length tests of the quadriceps, gastrocnemius, and soleus; (3) dynamic alignment during the SLS test and LSD; and (4) functional strength assessed through PPT ability during SLH for distance, triple hop for distance, crossover hop for distance, and timed step down. Treatment is delivered sequentially from the initial subgroup placement to the next. Piloting test results showed that 100% of patients who completed the PFPS algorithm intervention had clinically significant improvement in the AKPS and Global Rating of Change outcome measures. In addition, good interrater reliability was found with subgrouping using the algorithm (kappa = 0.90), and 100% of therapists who provided the intervention adhered to the treatment algorithm.

Table 10-13

EXAMPLE INTERVENTIONS FOR REHABILITATION OF PATELLOFEMORAL PAIN SYNDROME

PROBLEM	EXAMPLE INTERVENTIONS
Overtraining or rapid increases in training parameters	Education on active rest to manage high irritability; education on proper training loads with recognition of signs of tissue stress
Elevated fear avoidance	De-emphasis on anatomic findings; encourage active participation in rehabilitation process
Pain	Physical agents; tailor patella taping to pain relief with concordant sign
Peripatella soft tissue restrictions	Manual therapy of patella glides or tilts in the direction opposite of identified restriction
Flexibility deficits	Manual or self-stretching of quadriceps, hamstrings hip flexors, hip adductors, gastrocnemius, and soleus
Strength deficits	Hip/core/knee strengthening; progress from nonweightbearing to weightbearing; quadriceps strengthening within 90- to 45-degree range for OKC and 0- to 45-degree range for CKC
Alternations in gait creating elevated patellofemoral stress	Walking with reduced "noise" during stance phase; trial use of orthotic to control excessive pronation; running mechanics emphasizing increased step rate; noise reduction or use of midfoot-to-forefoot strike pattern
Dynamic malalignment during functional tasks	Provide tactile, visual, and verbal feedback to promote knee-over-toe position; maintain upright trunk in the frontal plane

Knee Stability Impairments

The most common physical therapy knee diagnosis of knee stability deficits is related to the health conditions or pathoanatomic diagnoses of patella instability and knee ligament tears. Patella instability can occur secondary to one macrotrauma event resulting in patella dislocation or can develop over time secondary to repetitive microtrauma.[237] Due to the biomechanics of the PFJ, lateral instability is most common. After an initial episode of patella dislocation, 15% to 44% of individuals experience recurrent patella instability.[238] Recurrent patella instability is a category of PFPS that develops after an initial episode of patella dislocation.[239] Recurrent patella instability occurs more frequently in women and in young individuals between the ages of 10 and 17 years.[18,239] Factors associated with recurrent patella instability include genu valgus, femoral anteversion, excessive tibial torsion, increased Q-angle, trochlea dysplasia, patella alta, generalized ligamentous laxity, VMO atrophy and insufficiency, tight lateral tissues (ITB, lateral retinaculum), or disruption of the MPFL.[18,237,239] Due to the many contributory factors for patella instability, the physical therapy diagnosis may be expanded to identify key impairments. For example, a physical therapy diagnosis of knee stability impairments with associated soft tissue dysfunction could appropriately classify patella instability related to tight lateral tissue or insufficient medial tissues.

In the absence of osteochondral defects or identified disruption of the MPFL, an initial episode of patella instability is usually treated conservatively. Due to high irritability and joint effusion, physical therapy examination following an acute initial patella dislocation may be limited to assessment of swelling, ROM, patella alignment, and palpation. Conservative management may involve a short period of immobilization, modalities for inflammation and pain relief, protected knee ROM to minimize adhesion formation, and use of patellofemoral bracing to protect against redislocation and to restore patellofemoral alignment.[18] When irritability levels subside or if the patient has recurrent patella instability, physical therapy examination should include assessment of tibiofemoral alignment for presence of genu valgus and the Q-angle for patellofemoral alignment; circumference measurements at the knee for signs of swelling and 10 cm proximal to the joint line to assess for VMO atrophy; patella mobility or glide test for evidence of hypermobility; patella apprehension test; passive and active patella tracking or J-sign; palpation of adductor tubercle for tenderness secondary to rupture of MPFL; assessment of knee, hip, and core strength; knee ROM; and muscle length tests of the hip, knee, and ankle.[237] Rehabilitation interventions in this phase are directed toward improving dynamic stability of the knee, establishing neuromuscular control, addressing soft tissue tightness that may contribute to patella instability (lateral retinaculum, ITB), and restoration of full knee ROM.[237]

Surgical management of recurrent patella instability is indicated when conservative management is unsuccessful.[18,240] Options for surgical management of patella instability target proximal soft tissues, such as repair or reconstruction of the MPFL or correction of altered osseous anatomy, such as tibial tubercle realignment. Lateral release is not recommended as the sole procedure for treatment of patella instability but may be used in conjunction with soft tissue repair or realignment procedures.[18] Given that the MPFL provides 50% to 60% restraint against lateral patella displacement when the knee is in 0 to 30 degrees of flexion, surgical management tends to focus on reconstruction of the MPFL.[18] Auto-graft options for MPFL reconstruction include the semitendinosus, gracilis, quadriceps tendon, adductor magnus, and tibial anterior.[18,237] Manske and Prohaska[237] present a 4 phase approach to rehabilitation following MPFL reconstruction with return to full activity at approximately 20 weeks postsurgery, dependent upon attainment of performance-based criteria. Phase 1 (protective phase) occurs day 1 postsurgery to 6 weeks. Interventions during phase 1 are directed toward pain control, minimization of swelling, controlled ROM to prevent postoperative stiffness per surgeon's protocol without disruption of the reconstructed tissue, passive patella mobility, weightbearing as tolerated in a locked brace, lower quarter muscle setting exercises, flexibility exercises for the hip and ankle, and NMES to manage quadriceps inhibition. Phase 2 (moderate protection [approximately weeks 7 to 12]), involves CKC strengthening of hip and thigh muscles, balance and proprioceptive exercises, and neuromuscular training. Phase 3 (minimum protection [approximately weeks 13 to 16]), involves loading progression of previous neuromuscular exercises to prepare for functional activities and introduction of plyometric activities. Phase 4 (return to activity [approximately weeks 17 to 20]), includes interval programs, SLH and functional drills to prepare for high-level sport demands. Manske and Prohaska[237] described discharge criteria as determined through the qualitative assessment of dynamic movement control during the single leg step down task, vertical jump ability (100% of height for men; 90% of height for women), and SLH distance (90% of height for men; 80% of height for women).

Knee ligament injury is primarily the result of a directionally applied contact or noncontact force to the knee with resulting impairments of pain, swelling, reports of or feeling of instability, laxity with ligamentous stress testing, balance/proprioception, and dynamic movement control of the trunk and lower quarter. Deficits in stability is a key impairment associated with knee ligament injury. In addition, movement coordination impairments contribute both to the occurrence of initial knee ligament injury and subsequent re-injury. Knee Stability and Movement Coordination Impairments is a clinical practice guideline published by the American Physical Therapy Association Orthopaedic Section in 2010 with a revision published in 2017.[7,177]

Of the 4 major ligaments at the knee, the ACL is the one most frequently injured. The incidence of ACL injuries is greatest in athletes between the ages of 15 and 40 years, in sports requiring pivoting, and in women.[241] Décary et al[242] identified clusters of history and physical examination tests to differentially diagnosis a complete or incomplete ACL tear. The likelihood of a complete ACL tear increases when the history involves the combination of a pivoting traumatic mechanism combined with a "popping" sensation (specificity = 94%; +LR = 9.80).[242] The likelihood of a partial ACL tear increases with the combination of pivoting traumatic mechanism and immediate effusion after trauma (history elements) with a positive Lachman test (physical examination tests; specificity = 95%; +LR = 17.5).[242] Two options exist for the management of individuals with ACL injury: conservative, nonoperative treatment or surgical reconstruction. Although approximately 65% of the individuals elect for surgery,[93] the rate of a second ACL injury in the reconstructed or contralateral lower extremity, incidence of premature knee osteoarthritis, and low rates of return to prior level of sports activity have led to increased consideration of conservative management and a reconsideration of procedures involved in the postsurgery rehabilitation.[243]

Conservative Management

Individuals electing the conservative rehabilitation approach after ACL injury do so in consideration of pursuing activity modification or having been determined to be a potential "coper." A potential coper is an individual who is likely to be successful in returning to activities requiring pivoting and cutting based on a screening tool examining hop performance, incidence of knee giving way, and self-report function on the KOS-ADL.[243] The screening tool to identify a potential coper includes hop test LSI of at least 80%, KOS-ADL score of greater than 80%, no more than 1 incidence of knee giving way, and greater than 60 on knee global rating of function.[244] Nonoperative rehabilitation proceeds as described in the section General Guidelines for Rehabilitation of Knee Dysfunction. Stage 1 involves aggressive management of knee hemarthrosis to prevent or minimize quadriceps reflex inhibition, restoration of full knee ROM, and attaining foundational quadriceps and hamstrings strength through both OKC and CKC therapeutic exercises. To reduce anterior shear of the tibia in the ACL deficient knee, OKC quadriceps strengthening is performed from 100 to 30 degrees of knee flexion ROM and CKC is performed from 0 to 45 degrees of knee flexion ROM.[243] Trunk control through core stabilization is instituted as a means to optimize components of neuromuscular control.[26] Stage 2 rehabilitation initiates when full knee ROM is achieved, swelling is resolved, and quadriceps strength is sufficient to allow ambulation without gait pattern deficits. This phase includes static and dynamic balance interventions; perturbation training; motor control training for dynamic lower extremity alignment during functional performance tasks; and strengthening of the core, hip, and thigh muscles.[26,209,212,243] Criteria to progress to stage 3 include no episode of knee giving way and quadriceps strength symmetry of greater than 90%.[243] Stage 3 rehabilitation focuses on agility and sport-specific skill training, incorporating direction and speed changes. Muscle performance exercises should be delivered in dosages to attain strength, endurance, or power requirements specific to the sport or functional activity. Use of a functional knee brace is recommended to enhance knee stability.[245] Throughout all stages of rehabilitation, cardiovascular training is utilized to prevent deconditioning and impairment-based interventions are provided to the uninvolved lower extremity. Discharge criteria include attainment of greater than 90% LSI in hop tests and quadriceps and hamstring strength. In addition, qualitative assessment of lower extremity dynamic alignment and postural orientation are recommended as a measure of neuromuscular control.[80,241,243]

Rehabilitation Post–Anterior Cruciate Ligament Reconstruction

The bone-patella tendon-bone (BPTB) autograft is the most common surgical procedure for ACLR followed by the hamstring autograft.[246] Survey response of orthopaedic surgeons for the National Football League and National Collegiate Athletic Association found 86% would use the BPTB autograft,[247] while an earlier survey conducted among Canadian orthopedic surgeons[248] reported 59% to use the BPTB autograft and 32% to use the hamstring tendon autograft. Results of a systematic review and meta-analysis comparing the BPTB autograft to the 4-strand hamstring tendon autograft found no significant differences for instrumented laxity measurements or clinical laxity measurements (Lachman's test), graft failure, ROM deficit, or IKDC outcome scores.[249] The better outcomes were found for the BPTB autograft on the pivot shift test and return to preinjury activity level, whereas the hamstring autograft had better outcomes related to anterior knee pain and kneeling pain. When comparing failure rate between the BPTB autograft to the 4-strand hamstring tendon autograft, higher failure rate was found for the hamstring autograft, although failure rates were low for both grafts (2.80% BPTB, 2.84% hamstring).[246] Current trends in reconstructive surgery are to preserve the ACL remnant to enhance the precision and acuity of neurosensory responses.[250]

Rehabilitation following ACLR has progressed from use of an extended period of immobilization and delayed strengthening to accelerated rehabilitation involving immediate ROM and weightbearing, early strengthening, and return to sport at 4 to 6 months. Current rehabilitation after ACLR continues to focus on immediate ROM, early weightbearing, and early strengthening; however, use of neuromuscular control interventions and restoring symmetrical, normal movement patterns is a priority and extending the time since injury to return to sport is recommended to prevent re-injury or contralateral injury.[251-253]

A preoperative rehabilitation program can positively affect outcomes after surgery. Preoperative treatment is directed toward attainment of full knee extension, 120 degrees or greater knee flexion, no or minimal effusion, ability to perform SLR without a quadriceps lag, normalized gait pattern with brace protection, and quadriceps strengthening in CKC in a protected ROM (0 to 45 degrees).[93,252] Patient education should also be provided in regard to rehabilitation goals postsurgery and the importance of compliance with postsurgical exercise, edema management, and weightbearing instructions.

Postoperative ACLR rehabilitation is divided into phases that are based on timelines related to healing tissues and criteria for progression to the next phase. The early or immediate postoperative phase typically spans weeks 0 to 4 with goals directed toward attainment of 0 to 120 degrees ROM with emphasis on achievement of full extension, quadriceps activation with superior patella glide, minimize effusion and pain, and ambulation with full knee extension.[93,254] Ambulation is progressed from weightbearing as tolerated with crutches and a brace locked at 0 degrees to full weightbearing without assistive device with the brace unlocked. Criteria for this progression is full knee extension and the ability to perform an SLR without a quadriceps lag.[252] CKC quadriceps strengthening is performed from 0 to 45 degrees using terminal knee extension, mini-squats, step-ups, and step-downs. OKC quadriceps strengthening is limited to 90 to 60 degrees to protect the graft and progresses from isometrics within this range to AROM.[251] Proprioceptive exercises can be initiated in nonweightbearing with passive and active joint repositioning, progressing to weightbearing for addition of balance training when quadriceps control is adequate to maintain knee extension in standing.[254] Weightbearing balance training proceeds from double leg activities to single leg stance with incorporation of vision and surface variations. Hamstrings and gluteal muscle strengthening should also be incorporated in the muscle performance interventions. If a hamstring autograft was performed, hamstring strengthening is delayed for the first 6 weeks.[251]

From 1 to 6 months, the emphasis is on attainment of full active and passive knee ROM progressive strengthening. Knee extension should be equal bilaterally and flexion greater than 100 degrees.[251] Stretching and manual therapy may be implemented if ROM deficits exist. Given that quadriceps asymmetry may persist at 6 months after ACLR and is a risk factor for ACL re-injury, strengthening focuses on achieving quadriceps symmetry greater than 80%. OKC strengthening range is increased to 90 to 45 degrees in weeks 10 to 16 and 90 to 0 degrees in weeks 16 to 20, and CKC range increases to 0 to 60/75 degrees.[251,255] As strengthening intensity and motion range progresses, the patient is cautioned to report any patella pain as well as persistent soreness as an indicator to adjust dosage parameters including rest. When the 80% quadriceps criteria is met in addition to a normal gait pattern, a straight line running progression program can be initiated.[251,256,257] Neuromuscular training is advanced to include perturbation training and use of unilateral functional tasks (see Table 10-7). Dynamic lower extremity alignment is emphasized with verbal, visual, and tactile feedback to prevent movement patterns of dynamic knee valgus.[26] Dynamic balance on the Y Balance Test should achieve 100% composite score.[251]

While return to play/sport after ACLR is a major goal of the injured athlete, it is estimated that 35% of athletes do not return to the preinjury level of sports participation.[258] Factors preventing return to sport at the preinjury level include negative psychological responses (fear of re-injury), prior ACLR on either lower extremity, deficits in hop test LSI, and low scores on patient-reported outcome measure.[113,259,260] ACL re-injury after ACLR occurs in 3% to 22% of athletes who return to sport and ACL injury in the contralateral lower extremity occurs in 3% to 24%.[241] Advances in ACLR rehabilitation protocols have moved from using time since ACLR as a criteria for return to sport to the consideration of both functional capacity and time since surgery.[253] Re-injury rates are highest in the first year after surgery, and risk of a second ACL injury in young athletes (less than 20 years) is greatest in the first 2 years after reconstruction.[251,253] Research findings show a delayed remodeling phase of the ACL autograft that extends 12 to 24 months for the hamstring autograft and 6 to 12 months for the BPTB autograft.[253] In addition, deficits in quadriceps strength and neuromuscular control in ACLR athletes have been found to persist at the 6- to 12-month period postsurgery.[253,261,262] Thus, for individuals desiring to return to high-level activity, the last phase rehabilitation should address both physical and psychological factors that may limit return to sport or contribute to re-injury or a second ACL injury. Interventions in this phase include agility, jumping, hopping, and cutting. Emphasis is placed on mechanics, trunk and lower extremity alignment, and the ability to perform agility, hopping, and cutting activities without compensation. For the high-level athlete, the time to acquire normalized neuromuscular control, strength symmetry, and allow adequate graft healing may necessitate delaying return to sport for 2 years.[253]

Quantitative criteria from PPT and strength testing can assist in determination of return-to-sport readiness. These criteria currently include 90% or greater LSI during hop testing and 90% or greater quadriceps strength symmetry.[93,94] Recent research, however, is questioning if this criteria overestimates knee function based on findings that bilateral strength deficits exist after ACL injury; strength tests do not reflect 90% estimated preinjury capacity and uninjured, healthy individuals have an LSI greater than 95%.[94,263,264] When examining hop performance of individuals 7 months post-ACLR, Gokeler et al[264] reported an LSI greater than 90%, yet significant differences existed in hop distances of the involved lower extremity compared to normative data and the uninvolved lower extremity compared to normative data. In this study, LSI for normal, healthy controls was 100.8% on SLH, 99.4% on triple hop, and 99.7% on the crossover hop. Additional criteria for return to sport is suggested to also include qualitative assessment of neuromuscular control of the trunk and lower extremity during landing tasks, self-report function, and self-report confidence.[260]

ACLR is often performed with concomitant procedures, such as meniscus repairs or chondral repair, or injuries, such as MCL tear, necessitating modifications to the postsurgery rehabilitation.[49,93,251] These modifications typically include a slower rate of progression, use of protective bracing, delayed weightbearing, restrictions in ROM, and targeted muscle performance exercises. For example, in the case of concomitant meniscal repair, the early phase of rehabilitation may include nonweightbearing to progressive weightbearing over the initial 6 to 8 weeks.[251] Therapeutic exercises are modified to limit knee flexion ROM to 90 degrees and to delay hamstring strengthening for the first 6 weeks. With a concomitant grade II to III MCL injury, sagittal plane knee flexion ROM restrictions are followed for 2 to 3 weeks and valgus forces are avoided during early muscle strengthening through positioning (use of tibial internal rotation) and use of a protective brace.[93] When the ACLR also includes chondral repair, weightbearing and ROM restrictions are followed specific to the type of chondral repair (eg, microfracture, autologous chondrocyte implantation, osteochondral autograft transfer system) and should be discussed with the surgeon.[93]

Knee Pain, Muscle Performance, and Mobility Impairments

Knee osteoarthritis is estimated to affect 19% of women and 14% of men in the United States and is the most common type of osteoarthritis.[153] The most predominant risk factors for knee osteoarthritis are advancing age, limb alignment, muscle weakness, and obesity.[265,266] Knee osteoarthritis is characterized by a progressive loss of articular cartilage resulting in pain, activity restriction, and disability. Physical therapy examination of an individual with knee osteoarthritis should consist of impairment-based measures (eg, pain, mobility, stability, alignment, proprioception/balance), functional performance measures (see Table 10-4), and self-report measures of function and disability (eg, Western Ontario and McMaster Universities Arthritis Index, 36-Item Short Form Survey, KOOS, PSFS; see Table 10-5).[267,268] Décary et al[268] identified 2 clusters of examination tests with 95% specificity and a 13.62 +LR for differentially diagnosing individuals with symptomatic knee osteoarthritis. Components of the first cluster were 50 to 58 years old and had a body mass index of 30 kg/m2 or greater combined with knee valgus or varus misalignment or limited passive knee extension ROM, while the second cluster included individuals over 58 years old and palpable crepitus in any knee compartment.

Primary impairments identified in the physical therapy examination of an individual with knee osteoarthritis are pain, knee ROM, and quadriceps muscle performance.[153] Of these impairments, addressing quadriceps muscle performance deficits has been stressed as a key component of osteoarthritis rehabilitation.[195,269,270] To mitigate the negative effect of pain on the tolerance of quadriceps exercise when delivered at effective dosages to improve muscle strength (greater than 60% maximal voluntary isometric contraction [MVIC][271]), NMES has been found effective when used independently and in combination with voluntary quadriceps contraction.[198,272] NMES delivered at a stimulation intensity of 40% maximal voluntary isometric contraction over an 8-week treatment intervention significantly increased knee extensor torque, muscle mass, and health status in individuals with knee osteoarthritis.[198,272]

Rehabilitation interventions found to be beneficial in the management of knee osteoarthritis include transcutaneous electrical nerve stimulation (short-term benefit for pain), strength and resistance training (short-term benefit for function), tai chi (moderate benefit for pain and function), whole-body vibration (moderate benefit for function), agility training and general exercise (long-term benefit for pain and function), manual therapy (long-term benefit for pain), and weight loss (moderate benefit for pain and function and long-term benefit for pain).[240] A review of the effectiveness of physical therapy interventions for knee osteoarthritis found aerobic and aquatic exercise to decrease disability, aerobic exercise and strengthening exercise to decrease pain and function, and proprioceptive exercise to decrease pain.[273] When investigating different types of strengthening exercises, both hip and leg strengthening exercises decrease pain and improve function and quality of life in individuals with knee osteoarthritis.[274,275] While both hip and leg strengthening showed similar improvements in pain, function, and quality of life, there was no change in hip or knee ROM or strength.[275] Based on the aforementioned research, physical therapy interventions recommended for the management of knee osteoarthritis include hip and knee strengthening exercises, transcutaneous electrical nerve stimulation, manual therapy, agility training, proprioceptive exercise, aerobic exercise, and education in weight loss strategies.[267]

Knee Pain and Mobility Impairments

Meniscal injury can occur traumatically or in association with degenerative changes in the tibiofemoral joint. Physical examination tests for meniscal pathology include joint line tenderness, McMurray's test, Apley's test, and the Thessaly test.[276,277] Damage to the menisci results in pain, inflammation, and limitation of movement during hyperextension or forced, maximum flexion. Subjective complaints commonly include catching or locking during ambulation or transitional movements.[278] Lowery et al[279] identified 5 tests (history or "catching" or "locking," pain with forced hyperextension, pain with maximum passive knee flexion, joint-line tenderness, and pain or audible click with McMurray's maneuver) to establish a meniscal pathology composite score. When 5/5 tests were positive, the specificity is 99.0% and sensitivity is 11.2% (11.2 +LR; 0.90 -LR), while 3/5 positive tests yielded a diagnostic accuracy of 90.2% specificity and 30.8% sensitivity (3.14 +LR; 0.77 -LR). More recently, Décary et al[280] identified a cluster of history and physical examination tests

to differentially diagnosis traumatic or degenerative symptomatic meniscal tears. Knee pain precipitated by a history of trauma (fall or pivot mechanism), isolated medial or diffuse knee pain, and positive medial joint line tenderness comprised a test cluster for traumatic meniscal tears (sensitivity 91%, specificity 90%, 8.92 +LR). Test components included in the clusters for diagnosis of degenerative knee meniscal tears were progressive onset of pain, isolated medial knee pain, mid-to-severe pain while performing activities or sports involving pivoting, no knee valgus/varus misalignment, and full passive knee flexion (sensitivity 58%, specificity 91%, 6.44 +LR).

Partial meniscal tears are usually treated conservatively utilizing interventions to target pain and inflammation reduction, restoration of ROM and muscle performance, and return to functional activities. When conservative management is unsuccessful or when the meniscal tear is significantly affecting function, surgical management is considered. The most common surgical options for a meniscal tear consist of partial meniscectomy or meniscal repair, which are largely dictated by location of the tear. When a meniscal lesion occurs in the central or nonvascular portion of the meniscus, a partial meniscectomy is most commonly conducted. Because a partial meniscectomy is performed arthroscopically and does not involve protection of healing tissues, the postsurgical rehabilitation commences immediately with early emphasis on control of postoperative swelling, regaining knee ROM, restoring quadriceps strength, and re-establishing neuromuscular control over 6 to 8 weeks.[177,215,280]

Because partial meniscectomies are associated with the development of knee osteoarthritis and preservation of the meniscus may enhance joint stability, meniscal repair is considered when the location of the tear is in the peripheral area where vascularization can promote healing of the repaired tissue.[281,282] In addition to peripheral location of the tear, meniscal repairs may also be considered for younger individuals or highly active individuals in whom the development of osteoarthritis after meniscectomy may occur at an earlier rate. Postoperative rehabilitation initially focuses on pain and edema reduction while establishing quadriceps control. Protective bracing locked in extension may be worn until quadriceps control for a nonantalgic gait pattern is attained. Knee flexion ROM is progressed slowly and hamstring strengthening is delayed until postoperative weeks 6 to 8 to prevent posterior translation forces on the meniscus.[177] Neuromuscular training begins with bilateral activities and advances to unilateral activities when adequate quadriceps control is achieved to provide knee stability. At 4 to 6 months postsurgery, if ROM and quadriceps strength are symmetrical, higher level functional activities may be instituted, such as return to running, plyometric, and agility training. Discharge criteria is attainment of 85% LSI with SLH tests and less than 15% deficit for quadriceps and hamstring strength.[282]

Conclusion

With a knowledge of knee anatomy and biomechanics combined with an understanding of a movement-based examination, the clinician is able to identify impairments of body function and the associated impact on activity and participation abilities resulting from presenting knee symptomology. The use of a classification-based diagnosis with staging of irritability and disability can assist the clinician in selecting and delivering condition-specific interventions for optimal outcomes in knee rehabilitation.

Case Studies

Case Study One

A 15-year-old adolescent girl, AF, reports anterior and lateral right knee pain that she relates to initiating summer practice for the high school cross-country team. Although she had not previously run cross-country, AF played soccer for 2 seasons and has been running up to 2 miles on a treadmill 3 times per week as part of self-structured conditioning program. The team had been practicing 2 weeks attaining a base millage of 15 miles per week over a 3 day per week practice when AF joined the team. The coach instructed AF to begin with 6 miles per week and progress by 0.25 miles each week. Desiring to run with her friends, AF ran 8 miles the first week, 10 miles the second week, and 12 miles the third week. Midweek of week 3, AF began experiencing knee pain that worsened over the rest of week 3 and into week 4. After cutting running back to 8 miles in week 4 without improvement in symptoms, AF's parents decided to seek physical therapy to help manage her pain.

Part One

- Outcome measures:
  - AKPS: 58/100
  - FABQ: 19/24
  - PSFS
    - Running: 2/10
    - Sitting more than 45 minutes: 4/10
    - Walking down stairs: 4/10
  - NPRS: 24-hour rating
    - Best: 2/10
    - Worst: 9/10
    - Current: 4/10

Questions

1. What is your initial clinical impression based on the subjective information provided?
2. What additional subjective information would you want to know?
3. Provide an initial staging of the condition.
4. How does the staging determination guide the objective component of the examination?

Part Two

- Observation
  - Static standing posture: Increased lordosis; bilateral genu recurvatum; calcaneal valgus; and inward facing patella (right greater than left)
  - Gait: No gait pattern deviations with walking
  - Dynamic posture: Single leg forward step down performed with pain (6/10) and a movement pattern of dynamic valgus, contralateral pelvic drop, and tibial tuberosity medial to second toe. This pattern was more apparent on right lower extremity than left.
- Active movement testing
  - Squat in standing: Full ROM, pain on descent
  - Knee flexion/extension: 130-0-10 pain at end flexion and extension with overpressure
- Passive movement testing
  - Tibiofemoral joint mobility: Within normal limits
  - PFJ mobility: Medial glide less than 25% patella width; inferior glide hypomobile
  - Thomas test: Right: full hip extension with knee flexion less than 45 degrees, hip in slight abduction; Left: full hip flexion with knee flexion less than 90 degrees
  - Gastrocsoleus flexibility: 0 degrees ankle dorsiflexion with knee extension; 5 degrees ankle dorsiflexion with knee flexed (right equal to left); weight-bearing ankle dorsiflexion 40 degrees (right equal to left)
- Resisted movement testing
  - Knee extension: Right 3+/5 (anterior knee pain); left 4/5
  - Knee flexion: 5/5 right and left
  - Hip abduction: Right 3+/5, left 4/5
  - Hip extension: Right 3+/5, left 4/5

Questions

1. What additional tests would you perform based on the findings provided?
2. What is your classification-based diagnosis considering all examination findings at this point?
3. Outline an impairment-based treatment intervention approach for this patient.

Case Study Two

BS is a 64-year-old woman referred to physical therapy with complaints of left lateral knee pain of 9 months duration. She retired in May of current year from 30 years as a first-grade teacher and began noticing knee pain in March of current year. Symptom onset was insidious and associated with sitting in low chairs used in the classroom, when running after children on the playground, and when going up/down stairs. She has pain at night when extending her leg straight and prefers to sleep on her side with her knees bent. Pain is best in the morning and increases during the day related to the amount of time she is on her feet. She has mild stiffness when sitting more than 15 minutes and mild pain when standing upright from sitting. Since retiring, she joined a women's golf league and has been golfing 3 to 4 times per week. She rides in a golf cart when playing and notes that pain is moderate on the downswing/impact to follow-through phases of her golf swing (she is right handed). She denies swelling in the knee. She is 5 feet and 2 inches and weighs 155 pounds (lbs), a weight she has maintained over the past 2 to 3 years.

Part One

- Outcome measures
  - KOOS: 55%
    - Symptoms/stiffness: 36%
    - Pain: 53%
    - Activities of daily living: 69%
    - Function in sport and recreation: 49%
    - Quality of life: 44%
  - PSFS
    - Golfing: 5/10
    - Standing: 4/10
    - Walking down stairs: 6/10
  - NPRS: 24-hour rating
    - Best: 1/10
    - Worst: 7/10
    - Current: 3/10

Questions

1. What is your initial clinical impression based on the subjective information provided?
2. What additional subjective information would you want to know?
3. Provide an initial staging of the condition.
4. How does the staging determination guide the objective component of the examination?

Part Two

- Observation
  - Static standing posture: Reduced lumbar lordosis; bilateral genu varum (left greater than right); slight knee flexion
  - Gait: Slight trunk inclination in stance
  - Dynamic posture: Partial bilateral squat performed with pain increase from 3/10 to 5/10
- Active movement testing
  - Partial squat in standing: Pain and crepitus during down and up phase
  - AROM: Knee flexion/extension: Left knee 128 to 12 degrees (right knee 130 to 0 to 0 degrees) pain at end available extension prior to overpressure
  - Hip flexion/extension: 120 to 5 degrees bilateral, no pain
- Passive movement testing
  - PROM: Left knee 130 to 7 degrees, tissue approximation end-feel flexion; hard capsular end-feel extension with crepitus palpable
  - Tibiofemoral joint mobility: Anterior glide of tibia hypomobile left
  - PFJ mobility: Within normal limits
- Resisted movement testing
  - Knee extension: Left 3+/5 (painful); right 4/5
  - Knee flexion: 4-/5 right and left
  - Hip abduction: Right 3+/5, right and left
  - Hip extension: Right 3+/5, right and left

Questions

1. What additional tests would you perform based on the findings provided?
2. What is your physical therapy classification-based diagnosis considering all examination findings at this point?
3. Outline an impairment-based treatment intervention approach for this patient.

REFERENCES

1. Sahrmann SA. The human movement system: our professional identity. *Phys Ther.* 2014;94(7):1034-1042. doi:10.2522/ptj.20130319

2. Manske RC, Prohaska D. Rehabilitation following medial patellofemoral ligament reconstruction for patellar instability. *Int J Sports Phys Ther.* 2017;12(3):494-511.

3. Hoogenboom BJ, Voight ML, Prentice WE. *Musculoskeletal Interventions Techniques for Therapeutic Exercise.* 3rd ed. McGraw-Hill; 2014.

4. Sueki DG, Cleland JA, Wainner RS. A regional interdependence model of musculoskeletal dysfunction: research, mechanisms, and clinical implications. *J Man Manip Ther.* 2013;21(2):90-102. doi:10.1179/2042618612Y.0000000027

5. Neumann D. *Kinesiology of the Musculoskeletal System.* 2nd ed. Elsevier; 2010.

6. Tetteh ES, Bajaj S, Ghodadra NS. Basic science and surgical treatment options for articular cartilage injuries of the knee. *J Orthop Sports Phys Ther.* 2012;42(3):243-253. doi:10.2519/jospt.2012.3673

7. Logerstedt DS, Scalzitti DA, Bennell KL, et al. Knee Pain and Mobility Impairments: Meniscal and Articular Cartilage Lesions Revision 2018. *J Orthop Sports Phys Ther.* 2018;48(2):A1-A50. doi:10.2519/jospt.2018.0301

8. Loudon JK. Biomechanics and pathomechanics of the patellofemoral joint. *Int J Sports Phys Ther.* 2016;11(6):820-830.

9. Moore K. *Clinically Oriented Anatomy.* 8th ed. Walters Kluwer; 2018.

10. Domnick C, Raschke MJ, Herbort M. Biomechanics of the anterior cruciate ligament: physiology, rupture and reconstruction techniques. *World J Orthop.* 2016;7(2):82-93. doi:10.5312/wjo.v7.i2.82

11. Butler DL, Noyes FR, Grood ES. Ligamentous restraints to anterior-posterior drawer in the human knee. A biomechanical study. *J Bone Joint Surg Am.* 1980;62(2):259-270.

12. Elkin JL, Zamora E, Gallo RA. Combined anterior cruciate ligament and medial collateral ligament knee injuries: anatomy, diagnosis, management recommendations, and return to sport. *Curr Rev Musculoskelet Med.* 2019;12(2):239-244. doi:10.1007/s12178-019-09549-3

13. Dold AP, Swensen S, Strauss E, Alaia M. The posteromedial corner of the knee: anatomy, pathology, and management strategies. *J Am Acad Orthop Surg.* 2017;25(11):752-761. doi:10.5435/JAAOS-D-16-00020

14. Lunden JB, Bzdusek PJ, Monson JK, Malcomson KW, Laprade RF. Current concepts in the recognition and treatment of posterolateral corner injuries of the knee. *J Orthop Sports Phys Ther.* 2010;40(8):502-516. doi:10.2519/jospt.2010.3269

15. Shon O-J, Park J-W, Kim B-J. Current Concepts of Posterolateral Corner Injuries of the Knee. *Knee Surg Relat Res.* 2017;29(4):256-268. doi:10.5792/ksrr.16.029

16. LaPrade MD, Kennedy MI, Wijdicks CA, LaPrade RF. Anatomy and biomechanics of the medial side of the knee and their surgical implications. *Sports Med Arthrosc Rev.* 2015;23(2):63-70. doi:10.1097/JSA.0000000000000054

17. Recondo JA, Salvador E, Villanúa JA, Barrera MC, Gervás C, Alústiza JM. Lateral stabilizing structures of the knee: functional anatomy and injuries assessed with MR imaging. *Radiographics.* 2000;20 Spec No:S91-S102. doi:10.1148/radiographics.20.suppl_1.g00oc02s91

18. Rhee S-J, Pavlou G, Oakley J, Barlow D, Haddad F. Modern management of patellar instability. *Int Orthop.* 2012;36(12):2447-2456. doi:10.1007/s00264-012-1669-4

19. Rhee S-J, Pavlou G, Oakley J, Barlow D, Haddad F. Modern management of patellar instability. *Int Orthop.* 2012;36(12):2447-2456. doi:10.1007/s00264-012-1669-4

20. Escala JS, Mellado JM, Olona M, Giné J, Saurí A, Neyret P. Objective patellar instability: MR-based quantitative assessment of potentially associated anatomical features. *Knee Surg Sports Traumatol Arthrosc.* 2006;14(3):264-272. doi:10.1007/s00167-005-0668-z

21. Di Stasi S, Myer GD, Hewett TE. Neuromuscular training to target deficits associated with second anterior cruciate ligament injury. *J Orthop Sports Phys Ther.* 2013;43(11):777-792, A1-11. doi:10.2519/jospt.2013.4693

22. Schmitt LC, Paterno MV, Hewett TE. The impact of quadriceps femoris strength asymmetry on functional performance at return to sport following anterior cruciate ligament reconstruction. *J Orthop Sports Phys Ther.* 2012;42(9):750-759. doi:10.2519/jospt.2012.4194

23. Willy RW, Meira EP. Current concepts in biomechanical interventions for patellofemoral pain. *Int J Sports Phys Ther.* 2016;11(6):877-890.

24. Vincent KR, Vincent HK. Resistance exercise for knee osteoarthritis. *PM R.* 2012;4(5 Suppl):S45-52. doi:10.1016/j.pmrj.2012.01.019

25. Noyes FR, Huser LE, Levy MS. Rotational knee instability in ACL-deficient knees: role of the anterolateral ligament and iliotibial band as defined by tibiofemoral compartment translations and rotations. *J Bone Joint Surg Am.* 2017;99(4):305-314. doi:10.2106/JBJS.16.00199

26. Ford KR, Nguyen A-D, Dischiavi SL, Hegedus EJ, Zuk EF, Taylor JB. An evidence-based review of hip-focused neuromuscular exercise interventions to address dynamic lower extremity valgus. *Open Access J Sports Med.* 2015;6:291-303. doi:10.2147/OAJSM.S72432

27. Deasy M, Leahy E, Semciw AI. Hip strength deficits in people with symptomatic knee osteoarthritis: a systematic review with meta-analysis. *J Orthop Sports Phys Ther.* 2016;46(8):629-639. doi:10.2519/jospt.2016.6618

28. Khayambashi K, Ghoddosi N, Straub RK, Powers CM. Hip muscle strength predicts noncontact anterior cruciate ligament injury in male and female athletes: a prospective study. *Am J Sports Med.* 2016;44(2):355-361. doi:10.1177/0363546515616237

29. Hewett TE, Myer GD, Ford KR, et al. Biomechanical measures of neuromuscular control and valgus loading of the knee predict anterior cruciate ligament injury risk in female athletes: a prospective study. *Am J Sports Med.* 2005;33(4):492-501. doi:10.1177/0363546504269591

30. Hollman JH, Ginos B, Kozuchowski J, Vaughn A, Krause DA, Youdas JW. Relationships between knee valgus, hip-muscle strength, and hip-muscle recruitment during a single-limb step-down. *J Sport Rehabil.* 2009;18(1):104-117. doi:10.1123/jsr.18.1.104

31. Van Cant J, Pineux C, Pitance L, Feipel V. Hip muscle strength and endurance in females with patellofemoral pain: a systematic review with meta-analysis. *Int J Sports Phys Ther.* 2014;9(5):564-582.

32. Prins MR, van der Wurff P. Females with patellofemoral pain syndrome have weak hip muscles: a systematic review. *Aust J Physiother.* 2009;55(1):9-15. doi:10.1016/s0004-9514(09)70055-8

33. Costa RA, Oliveira LM de, Watanabe SH, Jones A, Natour J. Isokinetic assessment of the hip muscles in patients with osteoarthritis of the knee. *Clinics (Sao Paulo).* 2010;65(12):1253-1259. doi:10.1590/s1807-59322010001200006

34. Kollock RO, Andrews C, Johnston A, et al. A meta-analysis to determine if lower extremity muscle strengthening should be included in military knee overuse injury-prevention programs. *J Athl Train.* 2016;51(11):919-926. doi:10.4085/1062-6050-51.4.09

35. de Moura Campos Carvalho-E-Silva AP, Peixoto Leão Almeida G, Oliveira Magalhães M, et al. Dynamic postural stability and muscle strength in patellofemoral pain: is there a correlation? *Knee.* 2016;23(4):616-621. doi:10.1016/j.knee.2016.04.013

36. Ferber R, Bolgla L, Earl-Boehm JE, Emery C, Hamstra-Wright K. Strengthening of the hip and core versus knee muscles for the treatment of patellofemoral pain: a multicenter randomized controlled trial. *J Athl Train.* 2015;50(4):366-377. doi:10.4085/1062-6050-49.3.70

37. Bloomer BA, Durall CJ. Does the addition of hip strengthening to a knee-focused exercise program improve outcomes in patients with patellofemoral pain syndrome? *J Sport Rehabil*. 2015;24(4):428-433. doi:10.1123/jsr.2014-0184

38. Fukuda TY, Melo WP, Zaffalon BM, et al. Hip posterolateral musculature strengthening in sedentary women with patellofemoral pain syndrome: a randomized controlled clinical trial with 1-year follow-up. *J Orthop Sports Phys Ther*. 2012;42(10):823-830. doi:10.2519/jospt.2012.4184

39. Flack NAMS, Nicholson HD, Woodley SJ. A review of the anatomy of the hip abductor muscles, gluteus medius, gluteus minimus, and tensor fascia lata. *Clin Anat*. 2012;25(6):697-708. doi:10.1002/ca.22004

40. Neumann D. *Kinesiology of the Musculoskeletal System. Foundations for Rehabilitation*. 2nd ed. Mosby Elsevier; 2010.

41. Bennell KL, Kyriakides M, Metcalf B, et al. Neuromuscular versus quadriceps strengthening exercise in patients with medial knee osteoarthritis and varus malalignment: a randomized controlled trial. *Arthritis Rheumatol*. 2014;66(4):950-959. doi:10.1002/art.38317

42. Chang A, Hayes K, Dunlop D, et al. Hip abduction moment and protection against medial tibiofemoral osteoarthritis progression. *Arthritis Rheum*. 2005;52(11):3515-3519. doi:10.1002/art.21406

43. Souza RB, Draper CE, Fredericson M, Powers CM. Femur rotation and patellofemoral joint kinematics: a weight-bearing magnetic resonance imaging analysis. *J Orthop Sports Phys Ther*. 2010;40(5):277-285. doi:10.2519/jospt.2010.3215

44. Myer GD, Ford KR, Di Stasi SL, Foss KDB, Micheli LJ, Hewett TE. High knee abduction moments are common risk factors for patellofemoral pain (PFP) and anterior cruciate ligament (ACL) injury in girls: is PFP itself a predictor for subsequent ACL injury? *Br J Sports Med*. 2015;49(2):118-122. doi:10.1136/bjsports-2013-092536

45. Powers CM, Ho K-Y, Chen Y-J, Souza RB, Farrokhi S. Patellofemoral joint stress during weight-bearing and non-weight-bearing quadriceps exercises. *J Orthop Sports Phys Ther*. 2014;44(5):320-327. doi:10.2519/jospt.2014.4936

46. Reinold MM, Wilk KE, Macrina LC, Dugas JR, Cain EL. Current concepts in the rehabilitation following articular cartilage repair procedures in the knee. *J Orthop Sports Phys Ther*. 2006;36(10):774-794. doi:10.2519/jospt.2006.2228

47. Wilk KE, Macrina LC, Reinold MM. Rehabilitation following microfracture of the knee. *Cartilage*. 2010;1(2):96-107. doi:10.1177/1947603510366029

48. Nho SJ, Pensak MJ, Seigerman DA, Cole BJ. Rehabilitation after autologous chondrocyte implantation in athletes. *Clin Sports Med*. 2010;29(2):267-282, viii. doi:10.1016/j.csm.2009.12.004

49. Mithoefer K, Hambly K, Logerstedt D, Ricci M, Silvers H, Della Villa S. Current concepts for rehabilitation and return to sport after knee articular cartilage repair in the athlete. *J Orthop Sports Phys Ther*. 2012;42(3):254-273. doi:10.2519/jospt.2012.3665

50. Escamilla RF, Fleisig GS, Zheng N, Barrentine SW, Wilk KE, Andrews JR. Biomechanics of the knee during closed kinetic chain and open kinetic chain exercises. *Med Sci Sports Exerc*. 1998;30(4):556-569. doi:10.1097/00005768-199804000-00014

51. Escamilla RF, Macleod TD, Wilk KE, Paulos L, Andrews JR. Anterior cruciate ligament strain and tensile forces for weight-bearing and non-weight-bearing exercises: a guide to exercise selection. *J Orthop Sports Phys Ther*. 2012;42(3):208-220. doi:10.2519/jospt.2012.3768

52. Wilk KE, Andrews JR. The effects of pad placement and angular velocity on tibial displacement during isokinetic exercise. *J Orthop Sports Phys Ther*. 1993;17(1):24-30. doi:10.2519/jospt.1993.17.1.24

53. Wilk KE, Escamilla RF, Fleisig GS, Barrentine SW, Andrews JR, Boyd ML. A comparison of tibiofemoral joint forces and electromyographic activity during open and closed kinetic chain exercises. *Am J Sports Med*. 1996;24(4):518-527. doi:10.1177/036354659602400418

54. Rosenthal MD, Rainey CE, Tognoni A, Worms R. Evaluation and management of posterior cruciate ligament injuries. *Phys Ther Sport*. 2012;13(4):196-208. doi:10.1016/j.ptsp.2012.03.016

55. Sahrmann S. *Diagnosis and Treatment of Movement Impairment Syndromes*. Mosby; 2002.

56. Tallroth K, Ristolainen L, Manninen M. Is a long leg a risk for hip or knee osteoarthritis? *Acta Orthop*. 2017;88(5):512-515. doi:10.1080/17453674.2017.1348066

57. Noll DR. Leg length discrepancy and osteoarthritic knee pain in the elderly: an observational study. *J Am Osteopath Assoc*. 2013;113(9):670-678. doi:10.7556/jaoa.2013.033

58. Harvey WF, Yang M, Cooke TD, et al. Associations of leg length inequality with knee osteroarhtritis: a cohort study. *Ann Intern Med*. 2010;152(5):287-295. doi:10.1059/0003-4819-152-5-201003020-00006

59. Harvey WF, Yang M, Cooke TDV, et al. Association of leg-length inequality with knee osteoarthritis: a cohort study. *Ann Intern Med*. 2010;152(5):287-295. doi:10.7326/0003-4819-152-5-201003020-00006

60. Woodfield HC, Gerstman BB, Olaisen RH, Johnson DF. Interexaminer reliability of supine leg checks for discriminating leg-length inequality. *J Manipulative Physiol Ther*. 2011;34(4):239-246. doi:10.1016/j.jmpt.2011.04.009

61. Jamaluddin S, Sulaiman AR, Imran MK, Juhara H, Ezane MA, Nordin S. Reliability and accuracy of the tape measurement method with a nearest reading of 5 mm in the assessment of leg length discrepancy. *Singapore Med J*. 2011;52(9):681-684.

62. McConnell J. The physical therapist's approach to patellofemoral disorders. *Clin Sports Med*. 2002;21(3):363-387. doi:10.1016/s0278-5919(02)00027-3

63. Loudon JK. Biomechanics and pathomechanics of the patellofemoral joint. *Int J Sports Phys Ther*. 2016;11(6):820-830.

64. Insall J, Salvati E. Patella position in the normal knee joint. *Radiology*. 1971;101(1):101-104. doi:10.1148/101.1.101

65. Dutton RA, Khadavi MJ, Fredericson M. Patellofemoral pain. *Phys Med Rehabil Clin N Am*. 2016;27(1):31-52. doi:10.1016/j.pmr.2015.08.002

66. Manske RC, Davies GJ. Examination of the patellofemoral joint. *Int J Sports Phys Ther*. 2016;11(6):831-853.

67. Takacs J, Carpenter MG, Garland SJ, Hunt MA. Factors associated with dynamic balance in people with knee osteoarthritis. *Arch Phys Med Rehabil*. 2015;96(10):1873-1879. doi:10.1016/j.apmr.2015.06.014

68. Powers CM, Witvrouw E, Davis IS, Crossley KM. Evidence-based framework for a pathomechanical model of patellofemoral pain: 2017 patellofemoral pain consensus statement from the 4th international patellofemoral pain research retreat, Manchester, UK: part 3. *Br J Sports Med*. 2017;51(24):1713-1723. doi:10.1136/bjsports-2017-098717

69. Powers CM, Bolgla LA, Callaghan MJ, Collins N, Sheehan FT. Patellofemoral pain: proximal, distal, and local factors, 2nd international research retreat. *J Orthop Sports Phys Ther*. 2012;42(6):A1-54. doi:10.2519/jospt.2012.0301

70. Mohammadpour S, Rajabi R, Minoonejad H, Sharifnezhad A. Association between preparatory knee muscle activation and knee valgus angle during single leg cross drop landing following anterior cruciate ligament reconstruction. *J Rehabil Res Dev*. 2019;6:15-20. doi:10.30476/JRSR.2019.44715

71. Ortiz A, Rosario-Canales M, Rodríguez A, Seda A, Figueroa C, Venegas-Ríos HL. Reliability and concurrent validity between two-dimensional and three-dimensional evaluations of knee valgus during drop jumps. *Open Access J Sports Med*. 2016;7:65-73. doi:10.2147/OAJSM.S100242

72. Paterno MV, Schmitt LC, Ford KR, et al. Biomechanical measures during landing and postural stability predict second anterior cruciate ligament injury after anterior cruciate ligament reconstruction and return to sport. *Am J Sports Med.* 2010;38(10):1968-1978. doi:10.1177/0363546510376053

73. Hewett TE, Myer GD, Ford KR, Paterno MV, Quatman CE. The 2012 ABJS Nicolas Andry award: the sequence of prevention: a systematic approach to prevent anterior cruciate ligament injury. *Clin Orthop.* 2012;470(10):2930-2940. doi:10.1007/s11999-012-2440-2

74. Hewett TE, Myer GD, Ford KR, Paterno MV, Quatman CE. Mechanisms, prediction, and prevention of ACL injuries: cut risk with three sharpened and validated tools. *J Orthop Res Off Publ Orthop Res Soc.* 2016;34(11):1843-1855. doi:10.1002/jor.23414

75. Munro A, Herrington L, Carolan M. Reliability of 2-dimensional video assessment of frontal-plane dynamic knee valgus during common athletic screening tasks. *J Sport Rehabil.* 2012;21(1):7-11. doi:10.1123/jsr.21.1.7

76. Munro A, Herrington L, Comfort P. The relationship between 2-dimensional knee-valgus angles during single-leg squat, single-leg-land, and drop-jump screening tests. *J Sport Rehabil.* 2017;26(1):72-77. doi:10.1123/jsr.2015-0102

77. Whatman C, Hume P, Hing W. Can 2D video be used to screen dynamic lower extremity alignment in young athletes? *New Zealand J Sports Med.* 2012:43-47.

78. Whatman C, Hing W, Hume P. Physiotherapist agreement when visually rating movement quality during lower extremity functional screening tests. *Phys Ther Sport.* 2012;13(2):87-96. doi:10.1016/j.ptsp.2011.07.001

79. Whatman C, Hume P, Hing W. The reliability and validity of physiotherapist visual rating of dynamic pelvis and knee alignment in young athletes. *Phys Ther Sport.* 2013;14(3):168-174. doi:10.1016/j.ptsp.2012.07.001

80. Nae J, Creaby MW, Cronström A, Ageberg E. Measurement properties of visual rating of postural orientation errors of the lower extremity - a systematic review and meta-analysis. *Phys Ther Sport.* 2017;27:52-64. doi:10.1016/j.ptsp.2017.04.003

81. Nae J, Creaby MW, Nilsson G, Crossley KM, Ageberg E. Measurement properties of a test battery to assess postural orientation during functional tasks in patients undergoing anterior cruciate ligament injury rehabilitation. *J Orthop Sports Phys Ther.* 2017;47(11):863-873. doi:10.2519/jospt.2017.7270

82. Willson JD, Davis IS. Utility of the frontal plane projection angle in females with patellofemoral pain. *J Orthop Sports Phys Ther.* 2008;38(10):606-615. doi:10.2519/jospt.2008.2706

83. Harris-Hayes M, Steger-May K, Koh C, Royer NK, Graci V, Salsich GB. Classification of lower extremity movement patterns based on visual assessment: reliability and correlation with 2-dimensional video analysis. *J Athl Train.* 2014;49(3):304-310. doi:10.4085/1062-6050-49.2.21

84. Mostaed MF, Werner DM, Barrios J. 2D and 3D kinematics during lateral step-down testing in individuals with anterior cruciate ligament reconstruction. *Int J Sports Phys Ther.* 2018;13(1):77-85.

85. Park K-M, Cynn H-S, Choung S-D. Musculoskeletal predictors of movement quality for the forward step-down test in asymptomatic women. *J Orthop Sports Phys Ther.* 2013;43(7):504-510. doi:10.2519/jospt.2013.4073

86. Shimokochi Y, Ambegaonkar JP, Meyer EG, Lee SY, Shultz SJ. Changing sagittal plane body position during single-leg landings influences the risk of non-contact anterior cruciate ligament injury. *Knee.* 2013;21(4):888-897. doi:10.1007/s00167-012-2011-9

87. Shimokochi Y, Ambegaonkar JP, Meyer EG. Changing sagittal-plane landing styles to modulate impact and tibiofemoral force magnitude and directions relative to the tibia. *J Athl Train.* 2016;51(9):669-681. doi:10.4085/1062-6050-51.10.15

88. Ford KR, Myer GD, Hewett TE. Longitudinal effects of maturation on lower extremity joint stiffness in adolescent athletes. *Am J Sports Med.* 2010;38(9):1829-1837. doi:10.1177/0363546510367425

89. Chang AH, Lee SJ, Zhao H, Ren Y, Zhang L-Q. Impaired varus-valgus proprioception and neuromuscular stabilization in medial knee osteoarthritis. *J Biomech.* 2014;47(2):360-366. doi:10.1016/j.jbiomech.2013.11.024

90. Freisinger GM, Schmitt LC, Wanamaker AB, Siston RA, Chaudhari AMW. Tibiofemoral osteoarthritis and varus-valgus laxity. *J Knee Surg.* 2017;30(5):440-451. doi:10.1055/s-0036-1592149

91. Duivenvoorden T, van Raaij TM, Horemans HLD, et al. Do laterally wedged insoles or valgus braces unload the medial compartment of the knee in patients with osteoarthritis? *Clin Orthop Relat Res.* 2015;473(1):265-274. doi:10.1007/s11999-014-3947-5

92. Hegedus EJ, McDonough SM, Bleakley C, Baxter D, Cook CE. Clinician-friendly lower extremity physical performance tests in athletes: a systematic review of measurement properties and correlation with injury. Part 2--the tests for the hip, thigh, foot and ankle including the star excursion balance test. *Br J Sports Med.* 2015;49(10):649-656. doi:10.1136/bjsports-2014-094341

93. Adams D, Logerstedt DS, Hunter-Giordano A, Axe MJ, Snyder-Mackler L. Current concepts for anterior cruciate ligament reconstruction: a criterion-based rehabilitation progression. *J Orthop Sports Phys Ther.* 2012;42(7):601-614. doi:10.2519/jospt.2012.3871

94. Wellsandt E, Failla MJ, Snyder-Mackler L. Limb symmetry indexes can overestimate knee function after anterior cruciate ligament injury. *J Orthop Sports Phys Ther.* 2017;47(5):334-338. doi:10.2519/jospt.2017.7285

95. Nae J, Creaby MW, Nilsson G, Crossley KM, Ageberg E. Measurement properties of a test battery to assess postural orientation during functional tasks in patients undergoing anterior cruciate ligament injury rehabilitation. *J Orthop Sports Phys Ther.* 2017;47(11):863-873. doi:10.2519/jospt.2017.7270

96. Nilstad A, Andersen TE, Kristianslund E, et al. Physiotherapists can identify female football players with high knee valgus angles during vertical drop jumps using real-time observational screening. *J Orthop Sports Phys Ther.* 2014;44(5):358-365. doi:10.2519/jospt.2014.4969

97. Adams D, Logerstedt DS, Hunter-Giordano A, Axe MJ, Snyder-Mackler L. Current concepts for anterior cruciate ligament reconstruction: a criterion-based rehabilitation progression. *J Orthop Sports Phys Ther.* 2012;42(7):601-614. doi:10.2519/jospt.2012.3871

98. Myers BA, Jenkins WL, Killian C, Rundquist P. Normative data for hop tests in high school and collegiate basketball and soccer players. *Int J Sports Phys Ther.* 2014;9(5):596-603.

99. Dobson F, Hinman RS, Hall M, et al. Reliability and measurement error of the Osteoarthritis Research Society International (OARSI) recommended performance-based tests of physical function in people with hip and knee osteoarthritis. *Osteoarthritis Cartilage.* 2017;25(11):1792-1796. doi:10.1016/j.joca.2017.06.006

100. Logerstedt D, Grindem H, Lynch A, et al. Single-legged hop tests as predictors of self-reported knee function after anterior cruciate ligament reconstruction. *Am J Sports Med.* 2012;40(10):2348-2356. doi:10.1177/0363546512457551

101. Dobson F, Hinman RS, Roos EM, et al. OARSI recommended performance-based tests to assess physical function in people diagnosed with hip or knee osteoarthritis. *Osteoarthritis Cartilage.* 2013;21(8):1042-1052. doi:10.1016/j.joca.2013.05.002

102. Panken AM, Heymans MW, van Oort L, Verhagen AP. Clinical prognostic factors for patients with anterior knee pain in physical therapy; a systematic review. *Int J Sports Phys Ther.* 2015;10(7):929-945.

103. Ferraz MB, Quaresma MR, Aquino LR, Atra E, Tugwell P, Goldsmith CH. Reliability of pain scales in the assessment of literate and illiterate patients with rheumatoid arthritis. *J Rheumatol.* 1990;17(8):1022-1024.

104. Williamson A, Hoggart B. Pain: a review of three commonly used pain rating scales. *J Clin Nurs.* 2005;14(7):798-804. doi:10.1111/j.1365-2702.2005.01121.x

105. Childs JD, Piva SR, Fritz JM. Responsiveness of the numeric pain rating scale in patients with low back pain. *Spine.* 2005;30(11):1331-1334. doi:10.1097/01.brs.0000164099.92112.29

106. Piva SR, Gil AB, Moore CG, Fitzgerald GK. Responsiveness of the activities of daily living scale of the knee outcome survey and numeric pain rating scale in patients with patellofemoral pain. *J Rehabil Med.* 2009;41(3):129-135. doi:10.2340/16501977-0295

107. Salaffi F, Stancati A, Silvestri CA, Ciapetti A, Grassi W. Minimal clinically important changes in chronic musculoskeletal pain intensity measured on a numerical rating scale. *Eur J Pain.* 2004;8(4):283-291. doi:10.1016/j.ejpain.2003.09.004

108. Tashjian RZ, Deloach J, Porucznik CA, Powell AP. Minimal clinically important differences (MCID) and patient acceptable symptomatic state (PASS) for visual analog scales (VAS) measuring pain in patients treated for rotator cuff disease. *J Shoulder Elbow Surg.* 2009;18(6):927-932. doi:10.1016/j.jse.2009.03.021

109. Jensen MP, Turner JA, Romano JM. What is the maximum number of levels needed in pain intensity measurement? *Pain.* 1994;58(3):387-392. doi:10.1016/0304-3959(94)90133-3

110. Spadoni GF, Stratford PW, Solomon PE, Wishart LR. The evaluation of change in pain intensity: a comparison of the P4 and single-item numeric pain rating scales. *J Orthop Sports Phys Ther.* 2004;34(4):187-193. doi:10.2519/jospt.2004.34.4.187

111. Logerstedt DS, Scalzitti D, Risberg MA, et al. Knee stability and movement coordination impairments: knee ligament sprain revision 2017. *J Orthop Sports Phys Ther.* 2017;47(11):A1-A47. doi:10.2519/jospt.2017.0303

112. Mueller MJ, Maluf KS. Tissue adaptation to physical stress: a proposed "physical stress theory" to guide physical therapist practice, education, and research. *Phys Ther.* 2002;82(4):383-403. doi:10.1093/ptj/82.4.383

113. Ardern CL, Österberg A, Tagesson S, Gauffin H, Webster KE, Kvist J. The impact of psychological readiness to return to sport and recreational activities after anterior cruciate ligament reconstruction. *Br J Sports Med.* 2014;48(22):1613-1619. doi:10.1136/bjsports-2014-093842

114. Ardern CL, Taylor NF, Feller JA, Whitehead TS, Webster KE. Psychological responses matter in returning to preinjury level of sport after anterior cruciate ligament reconstruction surgery. *Am J Sports Med.* 2013;41(7):1549-1558. doi:10.1177/0363546513489284

115. Maclachlan LR, Collins NJ, Matthews MLG, Hodges PW, Vicenzino B. The psychological features of patellofemoral pain: a systematic review. *Br J Sports Med.* 2017;51(9):732-742. doi:10.1136/bjsports-2016-096705

116. Barton CJ, Lack S, Hemmings S, Tufail S, Morrissey D. The "best practice guide to conservative management of patellofemoral pain": incorporating level 1 evidence with expert clinical reasoning. *Br J Sports Med.* 2015;49(14):923-934. doi:10.1136/bjsports-2014-093637

117. Academy of Orthopaedic Physical Therapy. Yellow flag assessment tool - about the tool. September 27, 2017. Accessed February 11, 2018. https://www.orthopt.org/content/s/yellow-flag-assessment-tool-about-the-tool

118. Watson CJ, Propps M, Ratner J, Zeigler DL, Horton P, Smith SS. Reliability and responsiveness of the lower extremity functional scale and the anterior knee pain scale in patients with anterior knee pain. *J Orthop Sports Phys Ther.* 2005;35(3):136-146. doi:10.2519/jospt.2005.35.3.136

119. Chatman AB, Hyams SP, Neel JM, et al. The patient-specific functional scale: measurement properties in patients with knee dysfunction. *Phys Ther.* 1997;77(8):820-829. doi:10.1093/ptj/77.8.820

120. Piva SR, Gil AB, Moore CG, Fitzgerald GK. Responsiveness of the activities of daily living scale of the knee outcome survey and numeric pain rating scale in patients with patellofemoral pain. *J Rehabil Med.* 2009;41(3):129-135. doi:10.2340/16501977-0295

121. Collins NJ, Mirsa D, Felson DT, Crossley KM, Roos EM. Measures of knee function. *Arthritis Care Res.* 2011;63(0 11):S208-S228. doi:10.1002/acr.20632

122. Greco NJ, Anderson AF, Mann BJ, et al. Responsiveness of the International Knee Documentation Committee Subjective Knee Form in comparison to the Western Ontario and McMaster Universities Osteoarthritis Index, modified Cincinnati Knee Rating System, and Short Form 36 in patients with focal articular cartilage defects. *Am J Sports Med.* 2010;38(5):891-902. doi:10.1177/0363546509354163

123. Irrgang JJ, Anderson AF, Boland AL, et al. Responsiveness of the International Knee Documentation Committee Subjective Knee Form. *Am J Sports Med.* 2006;34(10):1567-1573. doi:10.1177/0363546506288855

124. Crawford K, Briggs KK, Rodkey WG, Steadman JR. Reliability, validity, and responsiveness of the IKDC score for meniscus injuries of the knee. *Arthroscopy.* 2007;23(8):839-844. doi:10.1016/j.arthro.2007.02.005

125. Angst F, Aeschlimann A, Michel BA, Stucki G. Minimal clinically important rehabilitation effects in patients with osteoarthritis of the lower extremities. *J Rheumatol.* 2002;29(1):131-138.

126. Briggs KK, Lysholm J, Tegner Y, Rodkey WG, Kocher MS, Steadman JR. The reliability, validity, and responsiveness of the Lysholm score and Tegner activity scale for anterior cruciate ligament injuries of the knee: 25 years later. *Am J Sports Med.* 2009;37(5):890-897. doi:10.1177/0363546508330143

127. Woby SR, Roach NK, Urmston M, Watson PJ. Psychometric properties of the TSK-11: a shortened version of the Tampa Scale for Kinesiophobia. *Pain.* 2005;117(1-2):137-144. doi:10.1016/j.pain.2005.05.029

128. Waddell G, Newton M, Henderson I, Somerville D, Main CJ. A Fear-Avoidance Beliefs Questionnaire (FABQ) and the role of fear-avoidance beliefs in chronic low back pain and disability. *Pain.* 1993;52(2):157-168. doi:10.1016/030-3959(93)90127-B

129. Sullivan MJL, Bishop SR, Pivik J. The Pain Catastrophizing Scale: development and validation. *Psychol Assess.* 1995;7(4):524-532. doi:10.1037/1040-3590.7.4.524

130. Lentz TA, Beneciuk JM, Bialosky JE, et al. Development of a yellow flag assessment tool for orthopaedic physical therapists: results from the optimal screening for prediction of referral and outcome (OSPRO) cohort. *J Orthop Sports Phys Ther.* 2016;46(5):327-343. doi:10.2519/jospt.2016.6487

131. George SZ, Beneciuk JM, Lentz TA, Wu SS. The optimal screening for prediction of referral and outcome (OSPRO) in patients with musculoskeletal pain conditions: a longitudinal validation cohort from the USA. *BMJ Open.* 2017;7(6):e015188. doi:10.1136/bmjopen-2016-015188

132. Farrokhi S, O'Connell M, Fitzgerald GK. Altered gait biomechanics and increased knee-specific impairments in patients with coexisting tibiofemoral and patellofemoral osteoarthritis. *Gait Posture.* 2015;41(1):81-85. doi:10.1016/j.gaitpost.2014.08.014

133. Mehta SP, Barker K, Bowman B, Galloway H, Oliashirazi N, Oliashirazi A. Reliability, concurrent validity, and minimal detectable change for iPhone goniometer app in assessing knee range of motion. *J Knee Surg.* 2017;30(6):577-584. doi:10.1055/s-0036-1593877

134. Milanese S, Gordon S, Buettner P, et al. Reliability and concurrent validity of knee angle measurement: smart phone app versus universal goniometer used by experienced and novice clinicians. *Man Ther.* 2014;19(6):569-574. doi:10.1016/j.math.2014.05.009

135. Dos Santos RA, Derhon V, Brandalize M, Brandalize D, Rossi LP. Evaluation of knee range of motion: correlation between measurements using a universal goniometer and a smartphone goniometric application. *J Bodyw Mov Ther.* 2017;21(3):699-703. doi:10.1016/j.jbmt.2016.11.008

136. Reese NB, Bandy WD. *Joint Range of Motion and Muscle Length Testing.* 2nd ed. Saunders; 2010.

137. Joshi RP, Heatley FW. Measurement of coronal plane patellar mobility in normal subjects. *Knee Surg Sports Traumatol Arthrosc.* 2000;8(1):40-45. doi:10.1007/s001670050009

138. Kolowich PA, Paulos LE, Rosenberg TD, Farnsworth S. Lateral release of the patella: indications and contraindications. *Am J Sports Med.* 1990;18(4):359-365. doi:10.1177/036354659001800405

139. Boyle KL, Witt P, Riegger-Krugh C. Intrarater and interrater reliability of the beighton and horan joint mobility index. *J Athl Train.* 2003;38(4):281-285.

140. Boling MC, Padua DA, Marshall SW, Guskiewicz K, Pyne S, Beutler A. A prospective investigation of biomechanical risk factors for patellofemoral pain syndrome: the joint undertaking to monitor and prevent ACL injury (JUMP-ACL) cohort. *Am J Sports Med.* 2009;37(11):2108-2116. doi:10.1177/0363546509337934

141. Culvenor AG, Ruhdorfer A, Juhl C, Eckstein F, Øiestad BE. Knee extensor strength and risk of structural, symptomatic, and functional decline in knee osteoarthritis: a systematic review and meta-analysis. *Arthritis Care Res.* 2017;69(5):649-658. doi:10.1002/acr.23005

142. Øiestad BE, Juhl CB, Eitzen I, Thorlund JB. Knee extensor muscle weakness is a risk factor for development of knee osteoarthritis. A systematic review and meta-analysis. *Osteoarthritis Cartilage.* 2015;23(2):171-177. doi:10.1016/j.joca.2014.10.008

143. Sebastian D, Chovvath R, Malladi R. The sitting active and prone passive lag test: an inter-rater reliability study. *J Bodyw Mov Ther.* 2014;18(2):204-209. doi:10.1016/j.jbmt.2013.08.002

144. Bohannon RW, Kindig J, Sabo G, Duni AE, Cram P. Isometric knee extension force measured using a handheld dynamometer with and without belt-stabilization. *Physiother Theory Pract.* 2012;28(7):562-568. doi:10.3109/09593985.2011.640385

145. Kim S-G, Lee Y-S. The intra- and inter-rater reliabilities of lower extremity muscle strength assessment of healthy adults using a hand held dynamometer. *J Phys Ther Sci.* 2015;27(6):1799-1801. doi:10.1589/jpts.27.1799

146. Martins J, da Silva JR, da Silva MRB, Bevilaqua-Grossi D. Reliability and validity of the belt-stabilized handheld dynamometer in hip- and knee-strength tests. *J Athl Train.* 2017;52(9):809-819. doi:10.4085/1062-6050-52.6.04

147. Katoh M, Hiiragi Y, Uchida M. Validity of isometric muscle strength measurements of the lower limbs using a handheld dynamometer and belt: a comparison with an isokinetic dynamometer. *J Phys Ther Sci.* 2011;23(4):553-557. doi:10.1589/jpts.23.553

148. Chamorro C, Armijo-Olivo S, De la Fuente C, Fuentes J, Javier Chirosa L. Absolute reliability and concurrent validity of hand held dynamometry and isokinetic dynamometry in the hip, knee and ankle joint: systematic review and meta-analysis. *Open Med (Wars).* 2017;12:359-375. doi:10.1515/med-2017-0052

149. Dobson F, Hinman RS, Hall M, Terwee CB, Roos EM, Bennell KL. Measurement properties of performance-based measures to assess physical function in hip and knee osteoarthritis: a systematic review. *Osteoarthritis Cartilage.* 2012;20(12):1548-1562. doi:10.1016/j.joca.2012.08.015

150. Dobson F, Hinman RS, Hall M, et al. Reliability and measurement error of the Osteoarthritis Research Society International (OARSI) recommended performance-based tests of physical function in people with hip and knee osteoarthritis. *Osteoarthritis Cartilage.* 2017;25(11):1792-1796. doi:10.1016/j.joca.2017.06.006

151. Rikli R, Jones C. Functional fitness normative scores for community-residing older adults, ages 60-94. *J Aging Phys Act.* 7(2):162-181. doi:10.1123/japa.7.2.162

152. Wood LRJ, Blagojevic-Bucknall M, Stynes S, et al. Impairment-targeted exercises for older adults with knee pain: a proof-of-principle study (TargET-Knee-Pain). *BMC Musculoskeletal Disord.* 2016;17:47. doi:10.1186/s12891-016-0899-9

153. Iversen MD, Price LL, von Heideken J, Harvey WF, Wang C. Physical examination findings and their relationship with performance-based function in adults with knee osteoarthritis. *BMC Musculoskelet Disord.* 2016;17:273. doi:10.1186/s12891-016-1151-3

154. Selhorst M, Rice W, Degenhart T, Jackowski M, Tatman M. Evaluation of a treatment algorithm for patients with patellofemoral pain syndrome: a pilot study. *Int J Sports Phys Ther.* 2015;10(2):178-188.

155. Han J, Waddington G, Adams R, Anson J, Liu Y. Assessing proprioception: a critical review of methods. *J Sport Health Sci.* 2016;5(1):80-90. doi:10.1016/j.jshs.2014.10.004

156. Knoop J, Steultjens MPM, van der Leeden M, et al. Proprioception in knee osteoarthritis: a narrative review. *Osteoarthritis Cartilage.* 2011;19(4):381-388. doi:10.1016/j.joca.2011.01.003

157. Relph N, Herrington L, Tyson S. The effects of ACL injury on knee proprioception: a meta-analysis. *Physiotherapy.* 2014;100(3):187-195. doi:10.1016/j.physio.2013.11.002

158. Mir SM, Talebian S, Naseri N, Hadian M-R. Assessment of knee proprioception in the anterior cruciate ligament injury risk position in healthy subjects: a cross-sectional study. *J Phys Ther Sci.* 2014;26(10):1515-1518. doi:10.1589/jpts.26.1515

159. van der Esch M, Knoop J, Hunter DJ, et al. The association between reduced knee joint proprioception and medial meniscal abnormalities using MRI in knee osteoarthritis: results from the Amsterdam osteoarthritis cohort. *Osteoarthritis Cartilage.* 2013;21:676-681. doi:10.1016/j.joca.2013.02.002

160. Gribble PA, Hertel J, Plisky P. Using the Star Excursion Balance Test to assess dynamic postural-control deficits and outcomes in lower extremity injury: a literature and systematic review. *J Athl Train.* 2012;47(3):339-357. doi:10.4085/1062-6050-47.3.08

161. Lehmann T, Paschen L, Baumeister J. Single-leg assessment of postural stability after anterior cruciate ligament injury: a systematic review and meta-analysis. *Sports Med Open.* 2017;3(1):32. doi:10.1186/s40798-017-0100-5

162. Negahban H, Mazaheri M, Kingma I, van Dieën JH. A systematic review of postural control during single-leg stance in patients with untreated anterior cruciate ligament injury. *Knee Surg Sports Traumatol Arthrosc.* 2014;22(7):1491-1504. doi:10.1007/s00167-013-2501-4

163. Wikstrom EA, Song K, Pietrosimone BG, Blackburn JT, Padua DA. Visual utilization during postural control in anterior cruciate ligament- deficient and -reconstructed patients: systematic reviews and meta-analyses. *Arch Phys Med Rehabil.* 2017;98(10):2052-2065. doi:10.1016/j.apmr.2017.04.010

164. Yilmaz Yelvar GD, Çirak Y, Dalkilinç M, et al. Impairments of postural stability, core endurance, fall index and functional mobility skills in patients with patello femoral pain syndrome. *J Back Musculoskelet Rehabil.* 2016. doi:10.3233/BMR-160729

165. Lawson T, Morrison A, Blaxland S, Wenman M, Schmidt CG, Hunt MA. Laboratory-based measurement of standing balance in individuals with knee osteoarthritis: a systematic review. *Clin Biomech.* 2015;30(4):330-342. doi:10.1016/j.clinbiomech.2015.02.011

166. Takacs J, Garland SJ, Carpenter MG, Hunt MA. Validity and reliability of the community balance and mobility scale in individuals with knee osteoarthritis. *Phys Ther.* 2014;94(6):866-874. doi:10.2522/ptj.20130385

167. Smith MD, Bell DR. Negative effects on postural control after anterior cruciate ligament reconstruction as measured by the balance error scoring system. *J Sport Rehabil.* 2013;22:224-228. doi:10.1123/jsr.22.3.224

168. Herrington L, Hatcher J, Hatcher A, McNicholas M. A comparison of Star Excursion Balance Test reach distances between ACL deficient patients and asymptomatic controls. *Knee.* 2009;16(2):149-152. doi:10.1016/j.knee.2008.10.004

169. Zult T, Gokeler A, van Raay JJAM, Brouwer RW, Zijdewind I, Hortobágyi T. An anterior cruciate ligament injury does not affect the neuromuscular function of the non-injured leg except for dynamic balance and voluntary quadriceps activation. *Knee Surg Sports Traumatol Arthrosc.* 2017;25(1):172-183. doi:10.1007/s00167-016-4335-3

170. Clagg S, Paterno MV, Hewett TE, Schmitt LC. Performance on the modified star excursion balance test at the time of return to sport following anterior cruciate ligament reconstruction. *J Orthop Sports Phys Ther.* 2015;45(6):444-452. doi:10.2519/jospt.2015.5040

171. Aminaka N, Gribble PA. Patellar taping, patellofemoral pain syndrome, lower extremity kinematics, and dynamic postural control. *J Athl Train.* 2008;43(1):21-28. doi:10.4085/1062-6050-43.1.21

172. Gribble PA, Kelly SE, Refshauge KM, Hiller CE. Interrater reliability of the star excursion balance test. *J Athl Train.* 2013;48(5):621-626. doi:10.4085/1062-6050-48.3.03

173. Shaffer SW, Teyhen DS, Lorenson CL, et al. Y-balance test: a reliability study involving multiple raters. *Mil Med.* 2013;178(11):1264-1270. doi:10.7205/MILMED-D-13-00222

174. van Lieshout R, Reijneveld EAE, van den Berg SM, et al. Reproducibility of the modified star excursion balance test composite and specific reach direction scores. *Int J Sports Phys Ther.* 2016;11(3):356-365.

175. Pilsky P, Rauh MJ, Kaminski T, Underwood F. Star Excursion Balance Test as a predictor of lower extremity injury in high school basketball players. *J Orthop Sports Phys Ther.* 2006;36(12):911-919. doi:10.2519/jospt.2006.2244

176. Greenberg ET, Barle M, Glassmann E, Jung M-K. Interrater and test-retest reliability of the y balance test in healthy, early adolescent female athletes. *Int J Sports Phys Ther.* 2019;14(2):204-213.

177. Logerstedt DS, Scalzitti DA, Bennell KL, et al. Knee pain and mobility impairments: meniscal and articular cartilage lesions revision 2018. *J Orthop Sports Phys Ther.* 2018;48(2):A1-A50. doi:10.2519/jospt.2018.0301

178. Willy RW, Hoglund LT, Barton CJ, et al. Patellofemoral pain clinical practice guidelines linked to the international classification of functioning, disability and health from the Academy of Orthopaedic Physical Therapy of the American Physical Therapy Association. *J Orthop Sports Phys Ther.* 2019;49(9):CPG1-COG95. doi:10.2519/jospt.2019.0302

179. Academy of Orthopaedic Physical Therapy. Framework and History Clinical Practice Guidelines. June 13, 2016. Accessed March 24, 2018. https://www.orthopt.org/content/practice/clinical-practice-guidelines/cpg-framework-history

180. Kelley M, Shaefer M, Kuhn J, et al. Shoulder Pain and Mobility Deficits: Adhesive Capsulitis. *J Orthop Sports Phys Ther.* 2013;43(5):A1-A31. doi:10.2519/jospt.2013.0302

181. Smith BE, Thacker D, Crewesmith A, Hall M. Special tests for assessing meniscal tears within the knee: a systematic review and meta-analysis. *Evid Based Med.* 2015;20(3):88-97. doi:10.1136/ebmed-2014-110160

182. Meserve BB, Cleland JA, Boucher TR. A meta-analysis examining clinical test utilities for assessing meniscal injury. *Clin Rehabil.* 2008;22(2):143-161. doi:10.1177/0269215507080130

183. Hegedus EJ, Cook C, Hasselblad V, Goode A, McCrory DC. Physical examination tests for assessing a torn meniscus in the knee: a systematic review with meta-analysis. *J Orthop Sports Phys Ther.* 2007;37(9):541-550. doi:10.2519/jospt.2007.2560

184. Leblanc M-C, Kowalczuk M, Andruszkiewicz N, et al. Diagnostic accuracy of physical examination for anterior knee instability: a systematic review. *Knee Surg Sports Traumatol Arthrosc.* 2015;23(10):2805-2813. doi:10.1007/s00167-015-3563-2

185. van Eck CF, van den Bekerom MPJ, Fu FH, Poolman RW, Kerkhoffs GMMJ. Methods to diagnose acute anterior cruciate ligament rupture: a meta-analysis of physical examinations with and without anaesthesia. *Knee Surg Sports Traumatol Arthrosc.* 2013;21(8):1895-1903. doi:10.1007/s00167-012-2250-9

186. Benjaminse A, Gokeler A, van der Schans CP. Clinical diagnosis of an anterior cruciate ligament rupture: a meta-analysis. *J Orthop Sports Phys Ther.* 2006;36(5):267-288. doi:10.2519/jospt.2006.2011

187. Abruscato K, Browning K, Deleandro D, Menard Q, Wilhelm M, Hassen A. Diagnostic accuracy of the lever sign in detecting anterior cruciate ligament tears: a systematic review and meta-analysis. *Int J Sports Phys Ther.* 2019;14(1):2-13.

188. Nunes GS, Stapait EL, Kirsten MH, de Noronha M, Santos GM. Clinical test for diagnosis of patellofemoral pain syndrome: systematic review with meta-analysis. *Phys Ther Sport.* 2013;14(1):54-59. doi:10.1016/j.ptsp.2012.11.003

189. Cook C, Hegedus E, Hawkins R, Scovell F, Wyland D. Diagnostic accuracy and association to disability of clinical test findings associated with patellofemoral pain syndrome. *Physiother Can.* 2010;62(1):17-24. doi:10.3138/physio.62.1.17

190. Haim A, Yaniv M, Dekel S, Amir H. Patellofemoral pain syndrome: validity of clinical and radiological features. *Clin Orthop.* 2006;451:223-228. doi:10.1097/01.blo.0000229284.45485.6c

191. Sweitzer BA, Cook C, Steadman JR, Hawkins RJ, Wyland DJ. The inter-rater reliability and diagnostic accuracy of patellar mobility tests in patients with anterior knee pain. *Phys Sportsmed.* 2010;38(3):90-96. doi:10.3810/psm.2010.10.1813

192. Harvey LA, Brosseau L, Herbert RD. Continuous passive motion following total knee arthroplasty in people with arthritis. *Cochrane Database Syst Rev.* 2014;(2):CD004260. doi:10.1002/14651858.CD004260.pub3

193. Anemaet W, Hannerich AS. A framework for exercise prescription. *Top Geriatr Rehabil.* 2014;30(2):79-101. doi:10.1097/TGR.0000000000000011

194. Hart JM, Pietrosimone B, Hertel J, Ingersoll CD. Quadriceps activation following knee injuries: a systematic review. *J Athl Train.* 2010;45(1):87-97. doi:10.4085/1062-6050-45.1.87

195. Lewek MD, Rudolph KS, Snyder-Mackler L. Quadriceps femoris muscle weakness and activation failure in patients with symptomatic knee osteoarthritis. *J Orthop Res.* 2004;22(1):110-115. doi:10.1016/S0736-0266(03)00154-2

196. Hauger AV, Reiman MP, Bjordal JM, Sheets C, Ledbetter L, Goode AP. Neuromuscular electrical stimulation is effective in strengthening the quadriceps muscle after anterior cruciate ligament surgery. *Knee Surg Sports Traumatol Arthrosc.* 2018;26(2):399-410. doi:10.1007/s00167-017-4669-5

197. Laufer Y, Shtraker H, Elboim Gabyzon M. The effects of exercise and neuromuscular electrical stimulation in subjects with knee osteoarthritis: a 3-month follow-up study. *Clin Interv Aging.* 2014;9:1153-1161. doi:10.2147/CIA.S64104

198. Melo M de O, Pompeo KD, Brodt GA, Baroni BM, da Silva Junior DP, Vaz MA. Effects of neuromuscular electrical stimulation and low-level laser therapy on the muscle architecture and functional capacity in elderly patients with knee osteoarthritis: a randomized controlled trial. *Clin Rehabil.* 2015;29(6):570-580. doi:10.1177/0269215514552082

199. Palmieri-Smith RM, Thomas AC, Karvonen-Gutierrez C, Sowers M. A clinical trial of neuromuscular electrical stimulation in improving quadriceps muscle strength and activation among women with mild and moderate osteoarthritis. *Phys Ther.* 2010;90(10):1441-1452. doi:10.2522/ptj.20090330

200. Giggins O, Fullen B, Coughlan G. Neuromuscular electrical stimulation in the treatment of knee osteoarthritis: a systematic review and meta-analysis. *Clin Rehabil.* 2012;26(10):867-881. doi:10.1177/0269215511431902

201. Tate J, Suckut T, Wages J, Lyles H, Perrin B. The associations between hip strength and hip kinematics during a single leg hop in recreational athletes post acl reconstruction compared to healthy controls. *Int J Sports Phys Ther.* 2017;12(3):341-351.

202. Cronström A, Creaby MW, Nae J, Ageberg E. Modifiable factors associated with knee abduction during weight-bearing activities: a systematic review and meta-analysis. *Sports Med.* 2016;46(11):1647-1662. doi:10.1007/s40279-016-0519-8

203. Stearns KM, Powers CM. Improvements in hip muscle performance result in increased use of the hip extensors and abductors during a landing task. *Am J Sports Med.* 2014;42(3):602-609. doi:10.1177/0363546513518410

204. Di Stasi S, Myer GD, Hewett TE. Neuromuscular training to target deficits associated with second anterior cruciate ligament injury. *J Orthop Sports Phys Ther.* 2013;43(11):777-792, A1-11. doi:10.2519/jospt.2013.4693

205. Takacs J, Krowchuk NM, Garland SJ, Carpenter MG, Hunt MA. Dynamic balance training improves physical function in individuals with knee osteoarthritis: a pilot randomized controlled trial. *Arch Phys Med Rehabil.* 2017;98(8):1586-1593. doi:10.1016/j.apmr.2017.01.029

206. da Silva FS, de Melo FES, do Amaral MMG, et al. Efficacy of simple integrated group rehabilitation program for patients with knee osteoarthritis: single-blind randomized controlled trial. *J Rehabil Res Dev.* 2015;52(3):309-322. doi:10.1682/JRRD.2014.08.0199

207. Salsich GB, Graci V, Maxam DE. The effects of movement pattern modification on lower extremity kinematics and pain in women with patellofemoral pain. *J Orthop Sports Phys Ther.* 2012;42(12):1017-1024. doi:10.2519/jospt.2012.4231

208. Salsich GB, Yemm B, Steger-May K, Lang CE, Van Dillen LR. A feasibility study of a novel, task-specific movement training intervention for women with patellofemoral pain. *Clin Rehabil.* 2018;32(2):179-190. doi:10.1177/0269215517723055

209. Taylor JB, Nguyen A-D, Paterno MV, Huang B, Ford KR. Real-time optimized biofeedback utilizing sport techniques (ROBUST): a study protocol for a randomized controlled trial. *BMC Musculoskelet Disord.* 2017;18(1):71. doi:10.1186/s12891-017-1436-1

210. Sugimoto D, Myer GD, Barber Foss KD, Pepin MJ, Micheli LJ, Hewett TE. Critical components of neuromuscular training to reduce ACL injury risk in female athletes: meta-regression analysis. *Br J Sports Med.* 2016;50(20):1259-1266. doi:10.1136/bjsports-2015-095596

211. Sugimoto D, Myer GD, Foss KDB, Hewett TE. Specific exercise effects of preventive neuromuscular training intervention on anterior cruciate ligament injury risk reduction in young females: meta-analysis and subgroup analysis. *Br J Sports Med.* 2015;49(5):282-289. doi:10.1136/bjsports-2014-093461

212. Fitzgerald GK, Axe MJ, Snyder-Mackler L. The efficacy of perturbation training in nonoperative anterior cruciate ligament rehabilitation programs for physical active individuals. *Phys Ther.* 2000;80(2):128-140.

213. Fitzgerald GK, Childs JD, Ridge TM, Irrgang JJ. Agility and perturbation training for a physically active individual with knee osteoarthritis. *Phys Ther.* 2002;82(4):372-382. doi:10.1093/ptj/82.4.372

214. Fitzgerald GK, Piva SR, Gil AB, Wisniewski SR, Oddis CV, Irrgang JJ. Agility and perturbation training techniques in exercise therapy for reducing pain and improving function in people with knee osteoarthritis: a randomized clinical trial. *Phys Ther.* 2011;91(4):452-469. doi:10.2522/ptj.20100188

215. Brotzman BS, Manske RC. *Clinical Orthopaedic Rehabilitation An Evidence-Based Approach.* 3rd ed. Elsevier; 2011.

216. Cook C, Hegedus E, Hawkins R, Scovell F, Wyland D. Diagnostic accuracy and association to disability of clinical test findings associated with patellofemoral pain syndrome. *Physiother Can.* 2010;62(1):17-24. doi:10.3138/physio.62.1.17

217. Décary S, Frémont P, Pelletier B, et al. Validity of combining history elements and physical examination tests to diagnose patellofemoral pain. *Arch Phys Med Rehabil.* 2018;99(4):607-614.e1. doi:10.1016/j.apmr.2017.10.014

218. Sweitzer BA, Cook C, Steadman JR, Hawkins RJ, Wyland DJ. The inter-rater reliability and diagnostic accuracy of patellar mobility tests in patients with anterior knee pain. *Phys Sportsmed.* 2010;38(3):90-96. doi:10.3810/psm.2010.10.1813

219. Dye SF. The pathophysiology of patellofemoral pain: a tissue homeostasis perspective. *Clin Orthop Relat Res.* 2005;(436):100-110. doi:10.1097/01.blo.0000172303.744147d

220. Capin JJ, Snyder-Mackler L. The current management of patients with patellofemoral pain from the physical therapist's perspective. *Ann Jt.* 2018;3:40. doi:10.21037/aoj.2018.04.11

221. Witvrouw E, Callaghan MJ, Stefanik JJ, et al. Patellofemoral pain: consensus statement from the 3rd International Patellofemoral Pain Research Retreat held in Vancouver, September 2013. *Br J Sports Med.* 2014;48(6):411-414. doi:10.1136/bjsports-2014-093450

222. Crossley KM, Stefanik JJ, Selfe J, et al. 2016 patellofemoral pain consensus statement from the 4th International Patellofemoral Pain Research Retreat, Manchester. Part 1: terminology, definitions, clinical examination, natural history, patellofemoral osteoarthritis and patient-reported outcome measures. *Br J Sports Med.* 2016;50(14):839-843. doi:10.1136/bjsports-2016-096384

223. Petersen W, Rembitzki I, Liebau C. Patellofemoral pain in athletes. *Open Access J Sports Med.* 2017;8:143-154. doi:10.2147/OAJSM.S133406

224. Waryasz GR, McDermott AY. Patellofemoral pain syndrome (PFPS): a systematic review of anatomy and potential risk factors. *Dyn Med.* 2008;7:9. doi:10.1186/1476-5918-7-9

225. Salsich GB, Perman WH. Patellofemoral joint contact area is influenced by tibiofemoral rotation alignment in individuals who have patellofemoral pain. *J Orthop Sports Phys Ther.* 2007;37(9):521-528. doi:10.2519/jospt.2007.37.9.521

226. Rathleff MS, Rathleff CR, Crossley KM, Barton CJ. Is hip strength a risk factor for patellofemoral pain? A systematic review and meta-analysis. *Br J Sports Med.* 2014;48(14):1088. doi:10.1136/bjsports-2013-093305

227. Kwak SD, Ahmad CS, Gardner TR, et al. Hamstrings and iliotibial band forces affect knee kinematics and contact pattern. *J Orthop Res.* 2000;18(1):101-108. doi:10.1002/jor.1100180115

228. Merican AM, Amis AA. Iliotibial band tension affects patellofemoral and tibiofemoral kinematics. *J Biomech.* 2009;42(10):1539-1546. doi:10.1016/j.jbiomech.2009.03.041

229. Sigward SM, Ota S, Powers CM. Predictors of frontal plane knee excursion during a drop land in young female soccer players. *J Orthop Sports Phys Ther.* 2008;38(11):661-667. doi:10.2519/jospt.2008.2695

230. Rabin A, Kozol Z. Measures of range of motion and strength among healthy women with differing quality of lower extremity movement during the lateral step-down test. *J Orthop Sports Phys Ther.* 2010;40(12):792-800. doi:10.2519/jospt.2010.3424

231. Bolgla LA, Earl-Boehm J, Emery C, Hamstra-Wright K, Ferber R. Pain, function, and strength outcomes for males and females with patellofemoral pain who participate in either a hip/core- or knee-based rehabilitation program. *Int J Sports Phys Ther.* 2016;11(6):926-935.

232. Esculier J-F, Bouyer LJ, Roy J-S. The effects of a multimodal rehabilitation program on symptoms and ground-reaction forces in runners with patellofemoral pain syndrome. *J Sport Rehabil.* 2016;25(1):23-30. doi:10-1123/jsr.2014-0245

233. Lack S, Barton C, Sohan O, Crossley K, Morrissey D. Proximal muscle rehabilitation is effective for patellofemoral pain: a systematic review with meta-analysis. *Br J Sports Med.* 2015;49(21):1365-1376. doi:10.1136/bjsports-2015-094723

234. Nascimento LR, Teixeira-Salmela LF, Souza RB, Resende RA. Hip and knee strengthening is more effective than knee strengthening alone for reducing pain and improving activity in individuals with patellofemoral pain: a systematic review with meta-analysis. *J Orthop Sports Phys Ther.* 2018;48(1):19-31. doi:10.2519/jospt.2018.7365

235. Warden SJ, Hinman RS, Watson MA, Avin KG, Bialocerkowski AE, Crossley KM. Patellar taping and bracing for the treatment of chronic knee pain: a systematic review and meta-analysis. *Arthritis Rheum.* 2008;59(1):73-83. doi:10.1002/art.23242

236. Callaghan MJ, Selfe J. Patellar taping for patellofemoral pain syndrome in adults. *Cochrane Database Syst Rev.* 2012;(4):CD006717. doi:10.1002/14651858.CD006717.pub2

237. Manske RC, Prohaska D. Rehabilitation following medial patellofemoral ligament reconstruction for patellar instability. *Int J Sports Phys Ther.* 2017;12(3):494-511.

238. Khan M, Miller BS. Cochrane in CORR®: surgical versus nonsurgical interventions for treating patellar dislocation (review). *Clin Orthop Relat Res.* 2016;474(11):2337-2343. doi:10.1007/s11999-016-5014-x

239. Buchanan G, Torres L, Czarkowski B, Giangarra CE. Current concepts in the treatment of gross patellofemoral instability. *Int J Sports Phys Ther.* 2016;11(6):867-876.

240. Newberry SJ, FitzGerald J, SooHoo NF, et al. *Treatment of Osteoarthritis of the Knee: An Update Review.* Agency for Healthcare Research and Quality (US); 2017. Accessed March 12, 2018. http://www.ncbi.nlm.nih.gov/books/NBK447543/

241. van Melick N, van Cingel REH, Brooijmans F, et al. Evidence-based clinical practice update: practice guidelines for anterior cruciate ligament rehabilitation based on a systematic review and multidisciplinary consensus. *Br J Sports Med.* 2016;50(24):1506-1515. doi:10.1136/bjsports-2015-095898

242. Décary S, Fallaha M, Belzile S, et al. Clinical diagnosis of partial or complete anterior cruciate ligament tears using patients' history elements and physical examination tests. *PloS One.* 2018;13(6):e0198797. doi:10.1371/journal.pone.0198797

243. Paterno MV. Non-operative care of the patient with an ACL-deficient knee. *Curr Rev Musculoskelet Med.* 2017;10(3):322-327. doi:10.1007/s12178-017-9431-6

244. Fitzgerald GK, Axe MJ, Snyder-Mackler L. A decision-making scheme for returning patients to high-level activity with nonoperative treatment after anterior cruciate ligament. *Knee Surg Sports Traumatol Arthrosc.* 2000;8:76-82. doi:10.1007/s001670050190

245. Fitzgerald GK, Axe MJ, Snyder-Mackler L. Proposed practice guidelines for nonoperative anterior cruciate ligament rehabilitation of physically active individuals. *J Orthop Sports Phys Ther.* 2000;30(4):194-203. doi:10.2519/jospt.2000.30.4.194

246. Samuelsen BT, Webster KE, Johnson NR, Hewett TE, Krych AJ. Hamstring autograft versus patellar tendon autograft for ACL reconstruction: is there a difference in graft failure rate? A meta-analysis of 47,613 patients. *Clin Orthop Relat Res.* 2017;475(10):2459-2468. doi:10.1007/s11999-017-5278-9

247. Erickson BJ, Harris JD, Fillingham YA, et al. Anterior cruciate ligament reconstruction practice patterns by NFL and NCAA football team physicians. *Arthroscopy.* 2014;30(6):731-738. doi:10.1016/j.arthro.2014.02.034

248. Mirza F, Mai DD, Kirkley A, Fowler PJ, Amendola A. Management of injuries to the anterior cruciate ligament: results of a survey of orthopaedic surgeons in Canada. *Clin J Sport Med.* 2000;10(2):85-88. doi:10.1097/00042752-200004000-00001

249. Xie X, Liu X, Chen Z, Yu Y, Peng S, Li Q. A meta-analysis of bone-patellar tendon-bone autograft versus four-strand hamstring tendon autograft for anterior cruciate ligament reconstruction. *Knee.* 2015;22(2):100-110. doi:10.1016/j.knee.2014.11.014

250. Nyland J, Mattocks A, Kibbe S, Kalloub A, Greene JW, Caborn DNM. Anterior cruciate ligament reconstruction, rehabilitation, and return to play: 2015 update. *Open Access J Sports Med.* 2016;7:21-32. doi:10.2147/OAJSM.S72332

251. Joreitz R, Lynch A, Rabuck S, Lynch B, Davin S, Irrgang J. Patient-specific and surgery-specific factors that affect return to sport after ACL reconstruction. *Int J Sports Phys Ther.* 2016;11(2):264-278.

252. Malempati C, Jurjans J, Noehren B, Ireland ML, Johnson DL. Current rehabilitation concepts for anterior cruciate ligament surgery in athletes. *Orthopedics.* 2015;38(11):689-696. doi:10.3928/01477447-20151016-07

253. Nagelli CV, Hewett TE. Should return to sport be delayed until two years after anterior cruciate ligament reconstruction? Biological and functional considerations. *Sports Med Auckl NZ.* 2017;47(2):221-232. doi:10.1007/s40279-016-0584-z

254. Wilk KE, Macrina LC, Cain EL, Dugas JR, Andrews JR. Recent advances in the rehabilitation of anterior cruciate ligament injuries. *J Orthop Sports Phys Ther.* 2012;42(3):153-171. doi:10.2519/jospt.2012.3741

255. Fukuda TY, Fingerhut D, Moreira VC, et al. Open kinetic chain exercises in a restricted range of motion after anterior cruciate ligament reconstruction: a randomized controlled clinical trial. *Am J Sports Med.* 2013;41(4):788-794. doi:10.1177/0363546513476482

256. Di Stasi S, Myer GD, Hewett TE. Neuromuscular training to target deficits associated with second anterior cruciate ligament injury. *J Orthop Sports Phys Ther.* 2013;43(11):777-792, A1-11. doi:10.2519/jospt.2013.4693

257. Kruse LM, Gray B, Wright RW. Rehabilitation after anterior cruciate ligament reconstruction: a systematic review. *J Bone Joint Surg Am.* 2012;94(19):1737-1748. doi:10.2106/JBJS.K.01246

258. Ardern CL, Taylor NF, Feller JA, Webster KE. Fifty-five per cent return to competitive sport following anterior cruciate ligament reconstruction surgery: an updated systematic review and meta-analysis including aspects of physical functioning and contextual factors. *Br J Sports Med.* 2014;48(21):1543-1552. doi:10.1136/bjsports-2013-093398

259. Ardern CL, Taylor NF, Feller JA, Whitehead TS, Webster KE. Sports participation 2 years after anterior cruciate ligament reconstruction in athletes who had not returned to sport at 1 year: a prospective follow-up of physical function and psychological factors in 122 athletes. *Am J Sports Med.* 2015;43(4):848-856. doi:10.1177/0363546514563282

260. Paterno MV, Huang B, Thomas S, Hewett TE, Schmitt LC. Clinical factors that predict a second ACL injury after ACL reconstruction and return to sport: preliminary development of a clinical decision algorithm. *Orthop J Sports Med.* 2017;5(12):2325967117745279. doi:10.1177/2325967117745279

261. Hewett TE, Di Stasi SL, Myer GD. Current concepts for injury prevention in athletes after anterior cruciate ligament reconstruction. *Am J Sports Med.* 2013;41(1):216-224. doi:10.1177/0363546512459638

262. Lisee C, Lepley AS, Birchmeier T, O'Hagan K, Kuenze C. Quadriceps strength and volitional activation after anterior cruciate ligament reconstruction: a systematic review and meta-analysis. *Sports Health.* 2019;11(2):163-179. doi:10.1177/1941738118822739

263. Gokeler A, Dingenen B, Mouton C, Seil R. Clinical course and recommendations for patients after anterior cruciate ligament injury and subsequent reconstruction: a narrative review. *EFORT Open Rev.* 2017;2(10):410-420. doi:10.1302/2058-5241.2.170011

264. Gokeler A, Welling W, Benjaminse A, Lemmink K, Seil R, Zaffagnini S. A critical analysis of limb symmetry indices of hop tests in athletes after anterior cruciate ligament reconstruction: a case control study. *Orthop Traumatol Surg Res.* 2017;103(6):947-951. doi:10.1016/j.otsr.2017.02.015

265. Huleatt JB, Campbell KJ, Laprade RF. Nonoperative treatment approach to knee osteoarthritis in the master athlete. *Sports Health.* 2014;6(1):56-62. doi:10.1177/1941738113501460

266. Nicolella DP, O'Connor MI, Enoka RM, et al. Mechanical contributors to sex differences in idiopathic knee osteoarthritis. *Biol Sex Differ.* 2012;3(1):28. doi:10.1186/2042-6410-3-28

267. Peter WF, Jansen MJ, Hurkmans EJ, et al. Physiotherapy in hip and knee osteoarthritis: development of a practice guideline concerning initial assessment, treatment and evaluation. *Acta Reumatol Port.* 2011;36(3):268-281.

268. Décary S, Feldman D, Frémont P, et al. Initial derivation of diagnostic clusters combining history elements and physical examination tests for symptomatic knee osteoarthritis. *Musculoskeletal Care*. 2018;16(3):370-379. doi:10.1002/msc.1245

269. Brosseau L, Taki J, Desjardins B, et al. The Ottawa panel clinical practice guidelines for the management of knee osteoarthritis. Part two: strengthening exercise programs. *Clin Rehabil*. 2017;31(5):596-611. doi:10.1177/0269215517691084

270. Rabe KG, Matsuse H, Jackson A, Segal NA. Evaluation of the combined application of neuromuscular electrical stimulation and volitional contractions on thigh muscle strength, knee pain, and physical performance in women at risk for knee osteoarthritis: a randomized controlled trial. *PM R*. 2018;10(12):1301-1310. doi:10.1016/j.pmrj.2018.05.014

271. Mayer F, Scharhag-Rosenberger F, Carlsohn A, Cassel M, Müller S, Scharhag J. The intensity and effects of strength training in the elderly. *Dtsch Ärztebl Int*. 2011;108(21):359-364. doi:10.3238/arztebl.2011.0359

272. Vaz MA, Baroni BM, Geremia JM, et al. Neuromuscular electrical stimulation (NMES) reduces structural and functional losses of quadriceps muscle and improves health status in patients with knee osteoarthritis. *J Orthop Res*. 2013;31(4):511-516. doi:10.1002/jor.22264

273. Shamliyan TA, Wang S-Y, Olson-Kellogg B, Kane RL. *Physical Therapy Interventions for Knee Pain Secondary to Osteoarthritis*. Agency for Healthcare Research and Quality (US); 2012. Accessed April 1, 2018. http://www.ncbi.nlm.nih.gov/books/NBK114568/

274. Fransen M, McConnell S, Harmer AR, Van der Esch M, Simic M, Bennell KL. Exercise for osteoarthritis of the knee. *Cochrane Database Syst Rev*. 2015;1:CD004376. doi:10.1002/14651858.CD004376.pub3

275. Lun V, Marsh A, Bray R, Lindsay D, Wiley P. Efficacy of hip strengthening exercises compared with leg strengthening exercises on knee pain, function, and quality of life in patients with knee osteoarthritis. *Clin J Sport Med*. 2015;25(6):509-517. doi:10.1097/JSM.0000000000000170

276. Décary S, Fallaha M, Frémont P, et al. Diagnostic validity of combining history elements and physical examination tests for traumatic and degenerative symptomatic meniscal tears. *PM R*. 2018;10(5)472-482. doi:10.1016/j.pmrj.2017.10.009

277. Smith BE, Thacker D, Crewesmith A, Hall M. Special tests for assessing meniscal tears within the knee: a systematic review and meta-analysis. *Evid Based Med*. 2015;20(3):88-97. doi:10.1136/ebmed-2014-110160

278. Brody K, Baker RT, Nasypany A, Seegmiller JG. Meniscal lesions: the physical examination and evidence for conservative treatment. *Int J Athl Ther Train*. 2015;20(5):35-38. doi:10.1123/ijatt.2014-0103

279. Lowery DJ, Farley TD, Wing DW, Sterett WI, Steadman JR. A clinical composite score accurately detects meniscal pathology. *Arthroscopy*. 2006;22(11):1174-1179. doi:10.1016/j.arthro.2006.06.014

280. Zhang X, Hu M, Lou Z, Liao B. Effects of strength and neuromuscular training on functional performance in athletes after partial medial meniscectomy. *J Exerc Rehabil*. 2017;13(1):110-116. doi:10.12965/jer.1732864.432

281. Hudson Z, Darthuy E. Iliotibial band tightness and patellofemoral pain syndrome: a case-control study. *Man Ther*. 2009;14(2):147-151. doi:10.1016/j.math.2007.12.009

282. Cavanaugh JT, Killian SE. Rehabilitation following meniscal repair. *Curr Rev Musculoskelet Med*. 2012;5(1):46-58. doi:10.1007/s12178-011-9110-y

APPENDIX

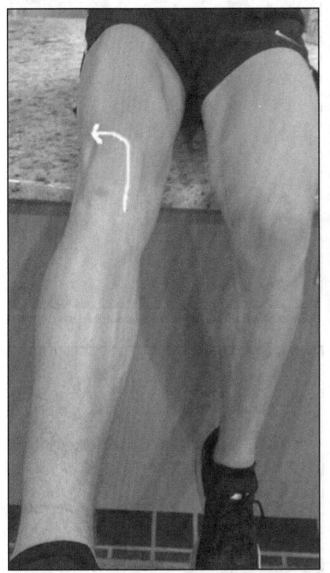

Figure 10-A1. Positive J-sign during active knee extension.

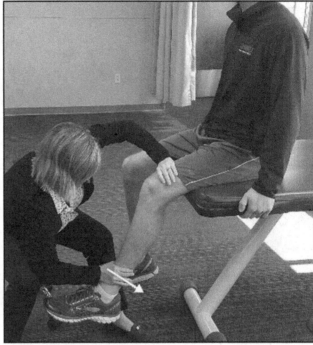

Figure 10-A2. Resisted isometric quadriceps test for patellofemoral pain.

Special Tests for the Patellofemoral Joint

Active and Passive Patella Tracking

Observation of patella tracking is performed with the patient seated, both knees flexed and lower legs hanging off the table. The patient leans backward slightly, supported by both hands to posteriorly tilt the pelvis and reduce hamstring passive tension. As the knee extends from a flexed position, the patella should track superiorly in a straight line or in a slight C curve from a lateral to medial to lateral position as full extension is attained.[1,2] Passive tracking involves the clinician passively extending one knee to assess the impact of osseous and noncontractile tissues. Active tracking involves the patient actively extending their knee to assess the impact of the dynamic stabilizers. A positive sign would be an abrupt lateral movement during the last 20 to 30 degrees of extension also described as a *J-sign* (Figure 10-A1).[2] Positive findings during active patella tracking may occur secondary to imbalances in dynamic medial stabilization while a positive finding during passive patella tracking may occur secondary to tight lateral static tissue restraints or weak medial static tissue restraints.

Patella Apprehension Test or Fairbank's Sign

The patient is positioned supine with the knee extended. The examiner palpates the medial border of the patella with both thumbs and glides the patella laterally as far as possible. Positive test findings are apprehension of the patient or quadriceps contraction in an attempt to control the patella, indicative of patella instability.[3]

Resisted Isometric Quadriceps Test

The patient is positioned seated with the knee flexed. The examiner resists knee extension (Figure 10-A2). A positive test is the presence of pain at the PFJ during resisted knee extension.[4]

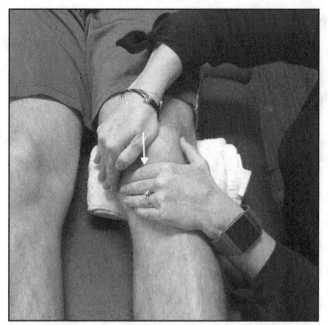

Figure 10-A3. Lateral tilt test for patellofemoral dysfunction.

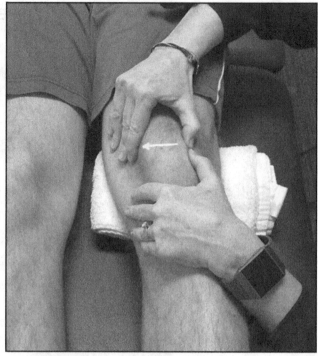

Figure 10-A4. Medial glide test for patellofemoral dysfunction.

Patella Tilt

The patient is positioned supine with the knee extended. The examiner attempts to lift the inferior border of the patella upward while pushing the superior border posteriorly without allowing gliding or rotation of the patella. A Positive test finding is the inability to lift the inferior patella border above the horizontal. Medial and lateral tilts are also assessed by palpating the medial and lateral patella borders with the knee relaxed in an extended position. The borders should be of equal height. The examiner then pushes the medial border posteriorly while lifting the lateral border anteriorly and by pushing the lateral border posteriorly while lifting the medial anteriorly (Figure 10-A3). There should be equal height when the medial and lateral patella borders are lifted. A positive lateral tilt is when the lateral border is palpated to be lower than the medial border and the height of the medial border when lifted passively is greater than passive lifting of the lateral border. Opposite findings exist for a medial tilt of the patella.[3,5]

Patella Glides

The patient is positioned supine with the knee in 30 degrees of flexion over a bolster or roll and the leg completely relaxed. The examiner places both thumbs on lateral border of the patella and glides the patella medially while maintaining the amount of patella tilt observed at rest (Figure 10-A4). The amount of patella glide can be compared to the width of the patella in such that normal patella glide should be about 25% of the width and excessive patella glide is 50% of the width.[3] Another method to estimate patella glide involves dividing the patella into longitudinal quadrants and visually estimating the number of quadrants. Mobility less than one quadrant is considered limited medial mobility, whereas 3 to 4 quadrants of mobility is considered hypermobility.[6] The amount of medial glide should be compared to the nonsymptomatic side. Glides

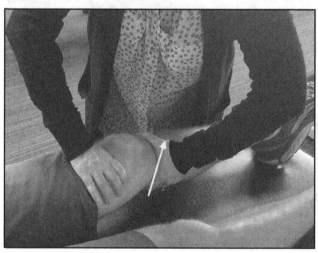

Figure 10-A5. Lachman's test.

are also performed in lateral direction (using the quadrant assessment method), superiorly and inferiorly.

Special Tests for Anterior Cruciate Ligament Sprain

Lachman Test

The patient is positioned supine with the involved knee flexed to 20 to 30 degrees. The examiner stabilizes the femur with one hand while applying an anterior directed force to the tibia with the other hand (Figure 10-A5). A positive test is excessive anterior translation of the tibia with a soft end-feel as compared to the uninvolved lower extremity.[7,8]

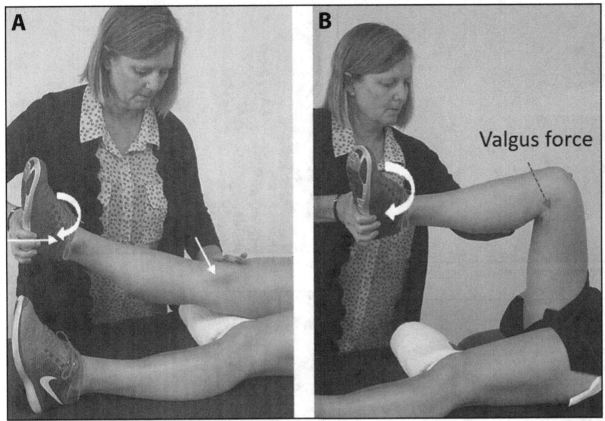

Figure 10-A6. Pivot shift test.

Pivot Shift

The patient is positioned supine with the involved knee in full extension. While holding the heel of the involved lower extremity with their distal hand and the lateral aspect of the lower leg at the fibula with the proximal hand, the examiner flexes the hip to approximately 45 degrees keeping the knee extended (Figure 10-A6A). The examiner then internally rotates the lower leg with the distal hand and applies a valgus force to the knee with the proximal hand while flexing the knee from the extended position (Figure 10-A6B). A positive test is an anterior subluxation of the lateral tibial plateau during the internal rotation and valgus forces followed by reduction as the knee is flexed at 30 to 40 degrees.[7,8]

Anterior Drawer Test

The patient is positioned supine with the involved knee flexed to 90 degrees with the foot flat on the table. The examiner sits on the foot, grasps around the posterior aspect of the proximal tibia with both hands, and applies an anterior force to the tibia (Figure 10-A7). A positive test is excessive anterior tibial translation with a soft end-feel as compared to the uninvolved lower extremity.[7,8]

Lever Sign

The patient is positioned supine with the involved knee extended and the heel resting on the table. The examiner places the fist of their distal hand under the proximal calf at the level of the tibial tuberosity to act as a fulcrum and to

position the knee in about 30 degrees of flexion. With the proximal hand, the examiner pushes from anterior to posterior on the distal aspect of the quadriceps. With an intact ACL, the heel will lift off of the table, indicating a negative test. If the ACL is disrupted, the heel will not lift off of the table, indicating a positive test.[9]

Tests for Posterior Cruciate Ligament Sprain

Posterior Drawer Test

The patient is positioned supine with the involved knee flexed to 90 degrees with the foot flat on the table. The examiner sits on the foot, places both hands on the anterior aspect of the proximal tibia and applies a posterior force to the tibia (Figure 10-A8). A positive test is excessive posterior tibial translation with a soft end-feel as compared to the uninvolved lower extremity.[7,10]

Posterior Sag Test

The patient is positioned supine and the examiner passively flexes both knees and hips to 90 degrees while comparing the position of the proximal tibia of the involved lower extremity to the uninvolved lower extremity (Figure 10-A9). A positive test is excessive sag of the proximal tibia of the involved lower extremity relative to the femoral condyles of the uninvolved lower extremity.[7]

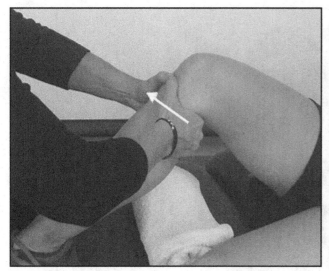

Figure 10-A7. Anterior drawer test.

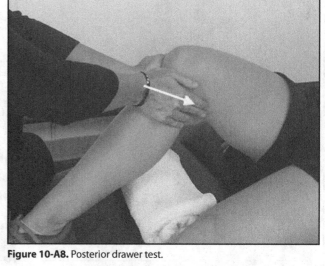

Figure 10-A8. Posterior drawer test.

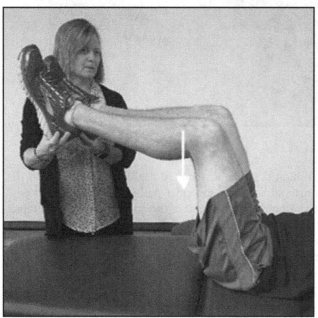

Figure 10-A9. Posterior sag test.

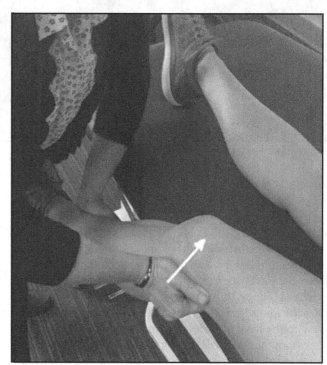

Figure 10-A10. Valgus stress test at 30 degrees knee flexion.

Tests for Sprain of the Medial and Lateral Collateral Ligaments

Valgus Stress Test at 0 and 30 Degrees

The patient is positioned supine with the involved knee extended. The examiner places the proximal hand on the lateral aspect of the knee and the distal hand on the lower leg just above the ankle. Apply a medially directed force (valgus) to the knee to gap the medial aspect of the knee. The test is repeated at 20 to 30 degrees of flexion (Figure 10-A10). A positive test is excessive medial gapping and pain as compared to the contralateral side. A positive test in full knee extension suggests implication of the ACL, PCL, posteromedial capsule, and posterior oblique ligament in addition to the MCL. A positive test in 20 to 30 degrees of flexion further implicates the MCL, potentially along with the posteromedial capsule and posterior oblique ligament.[11]

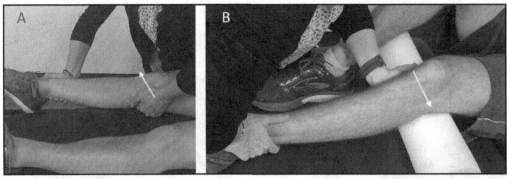

Figure 10-A11. Varus stress test.

Varus Stress Test at 0 and 30 Degrees

The patient is positioned supine with the involved knee extended. The examiner places the proximal hand on the medial aspect of the knee and the lateral aspect of the lower leg and applies a laterally directed force (varus) to the knee to gap the lateral aspect of the knee (Figure 10-A11A). The test is repeated at 20 to 30 degrees of flexion (Figure 10-A11B). A positive test is excessive lateral gapping and pain. A positive test in full knee extension suggests implication of the ACL, PCL, and posterolateral capsule in addition to the LCL. A positive test in 20 to 30 degrees of flexion further implicates the LCL.[12,13]

Tests for Meniscal Tears

Joint Line Tenderness

The patient is positioned in sitting with the knee flexed to 90 degrees. The medial and lateral tibiofemoral joint lines are palpated for tenderness (Figure 10-A12). Tenderness is assessed as present or absent.[4]

McMurray's Test

The patient is positioned supine with the involved knee in full passive flexion (Figure 10-A13A). The examiner's distal hand holds the heel of the foot and the proximal hand is on the knee. To test the lateral meniscus, the examiner medially rotates the tibia while extending the knee (Figure 10-A13B). To test the medial meniscus, the examiner laterally rotates the tibia while extending the knee. A positive test is an audible or palpable click that may be accompanied by report of pain.[7]

Apley's Test

The patient is positioned prone with the involved knee flexed to 90 degrees. The examiner uses their knee to stabilize the patient's thigh while holding the patient's lower leg at the ankle. The tibia is rotated internally and externally while a distraction force is applied to the tibia (Figure 10-A14A) followed by a compression force (Figure 10-A14B). Pain that

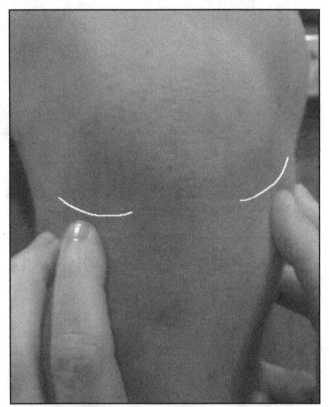

Figure 10-A12. Palpation of the medial and lateral tibiofemoral joint lines for tenderness.

occurs with compression more than with distraction is suggestive of a meniscal lesion, whereas pain that occurs with distraction more than with compression is suggestive of a ligamentous lesion.[7]

Thessaly Test

The patient is positioned in standing on the involved lower extremity with hand support for balance provided by the examiner. While maintaining the foot flat on the floor, the patient flexes their knee to 20 degrees and then rotates their knee and body internally and externally 3 times. A positive test is medial or lateral joint line pain during the maneuver.[14]

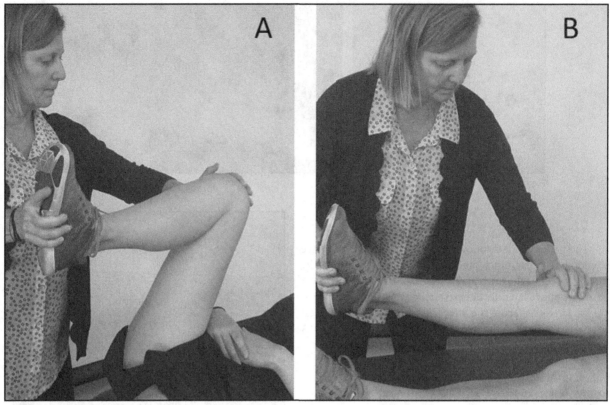

Figure 10-A13. McMurray's test.

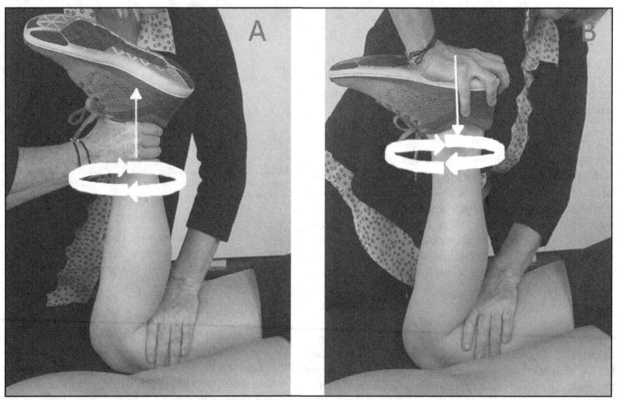

Figure 10-A14. (A) Apley's distraction and (B) compression test.

References

1. Loudon JK. Biomechanics and pathomechanics of the patellofemoral joint. *Int J Sports Phys Ther.* 2016;11(6):820-830.

2. Manske RC, Davies GJ. Examination of the patellofemoral joint. *Int J Sports Phys Ther.* 2016;11(6):831-853.

3. Nissen CW, Cullen MC, Hewett TE, Noyes FR. Physical and arthroscopic examination techniques of the patellofemoral joint. *J Orthop Sports Phys Ther.* 1998;28(5):277-285. doi:10.2519/jospt.1998.28.5.277

4. Cook CE, Hegedus EJ. *Orthopedic Physical Examination Tests: An Evidence-Based Approach.* 2nd ed. Pearson; 2013.

5. Dutton RA, Khadavi MJ, Fredericson M. Patellofemoral Pain. *Phys Med Rehabil Clin N Am.* 2016;27(1):31-52. doi:10.1016/j.pmr.2015.08.002

6. Kolowich PA, Paulos LE, Rosenberg TD, Farnsworth S. Lateral release of the patella: indications and contraindications. *Am J Sports Med.* 1990;18(4):359-365. doi:10.1177/036354659001800405

7. Malanga G, Andrus S, Nadler SF, McLean J. Physical examination of the knee: a review of the original test description and scientific validity of common orthopedic tests. *Arch Phys Med Rehabil.* 2003;84(4):592-603. doi:10.1053/apmr.2003.50026

8. Lange T, Freiberg A, Dröge P, Lützner J, Schmitt J, Kopkow C. The reliability of physical examination tests for the diagnosis of anterior cruciate ligament rupture--a systematic review. *Man Ther.* 2015;20(3):402-411. doi:10.1016/j.math.2014.11.003

9. Lelli A, Di Turi RP, Spenciner DB, Dòmini M. The "lever sign": a new clinical test for the diagnosis of anterior cruciate ligament rupture. *Knee Surg Sports Traumatol Arthrosc.* 2016;24(9):2794-2797. doi:10.1007/s00167-014-3490-7

10. Kopkow C, Freiberg A, Kirschner S, Seidler A, Schmitt J. Physical examination tests for the diagnosis of posterior cruciate ligament rupture: a systematic review. *J Orthop Sports Phys Ther.* 2013;43(11):804-813. doi:10.2519/jospt.2013.4906

11. Stannard JP. Medial and posteromedial instability of the knee: evaluation, treatment, and results. *Sports Med Arthrosc Rev.* 2010;18(4):263-268. doi:10.1097/JSA.0b013e3181eaf713

12. Devitt BM, Whelan DB. Physical examination and imaging of the lateral collateral ligament and posterolateral corner of the knee. *Sports Med Arthrosc Rev.* 2015;23(1):10-16. doi:10.1097/JSA.0000000000000046

13. Harilainen A. Evaluation of knee instability in acute ligamentous injuries. *Ann Chir Gynaecol.* 1987;76(5):269-273.

14. Karachalios T, Hantes M, Zibis AH, Zachos V, Karantanas AH, Malizos KN. Diagnostic accuracy of a new clinical test (the Thessaly test) for early detection of meniscal tears. *J Bone Joint Surg Am.* 2005;87(5):955-962. doi:10.2106/JBJS.D.02338

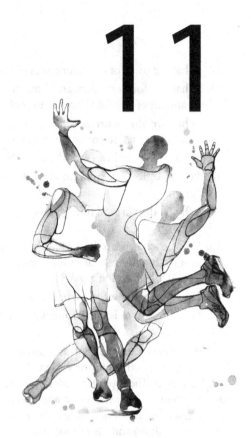

Foot and Ankle
Anatomy, Mechanics, and Rehabilitation

Robert Donatelli, PT, PhD; Georgeta Donatelli, PT, MS;
and Charles Baycroft, MD

Wallmann HW, Donatelli R, eds. *Foundations of Orthopedic Physical Therapy* (pp 309-338).
© 2024 Taylor & Francis Group.

KEY TERMS

Ankle joint arthrokinematics: Include internal rotation of the tibia, plantarflexion, and dorsiflexion of the talus.

Ankle joint movement: Described as dorsiflexion and plantarflexion.

Axis of motion of the ankle joint: Goes through both the tips of the malleoli (medial and lateral).

Lateral ligaments of the ankle: Are on the axis of motion; they include the anterior talofibular, calcaneal fibular, and posterior talofibular.

Pronation: Includes the collapse of the medial arch and calcaneal valgus.

Supination: Includes a high arch with plantar flexion of the first metatarsal and calcaneal varus.

CHAPTER QUESTIONS

1. What are the pronation and supination movements of the foot and ankle?

2. What is the function of the subtalar joint?

3. What is the function of the midtarsal joint?

4. What are the normal mechanics of the foot and ankle?

5. What is the difference between open and closed kinetic chain (CKC) movement of the foot and ankle?

6. What are the mechanics of the foot and ankle during gait?

7. How can we assess the movements of the foot and ankle and then apply them to treatment?

8. What is the function of the peroneus longus muscle?

9. What is the function of the toes during gait?

10. What is the windlass effect and how can it be evaluated?

11. Why is metatarsophalangeal (MTP) joint dorsiflexion so important to gait?

12. What are some of the deformities of the forefoot?

13. What are foot orthotics and how do they help in the treatment of foot and lower limb problems?

14. What are the neuromuscular changes when foot orthotics are used to correct mechanics?

15. What are the indicates for the use of foot orthotics?

16. What surgical intervention is needed with lateral ankle sprains?

17. What is the surgical intervention with Achilles tendon rupture?

18. What exercises are important in the rehabilitation of foot dysfunctions such as sprained ankle or postoperative Achilles tendon repair?

19. How important is the posterior tibialis to foot stability?

20. How important is the peroneus longus to foot stability?

This chapter on the foot and ankle is an overview of how the foot functions in the closed chain position such as weightbearing. The foot mechanics discussed in this chapter are important to the assessment and treatment of foot overuse injuries. In addition, a large part of this chapter is dedicated to definition and use of foot orthotics.

NORMAL ANATOMY AND FUNCTION OF THE FOOT AND ANKLE

The study of normal mechanics in the musculoskeletal system is the analysis of forces and their effects on anatomic structures such as bones, muscles, tendons, and ligaments. The study of forces acting on the musculoskeletal structures of the foot can be divided between the examination of bodies at rest (static) and bodies in motion (dynamic). Kinetics is the study of the relationship between the forces and the resulting movement of the musculoskeletal structures.

This chapter focuses on descriptions of movements and forces acting on the functional joints of the normal human foot and ankle that are important in the establishment of an organ of locomotion and a critical component of balance. The chapter includes normal foot postures and mechanics; abnormal postures; assessment of the foot and ankle; and treatment using foot orthotics, manual therapy, and exercise and will be demonstrated with patient case studies.

The foot is an important sensory organ of the somatosensory system. In addition to the vestibular system and vision, the foot serves as a sensory organ responsible for balance in standing and walking. What is a normal foot? Four of Cailliet's criteria for normalcy are absence of pain, normal muscle balance, central heel, and straight and mobile toes.[1] The authors of this chapter would add that adequate distributions of weightbearing forces on the foot while standing and during the stance phase of gait is also an important criterion of normalcy. This distribution of forces is a direct influence of the central nervous system (CNS) and plays a major role in balance.

The foot and ankle form a complex system that consists of 28 bones, 33 joints, and 112 ligaments, controlled by 13 extrinsic and 21 intrinsic muscles. The foot is the terminal joint in the lower kinetic chain that opposes external resistance. It is the first part of the lower kinetic chain that makes contact with the ground. Therefore, the foot needs to help attenuate the ground reaction forces and the compressive force of the body weight. Furthermore, the foot helps to convert the rotational forces that are initiated from the trunk and lower leg into 3 planes of human movement: sagittal, frontal, and horizontal (or transverse). Proper kinematics within the foot and ankle influence the ability of the lower limb to attenuate the forces of weightbearing. The combined effects of muscle and the unified effect of the soft tissues and proprioceptors within the foot, ankle, and lower extremity result in the most efficient posture that promotes force attenuation and balance.

The foot, for the purposes of this chapter, is divided into 3 sections: the midfoot, forefoot, and rearfoot. The rearfoot converts the torque of the lower limb. The transverse rotations of the lower extremity are converted into sagittal, horizontal, and frontal plane movement in the rearfoot. The rearfoot also influences the function and movement of the forefoot and midfoot. The midfoot and forefoot adapt to the ground as the terrain changes, adjusting to uneven surfaces. This important function of the midfoot and forefoot is dependent on the normal movement of the rearfoot.

EARLY DEVELOPMENT OF THE HUMAN FOOT

The rearfoot (hindfoot) is made up of the talus and calcaneus. The calcaneus is the first of the tarsal bones to begin ossification between the fifth and sixth fetal month. The talus is second to ossify, at about the eighth fetal month. The talus and calcaneus evolve into the body's primary weightbearing, balancing, and propulsive organ. The talus articulates with the calcaneus on facets parallel to the ground for additional balance and adaption. The calcaneus at 3 months represents an average of 25.3% of the total foot length; in adults, it is 35%.

The foot develops in a supinated position. Correction of the fetal supination is accomplished by changes of the rearfoot. As lateral rotation of the talar head and neck occurs, the forefoot varus is reduced. The ossification of the cuboid bone takes place from birth to 21 days of age. The navicular is one of the last of the tarsal bones to ossify, which it does between 2 and 5 years of age. At 2 years old, the ossification centers appear for the medial cuneiform and proximal phalanges. Between the ages of 2 and 3 years, the ossification centers of the middle cuneiform and middle phalanges appear. At the age of 10 years in girls and 12 years in boys, the foot is 90% of the adult size.

Clinical Note

Therefore, any treatment, such as foot orthotics, designed to make permanent changes in the medial arch height of the foot may be successful before the ages of 9 and 10 years, respectively. Collapse of the medial arch is a characteristic of excessive pronation or flatfeet. Dr. Bordelon reported significant long-lasting changes in the height of the medial arch by using foot orthotics in children several years younger than the ages noted earlier.

FUNCTIONAL ANATOMY AND MECHANICS OF THE ADULT FOOT

The functional joints of the foot and ankle are the ankle (talocrural), the subtalar, the midtarsal (transverse tarsal), the tarsometatarsal, and the MTP joints.

The rearfoot, midfoot, and forefoot function as a unit during the stance phase of gait. Alterations in any one of these structures influence the function of the entire foot and ankle during the stance phase. The interdependency and interrelationships of the rearfoot, midfoot, and forefoot are established by muscle and connective tissue structures. Movement of one joint influences movement of other joints in the foot and ankle. Therefore, alterations in the kinematics of the foot and ankle can influence the function of the lower limb. This section discusses the specific movements of the joints of the foot and ankle and their combined function during the stance phase of gait. Stability, muscle function, and proprioceptors of the foot and ankle are reviewed in this section.

Principles of Motion

Motion can be divided into 2 components: translation and rotation. Translation is movement of an object in a straight line that occurs when the line of force passes through the center of the object. Rotation is movement of an object in an arc around a fixed axis; it occurs when the line of force does not pass through the center of the object. The greater the distance between the line of force and the center of the object or center of mass, the greater the rate of rotation. Rotational movement is always perpendicular to the axis of rotation. When a door swings open, movement of rotation occurs around and perpendicular to the fixed axis of the hinge. Movement is also described according to the body plane in which it occurs (the plane of motion). As noted previously, the primary planes of motion in the foot and ankle are the frontal, sagittal, and transverse planes. The

frontal plane movements are inversion and eversion, the sagittal plane movements are dorsiflexion and plantarflexion, and the transverse plane movements are adduction and abduction. The joints of the foot and ankle function as hinges. Motion must occur perpendicular to the axis. If not, partial dislocation or impingement may occur. A true hinge joint provides 1 degree of freedom, or motion, in one plane. The interphalangeal joints of the toes provide 1 degree of freedom, or movement, in 1 body plane (dorsiflexion and plantarflexion in the sagittal). The MTP joints have 2 independent axes of motion. Each axis provides 1 degree of freedom, therefore giving the joints 2 degrees of freedom (dorsiflexion and plantarflexion in the sagittal plane and abduction and adduction in the transverse plane). The midtarsal, subtalar, and talocrural joints and the first and fifth rays (metatarsals) all provide movement in the 3 cardinal body planes, collectively known as *supination* and *pronation*.

Triplanar Movement of the Foot and Ankle

The ankle, subtalar, and midtarsal joints and the first and fifth rays have axes of motion that are oblique to the body planes. The axes of motion are at an angle to 3 body planes. The movement remains perpendicular to the axis, whereas the plane of movement occurs at an angle to all 3 body planes. If movement occurs in all 3 body planes simultaneously, it is referred to as *triplanar motion*. The triplanar movements of the foot and ankle are supination and pronation. The 3 body plane motions in pronation are abduction (transverse plane), dorsiflexion (sagittal plane), and calcaneal eversion (frontal plane). The talus moves in adduction and plantarflexion during weightbearing. Conversely, supination is a combined talar (dorsiflexion and abduction) and movements of plantarflexion, adduction, and calcaneal inversion, respectfully (Figure 11-1).

Ankle (Talocrural) Joint Mechanics

The tibiotalar, fibulotalar, and tibiofibular joints are 3 articulations that make up the ankle, or talocrural joint. The superior surface of the talus bone is wedge shaped and is referred to as the *trochlea*, which can be as much as 6 mm wider anteriorly. The mortise is formed by the distal end of the tibia, its medial malleolus, and the lateral malleolus of the fibula. Hicks, Barnett, and Napier[2,3] identified 2 axes of ankle joint motion. The dorsiflexion axis is oriented in a downward and lateral direction, and the plantarflexion axis is downward and medial. In the frontal plane, the axis of the ankle joint is observed as slightly distal to the medial and lateral malleoli, in a downward and lateral direction. The oblique anteroposterior inclination of the ankle axis as measured in the transverse plane is called *tibial torsion* or *malleolar torsion*. In the normal adult foot, the external tibial torsion is 23 degrees (Figure 11-2). Singh et al[4] describe an axis of rotation of the talocrural joint as a single constant axis

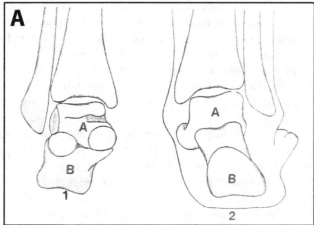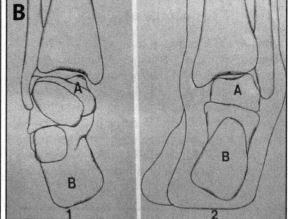

Figure 11-1. (A) Closed-chain pronation. (B) Closed-chain supination.

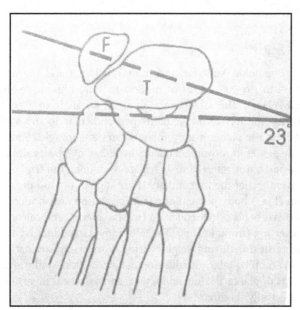

Figure 11-2. Tibial torsion.

of rotation, determined to be distal to the tips of the malleoli. The study by Singh et al further verifies that the talocrural joint is a triplane joint capable of assisting in torque conversion.[4] Although the triplanar movements of supination and pronation occur at the ankle joint because of the obliquity of the axes to the body planes, the functional movements of the ankle are considered dorsiflexion and plantarflexion in nonweightbearing and weightbearing postures. In weightbearing, the dorsiflexion and plantarflexion movements are described as CKC ankle movements. At heel contact to weight acceptance, medial rotation of the lower limb is accompanied by ankle joint plantarflexion. During midstance, anterior movement of the tibia on the talus is initiated as the foot is fixed against the ground. The anterior movement of the tibia on the talus in the CKC is referred to as *closed-chain dorsiflexion*. At heel-off, plantarflexion results in lateral rotation of the leg. The maximum amount of rotation of the tibia around the oblique axis of the ankle joint is 11 degrees and

the average amount of tibial rotation is 19 degrees. Inman describes reciprocal gait as rotations starting at the T5-T6 segment, which filters down to the lumbar spine, pelvis, femur, tibia, and then the talus as an extension of the tibia into the foot.[5,6] The subtalar joint must assist the ankle in accommodating the transverse rotations of the lower limb. There is a one-to-one relationship between talus adduction and tibial internal rotation.[5,6]

Ankle (Talocrural) Joint Stability

Stormont et al[7] determined that stability of the weightbearing ankle depends on several factors, including the congruity of articular surfaces, the orientation of ligaments, proprioceptor function, and the position of the ankle at the time of stress. McCullough and Burge[8] added muscle action to the dynamic stability of the weightbearing ankle. During loading of the ankle, or weightbearing, 100% of inversion and eversion ankle joint stability was accounted for by the joint articular surface. The 3 lateral collateral ligaments accounted for 87% of resistance to inversion in the unloaded position. The most important stabilizer was the calcaneofibular ligament. The anterior talofibular ligament was the second most significant stabilizer, resisting inversion of the ankle in the nonweightbearing position. The deltoid ligament afforded 83% of the ankle's joint stability during eversion in the unloaded condition. Internal and external rotation of the foot on the leg were generally more stable during weightbearing. The primary stabilizers for internal rotation included the anterior talofibular ligament and the deltoid ligament. External rotation is stabilized by the calcaneofibular ligament. The posterior talofibular ligament is the primary stabilizer during plantarflexion. Harper[9] has shown that the stability of the talus is afforded by the medial and lateral structures of the ankle. Tilting of the talus secondary to a valgus stress, anterior excursions, and lateral tilting were the 3 movements examined in the study. The lateral supporting structures of the joints of the ankle were the major restraint against anterior talar excursion. The anterior talofibular and calcaneofibular ligaments are synergistic, so when one is relaxed, the other is strained.

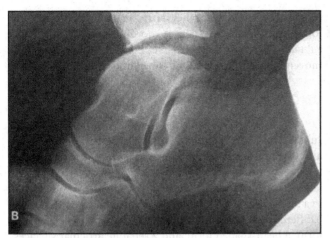

Figure 11-3. Anterior drawer.

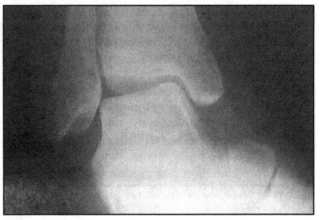

Figure 11-4. Talar tilt.

Clinical Note

It is important to note that the collateral ligaments of the ankle are stabilizers of the talus, provide proprioceptive input, and contribute to the transmission of rotational forces from the lower limb into the rearfoot. The rotational forces are converted into the 3 body plane movements by the action of the talus and calcaneus.

Clinically, a positive anterior draw sign (anterior position of the talus relative to the tibia (Figure 11-3) and talar tilt can be demonstrated roentgenographically (Figure 11-4), indicating torn lateral collateral ligaments. The deltoid ligament is the primary restraint to a valgus stress. It is an important factor in preventing rearfoot valgus, a component to rearfoot pronation. The final consideration regarding the ankle joint is its weightbearing capability and balance. The ankle joint is the first joint in the lower kinetic chain to accept weightbearing during gait. Frankel and Nordin[10] reported 11 to 13 cm of weightbearing surface in each ankle. Each ankle carries 49.3% of the body weight if the feet represent 1.4% of the total body weight. The weightbearing is shared by the tibiotalar and fibulotalar joints. Because of the large surface area, the load transmission across the ankle joint is less than that across either the hip joint or the knee joint. The talocrural joint is an efficient weightbearing structure. From heel strike to foot flat, the compressive forces increase within the ankle joint to approximately 3 times body weight. At heel-off, articular compressive forces reach 4.5 to 5.5 times body weight.

The ankle is in close proximity to the center of gravity and is, therefore, important for maintaining balance. Studies have shown that an unstable ankle reduces balance. The CNS uses sensory information to produce the appropriate muscle forces to maintain balance. Sensory systems contributing to balance include the visual, vestibular, and somatosensory systems. The role of each of these 3 systems in control of posture are important; however, the somatosensory system is considered to be the biggest contributor of feedback for postural control. Proprioceptors are the receptors in the muscles, tendons, and joint capsules that provide information about muscle length, contractile speed, muscle tension, and joint position. The ankle joint is located in close proximity to the body's base of support; therefore, the ankle plays an important role in maintaining balance. The ligaments of the ankle described earlier are not only important in the transfer of forces, but they are also richly endowed with proprioceptors that provide feedback of maintaining balance during functional activities such as standing, walking, and running.

Subtalar Joint Function

The talus and calcaneus are the bones that make up the subtalar joint. The subtalar joint has an important role as the distal component of the lower extremity and is responsible for the conversion of the rotatory forces of the lower extremity and shock absorption. The mechanics of the subtalar joint dictate the movements of the midtarsal joint and to a degree influence the forefoot. Movement between the talus and calcaneus occurs around an oblique axis. The axis of the subtalar joint extends anteromedially from the neck of the talus to the posterolateral portion of the calcaneus. The average inclination of the axis is 42 degrees from the horizontal and 23 degrees from the midline (Figure 11-5). The movement is perpendicular to the axis. Because the axis of the subtalar joint is oblique to 3 body planes, it is considered triplanar. The open kinetic chain pronation movement includes dorsiflexion, abduction, and eversion and for supination, plantarflexion, adduction, and inversion. Subtalar joint supination and pronation are measured clinically by the amount of calcaneal inversion and eversion, respectively. Root et al[11] describe an inversion to eversion ratio of 2:3, 20 degrees of inversion and 10 degrees of eversion. The midposition of the subtalar joint is referred to as *subtalar joint neutral*. However, there is no evidence that confirms that the subtalar neutral position actually exists. Bones and soft tissue structures limit the amount of calcaneal eversion and inversion. Inversion is

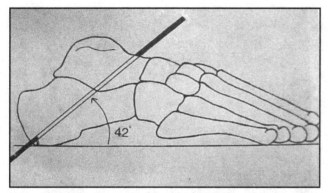

Figure 11-5. Inclination angle of the subtalar joint.

limited by the cervical ligament, calcaneofibular ligament, the peroneus longus and brevis, and the sustentaculum tali striking the talar tubercle. Eversion of the calcaneus is limited by the cervical ligament, lateral process of the talus striking the sinus tarsi surface of the calcaneus, tibiocalcaneal portion of the deltoid ligament, medial talocalcaneal ligament, posterior tibialis tendon and muscle, and the flexor digitorum longus tendon muscle.

SUBTALAR FUNCTION DURING THE STANCE PHASE OF GAIT

In the CKC, an important function of the subtalar joint is to act as a torque converter of the lower leg. As previously noted, the transverse plane rotations of the lower kinetic chain are attenuated at the subtalar joint. As demonstrated in Figure 11-6A, the cadaveric lower leg is in subtalar joint pronation, which produces internal rotation of the tibia, evidenced by the increased space between the tibia and fibula. Supination of the subtalar joint produces external rotation of the tibia (Figure 11-6B). The space between the fibula and tibia is reduced; the tibia is superimposed over the fibula indicating external rotation of the tibia.

During normal ambulation, Sarrafian[12] describes the anterior tibiotalar ligament as contributing to transmission of internal rotation of the tibia to the talus and the posterior talotibial ligament as contributing the transmission of external rotation of the tibia to the talus. The tibia has been found to rotate an average of 19 degrees. The foot cannot rotate by moving from a toe-in to a toe-out position during ambulation. Therefore, a mechanism must exist to permit the rotations of the lower limb to occur without movement of the foot (Boxes 11-1 and 11-2).

The combined CKC movement of the rearfoot is important for torque conversion and shock absorption. The obliquity of the ankle joint and subtalar joint axes allows the foot to accommodate for the transverse plane rotations of the lower limb. Talar movement is coordinated at the ankle and subtalar joint. As the foot makes contact with the ground, movement occurs around the subtalar joint axis.

Subtalar Joint Stability

The subtalar joint consists of the talus and calcaneus. The subtalar joint is made up of 2 articular areas. The posterior articulation consists of the convex calcaneus and the concave talus. The anterior articulations include medial, central, and lateral facets between the talus and calcaneus. Viladot et al,[13] in a dissection study demonstrated in 100 calcanei, identified 3 different anterior calcaneal facets of the talar joint: an ovoid form, a bean-shaped form, and 2 separate articular surfaces. The calcaneus forms an important part of the anteromedial subtalar joint. The sustentaculum tali is the anteromedial aspect of the calcaneus that supports the head and neck of the talus. When the calcaneus everts during pronation, the talus moves medially (adducts) and in plantarflexion. This motion is supported by the medial facet. In addition, the sustentaculum tali forms a fulcrum around which the tibialis posterior, flexor halluces longus, and flexor digitorum longus tendons pass. The contraction of these muscles provides the hindfoot (rearfoot) dynamic stability.

The talus has no muscle attachments; therefore, the ligaments of the subtalar joint are critical to joint stability. They can be divided into superficial and deep structures. The superficial ligaments include the lateral and posterior talocalcaneal ligaments. The deep ligamentous structures form a wall that divides the subtalar joint. The deep ligaments include the interosseous, cervical, and axial ligaments. Viladot et al[13] describes the cervical ligament as a portion of the interosseous structure that limits inversion and eversion. The tarsal canal separates the middle and posterior facets of the articulation between the talus and the calcaneus.[13] The ligament of the canal is sometimes referred to as the *cruciate ligament of the tarsus* or the *axial ligament*. The axial ligament is thick and strong dividing the anterior and posterior subtalar joint and is mainly responsible for limiting eversion. Figure 11-7 shows a dissection of the axial ligament, which divides the subtalar joint, the undersurface of the talus, and the superior surface of the calcaneus. Overstretching of the axial ligament can result in an acquired heel valgus deformity (Figure 11-8). Conversely, severe limitations in passive calcaneal eversion may be secondary to lack of extensibility of the axial ligament. In addition to mechanical function, as described previously, the ligaments of the subtalar joint are richly endowed with proprioceptors that contribute to balance. As described in the next section, one of the benefits of foot orthotics is the improvement in balance.

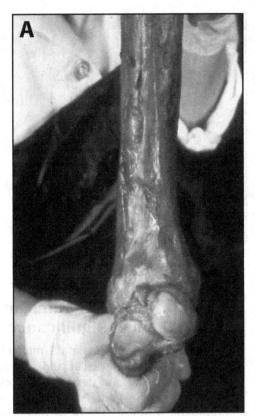 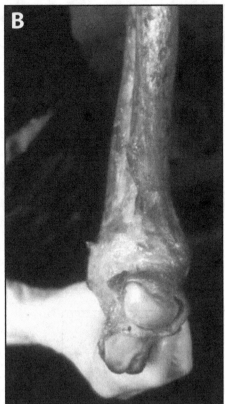

Figure 11-6. (A) Calcaneal eversion: Pronation of subtalar joint and internal rotation of the tibia. Observe the parallel position. (B) Calcaneal inversion: Subtalar supination. The tibia externally rotates—superimposed tibia over the fibula.

Box 11-1. Closed-Chain Pronation

After heel strike at footflat, the tibia rotates internally; the talus plantar flexes and adducts in the sagittal and transverse plane. The calcaneus simultaneously rolls into eversion to complete the torque conversion. This movement is referred to as *CKC pronation of the subtalar joint* (see Figure 11-1A).

Box 11-2. Closed-Chain Supination

As the heel lifts off the ground, the tibia rotates externally, pushing the talus into dorsiflexion and abduction. Simultaneously, the calcaneus inverts to complete the torque conversion. This is CKC supination (see Figure 11-1B).

In summary, the ankle and subtalar joints have the most important role in foot functional mechanics and balance. The ankle and subtalar joints are the first joints in the foot to hit the ground and provide stability during walking and running. The function of the ankle joint (talocrural) is plantarflexion and dorsiflexion of the foot, whereas the function of the subtalar joint ensures inversion and eversion of the foot. While walking and running, the ankle constantly adapts to terrain. The tarsal, metatarsal, and phalanx bones act as primary stabilizers and adjust the foot to each support surface for our movement style. In turn, these small movements affect the stabilizing adaptation of the heel bone, the talus bone, and the ankle joint, as the information is transmitted to the central balance analyzer in the medulla of the CNS. Thus, the ankle joint plays an important role in maintaining balance. An injury, lesion, or neuromuscular disorder of this complex system affects the interactions between muscles, bones, and ligaments and may cause instability and alterations in gait.

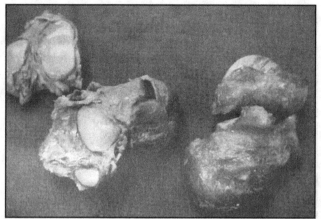

Figure 11-7. Dissection of the subtalar joint on the right talus on top of the calcaneus. Left is the talus and calcaneus articular surfaces. The axial ligament is between the large posterior joint surface and the smaller anterior joint surfaces. It is sometimes referred to as the *cruciate ligament of the ankle.*

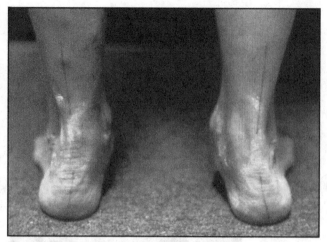

Figure 11-8. Calcaneal valgus (eversion) excessive pronation.

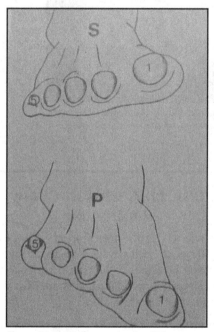

Figure 11-9. Forefoot supination (S)/ pronation (P) twist.

MIDFOOT STABILITY AND FUNCTION

The midtarsal, transverse tarsal, and Chopart's joint are synonymous with the articulations of the calcaneocuboid and the talonavicular joints. The rotational movement between the calcaneus and cuboid is described as pivotal. Rotational movements of the midtarsal joint allow the forefoot to twist on the rearfoot. Manter[14] describes this as supination and pronation twist (Figure 11-9). There is minor relative movement between the navicular and cuboid as

Box 11-3. Fulcrums and Clinical Significance

The rotational movements of the midtarsal, which include talus and navicular and calcaneus and cuboid in the CKC are described as locking and unlocking of the midtarsal joint. For example, during the push-off phase of gait, the pivotal movement of the calcaneus and cuboid (lock up the midtarsal) allows the cuboid to become fixed. A stable cuboid acts as a fulcrum for the peroneus longus muscle. The peroneus longus pulls around the cuboid and plantarflexes the first metatarsal in the push-off phase of gait. The posterior tibialis pulls around the navicular, stabilizing the midtarsal joint (Figure 11-10).

they move as a unit along with the forefoot. Manter[14] and Elftman[15] describe 2 axes of motion at the midtarsal joint. The first axis is longitudinal (extending lengthwise through the foot). Inversion and eversion are the movements occurring around the longitudinal axis. Clinically, inversion and eversion of the midtarsal joint can be observed in the normal rise and drop of the medial arch of the foot in the weightbearing position. Manter[14] describes this movement as a "screw-like" action of the cuboid and navicular rotating around the longitudinal axis. The screw-like action of the cuboid and navicular occurs during CKC inversion and eversion of the calcaneus. The second axis of the midtarsal joint is oblique or transverse. Several authors describe the transverse axis of the midtarsal joint as being inclined 52 degrees from the horizontal and 57 degrees from the frontal plane. Movement at the transverse axis is a combination of dorsiflexion and abduction and plantarflexion and adduction (Box 11-3).

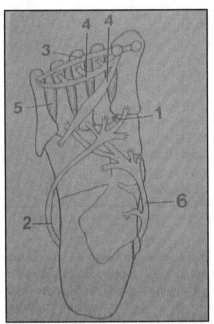

Figure 11-10. (1) Lesfranc's ligament. (2) Peroneus longus tendon fulcrum around the cuboid. (3) Transverse metatarsal ligament. (4) Adductor halluces. (5) Interosseous muscle. (6) Posterior tibialis tendon fulcrum around the navicular.

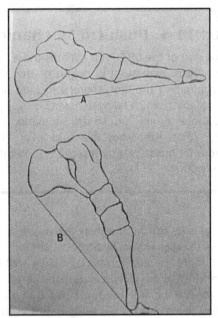

Figure 11-11. The windlass effect.

METATARSAL—TOES FUNCTION

Hicks[2,16] describes the metatarsals as beams supporting the longitudinal arches. The beams are tied together by a "tie rod" or plantar aponeurosis. On weightbearing, the metatarsals and calcaneus are forced apart, and tension develops within the tie rod.

Perry[17] describes the plantar fascia, or the aponeurosis, and the intrinsic musculature as the force transmitters from one end of the arch to the other. As the MTP joints are dorsiflexed in push-off, a "windlass effect" tightens the tie rod (plantar fasciae; Figure 11-11). The plantar fascia is a broad, dense band of longitudinally arranged collagen fibers. Collagen fibers are designed to resist tensile forces. As increased loads are applied, the plantar fascia becomes progressively stiffer or more capable to resist deformation. Hence, tension at one end of the tie rod is transmitted to the other end, pulling the ends closer together and raising the medial arch.

The plantar aponeurosis has 3 components: central, lateral, and medial. The central component originates from the posteromedial calcaneal tuberosity. The lateral or peroneal component originates from the lateral margin of the medial calcaneal tubercle and is connected with the origin of the abductor digiti minimi muscle. Finally, the medial or tibial component fibers originate distally and medially and are continuous with the abductor hallucis muscle. As noted

previously, the plantar aponeurosis originates predominantly from the medial aspect of the calcaneus; therefore, tension of the tissue promotes inversion of the calcaneus and supination of the subtalar joint. Thus, the windlass mechanism is important in establishing a rigid lever during push-off.

Numerous authors have demonstrated that the longitudinal arches are not supported by muscle. Lapidus[18] was one of the first to describe the concept of the foot functioning as a truss. A truss is a triangular structure with 2 beams connected by a tie rod. The vertical forces transmitted to the foot in weightbearing are attenuated by the truss mechanism. Therefore, intrinsic and extrinsic muscles are not used in static arch supports. Mann and Inman[19] report activity of the intrinsic muscles, abductor halluces brevis, flexor halluces brevis, flexor digitorum brevis, and abductor digiti minimi in stabilizing the transverse tarsal joint during the stance phase of gait. In normal feet, the onset of intrinsic muscle activity is initiated at approximately midstance, or after 35% of stance phase. In contrast, the onset of intrinsic muscle activity in flat-footed participants was within the first 25% of the stance phase. Huang et al[20] reported that the highest relative contribution to medial arch stability was provided by the plantar fascia, followed by the plantar ligaments and the spring ligament. The plantar fascia was a major factor in maintenance of the medial longitudinal arch. Cavanagh et al[21] reported that in a symptom-free population, the static peak pressures in the forefoot were 2.5 times lower than the peak pressures under the heel. Thus, about 60% of the weightbearing load is carried by the rearfoot, 8% by the midfoot, and 28% by the heads of the metatarsals. These peak pressures during standing are approximately 30% of those produced during walking and 16% of those during running. The second and third metatarsal heads bear the greatest forefoot pressures. The fact that the first ray does not bear the greatest pressure in

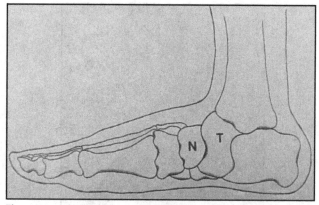

Figure 11-12. Vertical talus-convex pes valgus-flatfoot.

standing indicates that it has a more dynamic function during push-off. Earlier studies by Stokes et al[22] indicated that the forces under the first metatarsal during walking were found to be the highest. Hutton and Dhaneddran[23] reported that the first ray is the largest and strongest of all the metatarsals. The first metatarsal bone is twice as wide as the second metatarsal and 4 times as strong. Furthermore, the peroneus longus, posterior tibialis, and anterior tibialis muscles attach to the first ray (first metatarsal/first uniform) and function to stabilize it dynamically in the propulsive phase of gait. The head of the first metatarsal has a large joint surface and sesamoid bones to give the flexor halluces longus a mechanical advantage, minimizing joint forces. Finally, the inclination angle of the first metatarsal to the horizontal is greater than that of the other metatarsals, reducing the shearing and bending forces of weightbearing (Box 11-4).

The function of the toes is important to the biomechanics of the forefoot. During walking, the toes help to stabilize the longitudinal arch and maintain floor contact until the final phase of push-off. Approximately 40% of body weight is borne by the toes in the final stages of foot contact. During the stance phase of gait, the greatest load is through the first MTP joint. Weightbearing forces to the toes are attenuated by the tension in the toe flexor tendons during standing. Dorsiflexion of the toes, especially the first MTP joint, is important to the windlass mechanism. MTP joint movement occurs in 2 cardinal body planes. The sagittal plane of movement of the MTP joint is flexion and extension, and the transverse plane of movement is abduction and adduction. For tension to develop within the aponeurosis, 60 to 70 degrees of dorsiflexion is necessary.

The sesamoid bones are the attachment sites for several important soft tissue structures. Flexor halluces brevis, oblique head and transverse component of the adductor halluces, flexor halluces longus fibrous tunnel, and the deep transverse metatarsal ligament all insert into the borders of the medial and lateral sesamoid bones. The sesamoid bones maintain proper alignment of the flexor halluces longus tendon and are also responsible for absorbing vertical pressures in push-off. The flexor hallucis longus passes between the sesamoids.

The last 4 toes are attachment sites for the extensor digitorum tendon, flexor digitorum tendon, dorsal and plantar interossei, and lumbrical muscles. The interosseous and lumbrical muscles dynamically stabilize the toes on the floor in the tiptoe position. Failure of the lumbricals and interosseous muscles to function accounts for toe deformities, such as claw toes.

Human feet have evolved uniquely among primates, losing an opposable first digit in favor of a pronounced arch to enhance our ability to walk and run with an upright posture. Recent work suggests that the intrinsic muscles within our feet, lumbricals, and plantar interossei are key to how the foot functions during bipedal walking and running. Contrary to expectations, the intrinsic foot muscles contribute minimally to supporting the arch of the foot during walking and running. However, the intrinsic muscles do influence the ability to enhance forward propulsion from one stride into the next, highlighting their role in bipedal locomotion.

ABNORMAL PRONATION

There are many terms to describe abnormal pronation. *Flatfoot, pes planus, pes valgoplanus, pronated foot, calcaneovalgus foot, valgus foot,* and *talipes calcaneovalgus* are several of the terms found in the literature that describe or identify abnormal pronation. In this text, the term *abnormal pronation* is used to describe the flatfoot deformities.

The literature classifies the cause of abnormal pronation into 3 basic categories: congenital, acquired, and secondary to neuromuscular diseases (which is beyond the scope of this chapter). The term *congenital* means "to be born with" or "to have been present at birth." Congenital flatfoot can result from genetic factors or malposition of the fetus in the uterus. Congenital deformities can be further classified as rigid or flexible. The most common rigid flatfoot deformities with a possible genetic cause include convex pes valgus (congenital vertical talus; Figure 11-12), tarsal coalition, and congenital metatarsus varus. The most common congenital flexible flatfoot deformity is talipes calcaneovalgus.

Acquired flatfoot can result from abnormalities that are intrinsic or extrinsic (or both) to the foot and ankle. Intrinsic causes of acquired flatfoot include trauma and ligament laxity. Extrinsic factors causing abnormal pronation include rotational deformities of the lower extremity and leg length discrepancies.

Increased foot pronation compromises lower limb mechanics in the sagittal plane during the stance phase of gait. Resende et al[24] demonstrated that foot pronation increases foot segments flexibility and compromises foot lever arm function during the stance of gait.

CONGENITAL DEFORMITIES

Rigid Deformities

Convex pes valgus, or congenital vertical talus, is a dislocation of the talocalcaneonavicular joint that the fetus develops in the uterus within the first trimester of pregnancy, in addition to bony abnormalities of the subtalar joint, forefoot varus, and forefoot valgus. The cause is uncertain, and the deformity may occur either in isolation or in association with CNS abnormalities, such as spina bifida and arthrogryposis. The most striking characteristic of the convex pes valgus deformity visible on x-ray is plantar rotation of the talus toward a more vertical position (see Figure 11-12). The vertical position of the talus, however, is commonly observed in other flatfoot deformities, such as talipes calcaneovalgus. A distinguishing feature in a club foot deformity is the position of the navicular, which is completely dislocated, articulating with the dorsal surface of the neck of the talus.

Tarsal Coalitions

Tarsal coalition may be either a complete or incomplete fusion of the talus, calcaneus, cuboid, navicular, or cuneiforms. The joint fusion may be fibrous, cartilaginous, or osseous and can occur during the development of the fetus. Stormont and Peterson[25] found the most common tarsal coalition to be the calcaneonavicular followed by the talocalcaneal. The cause of tarsal coalitions strongly suggests a hereditary component.

Subtalar joint motion becomes progressively more limited with ossification of the coalition. The fusion can occur at the anterior, middle, or posterior facets of the subtalar joint. Limitations at the subtalar joint may be difficult for the clinician to determine. Limited mobility of the calcaneus may be concealed by movement at the midtarsal joint.

Rigid Metatarsal Deformities

McCrea[26] described 4 types of metatarsus deformities within the 3 body planes: metatarsus adductus (in the transverse plane); metatarsus varus (in the frontal plane), which is a subluxation at the tarsometatarsal joint; metatarsus adductovarus (combination of the transverse and frontal planes);

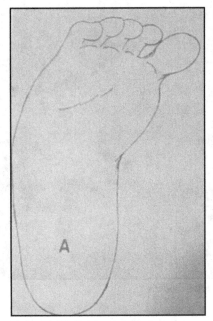

Figure 11-13. Metatarsus adductovarus.

and forefoot adductus (in the transverse plane), which is a deformity occurring at the midtarsal joint.

Kite observed in 300 cases that 94% (282) of the time congenital metatarsus varus was present at birth and is part of a clubfoot deformity.[27] In a rigid metatarsus varus, the forefoot cannot be abducted past midline. If there is a severe rigid metatarsus varus, the forefoot cannot be reduced from the in-toe position. Metatarsus adductus is a flexible transverse plane deformity that may develop into an in-toeing abnormality. The combination of metatarsus adductovarus is a rigid deformity, which also manifests as a toe-in gait (Figure 11-13). Abnormal pronation could develop as a compensation for the forefoot deformities.

ABNORMAL SUPINATION

Abnormal supination is the inability of the foot to pronate effectively during the stance phase of gait. This is commonly referred to as the *high-arched foot*, or *pes cavus*. Abnormal supination is a hypomobility of the joints of the foot and ankle that may result from muscle imbalances and soft tissue contractures. Abnormal supination usually is associated with a rigid structure that is unable to function as an efficient shock absorber or an adapter to changing terrain. A pes cavus deformity is plantarflexion of the forefoot on the rearfoot. Clinically, there are 3 important aspects of the pes cavus foot: increased height of the longitudinal arch, plantarflexion of the forefoot, and some amount of dorsal retraction of the toes (claw toes), hyperextension of the MTP, and flexion of the interphalangeal joints (Figure 11-14).

Pes cavus can be divided into 3 causes: neurologic, contracture of soft tissue structures, and idiopathic. The most clinical and scientifically documented article describing the

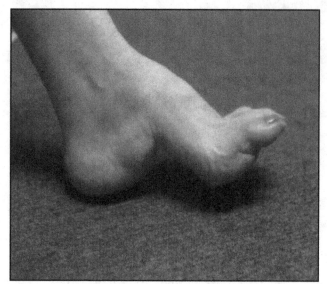

Figure 11-14. Pes cavus foot.

cause of pes cavus was presented in 1963 by Brewerton et al.[28] They reported evidence of CNS disorders in 66% of 77 patients followed in a pes cavus clinic over a 5-year period. The neurologic disorders included Friedreich's ataxia, peroneal muscular atrophy, poliomyelitis, spina bifida, cerebral palsy, spinal cord tumors, myelodysplasia, and monoplegia.

Muscle Imbalances and Pes Cavus

Etiology of pes cavus that may respond to physical therapy intervention include muscle imbalances and weakness of the intrinsic or extrinsic muscle groups of the foot and ankle. Several different muscle groups implicated in the mechanism producing pes cavus are:

1. Weakness of the dorsiflexors of the foot and ankle (anterior tibialis and extensor digitorum muscles), resulting in dropping of the forefoot, which causes contracture of the plantar fascia and shortening of the gastrocnemius and soleus muscle groups.

2. Overactivity of the peroneus longus muscle, producing plantarflexion of the first ray and forefoot pronation. The fixed plantarflexion of the first ray must be compensated by subtalar joint supination or inversion of the calcaneus.

3. Overactivity of the abductor halluces, flexor digitorum brevis, flexor halluces brevis, and quadratus plantae has been described as a deforming factor in pes cavus.

4. Weakness of the gastrocnemius soleus muscle group, producing a dorsiflexed calcaneus; this weakness may produce a calcaneocavus deformity.

ABNORMAL FOOT FUNCTION

For the purposes of this chapter, the etiology of abnormal function of the foot and ankle is the breakdown of the mechanisms designed to distribute and dissipate the normal forces of weightbearing. As previously discussed, closed chain pronation and supination are dynamic triplanar movements. In conjunction with ligament support and the assistance of muscle actions, triplane movements are essential for proper attenuation of compressive and rotatory forces during the stance phase of gait. For example, Mann[29] describes that a 150-pound (lbs) individual walking at a stride length of 2.5 feet, for 1 mile, would apply 127 tons of force to the feet. If that same individual ran 1 mile with the same stride length, the amount of force would increase to 220 tons. A long distance runner's feet contact the ground approximately 5000 times in a 1-hour run, with 2 to 3 times the body weight at every heel strike.

As noted earlier, these excessive forces are normally attenuated by the dynamic action of muscle, periarticular tissue strength, flexibility, and proper kinematics. For the purposes of this chapter, abnormal pronation and supination are acquired hyper- or hypomobilities, respectively, within the joints of the foot and ankle. Excessive motion or restricted motion reduces the ability of the foot to act as a shock absorber, torque convertor, mobile adaptor to the terrain, and a rigid lever at push-off. This could result in pathological conditions such as neuromas, hallux valgus, tailors bunions, keratosis, shin splints, nonspecific knee pain, plantar fasciitis, heel spurs, metatarsalgia, and Achilles tendinitis.

Acquired flexible flatfoot deformity occurs over time and can have different etiologies. However, it is most often associated with posterior tibialis tendon dysfunction. The posterior tibialis, like the peroneus longus, uses the ankle and tarsal bones as pulleys, changing direction twice. The medial malleolus is the first pulley and then the navicular bone, both acting as fulcrums. The anterior band of the posterior tibialis attaches to the navicular and medial cuneiform. The medial band inserts into the bones of the midfoot and the posterior band inserts into the calcaneus and cuboid.

The micromechanical overloading of the posterior tibialis tendon dysfunction can lead to chronic microtrauma to the posterior tibialis tendon. Microtears occur after 1500 to 2000 cycles per hour and trigger an inflammatory response. With advancing age, the tendon's elastic compliance decreases because of changes in collagen structure, thus creating a pathologic sequence where tendon weakening results in failure of the static stabilizers of the arch. Ligamentous support of the medial arch is important. If sufficient, then strength of the long and short plantar ligaments, the spring ligament (calcaneal/navicular), and the plantar fasciae good joint congruity and alignment are established. Thordarson et al[30] were able to demonstrate the relationship of medial soft tissue failure in cadaver models with sequential sectioning of the spring ligament complex and posterior-medial structures.

Two potential mechanical causes of an acquired flatfoot deformity include medial column instability and a contracture of the Achilles tendon or gastrocnemius fascia. With the former, medial column instability results in a compensatory hindfoot valgus. With the latter, a tight Achilles tendon or gastrocnemius fascia results in transmission of dorsiflexion forces from the ankle to the transverse tarsal joint and midfoot. This leads to midfoot collapse and hindfoot valgus.

Often the height of the medial arch provides the classification of whether the foot is pronated or supinated. Kitaoka et al[31] showed that the height changes of the normal arch loaded with 3 incremental physiologic loads were positively correlated with increased calcaneal eversion, a component of pronation. According to Mann and Inman,[19] pronation should occur directly after heel strike and continue until heel off. A lowered arch height in vivo has also been found to be correlated with increased calcaneal eversion between early to midstance and with internal leg rotation during locomotion, indicating that pronation is prolonged throughout the stance phase of gait. According to Root et al[11] and Donatelli[32] the most destructive forces on the foot and ankle are when the subtalar joint remains in pronation throughout the stance phase into push-off. A major etiology of overuse injuries to the foot and lower limb is prolonged pronation.

The hypermobility of the pes cavus foot can cause isolated problems such as chronic ankle sprains that result from the compensations that the forefoot and rearfoot make. Based on the experience of the authors of this chapter, the pes cavus foot is rarely seen in the clinic.

The most common pes cavus–type foot is the hypomobile first metatarsal or forefoot valgus. Hypomobility is usually described as a fixed plantarflexed first ray that is rigid. The rigid plantarflexed first metatarsal must be compensated for during the stance phase of gait. In midstance, the first metatarsal, which is in plantarflexion, strikes the ground first instead of all 5 metatarsals. Therefore, rapid supination of the subtalar joint occurs, immediately shifting the weight laterally onto the fifth metatarsal head. As a result of this compensated supination, the foot does not return to pronation during the stance phase of gait. The lack of pronation reduces the ability of the foot to absorb shock and adapt to changing terrain, causing ankle instability resulting in chronic ankle sprains. Mobilization of the first metatarsal is the most appropriate treatment if the first metatarsal is not in rigid plantarflexion. General treatment could be a combination of manual therapy and foot orthotics using a lateral wedge in the forefoot to reduce the need of the rearfoot to compensate.

TREATMENT: FOOT ORTHOTIC THERAPY

The authors of this chapter believe that foot orthotic therapy is an important aspect of rehabilitation. Treatment of the foot should be in conjunction with the assessment and treatment of the rest of the lower limb. Therefore, foot orthotic therapy should certainly be an important part of rehabilitation, which must include the foot and lower limb, in the overall treatment to improving balance and ambulation.

Foot Orthotics

The term *foot orthotics*, although possibly grammatically incorrect because orthotic is an adjective, is generally used because the original intent of the devices was to support the arches of the feet. A search in Google of the word "orthotics" generates 9,010,000 results in 0.62 seconds. Searching the word "orthosis" generates 2,200,000 results in 0.51 seconds.

The definition offered for the word orthosis is "a brace, splint, or other artificial external device serving to support the limbs or spine or to prevent or assist relative movement." Searching for the definition of "orthotic" reveals 272,000 results, among which is the following:

- Orthotic "Noun. (Also, orthosis). A device or support, especially for the foot, used to relieve or correct an orthopedic problem."
- An orthosis (or orthotic) is a type of medical device.
- The accepted use for such a medical device is: "to support, align, prevent, or correct deformities or to improve function of movable parts of the body."

For the purposes of this chapter, the definition of orthotics is medical devices that are inserted into the shoes to relieve or correct an orthopedic problem. Unfortunately, this tells us very little about what sort of devices we should use or what sort of orthopedic problems they can relieve or correct. Another confusing reality about this topic is that there are so many different types of inserts for footwear that claim to offer therapeutic benefits for innumerable medical problems. What can be stated quite confidently is that therapy with foot orthotic devices for many lower extremity problems is generally associated with patient satisfaction.

Anatomy of a Foot Orthotic Device

These devices consist of several parts:

1. An orthotic "shell" is produced by molding or machining a piece of material to match the shape and contours of the sole of the wearer's foot. To achieve the best results, one must also align the foot in a posture that is well balanced or neutral. This desirable foot posture and alignment is not as easy achieved in practice as it might seem in theory.

2. Wedges or "posts" are applied to the undersurface of the shell to apply specific forces to the foot and to compensate for deviations from a theoretically ideal alignment of lower extremity structures.

3. Additional features like top covers or shock absorbing materials can be incorporated into the design of the device as desired.

What Types of Devices Are Available?

Many products are presented as orthotics. They range from very inexpensive mass-produced insoles that are sold in shoe shops, pharmacies, and even convenience stores to very expensive rigid devices prescribed by podiatrists and other medical practitioners.

Most of these products claim to offer similar benefits such as curing and preventing overuse sports injuries, improving posture, relieving back pain, and controlling pronation.

Many of them claim that their effects are "scientifically proven" and some even refer to studies that supposedly support these claims. The majority of these claims are made in relation to some physical design feature or component material(s) that should in theory have a consistent and desired effect on the structure and function of a wearer's foot and leg.

Often, harder and more rigid materials are proposed to restrict pronation of the subtalar joint. Softer materials are proposed to reduce impact forces or shock. Technical features such as wedges, skives, and intrinsic posting technology are supposed to create superior outcomes.

Unfortunately, these claims have not been validated by independent research studies and the general consensus is that shoe inserts of various types can and do have beneficial effects in the treatment of various orthopedic conditions, but no specific product brand or type has been validated to be superior.

There are 3 main types or classes of foot orthotic devices:

1. Mass-produced insoles. These products are made by either injecting a thermoplastic material into a mold or heating and compressing a sheet of thermoplastic material in a mold. The materials used are generally EVA (ethylene-vinyl acetate) or polyurethane foams. These materials are readily available and inexpensive. In all cases, the material has been heated to a very high temperature, well in excess of 100 °C. These products might use design features and various colors to make them look technical, and they might claim some special features that enable them to control pronation. In reality, these products are insoles. Whether they are hanging on a rack in a shop or sold to therapists as medical devices makes no difference. These insoles can be modified by adding or removing some material, but they *cannot* be fully customized to suit a specific foot or problem.

2. Fully custom made (balanced) foot orthoses. These products were originally made by forming a piece of material to a plaster facsimile (cast) of the individual patient's foot to form what is called a *shell*. This shell was then modified by the addition of wedges or posts under specific areas of the foot and then shaped to fit into the patient's shoes. The theory and method of making these devices was developed in the late 1960s by podiatrists in the United States to control undesired movements of structures in the feet and legs that were presumed to be due to foot deformities. In recent times, technologies such as digital scanning and computer-controlled milling machines have been utilized in the process and new technologies like 3-dimensional printing will probably be used in the future. The materials used in these devices are generally hard, rigid plastic or carbon fiber to resist deformation from forces generated during gait. The devices are fabricated by trained technicians in a workshop called a *podiatry lab*. These products are expensive to reflect the cost of the technology, materials, and labor related to their fabrication from basic materials.

3. Partially prefabricated customizable (total contact) devices. These products were developed to combine the cost benefits of mass production with the potentially superior benefits of customization. Flexible, thermoplastic materials of various densities are cut and shaped by milling machines. The preferred material is polyethylene, which can be heated and thermoformed to a different shape at temperatures below 100 °C. These devices can be formed to provide a custom fitting shell either directly against the foot or by the pressure of the foot in the footwear that will be used. Postings or wedges are easily done by adding or removing material. An additional advantage of these products is that they enable the therapist to customize the device to suit the patient's needs in the office. The heating and remolding process can also be repeated if required.

Several research studies have indicated that these prefabricated devices are equally as effective as fully custom-made devices.

History of Foot Orthoses

In-Shoe Padding

It has been said that King Tut (1332–1333)[33] had a clubfoot deformity and wore padded sandals and that people had been known to put woollen padding in their shoes to improve comfort, but there is little recorded reference to the use of insoles before the time of the industrial revolution.

Industrial Revolution

Felt Insoles

In the mid to late 1800s, innkeepers are said to have provided insoles made from felt to relieve the weary, painful feet of their travelling guests. The earliest types of medical foot orthotics were custom contoured 18- to 20-gauge metal plates with medial and lateral flanges to stabilize the rearfoot. These were made popular around 1905 by an orthopedic surgeon named Dr. Royal Whitman. Their intended purpose was to stabilize and support weakened or fallen arches, and they were reported to have been very successful in 80% to 90% of patients.[34]

Balanced Foot Orthoses

In the 1960s, Chiropodist Merton Root and colleagues adapted the relatively new science of biomechanics to the understanding of the patient's foot problems.[11,35] Until that time, these problems had been ascribed to weakness of the structures that maintained the integrity of the medial longitudinal arches and were diagnosed as flat feet, weak feet, or fallen arches. Root and colleagues described a method of making a negative plaster case of the shape of the plantar surface of the foot with the foot placed in a specified posture (ie, the subtalar neutral position). A positive plaster of Paris facsimile of the foot was then formed within this negative cast and further modified according to a prescription based on measurements from the patient's feet. Additional "infill material" was usually applied to the medical longitudinal arch portion of the positive cast, and then a sheet of hard thermoplastic material was shaped to form the orthotic shell, and this was then adjusted with wedges under portions of the heel and forefoot. The theory was that the effectiveness of the device resulted from the effect of the wedges on the posture and movements of the forefoot rather than pressure against the arch as had been the case in the earlier, but similar, Whitman devices.

The "Running Revolution"

In the 1970s, people became very interested in running as a fitness and leisure activity. Jogging became very popular as a way of achieving and maintaining physical fitness and encouraged long distance running competitions, often to run a marathon. Running-related or overuse injuries did not respond well to medications and local physical therapy, and most patients were told to stop running as a therapy.

Patients objected to stopping their activity and sought assistance from other therapists including orthotists, chiropodists, and podiatrists who provided customized insoles that frequently solved running injury problems. Suddenly, people began to realize that foot orthotics could be used to treat many other lower limb problems and this created a very great interest in how the human foot functioned and how its function could affect other structures in the body. The science of biomechanics, the application of physical laws to the function of moveable parts of the human body, was also developing at this time, and scientists began to use new technologies like cinematography to study human movement. This gave rise to what we now know as sports science and sports medicine as well as an entire new industry related to sports equipment and therapy. Root and his colleagues[11,35] started to apply the principles of biomechanics to understanding how the foot functioned and how the function of the foot could be modified by customized shoe inserts in the treatment of lower extremity injuries.

Clinical Biomechanics

Root and colleagues developed a new and very detailed biomechanical theory (some of which has been described in the first section of this chapter), model, and method of examination and then therapy, which were published in 2 books. *Biomechanical Evaluation of the Foot*,[35] published in 1971, described the practical method of assessment and normal and abnormal function of the foot. A sequence of examination and measurements of the alignment of forefoot and rearfoot segments of the foot was proposed. Deviations from this ideal alignment were classified as structural deformities and given diagnostic labels that are quite specific to podiatry. It was theorized that the human foot and leg adapted or compensated for these structural deformities by excessive pronation of the subtalar joint and that precise devices could be prescribed to correct this compensation and overcome the foot deformities.

There are numerous alternatives that have been proposed, which are beyond the scope of this chapter, to Root and colleagues' theories.

What Does the Literature Tell Us?

There are large volumes of case studies, clinical trials, theoretical hypotheses, and reviews of the literature regarding foot orthotics, but in general, these are mainly of poor quality and provide little reliable evidence.

Most of the studies tend to be based on the belief that the effects of the devices on structure and function are mechanical, but some more recent research has indicated that in-shoe devices also have effects on postural stability and the electrical activity in various muscles.

Cochrane Collaboration

If one wishes to know how much opinion is validated by scientific research, the place to look is in the findings of the Cochrane Collaboration. If you search for foot orthoses or orthotics, you will find reviews of the literature in reference to the use of such devices in treating several types of problems, but overall there is very little "gold standard" validation.

Overall, the literature provides reassurance that foot orthotic devices of various types do provide beneficial outcomes for many patients and in relation to many common musculoskeletal problems. However, there is very little validation of the superiority of any particular class or brand of devices or for any one commonly believed theory of how the beneficial effects of these devices are achieved. There are many studies using sophisticated gait analysis technologies that validate the association between in-shoe devices and changes in lower extremity biomechanics, so it can be confidently believed that foot orthoses of various types do in fact alter the mechanics of gait even though the specific effects vary significantly between participants.

Sackett et al[36] reported that clinical evidence is also valid, and evidence-based medicine "is about integrating individual clinical expertise and the best external evidence." The majority of therapists and patients who have experience with foot orthoses do find these devices beneficial. It would seem that we can rely on the following statements:

- Foot orthoses/orthotics are frequently effective in relieving the symptoms of various musculoskeletal problems.
- They do alter the mechanics of gait, but these alterations are not consistent and vary significantly from person to person.
- The precise mechanism of action of this form of therapy is not known, and several conflicting and plausible theories have been proposed.
- Various types of devices have been shown to be effective, and no specific type is proven to be more effective than others.
- In particular, there is no validation for the opinion that expensive custom devices are more effective than less expensive, prefabricated ones.
- Foot orthoses are a noninvasive form of therapy that can be discontinued by the patient if desired.
- Foot orthotic therapy is safe, but there can be side effects such as foot, knee, and hip pain if the orthotic overcorrects the problem, which could cause aggravation of symptoms and postural instability.
- Foot orthoses are a relatively inexpensive form of therapy.

How Do Foot Orthoses Achieve Their Effects?

This is a subject that can stimulate very lively and heated debate because there are many plausible and popular theories. When people hold strong and divergent opinions about something, this tends to indicate a general lack of scientific knowledge in the field.

Biomechanics

Perhaps the most popular opinion is that foot orthoses relieve symptoms by altering the mechanical function of the foot and leg. This has been validated by gait analysis. We all know that we can reduce injury symptoms by altering the mechanics of gait. If foot orthoses are effective due to random change in the magnitude and orientation of forces within the body is likely to be effective. It is possible that, if the orthotics are comfortable, any randomly constructed devices that we put into a patient's shoes are likely to relieve symptoms.

Root Theory

Root and colleagues[11,35] proposed that their foot orthotic devices corrected the consequences of structural deformities in the patient's feet and legs. These deformities were assessed by taking measurements from segments of the foot and leg. Several studies have tried to validate these theories but have failed to do so.

One of the main problems with Root's biomechanical theories is that what he called the "ideal" or "normal" foot and leg does not exist. We defined normal earlier in the chapter as including no pain, normal muscle balance, central heel, and straight and mobile toes. In addition, adequate distributions of weight-bearing forces and a healthy nervous system should be included.

Johanson et al[37] was able to calculate through computerized gait analysis the amount of subtalar pronation movement while walking on a treadmill. The amount of pronation was determined by the calcaneal angles throughout the stance phase of gait. None of the participants had pain; however, they were determined to all have excessive calcaneal eversion angles, which caused a collapse of the medial arch height. An in-house prefabricated customizable foot orthotic was used. The study demonstrated that subtalar pronation could be controlled by using Root's concepts of heel and forefoot varus (medial) wedges applied to the bottom of the orthotics. The greatest control was when a combination of forefoot and rearfoot varus wedges were used. However, just the running shoe alone was able to control pronation to a minimal degree. As noted previously, how much control of pronation is needed to reduce pain in overuse injuries has not been conclusively determined.

Tissue Stress Model

The Tissue Stress Model is not a novel idea. It is based on the same ideas that are in current use in treatment of parts of the body other than the foot and lower extremity. The Tissue Stress Model does not rely on "unreliable measurement techniques." It is an accepted fact of physics that the application of forces to any material induces stress within the material and that excessively large or recurring forces cause structural damage to the material they act upon. Recurring forces acting on the soft tissues, bones, and joints of the lower extremities frequently cause sport-related overuse injuries, and foot orthoses have consistently been reported to be successful in the treatment of such problems.

Examination of the site of pain in overuse injuries generally reveals localized tenderness and possible swelling/inflammation or degeneration in an isolated portion of a structure, and this suggests that recurring forces acting on these sites have overstressed the tissues.

Inserting a device into the footwear alters the surface under the foot and thereby changes the distribution of forces throughout the lower extremities. If this redistribution of forces reduces the stress in the injured part of the structure, then symptoms should be relieved and the overuse injury should consequently heal and recover. The reduction of tissue stress does not have to be associated with an observable change in motion of segments of the foot or leg and does not indicate whether there has been an improvement or impairment of overall functional efficiency.

SUBTALAR JOINT AXIS LOCATION AND ROTATIONAL EQUILIBRIUM

Theory of Foot Function

Kirby,[38] a well-respected US podiatrist, proposed his theory in 2001. The central premise of this theory that relates to this chapter is that alterations in the subtalar joint axis can change the mechanical effect that both external forces (eg, ground reaction force) and internal forces (eg, ligamentous tensile forces, muscular tensile forces, joint compression forces) have on the structural components of the foot and lower extremity.

It is vitally important to point out that the simplification of the foot into this one model of foot function does not explain all of the complex interactions between the external and internal forces that act on the multiple joint axes of rotation that exist within the human foot and lower extremity.

Preferred Path of Motion

Nigg[39] proposed that each person has a somewhat unique sequence of ambulatory movements and that the various segments of the lower extremities had a preferred path of motion that contributed to efficient gait. It was determined that impact forces may not be important factors in the development of chronic and/or acute running-related injuries. This theory is a possible explanation for the findings that specific shoe modifications have varying effects on the biomechanics of gait in different participants. Nigg's theory concludes that impact forces are input signals that produce muscle tuning shortly before the next contact with the ground to minimize soft tissue vibration and/or reduce joint and tendon loading. However, more recent research tells us that shoe inserts can have an effect on increased motor unit activity.

OPTIMIZATION OF LOWER EXTREMITY FUNCTION

Function of the Lower Extremities

Because human bipedal gait must be efficient, then our anatomy must be compatible with and enable this, and the common variations that we see in the structure of human feet and legs cannot be pathological. There are congenital abnormalities, like club foot, and pathologies caused by trauma, disease, and degeneration. However, we should accept the fact that the majority of human beings have structurally normal feet and legs.

Efficient locomotion requires that the sequence of movements involved proceeds with minimal energy expenditure or stress within the system. There is evidence from gait analysis and some physiological studies that many people do have relatively inefficient gait and that the mechanical and metabolic efficiency can be improved with customized in-shoe devices. If we accept that this relative inefficiency is not due to the structures of the lower extremities, then it can only be due to the external environment. Here we have an observation that is frequently overlooked. Our human anatomy evolved to provide efficient locomotion in a primitive environment, *but* this environment does not exist as it did before. Our modern footwear and walking surfaces are exceptionally different than the natural ones of the past. The cause of lower extremity dysfunction must therefore be a consequence of our modern environment, and the results of therapy with foot orthotics are due to changing the environment in which our feet and legs are functioning.

Neuromuscular Influence on Function of the Lower Extremities

The process of achieving efficient bipedal gait is extremely complicated and poorly understood. Standing on 2 legs alone is an achievement that involves overcoming the inherent instability of supporting a large object on a small narrow base. Even a basic description of the complexity of walking would take up more than a chapter of this book.

Inman[5] describes reciprocal gait as a series of rotations that start from the fourth thoracic vertebra to the pelvis, femur, tibia, and then subtalar joint, which converts the rotations into 3 body plane movements, as described earlier. The most important structures are actually the muscles that control the dynamic posture and movement of the joints and the nervous system that orchestrates the sequencing and synchronization of the activity of the muscles. There is a structural framework of bones, and there are hinges or joints to enable movement and their function can be studied biomechanically; however, the achievement of this function is neuromuscular, not mechanical.

The nervous system contains millions of sensory nerve endings that monitor the state of all of the structures on the body. These neuroreceptors are constantly receiving information (stimuli) from the internal and external environment of the body and generating afferent signals to the CNS. There are estimated to be 100 billion neurons in the human brain and many more in other parts of the nervous system. These neurons are constantly receiving and processing signals from the entire body. They are processing and sharing this information via connections with other neurons and also generating efferent signals in response to the sensory input to control the function of all the structures in the body.

In essence, the human nervous system is like a computer that is far more powerful and complicated than any that we have managed to create. Unlike the static architecture of our computers, the nervous system has the attribute of plasticity and neurons can alter their function and their connections within the nervous system. This plasticity enables us to learn new skills and knowledge and store and access this information at any required moment.

The term *neuromotor* or *neuromuscular* is an adjective that means "pertaining to the relationship between the nervous system and movement." This is extremely relevant to optimizing the function of the lower extremities, which Collins et al[40] referred to in their definition of foot orthotics.

With this knowledge, we can begin to think of foot orthotics in a new, different, and better way:

1. Foot orthotics are custom-made, in-shoe medical devices that alter the environment under the foot and thereby change the forces acting on the foot.

2. These forces acting on the foot are transmitted up through the lower extremities and change the tension in the tissues that make up their structures.

3. These changes in forces and tissue tensions change the stimulation of neuroreceptors and generate new signals, which are then transmitted to the neurons in the nervous system.

4. The neurons process this information and generate new signals to the muscles.

5. The synchronization and sequencing of the activity of the muscles is controlled by these new signals, and this changes the movement of structures in the lower extremities, including those in the feet.

6. Movement is altered, and this is perceived as a biomechanical response to the forces exerted on the foot by the devices.

7. The function of the lower extremities has been changed.

8. This is a repeating and ongoing process.

Applying neuromotor principles to our understanding of foot orthotics does not conflict with the belief that they have kinetic effects. *Kinetic* is an adjective that means "pertaining to the relationship between the motion of material bodies and the associated forces and energy." The motion of the structures of the lower extremities is still related to the forces and energy applied by the devices, but this is achieved through the function of the nervous system and the efficiency of muscles function.

Kelly et al[41] demonstrated that a group of runners, while wearing Formthotics (Foot Science International; prefabricated and thermoformed to the participants' foot), had a significantly lower heart rate, and normalized electromyography (EMG) activity, which modified recruitment strategies in the vastus medialis and gluteus maximus. The study also reported increased control of knee and rearfoot kinematics. Lastly, the peroneus longus had increased activity, which promoted plantarflexion of the first ray, as described earlier, stabilizing the first metatarsal in push-off.

Clinical Note: How to Promote Cuboid—Navicular Fulcrums

The pivotal movement of the cuboid and calcaneus is accomplished by supination of the subtalar joint, which locks up the cuboid and navicular, establishing fulcrums. The navicular functions as a fulcrum for the posterior tibialis. The cuboid establishes a fulcrum for the peroneus longus. By use of an orthotic device, preferably prefabricated, customizable orthotics, it has been proven to increase the activation of the posterior tibialis and peroneus longus. The orthotic facilitates rigid fulcrums expediting plantarflexion of the first metatarsal and enhancing the windlass effect (see Figure 11-10).

In addition, Murley et al[42] demonstrated that prefabricated foot orthoses significantly altered tibialis posterior and peroneus longus EMG amplitude. However, only the modified, prefabricated orthoses that were heat-molded changed peroneus longus EMG amplitude toward a pattern observed with normal arched feet.

If we now agree that in-shoe devices can change the function of the lower extremities, we next have to be able to determine whether these changes are beneficial or detrimental to the goal of optimizing lower extremity function. As mentioned in relation to biomechanics and tissue stress, any change in the forces acting on a symptomatic site in a structure can relieve symptoms. Returning to the definition proposed by Collins et al,[40] foot orthotics (or orthoses) are in-shoe devices "shaped to match the plantar surface of the foot." This is more complicated than it might appear because we know that every person's foot is different and that the contours of the sole of the foot change as the posture of the foot changes.

In-shoe devices that have *not* been customized to conform accurately to the contours of the wearer's foot when the foot is in a posture related to optimal lower extremity function, would be more classified as insoles, whether custom made or mass produced. They might help to relieve symptoms and appear very technical or be very expensive, but unless they are specifically shaped to the contours of the individual patient's foot and, *most importantly*, can be shown to optimize the function of the patient's lower extremities, they are not foot orthoses (Box 11-5).

In order to provide this therapy, one would have to:

1. Understand lower extremity function

2. Understand the foot and ankle function

3. Be able to assess foot and lower extremity function

4. Recognize subjective and objective signs of lower extremity dysfunction

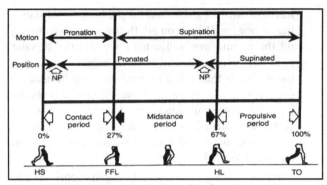

Figure 11-15. Pronation and supination of the foot during gait.

5. Appreciate the underlying cause of this dysfunction
6. Provide therapy to improve lower extremity function
7. Be able to assess the effectiveness of this therapy
8. Revise the therapy until lower extremity function has been optimized

LOWER EXTREMITY FUNCTION

Efficient gait should conserve energy and minimize potentially harmful stress in the lower extremities. Gait can be understood and analyzed in relation to what is called the *gait cycle*.

One cycle of gait consists of the events that occur from the time when one foot makes contact with the ground until it makes a second contact with the ground.

There are 2 phases of gait: Swing Phase (40%) when the foot is off the ground and Stance Phase (60%) when the foot is in contact with the ground. The events of the Stance Phase of gait are depicted in Figure 11-15.

There are 3 significant events, or periods, in the Stance Phase:

1. Contact Period is from heel contact until the foot is in full contact with the supporting surface.
2. Midstance Period is when the body is supported on one leg.
3. Propulsive Period is from heel lift to toe-off (see Figure 11-15)

The structures of the lower extremity should efficiently achieve 3 main objectives during the Stance Phase:

1. Make contact with the supporting surface, attenuate impact forces, and adapt to the physical characteristics of the contact surface to establish a base for one-legged stance.
2. Maintain a dynamically stable base of one-legged stance while the contralateral leg is swinging forward.
3. Enable energy generated by the muscles and the release of elastic energy from tendons and ligaments to be efficiently transmitted through dynamically stable forefoot structures.

FUNCTIONAL ASSESSMENT

Gait can be objectively assessed in a laboratory setting but this requires highly technical and expensive equipment and is very time consuming and costly. The facilities for doing this analysis are mainly in academic institutions and are for the use of academic researchers. They are not available or appropriate for clinical medicine. Lower budget systems are available, but they are not accurate diagnostic and assessment tools because they only allow for 2-dimensional analysis of motion. Force plates and pressure mapping systems can provide some objective information but are also very technical, expensive, and time consuming. Clinical assessment of function is still the most cost-effective and desirable option.

Visual gait analysis is admittedly very subjective and has poor interrater reliability, but with experience and practice, therapists can make very good use of this method. The patient can be observed while walking and even running from the front, rear, and sides. This analysis can be repeated to assess the effects of therapy.

There are 3 quite useful assessments related to the events of Stance Phase that can provide very useful information.

1. The relaxed standing posture of the feet. This indicates how the patient's foot has adapted itself to the supporting surface. In most cases, the subtalar joint will have assumed a pronated posture in order to try to flatten the foot to adapt to extrinsic factors and a collapse of the medial arch secondary to lack of ligament support. The physiological range of subtalar motion varies due to anatomical restraints and neuromotor function and whether the lower extremity muscles are reacting to reduce the stress in noncontractile tissues. There is a very large variation in the available range of motion (ROM) of normal joints from person to person. Some people have very cavus (high arched) feet with a limited ROM, and others have very flexible feet with a greater ROM. Arch height in itself is not a very relevant indicator of lower extremity function because there is a very great structural variation among normal people.
2. Postural stability/balance test. Having established stable contact with the supporting surface the lower extremity

has to maintain a stable base for the body while standing on one leg. When you ask the person to lift one leg off the ground, you will usually see that the subtalar joint tries to supinate and the arch height increases. If the patient is then asked to maintain their balance on one leg while closing the eyes, you will generally see the patient unable to maintain their balance secondary to vestibular system devices. Further discussion of the influences of the vestibular, somatosensory, and vision on balance is located in Chapter 21.

3. Forefoot stability/heel raise test. As gait progresses and the body's center of mass moves forward over the supporting foot, the tension in the posterior structures of the leg causes the heel to lift off of the ground. This is an important transition during which the function of the weightbearing lower extremity is transitioning from a dynamically stable base to a propulsive system. During this transition, there should be external rotation of the leg and supination of the subtalar joint. The efficiency of this transition can be assessed by having the patient stand on one leg (with the eyes open and then rise onto the toes). The Achilles tendon and gastrocnemius and soleus muscle are responsible for being able to lift the heel off the ground. The manual muscle test (MMT) for normal strength of these muscles is 10 repetitions without falling over.

SIGNS OF
LOWER EXTREMITY DYSFUNCTION

These are related to the assessments that one chooses to use.

Discomfort or pain is an indication of dysfunction. We mainly tend to think of pain as an indication of pathology, injury, or some structural damage or abnormality, but it can also be regarded as an indication of dysfunction, and hence, there is often pain without clinical or laboratory indications of structural pathology. When there is structural pathology, there will always be associated dysfunction, but there can be pain/discomfort with no evidence of a pathological cause. This commonly occurs in patients who develop chronic pain. Therapists search for structural pathology and recurring forces acting on the soft tissues, bones, and joints of the lower extremities, which frequently causes sports-related overuse injuries. However, sometimes chronic pain persists in spite of therapy directed to this structural and soft tissue diagnosis. Conversely, the relief of pain often indicates that function has been improved, and this is especially so if the patient perceives an awareness of "comfort."

Signs of dysfunction in relation to the 3 assessments described earlier are:

1. Persisting end of range subtalar pronation in relaxed stance
2. Impaired postural stability in one-legged stance
3. Difficulty in transitioning to forefoot stance

Other clinical tests will provide other indications of dysfunction such as:

- Being unable to run
- Impaired walking due to fatigue after a short distance
- Difficulty in getting out of a chair or out of the bath
- Falling or cautious walking related to a fear of falling
- A feeling of poorly coordinated gait
- Difficulty climbing stairs
- Inability to center the knee over the foot when doing a partial squat
- Loss of balance when changing direction
- Impaired ability to hop on one leg
- Instability when standing with the feet close together and eyes closed
- Widened base of gait when walking
- Reduction of vertical jumping height
- Increased instability in response to perturbations
- Persistent limping after injury symptoms have resolved

It is beyond the scope of this chapter to review the possible etiologies associated with the underlying causes of dysfunctional gait. Chapter 21 reviews and discusses several of the causes of the clinical tests noted above.

THERAPY TO IMPROVE
LOWER EXTREMITY FUNCTION

It is very important to realize that the most effective therapeutic approach for lower extremity problems is usually multimodal. In addition to the provision of customized in-shoe devices, there are often relevant joint restrictions, muscles imbalances, training errors, and other factors that require assessment and therapy. Of course, one must always be aware of the possibility of underlying neurological conditions that might be present, and this must always be considered as likely if and when a patient does not respond as expected to appropriate foot orthotic and physical therapy. Referral to an appropriate medical specialist should always be considered when more serious disorders are suspected.

ASSESSING THE EFFECTIVENESS OF THE ORTHOTIC THERAPY

This is achieved by repeating the functional assessments that were used to investigate the problem. In relation to the foot orthotic therapy, one would expect that there will be an improvement in static foot posture, postural stability, and forefoot stability as well as the other assessments that had been done.

Bonifácio et al demonstrated that foot orthoses change the joint mechanics in the foot, increasing lower limb stability and less work done by abductor hallucis and tibialis anterior muscles. These data support the use of foot orthoses to provide functional benefits during step descent, which may benefit patients with patellofemoral pain (PFP).

The patient should confirm that they can also perceive these improvements in function. Comfort is a very good indicator of function and in-shoe devices that optimize function should be perceived by the patient to feel comfortable. It was once thought that these devices were "controlling and correcting" pathology and that they were expected to feel uncomfortable and require a prolonged period of adaptation. What happened more often than not was that the patient could not tolerate wearing these overly aggressive and painful inserts and stopped using them after a very short time. Hopefully, therapists are now more aware that pain is an indication that something is wrong and that applies to therapy that hurts patients as well as the disorders that the therapists are supposed to be treating.

REVISION OF THERAPY

1. Functional therapy is a process rather than a prescription.
2. Each patient and their problem are somewhat different and unique and will respond in their own way to the modalities of therapy that are applied.
3. The therapy needs to be centered on the patient and finding the best and most appropriate and acceptable way to help them solve the problem.
4. The therapist must be prepared to listen carefully to understand how the patient perceives the problem and its effects on the patient's quality of life. There must be a clear understanding of what is being done and why and what outcome is expected by the therapist and the patient.
5. It is very important to show empathy, understanding, trust, and confidence, and avoid the use of terms and labels that imply that the problem cannot be solved as this increases the possibility of chronicity.
6. The choice of initial therapies is very important because those that provide prompt improvement in symptoms increase the patient's confidence in the therapist's ability

to understand and provide a solution for the problem. Modalities such as rest, analgesics, and exercises that do not have any immediate effects on maintaining and improving function are discouraging.

7. One of the most significant benefits of foot orthotic therapy is that there is usually a very immediate and significant improvement in symptoms and functional capacity. For this reason, it should be considered as part of the initial treatment instead of being held in reserve for use when other modalities have failed.
8. Appropriate foot orthotic therapy that optimizes lower extremity function is compatible with and should be routinely used in conjunction with other therapeutic modalities. This usually results in the efficient achievement of a desired patient outcome and that should always be the therapist's goal.
9. Perhaps the greatest problem related to foot orthotic therapy has been that it has been regarded as difficult and somewhat incompatible with other modalities. This has given therapists the impression that foot orthoses are expensive, uncomfortable, and restrictive devices that should only be used for patients with obvious structural defects or deformities in their feet. This has tended to overshadow the beneficial effects that this therapy has on lower extremity function and limit their potential for helping patients. Hopefully, this will change in the future.

ASSESSMENT OF THE FOOT AND ANKLE

The Seven Tests for the Foot and Ankle

The assessment of the foot and ankle should include testing for balance, mobility, ligamentous stability, and muscle strength. For the purposes of this chapter, we would like to introduce 7 tests for the foot and ankle. These tests will help determine the treatment approach, which includes manual therapy, eccentric loading, infrared light energy, balance training, and fabrication of foot orthotics.

Test 1: Closed-chain dorsiflexion—Open-chain dorsiflexion. The foot is fixed on the board, and the patient attempts to touch the knee on to the wall. A goniometer is used to measure the dorsiflexion of the ankle. Open chain dorsiflexion and plantarflexion passive and active (Figure 11-16).

Treatment: Limited dorsiflexion or plantarflexion of the ankle is successfully improved by mobilization, which is demonstrated in the chapter on mobilization.

Test 2: Windlass effect—Passive dorsiflexion of the MTP joint. The left demonstrates no increase in height of the medial arch, which could mean there is a torn or damaged plantar fascia (Figure 11-17).

Treatment: An overstretched or torn plantar fascia is best treated with foot orthotics.

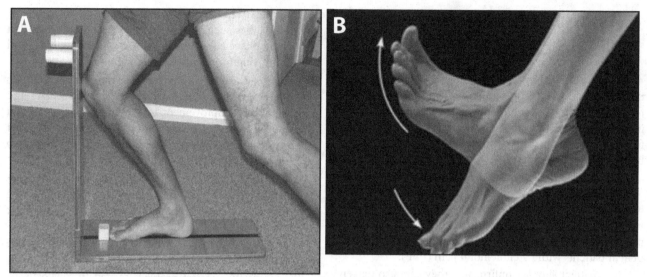

Figure 11-16. (A) Closed-chain dorsiflexion. (B) Open-chain dorsiflexion and plantarflexion.

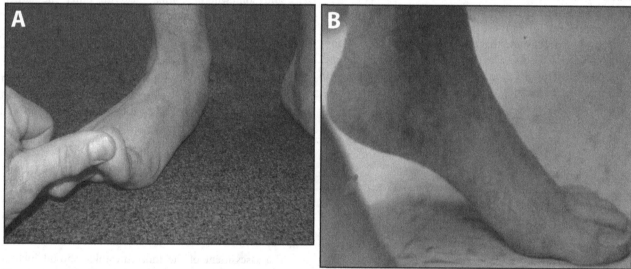

Figure 11-17. (A) Left is an abnormal windlass effect by MTP dorsiflexion. (B) Right is closed-chain dorsiflexion (heel lift) with the medial arch visible.

Test 3: Assessment of the subtalar joint mobility. Moving the calcaneus into inversion (left) and eversion (right). Static stance observe position of calcaneus—excessive calcaneal valgus, bilaterally.

Treatment: Approach for excessive calcaneal valgus is rearfoot medial (varus) post (Figure 11-18).

Test 4: Abduction and adduction of the forefoot—20 degrees of adduction and 10 degrees of abduction.

Treatment: Could include mobilization of the forefoot and a medial (varus) forefoot post (wedge; Figure 11-19).

Test 5: Inversion (supination twist)/eversion (pronated twist) of the forefoot.

Treatment: Using a customizable foot orthotic adding forefoot medial (varus) post (wedge; Figure 11-20).

Test 6: Supination resistance test—This test is designed to measure the amount of resistance into supination of the subtalar joint by pulling up on the medial arch. Scored 5 to 1, from 5 = maximum resistance to 1 = minimal resistance (Figure 11-21).

Treatment: Approach foot orthotic that is customizable and molds to the patients' foot. A rigid medial arch will cause pain and discomfort.

Test 7: Balance test single leg stance on hard surface eyes open, then eyes closed. The test is repeated while standing on foam, eyes open then eyes closed. The last part of this test is up on toes for balance and then to test the strength of the calf muscles.

Assessment and treatment of poor balance is reviewed in Chapter 21.

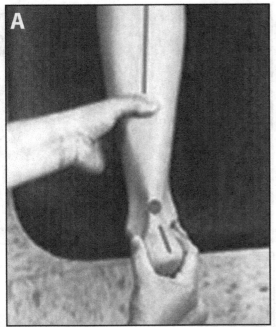

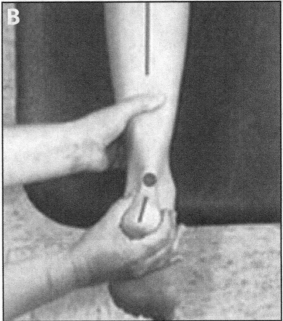

Figure 11-18. (A) Inversion. (B) Eversion. (C) Weight-bearing calcaneal valgus.

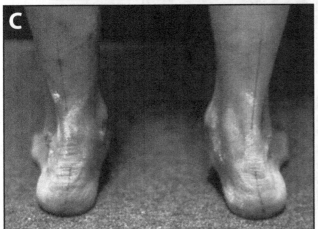

Figure 11-19. Forefoot adduction, neutral, and abduction.

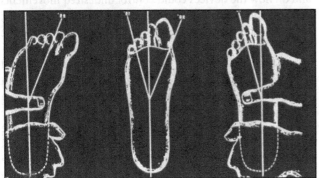

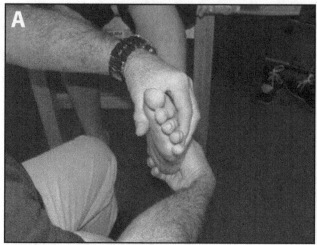 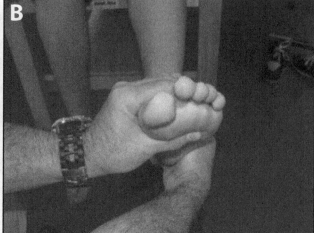

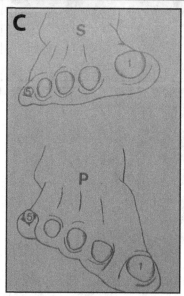

Figure 11-20. (A) Excessive supination twist or inversion of the foot. The right hand is stabilizing the heel to isolate the forefoot movement. (B) Photo demonstrates limited pronation twist/eversion of the forefoot. (C) Normal supination/pronation twist.

CONCLUSION

Foot orthotic inserts of various types have been used as medical therapy for about 150 years. They were initially used to provide comfort, but in the early 20th century, they were adopted by medical therapists and used for the treatment of foot pathologies related to the observation of flattening of the medial longitudinal arches of the feet. In the mid-20th century, this therapy was found to be effective in the treatment of many different lower extremity problems and several theories based on biomechanics were developed to explain how the devices worked. There was a great emphasis on identifying structural deviations from a theoretically ideal model and on how the devices could control undesired movements of structures related to these defects. In the current century, new paradigms have developed, which relate the therapeutic effects of foot orthotic therapy to the neuromotor mechanisms that determine the function of the musculoskeletal system. This enables us to shift our attention from the ability of the devices to control motion toward using them as a therapy to optimize function. As our understanding of the nervous system and the effects of the environment upon the function of the body increases, we may learn to understand this form of therapy better and become able to utilize it more effectively in the treatment of musculoskeletal disorders by optimizing the function of the lower extremities and the efficiency of bipedal gait.

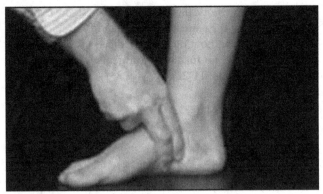

Figure 11-21. Supination resistance test.

CASE STUDIES

Case Study One: Knee Pain

Mr. Jones, an enthusiastic runner, arrived at the clinic late one Friday afternoon asking if someone might have a look at his sore knee.

History

The history was of generalized aching around the front of the left knee worse in the morning, when running, or when standing up after sitting for a while. Mr. Jones was an avid runner who trained 60 to 80 miles per week and completed 3 or 4 marathons each year. His training had been reduced to around 20 miles per week over the past 8 weeks since his knee became sore, and he had not been running for the past 5 days.

The past history was not remarkable. Mr. Jones said he was always in good health and had only suffered from occasional "aches and pains" related to his sport. He said that he had tried changing his shoes a couple of times and had been treated for 3 weeks by a physical therapist with ice, ultrasound, exercise, and some tape on his knee. He said the physical therapist had advised that he stop running until the knee felt better, but he had ignored this advice.

Examination

Examination revealed slight tenderness along the medial border of the left patella and some retropatellar crepitus.

Seven test assessment of lower extremity function—The following tests were positive:

- Test 2. Jack's test—Windlass mechanism. Jack's test assesses the force required to activate the windlass mechanism. The arch must rise to shorten the distance between the origin and insertion of the plantar fascia. Excessive resistance to dorsiflexion of the toes impedes the forward progression of gait and impairs the efficiency of

walking and running. Resupination of the subtalar joint and dorsiflexion of the toes are interrelated. In this case, the resistance to Jack's test was increased in the left foot. Once again indicating an overpronator. A medial forefoot wedge (varus post) is indicated to control pronation.

- Test 3. Inversion/eversion of the calcaneus (subtalar joint). Inversion was 20 degrees and eversion was 10 degrees. Static stand indicated excessive eversion/valgus position of the calcaneus. This test indicates an excessive pronated subtalar joint and the use of a rearfoot medial wedge (rearfoot varus post).

- Test 5. Supination/pronation twist demonstrated excessive inversion of the forefoot and limited eversion of the forefoot. The senior author of this chapter has observed that when there is excessive inversion with limited eversion, a forefoot medial wedge is important to increase the stability of the forefoot.

- Test 6. Supination resistance. Left = 4, right = 3, which indicated that the muscles of the left leg had to overcome more resistance to supinate the foot for efficient gait. During walking, there was prolonged pronation of both feet during the stance phase. Resupination of the left subtalar joint occurred at toe-off, which was substantially delayed. This test is positive for an overpronator.

- Test 7. The single leg stance eyes open is a quick balance test. The patient should be able to stand on one leg with hands on hips for 20 seconds without any movements that might compensate for loss of balance. This patient's balance was better on the right leg than the left. A quick test for forefoot stability is a single leg stance up on the forefoot. Once again, the patient should be able to stand up on his forefoot for 20 seconds. In this patient, forefoot stability was not normal bilaterally, indicating forefoot instability as demonstrated in test 5.

A provisional diagnosis of PFP syndrome was made.

All of the testing indicated excessive prolonged pronation throughout the stance phase of gait.

Mr. Jones was fitted with a pair of firm density Formthotics by heating them in the shoes and custom forming them to the feet (with the patient standing in a neutral position with the center of the patella in line with the second toe).

A forefoot varus post was added to the forefoot. The length of the post was from the toe break to the end of the metatarsal head; a rearfoot varus post was added to the heel. The posts were 3 to 4 mm in height.

He was advised to leave the orthotics in the rest of the day and to wear them as much as possible over the next 2 to 3 days to allow the orthotics to mold to his feet. He could also try some short runs over the weekend and to return for a full examination and further treatment the next week.

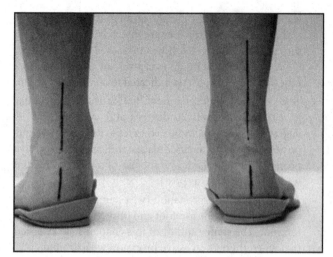

Figure 11-22. Rearfoot varus posts (wedges).

Mr. Jones returned to the clinic 5 years later. When asked why he had not come back as requested, he replied that there was no need because the pain had completely resolved over the first weekend of wearing the Formthotics and had not recurred. He said that the orthoses were now severely worn out and he would like some new ones. He said that he had been training and competing without problems and had also improved his marathon and 10K times. He had worn the Formthotics at all times, changing them from one pair of shoes to another. Figure 11-22 shows the orthotics while standing on them.

Comment: PFP is a common problem that responds well to treatment with foot orthoses. Simple flexible devices, like Formthotics (custom fitted by thermoforming and posting if required), reduce stress in the affected area and can improve lower extremity function without altering kinematics. Treating this condition without foot orthoses (eg, exercises, taping) can be a slow and frustrating process for the therapist and the patient. If inadequately treated, this condition can resolve over time but may also go on to cause chondromalacia patella, degeneration, and softening of the retropatellar cartilage.

In this case, the examination suggested that the orthotics should have been modified by the addition of wedges to make them more "theoretically" correct. A wedge or post applied under the heel on the medial side (rearfoot varus post) could have been used bilaterally to reduce the rearfoot eversion, reducing the supination resistance and also improving the balance.

However, the more recent literature about foot orthoses supports the opinion that total contact devices (of soft but resilient materials custom formed to the precise shape of the patient's foot in a neutral posture) are as effective as balanced orthotics, prescribed with wedges that are *assumed* to control motion of parts of the foot. There is also excellent evidence that custom thermoformed Formthotics are as effective as hard plastic prescribed devices with posts made in

a lab. Whatever orthotic theories might suggest, the reality in this case was that the patient had a rapid and extremely satisfactory outcome without further modifications of the orthoses, and therefore, no further adjustments were considered necessary (see Figure 11-22).

Case Study Two: Achilles Tendon Repair

Initial Evaluation and Findings

A 30-year-old professional basketball player ruptured his left Achilles tendon while playing basketball 8 weeks ago. The patient experienced some pain and episodes of Achilles tendonitis 1 year before the rupture. He continued to play through the pain attributing it to overuse and playing continuously for weeks at a time. This was at the end of the basketball season, and he wanted to finish it without indicating he had an injury. While running he heard a loud pop on the back of his heel. The intensity of the pain decreased but he was unable to walk without assistance. He underwent surgery to repair a type II rupture and end-to-end anastomosis 10 days following the injury.

Surgical Technique

1. An 8- to 12-cm posteromedial incision is made centered over the tear. Full-thickness skin flaps including the paratenon are then retracted to expose the tendon rupture (Figure 11-23).
2. The proximal tendon segment is then mobilized using a nonpenetrating clamp or grasping suture, and axial tension is applied to the tendon. The fascia of the posterior compartment is then incised anterior to the tendon rupture. The tendon is then repaired using a strong, nonabsorbable-braided suture.
3. The sutures enter the tendon anteriorly so that the knots sit along the anterior surface of the tendon and do not irritate the posterior closure. It is important to note that the entry point of the sutures partially determines the ultimate tension of the repair.
4. The final tension should mirror the resting position of contralateral side. With the knee bent, the ankle should rest in 10 to 15 degrees of equinus.
5. The core sutures are then tied together to complete the repair.

Following the surgery, the patient was put into a cast above the knee for 2 weeks and then below the knee for 2 weeks.

The rehabilitation goal is to return the patient to professional basketball within 6 months, with no restrictions.

At 4 weeks' postoperative, the initial evaluation demonstrated that passive dorsiflexion and plantarflexion were limited by 10 degrees into dorsiflexion and 20 degrees into plantarflexion.

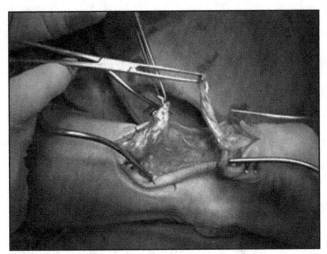

Figure 11-23. Torn Achilles.

Week One to Two—Postoperative Four to Five Weeks

Severe atrophy was noted within the left gastrocnemius/soleus muscles. The quadriceps and hamstring muscles also demonstrated weakness. MMT was performed on the left hip and weakness was detected within the posterior fibers of gluteus medius, gluteus maximus, and external rotators. MMT grade was -3 on all the previously mentioned muscle groups.

Treatment: Mobilize the scar, increase the ankle joint passive and active ROM. The initial treatment consisted of mobilization of the scar area using multiradiant LASER probe. The patient started using the stationary bike for active assistive ROM of the ankle.

Mobilization of the ankle: long axis mobilization and anterior-posterior glides of the tibia/fibula on the talus (see chapter on mobilization).

Start leg press with 50 pounds (lbs).

Start 2 way hip exercises using 10 lbs on a pulley. Hip extension and diagonal movement at 45 degrees of abduction.

Bilateral leg press to tolerance and progress to single leg press (Figure 11-24).

Week Three to Four—Seven to Eight Weeks Postoperative

Treatment: Continue the earlier treatment and initiate eccentric loading of the Achilles tendon by toe raises on a leg press with 25 lbs of force. Toe raises should be performed bilaterally with eccentric loading over the edge of a step as well as gentle hopping on a trampoline for several minutes.

Start balance activities.

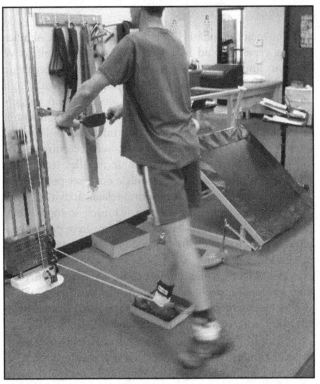

Figure 11-24. Two-way hip exercises on a box are used to help clear the foot from the ground without compensations at the trunk.

Week Five to Six—Nine to Ten Weeks Postoperative

Goal: Initiate more aggressive eccentric loading. The Eccentron (BTE Technologies) device uses only eccentric loading to the patient's tolerance.

Light jumping on the shuttle MVP with 50 lbs of resistance.

Continue eccentric loading off the side of a step, bilateral concentric and unilateral eccentric loading to patient tolerance.

Continue balance training single leg hops to gain control of closed-chain dorsiflexion angles.

Continue soft tissue mobilization.

Week Seven to Nine—Eleven to Thirteen Weeks Postoperative

Patient should initiate basketball activities of ball handling, light jump shots, and lateral movements with dribbling. Continue all of the earlier mentioned exercises and activities progressing in resistance for strength training of the hip and quadriceps. Eccentric loading and balance activities.

Week Ten and Beyond

The major emphasis in the rehabilitation of an Achilles rupture repair should be on remolding of the connective tissue to improve mobility and tensile strength. Eccentric strengthening exercises have been proven to provide high tendon strain in comparison to low tendon strain triggering an adaptive response in the Achilles tendon. Ohberg et al[43] found decreased Achilles tendon thickness and normal tendon structure in response to a 12-week eccentric training program in patients with chronic Achilles tendinosis. Stanish et al[44] suggested that eccentric exercises prepare patients for return to functional, sports-related activities better than those that emphasize concentric muscle strengthening. Eccentric strengthening exercise programs have been advocated as effective treatments for tendon overuse injuries and prevention of re-injury. Arampatzis et al[45] demonstrated that exercises involving high tendon strain were more effective than low tendon strain in human Achilles tendon. Multiple studies have demonstrated eccentric exercise regimens to be effective for the treatment of tendinopathy.

While the mechanism of action of eccentric exercise is poorly understood, it is theorized that eccentric exercise loads the tendon to a greater magnitude compared with concentric contraction, thereby stimulating a more effective repair response. Furthermore, eccentric exercise may facilitate remodeling by increasing the number of collagen cross-linkages.

REFERENCES

1. Cailliet R. *Foot and Ankle Pathology*. FA Davis; 1968.
2. Hicks JH. The mechanics of the foot. I. The joints. *J Anat*. 1953;87(4):345-357.
3. Barnett CH, Napier JR. The axis of rotation at the ankle joint in man: its influence upon the form of the talus and the mobility of the fibula. *J Anat*. 1952;86(Pt 1):1-9.
4. Singh AK, Starkweather KD, Hollister AM, Jatana S, Lupichuk AG. Kinematics of the ankle: a hinge axis model. *Foot Ankle*. 1992;13(8):439-446. doi:10.1177/107110079201300802
5. Inman VT. *The Joints of the Ankle*. Williams & Willkins; 1976
6. Inman VT, Rolston J, Todd F. *Human Walking*. Williams & Wilkins; 1981.
7. Stormont OM, Morrey BF, An KN, Cass JR. Stability of the loaded ankle. Relation between articular restraint and primary and secondary static restraints. *Am J Sports Med*. 1985;13(5):295-300. doi:10.1177/036354658501300502
8. McCullough CJ, Burge PD. Rotatory stability of the load-bearing ankle. An experimental study. *J Bone Joint Surg Br*. 1980;62B(4):460-464. doi:10.1302/0301-620X.62B4.7430225
9. Harper MC. Deltoid ligament: an anatomical evaluation of function. *Foot Ankle*. 1987;8(1):19-22. doi:10.1177/107110078700800104
10. Frankel VH, Nordin M. *Basic Biomechanics of the Skeletal System*. Lee & Febiger; 1980.
11. Root MR, Orien WP, Weed IN. *Normal and Abnormal Function of the Foot. Clinical Biomechanics, Volume II*. Clinical Biomechanics Corporation; 1977.
12. Kelkian SA, Sarrafian SK. Sarrafian's *Anatomy of the Foot and Ankle: Descriptive, Topographic, Functional*. Lippincott Williams & Wilkins; 2011.
13. Viladot A, Lorenzo JC, Salazar J, Rodríguez A. The subtalar joint: embryology and morphology. *Foot Ankle*. 1984;5(2):54-66. doi:10.1177/107110078400500203
14. Manter JT. Movements of the subtalar joint and transverse tarsal joints. Anat Rec. 1941;80(40):397-410.
15. Elftman H. The transverse tarsal joint and its control. *Clin Orthop*. 1960;16:41.
16. Hicks JH. The mechanics of the foot. IV. The action of muscles on the foot in standing. *Acta Anat (Basel)*. 1956;27(3):180-192.
17. Perry J. Anatomy and biomechanics of the hindfoot. *Clin Orthop*. 1983;(177):9-15
18. Lapidus PW. Kinesiology and mechanical anatomy of the tarsal joints. *Clin Orthop*. 1963;30:20-26.
19. Mann RA, Inman VT. Phasic activity of intrinsic muscles of the foot. *J Bone Joint Surg*. 1964;46:469-481.
20. Huang CK, Kitaoka HB, An KN, Chao EY. Biomechanical evaluation of the longitudinal arch stability. *Foot Ankle*. 1993;14(6):353-357.
21. Cavanagh PR, Rodgers MM, Iiboshi A. Pressure distribution under symptom-free feet during barefoot standing. *Foot Ankle*. 1987;7(5):262-276.
22. Stokes IA, Hutton WC, Stott JR. Forces acting on the metatarsals during normal walking. *J Anat*. 1979;129(Pt 3):579-590.
23. Hutton WC, Dhaneddran M. The mechanics of normal and hallux valgus feet—a quantitative study. *Clin Orthop*. 1981;(157):7-13.
24. Resende RA, Pinherio LSP, Orarino JM. Effects of foot pronation on the lower limb sagittal plane biomechanics during gait. *Gait Posture*. 2019;68:130-135.
25. Stormont DM, Peterson, HA. The relative incidence of tarsal coalition. *Clin Orthop Relat Res*. 1983;(181):28-36.
26. McCrea JD. *Pediatric Orthopaedics of the Lower Extremity*. Futura Publishing; 1985.
27. Kite JH. Congenital metatarsus varus. *J Bone Joint Surg Am*. 1967;49(2):388-397.
28. Brewerton DA, Sandifer PH, Sweetnam DR. "Idiopathic" pes cavus: an investigation into its aetiology. *Br Med J*. 1963;2(5358):659-661.
29. Mann RA. Biomechanics of running. In: Mack RP, ed. *Symposium on 619,1977 the Foot and Leg in Running Sports*. CV Mosby; 1982:1-29.
30. Thordarson DB, Schmotzer H, Chon J. Reconstruction with tenodesis in an adult flatfoot model. A biomechanical evaluation of four methods. *J Bone Joint Surg*. 1995;77(10):1557-1564.
31. Kitaoka HB, Alexander IJ, Adelaar RS, Nunley JA, Myerson MS, Sanders M. Clinical rating systems for the ankle–hindfoot, midfoot, hallux, and lesser toes. *Foot Ankle Int*. 1994;15(7):349-353.
32. Donatelli R. Abnormal biomechanics of the foot and ankle. *J Orthop Sports Phys Ther*. 1987;9(1):11-16.
33. Hawaa Z, Gad YZ, Ismail S, et al. Ancestry and pathology in King Tutankhamun's family. *JAMA*. 2010;303(7);638-647.
34. Whitman R. The importance of positive support in the curative treatment of weak feet and a comparison of the means employed to assure it. *Am J Orth Surg*. 1913;11:215-230.
35. Root M, Orien W, Weed J. *Biomechanical Evaluation of the Foot, Volume I*. Clinical Biomechanics Corporation; 1971.
36. Sackett DL, Rosenberg WMC, Muir Gray JA, Brian Haynes R, Scott Richardson W. Evidence based medicine: what it is and what it isn't. *BMJ*. 1996;312:71-72.
37. Johanson M, Donatelli R, Wooden MJ, Andrew P, Cummings GS. Effects of three different posting methods in controlling abnormal subtalar pronation. *Phys Ther*. 1994;74(2):149-158.
38. Kirby KA. Subtalar joint axis location and rotational equilibrium theory of foot function. *J Am Podiatr Med Assoc*. 2001;91(9):465-487.
39. Nigg BM. The role of impact forces and foot pronation: a new paradigm. *Clin J Sport Med*. 2001;11(1):2-9.

40. Collins N, Bisset L, McPoil T. Foot orthoses in lower limb overuse conditions: a systematic review and meta-analysis. *Foot Ankle.* 2007;28(3):396-412.

41. Kelly L, Kelly A, Girard O, Racinais S. Effect of orthoses on changes in neuromuscular control and aerobic cost of a 1-h run. *Med Sci Sports Exerc.* 2011;43(12):2335-2343.

42. Murley GS, Landorf KB, Menz HB, Do foot orthoses change lower limb muscle activity in flat-arched feet towards a pattern observed in normal-arched feet? *Clin Biomech (Bristol, Avon).* 2010;25(7):728-736.

43. Ohberg L, Lorentzon R, Alfredson H. Eccentric training in patients with chronic Achilles tendinosis: normalised tendon structure and decreased thickness at follow up. *Br J Sports Med.* 2004;38(1):8-11.

44. Stanish WD, Rubinovich RM, Curwin S. Eccentric exercise in chronic tendinitis. *Clin Orthop Relat Res.* 1986;(208):65-68.

45. Arampatzis A, Peper A, Bierbaum S, Albracht K. Plasticity of human Achilles tendon mechanical and morphological properties in response to cyclic strain. *J Biomech.* 2010;43(16):3073-3079.

BIBLIOGRAPHY

Alfredson H, Pietilä T, Jonsson P, Lorentzon R. Heavy-load eccentric calf muscle training for the treatment of chronic Achilles tendinosis. *Am J Sports Med.* 1998;26(3):360-366.

Barenfield PA, Wedely MS, Shea JM. The congenital cavus foot. *Clin Orthop Relat Res.* 1971;79:119-126.

Biomechanics of the subtalar joint and midtarsal joints. *J Am Podiatry Med Assoc.* 1975;65(8);756-764.

Blackburn J, Prentice W, Guskiewicz K, Busby M. Balance and joint stability: the relative contributions of proprioception and muscular strength. *J Sport Rehabil.* 2006;9:315-328.

Bloome DM, Marymont JV, Varner KE. Variations on the insertion of the posterior tibialis tendon: a cadaveric study. *Foot Ankle Int.* 2003;24:780-783.

Bonifácio D, Richards J, Selfe J, Curran S, Trede, R. Influence and benefits of foot orthoses on kinematics, kinetics and muscle activation during step descent task. *Gait Posture.* 2018;65:106-111.

Bordelon RL. Correction of hypermobile flatfoot in children by molded insert. *Foot Ankle.* 1980;1(3):143-150.

Broughton NS, Graham G, Memelaus MB. The high incidence of foot deformity in patients with high-level spina bifida. *J Bone Joint Surg Br.* 1994;76(4):548-550.

Brown LP, Yavorsky P. Locomotor biomechanics and pathomechanics: a review. *J Orthop Sports Phys Ther.* 1987;9(1):3-10. doi:10.2519/jospt.1987.9.1.3

Burston J, Richards J, Selfe J The effects of three quarter and full length foot orthoses on knee mechanics in healthy subjects and patellofemoral pain patients when walking and descending stairs. *Gait Posture.* 2018;62:518-522.

Coleman SS, Stelling FH III, Jarrett J. Pathomechanics and treatment of congenital vertical talus. *Clin Orthop Relat Res.* 1970;70:62-72.

Conroy GC, Rose MD. The evolution of the primate foot from the earliest primates to the Miocene hominoids. *Foot Ankle.* 1983;3(6):342-364. doi:10.1177/107110078300300604

Cowell HR, Elener V. Rigid painful flatfoot secondary to tarsal coalition. *Clin Orthop Relat Res.* 1983;(177):54-60.

Curran SA. Sagittal plane facilitation of motion model and associated foot pathologies. In: Albert SF, Curran SA, eds. *Lower Extremity Biomechanics: Theory and Practice.* Vol 1. Bipedmed, LLC; 2018:289-315.

DeRosa GP, Ahlfeld SK. Congenital vertical talus: the Riley experience. *Foot Ankle.* 1984;5(3):118-124.

Donatelli R, Hurlbert C, Conway D, St. Pierre R. Biomechanical foot orthotics: a retrospective study. *J Orthop Sports Phys Ther.* 1988;10:205-212.

Drennan JC, Sharrard WJ. The pathological anatomy of convex pes valgus. *J Bone Joint Surg Br.* 1971;53(3):455-461.

Dugan RC, D'Ambrosia RD. The effect of orthotics on the treatment of selected running injuries. *Foot Ankle.* 1986;6:313.

Dwyer FC. The present status of the problem of pes cavus. *Clin Orthop Relat Res.* 1975;(106):254-275.

Evans D. Calcaneo-valgus deformity. *J Bone Joint Surg Br.* 1975;57(3):270-278.

Farris DJ, Kelly LA , Cresswell AG, Lichtwark GA. The functional importance of human foot muscles for bipedal locomotion. *Proc Natl Acad Sci U S A.* 2019;116(5):1645-1650.

Galloway MT, Lalley AL, Shearn JT. The role of mechanical loading in tendon development, maintenance, injury and repair. *J Bone Joint Surg.* 2013;95(17):1620-1628.

Gieve DW, Rashdi T. Pressures under normal feet in standing and walking as measured by foil pedobarography. *Ann Rheum Dis.* 1984;43(6):816-818.

Green DR Carol A, Planal dominance. *J Am Podiatry Assoc.* 1984;74:98-103.

Gross CM. *Gray's Anatomy.* Lea & Febiger; 1968.

Hawke F, Burns J, Radford JA, du Toit V. Custom-made foot orthoses for the treatment of foot pain. *Cochrane Database Syst Rev.* 2008;(3):CD006801. doi:10.1002/14651858.CD006801.pub2.

Heiderscheit B, Hamill J, Tiberio D. A biomechanical perspective: do foot orthoses work?. *Br J Sports Med.* 2001;35(1):4-5. doi:10.1136/bjsm.35.1.4.

Herndon CH, Heyman CH. Problems in the recognition and treatment of congenital convex pes valgus. *J Bone Joint Surg Br.* 1963;45(2):413-429.

Hertel J, Denegar CR, Buckley WE, Sharkey NA, Stokes WL. Effect of rearfoot orthotics on postural control in healthy subjects. *Arch Phys Med Rehabil.* 2001;82(7):1000-1003.

Hierzenberg JE, Goldner JL, Martinez S, Silverman PM. Computerized tomography of talocalcaneal tarsal coalition: a clinical and anatomic study. *Foot Ankle.* 1986;6(6):273-288.

Hlavac H. Compensated forefoot varus. *J Am Podiatr Med Assoc.* 1970;60(6):229-233.

Houglum PA, Bertoti DB. *Brunnstrom's Clinical Kinesiology.* FA Davis; 2012.

Jaffe WL, Laitman JT. The evolution and anatomy of the human foot. In: Jahss MH, ed, *Disorders of the Foot, Vol 1.* WB Saunders; 1982:1.

Jahss MH, ed, *Disorders of the Foot.* Vol 1. WB Saunders; 1982.

Jahss MH. Evaluation of the cavus foot for orthopedic treatment. *Clin Orthop Relat Res.* 1983;(181):52-63.

Jayakumar S, Cowell HR. Rigid flatfoot. *Clin Orthop Relat Res.* 1977;(122):77-84.

Kapandji IA. *The Physiology of the Joints, Vol II, The Lower Limb.* Churchill Livingstone; 1970.

Kim E, Choi H, Cha J-H, Park J-C, Kim T. Effects of neuromuscular training on the rear-foot angle kinematics in elite women field hockey players with chronic ankle instability. *J Sports Sci Med.* 2017;16(1):137-146.

Kirby K, Fuller E. Subtalar joint equilibrium and tissue stress approach to biomechanical therapy of the foot and lower extremity. In: Albert SF, Curran SA, eds. *Lower Extremity Biomechanics: Theory and Practice.* Vol 1. Bipedmed, LLC; 2018:205-264.

Landorf K, Keenan A-M, Herbert RD. Effectiveness of foot orthoses to treat plantar fasciitis. A randomized trial. *Arch Intern Med.* 2006;166:1305-1310.

Landorf KB, Keenan AM. Efficacy of foot orthoses. What does the literature tell us? *J Am Podiatr Med Assoc.* 2000;90(3):149-158.

Leanderson J, Eriksson E, Nilsson C, Wykman A. Proprioception in classical ballet dancers. A prospective study of the influence of an ankle sprain on proprioception in the ankle joint. *Am J Sports Med.* 1996;24:370-374.

Leardini A, O'Connor JJ, Giannini S. Biomechanics of the natural, arthritic, and replaced human ankle joint. *J Foot Ankle Res.* 2014;7(1):8.

Lee WE. Podiatric biomechanics. An historical appraisal and discussion of the Root model as a clinical system of approach in the present context of theoretical uncertainty. *Clin Podiatr Med Surg.* 2001;18(4):555-684.

LeLièvre J. Current concepts and correction in the valgus foot. *Clin Orthop Relat Res.* 1970;70:43-55.

Maffulli N, Longo UG, Denaro V. Novel approaches for the management of tendinopathy. *J Bone Joint Surg Am.* 2010;92(15):2604-2613. Mann RA, Hag JT. The function of the toes in walking, jogging and running. *Clin Orthop.* 1979;(142):24-29.

McPoil TG, Cornwall MW. The relationship between subtalar joint neutral position and rearfoot motion during walking. *Foot Ankle Int.* 1994;15(3):141-45.

McPoil TG, Hunt GC. Evaluation and management of foot and ankle disorders: present problems and future directions. *J Orthop Sports Phys Ther.* 1995;21(6):381-388.

Miller CP, Chiodo CP. Open repair of Achilles tendon ruptures. *Tech Foot Ankle.* 2017;16(2):62-67.

Mündermann A, Nigg BM, Humble RN, Stefanyshyn DJ. Foot orthotics affect lower extremity kinematics and kinetics during running. *Clin Biomech.* 2003;18(3):254-262.

Mündermann A, Wakeling JM, Nigg BM, Humble RN, Stefanyshyn DJ. Foot orthoses affect frequency components of muscle activity in the lower extremity. *Gait Posture.* 2006;23(3):295-302.

Nawoczenski DA, Ludewig PM. Electromyographic effects of foot orthotics on selected lower extremity muscles during running. *Arch Phys Med Rehab.* 1999;80(5):540-544.

Nester CJ, van der Linden ML, Bowker P. Effect of foot orthoses on the kinematics and kinetics of normal walking gait. *Gait Posture.* 2003;17(2):180-187.

Nigg BM, Nurse MA, Stefanyshyn DJ. Shoe inserts and orthotics for sport and physical activities. *Med Sci Sports Exerc.* 1999;31(7 Suppl):S421-S428.

Panjabi MM. The Stabilizing system of the spine. Part II. Neutral zone and instability hypothesis. *J Spinal Disord.* 1992;5(4):390-396, discussion 397.

Payne CB. The past, present, and future of podiatric biomechanics. *J Am Podiatr Med Assoc.* 1998;88(2):53-63

Phillips RD, Christeck R, Phillips RL. Clinical measurement of the axis of the subtalar joint. *J Am Podiatry Med Assoc.* 1985;75:119-131.

Phillips RD, Phillips RL. Quantitative analysis of the locking position of the midtarsal joint. *J Am Podiatry Med Assoc.* 1983;73(10):518-522.

Purnell ML, Drummond DS, Engber WD, Breed AL. Congenital dislocation of the peroneal tendous in calcaneovalgus foot. *J Bone Joint Surg Br.* 1983;65(3):316-319.

Redmond AC, Landorf KB, Keenan A-M. Contoured, prefabricated foot orthoses demonstrate comparable mechanical properties to contoured, customised foot orthoses: a plantar pressure study. *J Foot Ankle Res.* 2009;2:20.

Rome K, Richie D Jr, Hatton AL. Can orthoses and insoles have an impact on postural stability? *Podiatry Today.* October 2010. Accessed April 25, 2022. https://www.hmpgloballearningnetwork.com/site/podiatry/can-orthoses-and-insoles-have-impact-postural-stability

Rose GK. Correction of the pronated foot. *J Bone Joint Surg.* 1982;44-B:642-647.

Samilson RL, Dillin W. Cavus, cavovarus, calcaneocavus. An update. *Clin Orthop Relat Res.* 1983;(177):125-132.

Sangeorzan A, Sangeorzan B. Subtalar joint biomechanics from normal to pathologic. *Foot Ankle Clin N Am.* 2018;23(3):341-352. doi:10.1016/j.fcl.2018.04.002

Shereff ML, Bejjani FJ, Kummer FJ. Kinematics of the first metatarsophalangeal joint. *J Bone Joint Surg.* 1986;68(3):392-398.

Shumway-Cook A, Woollacott MH. *Motor Control: Translating Research into Clinical Practice.* 3rd ed. Lippincott Williams & Wilkins; 2007.

Smidt GL. Biomechanics and physical therapy, a perspective. *Phys Ther.* 1984;64:1807.

Smith LS, Clarke TE, Hamill CL, Santopietro F. The effects of soft and semi-rigid orthoses upon rearfoot movement in running. *J Am Podiatr Med Assoc,* 76:227-232, 1986.

Stacoff A, Reinschmidt C, Nigg BM, et al. Effects of foot orthoses on skeletal motion during running. *Clin Biomech (Bristol, Avon).* 2000;15(1): 54-64. doi:10.1016/S0268-0033(99)00028-5.

Stiehl JB. Biomechanics of the ankle joint. In: Stiehl JB. *Inman's Joints of the Ankle.* 2nd ed. Williams & Wilkins; 1991:39.

Sutherland DB, Cooper L, Daniel D. The role of the ankle plantar flexors in normal walking. J Bone Joint Surg. 1980;62(3):354-363.

Tachdjian MO. *The Child's Foot.* WB Saunders; 1985.

Tynan MC, Klenerman L, Helliwell TR, Edwards RH, Hayward M. Investigation of muscle imbalance in the leg in symptomatic forefoot pes cavus: a multidisciplinary study. *Foot Ankle.* 1992;(9):489-501.

Van Deursen RW, Simoneau GG. Foot and ankle sensory neuropathy, proprioception, and postural stability. *J Orth Sports Phys Ther.* 1999;29:718-726.

Viladot A. The metatarsals. In: Jahss MH, ed. *Disorders of the Foot, Vol 1.* WB Saunders; 1982:659.

Whitney KA. Classification and treatment of congenital sagittal plane deformity. In: Albert SF, Curran SA, eds. *Lower Extremity Biomechanics: Theory and Practice.* Vol 1. Bipedmed, LLC; 2018:265-288.

Woo SL, Gomez MA, Woo YK, Akeson WH. Mechanical properties of tendons and ligaments. II. The relationships of immobilization and exercise on tissueremodeling. *Biorheology.* 1982;19(3):397-408.

12

The Effectiveness of Manual Therapy

Histological and Physiological Effects

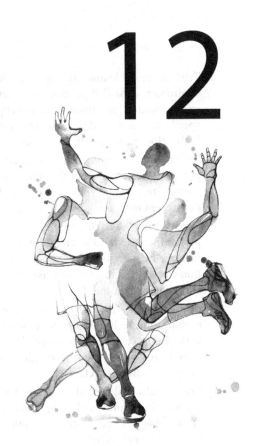

William H. O'Grady, PT, DPT, OCS, MA, FAPTA, FAAOMPT;
Mike Russell, DPT, CSCS; Robert Donatelli, PT, PhD; and Georgeta Donatelli, PT, MS

Wallmann HW, Donatelli R, eds. *Foundations of Orthopedic Physical Therapy* (pp 339-358).
© 2024 Taylor & Francis Group.

KEY TERMS

Enkephalin: This is a neurotransmitter in the brain, spinal cord, and other parts of the body that binds to opiate receptors and releases controlled levels of pain.

Joint dysfunction: This describes the reduced or lack of motion within a joint that prevents movement and/or causes pain with it.

Mechanoreceptors: These are sensory receptors in the joint that respond to mechanical pressure or distortion. There are 4 main types, which are activated primarily by light touch, stretch, and pain.

Mobilization/manipulation: It is described as a manual therapy technique comprising a continuum of skilled passive movements to the joints and/or related soft tissue that are applied at varying speeds and amplitudes, including a small-amplitude, high-velocity therapeutic movement.

Motion restriction: This is the barrier that is reached that prevents normal motion along the plane of a joint.

Periaqueductal gray matter (dPAG): This is located in the midbrain and activates the enkephalin and dynorphins. It is the primary control for descending pain modulation.

Proprioceptors: These are sensors that provide information about joint angle, muscle length, and muscle tension, which is integrated to give information about the position of the limb in space.

Substance P: P standing for "preparation" or "powder" is a first responder to most noxious/extreme stimuli (stressors; ie, those with a potential to compromise biological integrity). Substance P is thus regarded as an immediate defense, stress, repair, and survival system.

CHAPTER QUESTIONS

1. True or False—Manual therapy has been described as a specialized form of joint passive range of motion (PROM).

2. True or False—Manual therapy, which includes traditional mobilization, such as gliding, oscillations, and distractions, and manipulative therapy, which is described as thrust techniques, are methods used to restore mobility.

3. True or False—Manual therapy technique comprises a continuum of skilled passive movements to the joints and/or related soft tissue that are applied at varying speeds and amplitudes, including a small-amplitude, high-velocity therapeutic movement.

4. True or False—Manual therapy has been shown to improve muscle strength of the quadriceps directly after mobilization of the spinal segments. This change is a permanent increase in muscle strength.

5. True or False—The clinical message that manual therapy can increase muscle strength is that this immediate increase in strength can facilitate easier muscle activation when strengthening exercises are instituted shortly after manual treatment.

6. True or False—Another important physiological effect mobilization techniques have on soft tissue structures is the improvement in the normal extensibility of the capsule and stretching of the tightened soft tissues to induce beneficial effects.

7. True or False—Threlkeld[1] suggested that connective tissue mobility could also be improved by the restoration of the collagen fibers content of connective tissue structures to normal levels.

8. True or False—Maitland[2] and Kaltenborn[3] have suggested that joint mobilization may modulate proprioception input to joint structures.

9. True or False—Manual therapy to the knee demonstrated no improvement in balance and proprioception comparing 2 groups of patients with osteoarthritis in the knee.

10. True or False—Gillis et al[4] showed that manipulative therapy to the sacroiliac joint improved compensated Trendelenburg gait in patients with multiple sclerosis.

11. True or False—Courtney et al[5] in a review of manual therapy interventions in the lower quadrant, found that it was not effective in treating pain in the hips, knees, and ankles.

12. True or False—The different grades of mobilization are used to achieve different effects. Grade IV mobilization is performed at the middle of the joint range and increases joint mobility.

13. True or False—Grade II mobilization techniques are designed to modulate pain and muscle spasms.

14. True or False—Orthopedic manual physical therapy is any "hands-on" treatment provided by the physical therapist. Treatment may include moving joints in specific directions and at different speeds to regain movement (joint mobilization and manipulation), muscle stretching, passive movements of the affected body part, or having the patient move the body part against the therapist's resistance to improve muscle activation and timing. Selected specific soft tissue techniques may also be used to improve the mobility and function of tissue and muscles.

15. True or False—Manual therapy does not encompasses soft tissue mobilizations, muscle stretching, and scar tissue mobilizations.

16. True or False—Spinal manipulation improves muscle function through either excitation through motor pathways or by depressing sensory information from the muscle spindles.

17. True or False—The grade of manual therapy that the therapist decides to use is dependent upon where the pain presents itself along the continuum of motion.

18. True or False—There is no specific type of mobilization technique that has shown to be superior to others.

19. True or False—There are valid studies that show that subluxations are a cause of hypomobility in a joint.

20. True or False—Cervical spine meniscoids are intra-articular folds of synovial membrane that have been theorized to have potential clinical significance in neck pain. Manipulation techniques have been proposed as the method of releasing these meniscoids.

Manual therapy is an important part of rehabilitation. Restoring movement to a stiff and painful joint is critical for restoring function. Joint stiffness results from physiological changes. After periods of immobilization, the periarticular soft tissue structures surrounding the joints become stiff and limit the joint range of motion (ROM). Manual therapy has evolved as a specialized form of joint PROM.

Manual therapy, which includes traditional mobilization, such as gliding, oscillations and distractions, and manipulative therapy, which is described as thrust techniques, are methods used to restore mobility. The terms *manipulation* and *mobilization* have been used interchangeably separated by grades and speed of application. Nevertheless, manual techniques are just one component in the nonsurgical management of pain and joint dysfunction.

What is manual therapy? Manual therapy encompasses soft tissue mobilizations, muscle stretching, and scar tissue mobilizations. For the purposes of this chapter, we concentrate on the movement of joint surfaces such as gliding, oscillations, distractions, and manipulations. There will be some discussion regarding stretching of muscle and soft tissue mobilization.

The definition has been worked on over the years by various physical therapy, osteopathic, and chiropractic groups. Dr. Paris,[6] who felt mobilization and manipulation were interchangeable, originally defined manual therapy as "skilled passive movement of a joint." Grieve[7] described manual therapy as "the attempt at restoration of full, painless joint function by rhythmic, repetitive, passive movements within the patient's tolerance and within the voluntary and accessory range and graded according to examination findings." In the United States, the term *mobilization* has evolved among therapists. This was because it was the common term used in most of the state practice acts and because the term *manipulation* was so strongly associated with chiropractic. For example, manipulation was defined by Maitland[2] as a grade V. Maitland described 5 grades of mobilization 1 through 5.[2]

The *Guide to Physical Therapy Practice* defines manipulation/mobilization as:

> [A] manual therapy technique comprising a continuum of skilled passive movements to the joints and/or related soft tissue that are applied at varying speeds and amplitudes, including a small-amplitude/high-velocity therapeutic movement.[8]

The International Federation Orthopedic Manipulative Physical Therapists (IFOMPT) describe manual therapy as:

> Skilled hand movements intended to produce any or all of the following effects: improve tissue extensibility; increase range of motion of the joint complex; mobilize or manipulate soft tissues and joints; induce relaxation; change muscle function; modulate pain; and reduce soft tissue swelling, inflammation or movement restriction.[9]

According to the American Academy of Orthopedic Manual Physical Therapists' description of advanced clinical practice, orthopedic manual therapy is described as:

> [Orthopedic Manual Physical Therapy] is any "hands-on" treatment provided by the physical therapist. Treatment may include moving joints in specific directions and at different speeds to regain movement (joint mobilization and manipulation), muscle stretching, passive movements of the affected body part, or having the patient move the body part against the therapist's resistance to improve muscle activation and timing. Selected specific soft tissue techniques may also be used to improve the mobility and function of tissue and muscles.[10]

As noted earlier, manipulation/mobilization encompasses several active and passive techniques, grades, amplitudes, and speed to improve mobility and function. Thrust manipulation has been used interchangeably with the term *high-velocity, low-amplitude (HVLA)* manipulation. IFOMPT has offered a definition for manipulation as:

> A passive, high velocity, low amplitude thrust applied to a joint complex within its anatomical limit with the intent to restore optimal motion, function, and/or to reduce pain.[9]

Additionally, IFOMPT offered the following definition of mobilization as:

> A manual therapy technique comprising a continuum of skilled passive movements to the joint complex that are applied at varying speeds and amplitudes, that may include a small-amplitude/high velocity therapeutic movement (manipulation) with the intent to restore optimal motion, function, and/or to reduce pain.[9]

The terms *thrust manipulation* and *non-thrust manipulation* have been used in the literature. Thrust manipulation is used to describe interventions described as manipulation by the IFOMPT, and non-thrust manipulation would be synonymous with the term mobilization as proposed by the IFOMPT.[8]

The most common parameter associated with thrust and/or HVLA manipulation is the "pop" associated with it. For a long time, many clinicians judged the success of their treatment by the audible pop. Cleland et al[11] showed the number of pops had no clinical significance in the improvement of pain, ROM, or disability with manipulation in patients with mechanical neck pain. Sillevis et al[12] essentially came to the same conclusion with manipulation of the thoracic spine and Flynn et al[13] came to the same conclusion in the lumbar spine. The common denominator of manipulation/mobilization treatment therapy is that the anatomical part is under the control of the therapist. The exception to this is muscle energy treatment that requires active resistance by the patient. Both Maitland[2] and Kaltenborn[3] described grades of mobilization. Maitland[2] described 5 grades of mobilization, whereas Kaltenborn[3] described 3. The Maitland concept of treatment designated "The Maitland Concept of Manipulative Physiotherapy," as it came to be known, emphasized a specific way of thinking, continuous evaluation and assessment, and the art of manipulative treatment. He used the specific subjective and objective techniques in order to know when, how, and which techniques to perform, and adapt these to the individual patient. Maitland[2] used passive oscillatory techniques, whereas Kaltenborn[3] used sustained stretching techniques. Moon et al[14] compared both techniques in treating the shoulder. He found that both the Kaltenborn and Maitland techniques were equally effective treatments in respect to reducing pain and improving ROM. Maitland initially established 4 grades of treatment but added the fifth grade (manipulation). Below is a description of his grading system (Figure 12-1):

- Grade I: Small passive oscillatory movement at the beginning of the ROM. There is no loading of the connective tissue.
- Grade II: A slightly larger passive oscillatory motion is imparted from the beginning to the middle of the ROM.
- Grade III: A large passive oscillatory motion is imparted from the middle of the ROM to the beginning of the restriction.
- Grade IV: A small passive oscillatory motion is imparted against tissue resistance into the restricted part of the joint.
- Grade V: HVLA thrust at the end ROM.

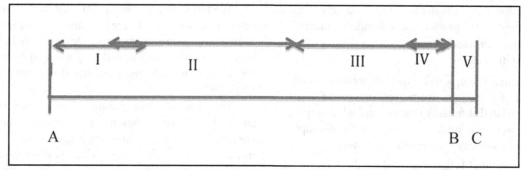

Figure 12-1. Maitland's 5 grades of manipulation/mobilization.

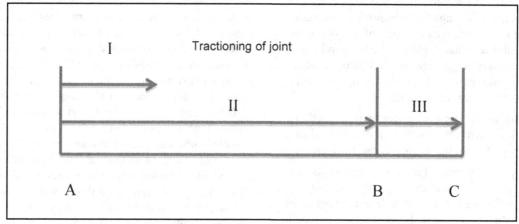

Figure 12-2. Kaltenborn's 3 grades of mobilization based on prolonged stretch or tractioning of the joint.

Kaltenborn divided his sustained stretch mobilization into 3 grades using tractioning force as follows (Figure 12-2):

- Grade I: The joint is unloaded neutralizing joint pressure without separating the joint surfaces.
- Grade II: The articulating surfaces are separated taking up the slack or eliminating play within the joint capsule.
- Grade III: The capsule and ligaments are stretched.

The different grades are used to treat different mechanoreceptors around the joint. Nevertheless, a thorough evaluation needs to be performed prior to applying a particular grade of mobilization. If pain is experienced *before* tissue limitation, gentle pain-inhibiting joint techniques may be used. *Stretching* under these circumstances is contraindicated. If pain is experienced *concurrently* with tissue limitation, the limitation is treated cautiously—gentle stretching techniques used. If pain is experienced *after* tissue limitation is met because of stretching of tight capsular tissue, the joint can be stretched aggressively.

So why are the various grades of mobilization/manipulation applied? Wyke's research in mechanoreceptors has helped us understand the effects of various manual therapies on them. Freeman and Wyke[15] described the 4 types of mechanoreceptors:

- Type I: Globular or ovoid

- Type II: Cylinidrical or tapered
- Type III: Spindle-like
- Type IV: nonmyelinized plexus and nonmyelinized free endings

Wyke[16] presented a logical argument as to the effects various passive movements had on the various mechanoreceptors that could be extrapolated to mobilization/manipulation.

Both Maitland[2] and Kaltenborn[3] have postulated that their mobilizations affected the mechanoreceptors based on their type and function. Sung et al[17] have presented a theoretical framework that suggests the impulse load of a spinal manipulation impacts proprioceptive primary afferent neurons from paraspinal tissues.

Maitland's mobilization/manipulation treatment[3] uses the various grades to modulate pain and/or to improve motion. The following list outlines the application of the grades and their functions:

- Grade I: Used to modulate pain and spasm.
- Grade II: Used to modulate pain and spasm.
- Grade III: Used to gain ROM within the joint.
- Grade IV: Used to gain ROM within the joint.
- Grade V: Thrust manipulation at the end of motion in a joint. Special training is needed.

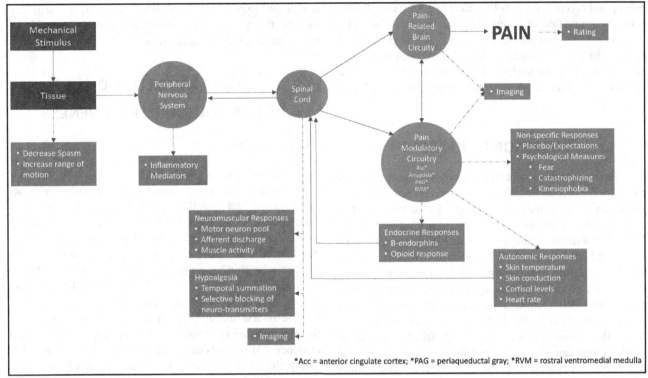

*Acc = anterior cingulate cortex; *PAG = periaqueductal gray; *RVM = rostral ventromedial medulla

Figure 12-3. Bialosky et al[38] model illustrating the comprehensive mechanism of manual therapy. (Reproduced with permission from Bialosky JE, Bishop MD, Price DD, Robinson ME, George SZ. The mechanisms of manual therapy in the treatment of musculoskeletal pain: a comprehensive model. *Man Ther.* 2009;14(5):531-538. doi:10.1016/j.math.2008.09.001.)

The Kaltenborn[3] graded mobilizations are also designed to modulate pain and to improve motion but differ in that they use sustained traction rather than oscillations:

- Grade I (loosen): Produces pain relief by reducing compressive forces. It neutralizes the joint pressure without separating the joints.
- Grade II (tightening): The slack is taken up separating the articular surfaces or to eliminate play within the capsule. Usually used to determine joint sensitivity.
- Grade III (stretch): Stretching of the soft tissue around the joint is involved. Used to increase the mobility in a hypomobile joint.

Mobilization/manipulation treatment has multiple effects on the joint and surrounding tissue. It has been well established that this treatment has multiple beneficial effects,[5,18-22] including neurophysiological, mechanical, and nutritional benefits.[23-33]

NEUROPHYSIOLOGICAL EFFECTS OF MOBILIZATION/MANIPULATION

There have been multiple studies that have illustrated the analgesic effect of mobilization and manipulation.[19,20] Coronado et al[34] in their meta-analysis examining the pain sensitivity testing used in these studies included chemical, electrical, mechanical, and thermal stimuli applied to various anatomical locations. This meta-analysis was appropriate for studies examining the immediate effect of spinal manipulation therapies (SMTs) on mechanical pressure pain threshold. SMT demonstrated a favorable effect over other interventions on increasing pressure pain threshold. There seems to be 2 main theories as to how pain is modulated with mobilization/manipulation. One is the gate theory,[35] which postulates that large myelinated fibers synapse onto the projection neuron. When pain is sensed, this projection neuron normally has increased activity, which activates a C fiber (ie, an unmyelinated type of fiber responsible for the transmission of prolonged, dull pain). If the large, myelinated fibers are stimulated, this causes an increase in their activity. They activate an inhibitory interneuron that inhibits the activity in the C fiber and the projection neuron, cutting the pain signal.

The second theory that explains pain reduction with mobilization/manipulation is the descending pathway inhibition via the dPAG. Stimulation of the dPAG of the midbrain activates enkephalin-releasing neurons that project to the raphe nuclei in the brainstem. Serotonin released from the raphe nuclei descends to the dorsal horn of the spinal cord where it forms excitatory connections with the "inhibitory interneurons" located in the substantia gelatinosa. When activated, these interneurons release endogenous opioid neurotransmitters, either enkephalin or dynorphin. These bind to mu-opioid receptors on the axons of incoming C and A-delta fibers carrying pain signals from nociceptors that are activated in the periphery. The activation of the mu-opioid receptor inhibits the release of substance P from these incoming first-order neurons and, in turn, inhibits the activation of the second-order neuron that is responsible for transmitting the pain signal up the spinothalamic tract to the ventroposteriolateral nucleus of the thalamus.[36,37] Bialosky et al[38] present a nice illustration of how this works in Figure 12-3.

NUTRITIONAL EFFECTS

Most researchers consider the synovial fluid to be the main source of joint nutrition. It has been shown that movement can improve nutrient exchange due to joint swelling and immobilization. Several animal studies verified the effects of mobilization and immobilization on the joints and their cartilage. Salter et al[27] demonstrated that there was cartilaginous healing with continuous passive motion in knees. It has been proposed that manual therapy via passive motion provides stimulation to the synovial fluid, which in turn provides nutrition to the cartilage.[25] Williams et al[28] have found that passive motion has a beneficial effect on minor cartilaginous damage experimentally in animals. Lederman and others have found that ligaments, tendons, and synovial fluid have all shown a better healing with passive motion.[25-28] Viidik[29] found that even slight degrees of motion or intermittent pressure on a joint are sufficient to stimulate the production of small amounts of cartilage. Lederman describes the positive responses from manual therapy by activating the trans-synovial pump that facilitates the drainage of the synovial fluid activated by movement of the joint. The nutrition of the cartilage is supplied partly by hydrokinetic transport as articular cartilage has no direct supply route from underlying bone. The nutrition and viability of the chondrocytes is totally dependent on synovial fluid. Movement produces smearing and agitation of the synovial fluid on the cartilage surface, which aids in this transport.[25]

MECHANICAL EFFECTS

One of primary and most obvious effects of the application joint mobilization/manipulation is its ability to improve ROM. There have been multiple studies both in the lumbar spine and other areas of the body that have substantiated this finding. Mobilization has been shown to maintain the extensibility and tensile strength of articular tissues.[1,19,39-41] Threlkeld[1] suggested that the research in connective tissue mechanical testing and connective tissue remodeling supports the use of manual therapy. He felt that physical forces can and do alter connective tissue. Mobilization has also been shown to improve muscle and ligament extensibility,[1,19,39-41] as well as increase lymph and blood flow.[25] Finally, it should be noted that motion increases muscle repair by restoring sarcomeres to the pre-immobilization state. Animal studies have shown that stretching muscle leads to increased muscle

length and hypertrophy.[25] Albina et al[42] demonstrated that mobilization caused relaxation of the gastrocnemius with the use of manual therapy techniques.

JOINT MOBILIZATION/ MANIPULATION EFFECTIVENESS

Joint Motion

Maitland,[2] Mennel,[43] Mennel,[44] Kaltenborn,[3] Cookson,[36] and Cookson and Kent[45] based their rationale for treatment on the fact that they can isolate accessory motions even though physiological joint motions are a combination of physiological and active or passive joint motions. The literature is replete with studies illustrating the benefit joint mobilization has on the shoulder, ankle, knee, and temporomandibular joints (TMJs).[46,47] The UK Evidence Report on Manual Therapies in 2009 was one of the most comprehensive review and analyses of the effectiveness of manual therapy in a variety of conditions. There appears to be good evidence that suggests that, aside from relief of pain and disability, the application of manual treatment has been shown to improve ROM in a variety of conditions especially in the extremities and TMJ.[46] This was further supported in the 2014 Update to the 2009 UK Evidence Report.[47]

Pain

Like restoration of motion, Mennell,[44] Cyriax,[48] Maitland,[2] Kaltenborn,[3] and other manual therapy pioneers[6,43] have based their principles of treatment on pain relief. The literature is replete with studies illustrating mobilization's/manipulation's effect on pain relief. Ali et al[18] demonstrated that Maitland's mobilization had a greater effect of reducing pain and stiffness than electrophysiological agents in patients with osteoarthritis of the knee.

A systematic review by the 2015 Ontario Protocol for Traffic Injury Management Collaboration[22] supported the available evidence that mobilization was effective in reducing nonspecific shoulder pain and ankle sprains. The 2009 UK Evidence Report on Manual Therapies provides thorough evidence in pain relief with the manual treatment of lumbar, cervical, shoulder, knee, and TMJ conditions.[46] Courtney et al,[5] in a review of manual therapy interventions in the lower quadrant, found that it was effective in treating pain in the hips, knees, and ankles. The 2014 Update to the 2009 UK Evidence Report further supports their findings of the success of manual therapy in pain reduction in the cervical spine, lumbar spine, and extremities.[47] Meneka et al[49] demonstrated a statistically significant improvement was found in the posttreatment Visual Analog Scale, Disabilities of the Arm, Shoulder, and Hand, and goniometer measurements for normal ROM following the Mulligan mobilization techniques.

Effects on Joint Locking

The chiropractic profession has long held out the idea of joint subluxations. There are no valid studies that show that subluxations are a cause of hypomobility in a joint. Theoretically, it has been suggested that the joint may be locked somewhere in the range. It has been proposed that either a meniscoid body in a facet joint can cause this or a positional fault caused by a loose body in the joint. Cervical spine meniscoids are intra-articular folds of synovial membrane that have been theorized to have potential clinical significance in neck pain. The joints that seem to lock have meniscoids.[50] The mechanism seems to be that a meniscoid is trapped in a groove in the articular cartilage. Additionally, this can be caused by a piece of meniscus breaking off forming a loose body. Loose bodies can also be caused by small pieces of bone that break off in the joint. Cyriax[48] has used loose body manipulations for the hip, knee, and ankle. He has even used manipulation for temporary unlocking of a meniscus in the knee. Although clinically good results have been reported with releasing meniscoids, we have a paucity of research in this area and have yet to find a way to measure the success of such manipulations.[50]

Effects on Muscle Guarding/Spasm

The gating of pain noticeably results in the reduction of pain and subsequently muscle guarding. Son et al[51] found that mobilization of the sacroiliac on college-aged women reduced their pain and hence reduced muscle guarding. Katavich,[52] in a review on the differential effects of SMT on acute and chronic muscle spasm, concluded the evidence seems to support the use of SMT on reflex muscle spasm. The author suggested that treatment this way may stimulate tissue receptors to modify neural activity within the central nervous system affecting muscles. This inhibition of the motor neuron pools may result in reducing muscle spasm. Agrawal and Karandikar-Agashe[53] demonstrated that mobilization of the asymptomatic cervical spine led to significant reduction of pain, significant increase in overall shoulder ROM, and a reduction in the functional disability after 5 days of treatment in individuals with shoulder pain.

MUSCLE STRENGTH

Ghanbari and Kamalgharibi[54] found that grade IV oscillations to the tibiofemoral joints of college-aged women increased isometric quadriceps strength. Grindstaff et al[55] performed lumbopelvic manipulation on healthy individuals (average age 28 years) and demonstrated increased quadriceps strength immediately after the intervention. However, the increase in quadriceps strength disappeared when measured 20 minutes later. Wang and Meadows[56] found similar results in the rotator cuff after manipulating C5-C6. Yerys et al[57] demonstrated an increase in isometric strength of the gluteus maximus post–grade IV mobilization of the anterior hip capsule on normal volunteers. One can speculate that this immediate increase in strength can facilitate easier muscle activation when strengthening exercises are instituted shortly after manual treatment. Pickar[18] suggested that the increased strength was a result of excitatory and inhibitory factors. In neurophysiological terms, spinal manipulation improves muscle function through either excitation through motor pathways or by depressing sensory information from the muscle spindles.

STRETCH/LENGTHEN TISSUE AROUND THE JOINT

Kaltenborn,[3] Maitland,[2] and Mulligan[58] advocated end-range mobilization, mid-range mobilization, and mobilization with movement, respectively, to improve joint capsule and soft tissue extensibility. Unfortunately, they did not base this on research. Yang et al[40] found that the use of end-range mobilization and mobilization with movement improved motion by lengthening soft tissue and stretching the capsule in patients with adhesive capsulitis. This was not true with mid-range mobilization. They found these mobilization techniques improved the normal extensibility of the shoulder capsule and stretched the tightened soft tissues to induce beneficial effects. Maher et al,[19] studying 13 patients with decreased tibiofemoral end-range flexion, found that traction compared to PROM of the joint was most successful in increasing ROM with less pain. This case series supports tibiofemoral joint traction as a means of stretching shortened articular and periarticular tissues without increasing reported levels of pain during or after treatment. Threlkeld[1] examined the theoretical mechanical effects on connective tissue. He suggested that manual therapy could increase the length and mobility of connective tissue. He added that the mobility of connective tissue could be changed by breaking some of the links between adjacent connective tissue bundles. He further suggested that connective tissue mobility could also be improved by the restoration of the interstitial fluid content of connective tissue structures to normal levels. This would thereby establish normal frictional resistance between the bundles and adjacent structures.

The behavior of loads on connective tissue and forces applied on tissues with manual therapy around the joint seem to provide a theoretical behavior for the use of this treatment. By comparing a spinal decompression apparatuses group to a manual therapy group, Choi and colleagues[59] found that they were able to increase the disk height with the latter.

PROPRIOCEPTION AND KINESTHETIC AWARENESS

Maitland[2] and Kaltenborn[3] have suggested that joint mobilization may modulate proprioception input to joint structures. In 2005, Deyle and colleagues[60] demonstrated improvement in balance and proprioception comparing 2 groups of patients with osteoarthritis in the knee. All interventions were the same with the home program and clinic group, except the latter group had manual therapy. In 2013, Rhon et al[61] conducted a similar study with the only difference being that manual therapy and perturbation were used to stimulate knee proprioception and balance. Again, they found that both interventions in the clinic obtained more positive outcomes than the identical home program sans manual therapy and perturbation. Wilder et al[62] compared thrust manipulation and mobilization and sham manual treatment groups. They found that mobilization and manipulation improved proprioception in the spine as measured by postural sway, repositioning accuracy, and response to sudden loads.

Lederman[25] has suggested that various groups of mechanoreceptors when maximally stimulated can increase proprioception from different musculoskeletal structures. He suggested that maximal stimulation of joint receptors can be achieved by articulation techniques such as joint oscillations.[25]

GAIT

There is an assumption that normalization of motion in the lower extremities more than likely improves gait. Deyle et al[60] showed that they could improve proprioception in patients with osteoarthritis in the knees with manual therapy. Additionally, as a result they were able improve their gait and walking distance with manual treatment. Gillis et al[4] showed that manipulative therapy to the sacroiliac joint improved compensated Trendelenburg gait in patients with multiple sclerosis. Landrum et al[63] found that using grade III mobilization on the talocrural joint not only improved dorsiflexion but helped to normalize gait in participants who had prolonged immobilization from ankle injuries.

CONCLUSION

As illustrated in this chapter, mobilization/manipulation is a viable method of reducing pain, improving ROM, improving gait, improving connective tissue extensibility, increasing muscle strength temporarily, and reducing muscle guarding/spasm. Understanding the mechanical, neurophysiological, and nutritional values of mobilization/manipulation will allow the clinician a lot of latitude in choice of manual treatment. It is up to the clinician to determine the appropriate grade with which to treat the patient most effectively. Where the pain presents itself along the continuum of motion will guide the clinician as to what appropriate grade should be used. Understanding the clinical value of manual therapy and the multiple advantages it presents in your patient's specific diagnoses will go a long way in obtaining the best outcomes. While some in the profession hold the ability to perform thrust manipulation as requiring exceptional skill, the authors of this chapter believe that performing mobilization properly presents a greater challenge and perhaps greater skill. It is important to understand what the specific treatment goal is and what structures to effect in order to ensure the best outcomes.

CASE STUDIES

Case Study One

The patient is a 23-year-old man who while running stepped in a hole and sprained his left ankle 4 weeks ago. The patient was not having much pain but had limited dorsiflexion. He saw a therapist who performed a talocrural thrust technique, heel cord stretching, and active ROM exercises. The dorsiflexion improved some but was not equal to the noninvolved side. The patient still had some discomfort in the distal lateral condyle. Further examination revealed loss of motion in the proximal tibiofibular joint. Examination revealed the tibia was stuck anteriorly and inferiorly in relation to the tibia. This prevents the ankle from achieving full dorsiflexion as the distal end of the fibula is translated inferiorly onto the talus, restricting the ability of the ankle to dorsiflex fully. A thrust technique moving the proximal fibular head posteriorly produced increased ankle dorsiflexion allowing the fibula to move posterior and superior into the underside of the lateral tibial condyle when dorsiflexion was introduced.

Case Study Two

The patient is 17-year-old high school football player who, at the end of practice, injured his right wrist. He dove for a pass in the end zone and fell on an outstretched left hand while attempting to catch the ball. Radiographs ruled out a fracture in his wrist. There was no snuffbox pain noted upon palpation. He had some mild swelling in the wrist, which was rapidly subsiding with treatment. However, he still complained of nonspecific pain in his left wrist and noted some loss of ulnar deviation. Gentle graded mobilization was performed to the radiolunate and radioscaphoid joints to restore extension and for pain control. Further examination revealed he also had an increased carrying angle in his left forearm compared to the right with some loss of supination motion in the proximal radioulnar joint. The radial head appeared jammed proximally into the distal humerus resulting in forearm abduction producing an increased carrying angle. A thrust manipulation to reduce abduction at the elbow/forearm was applied to the medial radioulnar joint to correct this. This eliminated the discomfort in the left wrist, allowed full supination of the forearm, and restored ulnar deviation of the wrist.

REFERENCES

1. Threlkeld AJ. The effects of manual therapy on connective tissue. *Phys Ther.* 1992;72(12):893-904. doi:10.1093/ptj/72.12.893

2. Maitland GD. *Vertebral Manipulation.* 4th ed. Buttersworth Inc.; 1997.

3. Kaltenborn FM. *Manual Mobilization to the Joints: The Kaltenborn Method of Joint Examination and Treatment - Vol. 1: The Extremities.* 8th ed. Orthopedic Physical Therapy Products; 2014.

4. Gillis AC, Swanson RL, Jenora D, Venkataraman V. Use of osteopathic manipulative treatment to manage compensated trendelenburg gait caused by sacroiliac somatic dysfunction. *J Am Osteopath Assoc.* 2010;110(2):81-86. doi:10.7556/jaoa.2010.110.2.81

5. Courtney CA, Clarke JD, Duncombe AM, O'Hearn MA. Clinical presentation and manual therapy for lower quadrant musculoskeletal conditions. *J Man Manip Ther.* 2011;19(4):212-222. doi:10.1179/106698111X13129729552029

6. Paris SV. Spinal manipulative therapy. *Clin Orthop Relat Res.* 1983;(179):55-61.

7. Grieve G. *Grieve's Modern Manual Therapy.* Harcourt Publishers; 1994.

8. American Physical Therapy Association. *Guide to physical therapist practice second edition.* Phys Ther. 2001;81(1):9-746.

9. International Federation of Orthopedic Manipulative Therapists. Standards Document. 2016. Accessed September 4, 2007. http://www.ifomt.org/Educational+Standards.html.

10. Mintken PE, DeRosa C, Little T, Smith, B, American Academy of Orthopaedic Manual Physical Therapists. AAOMPT clinical guidelines: a model for standardizing manipulation terminology in physical therapy practice. *J Orthop Sports Phys Ther.* 2008;38(3):A1-A6. doi:10.2519/jospt.2008.0301

11. Cleland JA, Flynn TW, Childs, JD, Eberhart, S. The audible pop from thoracic spine thrust manipulation and its relation to short-term outcomes in patients with neck pain. *J Man Manip Ther.* 2007; 15(3): 143-154. doi:10.1179/106698107790819828

12. Sillevis R, Cleland J, Hellman M, Beekhuizen K. Immediate effect of a thoracic spine thrust spine thrust manipulation on the autonomic nervous system: a randomized clinical trial. *J Man Manip Ther.* 2010; 18(4): 181-190. doi:10.1179/106698110X1280499347126

13. Flynn TW, Childs JD, Fritz JM. The audible pop from high-velocity thrust manipulation and outcome in individuals with low back pain. *J Manipulative Physiol Ther.* 2006;29(1):40-5. doi:10.1016/j.jmpt.2005.11.005

14. Moon GD, Lim JY, Kim DY, Kim TH. Comparison of Maitland and Kaltenborn mobilization techniques for improving shoulder pain and range of motion in frozen shoulders. *J of Phys Ther Sci.* 2015;27(5):1391-1395. doi:10.1589/jpts.27.1391

15. Freeman MA, Wyke B. The innervation of the knee joint. An anatomical and histological study in the cat. *J Anat.* 1967;101(Pt 3):505-532.

16. Wyke B. Articular neurology: a review. *Physiotherapy,* 1972;58(3):94-99.

17. Sung PS, Kang Y-M, Pickar JG. Effect of spinal manipulation duration on low threshold mechanoreceptors in lumbar paraspinal muscles: a preliminary report. *Spine J.* 2004;30(1):115-122. doi:10.1097/01.brs.0000147800.88242.48

18. Pickar JG. Neurophysiological effects of spinal manipulation. *Spine J.* 2002;2(5):357-371. doi:10.1016/s1529-9430(02)00400-x

19. Maher S, Creighton D, Kondratek M, Krauss J, Qu X. The effect of tibio-femoral traction mobilization on passive knee flexion motion impairment and pain: a case series. *J Man Manip Ther.* 2010;18(1): 29–36. doi:10.1179/106698110X12595770849560

20. Medlicott MS, Harris SR. A systematic review of the effectiveness of exercise, manual therapy, electrotherapy, relaxation training, and biofeedback in the management of temporomandibular disorder. *Phys Ther.* 2006;86(7):955-973.

21. Ali SS, Ahmed SI, Kahn M, Soomro RR. Comparing the effects of manual therapy versus electrophysical agents in the management of knee osteoarthritis. *Pak J Pharm Sci.* 2014;27(4 Suppl):1103-1106.

22. Southerst D, Yu H, Randhawa K, et al. The effectiveness of manual therapy for the management of musculoskeletal disorders of the upper and lower extremities: a systematic review by the Ontario Protocol for Traffic Injury Management (OPTIMa) Collaboration, *Chiropr Man Therap.* 2015;23:30. doi:10.1186/s12998-015-0075-6

23. Akeson WH, Amiel D, Woo SL-Y. Physiology and therapeutic value of passive motion. In: Helminen HJ, KivarendaI Tammi M, eds. *Joint loading, biology and health of articular structures.* John Wright; 1987:375-394.

24. Levick JR. Synovial fluid and trans-synovial flow in stationary and moving normal joints, In: Helminen HJ, KivarendaI Tammi M, eds. *Joint loading, biology and health of articular structures.* John Wright;1987:149-186.

25. Lederman E. *The Science and Practice of Manual Therapy.* 2nd ed. Churchill Livingstone;2005:9-68.

26. Wolf J. Blood supply and nutrition of articular cartilage. *Folia Morphol (Praha).* 1975;23(3):197-209.

27. Salter RB, Simmonds DF, Malcolm BW, Rumble EJ, MacMichael D, Clements ND. The biological effect of continuous passive motion on the healing of full-thickness defects in articular cartilage. An experimental investigation in the rabbit. *J Bone Joint Surg Am.* 1980;62(8):1232-1251.

28. Williams JM, Moran M, Thonar EJ, Salter RB. Continuous passive motion stimulates repair of rabbit knee articular cartilage after matrix proteoglycan loss. *Clin Orthop Relat Res.* 1994;(304):252-262.

29. Viidik A. Functional properties of collagenous tissues. *Int Rev Connect Tissue Res.* 1973;6:127-215. doi:10.1016/b978-0-12-363706-2.50010-6

30. Tuttle N, Barrett RS, Laakso L. Relation between changes in posteroanterior stiffness and active range of movement of the cervical spine following manual therapy treatment. *Spine.* 2008;33(19):E673-E679. doi:10.1097/BRS.0b013e31817f93f9

31. Campbell BD, Snodgrass SJ. The effects of thoracic manipulation on posteroanterior spinal stiffness. *J Orthop Sports Phys Ther.* 2010;40(11):685-693. doi:10.2519/jospt.2010.3271

32. Johnson AJ, Godges JJ, Zimmerman GJ, Ounanian LL. The effect of anterior versus posterior glide joint mobilization on external rotation range of motion in patients with shoulder adhesive capsulitis. *J Orthop Sports Phys Ther.* 2007;37(3):88-99. doi:10.2519/jospt.2007.2307

33. Randall T, Portney L, Harris BA. Effects of joint mobilization on joint stiffness and active motion of the metacarpal-phalangeal joint. *J Orthop Sports Phys Ther.* 1992;16(1):30-36. doi:10.2519/jospt.1992.16.1.30

34. Coronado RA, Gay CW, Bialosky JE, Carnaby GD. Changes in pain sensitivity following spinal manipulation: a systematic review and meta-analysis. *J Electromyogr Kinesiol.* 2012;22(5):752-767. doi:10.1016/j.jelekin.2011.12.013

35. Melzak RP, Wall PD. Pain mechanisms: a new theory. *Science.* 1965;150(3699):971-979. doi:10.1126/science.150.3699.971

36. Cookson JC. Orthopedic manual therapy-an overview. Part II: the spine. *Phys Ther.* 1979;59(3):259-567. doi:10.1093/ptj/59.3.259

37. Wright A. Hypoalgesia post-manipulative therapy: a review of a potential neurophysiological mechanism. *Man Ther.* 1995;1(1):11-16. doi:10.1054/math.1995.0244

38. Bialosky JE, Bishop MD, Price DD, Robinson ME, George SZ. The mechanisms of manual therapy in the treatment of musculoskeletal pain: a comprehensive model. *Man Ther.* 2009;14(5):531-538. doi:10.1016/j.math.2008.09.001

39. Norkin CC, Levangie PK. *Joint Structure and Function: A Comprehensive Analysis.* 2nd ed. F. A. Davis;1992:7-73.

40. Yang J-I, Chang C, Chen S, Wang S-F, Lin J. Mobilization techniques in subjects with frozen shoulder syndrome: randomized multiple-treatment trial. *Phys Ther.* 2007;87(10):1307-1315. doi:10.2552/ptj.20060295

41. Yang J-I, Jan M-H, Chang C, Lin J. Effectiveness of the end-range mobilization and scapular mobilization approach in a subgroup of subjects with frozen shoulder syndrome: a randomized control trial. *Man Ther.* 2012;17(1):47-52. doi:10.1016/j.math.2011.08.006

42. Albina SR, Koppenhaver SL, Bailey B, et al. The effect of manual therapy on gastrocnemius muscle stiffness in healthy individuals. *Foot (Edinb).* 2019;38:70-75. doi:10.1016/j.foot.2019.01.006

43. Mennell JB. *Massage, Its Principles and Practice.* 2nd ed. P. Blakiston's Son & Co; 1920.

44. Mennell JM. *Joint Pain: Diagnosis and Treatment Using Manipulative Techniques.* Williams and Wilkins; 1964.

45. Cookson JC, Kent BE. Orthopedic manual therapy- an overview. Part I: the extremities. *Phys Ther.* 1979;59(2):136-146. doi:10.1093/ptj/59.2.136

46. Bronfort G, Haas M, Evans R, Leininger B, Triano J. Effectiveness of manual therapies: the UK evidence report. *Chiropr Osteopat.* 2010;18:3. doi:10.1186/1746-1340-18-3

47. Clar C, Tsertsvadze A, Court R, Lewando Hundt G, Clarke A, Sutcliffe P. Clinical effectiveness of manual therapy for the management of musculoskeletal and non-musculoskeletal conditions: systematic review and update of UK evidence report. *Chiropr Man Therap.* 2014;22(1):12. doi:10.1185/2045-709X-22-12

48. Cyriax JH. *Textbook of Orthopaedic Medicine: Volume 1: Diagnosis of Soft Tissue Lesions.* 8th ed. Bailliere Tindall; 1982.

49. Meneka B, Tarakci D, Alguna ZC. The effect of Mulligan mobilization on pain and life quality of patients with rotator cuff syndrome: a randomized controlled trial. *J Back Musculoskelet Rehabil.* 2019;32(1):171-178. doi:10.3233/BMR-181230

50. Jones TR, James JE, Adams JW, Garcia J, Walker SL, Ellis JP. Lumbar zygapophyseal joint meniscoids: evidence of their role in chronic intersegmental hypomobility. *J Manipulative Physiol Ther.* 1998;12(5):374-385.

51. Son J-H, Park GD, Park HS. The effect of sacroiliac joint mobilization on pelvic deformation and the static balance ability of female university students with SI joint dysfunction. *J Phys Ther Sci.* 2014;26(6):845-848. doi:10.1589/jpts.26.845

52. Katavich L. Differential effects of spinal manipulative therapy on acute and chronic muscle spasm: a proposal for mechanisms and efficacy. *Manual Therapy.* 1998;3(3):132-139. doi:10.1016/S1356-689X(98)80003-9

53. Agrawal R, Karandikar-Agashe G. The effect of mobilization of an asymptomatic cervical spine on shoulder pain, shoulder range of motion and shoulder disability in patients with shoulder pain. *Indian J Physiother Occup Ther.* 2020; 14(1):196-201. doi:10.5958/0973-5674.2020.000655.0

54. Ghanbari A, Kamalgharibi S. Effect of knee joint mobilization on quadriceps muscle strength. *Int J Health Rehabil Sci.* 2013;2(4):186-191.

55. Grindstaff TL, Hertel J, Beazell JR, Magrum EM, Ingersoll CD. Effects of lumbopelvic joint manipulation on quadriceps activation and strength in healthy individuals. *Man Ther.* 2009;14(4):415-420. doi:10.1016/j.math.2008.06.005

56. Wang SS, Meadows J. Immediate and carryover changes of C5-6 joint mobilization on shoulder external rotator muscle strength. *J Manipulative Physiol Ther.* 2010;33(2):102-108. doi:10.1016/j.jmpt.2009.12.006

57. Yerys S, Makofsky H, Byrd C, Pennachio J, Cinkay J. Effect of mobilization of the anterior hip capsule on gluteus maximus strength. *J Manual Manipulative Ther.* 2002;10(4):218-224. doi:10.1179/106698102790819085

58. Mulligan BR. *Manual Therapy: Nags, Snags, MWMs, etc.* 6th ed. Orthopedic Physical Therapy Products; 2010.

59. Choi J, Hwangbo G, Park J, Lee S. The effects of manual therapy using joint mobilization and flexion-distraction techniques on chronic low back pain and disc heights. *J Phys Ther Sci.* 2014;26(8): 1259–1262. doi:10.1589/jpts.26.1259

60. Deyle GD, Allison SC, Matekel RL, et al. Physical therapy treatment effectiveness for osteoarthritis of the knee: a randomized comparison of supervised clinical exercise and manual therapy procedures versus a home exercise program. *Phys Ther.* 2005;85(12):1301–1317.

61. Rhon D, Deyle G, Gill N, Rendeiro D. Manual physical therapy and perturbation exercises in knee osteoarthritis. *J Man Manip Ther.* 2013;21(4):220–228. doi:10.1179/2042618613Y.0000000039

62. Wilder DG, Vining RD, Pohlman KA, et al. Effect of spinal manipulation on sensorimotor functions in back pain patients: study protocol for a randomised controlled trial. *Trials.* 2011;12:161. doi:10.1186/1745-6215-12-161

63. Landrum EL, Kellin BM, Parente WR, Ingersoll CD, Hertel J. Immediate effects of anterior-to-posterior talocrural joint mobilization after prolonged ankle immobilization: a preliminary study. *J Man Manip Ther.* 2008;16(2):100-105. doi:10.1179/106698108790818413

Appendix: Examples of Different Types of Mobilizations

Distraction and Depression

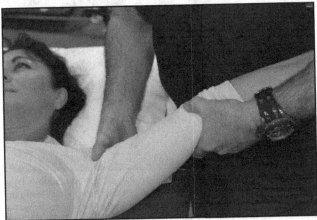

Figure 12-A1. Inferior capsule glide (depression) in abduction. Patient position: Supine. Contacts: Grasp the arm near the elbow to stabilize in 90 degrees of abduction. The web space of the other hand contacts the head of the humerus. Direction of movement: Depress the head of the humerus inferiorly.

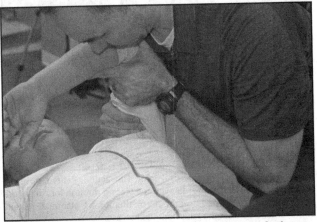

Figure 12-A2. Lateral glide (distraction). Patient position: Supine arm in 90 degrees of flexion. Contacts: Grasp near the elbow to stabilize; the other hand grasps the proximal humerus near the axilla. Direction of movement: Distract the humeral head laterally.

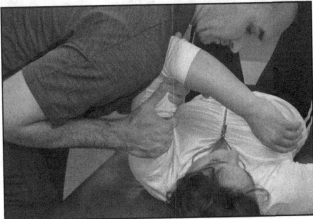

Figure 12-A3. Lateral glide (distraction) alternate angle.

Foot and Ankle

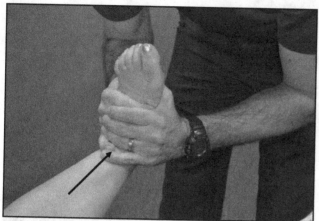

Figure 12-A4. Talocrural (mortise) joint. Distraction. Patient position: Supine. Contacts: Grasps the foot with the second through fourth fingers of both hands overlapped over the dorm; thumbs are plantar. Direction of movement: Distract the talus from the mortise.

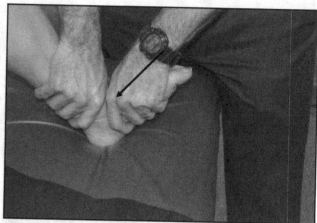

Figure 12-A5. Talocrural posterior glide. Patient position: Supine, knee flexed, with the heel rested on the table. Contacts: Web contact along the anterior surface of the talus; the other hand grasps the anterior aspect of the lower leg above the malleoli. Direction of movement: Glide the talus posterior.

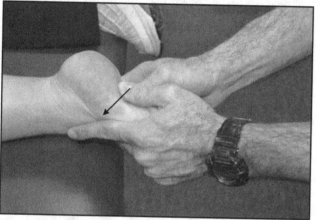

Figure 12-A6. Cuboid whip. Patient position: Supine with foot off the table. Contacts: Grasp the forefoot with overlapping fingers at the dorsum of the foot. Thumbs overlapped over the cuboid. Direction of movement: Combine plantarflexion of the forefoot and force through the cuboid.

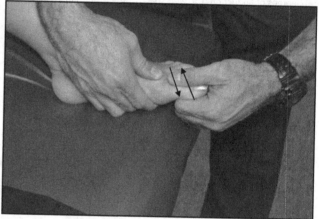

Figure 12-A7. Intermetatarsal joint dorsoplantar glides. Patient position: Supine. Contacts: Stabilize the first metatarsal head; the other hand grasps the dorsal and plantar aspects of the proximal phalanx. Direction of movement: Glide the phalanx in dorsal and plantar directions.

Hip Mobilizations

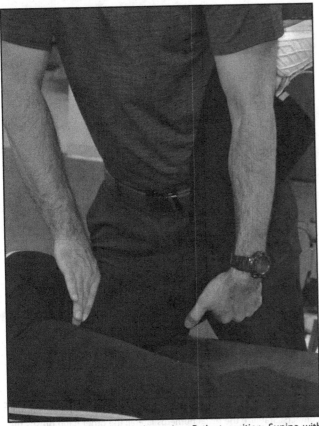

Figure 12-A8. Hip long axis distraction. Patient position: Supine with the involved leg extended. Contacts: Grasp the lower leg and hold in slight flexion and abduction. Direction of movement: The therapist leans backward and pulls along the long axis of the leg.

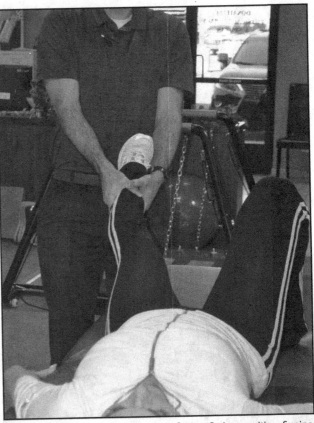

Figure 12-A9. Hip lateral distraction in flexion. Patient position: Supine, hip and knee flexed to 90 degrees. Contacts: The back of the knee rests on the therapist's shoulder, hands grasp the medial aspect of the proximal thigh with hands overlapping. Direction of movement: The femoral head is distracted laterally.

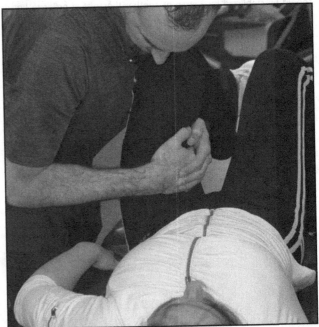

Figure 12-A10. Hip anterior capsule stretch. Patient position: Prone, slight knee bent. Direction of movement: Simultaneously lift the knee while pushing the femoral head anterior.

Humeroulnar Mobilizations

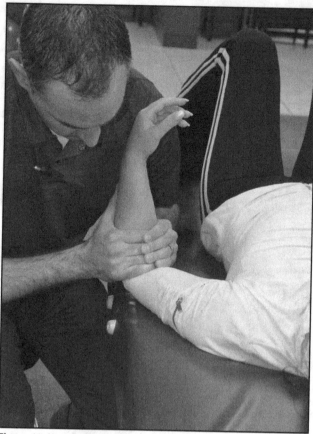

Figure 12-A11. Humeroulnar joint distraction. Patient position: Supine, elbow flexed to 90 degrees. Contacts: The patient's forearm is stabilized against the therapist's shoulder; the therapist's hands grasp the proximal aspect of the forearm, with the fingers interlocked or stacked. Direction of the movement: Distract the forearm from the humerus. The shoulder should be stabilized by a strap or another therapist in order to better isolate the treatment.

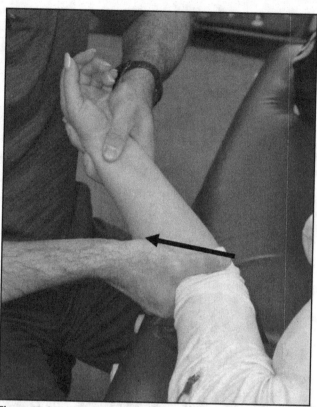

Figure 12-A12. Humeroulnar joint abduction. Patient position: Supine. Contacts: Stabilize the distal humerus lateral; the other hand grasps the proximal forearm. Direction of movement: The forearm is abducted on the humerus.

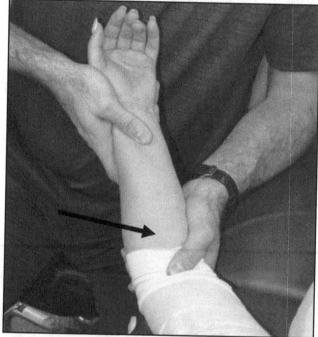

Figure 12-A13. Humeroulnar joint adduction. Patient position: Supine. Contacts: Stabilize the distal humerus medially; the other hand grasps the radial aspect of the forearm above the wrist. Direction of movement: The forearm is adducted on the humerus.

Metacarpal Joints

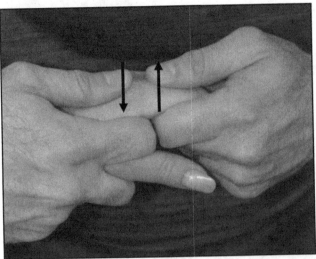

Figure 12-A14. Metacarpophalangeal joint glide. Anterior posterior glide. Patient position: Supine or sitting. Contacts: Stabilize the shaft of the second metacarpal; the other hand grasps the shaft of the proximal phalanx. Direction of movement: Glide the proximal phalanx anterior and posterior.

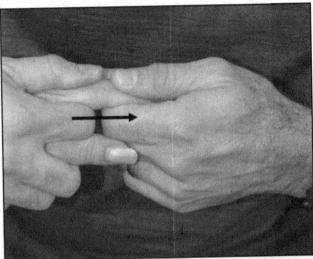

Figure 12-A15. Metacarpophalangeal joint distraction. Patient position: Supine or sitting. Contacts: Stabilize the shaft of the second metacarpal; the other hand grasps the shaft of the proximal phalanx. Direction of movement: Distract the phalanx from the metacarpal.

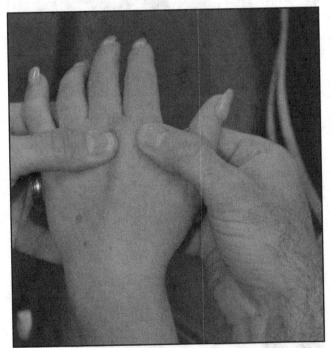

Figure 12-A16. Intermetacarpophalangeal joint glide. Patient position: Supine or sitting. Contacts: Stabilize the head of the intended metacarpal with the thumb and forefinger; the other hand grasps the head of the adjacent metacarpal. Direction of movement: Glide the metacarpal anterior and posterior; repeat for each metacarpal.

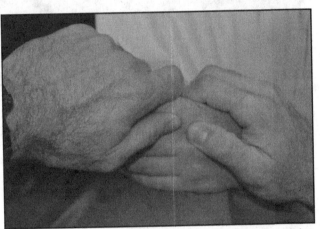

Figure 12-A17. Mediolateral glide. Patient position: Supine or sitting. Contacts: Stabilize the shaft of the second metacarpal; the proximal phalanx is grasped on the medial and lateral aspects of the shaft. Direction of movement: Glide the phalanx medially and laterally.

Radioulnar

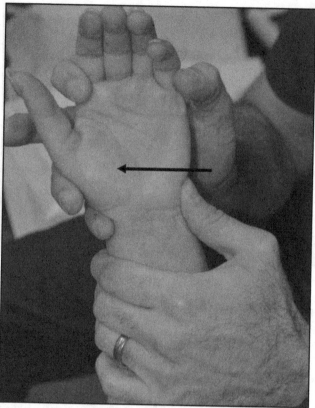

Figure 12-A18. Pisiform glide. Lateral glide of the pisiform joint. Patient position: Supine or sitting. Contacts: Grasp the patients hand firmly to stabilize; contact the thumb tip of the opposite hand against the pisiform bone while grasping the distal forearm with the fingers. Direction of movement: Lateral.

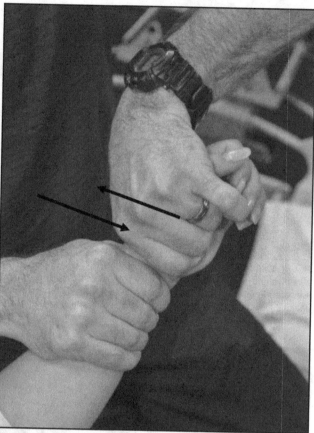

Figure 12-A19. Radiocarpal joint glides. Patient position: Supine or sitting. Contacts: Proximal thumb, index finger, and first web space stabilize the radius and ulna; the distal hand grasps the proximal row of carpal bone. Direction of movement: Volar and dorsal glide with wrist in pronation.

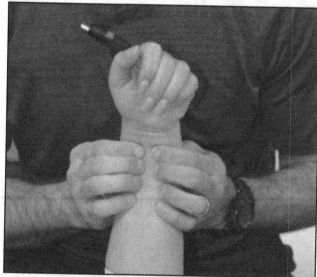

Figure 12-A20. Distal radioulnar joint. Inward and outward roll. Patient position: Supine or sitting. Contacts: Grasp the distal aspect of the radius and ulna with pads of fingers contacting the volar surface and thenar eminences contacting the dorsal surfaces. Direction of movement: Roll the radius and ulna inward and outward on one another.

Subscapular Tilt Technique

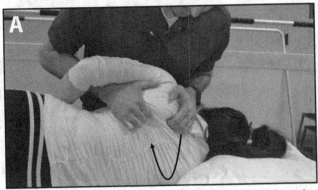
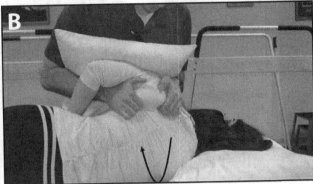

Figure 12-A20. (A) Scapular distraction. Patient position: Side lying close to the edge of the table, involved arm side up, and the arm is supported by the clinician. Therapist position: Facing the patient with the caudal hand underneath the inferior angle of the scapula, and the cephalad hand grasping the vertebral boarder of the scapula. The clinician's sternum is the third contact point at the anterior aspect of the shoulder. Both hands tilt the scapula away from the thoracic wall. (B) Alternative technique with barrier (pillow) between the clinician and patient. Hand position is the same and the technique is unaltered.

Shoulder Techniques

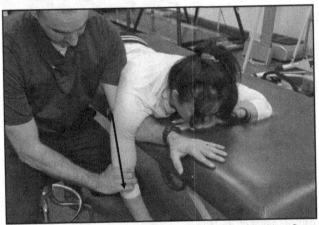
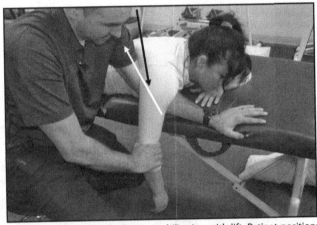

Figure 12-A22. Prone oscillation mobilization. Patient position: Prone lying with involved extremity hanging off the edge of the table. Therapist position: Seated next to the patient with bent elbow at the axilla of the patient. Mobilize the arm at the elbow, directing the force down toward the table in an oscillatory fashion. Caution to not cause pain at the anterior arm of the patient.

Figure 12-A23. Prone oscillation mobilization with lift. Patient position: Prone lying with involved extremity hanging off the edge of the table. Therapist position: Seated next to the patient with bent elbow at the axilla of the patient. Mobilize the arm at the elbow, directing the force down toward the table using oscillations. The therapist's arm lifts during the mobilization to increase posterior capsule stretch. Caution to not cause pain at the anterior arm of the patient.

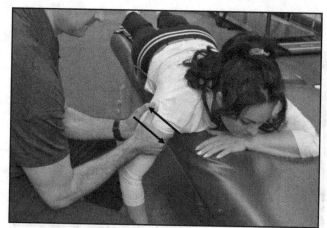

Figure 12-A24. Posterior capsule mobilization. Patient position: Prone with the involved extremity hanging off the edge of the table. Therapist position: Facing the patient in a sitting position; the therapist grasps the humeral head and performs a posterior-anterior mobilization. The movement is anterior and posterior glides.

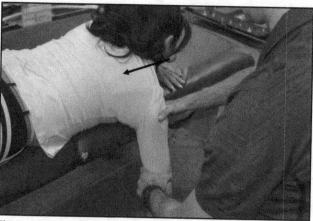

Figure 12-A25. Inferior mobilization. Patient position: Prone lying on the table with involved arm off the table. Therapist position: Facing the patient in a seated position. Contacts: Web space of the first hand at the head of the humerus and performs an inferiormobilization. The opposite arm stabilizes the patient's arm off the table.

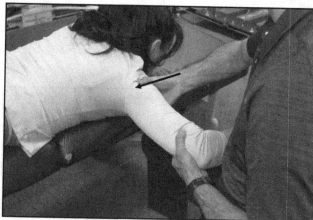

Figure 12-A26. Inferior mobilization with shoulder abducted and external rotation. Patient position: Prone with involved extremity off the table. Patient's shoulder abducted 90 degrees with external rotation, resting on the therapist's knee. Therapist position: Sitting facing the patient. Contacts: Web space of the first hand at the head of the humerus and performs an inferior mobilization. The opposite arm stabilizes the patient's elbow off the table.

Subscapular Release

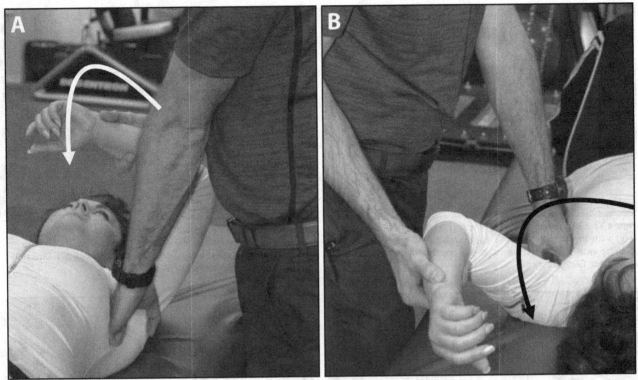

Figure 12-A27. (A) Subscapularis release. Patient position: Supine with involved extremity toward therapist. Contacts: Flexed interphalangeal joints pinning the subscapularis of the involved extremity. Opposite hand resisting the patient's attempt to internally rotate. Contract relax 6 seconds on then off as needed to produce motion. (B) Subscapularis release. Contract relax technique. Second position: Rotating the shoulder into external rotation while maintaining the pin stretch of the subscapularis muscle. Repeat as necessary to increase ROM.

Tibiofemoral

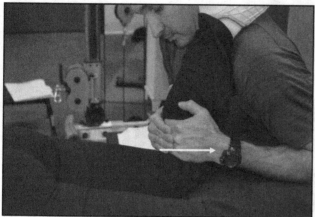

Figure 12-A28. Tibiofemoral joint anterior glide. Patient position: Prone lying with involved knee flexed approximately 45 degrees. Contacts: Stabilize with overlapped hands at the popliteal region. Direction of movement: Glide anterior.

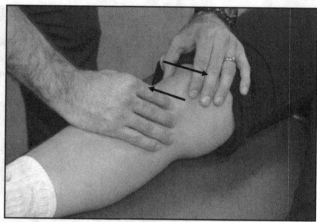

Figure 12-A29. Patellofemoral joint medial and lateral glide. Patient position: Supine with leg extended. Contacts: Use the thumb and index finger against the medial or lateral patellar boarders. Direction of movement: Glide medial and lateral.

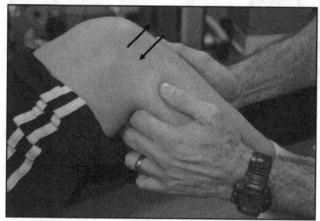

Figure 12-A30. Superior tibiofibular joint anteroposterior glide. Patient position: Supine, knee flexed to 90 degrees. Contacts: Stabilize the medial aspect of the tibia; grasp the fibular head with the thumb and forefinger. Direction of movement: Glide the fibular head anteriorly and posteriorly.

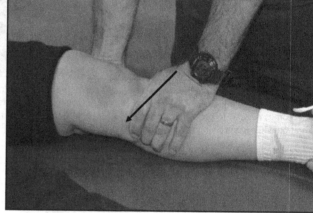

Figure 12-A31. Tibiofemoral joint posterior glide. Patient position: Supine, knee extended with slight flexion. Contacts: Stabilize the posterior aspect of the distal femur; grasp over the tibial tuberosity. Direction of movement: Glide the tibia posterior.

PART IV

Spinal Column

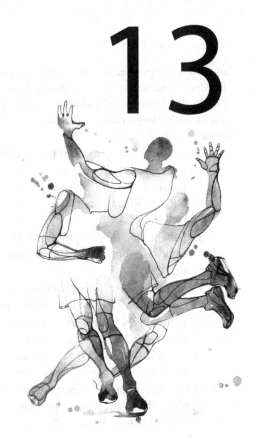

Differential Diagnosis and Treatment of the Cervical and Upper Thoracic Spine

Jeevan Pandya, PT, PhD, DPT, MHS, OCS, COMT;
Mary Beth Geiser, PT, DPT, OCS; and Jena Cleary, PT, DPT, OCS

KEY TERMS

Clinical prediction rule (CPR): A cluster of tests and assessments that has been researched and validated to help a clinician with the diagnosis process.

Clinical reasoning: A process by which a clinician gathers information, creates, and tests hypotheses and determines optimal diagnosis and treatment based on the information collected.

Coupling mechanics: The description used for paired biomechanics in the cervical and thoracic spine that create a functional movement.

Differential diagnosis: The process of distinguishing between 2 or more diseases with similar signs and symptoms.

Radiculopathy: An injury or irritation of a nerve or nerve root that can lead to the symptoms of pain, numbness, and/or weakness in the part of the body innervated by the nerve or nerve root.

Sensitivity of test: The ability of the test to correctly identify patients with the disease.

Specificity of test: The ability of the test to correctly identify patients without the disease.

CHAPTER QUESTIONS

1. Functional movements in the cervical spine are not uniplanar. These segmental motions are called *coupling* and are important for manual therapy treatment. Right rotation of C4 on C5 is coupled with which motion?

   A. Right side-bending of C4 on C5

   B. Left side-bending of C4 on C5

   C. Right rotation of C5 on C6

   D. Left rotation of C5 on C6

2. How much cervical rotation is the atlantoaxial (A-A; C1-C2) joint responsible for?

   A. 10 degrees

   B. 25 degrees

   C. 45 degrees

   D. 80 degrees

   Case scenario—A 28-year-old man reports to physical therapy for evaluation and treatment of a cervical strain from slipping on the ice 2 weeks ago and hitting his head on the ground. The patient reports headaches, head heaviness, and neck stiffness. He can rotate his neck to 20 degrees in either direction. Pain increases with prolonged vertical positions

Wallmann HW, Donatelli R, eds. *Foundations of Orthopedic Physical Therapy* (pp 361-401).
© 2024 Taylor & Francis Group.

and bilateral upper extremity activity. At present, he is only able to sit and drive for 15 minutes. Pain on the Numeric Pain Rating Scale is 2/10 and at worst is 9/10. The patient has not been able to go back to work due to constant complaint of pain.

3. What is the next most appropriate step to take?

   A. Patient should have radiographs before initiating physical therapy interventions as per Canadian C-Spine Rule to limited cervical spine range of motion (ROM).

   B. Patient can initiate physical therapy intervention, as he does not report any paresthesias in the upper extremity.

   C. Patient cannot initiate physical therapy interventions at this time due to increased pain.

   D. Patient does not report of any paresthesias and his current pain is 2/10, his symptoms are mechanical in nature. Hence, educate the patient about pain and discharge with a home exercise program.

4. If the radiographs are negative, based on the patient's history, what is the most important assessment to perform to screen for upper cervical spine ligament laxity prior to initiating treatment?

   A. Spurling test

   B. Vertebrobasilar insufficiency (VBI) testing

   C. Sharp-Purser test

   D. Distraction test

5. What 2 structures are palpated during a Sharp-Purser test?

   A. Forehead and transverse process of C1

   B. Forehead and spinous process of C2

   C. Forehead and transverse process of C2

   D. Mandible and spinout process of C2

6. Which of the following symptoms are more commonly associated with cervicogenic dizziness (CGD) and would lead a physical therapist to believe that the dizziness is of musculoskeletal origin?

   A. Dysphasia

   B. Vertigo associated with position changes (ie, sit to supine)

   C. Drop attacks

   D. Neck pain

7. Which special test is used to assess for dizziness due to benign paroxysmal positional vertigo (BPPV)?

   A. Dix Hallpike test

   B. Neck torsion nystagmus test

   C. Cervical relocation test

   D. DeKleyn test

8. What are the 3 main pillars of evidence-based practice (EBP)?

   A. Expert opinion, clinical experience, and patient values

   B. Clinical experience, best available literature, and patient values

   C. Personal values, expert input, and best available literature

   D. Personal values, patient values, and clinical experience

9. A 40-year-old woman reports a 3-week history of right-sided neck pain and stiffness. She thinks she just slept on it wrong one night and reported no new injury. Your physical examination reveals cervical spine flexion to 60 degrees, extension to 55 degrees, left rotation to 70 degrees, and right rotation to 40 degrees. All movements produce pain at the end of active range of motion (AROM), and you note the C6 and C7 spinal segments to be hypomobile. Tests of cervical spine ligamentous insufficiency are negative, and she has no limitation in right and left upper extremity mobility. Based on your patient's history and observation you suspect for cervical radiculopathy. What other tests would you like to conduct to improve your hypothesis?

   A. Arm squeeze test, upper limb tension test (ULTT), and shoulder abduction test

   B. Arm squeeze test, Spurling test, and distraction test

   C. Shoulder abduction test, Spurling test, and ULTT

   D. ULTT, Spurling test, and distraction test

10. A 67-year-old woman presents to your clinic with neck pain and mobility deficits. Your physical examination reveals a shortened right anterior scalene. As a treatment you have decided to stretch the muscle. You start by stabilizing the patient's right clavicle and first rib. Knowing your anatomy, what are the other movements you need to add to stretch the anterior scalene?

   A. Left side-bending and right rotation of cervical spine

   B. Left side-bending and left rotation of cervical spine

   C. Right side-bending and left rotation of the cervical spine

   D. Right side-bending and right rotation cervical spine

11. When an injury to the cervical spine is a concern, which of the following factors signifies that cervical spine radiography is indicated in alert and stable trauma patients?

    A. 61-year-old man

    B. No midline C-spine tenderness

    C. Ability to rotate the neck 55 degrees to the right and 63 degrees to the left

    D. Fall from a 4-foot stepladder

12. John, a 72-year-old man, visits your clinic without referral and reports a 3-week history of right-side upper back pain and chest pain, morning stiffness, and difficulty sleeping on the right side. Upon further questioning, he reveals that he often wakes up in the middle of the night because of the pain. During your examination, you ask him to take a deep breath while palpating his ribs. You note that he has limited chest expansion and hear crackling noise. Based on your findings, you decide to refer him to his physician with a suspicion of?

    A. Lung Cancer

    B. Rheumatoid arthritis

    C. Fracture of ribs

    D. Intercostal muscle strain

13. You are attempting to palpate the right transverse process of T9. What anatomical landmark can help you accomplish that?

    A. Palpating right of the T7 spinous process

    B. Palpating right of the T8 spinous process

    C. Palpating right of the T9 spinous process

    D. Palpating right of the T6 spinous process

14. While observing your patient in standing, you ask her to take in a deep breath. Which of the following best describes the expected motion of her ninth rib during this activity?

    A. Anterior aspect moves inferiorly and anteriorly

    B. Anterior aspect moves superiorly and anteriorly

    C. Lateral aspect moves inferiorly and laterally

    D. Lateral aspect moves superiorly and laterally

Case Scenario—A 49-year-old schoolteacher presents to clinic with a primary complaint of upper thoracic stiffness and intermittent numbness and tingling in both hands and upper anterior thighs. The patient reports insidious onset over the past several months. The patient reports that symptoms are aggravated in the hands and thighs with looking up. Also, driving and running aggravates her symptoms. The patient also reports of occasional loss of balance over the past several months. Otherwise, she is in good health and exercises regularly. There are no complaints of night pain, any recent history of weight loss, and general sickness.

15. Given this patient's history and symptoms, what is the most likely pathoanatomical diagnosis that should be ruled out?

    A. Cervical radiculopathy

    B. Cervical myelopathy

    C. Primary or secondary vertebral bone tumor

    D. Thoracic disk herniation

16. Which cluster of positive special tests would help you to rule in the diagnosis of cervical myelopathy?

    A. Spurling test, Hoffmann test, and distraction test

    B. Spurling test, Hoffmann test, and Babinski test

    C. Babinski test, Hoffmann test, and inverted supinator test

    D. Inverted supinator test, Babinski test, and ULTT

17. True or False—Adson's test and Wright's test are the most accurate and specific special tests to rule in the diagnosis of thoracic outlet syndrome (TOS).

18. The patient is a 30-year-old nurse, who reports to you with severe burning pain in their right arm and neck region. They do not recall any injury. However, they did report some "kink" in their neck 2 weeks ago. They report that they have constant pain around their neck, which radiates down the inside their arm and shoulder blade region. They report wakening 4 to 5 times throughout the night due to pain and can not lie on their back. They are unable to lift their right arm due to pain. What other information do you need to rule out possible red flags?

    A. Any report of headaches or dizziness

    B. Any episodes of low back pain (LBP)

    C. Any history of cancer

    D. Any history of heart disease

19. Which one of these is a yellow flag that might alter the course of treatment or necessitate a referral?

    A. Feeling unappreciated and unsupported at workplace

    B. Belief that work is the cause of pain and would further aggravate pain

    C. Bowel and bladder incontinence

    D. Fear of movement and re-injury and catastrophizing beliefs

20. A patient with neck pain comes to your clinic for an evaluation. You immediately notice that the patient had a sense of caution when turning her neck. She describes her neck pain extremely vaguely on both sides of her cervical spine and upper trapezius. As part of your screening process for upper quarter patients, you ask about dizziness, nausea and vomiting, and a few other questions that are linked to various pathologies. The patient reported she did have some dizziness when turning her head and changing positions. Also, the patient reported that she has noticed difficulty with her speech and has fainted few times. Her other medical history is significant for hypertension (HTN) and diabetes mellitus. Based on the given information, what would you suggest the primary cause of her symptoms?

    A. CGD

    B. VBI

    C. Vestibular dysfunction

    D. Cervical myelopathy

EVIDENCE-BASED PRACTICE

The profession of physical therapy benefited from the impulse to integrate EBP. The movement forced the profession to accept responsibility for physical therapist's actions, challenged their clinical decision-making skills, and obligated them to critically examine the educational structure of future physical therapy programs. One cannot fully comprehend the impact of EBP on all health care professions without first acknowledging the physician, Gordon Guyatt, who coined the term's predecessor, "evidence-based medicine."[1] Claimed as "one of modern medicine's greatest intellectual achievements," evidence-based medicine is now a worldwide phenomenon.[2]

For EBP to be complete, it must encompass 3 essential pillars: (1) clinical experience, (2) best available literature, and (3) the value patients place on the intervention as well as the expectations they have for the intervention's success or failure.[3] When all 3 pillars are present, the therapist has the necessary tools to make an informed decision about an optimal treatment or diagnostic test selection and uses the information acquired to influence the plan of care for the patient. In a perfect world, an experienced therapist finds strong evidence for the desired intervention or procedure, and the patient recognizes the value of what is being performed and as well as possesses high expectations that this interaction with the clinician will improve their symptoms.

Before an informed decision by the physical therapist is made, key steps should be completed to arrive at a conclusion. One must first ask or formulate a clinical question and then try to acquire all necessary data to appraise the evidence in front of a clinician and grade its merit. The final steps require a therapist to apply what has been learned in clinical decision making and integrate the evidence into the patient's performance, evaluating the outcome and process.[4] However, it is essential that the data is properly analyzed for efficacy.

DIFFERENTIAL DIAGNOSIS

Differential diagnosis is a systemic method of distinguishing diseases of similar characteristics from another.[5,6] Identifying a particular diagnosis is a process of carefully evaluating the data collected during subjective and objective examinations. The collected data are then used to categorize the most appropriate or closely related pathological diagnosis that represents a patient's present pathological condition and clinical presentation.[6,7] However, for a physical therapist, it is equally important to identify a functional or treatment diagnosis based on movement impairments and EBP to accurately treat the person and disorder.

It is important that each body region or body system receive proper screening during the examination process. Merely positive or negative clinical tests cannot completely confirm or exclude the presence of disease. Hence, physical therapists must carefully examine the individual elements of collected data from the examination. Each element of examination—history taking, clinical observation, tests, and re-tests—are equally important in the differential diagnosis process. Furthermore, the evaluation and accurate diagnosis requires astute inspection and clinical reasoning to recognize essential elements of the examination that can be the leading cause of a patient's impairments. A physical therapist's differential diagnostic abilities are particularly challenged when a patient presents with signs and symptoms that arise from multiple segments or systems. It is imperative that multiple systems are appropriately tested prior to confirming a differential diagnosis.[8]

It is important to distinguish differential diagnosis from screening. Differential diagnosis is composed of 4 key elements:

1. Taking a thorough history and collecting subjective information. Knowing a patient's medical and detailed history related to their present symptoms is one of the most important aspects of evaluation, and thus, is helpful for formulating the differential diagnosis. The information garnered from the patient history helps direct and then tailor the rest of the clinical assessment. It is important to ask the patient about pain, stiffness, or spasms, as these may represent "asterisk signs" that lead the patient to seek help. Finding asterisk signs (reproducible and important motions, actions, or characteristics) pertinent to the patient's story or cause of concern allows physical therapists opportunities to test treatment effectiveness. All of these cues collected from the patient's subjective history will guide physical therapists to the next steps in the evaluation process.[9,10,11]

2. Screening (performing tests with high sensitivity). Differentiating between mechanical and systemic conditions can be occasionally difficult. Therefore, it is important that physical therapists perform thorough screening before initiating the physical examination. The most important goal of screening is to identify if the patient has a need for physical therapy treatment or if a referral back to the physician for a consultation or another medical professional for testing is required. Screening should be followed immediately after history taking to identify suspected red flags, yellow flags, and risk factors prior to initiating and continuing treatment.[6,9,10]

3. Performing a physical examination and special tests. Examination is the process of assessing for a suspected diagnosis hypothesized based on the data obtained from the subjective history and screening.[6,11] Different measures and tests (sensitive and specific tests) are used to strengthen or refute the clinical theories, essential for differential diagnosis, until a single or more predominant theory immerges as a winner. A highly sensitive test has the ability to detect patients with the presence of disorder or disease. Hence, sensitive tests are better to rule out a specific disease or disorder. For the cervical

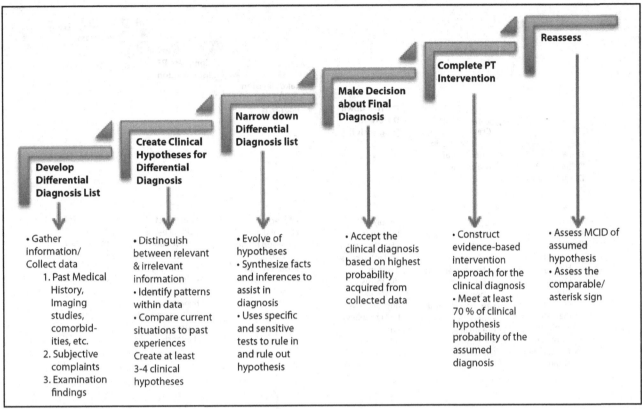

Figure 13-1. Decision-making process used by physical therapists. (MCID = minimal clinically important difference.)

spine, many clinical tests such as reflex testing and sensibility testing are used for screening. However, these tests might yield very little useful information as they demonstrate poor sensitivity. Findings from a single special test may not be of a great significance but may be helpful when used in cluster and interpreted with other gathered information.[8] On the other hand, highly specific tests help to detect those patients who actually do not have the disorder or disease and provide physical therapists the opportunity to consider alternative theories during the examination. In summary, sensitive tests help in ruling out the disorder and specific tests help in ruling in the disorder. High levels of sensitive and specific tests are used to confirm the diagnosis or identify the specific tissue or body region of movement dysfunction.

4. Clinical reasoning. This is the final and most important piece of the differential diagnosis evaluation process. It is a decision-making process used by physical therapists to make wise judgments about the final diagnosis and implement an appropriate plan of care based on collected data from the evaluation (Figure 13-1).[9] Judicious clinical reasoning will help to improve patient outcomes and prevent misdiagnosis. Continuous self-reflection of clinical decisions and analysis of patient outcomes will help physical therapists to recognize patterns and thus will improve their overall clinical reasoning abilities. Clinical reasoning is an unceasing

process that starts as soon the physical therapist meets the patient and continues throughout each session of therapy until the final goals are obtained. Hypothetico-deductive is the most common form of clinical reasoning used in physical therapy settings.[12] In this form, the therapist configures the initial hypothesis based on the collected data, which continues to get refined throughout the evaluation process. The hypotheses should be confirmed by responses to treatment, which involves a process of repeated reassessment.

The result obtained from the clinical reasoning process is also used as data. Next, the patient's own personal hypothesis, understanding, and reaction to the underlying problem are an essential and integral part of the clinical reasoning process (Figure 13-2). The physical therapist's capability to use clinical reasoning and incorporate the patient experience is an ideal form of patient-centered practice. This patient-centered approach to practice involves valuing the individual needs and rights of the patient, understanding a patient's illness, and involving the patient in the decision-making process.[9] Thus, incorporating a patient into the treatment and decision making leads to better outcomes.

When considering a patients' differential diagnosis, physical therapists must decide which disorder to pursue first. Pursuing too many disorders at the same time may lead to unnecessary testing. It is important to remember that defining a clinical diagnosis is a dynamic process; new information can decrease or increase the probability of a different

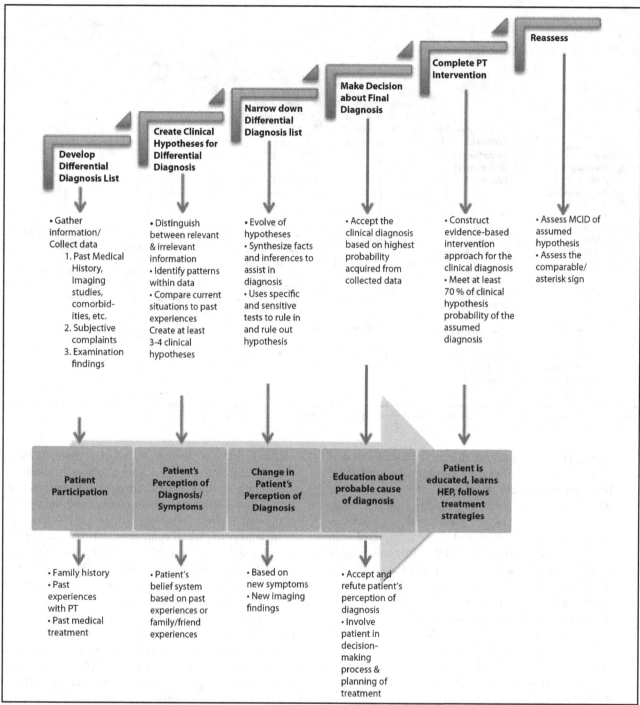

Figure 13-2. Overlap of patient's personal hypothesis and subsequent reactions. (MCID = minimal clinically important difference.)

diagnosis to emerge (Figures 13-3 and 13-4). Significant differences have been noted between novice and experienced therapists in their clinical reasoning abilities.[9] This is primarily due to a lack of experience, deficiency of skill sets, and inadequate knowledge for the novice.[9,12] Clinical skills and knowledge that promote clinical decisions are first learned in the classroom; however, understanding how individual characteristics influence clinical decision making will develop with experience and over time. With experience, newer clinicians should be able to recognize and prioritize

differential diagnosis based on whether they are (1) probabilistic (ie, considering disorders that are more likely and with high probability based on history and objective findings), (2) prognostic (ie, recognizing disorders that may get serious over time if left untreated or undiagnosed but does not need immediate attention), or (3) pragmatic (ie, identifying disorders that will be more responsive to physical therapy treatment and the ones that may not or are unlikely to respond to physical therapy treatment.)[10,11,13-15]

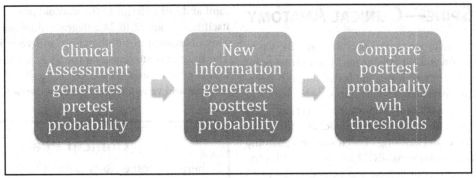

Figure 13-3. Probabilistic diagnostic reasoning.

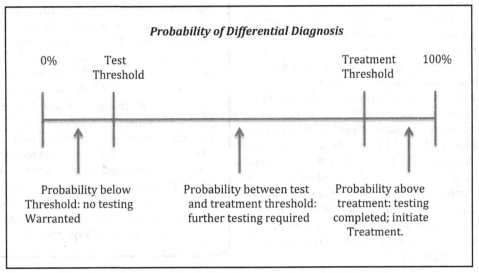

Figure 13-4. Use of test and treatment thresholds in the diagnostic process.[10,11,13-15]

This section presents a more evidence-based method to approach differential diagnosis and clinical reasoning. To start, a clinician must ask a few very important questions.

Questions to Ask for Differential Diagnosis

Questions physical therapists should ask themselves to improve clinical reasoning during a patient assessment[9,12]:

1. Did I gather complete and necessary subjective information by asking pertinent and applicable questions?

2. Is the patient appropriate for physical therapy?

3. Did I create 3 plausible differential diagnoses based on subjective information?

4. Did I receive any clues from the patient's presentation (eg, posture, swelling, gait, transitional motions, extremity movements) that might sway my hypothesis?

5. From my screening, are there any red flags (avoid physical therapy) or yellow flags (be cautious) identified during the clinical examination (both subjective and objective)?

6. What are the benefits from the tests I am going to perform? Are these tests highly sensitive or specific?

7. Would this cluster of tests aide me in developing or refuting my hypothesis?

8. Is there a comparable sign or asterisk sign present and will they assist me in my ability to judge changes in the patient's status or my treatment efficacy?

9. Would knowing additional information change my hypothesis, assessment, or alter my original treatment plan?

10. What is the best EBP treatment approach recommended for my hypothetical diagnosis?

11. Does the patient understand the diagnosis and plan of care I have proposed?

12. Is the patient ready to participate in treatment?

By integrating all components mentioned in this chapter thus far (EBP, screening, examinations, clinical reasoning, and self-reflection), physical therapists should be able to arrive at the most likely clinical diagnosis for their patients.

CERVICAL SPINE—CLINICAL ANATOMY

Cervical spine disorders are as prevalent as LBP. Up to 70% of the population will experience neck pain at one point in their lifetime.[16-23] The cervical spine is divided into 2 distinct sections: the cervicoencephalic (upper cervical) and cervicobrachial (lower cervical) regions. Each section of the cervical spine varies in terms of biomechanics and functionality. Therefore, the understanding of each section's anatomy is paramount. Suggested normal ROM for the cervical spine includes 70 to 90 degrees of flexion and extension, 20 to 45 degrees of side-bending bilaterally, and 80 to 90 degrees rotation bilaterally.[24-28]

With the exception of C1-C2, each vertebral segment consists of 5 articular regions, including the intervertebral joint, 2 superior zygapophyseal joints, and 2 inferior zygapophyseal joints.[29] The zygapophyseal, or facet, joints are the articulations between 2 vertebrae that are designed to assist with movement in a specific plane and also to restrict segmental movement in other planes.[30,31] It is important to study the anatomy and mechanics of these facet joints due to their close proximity to the nerve roots. The nerve root exits the spinal cord and travels just anterior to the facet joints through the neural foramen. The alignment of the facet joints varies throughout the cervical and thoracic spine. At the upper cervical spine, the superior facets face posteromedial, whereas in lower cervical and upper thoracic spine they face posterolateral.[32] The cervical spine also possesses special foramens for vertebral arteries.[32]

UPPER CERVICAL SPINE (C0-C3)

The upper cervical spine is made up of the joints between the occiput, C1, and C2; these joints are commonly referred to as the *atlanto-occipital (O-A)* and *A-A joints*. The mobility and stability of these joints is very important because the O-A and A-A joints are responsible for the protection of fundamental nerves and vessels while allowing the greatest ROM compared to the entire cervical spine as a whole.[33-37] Information on these specific vessels and neural structures will be discussed later in this section.

Specific Osteology/Arthrology

Atlanto-Occipital Joint

Structurally, the O-A joint is composed of the convex-concave articulations between the occipital condyles and first cervical vertebra (C1). The convex right and left condyles of the occiput move with good congruency along the concave surfaces of the right and left transverse processes of the atlas (C1) vertebrae. Palpation of the C1 transverse processes can be found immediately inferior-posterior to the mandibular

joint and just anterior to the mastoid process. The O-A joint itself has about 23 to 24.5 degrees of flexion and extension, a small amount of side-bending, and very little rotation.[33,38] The ligaments surrounding the O-A joint increase stability for the protection of the surrounding vital structures (nerves, arteries, and veins) in this region of the neck.

Clinical Pearl

There is another joint often affected because of upper cervical spine dysfunction, which is the temporomandibular joint. In more than 90% of cases, temporomandibular dysfunctions (TMD) will have significant connection to the upper cervical spine. Hence, it becomes paramount to check for upper cervical spine dysfunction for all patients with clinical signs of TMD problems. A patient may report jaw pain with TMD-like symptoms, ear pain or fullness in the ear, and/or headaches. Upon visual examination, a forward head with upper cervical extension may be evident. Although a diagnosis of TMD is likely coexistent, O-A mobility should be evaluated. Upon examination, palpation of the C1 transverse process, which is immediately inferoposterior to the mandibular joint and just anterior to the mastoid process, can sometimes reproduce the patient's symptoms.

Atlantoaxial Joint

The A-A joint is very unique and does not resemble any other joint in the spine. The atlas (C1), the most superior cervical vertebra, does not possess a formal vertebral body. The axis (C2) has the odontoid process (or dens) that extends vertically from its vertebral body. C1 and C2 articulate at both the dens as well as the facet joints.[39,40] The A-A joint functions as the primary weightbearing joint for the occiput on the cervical spine. The A-A joint is responsible for a significant amount of rotation.[41] Normal rotation ROM for this joint has been documented to be anywhere from 40 to 50 degrees.[38,42] Cervical rotation at the A-A joint moves just as an airplane would while taking a turn. For instance, right cervical rotation includes the "right lateral mass" moving posterior-inferiorly, while the "left lateral mass" moves anterior-superiorly. Literature also supports a small amount of side-bending, about 6 to 7 degrees occurring at this A-A joint.[33]

Although the special architecture of this joint allows for significant mobility, it does not have structural stability when compared to the O-A joint, which leads the A-A joint to be more susceptible to instability. C1 and C2 rely on ligamentous structures to provide stability. The transverse and alar ligaments are the primary stabilizing ligaments of the A-A joint. The transverse ligament laterally holds the dens in place to prevent it from contacting the spinal cord during cervical flexion.[43] The alar ligaments originate from the dens and attach to the occipital condyles to limit cranial rotation. Furthermore, the alar ligaments only allow a small amount of side-bending at this joint.[44,45]

Clinical Pearl

When a patient is presenting with clinical signs of cervical instability, it is vital to assess upper cervical stability, especially if this patient's symptoms are associated with trauma. The alar ligament test and the Sharp-Purser test are the 2 most common tests for ligamentous instability. However, the validity and accuracy of these tests are not well documented, and the sensitivity is low. It is important to take into consideration the subjective information and other objective findings, rather than simply relying on the test to rule out instability. The best way to rule out ligamentous instability is with imaging.[1]

Although instability is more commonly associated with trauma, it can also be related to disorders that affect connective tissue structure, such as Down syndrome and Ehlers-Danlos syndrome.

LOWER CERVICAL SPINE

The lower cervical spine consists of vertebrae from C3 through C7. The key function of the lower cervical spine is to support the head, keep it upright, yet allow mobility. The vertebrae accordingly exhibit features that reflect these load bearing, stabilizing, and mobility functions.[46,47]

Specific Osteology/Arthrology

Each vertebra in the lower cervical spine consists of 3 pillars. These 3 pillars form a triangular arrangement in such a way that when vertebrae are stacked on top of each other, they form 3 parallel columns that help in the load-bearing function of the lower cervical spine.[48] The anterior pillars are formed by the vertebral bodies, which are connected by intervertebral disks. The 2 posterior columns are formed by the articular pillars of the cervical vertebrae. The superior and inferior articular processes of consecutive vertebrae are opposed to one another and united by a joint capsule to form the zygapophyseal joints. The articular facet of each superior articular process faces superiorly and posteriorly at an angle of about 45 degrees, which allows them to bear the weight of the proximal pillar. The key difference between the superior articular surfaces of the upper and lower cervical spine is that they are shorter at the upper cervical spine and are taller

at the lower cervical spine. Because of the taller articular surfaces at the lower cervical spine, the axes of flexion-extension movement at these levels lie closer to the intervertebral disk of the segment. Furthermore, their movements in transverse plane are very limited between these articular surfaces. Hence, any biomechanical changes in this alignment can lead to the reduction of space of the spinal canal and cause the symptoms of the cervical spinal stenosis.[48-50]

The lower cervical spine is mostly responsible for flexion and extension, although it does contribute about 30 degrees to the total amount of cervical rotation.[23] The greatest amount of flexion-extension occurs at the C4-C5 level, and studies have found a range between 16 and 23 degrees at this level.[46,47,51,52] C7 has the most limited flexion-extension ROM, mostly because this segment acts as a transition to the thoracic spine. Clinically, lower cervical spine dysfunction can present in a variety of ways. For instance, pain and paresthesia stemming from a cervical radiculopathy or nerve root irritation can cause symptoms in a specific dermatome and/or myotome pattern. However, the lower cervical spine can sometimes refer pain to the scapular region and present as a thoracic dysfunction. For instance, a C5-C7 facet dysfunction can cause pain or symptoms along the medial border of the scapula or to the midthoracic spine, presenting as a thoracic dysfunction.[53,54]

Clinical Pearl

C5-C6 is the most common level for cervical radiculopathy. One of the reasons suggested for increased prevalence at this level is that C5-C6 is the most unstable joint in the cervical spine and is commonly hypermobile. The facet joints at this level face posterolateral, which has the least resistance to cervical flexion. This slight difference causes poor stability at this joint.[32]

THORACIC SPINE

Specific Osteology/Arthrology

Understanding the anatomy and biomechanics of the thoracic spine is very important for evaluation and manual therapy treatment. The thoracic spine is unique compared to the cervical and lumbar spines because of the vertebral articulations with the ribs. A thoracic vertebra contains the same components as a cervical vertebra, including the vertebral body, vertebral arch, transverse process, and spinous process.[55,56] However, the addition of the ribs changes the structure of the vertebra. Therefore, knowledge of these differences is important.

The thoracic spine can be divided into 3 separate parts: the upper, middle, and lower thoracic spine. The upper thoracic spine acts more like the cervical spine in terms of movement. The segment C7-T3 is a transitional zone between cervical lordosis and thoracic kyphosis. The first thoracic vertebra is considered the transitional vertebra. The second thoracic vertebra, identified by its enlarged pedicle, carries the weight borne by the articular surfaces into a more forward position. Hence, the movements at the upper thoracic spine are very limited, except the movements in the sagittal plane. It demonstrates approximately 3 to 5 degrees of flexion and extension. At each intervertebral level below the second vertebra, the vertebral bodies and disks essentially carry the weight. Movements between segments T3-T10 are also limited due to the articulation of the thorax. The segments between T3-T7 have the least physiological and segmental mobility.[57] The midthoracic spine, along with the rib cage, acts independently and demonstrates anywhere from 2 to 7 degrees of flexion and extension. Also, the thoracic spine has the narrowest foramen canal space, with the cross sectional area being the smallest between T3 and T8, thus making it more susceptible to conditions such as T4 syndrome.[57] The lower thoracic spine acts more like the lumbar spine and has the most ROM of the entire thoracic spine. T12 to L1 has up to 20 degrees of flexion and extension.[58]

The vertebral bodies throughout the thoracic spine are made to withstand significant weightbearing. The shape of each vertebral body is greater posteriorly than anteriorly, which gives the spine a slight thoracic kyphosis.[59,60] The arch of the thoracic spine is smaller than that of the cervical spine, creating a narrower vertebral foramen. In the thoracic spine, the pedicles are thin, whereas the laminas are thick. The transverse processes are thicker and decrease in length caudally throughout the thoracic spine.[61] With the exception of T1, T11, and T12, the ribs articulate with the thoracic vertebrae via the costovertebral joints on the lateral tip of the transverse process.[61] Anteriorly, ribs 1 through 7, the true ribs, articulate with the sternum by the sternocostal joints.[55]

The spinous processes are thin and angle downward at varying degrees.[40] The "Rule of 3s" is an easy way to remember the spinous process orientation and can assist in correctly identifying the vertebral levels with palpation.[56] T1-T3 spinous processes are oriented in line with the corresponding vertebrae. T4-T6 spinous processes are one-half a vertebra below the corresponding level. T7-T9 spinous processes are one full vertebra below, and T10-T12 again are at the same level to which they correspond.[56,62]

The facet joints in the thoracic spine control and restrict movement in specific directions. The alignment of the facet joints changes the mobility of the thoracic spine and differs cranially to caudally. Clinically, for most of the thoracic spine, the facet joints are aligned to limit thoracic flexion and extension.[61,63] Therefore, this movement will be painful for a patient with facet joint dysfunction. Flexion-extension and side-bending increases from T1 to T12 as the facet joint orientation changes to resist rotation, whereas rotation decreases from T1 to T12.[61-64] In the lowest part of the thoracic spine, the T11 and T12 segments mimic the form of the lumbar vertebrae.[61,63,65]

DISKS

Each vertebral body is connected to another through an intervertebral disk, as it forms a fibrocartilaginous joint between 2 adjacent vertebrae.[66] However, there is no disk between the atlas (C1), axis (C2) in the cervical spine. Like so many structures in the body, disks are multifunctional.[67] Three main functions of the disk are: (1) force (shock absorption), (2) act as a symphysis between the vertebrae, and (3) provide physical expression of posture (lordosis or kyphosis). However, there are no disks between the occiput and atlas and between the atlas and axis. The cervical disks are mainly responsible for providing normal cervical lordosis in the upper and middle cervical spine. As opposed to that, the normal curvature of kyphosis in the thoracic spine is caused entirely due to the shape of the vertebral bodies of each vertebra. The key difference to remember is the intervertebral disks in the cervical spine are thicker in relative to the size of its vertebral bodies, which then make them more susceptible for disk herniation and related radiculopathy. On the contrary the intervertebral disks in the thoracic spine are thin relation to the size of its vertebral bodies.[66,67] The disk height in the thoracic region is less than the cervical and lumbar regions. A cervical disk is about two-fifths the height of the vertebral body, whereas a thoracic disk is only one-fifth the height of the vertebral body.[62] With a slimmer disk, the nucleus pulposus is smaller as well.[68] Another anatomical feature of the thoracic disk is the annulus fibrosis. The annulus is important for stability and assists in limiting hyperflexion of the thoracic spine.[61] Disk herniation in the thoracic region is less frequently reported in part due to the smaller disk and nucleus as well as the anatomy of the facet joints.[59]

Clinical Pearl

As discussed earlier, true injury to the thoracic disk, such as disk herniation, is rare. However, increased loading on the thoracic spine and disks can lead to degeneration. This degenerative damage is typically seen at the microscopic level, and therefore will not typically show up on radiographic images. At times, the cause of pain is difficult to distinguish because the damage to the disk occurs gradually and pain will not occur immediately. As the damage progresses and becomes greater, osteophytes may form and can lead to a narrowed spinal canal and neural compression.[60,61] Sudden onset of pain in the thoracic region, especially in an older person, should be closely monitored for presence of a compression fracture.

BIOMECHANICS AND COUPLING MECHANISMS OF THE SPINE

Cervical Coupled Mechanics

Movement at specific levels has been discussed up to this point, but realistically, movements in the cervical spine are paired, or coupled, to create functional movements. Understanding the coupled cervical motion is important for evaluation and manual therapy treatment of cervical spine dysfunction. Coupling biomechanics involves the concept that specific vertebral levels will rotate or translate along one axis in order to complete a general movement upon another axis. When the orientation of the cervical facet joints in the cervical spine is in an oblique plane, side-bending and rotation will occur simultaneously. Many studies have been conducted to identify the coupled motions at each cervical level. The initiation of either side-bending or rotation from C3 to T1 is coupled with ipsilateral rotation and side-bending, respectively. However, C1-C2 had variable results. With side-bending, some studies found ipsilateral rotation as the couple movement, while other studies found contralateral rotation as the couple movement. With rotation as the first initiated movement, studies found that C0-C2 will be coupled with contralateral side-bending.[69]

Thoracic Coupling Mechanics

It is generally said that coupling motions in the thoracic spine occur in opposite directions.[70] Clinically, thoracic movements are observed to have contralateral side-bending or rotation. However, coupled motions in the thoracic spine are not as definitive as in the cervical spine, and there is more discrepancy and variability recorded in the literature for coupled motion in the thoracic region.[64,71] Although this variation exists, in the thoracic region, flexion and extension are typically coupled with segmental translation and rotation.[70]

Rib Joint Mechanics and Dysfunction

When a thoracic segment moves, so do the adjacent ribs. With flexion, the rib will translate forward and rotate anteriorly. The opposite movement happens with extension.[64] In rotation, the superior vertebra will rotate in the contralateral direction (rotation is named by direction of movement of the vertebral body), the ipsilateral rib head will posteriorly rotate, and the contralateral rib will anteriorly rotate. For example, with right rotation, the superior vertebra will rotate to the left, the right rib will rotate backward, and the left rib will rotate forward.[64]

The rib cage must allow for motion during respiration. Here, rib motion is often described as either a "pump handle," "bucket handle," or "caliper motion." Motion in the upper ribs occurs in the anterior-posterior direction around a horizontal axis is called *pump handle motion*. This is most common in the upper ribs. Motion in the mid to lower ribs occurs in the lateral direction through an anterior-posterior axis and is called *bucket handle motion*. The floating ribs at T11 and T12 have more of an opening and closing motion around a vertical axis, called *caliper motion*.[29,72-76]

Many times, dysfunction of the thoracic spine often also involves the ribs because the motion in the region is dependent on all segments moving appropriately. In the upper thoracic region, the first rib elevates, causing superior and posterior translation during inspiration and relaxes to its normal position with expiration.[29]

Dysfunction of the first rib occurs quite often with TOS. The elevation and translation of this rib is reduced during respiration, causing compression of the neural and vascular structures near this region. Full motion at the first rib is limited due to the strong attachment to the manubrium. Dysfunctions in the middle thoracic spine region are also frequently seen in the clinic.[77] The middle thoracic spine is commonly restricted into flexion. Along with this restriction of the vertebrae, an adjacent rib can become restricted in an external torsion, where the rib gets stuck posteriorly and cannot move into anterior rotation and forward translation during thoracic flexion.[72,74,75] A rib can also be subluxed either anteriorly or posteriorly when trauma occurs to the body.[55]

Clinical Pearl

It is important to screen the ribs whenever a patient reports thoracic region pain, posterior rib discomfort, scapular pain, or anterior chest pain that is worsened with breathing, especially if there has been direct trauma or impact to the thorax. This pain pattern can be due to an anteriorly subluxed rib. Clinically, palpation to this rib will demonstrate an anteriorly protruding rib with associated point tenderness. Manual therapy and muscle energy techniques can be used to move the rib posteriorly to its normal position. (Physical therapists should also screen for a posteriorly subluxed rib after an anteriorly directed force or a blunt trauma to the chest.)

MUSCULATURE OF THE CERVICAL AND THORACIC REGION

Cervical Musculature

Several key muscles of the upper quadrant influence movement in the cervical spine and lend to its stability. Structure is important, but without the activation of muscles, the cervical spine will not move. About 80% of the stability in the cervical spine is due to musculature surrounding the cervical spine.[70,78] Muscles of the upper cervical spine tend to provide movements to a single segment, whereas muscles of the lower cervical region tend to act on the spine as a whole.[38]

Deep cervical flexors and superficial cervical flexors are the most common muscle groups for the cervical spine. These muscles provide important joint stability and postural control and include the longus capitis, longus colli, and rectus capitis anterior and lateralis.[79] The sternocleidomastoid (SCM) and anterior scalenes are considered the superficial flexors for the cervical region. The SCM assists with cervical flexion with bilateral activation and contralateral cervical rotation with ipsilateral side-bending when a unilateral muscle is activated. Studies have shown that in patients with neck pain, the deep neck flexors tend to have poor activation and endurance, whereas the superficial flexors (mostly the SCM) have increased activation compared to those without neck pain.[80,81] The deep cervical flexors are comparable to the transverse abdominus in terms of stability. Just as the transverse abdominus muscle has been found to have delayed activation with overhead movements in patients with chronic LBP, the deep cervical flexors have been found to be delayed in activation with overhead movements in patients with neck pain.[82,83] A study conducted by Falla[83] found a significant delay in deep cervical flexor activation leading to poor cervical stability with postural movements and increased likelihood of injury.

Other muscles, such as the upper trapezius and levator scapulae originate from the cervical spine and work synergistically to elevate and upwardly rotate the scapula. Both muscles play an important role around the cervical spine. When acting bilaterally, these muscles can cause extension of the cervical spine. And, when acting unilaterally, they can contribute to the side-bending of the cervical spine to the same side.[56,61] Usually during forward head posture, both levator scapulae and upper trapezius muscles are put under significant stretch, which in turn increases tightness in these muscles. Prolonged increased activity in these muscles can lead to cervicogenic headaches (CGHs).

Thoracic Musculature

Key muscles that attach to the thoracic spine and ribs include the diaphragm, pectoralis major and minor, scalenes, serratus anterior, and trapezius. Other muscles influence the movement of the spinal column and are oriented posteriorly, laterally, and superficially. Of these, the posterior musculature is most important, as these muscles affect postural control as well as assisting in rotation of the spine. The posterior muscles include erector spinae, iliocostalis, longissimus, spinalis, and multifidus.[56,61,62] The multifidi are more prominent in the thoracic spine than the cervical spine but are thickest in the lumbar spine region; they play an important function in providing postural stability.[61] Superficially, the latissimus dorsi originates from the spinous processes in the lower thoracic spine. Laterally, the quadratus lumborum, psoas, and intertransverse muscles originate from the lower thoracic spine as well and have various actions on thoracic and lumbar movements.[61]

Ligaments of the Cervical and Thoracic Spine

Along with muscles, the ligaments surrounding the spine play an important role in stabilization, more so in the cervical region than the thoracic spine. The ligaments are more important for stability in the cervical spine, whereas in the thoracic spine, they are primarily designed to limit excessive flexion and extension movements.

Key ligaments in the cervical and thoracic spine include the apical ligament, the anterior-atlanto-occipital membrane, the nuchal ligament, the tectorial membrane, anterior longitudinal ligament (ALL), posterior longitudinal ligament (PLL), and ligamentum flavum.[84] The main ligaments for the O-A joint include the apical ligament, the anterior O-A membrane, and the tectorial membrane (located posteriorly to the joint).[85,86] In theory, the tectorial membrane, which is the origination of the PLL, is specific to the upper cervical spine. It originates on the body of C2 and travels horizontally to cover the dens and the cruciform ligament. It is likely that the tectorial membrane stabilizes the upper cervical spine to reduce flexion and extension; however, the entire role of this membrane is not completely known.[87-89] The transverse and alar ligaments are the primary stabilizing ligaments of the A-A joint. The thick transverse ligament anteriorly holds the dens in place and acts as a restraint to prevent it from contacting the spinal cord during cervical flexion. The right and left alar ligaments originate from the dens and attach superiorly to the medial side of each occipital condyle to limit cranial rotation. Based on their attachments, the alar ligaments only allow a small amount of side-bending at the A-A joint.[44,45]

The ALL, which is located on the anterior portion of all vertebral bodies, extends from the cervical spine and restricts hyperextension and distraction.[90,91] When the ALL reaches the thoracic spine, it becomes thicker and stronger as it descends from T1 to T11. This increase in thickness is important as the thoracic spine transitions into the lumbar spine, and the facet joints no longer restrict flexion and extension.[92-94] Opposite this, the PLL extends from the cervical spine to the sacrum and limits flexion. The PLL is thickest as it courses over the thoracic spine.[61,92] Another important ligament in the spine is the ligamentum flavum, it extends from the anterior superior borders of the lamina to the anterior inferior borders of the lamina above. This ligament is very elastic and vertically connects one lamina to the next. It has tension even when the spine is in neutral; it is stretched with flexion and assists with return to the neutral position.[58,95]

Neural and Vascular Structures

The cervical spine consists of 8 paired spinal nerves, and the thoracic spine consists of 12 paired spinal nerves. In the cervical spine, all nerve roots exit the foramen above the named vertebral level with the exception of the C8 nerve root, which exits below the C7 vertebrae. However, all nerve roots at the thoracic and lumbar levels exit inferior to the named spinal level.

At the level of first cervical vertebrae, the C1 nerve root exits the spinal canal along with the vertebral artery. The wide transverse processes at C1 create an interesting path for these structures. As the cervical spine is moved into side-bending or rotation the vertebral artery on the contralateral side undergoes tension and is lengthened.[38] As a result of this change, the vascular and neural structures could be compromised.

During the assessment and treatment, the therapist needs to be aware of potential physiological changes, pathologies, or stressors that can influence the efficiency of neural and vascular structures. It is important to clear VBI as a differential diagnosis in all cervical spine evaluations prior to placing a patient's cervical spine into a terminal or more compromising position.[16] In regard to testing for VBI, a couple of key differences will help distinguish between VBI and other dizziness disorders. With VBI, a patient's symptoms tend to worsen the longer the provocative position is held; however, a patient's symptoms tend to subside or improve if peripheral vestibular disorders or CGD is present.[96] Specific testing for VBI will be discussed later in this chapter.

When the second and third cervical spinal nerves exit the spinal canal, they become the occipital nerves. These nerves innervate the occiput and the temporal region. Fibers of the dorsal primary ramus of the second cervical nerve and, to a lesser extent, fibers of the third cervical nerve combine to form the greater occipital nerve, which innervates the musculature in the occipital region. Hypomobility or dysfunction of the O-A joint can cause compression of the occipital nerves or spinal cord, which can lead to CGHs or cervical myelopathy.[97,98]

The sympathetic chain is unique to the thoracic spine and is located just anterior to the costovertebral joints. The vertebral canal in the midthoracic spine (T4-T9) is smaller in comparison to the rest of the thoracic spine. Therefore, the spinal cord does not have as much mobility through this area, and this region of the thoracic spine sometimes is referred to as the *critical zone*.[99] Because of this narrow region, thoracic hypomobility of the midthoracic spine can affect the overall mobility nervous system (in both upper and lower quadrants of the body) and cause neural tension.

DIFFERENTIAL DIAGNOSIS FOR DIZZINESS

Incidence and Prevalence

Dizziness is a symptom of many different medical conditions but not a disease. The term *vertigo* refers to the sensation of spinning or whirling that occurs as a result of a disturbance in balance (equilibrium). Patients may describe a feeling of dizziness as a lightheadedness, faintness, and unsteadiness. Dizziness is sometimes referred to as *vertigo*, but they are different in presentation and pathophysiology. Dizziness is one of the most common health problems in adults. According to the National Institute of Health, about 40% of the US population will experience dizziness at least once in their lifetime.[100] The prevalence of dizziness is higher in women and adults over the age of 45 years and increases with age.[101,102]

Because of such a high prevalence of dizziness many patients are referred to physical therapy. Hence, developing a list of differential diagnoses is important to identify the reason behind a patient's symptom. Specifically, dizziness can be a symptom of cardiovascular, metabolic, musculoskeletal, neurologic, psychiatric, or vestibular disorders.[102] In approximately 50% of cases, dizziness is due to vestibular dysfunction.[103-105] Therefore, taking an accurate and detailed subjective history is very important for differential diagnosis.

Subjective Examination for Dizziness

Generally, a patient with CGD will report an acute onset of symptoms, possibly after a trauma such as a fall, head injury, or whiplash injury. However, the onset of symptoms from trauma is variable and can develop anywhere from days to months after the initial injury.[106] Although many times CGD is often acute, patients with chronic neck pain may also report a gradual onset of dizziness. Symptoms of CGD are usually experienced with turning the head side to side, such as turning to look behind them while driving. Patients may also complain of dizziness with looking up and down.

Some patients may describe the dizziness as if they are spinning inside the room, whereas others may describe their symptoms as "lightheadedness" or "drunkenness."[107] Although patients with CGD may complain of vertigo, symptoms of this diagnosis rarely cause true vertigo.[106] True vertigo, however, is related to a vestibular disorder. A patient's initial complaint may be dizziness, but they can also complain of neck pain, decreased cervical ROM, radicular upper extremity pain, vertigo, nausea, headaches, tinnitus or hearing loss, visual disturbances, and/or ataxia. Patients complaining of neck pain will frequently demonstrate tenderness to cervical musculature, poor postural control, and reduced proprioception. Dizziness symptoms associated with and exacerbated by cervical movements can last anywhere from a couple minutes to a few hours.[106]

Table 13-1

SPECIFIC QUESTIONS TO ASK A PATIENT WITH A COMPLAINT OF DIZZINESS

- How did the symptoms begin?—Gradual, sudden, or injury or trauma related?

- When do the symptoms come?—At rest? After movement? With a specific set of activities?

- How long do the symptoms last?—Duration of symptoms?

- Does the head position change the symptoms?—Improve, worsen, no change?

- Do you have neck pain?—Where, what aggravates it, what relieves it?

- Do you have a history of balance deficits or falls?—How frequent?

- What helps to relieve the symptoms?—Positions, medications, exercise?

- Any past history of interventions for your problem?—Medical or therapy related?

Patients with CGD will often report a sensation of spinning. Conversely, patients with vestibular dizziness will often report that the room is spinning around them. Patients with vertigo from a vestibular origin (primarily of BPPV origin) will likely complain of dizziness while trying to lie down or when turning over in bed. These symptoms often do not usually last long, but they can be intense when they occur. Irrespective of the type of dizziness reported, a therapist should be careful in interpreting data solely based on subjective information, as a lot of these symptoms can overlap. In Table 13-1 are a few specific questions to ask a patient with a complaint of dizziness:

Objective Measures and Findings

Like any evaluation, after clearing the patient of major disease, the patient should be screened for red flags and appropriateness for physical therapy before initiating the physical therapy examination. If the patient has a history of whiplash and/or head injury, the Canadian C-Spine Rule (https://www.physio-pedia.com/Canadian_C-Spine_Rule) should be performed, along with ligamentous integrity and VBI testing. Any patient experiencing dizziness with cervical ROM that cannot be explained by any other comorbidity should be referred to a physician for further screening prior to continuing the physical therapy evaluation.[108,109]

Once the patient is found appropriate for physical therapy, assess for cervical ROM; segmental cervical joint limitations, especially in the upper cervical spine region; and strength and endurance of cervical, thoracic, and shoulder muscles. Also, assess for any impairments in proprioception of cervical spine, vestibular function, oculomotor, and neurological functions.[110-113] Hypertonic muscles such as levator scapula, trapezius, and suboccipitals can be tender and painful. It is likely that poor muscle endurance is contributing to the patient's symptoms.[114] A general approach to

a patient with dizziness is illustrated in Figure 13-5. Along with a thorough subjective and objective examination, recommended special tests can further increase the probability of your differential diagnosis.

VERTEBRAL BASILAR INSUFFICIENCY TESTING

VBI testing (seated and AROM): Sensitivity = 0.50, specificity = 0.13 and supine and passive ROM: Sensitivity = 0.90, specificity = 0.77. Important: VBI testing has weak sensitivity. Therefore, if a patient tests positive, they may have VBI but testing negative *does not* completely rule out VBI.[115]

The initial examination should first and foremost begin with a screening for symptoms of VBI. The clinical practice rule was created by the Australian Physiotherapy Association to help therapists screen for VBI symptoms; however, the VBI tests lack evidence and are sometimes considered controversial. However, it is essential to assess and document the results so as not to overlook a patient who may actually be experiencing these symptoms.[116] The theory behind the testing is to maximally stress the contralateral vertebral artery by stretching it to reduce the lumen of the artery. The position of cervical extension with contralateral rotation has been shown to reduce the diameter of the artery. The more common tests include the minimized deKleyn test and the premanipulative hold technique.[117] A typical screening process involves several components. First assessed, cervical spine active motion in a seated position, where the patient actively rotates and/or extends the cervical spine to end range. The minimized deKleyn test, or modified VBI test, is performed with the patient placed in supine and the therapist passively brings the patient's cervical spine into end-range rotation, then extension, and then rotation and extension combined

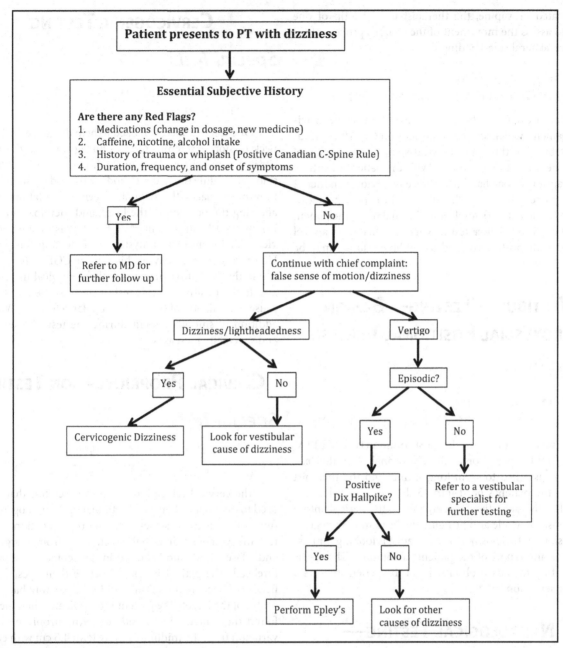

Figure 13-5. How to approach a patient with dizziness.

on each side. The patient is to count backward from 15 while maintaining this position.[117] In the premanipulative hold technique, the therapist brings the patient into the position in which the manipulation will be performed, and then holds this position while the patient counts backward from 15. Then, with the patient in supine, the therapist passively moves the patient's head into rotation and/or extension. During this screening, the therapist should continually watch for cranial nerve (CN) symptoms. If a patient complains of VBI symptoms and tests positive for VBI, referral to the patient's primary care physician is warranted.[118] VBI is a clinical reasoning process and not a complete diagnosis; therefore, further testing is paramount.

LIGAMENTOUS TESTING FOR SUSPECTED SPINAL INSTABILITY

Special Tests

Alar Ligament Test (Sensitivity = 0.98, Specificity = 0.70)

As discussed earlier in this chapter, the alar ligament stabilizes the O-A joint. If a patient is reporting symptoms of dizziness after a trauma, the alar ligament should be tested to ensure there is no injury to this ligament. With the patient either seated or supine, the therapist uses the tip of one thumb to assess the movement of the spinous process of C2 with contralateral side-bending.[119-121]

Sharp Purser Test
(Sensitivity = 0.69, Specificity = 0.96)

This test evaluates the transverse portion of the cruciform ligament, which stabilizes the dens on C1. After a trauma, instability of the upper cervical spine due to injury of this ligament must be ruled out. With the patient in sitting, the therapist uses one hand to stabilize posteriorly on the C2 spinous process. The other hand is used to apply posterior pressure to the patient's forehead. Minimal to no movement should be felt. A positive test is when the therapist can feel the head shift posteriorly, and an audible "clunk" may be present.[119-121]

VESTIBULAR TESTING—BENIGN PAROXYSMAL POSITIONAL VERTIGO

Special Tests

Dix Hallpike Test
(Sensitivity = 0.79, Specificity = 0.75)

This maneuver tests for the most common type of BPPV, which affects the posterior semicircular canal. With this test, the patient is asked to sit in long sitting, and the therapist positions the patient's head into 45 degrees of cervical rotation. The therapist then quickly moves the patient into a supine position while also bringing the head into 30 degrees of extension. In this position, the therapist is looking for nystagmus or any report of the patient's symptoms. The test is positive if nystagmus is observed and the patient reports a spinning sensation.[122-124]

NEUROLOGICAL TESTING— ACUTE STROKE

Special Tests

Head-Impulse Test, Nystagmus Test
(Sensitivity = 0.96, Specificity = 0.84)

This is a 3-step bedside test that is conducted to diagnose a patient with acute vestibular syndrome due to stroke. Head Impulse Test, Nystagmus Test (HINT) includes the horizontal head impulse test of vestibulo-ocular reflex function, observation of nystagmus, and testing for skew deviation. Skew is in reference to ocular alignment, where the alignment of the gaze is altered when alternating covering the right and left eye.[125,126]

CERVICOGENIC TESTING

Special Tests

Neck Torsion Nystagmus Test
(Specificity = 0.91, Sensitivity = 0.90)

One test that has been used to help diagnose CGD is the neck torsion nystagmus test.[127] During this test, the patient sits in a swivel chair. The clinician holds the patient's head to stabilize it while the patient's body is rotated to the side. This movement places the patient in cervical rotation without affecting the position of the head, and therefore not affecting the vestibular system.[128,129] This test is positive for cervicogenic involvement if nystagmus is seen in this position. However, the specificity of this test for CGD is low. During the study, 50% of participants without cervical involvement also tested positive for this test. It may just be that this test causes stimulation of the cervical ocular reflex.[129,130] With the addition of smooth pursuit during the test, the sensitivity and specificity increases.[131]

CERVICAL PROPRIOCEPTION TESTING

Special Tests

Cervical Relocation Test
(Specificity = 0.93, Sensitivity = 0.86)

The cervical relocation test is another test that can be used to distinguish between vestibular and cervicogenic dysfunction. This test assesses cervical proprioception. For this test, the patient sits in a chair 90 cm away from a target map, and a laser headlamp is placed in the center of the patient's forehead. The patient is asked to close their eyes, turn the head in a specific direction, and find their way back to the center of the target. The patient is to indicate when they have found the center.[107,132] In patients with chronic neck pain, variation from the midline of more than 4.5 cm with cervical rotation is said to be abnormal.[132]

DIFFERENTIAL DIAGNOSIS REASONING

The goal of the previously mentioned information is to assist in differentiating different forms of dizziness or vertigo. As described earlier, there is a distinct difference between vestibular dizziness/vertigo and other types of dizziness.

Vestibular vertigo can have a central or peripheral origin. The most common causes of peripheral vestibular vertigo include BPPV, labyrinthine concussion, and Meniere's disease.[113] Central disorders are caused by infection or illness, head injury, multiple sclerosis (MS), or migraines. CGD can be defined as dizziness that results from abnormal mechanics of the cervical spine. However, there is not a "gold standard" definition for CGD, and it is usually treated as a diagnosis of exclusion.[111-113,133-135] CGD is separate from and does not occur due to vestibular dysfunction.[7] Although CGD is still not fully understood, it is thought that it occurs due to vascular compression (VBI), vasomotor changes, or "altered proprioceptive input."[110,111,133]

Altered cervical proprioceptive input can be caused by hypomobility in the thoracic or cervical spine and altered muscle activity. Quite often, people with whiplash injuries experience CGD due to trauma to the cervical spine.[14] Often the altered muscular activity and reduced joint mobility after whiplash can alter the cervical spine proprioception, which in turn affects the cervico-ocular and cervical vestibular reflexes, thus leading to dizziness.[113,135-141] Further details for differential diagnosis are mentioned in Table 13-2.

TREATMENT FOR CERVICOGENIC DIZZINESS

Research about specific interventions for CGD is minimal. However, most of the studies have shown that treatment for specific musculoskeletal impairments reduces a patient's symptoms.[114,141] Interventions may include manual therapy techniques, postural strengthening and endurance, neuromuscular reeducation, balance training, and modalities.[113,114] The addition of vestibular rehabilitation and eye exercises may also be beneficial to reduce a patient's symptoms of dizziness.[113]

Manual therapy techniques such as joint mobilizations, manipulation, soft tissue mobilizations, and muscle energy techniques have been used clinically to help reduce pain and improve mobility. Also, manual therapy has shown effectiveness in reducing symptoms of dizziness associated with cervicogenic impairments.[117] However, manual therapy has been proven to reduce symptoms of dizziness associated with cervicogenic involvement. Therefore, familiarization of the symptoms, tests, and differential diagnosis for dizziness is essential for proper treatment and safety of the patient.[117]

Deep cervical flexor and postural strengthening should be another primary goal. Proprioception therapy using a laser pointer is another promising treatment technique that can be used for CGD. Because these patients have increased sensitivity to proprioceptive input, it is important to retrain the cervical spine to move correctly. The patient could be asked to relocate the laser to a marked target with eyes closed, or simply to follow specific lines on a map with the laser.

HEADACHES

Headache is a common complaint that can affect much of the population at some point in their lives. Headache is the most prevalent pain disorder, affecting 66% of the global population[142]; thereby, it represents a major health problem, often disturbing both quality of life and work productivity.[143,144] The most common form of headache is a tension-type headache with a global prevalence of 38%, whereas migraines have a prevalence of 10%, chronic daily headache 3%, CGH 2.5% to 4.1%, and cluster headaches only 2% to 3%.[142,145,146] The underlying pathological bases for headache symptoms are many, diverse, and often difficult to distinguish.

Classification of headache is principally based on both the evaluation of headache symptoms as well as clinical testing. The International Classification of Headache Disorders has identified 14 different types of headaches. They have divided headaches into 2 categories: (1) primary, includes those of vascular and muscular origin (cluster, migraine, and tension-type headaches), and (2) secondary, mainly results from other sources, such as inflammation, or from head and neck injuries.[147] The International Classification of Headache Disorders defines CGH as a secondary headache, where the source for the headache is caused by a disorder of the cervical spine and its component bony, disk, and/or soft tissue elements, which can or cannot be accompanied with neck pain.[147]

Some headaches are easy to differentiate from CGH due to their distinctive subjective characteristics. For example, cluster headaches, paroxysmal hemicranias, and other trigeminal autonomic cephalalgias typically present with very severe unilateral but short-lasting headache complaints. According to the International Headache Society,[147] headache duration may be as short as 2 minutes with a frequency of 5 per day for paroxysmal hemicrania. Typically, the pain is associated with autonomic features of eye tearing, nasal stuffiness, facial sweating, and ptosis. Taken as a whole, these characteristics are not consistent with CGH, and patients presenting with such symptoms should seek medical consultation, as they are unlikely to respond to physical therapy.

Clinical Anatomy

CGH arises primarily from musculoskeletal dysfunction in the upper 3 cervical segments.[150] The anatomic basis for CGH lies in the relationship between afferents of the upper 3 cervical nerves and the afferents of the trigeminal nerve.[143] Any structure innervated by the C1-C3 spinal nerves could be a source of CGH.[151] The other possible sources for CGH could be the dorsal roots from C1 through C7, the intervertebral disks down to the C7 level, the zygapophyseal joints from C2-C3 to C6-C7, and any of the following nerves: greater and lesser occipital nerve, the third occipital nerve, and the major auricular nerve.[152] One author speculates that CGH may be caused by structures in the mid- and lower cervical spine; however, research is limited and additional research for this theory is still under investigation.[152]

Table 13-2

CLINICAL PRESENTATIONS OF DIZZINESS[113,135-141,148,149]

	MUSCULOSKELETAL (CERVICOGENIC DIZZINESS)	VESTIBULAR (BPPV)	CARDIOVASCULAR (VBI)	NEUROLOGICAL (STROKE)
SIGNS AND SYMPTOMS	Dizziness, associated neck pain, reduced cervical ROM, suboccipital headaches	Vertigo with positional changes, worse in the morning	Dizziness, diplopia, dysphasia, dysarthria, drop attacks, ataxia, anxiety, nystagmus, nausea, numbness	(Facial dropping, arm weakness, speech difficulties, and time to call) FAST acronym, dysphasia, balance deficits, tingling
FREQUENCY AND DURATION OF SYMPTOMS	Minutes to hours, fatigable with repeated motions	Seconds	Symptoms increase as position is held	Varying symptoms and duration
POSSIBLE CAUSES	Whiplash or trauma, altered cervical proprioceptive input, decreased cervical or thoracic ROM	Head trauma, head held in one position for prolonged period, high-intensity aerobics, Meniere's disease, vestibular neuritis, ear infection, labyrinthine conditions	Atherosclerosis, HTN, cardiovascular disease, diabetes mellitus, family history of disease, obesity, elevated lipids, or fats in blood	HTN, cardiovascular disease, obesity, coronary artery disease, peripheral artery disease, obesity, heavy smoking and/or drinking, prior history, family history
TESTING AND OBJECTIVE MEASURES	Sharp-Purser, alar ligament, upper cervical segmental mobility, cervical flexion-rotation test	Dix-Hallpike	Seated rotation, passive cervical rotation test	HINTS test—test for skew
TREATMENT APPROACH	Can be treated by physical therapy	Can be treated by vestibular therapy	Refer to doctor—further testing warranted	Referral to emergency department—emergency testing warranted

Subjective Complaints

CGH is often challenging to diagnose due to its variability in the symptoms. Hence, it is essential to take a detailed history of the client's complaints. Table 13-3 provides physical therapists with essential information they should gather during the subjective examination process when assessing someone for a CGH.

Key characteristics of CGH according to the Cervicogenic Headache International Study Group[147,153] are shown in Table 13-4.

Examination

Examination includes history, review of systems, and physical examination. The first goal of the examination is to identify potentially serious pathologies that require referral to a physician for diagnosis (eg, central nervous system disease, check for red flags; Table 13-5). Examination is also necessary to identify conditions that necessitate consultation for additional treatment such as medications or psychotherapy in combination with physical therapy. Third, examination should help clarify the source of the symptoms arising within the musculoskeletal structures. In many cases, precise diagnosis may not be possible, but the examination provides a baseline level of function from which to assess the effects of intervention.

Table 13-3

ESSENTIAL INFORMATION TO COLLECT FROM SUBJECTIVE HISTORY TO DIFFERENTIATE SYMPTOMS

DIFFERENT TYPES OF HEADACHES

- Current symptoms
  - Location of symptoms (record on body chart)
  - Intensity of symptoms
  - Character and quality of headache
  - Constant vs intermittent
  - Duration of episodes or exacerbations
  - Frequency of episodes or exacerbations
  - Aggravating and easing factors
  - Variations with time of day
  - Night pain, effect on sleep
  - Medications and their effects on headache
- Previous history
  - Date of onset
  - Predisposing factors, injuries, trauma, falls
  - Progression or regression of symptoms since onset
  - Previous treatment including drugs, injections, surgery, therapy, etc
  - Frequency and duration of any recurrences
- Questions to ask for any CN involvement
  - Any loss of smell (test each nostril)? CN I
  - Any loss of taste? CNs VII, IX
  - Any loss of hearing or ringing in the ears? CN VIII
  - Any loss of vision or visual acuity? CN II
  - History of blurred vision? CN III
  - History of double vision? CNs III, IV, VI
  - Numbness of face or frontal scalp? CN V
  - Hypersensitivity to sound? CN VII
  - Difficulty swallowing? CNs IX, X
  - Can the patient say "ahhh"? CN IX
  - Can the patient make a smile? CN VII
  - Chronic cough, loss or impairment of voice? CN X
  - Is there an inability to shrug shoulders? CN XI

Table 13-4

CERVICOGENIC HEADACHE: CERVICOGENIC HEADACHE INTERNATIONAL STUDY GROUP DIAGNOSTIC CRITERIA[147,153,158,159]

- Major criteria
  - Symptoms and signs of neck involvement. Precipitation of comparable symptoms by:
    - Neck movement and/or sustained, awkward head positioning
    - External pressure over the upper cervical or occipital region
    - Restriction of ROM in the neck
    - Ipsilateral neck, shoulder, or arm pain
  - Confirmatory evidence by diagnostic anesthetic block
  - Unilaterality of the head pain, without side shift
- Main head pain characteristics
  - Moderate-severe, nonthrobbing pain, usually starting in the neck
  - Episodes of varying duration, or fluctuating, continuous pain
- Other characteristics of some importance
  - Effects of medications:
    - Only marginal or lack of effect of indomethacin
    - Only marginal or lack of effect of ergotamine and sumatriptan
  - Female sex
  - Not infrequent history of head or indirect neck trauma, usually of more than medium severity
- Other features of lesser importance
  - Various attack-related phenomena, only occasionally present, and/or moderately expressed when present:
    - Nausea
    - Phonophobia and photophobia
    - Dizziness
    - Ipsilateral blurred vision
    - Difficulties swallowing
    - Ipsilateral edema, mostly in the periocular area
  - Ipsilateral edema, mostly in the periocular area

Adapted from Headache Classification Committee of the International Headache Society. The international classification of headache disorders, 3rd edition (beta version). *Cephalalgia.* 2013;33(9):629-808. doi:10.1177/0333102413485658

Table 13-5
RED FLAGS DURING HEADACHE SCREENING
• New onset of headache or change in existing pattern of headache, especially in patients more than 50 years of age
• Onset of headache after trauma or accident
• Sudden onset of severe, constant, and unrelenting headache
• Headache associated with history of any systemic illness, cancer, or seizure
• Headache associated with focal neurologic signs and symptoms
• New onset of a headache during or following pregnancy
• Persistent and/or progressive worsening of headache
• Headache triggered by changes in posture
• No effect to seemingly appropriate treatment
• Headache that awakens patient from night sleep, especially in children
• Uncontrolled HTN
Patients with one or more red flags should be referred for an immediate medical consultation and further investigations.
Adapted from Huijbregts PA. Clinical reasoning in the diagnosis: history taking in patients with headache. In Fernandez-de-Las-Penas C, Arendt-Nielsen L, Gerwin RD, eds. Tension-type and Cervicogenic Headache. Pathophysiology, Diagnosis and Management. Jones and Bartlett Publishers; 2010:133-151.

Special Tests

Passive Physiological Intervertebral Movements (Sensitivity = 0.05, Specificity = 0.99)

A good reliable differential test, in combination with other tests, is Passive Physiological Intervertebral Movements (PPIVMs). PPIVMs are used to determine available ROM at the spine. PPIVMs test the available movement at each spinal segment through passive physiological motion while palpating between adjacent spinous processes and articular facets. During the passive assessment of the spine, it is not only important to analyze the ROM of the spinal segment (hypo- or hypermobility), but also to check for the presence of any muscle spasms or provocation of pain. Furthermore, by providing manual overpressure to the spine, the physical therapist can assess the end-feel of the movement. This technique helps therapists identify location, nature, severity, and irritability of symptoms at each spinal segment.[154]

Cervical-Flexion Rotation Test (Kappa = 0.81, Sensitivity = 0.91, Specificity = 0.90)

In this test, the neck of the patient is passively held in end-range flexion. The physical therapist rotates the patient's neck to each side until resistance is felt or until the patient complains of pain. At this end point, the therapist makes a visual estimate of the rotation range to each side and documents on which side the cervical-flexion rotation test was positive or negative. The test is positive if pain is reported for either direction or when the estimated range was reduced by more than 10 degrees from the anticipated normal ROM (40 to 45 degrees).[154]

Cranial Cervical Flexion Test (Inter-Examiner Kappa = 0.72)

With the patient in supine, a pressure biofeedback unit is placed suboccipitally. The patient performs a gentle head-nodding action of craniocervical flexion for 5 different 10-second incremental stages of increasing pressure ranges (22, 24, 26, 28, and 30 mm Hg). Performance is measured as the highest level of pressure the patient can hold and sustain for 10 seconds.[155,156]

Neck Flexor Endurance Test (Inter-Examiner Kapper = 0.96)

In supine, with the patient's knees flexed in hook-lying, the patient begins by holding the tongue on the roof of the mouth and breathes normally. The physical therapist cues the patient to lift their head off the table and hold it as long as possible with the neck in a neutral position. The test is timed with a stopwatch and terminated when the head moves more than 5 degrees in any direction or skin folds begin to separate due to loss of chin tuck or the patient's head touches the

Table 13-6

International Classification of Headache Disorders Criteria[158]

CLINICAL FEATURES	CERVICOGENIC HEADACHE	MIGRAINE HEADACHE	TENSION-TYPE HEADACHE	CLUSTER HEADACHE
Female:male	Female = male	Female > male	Female > male	Female < male
Lateralization	Unilateral	Mostly unilateral	Diffuse bilateral	Unilateral
Location	Unilateral and does not change sides; frontal, retro-orbital, temporal, occipital	Unilateral and can change sides; frontal, retro-orbital, temporal, occipital	Bilateral; frontal, retro-orbital, temporal, occipital	Orbital, supraorbital, temporal
Frequency	Chronic, episodic 2 to 3 per week	Once per year to several per week	1 to 30 per month	2 to 3 times per day
Severity	Moderate/severe	Moderate/severe	Mild/moderate	Moderate/severe
Duration	May last hours to days	24 to 72 hours	May last hours to days	15 minutes to 3 hours
Pain characters	Nonthrobbing, and nonlacerating, pain usually starts in the neck	Throbbing, pulsating	Dull	Throbbing, pulsating
Triggers	Sustained postures, limited cervical ROM, pressure over or around cervical spine, trauma	Physical exertion, certain foods, environmental stresses (light or noise)	Emotional stress, muscle tension	Vascular, autonomic nervous system, increased levels of histamine
Associated symptoms	Decreased ROM, neck pain and stiffness, phonophobia, photophobia	Aura, nausea, vomiting, visual changes, phonophobia, photophobia	Occasionally decreased appetite, phonophobia, photophobia	Conjunctival injection, lacrimation, nasal congestion, rhinorrhea, forehead or facial sweating, meiosis ptosis, eyelid edema

clinician's hand for more than 1 second. It is suggested that this test is more likely to demonstrate the strength of the deep neck flexor muscles.[155,156]

Differential Diagnosis Reasoning

CGH is a syndrome that refers to the symptoms of pain perceived in any part of the head region, which arises as a result of dysfunction or inflammation of the structures originating from the cervical spine.[157] These structures can be nerves, nerve root ganglia, facet joints, intervertebral disks, ligaments, muscles, etc. Primarily, CGH is defined as a unilateral headache with associated neck pain and stiffness. However, the criteria of unilaterality have been debated,[157] as patients with bilateral headache have also been diagnosed with CGH. When symptoms of CGH become more chronic and severe, unilateral headaches can spread to the opposite

side.[157] Other important features of CGH are signs and symptoms of neck involvement, such as mechanical exacerbation of attacks with neck movements, reduced cervical ROM, ipsilateral referred pain in the neck/shoulder/arm region (can be radicular or nonradicular in nature). CGH also may be provoked with direct external palpation pressure over the structures in the upper cervical region. Pressure along the course of the greater occipital nerve, over the groove immediately behind the mastoid process, and over the upper part of the SCM muscle may exacerbate the symptoms on the same side. Furthermore, CGH may be activated by neck movements sustained in one position, awkward head positioning during sleep or during repetitive functional activities (eg, washing the ceiling, sitting in front of a computer, watching TV). The International Headache Society has recommended set criteria for differential diagnosis of a patient with CGH (Tables 13-6 and 13-7).

Table 13-7

DIFFERENTIATIONS BETWEEN DIFFERENT TYPES OF HEADACHES[158,166-170]

- Pain originating from neck and experienced in one or more head, neck, or face, fulfilling criteria of evidence of causation and pain and symptoms.
- Clinical, laboratory, and/or imaging evidence of a disorder or lesion at cervical spine or within the soft tissues surrounding the neck, suspected as the cause of the headache.
- Evidence of causation demonstrated by at least 2 of the following:
  - Headache has developed in temporal relation to the onset of the cervical disorder or appearance of the lesion.
  - Headache has significantly improved or resolved in parallel with improvement in or resolution of the cervical disorder or lesion.
  - Cervical ROM is reduced and headache is made significantly worse by provocative maneuvers.
  - Headache is abolished following diagnostic blockade of a cervical structure or its nerve supply.
- Pain and symptoms generally resolve within 3 months after successful treatment of the lesion and disorder.

DIFFERENTIAL DIAGNOSIS OF THE UPPER QUADRANT

Differential diagnosis of pain in the upper quarter is often challenging for the physical therapists because it can have many pathological sources. Pain experienced in the shoulder, upper, and forearm can be as a result of a myriad of medical conditions,[160,161] including mechanical pain from nearby musculoskeletal structures such as the cervical spine or shoulder,[161] or from regional structures such as the thoracic spine or neighboring brachial plexus.[160] Nonmechanical tissues such as metastasis of surrounding bones or referred pain from the viscera can also cause arm pain.[161] Appropriate questioning during the subjective history and selected physical measurements can assist in determining whether the pain is mechanical or nonmechanical in nature.

Murphy and Hurwitz[162] advocate the use of 3 diagnostic questions as a conceptual basis for a clinical decision-making rule in the management of mechanical and nonmechanical musculoskeletal pain. The first question is "Are the patient's symptoms reflective of a visceral disorder or a serious or potentially life-threatening illness?"[162] This question urges the therapist to consider if the signs and symptoms could be arising from nonmechanical conditions such as cancer of the surrounding bone or soft tissues, visceral pathology, fracture, disease of the gastrointestinal tract, or seronegative spondyloarthropathy. The second question is "From where is the patient's pain arising?"[162] It does not involve narrowly identifying one structural source of the pain; rather, the therapist tries to understand the characteristics about the pain source. This leads the therapist to use the appropriate tests and measures early in the physical examination to rule out conditions. The third and final question is "What has gone wrong with this person as a whole that would cause the pain experience to develop and persist?"[162] This final question encourages the therapist to consider what other variables are present that serve to maintain or perpetuate the pain experience. Possible factors for consideration are depression, passive coping, central pain hypersensitivity, and fear. The use of these 3 questions in the management of mechanical and nonmechanical musculoskeletal pain allows recognition of different conditions, likely the cause of symptoms. Special tests should be chosen based on the information gleaned in the second question, which can help in confirming the diagnosis.[5,6] Other contributory conditions that may affect prognosis should be recognized and management should be altered to affect these conditions as well.

CERVICAL RADICULOPATHY

Simply defined, cervical radiculopathy is a dysfunction of a nerve root in the cervical spine, more commonly associated with a compressive mechanism. This disorder is broad with several mechanisms of pathology present, and people of any age can be affected.[163] Peak prominence occurs between the ages of 40 to 50 years with an annual incidence 107.3 men and 63.5 women per 100,000, with a 1.7:1 ratio of men to women.[163,164]

To understand the clinical presentation of cervical radiculopathy, therapists must have a functional understanding of the relevant anatomy of the head, neck, and upper quadrant region. Since the nerve root is the primary reason for the presence of radiculopathy, any source affecting its integrity can be a culprit. Nerve roots can become compressed, inflamed, pinched, obstructed, tensioned, or mechanically sensitized from certain anatomical structures (disk herniation, or osteophytes at the zygapophyseal joints, uncovertebral joints, and vertebral end plates), certain movements of the neck or arm, and sustained positions of the neck or arm. Certain medical conditions such as changes in metabolic activity (diabetes), infection (Lyme's disease or herpes zoster), demyelination, avulsion, or neoplastic sources could also affect nerve root integrity.[165] Radicular symptoms in the C7 (70%) and C6 (20%) nerve roots are most frequently reported and can occur with or without sensory or motor changes or both. Symptoms arising in C5, C8, and T1, although rarer (10%), also require shrewd investigation.

Subjective Complaints

During the subjective history, the therapist needs to be mindful of how different anatomical structures contribute to the symptoms.

Typical symptoms of cervical radiculopathy that patients complain about are:

- Irradiating arm pain—Mostly unilateral (sometimes more specific to a particular dermatome when a single root is involved)
- Neck pain
- Paresthesia (tingling/numbness)—Mostly unilateral
- Shoulder and scapular pain
- Muscle weakness (can be arm/forearm/hand/fingers)
- Occasionally headaches can be reported

Atypical symptoms over the chest (mimicking angina), breast, or face must be carefully screened for other possible underlying pathologies. Discrete analyses of patterns associated with cervical myelopathy are pertinent because nerve root compression or spinal cord compression can both occur from the presence of cervical spondylosis.

Symptoms are generally amplified with side flexion toward the side of pain, and when an extension or rotation of the neck takes place because these movements reduce the space available for the nerve root to exit the foramen, it causes impingement or compression.[163] This often causes the patient to present with a stiff neck and a decrease in cervical spine ROM as movement may activate their symptoms. This in turn results in secondary musculoskeletal problems, which can manifest as a decrease in muscle length of the cervical spine musculature (upper fibers of trapezius, scalenes, levator scapulae); weakness; joint stiffness; capsule tightness; and postural compensations, which can affect movement strategies of other adjacent or remote areas of the body.

Finding (Red, Yellow, and Blue) Flags and Red Herrings

A detailed examination is necessary to diagnose the patient with cervical radiculopathy. Prior to performing any specialized testing, therapists need to perform a thorough medical history evaluation and a full screening of red flags should also be performed before commencing cervical examination; these steps only enhance the therapist's ability to formulate a proper diagnosis.[171] The presence of a lone red flag would not necessarily provide a strong indication of serious pathology. Its existence should be evaluated in the context of the person's subjective and medical history and then combined with the clinical findings of the examination process.[172] Provocative tests of various utilities are performed to confirm, negate, or aggravate the symptoms in the neck region or affected arm. Therapists combine clinical reasoning with these results to determine the likelihood that a cervical radiculopathy is present. Some authors promote using a clustering of clinical tests to determine if cervical radiculopathy exists; this method offers a potentially reliable and more cost-effective model to diagnostic imaging and electrophysiological testing.[173]

Patients' inappropriate misattribution of insidious symptoms to a traumatic event is common and can be misleading. Clinical reasoning is only as good as the information that it is based on indicating the importance of thorough questioning in the subjective assessment. The customary 3 types of errors that can occur in clinical reasoning include:

1. Faulty perception or elicitation of cues
2. Incomplete factual knowledge
3. Misapplication of known facts to a specific problem

Within the clinical reasoning process, physical therapists should determine if there are logical inferences for the information they are receiving from the patient. Therapists should evaluate each encounter with the patient as relevant and not be swayed by previous investigations being reported on as normal or become complacent because of the client's familiarity to the treating clinician. In the early stages, serious spinal pathology is difficult to detect. For example, weight loss is not always evident in the early stages of cancer.[172,174]

Although most therapists are familiar with red and yellow flag identification, the concept of teasing out red herrings (ie, information that is distracting, misleading or irrelevant or illogical that leads to a false conclusion) must also be part of the differential diagnosis process.[175] Misidentifying red herring signs could bias the therapist to think a radiculopathy is present when in fact there are signs that a more serious spinal pathology (eg, spinal stenosis, lower limb edema, peripheral neuropathy, cervical myelopathy, alcoholism, diabetes, MS, upper motor neuron disease) exists instead.[175] When completing a self-assessment of one's own personal assessment and examination style, it is important for therapists to encompass all information obtained (subjective information, threats of red flags or red herrings, provocative testing, and clinical presentation) in the context of the patient's current presenting condition and not rely on any one finding to determine the diagnosis outcome.[174,175]

There are certain signs and symptoms that when observed in a patient's examination or history, alerts us to the fact that something could be seriously wrong. Red flags are indicators of possible serious pathology that requires urgent further investigation and physician referral. These indicators are inflammatory or neurological conditions, structural musculoskeletal damage or disorders, circulatory problems, suspected infections, tumors, or systemic disease. Thus, every physical therapist should be aware and trained in identifying red flags.

Some examples of red flags[172,175]:

- Systemic disease or inflammatory condition—Resting pulse greater than 100 beats per minute, resting respiration greater than 25 beats per minute, fatigue
- Cauda equine syndrome
- Suspicion of fracture
- Sudden weight loss greater than 10 pounds over 3 months (suspect for cancer)
- Previous history of cancer
- Bowel and bladder incontinence

Yellow flags are the psychosocial flags responsible for and associated with poor outcomes to the intervention and prognosis.[174,176] Yellow flags are factors that increase a patient's risk for developing a long-term disability.[176] Ideally, yellow flags include aspects of thoughts, feelings, and behaviors.

Some examples of yellow flags[174,176]:

- Beliefs, appraisals, and judgments—Catastrophizing; thinking the worst; expectations of poor outcome from treatment; etc
- Pain behavior—Fear of movement and re-injury; over-reliance on passive treatment approach
- Emotional response—Fear, anxiety, low moods, being too preoccupied with health

Blue flags indicate a patient's perception toward work/job duties and concerns about the ability to do those activities.

Examples of blue flags[177]:

- Belief that work is the cause of injury and will further aggravate injury
- Feeling unappreciated and unsupported at workplace

Tests to Assess Yellow Flags

Depression Screening

Screening tools such as the Beck Depression Inventory or the Depression Anxiety Screening Scale are useful in screening patients for depression. Psychometric properties of the Beck Depression Inventory show a cut-off score of 5 or more for screening (sensitivity = 0.90, specificity = 0.17) and a cut-off score of 22 or more for diagnostic utility (sensitivity = 0.27, specificity = 0.90).[178,179]

Pain Catastrophizing

The Pain Catastrophizing Scale (PCS) helps determine if the patient is exaggerating their pain and/or symptoms and the severity of the situation as a whole. Cronbach alpha values reported for the total PCS (α = .87) and factor scales (rumination α = .87; magnification α = .60; helplessness α = .87) were found to be satisfactory. The total PCS score showed strong temporal validity.[180] In a patient population with a different type of condition (acute whiplash vs radiculopathy), there is a significant and moderate correlation between pain pressure threshold and the PCS as well as cold pain threshold and the PCS.[181]

Application of Rules and Provocative Tests

Therapists should initiate their screening with the Canadian C-Spine Rule if any type of trauma is reported or suspected. These rules (sensitivity = 0.99, specificity = 0.45),[182] which have undergone rigorous testing, display high reliability, validity, and sensitivity for clinical use.

Differential Diagnosis— Provocation Tests

The next phase of differential diagnosis should include provocative testing and application of CPRs or clinical guidelines. Therapists should familiarize themselves with the literature surrounding these options and make critical decisions about including them into their development of a proper diagnosis.

As mentioned earlier, reflex testing, sensory testing, and manual muscle testing are habitually completed by therapists attempting to find a neurological component to a patient's complaints; however, the helpfulness of these tests have been questioned. Testing of reflexes are described in Table 13-8.

SENSORY TESTING

Typically, sensory testing includes 3 components: pin prick, dull, and light touch testing methods. Common objects found in any clinic can be used for this aspect of the examination: a thumb tack/pin, round edge of a paper clip or eraser tip, and a swipe of a fingertip, respectively. Although reliability for sensation testing has been completed, kappa values are varied (kappa = 0.16 for C8 pin prick[173] to kappa = 0.90 for light touch along the medial cutaneous nerve); the data on sensitivity and specificity testing are lacking.[183] Wainner et al[173] is one of the few researchers to study pin prick across the cervical dermatomes in isolation from C5-T1. Pin prick testing to the C5 dermatome has the greatest reliability (kappa = 0.67, sensitivity = 0.29, specificity = 0.86), T1 testing is next (kappa = 0.46, sensitivity = 0.18, specificity = 0.79), with more pertinent testing for radiculopathy (C7: kappa = 0.40, sensitivity = 0.28, specificity = 0.77 and C6: kappa = 0.28, sensitivity = 0.24, specificity = 0.66), trailing behind in utility.[173] Variations in patterns or overlapping patterns in dermatomes may skew the clinical reasoning processes of some therapists, but combining this aspect of the examination with other more useful tests may help them come to the correct conclusion. Table 13-9 represents typical body regions where each dermatome is tested.

Table 13-8

DEEP TENDON REFLEXES[173,184,185]

BODY REGION	TEST PROCEDURE	CERVICAL MYELOPATHY	CERVICAL RADICULOPATHY
Biceps (C6)	The patient is seated with the arm supported, relaxed and in small amount of supination. The therapist places thumb over the tendon at the elbow and briskly hits the thumb with the reflex hammer. Testing should produce the reflex reaction of elbow flexion.	Intraclass correlation coefficient (ICC) = 89%, sensitivity = 0.44, specificity = 0.71, sensitivity = 0.18, specificity = 0.96 Positive test: Hyperreflexia	kappa = 0.73, sensitivity = 0.24, specificity = 0.95 Positive test: A decline in the reflex when assessed against the opposite limb. Baseline is normal.
Brachioradialis (C6)	The patient is seated with the arm supported, relaxed and in small amount of pronation. The therapist places thumb over the junction where the muscle meets the tendon and briskly hits this location with the reflex hammer. Testing should produce the reflex reaction of elbow flexion with some pronation.	Not used	kappa = 0.73, sensitivity = 0.24, specificity = 0.95 Positive test: A decline in the reflex when assessed against the opposite limb. Baseline is normal.
Triceps (C7)	The patient is seated with the arm supported, relaxed, and placed in 90 degrees of shoulder extension and 90 degrees of elbow flexion. The therapist places the thumb over the distal tendon at the elbow and briskly hits the thumb with the reflex hammer. Testing should produce the reflex reaction of elbow extension.	ICC = 89% sensitivity = 0.44, specificity = 0.71, sensitivity = 0.18, specificity = 0.96 Positive test: Hyperreflexia	ICC = not reported, sensitivity = 0.03, specificity = 0.93 Positive test: A decline in the reflex when assessed against the opposite limb. Baseline is normal.

Table 13-9

CERVICAL LEVELS AND ASSOCIATED DERMATOMES, MYOTOMES, AND DEEP TENDON REFLEXES[163-165,187-189]

NERVE ROOTS	SENSORY TESTING	MOTOR TESTING	REFLEX
C1-C2	Front of the face	Neck flexion	No reflexes
C3	Lateral face and skull	Lateral flexion of cervical spine	No reflexes
C4	Upper shoulder/ acromioclavicular joint area	Diaphragm, shoulder shrugs	No reflexes
C5	Lateral shoulder/upper arm	Shoulder abduction	Biceps (musculocutaneous)
C6	Lateral lower arm and hand (thumb and index finger)	Elbow flexion and wrist extension	Brachioradialis (musculocutaneous)
C7	Palmer aspect of hand— middle 3 fingers	Elbow extension and wrist flexion	Triceps (radial)
C8	Little finger and medial lower arm	Finger flexion and thumb extension	No reflexes
T1	Upper arm and medial elbow region	Finger abduction	No reflexes

MANUAL MUSCLE TESTING/ STRENGTH TESTING

Cook and Hegedus[186] offer insightful data on the usefulness of a variety of manual muscle tests for cervically innervated musculature (C1-T1). A review of this literature shows a high variance in kappa values (kappa = 0.23 for the flexor carpi radialis to kappa = 0.69 for the biceps) with high specificity ranges (specificity = 0.89 for the deltoid and flexor carpi radialis and specificity = 0.94 for the biceps), but unfortunately the data have low sensitivity numbers (ranging from 3% to only 24%). Caution should be used for any of these tests, especially if used in isolation or as a final confirming test. Therapists screening patients with suspected radiculopathy should also consider assessing other muscles of the upper extremity and cervical and thoracic spine, as a part of comprehensive examination.

Special Tests

Spurling Test

The test is first assessed at rest with the patient in sitting for signs of any pain. If there is no pain at rest, then the patient is asked to perform active side-bending toward the limb with the complaints. The test is positive if any pain down the limb is experienced during this active motion. If there are no reproductions of symptoms, the examiner must then merge a combination of passive compression and additional side-bending toward the side of the body with symptoms. Reproduction of familiar radicular pain indicates a positive test as well. Provoked symptoms for this test can include paresthesia or pain into the limb. Some authors report a negative finding if only neck pain is produced. Some discrepancies are noted in the sensitivity and specificity of this test. Spurling A—(kappa = 0.60, sensitivity = 0.50, specificity = 0.86)[186] and Spurling B (side-bending, rotation and extension; kappa = 0.62, sensitivity = 0.50, specificity = 0.74).[173] Clinical variations of the Spurling test include adding in rotation or extension to the testing protocol.[190,191]

Cervical Distraction Test (Kappa = 0.88, Sensitivity = 0.44, Specificity = 0.90)

This test is typically performed on patients who are already symptomatic. If during the technique, the patient reports a reduction in symptoms, the test response is positive and helps the therapist rule in the presence of radicular pain. With the patient supine and head well supported, the physical therapist employs a long axis traction force directly through the cervical spine. Typically, 3 different conditions of distraction are performed: an initial gentle traction pull, a controlled traction pull past the point of pain, and the use of repeated trials. If partial or full relief of symptoms is noted, the therapist could consider this a viable option for treatment.[173]

Upper Limb Tension Tests (Kappa = 0.75, Sensitivity = 0.97, Specificity = 0.22)

Performing tests with good sensitivity early in the examination helps enhance therapists' ability to rule out a condition that is being considered as a potential diagnosis, such as radiculopathy. Along with its high kappa value and robust sensitivity rating, a lack of symptoms with median nerve upper limb testing (negative response to the provocation positioning), make this test a clear choice for all clinicians. The radial nerve is another structure commonly tested when radiculopathy is suspected; however, even though it possesses better interrater reliability testing (kappa = 0.83)[186] than the median nerve, its lower sensitivity value (sensitivity = 0.72, specificity = 0.33)[186] makes this a less compelling test for clinical use. Other tests for the ulnar nerve have not been studied enough and carry little weight for confirming or refuting the presence of cervical radiculopathy. In simplified terms, passive median nerve testing progressively moves the patient's arm through a series of different positions and assesses the patient's response or lack of response at each step. An example of median nerve progression is listed here:

1. Lying supine and at rest
2. After the initiation of shoulder abduction to approximately 90 degrees (this requires manual pressure or a blocking maneuver over the shoulder girdle; the patient's elbow is typically flexed to approximately 90 degrees, wrist is secured, and slight tension is placed on the thumb into extension)
3. After shoulder abduction to 110 degrees and slight extension
4. After introducing forearm supination, wrist flexion, and finger flexion
5. After shoulder external rotation to approximately 90 degrees
6. After elbow extension
7. After cervical lateral flexion away (or toward) the involved limb[173]

Valsalva Test (Kappa = 0.63, Sensitivity = 0.22, Specificity = 0.94)

While seated, the client performs a bearing down maneuver while simultaneously holding their breath. If pain is reported during the maneuver, the therapist would assign a positive rating to the test. If a client is unfamiliar with the term *bearing down*, a therapist would explain that this maneuver is similar to actions needed to pass a bowel movement.[173,186]

Shoulder Abduction Test (Kappa = 0.22, Sensitivity = 0.17, Specificity = 0.92)

The shoulder abduction test is commonly performed for ruling in the presence of radicular pain due its simplicity. Here, the therapist directs the patient to position the hand on the top of the head; an improvement in symptoms (typically pain) is assessed and considered a positive test. Performing this posture a few times each day could promote temporary changes in symptoms for a client suffering from radicular pain. Unfortunately, this test provides therapists with dichotomous data (yes or no, there is a change in symptoms) but offers no insight on which cervical nerve root is the source.[192]

Importance of Clustered Testing

Wainner et al[173] devised a CPR for radiculopathy with 4 main criteria best suited to assist therapists during their differential diagnosis process (Spurling, Cervical Distraction Test, ULTT for the median nerve and involved cervical rotation less than 60 degrees). The last criterion—involved cervical rotation less than 60 degrees (sensitivity = 0.89, specificity = 0.49)—is an easy clinical test to perform. A few other helpful CPRs used to help differentiate different diagnoses in the upper quadrant are summarized in Table 13-10. Unfortunately, all of these diagnostic CPRs for the cervical spine and upper quadrant testing are in the derivation stage.

Clinical Prediction Rules

Yes Rationale, Once Validated

- Step 1: Development or derivation phase, caution with widespread use
- Step 2: Validation, across other population, randomized control trial, more generalizability, widespread clinical use
- Step 3: Utility and impact effect

Cervical Myelopathy

Background

Myelopathy can result from congenital narrowing, progressive spondylolitic changes in the cervical spine structure, and/or increased degenerative changes in the intervertebral disks. Patients aged 45 years or more are more likely to be diagnosed with this condition than younger individuals.[193-196] Past history of radiculopathy or previous symptoms from signs of cervical spondylosis are associated with myelopathy. Patients with myelopathy can experience changes in mobility, ataxic gait, altered function, differing levels of disability, and can report a reduced quality of life. Upper motor neuron signs (Babinski sign, Hoffmann test, and clonus) occur as pressure on the spinal cord increases or structural changes progress causing more central stenosis narrowing.[193] Later signs of progression can exhibit both lower motor neuron signs (reduced reflexes, segmental weakness, and atrophy) often at the level of compression and upper motor neuron signs and below the level of compression during clinical setting.[193,194] Common sites for lower motor neuron signs tend

Table 13-10 ———————————————————————————

CLINICAL PREDICTION RULES[173,184,185,192,193,197]

POSSIBLE DIAGNOSIS	CLINICAL PREDICTION RULE TESTS
Cervical radiculopathy	1. + Upper Limb Tension Test A (ULTTA) 2. + Spurling test 3. + Distraction test 4. Cervical rotation less than 60 degrees on the ipsilateral side All 4 tests + (sensitivity = 0.24, specificity = 0.99) Any 3 tests + (sensitivity = 0.39, specificity = 0.94) Any 2 tests + (sensitivity = 0.39, specificity = 0.56)
Cervical myelopathy	1. Gait deviations 2. + Hoffmann test 3. + Inverted supinator sign 4. + Babinski test 5. Age more than 45 years Any 4 of 5 + (sensitivity = 0.90, specificity = 1.00) Any 3 of 5 + (sensitivity = 0.19, specificity = 0.99) Any 2 of 5 + (sensitivity = 0.39, specificity = 0.88) Any 1 of 5 + (sensitivity = 0.94, specificity = 0.31)
Carpal tunnel	1. Handshaking does not improve symptoms 2. Wrist-ratio index greater than 0.67 3. Symptom severity scale score greater than 1.9 4. Diminished sensation in median sensory field 1 (thumb) 5. Age more than 45 years All 5 of 5 + (sensitivity = 0.18, specificity = 0.95) Any 4 of 5 + (sensitivity = 0.77, specificity = 0.83) Any 3 of 5 + (sensitivity = 0.98, specificity = 0.54) Any 2 of 5 + (sensitivity = 0.98, specificity = 0.14)
Shoulder (subacromial) impingement	1. + Hawkins-Kennedy test 2. + Painful arc sign 3. + Infraspinatus muscle test Cluster (sensitivity = 0.33, specificity = 0.98)
Rotator cuff pathology	1. + Hawkins-Kennedy test 2. + Drop arm test 3. + Full can test 4. + External rotation lag sign 5. Weakness in external rotation movement (Sensitivity = 0.30, specificity = 0.86)

to occur between levels C5-C7, possibly causing bias to the distracted or rushed examiner. Spinal cord ischemia, from compression over the blood supply to the cord, can occur during the natural course of progression. Severe signs of compression can lead to signs of paralysis in the limbs, loss of hand function or fluctuations, or loss in control of bowel or bladder function. All therapists need to be aware that immediate medical management is recommended for any patient presenting with rapid or progressive onset of sphincter or elimination issue for any bowel and bladder, regardless of diagnosis. Therapists need to use solid clinical reasoning and research-based clinical diagnostic tests to help differentiate signs and symptoms of other conditions such as cervical radiculopathy (common C5-C7 origin), MS (gait and balance disturbances), amyotrophic lateral sclerosis (onset of disease, mixed upper and lower motor neuron signs), cauda equina (bowel and bladder deficits, lower extremity findings), stroke (upper and lower limb presentation, balance concerns), Guillain-Barré syndrome (presence of quadriparesis or paraparesis, but additional CN signs that are absent in myelopathy) all of which can present with overlapping or similar clinical presentations or symptoms to myelopathy.[194-196]

Presentation of nondermatomal sensory patterns, spreading of pain in other extremities, pain that is disproportionate to an injury or pain lasting longer than expected are likely signs of central mediated pain vs myelopathy. Since progression of myelopathy produces more destructive and potentially life-altering effects than cervical radiculopathy, referrals to other medical professionals may be needed to best manage care for these patients. Early operative management of myelopathy can help prevent progression of symptoms. Although cord compressions can occur in other areas of the spine (thoracic and lumbar region), this chapter focuses only on the myelopathy found in the cervical spine region.

Subjective Complaints

The first subtle sign often reported in patients with myelopathy signs is a change in gait quality or stiffness symptoms in the lower extremities. Mild cases may also report slight dizziness and occasionally neck discomfort. Once progression occurs, patients can experience a fluctuation or worsening of symptoms with different neck positions. Signs of spastic-like gait are both reported and observed. Functional limitation can be expressed as lower extremity weakness, antalgic gait, fatigue during gait, balance disturbances, and hand clumsiness.

Special Tests

Hoffmann Test (ICC = 89%, Sensitivity = 0.44, Specificity = 0.75)

During this test, the middle finger of the patient first must be passively stabilized above the distal interphalangeal joint, then a quick downward flick is applied to the distal tip of the patient's finger. If the patient demonstrates movement in the thumb (opposition and adduction) and slight flexion in the fingers, the test is considered positive. Several other authors have claimed sensitivity scores between 0.81 and 0.94; however, these studies possess a higher level of bias in their methodology.[184,198,199]

Babinski Sign (ICC = 89%, Sensitivity = 0.33, Specificity = 0.92)

The therapist, using a blunt edge, applies an upward stroke along the lateral plantar surface of the patient's neutrally positioned foot (preferably while the patient is supine). When negative, slight toe flexion is seen. Great toe extension can be seen when the test is positive.[184]

Clonus Testing (ICC = 98%, Sensitivity = 0.11, Specificity = 0.96)

This technique is commonly performed on a patient's ankle in sitting or supine while in passive dorsiflexion; however, as an alternative, it can be performed on the wrist (into passive extension) as well. The therapist first utilizes a swift overpressure maneuver into dorsiflexion (wrist extension) and then maintains pressure through the joint. When 3 or more involuntary "beats" of movement are seen, the test is considered positive. It is important for the therapist to remember that 1 or 2 beats of movement is still considered a normal response.[184]

Inverted Supinator Sign (ICC = 78%, Sensitivity = 0.61, Specificity = 0.78)

With the patient's elbow held in flexion, slightly pronated, and fully relaxed, the therapist rapidly taps or hits the distal attachment of the brachioradialis (tendon) repeated times. The test is considered positive if finger flexion or a small amount of elbow extension is seen.[184]

Gait Deviations (Sensitivity = 0.19, Specificity = 0.94)

After observing a patient's gait, the therapist makes a judgment call if any of these abnormalities are observed: ataxia, wide-based gait, or signs of spastic gait. A kinematic study analyzing gait mechanics during walking and treadmill activities (N = 12) of patients with myelopathy revealed that, prior to surgical correction and decompression, these patients ambulated with increased step width, longer than normal double limb support, reduced ankle motion, and significant difference in gait velocity and step length.[185,200]

Lhermitte's Sign or Phenomenon (Sensitivity = 0.03, Specificity = 0.97)

Performed sitting or standing, the patient is asked to move the neck into flexion and asked if any symptoms are reproduced. The test is considered positive if the client reports the sensation of an "electric" shock in the middle of the spinal region, but evidence on the utility of this test is limited.

Table 13-11

THORACIC OUTLET SYNDROME[204-208]

TYPE	COMPRESSION	PERCENT OF CASES	TYPICAL SYMPTOMS	OTHER
Neurogenic	Brachial plexus	95%	Numbness Weakness Dysesthesia	Vague, nonanatomic, not always in particular peripheral nerve distribution Motor greater than sensory Median vs ulnar nerve bias
Vascular	Subclavian vein	3%	Extremity swelling Deep vein thrombosis	Extremity swelling—changes in girth measurement Deep vein thrombosis—possible limb discoloration
Arterial	Subclavian artery	1%	Arm pain with exertion Thromboembolism Acute arterial thrombosis Possible temperature changes Pallor distal extremity or hand	Diminished pulses

Hypothetically, therapists could rationalize the presence of other serious pathology within in the cervical region (possibly presence of MS plaque or spinal nerve trauma) with this test, but research solidifying this finding is inadequate.[193,201]

THORACIC OUTLET SYNDROME

Background

The term *TOS* can represent a variety of symptoms in the upper quadrant and has been linked to a large array of different terms.[202,203] Unwanted compression that is adjacent to or involving the scalene triangle, pectoralis minor, or costoclavicular space are common sources.[204-207] Traditionally, TOS is classified into 3 categories: neurogenic, vascular, and arterial. The neurogenic form represents 95% of all cases (Table 13-11).[202,203,207] Occurrence is 1:1,000,000 for true neurogenic TOS with higher ratios (9:1) for women.[204,205]

Clinical Anatomy

From a muscular standpoint, the scalene group, with attachments to both the cervical spine and upper ribs, should be the primary site the physical therapist examines followed by the pectoralis minor. Shortening of the pectoralis minor can lead to a narrowing of subcoracoid or subpectoralis minor space, thus leading to compression of the neurovascular structures with hyperabduction movements.[206] Other pertinent muscles to assess include the subclavius and SCM.

All muscles should be assessed for irritability to palpation, presence of trigger points, symptom provocation during contraction, hypertrophy, muscle length flexibility, and any abnormalities in origins or insertions that are variants or congenital.

The structure can also be compressed in the costoclavicular triangle, which is bordered anteriorly by the middle third of the clavicle, posteromedially by the first rib, and posterolaterally by the upper border of the scapula.[204,206]

Hence, assessments of tissues and other structures of the upper quadrant including clavicle, first 2 intercostal spaces, cervicothoracic junction, and structures attaching to the sternoclavicular region should not be ignored.

Anatomical abnormalities can also be a potential cause for compromising the thoracic outlet as well. This can include abnormal C7 vertebrae, presence of cervical rib, upper thoracic spine hypomobility, clavicular hypomobility, and abnormal soft tissue changes around lower cervical and upper thoracic spine.[206]

Subjective Complaints

Careful delineation of symptom location (eg, specific to neck, upper arm, forearm, hand, fingers), type of symptoms reported (eg, numbness, tingling, weakness, pain, fatigue, sensation of limb "falling asleep," temperature changes), and frequency of symptoms (eg, constant, intermittent, only with positional or overhead maneuvers) may help refine where the chief complaint is.

Injuries to the upper quadrant such as a past history of a motor vehicle accident (hyperflexion-extension mechanisms), bike collision (head, shoulder, or clavicular trauma), fall or slip (strike to the head, outstretched arm, fractures in the upper quadrant), or musculoskeletal overuse from occupational (lifting, reaching) or sports/recreational (throwing, pitching, swimming, racquet sports, weight lifting) activities could enhance suspicions that a particular body region is inflamed or requires closer examination.[209,210]

Probable causes of the injury could be[204,205,211,212]:

- Neurapraxia and/or brachial plexus irritation (eg, Was this caused from carrying a backpack? Did the client report a recent hiking trip?)

- Other sources of injury (eg, Past history of scalene blocks? Past or recent surgery where the arm was placed in traction during the procedure? Was there neonatal trauma or stress to the arm during delivery?)

Associated symptoms of neurogenic compression can include pain, numbness, dysesthesia, and weakness. In the later stages, there might be thenar-biased hand intrinsic weakness (median nerve), especially with overhead activities; swelling in upper extremity (most commonly in hand and forearm); and ulnar sensory changes.[208]

Arterial compression is the most rare form; however, if severe, an urgent diagnosis is needed. Changes in temperature (typically cooler), paresthesia, pain, and limb color changes (pallor) can occur. For the younger population or someone with persistent symptoms, the presence of a cervical rib needs to be ruled out.[203,207,210]

Special Tests

There is moderate evidence to support the use of clinical diagnostic tests in the differential diagnosis of upper-extremity pathology. However, these clinical diagnostic tests do not allow for the differential diagnosis of TOS exclusively. Most of the special tests used for differential diagnosis of TOS have poor reliability and have been inconsistent.[186,192] Hence, clinicians should be careful and use caution in diagnosing a patient for TOS just based on these special tests. Diagnosis of TOS should be made based on a strong correlation and should be developed between subjective complaints, objective findings, and special tests.

Elevated Arm Stress Test (Sensitivity = 0.52 to 0.84, Specificity = 0.30 to 0.100)

Patient is seated with arms above 90 degrees of abduction and full external rotation with head in neutral position. Patient opens and closes hands into fists while holding the elevated position for 3 minutes. Positive test: pain and/or paresthesia and discontinuation with dropping of the arms for relief of pain.[186,213]

Adson's Test (Sensitivity = 0.79, Specificity = 0.74 to 0.100)

Patient is seated with arms at the side. The radial pulse is palpated. Patient inhales deeply, holds the breath, extends, and rotates the neck toward the side being tested. Positive test: change in radial pulse and/or pain, paresthesia reproduction.[186,213]

Wright's Test (Sensitivity = 0.70 to 0.90, Specificity = 0.29 to 0.53)

Patient is seated with arms at the side. The radial pulse is palpated. Examiner places the patient's shoulder into abduction above the head. The position is held for 1 to 2 minutes. Positive test: change in radial pulse and/or symptom reproduction.[213]

Costoclavicular Maneuver (Sensitivity = Not Tested, Specificity = 0.53 to 1.00)

Patient sits straight with arms at the side. Radial pulse is assessed. Patient retracts and depresses shoulders while protruding the chest. Position is held for up to 1 minute. Positive test: change in radial pulse and/or pain and paresthesia.[213]

Supraclavicular Pressure (Sensitivity = Not Tested, Specificity = 0.85 to 0.98)

Patient is seated with arms at the side. Examiner places fingers on the upper trapezius, and the thumbs contact the anterior scalene muscle near the first ribs. The examiner squeezes the fingers and thumb together for 30 seconds. Positive test: reproduction of pain or paresthesia.[204]

Cyriax Release (Sensitivity = Not Tested, Specificity = 0.77 to 0.97)

Patient is seated or standing. Examiner stands behind patient and grasps under the forearms, holding the elbows at 80 degrees of flexion with the forearms and wrists in neutral. Examiner leans the patient's trunk posteriorly and passively elevates the shoulder girdle. The position is held for up to 3 minutes. Positive test: paresthesia and/or numbness (release phenomenon) or symptom reproduction.[204]

T4 Syndrome

T4 syndrome is a relatively uncommon condition in which spinal injury and/or significant hypomobility at the T4 vertebra can cause a set of symptoms such as diffuse arm pain and pins and needles or numbness in the upper arm associated with or without headaches and upper back stiffness.[214,215]

Subjective Complaints

Patients generally complain of a peculiar glove-like distribution of pain in their hand or forearm, which can often lead to a mistaken diagnosis, including psychogenesis.[216] Referred pain into the neck and scapular regions may also be associated with T4 syndrome. T4 syndrome is more common in women than men and in patients who work with a flexed posture (ie, at a computer, cash register, assembly line).[214,217]

Cause

The cause of T4 syndrome is unknown but may be linked with joint hypomobility and faulty postural alignment. Both the thoracic intervertebral disks and thoracic zygapophyseal joints are thought to be primary pain generators in T4 syndrome based on their pain patterns.[217,218] The upper-mid thoracic spine tends to be hypomobile with the T2-T7 region of the sympathetic chain supplying the upper extremity. Thus, it is hypothesized that sympathetic dysfunction, somehow related to vertebral dysfunction in the upper thoracic region (T2-T7), causes a referred or reflex phenomenon in the arm or hands due to the close proximity of the sympathetic chain to the thoracic spine.[209-219]

Examination

To start, a thorough neurological examination should also be conducted to rule out any neural involvement as the neurological examination presents normal in patients with T4 syndrome.[213,217] Palpation and segmental assessment of the thoracic vertebrae will display tenderness and hypomobility at and around the T2-T7 segments with the T4 segment being the most involved.[217,218] Unfortunately, there are no special tests available to diagnose T4 syndrome.

Differential Diagnosis

T4 syndrome is a fairly uncommon diagnosis, and it can be misdiagnosed because of this.[214,216] It is a diagnosis of exclusion. Diagnoses such as myelopathy, cardiac pain, TOS, systemic illness, thoracic tumor, polyneuritis, fibromyalgia, nerve root compression, and complex regional pain syndrome should be ruled out before considering T4 syndrome as the diagnosis.

Case Studies

To help integrate what was presented in this chapter let us examine these case studies to test your knowledge.

Key factors to consider:

- Subjective history
- Red and yellow flags and red herrings
- Screening process using tests with high sensitivity
- Physical examination and testing
- Clinical reasoning
- Implementing EBP
- Differential diagnosis

Based only on the data in Table 13-12 and the information presented in this chapter, try to determine which diagnosis is present. Does the data in the table support a certain diagnosis? What information is missing in the subjective or objective portions? What red flags or red herrings would have swayed the therapist's decision?

Other Questions to Ponder

1. How significant is the age of these patients in the case studies? What if all these patients were between 25 and 35 years of age or all of them were more than 65 years of age? How differently would you have processed the information given?

2. How influential was sex in your clinical reasoning? Would you have come up with the same diagnoses if the sex was switched?

3. At what point during your examination and screening process would you consider getting additional medical screening, imaging, or lab work?

Table 13-12

CASE STUDIES' DATA

INFORMATION	PATIENT 1	PATIENT 2	PATIENT 3
Onset	Progressive 1 month	Sudden 1 day	Insidious 3 months
Gender	Woman	Woman	Woman
Age (years)	45	50	55
Subjective information	Worse after overhead painting No headache Throbbing pain Enjoys cycling	Slipped down steps and hit her head Intermittent headache	Nontraumatic Dizziness reported Photo sensitivity Nonthrobbing
Pain	Ipsilateral neck pain and middle finger tingling	Bilateral head pain Neck pain	Ipsilateral shoulder pain and unilateral head pain
Severity	Moderate to mild	Moderate	Severe
Palpation	Tenderness in the upper quadrant, vague	Tenderness over central spine	Tenderness over upper cervical region (C0-C3) and mastoid process
ROM	Backward bending worsens pain, ipsilateral side-bending Rotation less than 60 degrees Repetitive reaching overhead provokes pain	Rotation is less than 45 degrees	Some neck motions are limited and worse with awkward positioning and/or repetitive motions
PPIVMs	Limited C5-C6, C6-C7	Not tolerated	Restricted C1-C3
Strength	Weak triceps Weak wrist flexion	None	Low endurance for craniocervical flexors Deep neck flexors
Sensory testing	Reduced pin prick middle finger	No deficits	Sensitive over occipital nerve region
Possible screening to consider	Wainner's CPR for radiculopathy	Cervical spine rules to assess for fracture	CNs must be clear, rule out serious pathology related to central nervous system

(continued)

Table 13-12 (continued)

CASE STUDIES' DATA

INFORMATION	PATIENT 1	PATIENT 2	PATIENT 3
Which diagnosis is correct?	Radiculopathy involving C6 or C7?	Mechanical neck pain or cervical fracture?	CGH or migraine?
Supporting evidence used and strength of evidence	Wainner et al[173] (moderate) American Physical Therapy Association (APTA) Neck Guidelines	Sterling et al (strong) International Federation Orthopedic Manipulative Physical Therapists (IFOMPT) Screening (clinical guideline) APTA Neck Pain Clinical Practice Guidelines	International Headache Criteria (clinical guideline), IFOMPT screening (clinical guideline) APTA Neck Pain Clinical Practice Guidelines
Most sensitive and specific tests used in screening process	+ ULTTA + Spurling test + Distraction test Cervical rotation less than 60 degrees on the ipsilateral side	(-) ULTTA (-) Hoffmann test (-) Spurling test (-) Distraction test + Hypomobility at cervical and thoracic spine	Supine and cervical passive ROM (premanipulative hold test) Seated and cervical AROM (minimized deKleyn test)
What if the following additional information was added to the case study or replaced some of the following data	Pain was reported in the upper arm or scapular region and biceps weakness was significant	Full neck motion Vague tenderness over upper quadrant	Presence of fever chills, weight loss, systemic change in health, new head pain that started after 50 years old
Possible new or completing diagnosis	C6 radiculopathy	Mechanical neck pain	Cancer with metastasis to the head or brain
What data or information would need to change or be added to the case study to support this alternative diagnosis?	Cervical myelopathy	Upper cervical instability	Vertebral artery insufficiency
How influential would these red flags or red herring signs affect the clinical-reasoning process for the final diagnosis?	• No arm weakness but complaints of chest pain, left arm pain, and indigestion • Nonanatomic distribution of pain or dysesthesia • Hand intrinsic weakness, cervical rib, playing a racquet sport vs cycling • History of Raynaud's or diabetes	• Clinical depression • Difficulty swallowing • A bike collision or motor vehicle accident • Inability to hold the arm in abduction and weakness of shoulder external rotation	• Difficulty swallowing • Presence of aura and sensitivity to noises • Worsening pain when performing Valsalva (bearing down) maneuver • Rapid sudden onset of head pain, "headache like none other"
Answers	C7	Cervical fracture	CGH

REFERENCES

1. Guyatt G, Rennie D, Meade M, Cook D. *Users' Guide to the Medical Literature: A Manual for Evidence-Based Clinical Practice.* 2nd ed. McGraw-Hill; 2008.

2. Smith R, Rennie D. Evidence-based medicine- an oral history. *BMJ.* 2014;384;g371. doi:10.1136/bmj.g371

3. Dawes M, Summerskill W, Glasziou P, et al. Sicily statement on evidence-based practice. *BMC Med Educ.* 2005;5:1. doi:10.1186/1472-6920-5-1

4. Tilson JK, Kaplan SL, Harris JL, et al. Sicily statement on classification and development of evidence-based practice learning assessment tools. *BMC Med Educ.* 2011;11:78. doi:10.1186/1472-6920-11-78

5. Richardson WS, Wilson MC, Guyatt GH. Users' guides to the medical literature XV. How to use an article about disease probability for differential diagnosis. *JAMA.* 1999;281(13):1214-1219. doi:10.1001/jama.281.13.1214

6. Cook C, Hegedus E. *Orthopedic Physical Examination Tests: An Evidence-Based Approach.* Prentice-Hall Publishing; 2007.

7. American Physical Therapy Association. *Guide to Physical Therapist Practice 4.0.* 2023. Accessed April 27, 2023. https://guide.apta.org/

8. Tversky A, Kahneman D. Judgement under uncertainty: heuristics and biases. *Science.* 1974;185(4157):1124-1131. doi:10.1126/science.185.4157.1124

9. Doody C, McAteer M. Clinical reasoning of expert and novice physiotherapists in an outpatient orthopaedic setting. *Physiotherapy.* 2002;28(5):258-268. doi:10.1016/S0031-9406(05)61417-4

10. Guyatt GH, Sackett DL, Cook DJ. Users' guide to the medical literature: II. How to use an article about therapy and prevention: A. Are the results of the study valid? Evidence-based medicine working group. *JAMA.* 1993;270:2598-2601.

11. Guyatt GH, Sackett DL, Cook DJ. Users' guide to the medical literature: II. How to use an article about therapy and prevention: B. What were the results and will they help me in caring for my patients? Evidence-based medicine working group. *JAMA.* 1994;271(1):59-63. doi:10.1001/jama.271.1.59

12. Higgs J, Jones M. Clinical decision making and multiple problem spaces. In: Higgs J, Jones MA, Loftus S, Christensen N. *Clinical reasoning in health professions.* Elsevier; 2008:4-19.

13. Pauker SG, Kassirer JP. The threshold approach to clinical decision making. *N Engl J Med.* 1980;302(20):1109-1117. doi:10.1056/NEJM198005153022003

14. Jaeschke R, Guyatt GH, Scakett DL. Users' guides to the medical literature: III. How to use an article about a diagnostic test: A. Are the results of the study valid? Evidence-based medicine working group. *JAMA.* 1994;271(5):389-391. doi:10.1001/jama.271.5.389

15. Jaeschke R, Guyatt GH, Scakett DL. Users' guides to the medical literature: III. How to use an article about a diagnostic test: B. What are the results and will they help me in caring for my patients? Evidence-based medicine working group. *JAMA.* 1994;271(9):703-707. doi:10.1001/jama.1994.03510330081039

16. Cleland JA, Markowski AM, Childs JD. *Current Concepts of Orthopedic Physical Therapy. The Cervical Spine: Physical Therapy Patient Management Utilizing Current Evidence.* 2nd ed. American Physical Therapy Association; 2006.

17. Bovim G, Schrader H, Sand T. Neck pain in the general population. *Spine.* 1994;19(12):1307-1309. doi:10.1097/00007632-199406000-00001

18. Elnagger IM, Nordin M, Sheikhzadeh A, Parnianpour M, Kahanovitz N. Effects of spinal flexion and extension exercises on low-back pain and spinal mobility in chronic mechanical low-back pain patients. *Spine.* 1991;16(8):967-972. doi:10.1097/00007632-199108000-00018

19. Cote P, Cassidy J, Carroll L. The factors associated with neck pain and its related disability in the Saskatchewan population. *Spine.* 2000;25(9):1109-1117. doi:10.1097/00007632-200005010-00012

20. Cote P, Cassidy JD, Carroll L. The Saskatchewan Heath and Back Pain Survey. The prevalence of neck pain and related disability in Saskatchewan adults. *Spine.* 1998;23(15):1689-1698. doi:10.1097/00007632-199808010-00015

21. Linton SJ, Ryberg M. Do epidemiological results replicate? The prevalence and health-economic consequences of neck and back pain in the general population. *Eur J Pain.* 2000;4(4):347-354. doi:10.1053/eujp.2000.0190

22. Palmer KT, Walker-Bone K, Griffin MJ, et al. Prevalence and occupational associations of neck pain in the British population. *Scand J Work Environ Health.* 2001;27(1):49-56. doi:10.5271/sjweh.586

23. Brattberg G, Thorslund M, Wikman A. The prevalence of pain in a general population. The results of a postal survey in a county of Sweden. *Pain.* 1989;37(2):215-222. doi:10.1016/0304-3959(89)90133-4

24. Bennett JG, Bergmanis LE, Carpenter JK, Skowlund HV. Range of motion of the neck. *J Amer Phys Ther Arroc.* 1963;43:45-47. doi:10.1093/ptj/43.1.45

25. Buck CA Darneron FB, Dew MJ, Skowlund HV. Study of range of motion in the neck utilizing a bubble goniometer. *Arch Phys Med Rehabil.* 1959;40:390-392.

26. Defibaugh JJ. Measurement of head motion, part II: an experimental study of head motion in adult males. *Phys Ther.* 1964;44:163-168.

27. Windle WF. *The Spinal Cord and its Reaction to Traumatic Injury: Anatomy, Physiology, Pharmacology, Therapeutics.* Marcel Deker; 1980.

28. Youdas JW, Garrett TR, Suman VJ, Bogard CL, Hallman HO, Carey JR. Normal range of motion of the cervical spine: an initial goniometric study. *Phys Ther.* 1992;72(11):770-780. doi:10.1093/ptj/72.11.770

29. Levangie PK, Norkin CC. *Joint Structure and Function: A Comprehensive Analysis.* 3rd ed. F.A. Davis; 2001.

30. van Shaik JP, van Pinxteren B, Verbiest H, Crowe A, Zuiderveld KJ. The facet orientation circle A new parameter for facet joint angulation in the lower lumbar spine. *Spine.* 1997;22(5):531-536. doi:10.1097/00007632-199703010-00014

31. Pal GP, Routal RV. A study of weight transmission through the cervical and upper thoracic regions of the vertebral column in man. *J Anat.* 1986;148:245-261.

32. Pal GP, Routal RV, Saggu SK. The orientation of the articular facets of the zygapophyseal joints at the cervical and upper thoracic region. *J Anat.* 2001;198(4):431-441. doi:10.1046/j.1469-7580.2001.19840431.x

33. Lopez AJ, Scheer JK, Leibl KE, Smith ZA, Dlouhy BJ, Dahdaleh NS. Anatomy and biomechanics of the craniovertebral junction. *Neurosurg Focus.* 2015;38(4):E2. doi:10.3171/2015.1.FOCUS14807

34. Panjabi M, Dvorak J, Duranceau J, et al. Three-dimensional movements of the upper cervical spine. *Spine.* 1988;13(7):726–730. doi:10.1097/00007632-198807000-00003

35. Selecki BR. The effects of rotation of the atlas on the axis: experimental work. *Med J Aust.* 1969;1(20):1012–1015.

36. White AA III, Panjabi MM. The clinical biomechanics of the occipitoatlantoaxial complex. *Orthop Clin North Am.* 1978;9(4): 867-878.

37. Wolfla CE. Anatomical, biomechanical, and practical considerations in posterior occipitocervical instrumentation. *Spine J.* 2006;6(6):225S-232S. doi:10.106/j.spinee.2006.06.001

38. Penning L. Normal movements of the cervical spine. *Am J Roentgenol.* 1978;130(2):317-326. doi:10.2214/ajr.130.2.317

39. Crisco JJ III, Oda T, Panjabi MM, Bueff HU, Dvorák J, Grob D. Transections of the C1-C2 joint capsular ligaments in the cadaveric spine. *Spine.* 1991;16(10):S474-S479. doi:10.1097/00007632-199110001-00003

40. von Torklus D, Gehle W. *The Upper Cervical Spine. Regional Anatomy, Pathology, and Traumatology. A Systemic Radiological Atlas and Textbook.* Buttersworths; 1972.

41. Bogduk N, Mercer S. Biomechanics of the cervical spine. I: normal kinematics. *Clin Biomech.* 2000;15(9):633-648. doi:10.1016/s0268-0033(00)00034-6

42. Swartz EE, Floyd RT, Cendoma M. Cervical spine functional anatomy and the biomechanics of injury due to compressive loading. *J Athl Train.* 2005;40(3): 155-161.

43. Oda T, Panjabi MM, Crisco JJ III, Oxland TR, Katz L, Nolte LP. Experimental study of atlas injuries. II. Relevance to clinical diagnosis and treatment. *Spine.* 1991;16(10):S466–S473. doi:10.1097-00007632-199110001-00002

44. Clark CR, White AA III. Fractures of the dens. A multicenter study. *J Bone Joint Surg Am.* 1985;67(9):1340–1348.

45. Dvorak J, Schneider E, Saldinger P, Rahn B. Biomechanics of the craniocervical region: the alar and transverse ligaments. *J Orthop Res.* 1988;6(3):452–461. doi:10.1002/jor.1100060317

46. Bhalla SK, Simmons EH. Normal ranges of intervertebral-joint motion of the cervical spine. *Can J Surg.* 1969;12(2):181-187.

47. Dvorak J, Froehlich D, Penning L, Baumgartner H, Panjabi MM. Functional radiographic diagnosis of the cervical spine: flexion/extension. *Spine.* 1988;13(7):748-755. doi:10.1097/00007632-1988070000-00007

48. Nowitzke A, Westaway M, Bogduk N. Cervical zygapophyseal joints: geometrical parameters and relationship to cervical kinematics. *Clin Biomech.* 1994;9(6):342-348. doi:10.1016/0268-0033(94)90063-9

49. Penning L. Differences in anatomy, motion, development and aging of the upper and lower cervical disk segments. *Clin Biomech.* 1988;3(1):37-47. doi:10.1016/0268-0033(88)90124-6

50. Penning L. Normal movements of the cervical spine. *Am J Roentgenol.* 1978;130(2):317-326. doi:10.2214/ajr.130.2.317

51. Aho A, Vartiainen O, Salo O. Segmentary mobility of the lumbar spine in antero-posterior flexion. *Ann Med Intern Fenn.* 1955;44(4):275-285.

52. Lind B, Sihlbom H, Nordwall A, Malchau H. Normal ranges of motion of the cervical spine. *Arch Phys Med Rehabil.* 1989;70(9):692-695.

53. Hurwitz EL, Aker PD, Adams AH, Meeker WC, Shekelle PG. Manipulation and mobilization of the cervical spine. A systematic review of the literature. *Spine.* 1996;21(15):1746-1759. doi:10.1097/00007632-199608010-00007

54. Kjellman GV, Skargren El, Oberg BE. A critical analysis of randomized clinical trials on neck pain and treatment efficacy. A review of the literature. *Scand J Rehabil Med.* 1999;31(3):139-152. doi:10.1080/003655099444489

55. Egan W, Flynn TW. *The Thoracic Spine and Rib Cage: Physical Therapy Patient Management Utilizing Current Evidence. Current Concepts of Orthopaedic Physical Therapy.* 2nd ed. American Physical Therapy Association; 2006.

56. Greenman PE. *Principles of Manual Medicine.* 3rd ed. Williams & Wilkins; 2003.

57. Paris SV. Anatomy as related to function and pain. *Orthop Clin North Am.* 1983;14(3):475-489.

58. White AA III, Panjabi MM. *Clinical biomechanics of the spine.* 2nd ed. JB Lippincott; 1990.

59. Mainman DJ, Larson SJ, Luck E, El-Ghatit A. The lateral extracavitary approach to the spine for thoracic disc herniation: report of 23 cases. *Neurosurg.* 1984;14(2):178-182. doi:10.1227/00006123-198402000-00010

60. Yoganandan N, Myklebust JB, Cusick JF F, Wilson CR, Sances Jr A. Functional biomechanics of the thoracolumbar vertebral cortex. *Clin Biomech.* 1988;3(1):11-18. doi:10.1016/0268-0033(88)90119-2

61. Mainman DJ, Pintar FA. Anatomy and clinical biomechanics of the thoracic spine. *Clin Neurosurg.* 1992;38:296-324.

62. Cropper JR. Regional anatomy and biomechanics. In: Flynn TW, ed. *The Thoracic Spine and Rib Cage.* Butterworth-Heinemann; 1996:3-30.

63. el-Khoury GY, Whitten CG. Trauma to the upper thoracic spine: anatomy, biomechanics, and unique imaging features. *Am J Roentgenol.* 1993;160(1):95-102. doi:10.2214/ajr.160.1.8416656

64. Lee D. Biomechanics of the thorax. In: Grant R, ed. *Physical Therapy of the Cervical and Thoracic Spine.* 3rd ed. Elsevier; 2002:45-60.

65. White AA III, Panjabi MM. The basic kinematics of the human spine: a review of past and current knowledge. *Spine.* 1978;3(1):12-20. doi:10.1097/00007632-197803000-00003

66. Morris JM. Biomechanics of the spine. *Arch Surg.* 1973;107(3):418-423. doi:10.1001/archsurg.1973.01350210054017

67. Morris JM, Lucas DB, Bresler B. Role of the trunk in stability of the spine. *J Bone Joint Surg Am.* 1961;43(3):327-351. doi:10.2106/00004623-196143030-00001

68. Galante JO. Tensile properties of the human lumbar annulus fibrosis. *Acta Orthop Scand.* 1967;38(100):1-91. doi:10.3109/ort.1967.38.suppl-100.01

69. Cook C, Hegedus E, Showalter C, Sizer PS Jr. Coupling behavior of the cervical spine: a systematic review of the literature. *J Manipulative Physiol Ther.* 2006:29(7)570-575. doi:10.1016/j.jmpt.2006.06.020

70. Panjabi MM, Brand RA, White AA III. Three-dimensional flexibility and stiffness properties of the thoracic spine. *J Biomech.* 1976;9(4):185-192. doi:10.1016/0021-9290(76)90003-8

71. Sizer PS Jr, Brismee JM, Cook C. Coupling behavior of the thoracic spine: a systematic review of literature. *J Manipulative Physiol Ther.* 2007;30(5): 390-399. doi:10.1016/j.jmpt.2007.04.009

72. Grieve GP. *Common Vertebral Joint Problems.* 2nd ed. Churchill Livingstone; 1988.

73. Kapandji IA. *The Physiology of the Joints.* 2nd ed. Churchill Livingstone; 1974.

74. Williams PL, Warwick R. *Gray's Anatomy.* 37th ed. Churchill Livingstone; 1989.

75. Wilson TA, Rehder K, Krayer S, Hoffman EA, Whitney CG, Rodarte JR. Geometry and respiratory displacement of the human ribs. *J Appl Physiol.* 1987;62(5):1872-1877. doi:10.1152/jappl.1987.62.5.1872

76. Winkel D. *Diagnosis and Treatment of the Spine.* Aspen Publishing; 1996.

77. Lindgren KA, Leino E, Manninen H. Cineradiography of the hypomobile first rib. *Arch Phys Med Rehabil.* 1989;70(5):408-409.

78. Panjabi MM, Cholewicki J, Nibu K, Grauer J, Babat LB, Dvorak J. Critical load of the human cervical spine: an in vitro experimental study. *Clin Biomech.* 1998;13(1):11-17. doi:10.1016/s0268-003(97)00057-0

79. Patwardhan AG, Havey RM, Ghanayem AJ, et al. Load-carrying capacity of the human cervical spine in compression is increased under a follower load. *Spine.* 2000;25(12):1548-1554. doi:10.1097/00007632-200006150-00015

80. Jull G, Kristjansson E, Dall'Alba P. Impairments in the cervical flexors: a comparison of whiplash and insidious onset neck pain patients. *Man Ther.* 2004;9(2):89-94. doi:10.1016/S1356-689X(03)00086-9

81. Jull GA. Deep cervical flexor muscle dysfunction in whiplash. *J Musculoskelet Pain.* 2000;8(1-2):143-154. doi:10.1300/J094v08n01_12

82. Hodges PW, Richardson CA. Inefficient muscular stabilization of the lumbar spine associated with low back pain. A motor control evaluation of transversus abdominis. *Spine.* 1996;21(22):2640-2650. doi:10.1097/00007632-199611150-00014

83. Falla D. Unravelling the complexity of muscle impairment in chronic neck pain. *Man Ther.* 2004;9(3):125–133. doi:10.1016/j.math.2004.05.003

84. Debernardi A, D'Aliberti G, Talamonti G, Villa F, Piparo M, Collice M. The craniovertebral junction area and the role of the ligaments and membranes. *Neurosurgery.* 2011;68(2):291–301. doi:10.1227/NEU.0b013e3182011262

85. Jea A, Tatsui C, Farhat H, Vanni S, Levi AD. Vertically unstable type III odontoid fractures: case report. *Neurosurgery.* 2006;58(4):E797. doi:10.1227/01.NEU.0000208555.34661.CD

86. Tubbs RS, Grabb PA, Spooner A, Wilson W, Oakes WJ. The apical ligament: anatomy and functional significance. *J Neurosurg.* 2000;92(2):197–200. doi:10.3171/spi.2000.92.2.0197

87. Steinmetz MP, Mroz TE, Benzel EC. Craniovertebral junction: biomechanical considerations. *Neurosurgery.* 2010;66(3):7–12. doi:10.1227/01.NEU.0000366109.85796.42

88. Tubbs RS, Kelly DR, Humphrey ER, et al. The tectorial membrane: anatomical, biomechanical, and histological analysis. *Clin Anat.* 2007;20(4):382–386. doi:10.1002/ca.20334

89. Werne S. Studies in spontaneous atlas dislocation. *Acta Orthop Scand Suppl.* 1957;23:1–150. doi:10.3109/ort.1957.28.suppl-23.01

90. King AI, Vulcan AP. Elastic deformation characteristics of the spine. *J Biomech.* 1971;2(5):413–416. doi:10.1016/0021-9290(71)90061-3

91. Sances A, Myklebust J, Mainman D, Larson S, Cusick J, Jodat R. The biomechanics of spinal injuries. *Crit Rev Bioeng.* 1984;11(1):1–76. doi:10.4271/902309

92. Myklebust JB, Pintar F, Yoganandan N, et al. Tensile strength of spinal ligaments. *Spine.* 1988;13(5):526–531.

93. Myklebust JB, Sances A, Mainman D, et al. Experimental spinal trauma studies in the human and monkey cadaver. In: Society of Automotive Engineers. *Proceedings of the 27th Stapp Car Crash Conference.* 1983:149-161.

94. Pintar F, Myklebust JB, Yoganandan N, et al. Biomechanics of human spinal ligaments. In: Sances A, Thomas DJ, Ewing CL, Larson SJ, Unterharnscheidt, eds. *Mechanisms of Head and Spine Trauma.* Aloray Publishers; 1986: 505-530.

95. Nachemson AL, Evans JH. Some mechanical properties of the third lumbar interlaminar ligament (ligamentum flavum). *J Biomech.* 1968;1(3):211-220. doi:10.1016/0021-9290(68)90006-7

96. van der Velde, GM. Benign paroxysmal positional vertigo. Part I: background and clinical presentation. *J Can Chiropr Assoc.* 1999;43(1):31-40.

97. Rennie C, Haffajee MR, Ebrahim MAA. The sinuvertebral nerves at the craniovertebral junction: a microdissection study. *Clin Anat.* 2013;26(3):357–366. doi:10.1002/ca.22105

98. Cesmebasi A, Muhleman MA, Hulsberg P, et al. Occipital neuralgia: anatomical considerations. *Clin Anat.* 2015;28(1):101-108. doi:10.1002/ca.22468

99. Butler DS. *The Sensitive Nervous System.* OPTP; 2000.

100. Center for Neurological Treatment and Research. Vertigo overview, incidence, and prevalence. Center for Neurological Treatment and Research. December 31, 1999. Accessed January 22, 2017. www.neurocntr.com/vertigo-dizziness.php

101. Horn LB. Differentiating between vestibular and non-vestibular balance disorders. *Neurology Report.* 1997;21(1):23-27.

102. Hoffman RM, Einstadter D, Kroenke K. Evaluating dizziness. *Am J Med.* 1999;107(5):468-478. doi:10.1016/s0002-9343(99)00260-0

103. Hall CD, Clarke Cox L. The role of vestibular rehabilitation in the balance disorder patient. *Otolaryngol Clin N Am.* 2009;42(1):161–169. doi:10.1016/j.otc.2008.09.006

104. Marchetti GF, Whitney SL. Older adults and balance dysfunction. *Neurol Clin.* 2005;23(3):785–805. doi:10.1016/j.ncl.2005.01.009

105. Polensek SH, Sterk CE, Tusa RJ. Screening for vestibular disorders: a study of clinicians' compliance with recommended practices. *Med Sci Monit.* 2008;14(5):CR238–CR242.

106. Brown JJ. Cervical contributions to balance: cervical vertigo. In: Berthoz A, Vidal PP, Graf W, eds. *The Head-Neck Sensory Motor System.* Oxford University Press; 1992:644-647.

107. L'Heureux-Lebeau B, Godbout A, Berbiche D, Saliba I. Evaluation of paraclinical tests in the diagnosis of cervicogenic dizziness. *Otol Neurotol.* 2014;35(10):1858-1865. doi:10.1097/MAO.0000000000000506

108. Australian Physiotherapy Association. Protocol for pre-manipulative testing of the cervical spine. *Aust J Physiother.* 1988;34:97-100.

109. Magarey M, Coughlan B, Rebback T. *Clinical Guidelines for Pre-Manipulative Procedures for the Cervical Spine.* Australian Physiotherapy Association; 2000.

110. Biesinger E. Vertigo caused by disorders of the cervical vertebral column. Diagnosis and treatment. *Adv Otorhinolaryngol.* 1988;39:44-51. doi:10.1159/000415654

111. Bracher ES, Almeida CI, Almeida RR, Duprat AC, Bracher CB. A combined approach for the treatment of cervical vertigo. *J Manip Phys Ther.* 2000;23(2):96-100. doi:10.1016/s0161-4754(00)90074-5

112. Herdman SJ. *Vestibular Rehabilitation.* 3rd ed. F. A. Davis; 2007.

113. Wrisley DM, Sparto PJ, Whitney SL, Furman JM. Cervicogenic dizziness: a review of diagnosis and treatment. *J Orthop Sports Phys Ther.* 2000;30(12):755-766. doi:10.2519/jospt.2000.30.12.755

114. Malmstrom E-M, Karlberg M, Melander A, Magnusson M, Moritz U. Cervicogenic dizziness – musculoskeletal findings before and after treatment and long-term outcome. *Disabil Rehabil.* 2007;29(15):1193-1205. doi:10.1080/09638280600948383

115. Hutting N, Verhagen AP, Vijverman V, Keesenberg MDM, Dixon G, Scholten-Peeters GGM. Diagnostic accuracy of premanipulative vertebrobascilar insufficiency tests: a systematic review. *Man Ther.* 2013;18(3):177-182. doi:10.1016/j.math.2012.09.009

116. Côté P, Kreitz BG, Cassidy JD, Thiel H. The validity of the extension-rotation test as a clinical screening procedure before neck manipulation: a secondary analysis. *J Manipulative Physiol Ther.* 1996;19(3):159-164.

117. Meadows J. *Orthopedic Differential Diagnosis in Orthopedic Physical Therapy: A Case Sudy Approach.* McGraw-Hill; 1999.

118. Miller MB. The cervical spine: physical therapy patient management using current evidence. In: *Current Concepts of Orthopaedic Physical Therapy.* 4th ed. American Physical Therapy Association; 2016:1-73.

119. Magee D. *Orthopedic Physical Assessment.* 4th ed. Saunders; 2002.

120. Sharp J, Purser DW. Spontaneuous atlanto-axial dislocation in ankylosing spondylitis and rheumatoid arthritis. *Ann Rhem Dis.* 1961;20(1):47-77. doi:10.1136/ard.20.1.47

121. Uitvlugt G, Indenbaum S. Clinical assessment of atlantoaxial instability using the Sharp-Purser test. *Arthritis Rheum.* 1988;31(7):918-922. doi:10.1002/art.1780310715

122. Baloh RW. *Dizziness, Hearing Loss, and Tinnitus.* F. A. Davis; 1998.

123. Dix MR, Hallpike CS. The pathology, symptomology, and diagnosis of certain common disorders of the vestibular system. *Ann Otorhinolaryngol.* 1952;61(4):987-1016. doi:10.1177/000348945206100403

124. Halker RB, Barrs DM, Wellik KE, Wingerchuk DM, Demaerschalk BM. Establishing a diagnosis of benign paroxysmal positional vertigo through the Dix-Hallpike and side-lying maneuvers: a critically appraised topic. *Neurologist.* 2008;14(3):201-204. doi:10.1097/NRL.0b013e31816f2820

125. Kattah JC, Talkad AV, Wang DZ, Hsieh Y-H, Newman-Toker DE. HINTS to diagnose stroke in the acute vestibular syndrome: three-step bedside oculomotor examination more sensitive than early MRI diffusion-weighted imaging. *Stroke.* 2009;40:3504-3510. doi:10.1161/STROKEAHA.109.551234

126. Newman-Toker DE, Kerber KA, Hsieh Y-H, et al. HINTS outperforms ABCD2 to screen for stroke in acute continuous vertigo and dizziness. *Acad Emerg Med.* 2013;20(10):986-996. doi:10.1111/acem.12223

127. Phillipszoon AJ, Bos J. Neck torsion nystagmus. *Pract Oto-Rhino-Laryngologist.* 1963;25:339-344. doi:10.1159/000274540

128. Fitz-Ritson D. Assessment of cervicogenic vertigo. *J Manipulative Physiol Ther.* 1991;14(3):193-198.

129. Norré ME. Cervical vertigo. Diagnostic and semiological problem with special emphasis upon "cervical nystagmus." *Acta Otorhinolaryngol Belg.* 1987;41:436-452.

130. Oosterveld WJ, Kortschot HW, Kingma GG, de Jong HA, Saatci MR. Electronystagmographic findings following cervical whiplash injuries. *Acta Otolaryngol.* 1991;111(2):201-205. doi:10.3109/00016489109137375

131. Tjell C, Rosenhall U. Smooth pursuit neck torsion test: a specific test for cervical dizziness. *Am J Otol.* 1998;19(1):76-81.

132. Revel M, Andre-Deshays C, Minguet M. Cervicocephalic kinesthetic sensibility in patients with cervical pain. *Arch Phys Med Rehabil.* 1991;72(5):288-291.

133. Reid SA, Rivett DA. Manual therapy treatment of cervicogenic dizziness: a systematic review. *Man Ther.* 2005;10(1):4-13. doi:10.1016/j.math.2004.03.006

134. Furman JM, Whitney SL. Central causes of dizziness. Phys Ther. 2000; 80:179-187. doi:10.1093/ptj/8020179

135. Morinaka S. Musculoskeletal diseases as a causal factor of cervical vertigo. *Auris Nasus Larynx.* 2009;36(6):649-654. doi:10.1016/j.anl.2009.04.009

136. Hinoki M. *Vertigo Viewed from Neurotology.* 1st ed. Kanahara & Co; 2003.

137. Hinoki M. *Vertigo – Theoretical and Clinical Considerations.* 1st ed. Kanehara & Co; 1997.

138. Hinoki M, Niki H. Neurotological studies on the role of the sympathetic nervous system in the formation of traumatic vertigo of cervical origin. *Acta Otolaryngol Suppl.* 1975;330:185-196. doi:10.3109/00016487509121290

139. Hinoki M. Vertigo due to whiplash injury: a neurotological approach. *Acta Otolaryngol Suppl.* 1984;419:9-29.

140. Norré ME. Neurophysiology of vertigo with special reference to cervical vertigo: A review. *Acta Belg Med Phys.* 1986;9(3):183-194.

141. Karlberg M, Magnusson M, Malmström EM, Melander A, Moritz U. Postural and symptomatic improvement after physiotherapy in patients with dizziness of suspected cervical origin. *Arch Phys Med Rehabil.* 1996;77(9):874-882. doi:10.1016/s003-9993(96)90273-7

142. Stovner L, Hagen K, Jensen R, et al. The global burden of headache: a documentation of headache prevalence and disability worldwide. *Cephalalgia.* 2007;27(3):193-210. doi:10.1111/j.1468-2982-2007-01288.x

143. Diener I. The impact of cervicogenic headache on patients attending a private physiotherapy practice in Cape Town. *S Afr J Physiother.* 2001;57:35-39. doi:10.4102/sajp.v57i1.493

144. Lipton RB, Stewart WF. The epidemiology of migraine. *Eur Neurol.* 1994;34(Suppl 2):6-11. doi:10.1159/000119525

145. Haldeman S, Dagenais S. Cervicogenic headaches: a critical review. *Spine J.* 2001;1(1):31-46. doi:10.1016/s1529-9430(01)00024-9

146. Sjaastad O, Bakketeig LS. Prevalence of cervicogenic headache: Vågå study of headache epidemiology. *Acta Neurol Scand.* 2008;117(3):170-183. doi:10.1111/j.1600-0404.2007.00962.x

147. Sjaastad O, Fredriksen TA, Pfaffenrath V. Cervicogenic headache: diagnostic criteria. The Cervicogenic Headache International Study Group. *Headache.* 1998;38(6):442-445. doi:10.1046/j.1526-4610.199813806442.x

148. Huijbregts PA. Clinical reasoning in the diagnosis: history taking in patients with headache. In Fernandez-de-Las-Penas C, Arendt-Nielsen L, Gerwin RD, eds. *Tension-type and Cervicogenic Headache. Pathophysiology, Diagnosis and Management.* Jones and Bartlett Publishers; 2010:133-151.

149. Rushton A, Rivett D, Carlesso L, Flynn T, Hing W, Kerry R. International framework for examination of the cervical region for potential of cervical arterial dysfunction prior to orthopaedic manual therapy intervention. *Man Ther.* 2014;19(3):222-228. doi:10.1016/j.math.2013.11.005

150. Bogduk N. Headache and the neck. In: Goadsby P, Silberstein S, eds. *Headache.* Butterworth-Heinemann; 1997.

151. Page P. Cervicogenic headaches: An evidence-led approach to clinical management. *Int J Sports Phys Ther.* 2011;6(3):254-266

152. Fredriksen TA, Sjaastad O: Cervicogenic headache: current concepts of pathogenesis related to anatomical structure. *Clin Exp Rheumatol.* 2000;18(2 suppl 19):S16–S18.

153. Sjaastad O, Fredriksen TA, Pfaffenrath V. Cervicogenic headache: diagnostic criteria. *Headache.* 1990;30(11):725–726. doi:10.1111/j.1526-4610.1990.hed.3011725.x

154. Rubio-Ochoa, J, Benítez-Martínez J, Lluch E, Santacruz-Zaragoza, Gómez-Contreras P, Cook CE. Physical examination tests for screening and diagnosis of cervicogenic headache: a systematic review. *Man Ther.* 2016;21:35-40. doi:10.1016/j.math.2015.09.008

155. Childs JD, Cleland JA, Elliott JM, et al. Neck pain: clinical practice guidelines linked to the international classification of functioning, disability, and health from the orthopaedic section of the American Physical Therapy Association. *J Orthop Sports Phys Ther.* 2008;38(9):A1-A34. doi:10.2519/jospt.2008.0303

156. Blanpied PR, Gross AR, Elliott JM, et al. Neck pain: revision 2017: clinical practice guidelines linked to the international classification of functioning, disability and health from the orthopaedic section of the American Physical Therapy Association. *J Orthop Sports Phys Ther.* 2017;47(7):A1–A83. doi:10.2519/jospt.2017.0302

157. Yi X., Cook AJ, Hamill-Ruth RJ, Rowlingson JC. Cervicogenic headache in patients with presumed migraine: missed diagnosis or misdiagnosis?. *J Pain.* 2005;6(10):700-703. doi:10.1016/j.jpain.2005.04.005

158. Headache Classification Committee of the International Headache Society. The international classification of headache disorders, 3rd edition (beta version). *Cephalalgia.* 2013;33(9):629-808. doi:10.1177/0333102413485658

159. Headache Classification Committee of the International Headache Society. The international classification of headache disorders, 3rd edition (beta version). *Cephalalgia.* 2013;33(9):629-808. doi:10.1177/0333102413485658

160. Eubanks J. Cervical radiculopathy: nonoperative management of neck pain and radicular symptoms. *Am Fam Physician.* 2010;81(1):33-40.

161. Olson KA. *Manual Physical Therapy of the Spine.* Elsevier; 2009:253-258.

162. Murphy DR, Hurwitz EL. Application of a diagnosis-based clinical decision guide in patients with low back pain. *Chiropr Man Therap.* 2011;19:26. doi:10.1186/2045-709x-19-26

163. Ellenberg MR, Honet JC, Treanor WJ. Cervical radiculopathy. *Arch Phys Med Rehabil.* 1994;75:342-352. doi:10.1016/0003-9993(94)90040-x

164. Radhakrishnan K, Litchy WJ, O'Fallon WM, Kurland LT. Epidemiology of cervical radiculopathy. A population-based study from Rochester, Minnesota, 1976 through 1990. *Brain.* 1994:117(Pt 2);325-335. doi:10.1093/brain/117.2.325

165. Bogduk N, Twomey CT. *Clinically Relevant Anatomy for the Lumbar Spine.* 2nd ed. Churchill Livingston; 1991.

166. Dwyer A, Aprill C, Bogduk N. Cervical zygapophyseal joint pain patterns. I: A study in normal volunteers. *Spine.* 1990;15(6):453-457. doi:10.1097/00007632-199006000-00004

167. Hanten WP, Oslon SL, Ludwig GM. Reliability of manual mobility testing of the upper cervical spine in subjects with cervicogenic headache. *J Man Manipulative Ther.* 2002;10(2):76-82. doi:10.1179/106698102790819328

168. Pfaffenrath V, Kaube H. Diagnostics of cervicogenic headache. *Funct Neurol*. 1990;5(2):159–164.

169. Petersen SM. Articular and muscular impairments in cervicogenic headache: a case report. *J Orthop Sports Phys Ther*. 2003;33(1):21–30. doi:10.2519/jospt.2003.33.1.21

170. Nicholson GG, Gaston J. Cervical headache. *J Orthop Sports Phys Ther*. 2001;31(4):184-193. doi:10.2519/jospt.2001.31.4.184

171. Main CJ, Sullivan MJ, Watson PJ. Risk identification and screening. In: Main CJ, Sullivan MJ, Watson PJ, eds. *Pain Management: Practical Applications of the Biopsychosocial Perspective in Clinical and Occupational Settings*. Churchill Livingstone; 2008:97–134.

172. Leerar PJ, Boissonnault W, Domholdt E, Roddey T. Documentation of red flags by physical therapists for patients with low back pain. *J Man Manip Ther*. 2007;15(1):42–49. doi:10.1179/106698107791090105

173. Wainner RS, Fritz JM, Irrgang JJ, Boninger ML, Delitto A, Allison S. Reliability and diagnostic accuracy of the clinical examination and patient self-report measures for cervical radiculopathy. *Spine*. 2003;28(1):52-62. doi:10.1097/00007632-200301010-00014

174. Nicholas MK, Linton SJ, Watson PJ, Main CJ, "Decade of the Flags" Working Group. Early identification and management of psychological risk factors ("yellow flags") in patients with low back pain: a reappraisal. *Phys Ther*. 2011;91(5):737-753. doi:10.2522/ptj.20100224

175. Greenhalgh S, Selfe J. Margaret: a tragic case of spinal red flags and red herrings. *Physiotherapy*. 2004;90(2):73-76. doi:10.1016/S0031-9406(03)00008-7

176. Kendall NAS, Linton SJ, Main CJ. *Guide to Assessing Psychosocial Yellow Flags in Acute Low Back Pain: Risk Factors for Long-Term Disability and Work Loss*. Accident Rehabilitation and Compensation Insurance Corporation of New Zealand and the National Health Committee; 1997.

177. Shaw WS, van der Windt DA, Main CJ, Loisel P, Linton SJ, "Decade of the Flags: Working Group. Early patient screening and intervention to address individual level occupational factors ("blue flags") in back disability. *J Occup Rehabil*. 2009;19(1):64-80. doi:10.1007/s10926-008-9159-7

178. Arroll B, Goodyear-Smith F, Kerse N, Fishman T, Gunn J. Effect of the addition of a "help" question to two screening questions on specificity for diagnosis of depression in general practice: diagnostic validity study. *BMJ*. 2005;331(7521):884. doi:10.1136/bmj.38607.464537.7C

179. Ski CF, Thompson DR, Hare DL, Stewart AG, Watson R. Cardiac depression scale: mokken scaling in heart failure patients. *Health Qual Life Outcomes*. 2012;10:141. doi:10.1186/1477-7525-10-141

180. Sullivan M, Bishop SR, Pivik JR. The pain catastrophizing scale: development and validation. *Psychol Assess*. 1995;7(4):524-532. doi:10.1037/1040-3590.7.4.524

181. Osman A, Barrios FX, Kopper BA, Hauptmann W, Jones J, O'Neill E. Factor structure, reliability, and validity of the pain catastrophizing scale. *J Behav Med*. 1997;20(6):589-605. doi:10.1023/a:1025570508954

182. Stiell IG, Wells GA, Vandemheen KL, et al. The Canadian C-spine rule for radiography in alert and stable trauma patients. *JAMA*. 2001;286(15):1841–1848. doi:10.1001/jama.286.15.1841

183. Jepsen JR, Laursen LH, Hagert C-G, Kreiner S, Larsen AI. Diagnostic accuracy of the neurological upper limb examination I: inter-rater reproducibility of selected findings and patterns. *BMC Neurol*. 2006;6:8. doi:10.1186/1471-2377-6-8

184. Cook C, Roman M, Stewart KM, Leithe LG, Isaacs R. Reliability and diagnostic accuracy of clinical special tests for myelopathy in patients seen for cervical dysfunction. *J Orthop Sports Phys Ther*. 2009;39(3):172-178. doi:10.2519/jospt.2009.2938

185. Cook C, Brown C, Isaacs R, Roman M, Davis S, Richardson W. Clustered clinical findings for diagnosis of cervical spine myelopathy. *J Man Manip Ther*. 2010;18(4):175-180. doi:10.1179/1066981X12804993427045

186. Cook CE, Hegedus EJ. *Orthopedic Physical Examination Tests: An Evidence-Based Approach*. 2nd ed. Pearson; 2012.

187. Young IA, Michener LA, Cleland JA, Aguilera AJ, Snyder AR. Manual therapy, exercise, and traction for patients with cervical radiculopathy: a randomized clinical trial. *Phys Ther*. 2009;89(7):632-642. doi:10.2522/ptj.20080283

188. Lindsay KW, Bone I. *Neurology and Neurosurgery Illustrated*. 4th ed. Churchill Livingstone; 1994.

189. Kuijper B, Tans JTJ, Beelen A, Nollet F, de Visser M. Cervical collar or physiotherapy versus wait and see policy for recent onset cervical radiculopathy: randomised trial. *BMJ*. 2009;339:b3883. doi:10.1136/bmj.b3883

190. Wainner RS, Gill H. Diagnosis and nonoperative management of cervical radiculopathy. *J Orthop Sports Phys Ther*. 2000;30(12):728–744. doi:10.2519/jospt.2000.30.12.728

191. Tong HC, Haig AJ, Yamakawa K. The Spurling test and cervical radiculopathy. *Spine*. 2002;27(2):156-159. doi:10.1097/00007632-200201150-0007

192. Cleland J, Koppenhaver S. *Netter's Orthopaedic Clinical Examination: An Evidence-Based Approach*. 2nd ed. Saunders; 2010.

193. Cook CE, Hegedus E, Pietrobon R, Goode A. A pragmatic neurological screen for patients with suspected cord compression myelopathy. *Phys Ther*. 2007;87(9):1233-1242. doi:10.2522/ptj.20060150

194. Montgomery DM, Brower RS. Cervical spondylotic myelopathy. Clinical syndrome and natural history. *Orthop Clin North Am*. 1992;23(3):487-493.

195. Ogino H, Tada K, Okada K, et al. Canal diameter, anteroposterior compression ration, and spondylitic myelopathy of the cervical spine. *Spine*. 1976;8(1):1-15. doi:10.1097/00007632-198301000-00001

196. Montgomery DM, Brower RS. Cervical spondylotic myelopathy. Clinical syndrome and natural history. *Orthop Clin North Am*. 1992;23(3):487-493.

197. Wainner RS, Fritz JM, Irrgang JJ, Delitto A, Allison S, Boninger ML. Development of a clinical prediction rule for the diagnosis of carpal tunnel syndrome. *Arch Phys Med Rehabil*. 2005;86(4):609–618. doi:10.1016/j.apmr.2004.11.008

198. Sung RD, Wang JC. Correlation between positive Hoffmann's reflex and cervical pathology in asymptomatic individuals. *Spine*. 2001;26(1):67-70. doi:10.1097/00007632-200101010-00013

199. Wong TM, Leung HB, Wong WC. Correlation between magnetic resonance imaging and radiographic measurement of cervical spine in cervical myelopathic patients. J Orthop Surg. 2004;12(2):239-242. doi:10.1177/230949900401200220

200. Kuhtz-Buschbeck JP, Jöhnk K, Mäder S, Stolze H, Mehdorn M. Analysis of gait in cervical myelopathy. *Gait Posture*. 1999;9(3):184-189. doi:10.1016/s0966-6362(99)00015-6

201. Uchihara T, Furukawa T, Tsukagoshi H. Compression of brachial plexus as a diagnostic test of cervical cord lesion. *Spine*. 1994;19(9):2170-2173. doi:10.1097/00007632-199410000-00007

202. Laulan J, Fouquet B, Rodaix C, Jauffret P, Roguelaure Y, Descatha A. Thoracic outlet syndrome: definition, aetiological factors, diagnosis, management, and occupational impact. *J Occup Rehabil*. 2011;21(3):366–373. doi:10.1007/s10926-010-9278-9

203. Talu GK. Thoracic outlet syndrome. *Derleme*. 2005;17(2).

204. Hooper TL, Denton J, McGalliard MK, Brismée J-M, Sizer PS. Thoracic outlet syndrome: a controversial clinical condition. Part 1: anatomy, and clinical examination/diagnosis. *J Man Manip Ther*. 2010;18(2):74-83. doi:10.1179/10669811X12640740712734

205. Laulan J, Fouquet B, Rodaix C, Jauffret P, Roquelaure Y, Descatha A. Thoracic outlet syndrome: definition, aetiological factors, diagnosis, management and occupational impact. *J Occup Rehabil*. 2011;21(3):366-373. doi:10.1007/s10926-010-9278-9

206. Atasoy E. Thoracic outlet syndrome: anatomy. *Hand Clin*. 2004;20(1):7-14. doi:10.1016/s0749-0712(03)00078-7

207. Lindgren K-A. Thoracic outlet syndrome. *Int Musculoskelet Med.* 2010;32(1):17-24. doi:10.1179/175361410X12652805807792

208. Christo PJ, McGreevy K. Updated perspectives on neurogenic thoracic outlet syndrome. *Curr Pain Headache Rep.* 2011;15(1):14-21. doi:10.1007/s11916-010-0163-1

209. Rayan GM, Jensen C. Thoracic outlet syndrome: provocative examination maneuvers in a typical population. *J Shoulder Elbow Surg.* 1995;4(2):113-117. doi:10.1016/s1058-2746(05)80064-3

210. Winsor T, Brow R. Costoclavicular syndrome: its diagnosis and treatment. *JAMA.* 1966;196(8):697-699. doi:10.1001/jama.1966.03100210067017

211. Shultz SJ, Houglum PA, Perrin DH. *Examination of Musculoskeletal Injuries.* 3rd ed. Human Kinetics; 2010.

212. Donatelli RA. *Physical Therapy of the Shoulder.* 2nd ed. Churchill Livingstone; 1991.

213. Fernández-de-las-Peñas C, Cleland J, Dommerholt J. *Manual Therapy for Musculoskeletal Pain Syndromes: An Evidence- and Clinical-Informed Approach.* Elsevier; 2015.

214. Evans P. The T4 syndrome some basic science aspects. *Physiotherapy.* 1997;83(4):186-189. doi:10.1016/S0031-9406(05)66077-4

215. Conroy JL, Schneiders AG. The T4 syndrome. *Man Ther.* 2005;10(4):292-296. doi:10.1016/j.math.2005.01.007

216. DeFranca GG, Levine LJ. The T4 syndrome. *J Manipulative Physiol Ther.* 1995;18(1):34-37.

217. Mellick GA, Mellick LB. Clinical presentation, quantitative sensory testing, and therapy of 2 patients with fourth thoracic syndrome. *J Manipulative Physiol Ther.* 2006;29(5):403-408. doi:10.1016/j.jmpt.2006.04.003

218. Fruth SJ. Differential diagnosis and treatment in a patient with posterior upper thoracic pain. *Phys Ther.* 2006;86(2):254-268.

219. Jowsey P, Perry J. Sympathetic nervous system effects in the hands following a grade III postero-anterior rotatory mobilisation technique to T4: a randomised placebo-controlled trial. *Man Ther.* 2010;15(3):248-253. doi:10.1016/j.math.2009.12.008

14

Physical Therapy Management of Temporomandibular Disorders With Cervical Spine Considerations

Steven L. Kraus, PT, OCS Emeritus, MTC, CCTT, CODN

KEY TERMS

Active myofascial trigger point: Produces spontaneous pain and/or referred pain and always evokes symptoms.

Anterior guidance (protrusive guidance or canine guidance): Is the relationship of any of the anterior 6 mandibular teeth maintaining contact with any of the anterior 6 maxillary teeth during protrusive and lateral excursions. When a person moves their jaw forward, the posterior teeth should separate. When a person moves their jaw into lateral excursion, the posterior teeth on the contralateral side should separate.

Behavioral modification: The process of changing unwanted behaviors that contribute to an overuse, disuse, and/or abuse of the muscles of mastication, temporomandibular joint (TMJ), and/or cervical spine.

Bruxism: A repetitive jaw-muscle activity characterized by clenching or grinding of the teeth and/or by bracing or thrusting of the mandible.

Cervicogenic headache (CGH): A headache whose origin is the cervical spine.

Click: A distinct sound (eg, click, pop, snap) that is of a brief and very limited duration with a clear beginning and end that emanates from the TMJ.

Crepitus: A noise, like sandpaper moving over a surface, that is longer in duration that emanates from the TMJ.

Dislocation: Joint is outside its physiological and anatomical boundary.

Familiar symptom: A symptom that the patient has experienced in the past 30 days and not a symptom that was experienced only as a result of the physical examination (false positive).

Latent myofascial trigger point: Is asymptomatic and can be quiescent for months or years but becomes painful when stretched or compressed (palpated) during the physical examination.

Modify: To reproduce, increase, or decrease the patient's symptoms.

Occlusion: How the teeth come together.

Provocation test: Tests performed to modify the patient's familiar symptom(s)

Psychosocial distress: Involves, but is not limited to, fear, anxiety, anger, and depression.

Wallmann HW, Donatelli R, eds. *Foundations of Orthopedic Physical Therapy* (pp 403-435).
© 2024 Taylor & Francis Group.

- 403 -

Subluxation: Joint is outside its physiological boundary but inside its anatomical boundary.

Temporomandibular disorders (TMD): A cluster of symptoms and signs involving masticatory muscles, the TMJs, or both.

CHAPTER QUESTIONS

Answers to questions can be found at https://www.tmd-stevekraus.com/. Go to tab "Links."

1. What percent of the US population have a malocclusion?
   A. Less than 25%
   B. 25% to less than 50%
   C. 50% to less than 75%
   D. 75% to 100%

2. Which of the following disk displacements is always associated with pain?
   A. Disk displacement with reduction (DDwR)
   B. Disk displacement without reduction with limited opening (DDwoR wLO)
   C. Disk displacement without reduction without limited opening (DDwoR woLO)
   D. None of the above

3. Which of the following findings of the clinical examination of TMD requires treatment?
   A. Click greater than 30 mm without pain
   B. Crepitus greater than 30 mm without pain
   C. Deflection equal to or less than 30 mm without pain
   D. Deflection greater than 30 mm without pain

4. Which of the following clinical findings will help to diagnose subluxation?
   A. Late opening click with mouth opening and late closing click with mouth closing
   B. Early opening click with mouth opening and late closing click with mouth closing
   C. Late opening click with mouth opening and early closing click with mouth closing
   D. Early opening click with mouth opening and early closing click with mouth closing

5. Using the kinesiograph can _____.
   A. Make and accurate diagnosis of TMD
   B. Separate normal patients from patients with TMD
   C. Analyze mandibular movements three dimensionally
   D. Use the data to make an evidence based oral appliance

6. Which one of the following is a common finding with patients with a displaced disk?
   A. Facial asymmetry on the side of the displaced disk
   B. Clicking with or without locking related to a displaced disk
   C. Neck pain on the opposite side of the displaced disk
   D. Posterior open bite on side of the displaced disk

7. Which of the following should be included routinely as part of a TMD examination?
   A. Imaging studies
   B. Occlusal studies
   C. Sleep apnea studies
   D. None of the above

8. Which diagnostic subset of TMD is always associated with a click?
   A. Disk displacement without reduction (DDwoR)
   B. Degenerative joint disease (DJD)
   C. DDwR
   D. Subluxation

9. Which of the following applies to the Diagnostic Criteria of Temporomandibular Disorders (DC/TMD)
   A. Sensitivity and specificity values unknown
   B. Does not account for concurrent diagnostic subsets
   C. Is seldom used in academic and clinical research
   D. Unable to differentiate between myalgia and arthralgia

10. According to the DC/TMD, familiar symptom(s) are symptoms that the patient has experienced in the past _____.
    A. 30 days
    B. 60 days
    C. 90 days
    D. 120 days

11. Which of the following is true about the DC/TMD?
    A. Does consider latent myofascial trigger points
    B. Does not consider latent myofascial trigger points
    C. Does not consider active myofascial trigger points
    D. Does not consider active or latent myofascial trigger points

12. The probability that a malocclusion can cause TMD problems:
    A. Very high
    B. High
    C. Moderate
    D. Low

13. To be clinically meaningful, a noise associated with a DDwR must be _____.
    A. Palpated by the clinician but not heard by the patient
    B. Palpated by the clinician and heard by the patient
    C. Not palpated by the clinician and not heard by the patient
    D. Not palpated by the clinician but heard by the patient

14. Which of the following is not an indication for wearing an oral appliance?

    A. To reduce morning jaw muscle pain and/or headache triggered by sleep bruxism

    B. To establish a centric relation and centric occlusion of the condyle to minimize sleep bruxism

    C. To reduce morning locking/catching associated with a disk displacement related to sleep bruxism

    D. To protect occlusal surfaces of teeth and dental restorations from sleep bruxism

15. Reducing TMJ loading over time is best achieved by _____.

    A. Intraoral joint distraction grade 3

    B. Normalize head and neck posture

    C. Reduce parafunctional activity

    D. Patient wears a pivotal appliance

16. The cause of nocturnal bruxism is _____.

    A. Malocclusion

    B. Sleep apnea

    C. Psychosocial distress

    D. Multifactorial

17. The trigeminocervical nucleus is located in the upper cervical spinal cord within the _____.

    A. Par oralis

    B. Pars cranialis

    C. Pars caudalis

    D. Pars intermedius

18. Subjective tinnitus, subjective fullness, and subjective hearing loss may be related to an increase in activity of which of the following muscles?

    A. Auricular levator and labii superioris

    B. Tensor veli palatine and tensor tympani

    C. Musculus uvulae and palatopharyngeus

    D. Palatoglossus and laryngopharynx

19. What percentage of asymptomatic participants greater than 40 years old have positive imaging findings of cervical spondylitis and cervical disk herniation?

    A. 20%

    B. 40%

    C. 60%

    D. 80%

20. The American Board of Physical Therapy Specialties was established to provide formal recognition for physical therapists with advanced clinical knowledge, experience, and skills in 9 specialty areas of practice. The field of TMDs and orofacial pain falls into which specialty area?

    A. Neurology

    B. Orthopedics

    C. Clinical electrophysiology

    D. None of the above

INTRODUCTION

The International Classification of Headache Disorders (ICHD) identified more than 284 sources for headache and facial pain (HFP), making the evaluation and treatment of HFP a daunting task.[1] Dental, neurologic, musculoskeletal, otolaryngologic, vascular, metaplastic, infectious disease, neuropathic, and neurogenic are potential sources for HFP. The management of HFP can involve several health care professionals, which may include a dentist, oral surgeon, physical therapist, and physicians of different specialties. The ICHD lists TMD and neck pain as 2 sources for HFP. TMD and neck pain are musculoskeletal disorders that will be the focus of this chapter and best managed by a physical therapist.

TMD is divided into myogenous disorders involving the muscles of mastication and arthrogenous disorders involving the TMJ.[2] Myogenous and arthrogenous each have additional diagnostic subsets that are listed in Appendix A. It is estimated that up to 12% of the population experience signs and symptoms of TMD.[3] Common sources for neck pain consist of any one or combination of cervical disks, nerve roots, facet joints, and associated muscles. Generic terms used to describe involvement of the previous cervical tissues are *chronic uncomplicated neck pain, nonspecific neck pain, mechanical neck pain, cervical spine disorders (CSD)*, and *neck pain*. In this chapter, neck pain and CSD will be interchanged to indicate symptoms originating from the cervical spine. It is estimated that up to 14% of the population experience signs and symptoms related to neck pain.[4]

Little information is available for costs of services related to TMD. In 1995, the annual cost for treating TMD and orofacial pain was estimated to be $32 billion.[5] In 1994, neck and back pain estimated medical expenditures was $33.6 billion.[6] One can only imagine what the annual costs for TMD and neck pain treatment may be composed of in today's dollars. In contrast to other medical conditions, the National Heart, Lung, and Blood Institute estimated in 2002 that the cost of treatment for diabetes was $98.1 billion, and in 2007, the cost of treatment for cancer was $89.0 billion.[7]

The emphasis of this chapter is on physical therapists as a health care provider that offers a conservative, evidence-based, and cost-effective treatment for TMD and CSD. The first part of this chapter discusses the diagnostic criteria and management for TMD followed by a discussion on predoctoral education for health care professionals pertaining to TMD. The last part of the chapter is an overview of cervical spine considerations for patients with TMD and HFP. Mechanisms by which the cervical spine contributes to TMD myalgia, headache, and ears symptoms will be reviewed. Cervical spine evaluation and management will be highlighted.

Table 14-1

RED FLAGS

Suspect pathology with any of the following red flags:

- Blunt trauma to jaw and/or neck

- Osteoporosis with minor or no trauma

- Neurologic signs (cranial nerve examination positive)

- Dysarthria, dysphagia, diplopia, drop attacks

- Less than 17 years old with stiff neck, headache, and fever in the absence of trauma suggest meningitis

- Unremitting night pain, fever, unexplained weight loss within 6 months or night sweats

Imaging studies and erythrocyte sedimentation rate are highly sensitive and specific to diagnose fracture, instability, infections, and cancer to rule out such pathology.[10]

TEMPOROMANDIBULAR DISORDERS

Diagnosing Temporomandibular Disorders

Imaging

Imaging studies of TMJ include, but are not limited to, a panoramic radiograph, computed tomography, and magnetic resonance imaging (MRI).[2] The panoramic radiograph is the most widely used imaging in the dental office. The panoramic radiograph provides a broad view of the mandible, teeth, sinuses, nasal area, and TMJ. Computed tomography scanning provides detail of bony structures. The cone beam allows for viewing the condyle in multiple planes so all surfaces can be visualized. Cone beam tomography can image both hard and soft tissues.[8] MRI evaluates the soft tissue of TMJ. MRI has become the gold standard to diagnose TMJ disk displacements.[9]

The primary advantage of imaging studies is to rule out fractures and disease that are suspected with red flags (Table 14-1).[10] Pertinent to TMD, imaging cannot differentiate patients who are in pain from those who are not in pain.[9] Technology has allowed us to see in detail TMJ and adjacent tissues, but seldom does it change the initial treatment plan or lead to a better treatment outcome. Routine imaging of TMJ will overdiagnose arthrogenous conditions that may not be related to the patient's pain and would therefore not require treatment.[9] An example is a disk displacement, which is a common TMJ diagnosis. MRI studies have repeatedly been shown to identify one-third of asymptomatic volunteers with disk displacement of their TMJ.[11,12] Imaging of TMJ is mainly indicated when red flags (see Table 14-1) are present or if the patient's pain stemming from the TMJ has not responded to conservative care and TMJ surgery is being considered.[12]

Computerized Instruments

Computerized instruments include sonography to measure vibration stemming from TMJ, electromyography to measure the activity of jaw muscles, and electronic tracking instruments to record mandibular position and movement 3-dimensionally.[13] Data produced from the computerized instruments are used to make a TMD diagnosis and the structural design of an oral appliance.[13-15] Unfortunately, computerized instruments overdiagnose patient's with TMD and any subsequent treatments would likely be unnecessary.[13-15] According to the American Association for Dental Research's Policy Statement on Temporomandibular Disorders:

> [T]he consensus of recent scientific literature about currently available technological diagnostic devices for TMDs is that except for various imaging modalities, none of them shows the sensitivity and specificity required to separate normal subjects from TMD patients or to distinguish among TMD subgroups.[16]

Occlusal Studies

Occlusion as it relates to TMD is one of the most debated topics in dentistry. In 1934, Costen made an observation that certain symptoms, such as loss of hearing, tinnitus, dizziness, headache, and a burning sensation of the throat and tongue was the result of a dental malocclusion.[17] Ninety five percent of the population have some form of malocclusion (eg, crowding, malalignment, structural abnormality).[18] Costen's fundamental observation of cause and effect was extended by many dentists to include malocclusion as an etiology for TMD, to justify occlusal equilibration, prosthodontics, and orthodontics in the diagnosis, prevention, and treatment of TMD.[19-25] Studies have concluded that a malocclusion is not an etiology of TMD; malocclusion cannot diagnose TMD, and occlusal treatment cannot prevent or treat TMD.[20-26] Although a very limited number of patients diagnosed with

TMD could benefit from occlusal treatment, the author of this chapter is not aware of any published guidelines that have a broad consensus among academic and clinical dentists that clearly identifies the criteria for when occlusal therapy should be offered for patients suffering from TMD. Okeson summarizes the state of the occlusion and TMD in the following way:

> One might conclude that if occlusion were the major etiologic factor in TMD, the profession would have confirmed this many years ago. On the other hand, if occlusion has nothing to do with TMD, the profession would have also likewise already confirmed this conclusion. Apparently neither of these conclusions is true. Instead, the confusion and controversy concerning the relationship between occlusion and TMD continues. The general message is that there is no simple cause-and-effect relationship explaining the association between occlusion and TMD.[27]

Clinical Examination

In 1992, the Research Diagnostic Criteria for Temporomandibular Disorders (RDC/TMD) was established and has become the most widely used diagnostic criterion for TMD in academic and clinical research.[28] RDC/TMD diagnostic criterion is divided into axis I, which consists of the history and physical examination, and axis II, which assesses psychosocial distress.[28] In 2014, the RDC/TMD was updated and renamed to the DC/TMD.[29] The 12 diagnostic subsets of TMD consist of 5 myogenous and 7 arthrogenous diagnostic subsets. For the purpose of this chapter, local myalgia, myofascial pain, and myofascial pain with referral will be placed under the diagnostic subset of myalgia. Myalgia and headache attributed to temporomandibular disorder (HTMD) will be the 2 myogenous diagnostic subsets discussed in this chapter. History and physical examination along with sensitivity and specificity values for all myogenous and arthrogenous diagnostic categories can be found in Appendix A.

Many patients present with one or more TMD diagnostic subsets.[2,30,31] The DC/TMD does not account for patients having concurrent diagnostic subsets of TMD. Clinicians may need to modify the DC/TMD, using their clinical experience and clinical reasoning to arrive at a valid diagnostic subset of TMD. With several exceptions, the author of this chapter closely follows the DC/TMD.[30,32] Clinical Examination forms used by the author to document the history and physical examination for TMD can be found in Box 14-1.

History

Common TMD symptoms are:
- Facial, jaw, and/or ear symptoms
- Headache of any type located in the temple(s)
- The following symptoms may or may not be accompanied by pain:
  - Joint sounds with jaw movement
  - Intermittent locking on opening

  - Intermittent locking on closing from a wide-open mouth position
  - Unable to bring back teeth into full occlusion
  - Unable to close from a wide-open mouth position
  - Limited mouth opening but not severe enough to interfere with opening of the mouth to eat and yawn
  - Limited mouth opening that is severe enough to interfere with opening of the mouth to eat and yawn

Pain and symptom will be interchanged throughout this chapter. The history portion of axis I documents functional or parafunctional activities that may modify common TMD symptoms. Symptom frequency (constant, daily, or weekly) and pain intensity, using the Visual Analog Scale 0 to 10, will be documented. Documentation will include, but is not limited to, functional limitations associated with chewing, talking, and/or yawning. Functional limitations can be documented by completing the JFLS (see Box 14-1).[33] The JFLS assesses the patient's limitation in mastication, mobility, and communication. On subsequent visits, reassessing patient's symptoms (change in frequency and intensity) and functional limitations can provide information regarding patient's progress with treatments.

The history portion of the examination will also include axis II. Axis II assesses psychosocial distress. Psychosocial distress involves, but is not limited to, fear, anxiety, anger, and depression. Psychosocial distress can affect treatment outcomes by enhancing a patient's perception of pain contributing to an allodynia or hyperalgesia response to nociceptive input.[34] The PHQ is a short, reliable, and valid screening instrument for detecting "psychological distress"–related anxiety and/or depression (see Box 14-1).[35] The GCPS measures pain intensity and disability (see Box 14-1).[36] Kotiranta et al[37] did a study of 399 patients diagnosed with TMD to determine how often pain disability was magnified by psychosocial distress. The majority (61%) of patients fell into

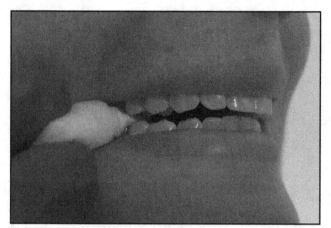

Figure 14-1. Bite Test. Patient bites on a dental roll or rolled up gauze that is placed between 2 opposing mandibular and maxillary molars. Biting with a firm force results in joint loading of the contralateral side. Joint loading does occur on the ipsilateral side but not to the same degree. A positive response is reproduction of the patient's familiar pain on the contralateral side stemming from the TMJ. Figure depicts joint loading of the left TMJ. Bite test requires jaw-closing muscles to contract. Although the bite test is used to assist in diagnosing arthralgia, if myalgia is also present, the bite test may elicit a myalgia response. Location of the familiar pain along with other tests used to diagnose arthralgia and myalgia will assist in making the diagnosis of arthralgia and/or myalgia.

the no-disability group, 27% to the low-disability group, with only 12% in the high-disability group. Myalgia is associated with bruxism, and bruxism is often found to be associated with psychosocial distress.[38] Patients with no disability to low disability often respond well to a conservative treatment program offered by a physical therapist and if indicated, an evidence-based oral appliance from a dentist. Patients with high psychosocial distress may not reach full potential regardless of treatments offered. Psychosocial distress is a complex topic. Incorporating the PHQ and GCPS or other methods to assess psychosocial distress can assist the clinician to identify patients with high psychosocial distress who may need to be referred to the appropriate health care professional.

Physical Examination

The physical examination consists of 3 parts: provocation tests, assessing mandibular dynamics, and assessing joint noises. The primary focus of the physical examination is to modify common familiar symptoms of TMD.

Provocation Tests. Provocation tests are done to modify the patient's familiar symptom(s). Provocation tests include palpation of the masseter and temporalis muscles, palpation over the lateral pole of the TMJ, maximum unassisted and maximum assisted mouth opening, mandibular protrusive and lateral excursions, and bite test. Active or latent myofascial trigger points can only be diagnosed with palpation. Active myofascial trigger points are a common source of TMD symptoms to include, but are not limited to, facial, jaw, ear, and headache pain. When an active trigger point is palpated, the patient's familiar symptoms would be modified (ie, increased).[39,40] An exception of reproducing familiar pain

during the examination are latent myofascial trigger points. A latent myofascial trigger point is asymptomatic and can be quiescent for months or years but only becomes painful when stretched or compressed (palpated) during the physical examination.[39] Latent myofascial trigger points may be a source of referred pain and/or can perpetuate adjacent active myofascial trigger points (satellite myofascial trigger points).[40] Active satellite myofascial trigger points may become resistive to treatment unless the latent myofascial trigger points are first treated.[40] The definition of familiar pain would not apply to latent myofascial trigger points because latent myofascial trigger points are not painful at the time of the examination unless palpated. The DC/TMD does not account for latent myofascial trigger points in their diagnostic criterion for myalgia.

Bite test is described in Figure 14-1.[41] Knowledge of the anatomy will assist the clinician to determine what tissue is provoked and whether the involved tissue correlates to the patient's familiar symptoms and functional limitations. There are other provocation tests that the reader may find useful,[42] but at this time, they have not been incorporated into the DC/TMD. Regardless of the provocation tests used, the clinician needs to understand the strengths and limitations of each test.

Mandibular Dynamics. Mouth opening or interincisal opening (IO) is measured using a millimeter (mm) ruler. IO is the distance from the tip of an upper central incisor to the tip of the lower central incisor (Figure 14-2). DC/TMD includes overbite in their IO measurement. The author of this chapter does not add vertical incisal overlap (overbite) to the IO measurement. The rationale for not including overbite is that this relationship between the central incisors is constant and does not change during the time that a patient is receiving treatment. Measuring IO is a useful clinical measurement because it is the variable that is expected to change in response to intervention.[32] Not correcting for overbite reduces reliability concerns when measuring IO.[32]

Functional maximum unassisted IO ranges from greater than 30 mm to 40 mm or more. Maximum unassisted IO that is 30 mm or less represents a significant limitation in mouth opening.[30,32] Objectives for measuring maximum unassisted IO and maximum assisted IO mouth opening are listed in Figures 14-2 and 14-3. Opening of the mouth can occur in midline or the mandible can deflect (movement away from midline but does not return) or deviate (movement away from midline but then returns to midline). Boney asymmetries are common in the TMJ. Boney asymmetries consist of, but are not limited to, the shape of the mandibular condyles, variations of the long axis of the condyles, and angle of the articular eminences. If IO is functional, any associated deflection or deviation of the mandible may be the result of boney asymmetry and would not require treatment.

The DC/TMD recommends using a millimeter ruler to measure lateral and protrusive mandible movements. However, there are also reliability concerns in obtaining

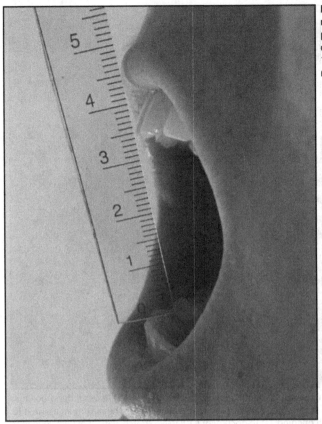

Figure 14-2. Measuring Maximum Unassisted IO. Objectives for measuring maximum unassisted IO: (1) to document maximum unassisted IO without pain, (2) to document maximum unassisted IO with pain, and (3) if pain on opening is present, assess if #2 modifies patient's familiar pain. Objectives 1, 2, and 3 are used as a baseline documentation to reassess the patient's response to treatments.

such measurements using a millimeter ruler.[30] The author of this chapter prefers to assess functional lateral excursions and functional protrusion by observing how the mandibular canines and central incisors move in relationship to the maxillary canines and central incisors (Figures 14-4 and 14-5). Ultimately, what the patient believes and feels with mouth opening, lateral excursions, and protrusion is as important as what the clinician can measure and observe.

Joint Noises. A noise originating from the TMJ will be heard by the patient. The clinician may or may not hear the noise. The clinician will palpate over the lateral pole of the condyle as the patient moves their mandible. If a noise is present, the clinician will feel a vibration created by friction between the tissues causing the noise. A click or crepitus are 2 noises associated with TMD. A click is required to diagnose a DDwR (Figure 14-6) and crepitus is required to diagnose DJD. Without a click or crepitus, a DDwR and DJD cannot be diagnosed by the clinical examination (Appendix A). A click may or may not occur with subluxation (see Appendix A). A noise that cannot be associated with a DDwR, DJD, or subluxation is an unclassified noise. An unclassified noise is likely related to a *deviation in form*, referring to any change in the articular surfaces of the TMJ that may result in a noise.[26]

In summary, imaging studies, computerized instruments, and occlusal studies are not necessary to make the diagnosis or determine treatment for all common TMD diagnostic subsets. These previous procedures will overdiagnose

TMD, resulting in treatments that are not necessary and will only drive up the cost of care. What is available to medical, dental, and physical therapy professionals is a reasonably reliable and valid clinical examination that can diagnose all common diagnostic subsets of TMD (see Appendix A).[28,30,32] An accurate diagnosis that factors in psychosocial distress often leads to a better treatment plan and treatment outcomes.[28,43,44]

Treatment Guidelines for Temporomandibular Disorder

The first treatment guideline for TMD was published in 1982 by The President's Conference on the Examination, Diagnosis, and Management of Temporomandibular Disorders.[45] Since 1982, the American Academy of Oral Facial Pain (AAOP) has published 7 treatment guidelines for orofacial pain. The most recent guideline was published in 2023.[2] All guidelines agree that treatments are to be conservative and cost effective for all common diagnostic subsets of TMD. Conservative care consists of medication, oral appliance, behavioral modification, and physical therapy. However, this author believes that physical therapy is underrepresented in the AAOP guidelines, position papers, policy statements, and other scientific literature.

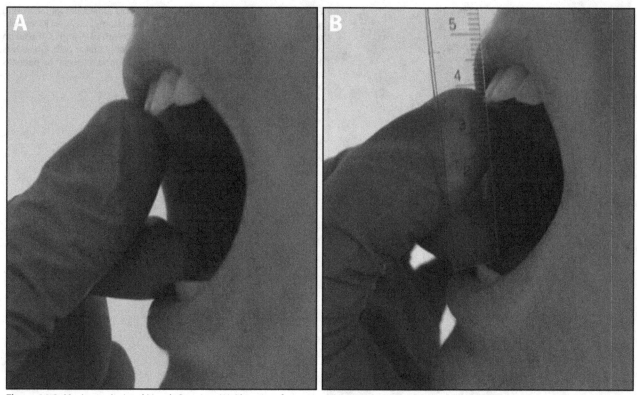

Figure 14-3. Maximum Assisted Mouth Opening. (A) Objectives for maximum assisted mouth opening (passive stretch): (1) Assess if this procedure modifies the patient's familiar pain and (2) assess end-range feel (ie, firm or springy). (B) With passive stretch, measure the maximum assisted IO using a millimeter ruler. Objective for measuring maximum assisted mouth opening: (1) to document IO. Passive stretch: Patient actively opens as wide as possible followed by the clinician pressing down on the patient's mandibular central incisors with the index finger as the thumb presses up on the maxillary central incisors. Objectives listed in A and B are used as baseline documentation to reassess the patient's response to treatments. Clinical points: (1) Maximum assisted opening should only be done if the patient has limited opening as determined by measuring maximum unassisted opening, and (2) maximum assisted opening should not be done if TMJ surgery or orthognathic surgery was recently done (depending on the surgery, this may vary between 1 to 3 months).

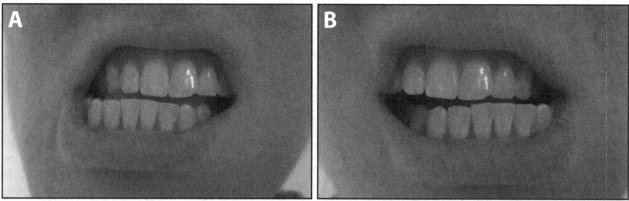

Figure 14-4. Functional Lateral Excursions. (A) Functional right lateral excursion. (B) Functional left lateral excursion. Functional lateral excursions are assessed by observing if the patient can move their mandibular canine past their maxillary canine on the ipsilateral side. Functional lateral excursions are necessary to chew food. If the patient cannot achieve an end-to-end position of their mandibular and maxillary canines, this is considered limited lateral excursion. Objectives for observing lateral excursions: (1) assess if lateral excursion(s) modify patient's familiar pain and (2) assess if patient has limited lateral excursion(s). Objectives are used as baseline documentation to reassess patient's response to treatments.

Clinical Point of the Clinical Examination

The DC/TMD requires pain to be present to make the diagnosis for myalgia and arthralgia. The DC/TMD does not require pain to be present to make the diagnosis for all other TMD arthrogenous diagnoses (ie, all disk displacements, DJD, dislocation, and subluxation). Knowing that arthrogenous diagnosis subsets may not be painful (exception is arthralgia) will guide treatment options and provide realistic expectations for treatment outcomes. Myalgia and/or arthralgia may represent separate mutually independent manifestations from other coexisting TMD arthrogenous conditions.[28,30]

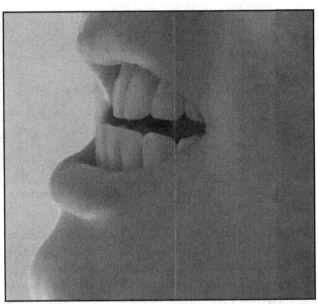

Figure 14-5. Functional Protrusion. Functional protrusion is assessed by observing if the patient can move their mandibular central incisors past the maxillary central incisors. Functional protrusion is necessary to bite and for phonetics. If the patient cannot achieve an end-to-end position of their mandibular and maxillary central incisors, this is considered limited protrusion. Objectives for observing protrusion: (1) assess if protrusion modifies patient's familiar pain and (2) assess if protrusion is limited. Objectives are used as baseline documentation to reassess patient's response to treatments.

Medication

Over-the-counter medications are available to patients. Although cost effective, over-the-counter medication taken for pain control has associated complications. Prolonged use of a nonsteroidal anti-inflammatory drug can cause gastrointestinal irritation.[46] Excessive use of acetaminophen, especially coupled with alcohol, can lead to liver damage.[46] Prescription medication such as a muscle relaxant have known complications such as dependency or can have severe interactions if taken with antihistamines or alcohol. Narcotics should seldom be given, and if given, the clinician must take ownership of overseeing the distribution, complications, abuse, and addiction that may arise. For more information on medication for TMD and HFP, the reader is referred to Kraus et al.[46]

Oral Appliance

The primary treatment offered by the dental profession for TMD is an oral appliance. An oral appliance is referred to by many different names with many different designs. Regardless of design, all oral appliances have some evidence as to their effectiveness but for reasons that are not known.[47] Evidence to justify the use of any oral appliance for any diagnostic subset of TMD is mixed.[48-50] All oral appliances have potential complications, which may include an increase in pain and/or movement of teeth.[47] Should a patient respond to wearing an oral appliance, it should not be assumed that a malocclusion was the etiology of the patient's symptoms and occlusal treatment is required.

Indications for an oral appliance are[50]:

- To reduce morning jaw muscle pain and/or headache (temples) related to myalgia and/or arthralgia triggered by sleep bruxism

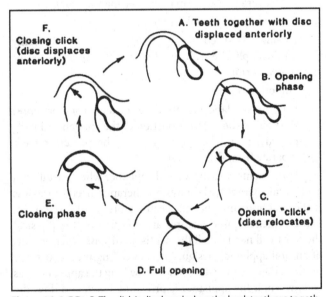

Figure 14-6. DDwR. The disk is displaced when the back teeth are together. As the mouth opens, an opening click occurs, indicating the disk has relocated on the condyle. As the mouth closes, bringing back teeth together, a closing click occurs. The closing click indicates the disk is displacing anterior or anteromedially to the condyle. (Reproduced with permission from Steve L Kraus. Evaluation and Management of Temporomandibular Disorders. Copyright 1993 by Steven L Kraus PT OCS. Reprinted with permission from: Evaluation, Treatment and Prevention of Musculoskeletal Disorders by H Duane Saunders, MS PT and Robin Saunders, MS PT. The Saunders Group Minneapolis, MN 55439.)

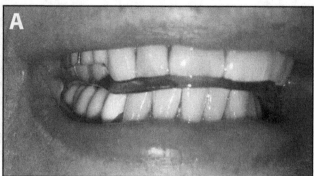

Figure 14-7. Examples of 2 oral appliances with evidence-based features.

- To reduce limited mouth opening in the morning due to myalgia or intermittent locking/catching associated with a disk displacement, both triggered by sleep bruxism
- To protect occlusal surfaces of teeth and dental restorations from sleep bruxism forces

To choose one oral appliance design over another may be based on minimizing complications from wearing an oral appliance than the effectiveness from wearing the oral appliance. An oral appliance with the following features has the best evidence for reducing myalgia and minimizing complications from prolong use (Figure 14-7)[47]:

- Made of hard acrylic
- Full coverage (can be maxillary or mandibular)
- Thin posteriorly (molar region)
- During unassisted closing, all opposing teeth hit evenly on the appliance with slightly heavier contact posterior than anterior
- Smooth (flat)
- Anterior guidance: As the anterior teeth (one or more) slide along the anterior portion of the appliance during protrusive and lateral excursions, the posterior teeth separate from the appliance

For patients wearing an oral appliance who consult with a physical therapist, the physical therapist needs to assess if the oral appliance has the features previously described. If the evidence-based features are not present, the physical therapist will need to call the dentist to discuss other options of an oral appliance design. Prior to calling the dentist, the physical therapist needs to assess how long the appliance has been worn, if the appliance is providing relief, and does the patient believe the appliance is changing their bite.

Physical Therapy

Treatment for all common diagnostic subsets for TMD should begin with a physical therapist, unless red flags are present or the examination is inconclusive. Physical therapy is cost effective and conservative.[30] Patient's TMD signs and symptoms often improve with physical therapy alone. After 4 to 6 physical therapy treatments, if the patient's signs and symptoms are not improving and there are indications for an

oral appliance, the patient can be referred to a dentist for an oral appliance. Pain that is confined to the joint and is refractory to both physical therapy treatment and an oral appliance, a referral to an oral surgeon would be indicated.

Physical therapy treatment objectives for TMD are to eliminate or reduce pain with a return to unrestricted mandibular function regardless of joint noise, DJD, and disk displacement. Conventional physical therapy treatments for TMD are listed in Appendix C. Indications of modalities and procedures can be found in the references.[43,51-53] The following highlights several of the conventional physical therapy treatments.

Patient Education

Patients will be educated on their TMD diagnosis, treatment objectives, other treatment options, and treatment expectations. Patient education will address inaccurate or misleading information regarding the etiology, diagnosis, and treatment of TMD. Misinformation may come from family members, friends, the internet, and, unfortunately, from health care professionals. Patient's psychosocial distress may be unnecessarily enhanced or be the result of misinformation.[48] It is essential that the physical therapist addresses misinformation and provides a "biopsychosocial message" of encouragement to the patient that will assure and reassure that a positive treatment outcome can be achieved.[54]

Behavioral Modification

Behavioral modification is defined as the process of changing unwanted behavior that contributes to an overuse, disuse, and/or abuse of the muscles of mastication and/or TMJ. Treatment success is largely dependent on reducing or eliminating oral parafunctional activity. Oral parafunctional activity includes habitual use of the mouth unrelated to eating, drinking, yawning, or talking. A significant oral parafunctional activity is bruxism. Bruxism is believed to be the most common trigger for TMD myalagia. Bruxism can be diurnal or nocturnal that consists of repetitive jaw-muscle activity characterized by clenching or grinding of the teeth and/or by bracing or thrusting of the mandible.[55] The etiology of bruxism is unknown.[55]

Diurnal Bruxism. Diurnal bruxism is best managed by educating the patient to be mindful that their teeth should not come into contact during their waking hours unless they are chewing or swallowing. The patient is instructed on keeping their tongue up and back teeth apart (TUTA).[51] TUTA is a very simple and effective self-awareness exercise to control diurnal bruxism. There continues to be discussions pertaining to the rest position of the tongue. Is the resting tongue position up against the palate of the mouth or down on the floor of the mouth? Wherever the resting position of the tongue is located, it should be a position that is maintained by the patient without effort and with back teeth slightly apart.

Bruxism also consists of bracing or thrusting of the mandible. This unwanted behavior is avoided by the "wiggle at will" (WW) exercise.[51] WW is performed by the patient moving their mandible left and right in a low amplitude movement. Only a few repetitions are necessary but performed many times throughout the day. Any pain or repetitive clicking is to be avoided. WW will be discontinued for patients who are not coordinated moving their mandible from side to side.

Patients must recognize triggers that may lead to bruxism. Common triggers consist of physical triggers (eg, lifting, reaching, pushing, pulling), focus triggers (eg, computer, driving, reading), emotional stress (eg, mental demands of work and home, interpersonal relationships, work pace), and psychosocial distress triggers (eg, fear, anxiety, anger, depression). When confronted with triggers, patients must focus on TUTA and WW.

Patients must eliminate oral parafunctional activities consisting of, but not limited to, nail biting, biting the inside of the cheek, or chewing gum or ice. Other activities to reduce, modify, or eliminate include chin leaning, eating hard/chewy food, singing, playing a musical instrument that involves pressure on the mandible, and sucking thick liquid through a straw.

Patients with TMD may concurrently have sleep apnea. Sleep apnea is considered to be one of many comorbidities of TMD myalgia. Sleep apnea may be treated by a sleep apnea appliance that repositions the mandible forward or by wearing a full-face continuous positive airway pressure (CPAP) mask that may apply retrusive pressure on the mandible. The sleep apnea appliance, or CPAP, can trigger bruxism and/or joint pain. Such devices may have to be modified or discontinued until the TMD symptoms become more manageable. Patients diagnosed with a disk displacement may be treated with an anterior repositioning appliance (ARA). As the name implies, an ARA repositions the mandible in a protrusive position. Like the sleep apnea appliance, an ARA can trigger bruxism and/or joint pain. If an ARA is worn for an extended period of time, the ARA can change the patient's occlusion, committing the patient to having orthodontic treatment.

Nocturnal Bruxism. Nocturnal bruxism is a challenge to control because the patient performs this unwanted behavior at night. Awake and sleep bruxism are not independent but interact additively.[56] Reducing diurnal pain and bruxism may help to reduce nocturnal bruxism.[56] Patients must avoid stomach sleeping and placing their hands under their mandible when sleeping on their side. Patients are encouraged to use a soft yet supportive pillow. A reduction in nocturnal bruxism may be helped if the patient were to increase aerobic exercise,[57] reduce caffeine, improve diet,[58] and avoid irregular sleep patterns due to lifestyle.[59] Although managing daytime pain and bruxism and improving sleeping postures may help reduce nocturnal bruxism, patients often require an evidence-based oral appliance (see Figure 14-7).

Manual Therapy, Therapeutic Exercise, and Modalities

There are a number of systematic and meta-analysis publications summarizing the evidence for physical therapy treatment for TMD patients.[60-64] A universal conclusion reached by the reviewers is that most randomized clinical trials reviewed were of poor methodological quality, investigated more than one physical therapy procedure or modality, investigated other treatments (oral appliance and medication) at the same time a physical therapy modality or procedure was investigated, and the definition of physical therapy in some studies included chiropractic, osteopathic, and massage therapists. The reviewers of this literature suggested conclusions be interpreted with caution. A generalization of all these studies suggests that active and passive exercise for the mandible, manual therapy, postural exercises, and neck exercises appear to have favorable effects for patients with TMD in the reduction of pain and improved IO.[60-64]

A systematic review and meta-analysis article published in 2016 looked at interventions of manual therapy, dry needling, and exercise therapy that were administered only by physical therapists.[65] The search identified 7 articles that met the inclusion criteria that were used in the analysis. The conclusion was manual therapy, dry needling, and exercise performed by physical therapists are more effective than other treatment modalities and sham treatments in reducing TMD pain and improving active mandibular ROM.[65] Conclusions were not definitive and should be reviewed with caution due to a small number of studies and variability of instruments used to assess the outcomes.

Clinical Points Pertaining to Temporomandibular Disorder Treatment

Point One

The TMJ is a load bearing joint.[66] Excessive and prolonged joint loading places stress on all components of the TMJ. Joint loading is reduced by eliminating or reducing parafunctional activities. Reducing TMJ loading often has a positive effect on concurrent arthrogenous diagnostic subsets. Reducing joint loading often results in arthralgia being reduced or eliminated, clicking related to a DDwR or subluxation becomes faint or undetectable, crepitus associated with DJD becomes faint or undetectable, and intermittent locking associated with a DDwR decreases in frequency or is eliminated. At the risk of oversimplification, focusing on reducing joint loading by managing parafunctional activities will help many patients with concurrent arthrogenous disorders.

Point Two

If reducing joint loading does not help to reduce the frequency or eliminate intermittent locking associated with a DDwR, a change in treatment protocol is required. Therapeutic exercises and intraoral mobilization techniques can be offered for the purpose of increasing mouth opening while preventing the disk to relocate during mouth opening. The objective of these techniques is to progress a DDwR with intermittent locking to a DDwoR woLO. This is acceptable for the following reasons:

- MRI studies of the TMJ have identified one-third of asymptomatic volunteers have unilaterally or bilaterally a DDwoR woLO.[10,11]

- In their simplest application, arthrocentesis and arthroscopy are successful in the reduction of TMJ pain and improving mouth opening in patients diagnosed with a disk displacement. However, the success of these 2 procedures is not dependent on relocating a displaced disk. Following these 2 surgical procedures, patients often have a DDwoR woLO[67,68]

Point Three

Patients with a DDwoR wLO (Figure 14-8) can, over time, improve their mouth opening without any treatment.[69,70] Patients often pursue treatment because this condition severely limits mouth opening while brushing teeth, eating, and yawning. A systematic review examined 20 studies that utilized different treatment options for a DDwoR wLO.[71] Treatment options were divided into 3 groups: noninvasive, consisting of patient education, self-management, physical therapy, and splint therapy; minimally invasive, consisting of arthrocentesis; and invasive, consisting of arthroscopy and arthrotomy. The comparable therapeutic effects of the 3 groups of interventions identified physical therapy as one of the simplest, least costly, and least invasive interventions for the management of a DDwoR wLO. Kraus and Prodoehl[72] investigated physical therapy treatment outcomes for 97 patients diagnosed with a DDwoR wLO. This study concluded that physical therapy treatment provided a positive trend for long-term benefits of pain reduction, improved active IO, and patient satisfaction for patients diagnosed with a DDwoR wLO.[72]

Point Four

DJD (osteoarthrosis) has been identified in patients whose disks are displaced and in patients whose disks are not displaced.[73,74] Degenerative changes of the TMJ may be dependent on the balance between a patient's adaptive capacity and functional loading or excessive loading with or without a disk displacement.[74] The message to communicate to patients is that the disk does not have to be in place to have successful treatment outcomes of pain reduction and a return to function.[75]

PRE- AND POSTDOCTORAL EDUCATION OF HEALTH CARE PROVIDERS FOR TEMPOROMANDIBULAR DISORDERS

Clinician's knowledge of anatomy, physiology, mechanics, etiology, and pathophysiology will help in all aspects of the examination and treatment for TMD. A clinician's knowledge is dependent on their educational experiences.

Unfortunately, at the time of this writing, there is no standardized curricula to guide predoctoral teaching across the dental, physical therapy, and medical professions. A 2007 study of predoctoral dental education on TMD found that only 3 dental schools described their TMD-related teaching situation as ideal.[76] The study concluded that dental professionals may not receive any entry-level training on diagnosing or managing TMD. It was not until 2020 that the Commission for Dental Accreditation (CODA) approved the teaching of TMDs in the predoctoral curriculums of all US dental schools by 2022.[77,78] The American Dental Association (ADA) did not recognize orofacial pain (to include TMD) as one of the 12 dental specialties until 2020.[79] With these changes made only recently by CODA and the ADA, it should not be a surprise there is a shortage of trained dental professionals who are competent in the management of TMD.[80]

A recent study examined self-perceived adequacy of entry-level TMD education of physical therapists from Florida.[81] This pilot study shows the lack of confidence of physical therapists in Florida to treat patients with TMD. A recent study investigated the status of entry level physical therapy education in the United States related to the diagnosis and management of TMD.[82] An email survey was sent to 224 accredited, entry-level US physical therapy programs. Of the programs that responded, this survey identified several barriers of the entry-level physical therapy programs suggesting not all entry-level physical therapists are ready to work with patients with TMD.[82]

Post-graduation, there are various avenues by which physical therapists can obtain professional development. Physical therapists can review the American Physical Therapy Association *Guide to Physical Therapy Practice*. The guide mentions TMD as a musculoskeletal condition causing pain but it does not provide any specific protocols for diagnosis or management of TMD.[83] The Orthopedic Clinical Specialist (OCS) certification is recognized by The American Board of Physical Therapy Specialties.[84] The OCS status is achieved by passing a multiple-choice format with no oral or practical testing. Only 3% of the questions on the OCS examination are related to the head, maxillofacial, or craniomandibular areas.[84] Orthopedic residency and fellowship programs in the United States and internationally provide limited educational experiences on the diagnosing and management of TMD.[85,86] There are a few postdoctoral educational opportunities for the physical therapist that leads to specialization in TMD.[87] The most common avenue physical therapists rely on for professional development are continuing education courses to maintain their clinical competency.[88] Peterson et al concluded that most continuing education courses (regardless of topic) do not incorporate current best evidence but may instead teach outdated or misaligned concepts, riddled with inefficiencies.[88] Physical therapists incorporating continuing education courses should take note of the concerns raised by Peterson et al when choosing continuing education courses on TMD management. To help in this short coming of professional development opportunities on TMD management, the American Physical Therapy Association is sponsoring the first TMD clinical practice guidelines to be published early in 2024.[89]

The consumer should know what to expect of the medical and other health care providers regarding their education on TMD. Medical doctors receive little to no training on

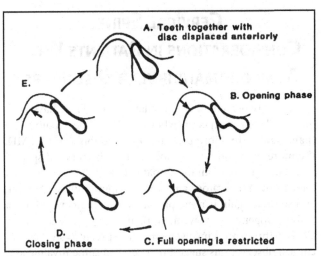

Figure 14-8. DDwoR. The disk is displaced when the back teeth are together. As the mouth opens, the disk remains displaced during full mouth opening and closing. Active IO less than or equal to 30 mm is associated with a DDwoR wLO. Active IO greater than 30 mm is associated with a DDwoR woLO. See Appendix A for additional diagnostic criteria. (Reproduced with permission from Steve L Kraus. Evaluation and Management of Temporomandibular Disorders. Copyright 1993 by Steven L Kraus PT OCS. Reprinted with permission from: Evaluation, Treatment and Prevention of Musculoskeletal Disorders by H Duane Saunders, MS PT and Robin Saunders, MS PT. The Saunders Group.)

the classification and management of TMD.[90,91] Greene and Bertagna[92] in their web search, found no evidence that TMD is taught as part of the regular curriculum in all medical and allied practitioners with professional degrees and clinicians with training in complementary alternative therapy. Greene and Bertagna concluded "physical therapists emerged as the only ancillary health care professionals with some positive aspects with regard to their training as well as their treatment approaches for TMDs."[92]

Predoctoral education on TMD for health care professionals is sobering. Postdoctoral TMD education becomes the responsibility of the dentist, physician, and physical therapist to be kept informed by attending scientific forums with an inquisitive mind and to read current scientific publications in peer-reviewed journals and textbooks on TMD. Despite the lack of continuity of the health care professional's education on TMD, the majority of patients with acute and chronic TMD do respond well to an evidence-based diagnostic and treatment approach offered by physical therapy and dental professionals. However, some patients continue to experience TMD and HFP. For nonresponding patients, investigating TMJ pathology, high pain disability, psychosocial distress, comorbidities, and other diagnoses contributing to HFP need to be considered. However, a very common missed or misdiagnosis for patients suffering from TMD and HFP is a CSD. Cervical spine influences on TMD and HFP will be discussed next.

CERVICAL SPINE CONSIDERATIONS IN PATIENTS WITH TEMPOROMANDIBULAR DISORDERS

Seventy percent of the population with TMD have neck pain.[30,93] Women experience both TMD and neck pain more than men.[30] The more pain and dysfunction due to TMD, the more pain and dysfunction exist in the cervical spine.[94] Bruxism is more common in patients who have myofascial pain in the masticatory and cervical spine muscles.[95] Neck and shoulder pain is more prevalent in patients who have a TMD myogenous involvement, than in patients who have a TMD arthrogenous involvement.[96] The previous studies and clinical observations suggest that cervical spine myalgia and masticatory myalgia may interact with each other and not just coexist with each other.

Cervical Neck Reflexes

The trigeminal cervical reflex (TCR) and asymmetric/symmetric tonic neck reflexes (TNR) are an elaborate set of reflexes between trigeminal and cervical areas. The TCR is mediated by a pathway comprising the trigeminal nerve and trigeminal spinal tract, which projects to motor neurons of the sternocleidomastoid muscle and posterior neck muscles.[97] The reflex is a defensive withdrawal of the head by contraction of neck muscles in response to facial stimuli.[98] Neck muscles are constantly providing orientation of the face in response to posture and movement.[99]

The TNR is a primitive reflex that exists in newborn babies and is still present in adults.[100] The origin of the TNR is in the upper 3 cervical segments (muscles and facet joints).[101] The TNR, in response to movement of the head and neck, modifies masticatory muscle activity. Funakoshi and Amano[101] observed the effects of the TNR on the tone of jaw muscles in rats. Muscle tone of the jaw muscles varied with flexion, extension, and rotation of the neck. When the first 3 cervical nerves were cut, the effects of head/neck movement on the jaw activity were abolished.[101] Other studies have demonstrated the TNR effects on jaw muscle activity.[102,103]

Functional Jaw Movements

A synergistic relationship exists between the cervical spine muscles and the muscles of mastication. Movement of the head-neck occurs with oral functions involving chewing, talking, swallowing, and yawning.[104] The TCR and TNR likely play an integral role in this synergistic relationship. Coordinated mandibular and head-neck movements during jaw opening/closing activities has been observed during chewing.[105] Each chewing cycle was accompanied not only by mandibular movements but also by head extension-flexion movements suggesting a close functional linkage between the jaw and the neck regions.[105] Zafar and colleagues completed 2 studies that found a high degree of temporal coordination between concomitant mandibular and head and neck movements during maximum jaw opening and closing tasks at both fast and slow speeds.[106,107] Ericksson and colleagues[108] describe this synergistic relationship between the cervical spine and muscles of mastication as "functional jaw movements" (FJMs). Functional jaw movements are the result of activation of jaw and neck muscles, leading to simultaneous movements in the temporomandibular, atlanto-occipital, and cervical spine joints.[108] When the head is fixated, reduced mandibular movements and shorter duration of jaw opening/closing cycles were observed.[109] The findings suggest a recruitment of neck muscles during jaw activities exists and head fixation can impair jaw function.[109,110] In a non-patient population, different head and neck postures have been shown to affect genioglossus muscle activity during swallow.[111] In a pilot study of 8 partipants, a change in head and neck posture affects the rest position of the mandible.[112] Other studies have shown that head and neck posture can affect the rest position of the mandible, resulting in a change in the trajectory of jaw closure and subsequently a change in the initial tooth/teeth contact.[113-115] Clinically, altered masticatory muscle activity occurs in response to diminished cervical movement and changes in head and neck posture.[116]

Neck Pain and Masticatory Muscle Activity

Myalgia is the most common diagnostic subset for acute or chronic TMD and CSD.[117] Patients with jaw and neck pain share common risk factors. Psychosocial distress is one of the most common risk factors contributing to an increase in myalgia of the cervical spine and jaw.[118,119] Another risk factor, often overlooked, that increases masticatory muscle activity is neck pain. Komiyama and colleagues induced experimental pain by injecting 0.5 ml of hypertonic (6%) saline in the trapezius muscle of 12 participants, 25 to 35 years of age.[120] In addition to pain referral over a wide area to include the temporomandibular region, there was a reduction in mouth opening.[120] Hu and colleagues[121] injected an inflammatory irritant into deep neck muscles surrounding C1-C3 of 19 anaesthetized rats, resulting in a sustained and reversible activation of both jaw and neck muscles. Carlson and colleagues[122] investigated 20 patients with upper trapezius myofascial trigger points and ipsilateral masseter muscle pain. Each patient received a single trigger point injection of 2% lidocaine solution in the upper trapezius muscle. After trapezius injection, there was a significant reduction in pain intensity and electromyography activity of the masseter muscle.[122] Myofascial trigger points in the muscles of mastication may be satellite trigger points and may be resistive to treatment until the primary myofascial trigger points in the cervical spine muscles are first treated.[40,123] A recent study using rats showed that by activating nociceptors of the trapezius muscle increased the level of calcitonin gene-related peptide in the trigeminal ganglion, which led to sensitization of the trigeminal system, concluding neck pain is a risk for masticatory muscle pain.[124]

Considering the previous studies, it should come as no surprise that there is a strong association between jaw disability and neck disability. Using the Jaw Functional Scale and the Neck Disability Index, Olivo and colleagues demonstrated that patients having more disability in the neck also have more jaw disability and vice versa.[125] Other studies have shown patients with TMD that had more limited mouth opening and tender points on palpation also exhibited significantly more cervical spine limitations and more tender points upon palpation of neck and shoulder muscles.[126-128]

Patients with myalgia of the muscles of mastication can no longer be viewed as a local disorder of the jaw. The cervical spine must be evaluated in patients with simple to complex symptoms stemming from the muscles of mastication and/or TMJ. Postural reeducation, manual therapy, and exercise directed at the cervical spine improves pain intensity, pressure pain sensitivity, as well as limited mouth opening in patients with masticatory muscle pain.[129-131]

Cervical Spine and Headache and Facial Pain

The ICHD identifies the cervical spine as a second of 2 musculoskeletal sources for HFP.[1] A high occurrence of neck pain has been found in patients with HFP. Two hundred consecutive female patients referred to a university facial pain clinic were asked to mark all painful sites on sketches that showed contours of a human body in frontal and rear views.[132] Analysis of the pain distribution according to the arrangements of dermatomes revealed pain was not confined only to the region innervated by the trigeminal nerve. One hundred thirty-one patients had pain in the trigeminal area but also had widespread pain to include spinal dermatomes C2, C3, and C4. Patients with HFP often experience pain in the neck and shoulder areas.[133,134]

Cephalic symptoms such as headache, ear, and jaw symptoms can originate from the cervical spine. This referral mechanism is based on the established neurophysiological relationship of the upper 3 cervical nerves converging onto neurons of cranial nerve V as well as neurons from cranial nerves VII, IX, and X.[135-138] This region of convergence is in the upper cervical spinal cord within the pars caudalis portion of the spinal nucleus of the trigeminal nerve and is referred to as the *trigeminocervical nucleus* (Figure 14-9).[139] All pain and temperature originating from the head and face terminates in the trigeminocervical nucleus.[140] Cervical spine tissues innervated by C1, C2, and C3 spinal nerves that are responsible for cephalic symptoms are listed in Figure 14-10.[141]

Cervicogenic Headache

Sjaastad et al first identified CGH in 1983.[142] Cervicogenic symptoms are symptoms originating from the cervical spine and are felt by the patient in the head, face, jaw, and ear areas.

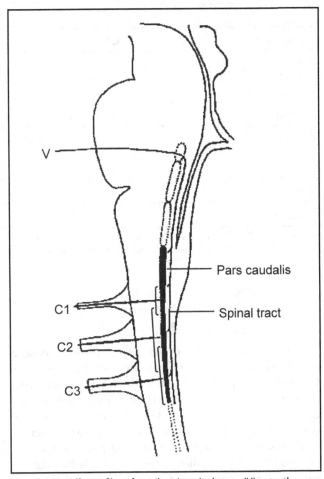

Figure 14-9. Afferent fibers from the trigeminal nerve (V) enter the pons and descend within the spinal tract of the trigeminal nerve to the upper cervical levels C1, C2, and C3. Trigeminal and cervical afferents constitute the trigeminocervical nucleus. (Reproduced with permission from Haldeman S, Dagenais S. Cervicogenic headaches: a critical review. *Spine J.* 1[2001]:31-46.)

Tissues innervated by C1, C2, and/or C3 can be the source of CGH. The prevalence of a CGH estimates range from 0.4% to 2.5% of the general population to 15% to 20% of patients with chronic headaches.[139] CGH is 1 of the 3 large headache groups; the other 2 are tension-type headache (TTH) and common migraine without aura.[143]

The clinical examination used to diagnose CGH is[144]:

1. Pain can be unilateral, but can be bilateral, localized to neck and occipital region. May project to forehead, orbital region, temples, vertex, or ears. ICHD indicates that "Migrainous features such as nausea, vomiting and photo/phonophobia may be present with [CGH]"[1]

2. Headache modified by at least one of the following:

   A. Neck movement and/or sustained head position

   B. Palpation of neck muscles (upper cervical, trapezius, and sternocleidomastoid muscles)

3. Restricted active or passive cervical ROM

	Innervation		
Structure	C1	C2	C3
Joints	Atlanto-occipital	Median atlantoaxial Lateral atlantoaxial	C2-3 zygapophyseal C2-3 disc
Ligaments		Transverse atlantoaxial and alar; membrana tectoria	
Muscles	Suboccipital	Prevertebral; sternocleidomastoid, trapezius Semispinalis, splenius Multifidus; semispinalis	
Dura		Upper spinal cord; posterior cranial fossa	
Arteries		Vertebral; internal carotid	

Figure 14-10. Possible sources of CGH listed according to innervation and type of structures. (Reproduced with permission from Bogduk N. Cervicogenic headache: anatomic basis and pathophysiologic mechanisms. *Curr Pain Headache Rep.* 2001;5:382-386.)

Cervicogenic Headache and Headache Attributed to Temporomandibular Disorder

There is considerable overlap of symptoms associated with CGH and HFP. Cervical spine tissues listed in Figure 14-10 can refer pain cephalically. The cervical spine tissue responsible for the majority of HFP originates from myofascial trigger points.[139] Myofascial trigger points located in the semispinalis capitis, longissimus and splenius capitis, sternocleidomastoid, and trapezius can all refer pain into the temple area.[145] As stated earlier, HTMD is a headache originating from the temporalis muscle and felt by the patient in the temporalis muscle.[28] A differential diagnosis will be required to know if the patient's headache located in the temple area is referred from the cervical spine or originating from the temporalis muscle. Treatment would then be directed toward the cervical spine muscles or temporalis muscle or both.

The next section highlights the overlap of CGH and HTMD with TTH and migraine

Tension-Type Headache

TTH is the most common of all headaches.[1] In 1972, Wolff believed that TTH was due to sustained contraction of the pericranial muscles contributing to ischemia of the muscle, and pain causing a pressure or band-like tightness in the head.[146] The ICHD states "[i]ncreased pericranial tenderness recorded by manual palpation is the most significant abnormal finding in patients with [TTH]."[1] To diagnose TTH, the ICHD recommends the following muscles be palpated: frontalis, temporalis, masseter, pterygoid, and cervical muscles to include sternocleidomastoid, splenius, and trapezius muscles.[1] Patient's description of a pressure or band-like tightness and increased tenderness on palpation of jaw and neck/shoulder muscles resemble the descriptions of referred pain originating from myofascial trigger points.[146] Clinically, the majority of TTH are reproduced by palpating myofascial trigger points located in key muscles such as the temporalis, sternocleidomastoid, splenius, and trapezius.[147]

Tension-Type Headache and Cervical Spine. Sakai and colleagues[148] diagnosed 60 patients with TTH, and Ashina and colleagues[149] diagnosed 20 patients with TTH. Both studies concluded that tension in the trapezius muscle of patients with TTH was significantly greater than that in age-matched normal participants. In a controlled study of 20 participants diagnosed with TTH, all participants had myofascial trigger points in the suboccipital muscles.[150] Active myofascial trigger points in suboccipital muscles of 13/20 (65%) were associated with referred pain that reproduced the participants' TTH. Latent myofascial trigger points were identified in 7/20 (35%) participants with TTH. Headache intensity and frequency was greater in participants with TTH who had active myofascial trigger points compared to those with only latent myofascial points.[150]

Tension-Type Headache and Headache Attributed to Temporomandibular Disorder. There is a significant overlap between TTH and HTMD.[151,152] Forty percent of patients diagnosed with TTH will have a TMD myalgia (temporalis) diagnosis.[153] HTMD and/or TMD myalgia may be a pathogenesis for TTH.[154] Management of TTH will need to incorporate treatment of the myofascial trigger points located in the muscles of mastication, especially the temporalis.[153]

Migraine

Woman are diagnosed more with migraine than men.[155] Migraine with or without aura is an episodic headache lasting 4 to 72 hours with aura as the defining feature of migraine.[1] Migraine can be diagnosed with a certain degree of confidence if the patient responds positively to 2 or more of the following 3 items[156]:

1. Has a headache limited your activities for a day or more in the last 3 months? (disability)
2. Are you nauseated or sick to your stomach when you have a headache? (nausea)
3. Does light bother you when you have a headache? (photophobia)

Migraine and Cervical Spine. As stated earlier, "Migrainous features such as nausea, vomiting and photo/phonophobia may be present with [CGH]."[1] Up to 75% of patients with migraine report having neck pain or stiffness associated with their migraine attack.[157] Regardless of the intensity of an episodic or chronic migraine, the migraine is more likely to be accompanied by neck pain than by nausea.[158] Myofascial trigger points located in cervical spine muscles can trigger a migraine and have been considered to be a pathogenesis for migraine.[124,159-167] Patients with migraine should have their cervical spine evaluated and if indicated treated.

Migraine and Headache Attributed to Temporomandibular Disorder. Tenderness of the pericranial muscles (temporalis) during a migraine attack has been known for more than 70 years.[168] TMD myalgia (HTMD) is a risk factor for increased frequency of migraine and often leads to chronic migraine, whereas TMD arthrogenous diagnostic subsets are not a risk factor to migraine.[169] Although they may be separate problems, TMD myalgia and migraine might aggravate or sustain each other.[170] Garrigos-Pedron and colleagues[171] looked at 45 participants diagnosed with chronic migraine and TMD. Patients were randomized in 2 groups: a cervical group that received only physical therapy to the cervical region, and the orofacial group that received physical therapy to both the cervical and orofacial regions. Results showed that both groups reported significant improvement in pain and disability, but cervical and orofacial treatment was more effective than cervical treatment alone. Clinical implication is patients with migraine may benefit by treating coexisting TMD myalgia and cervical myalgia by a physical therapist.

Clinical Points

Peripheral and central mechanisms have been suggested as important components of TTH and migraine. Evidence suggests a strong myofascial component associated with TTH and migraine. What has yet to be determined is if the masticatory and cervical spine muscles are the result of a TTH or migraine or the pathogenesis of a TTH or migraine. If the latter is true, this would have strong implications for treatment directed toward the muscles of mastication and cervical spine for patients suffering from TTH or migraine.

Cervicogenic Somatosensory Ear Symptoms

Ear symptoms include ear pain, tinnitus, fullness, and subjective hearing loss. Ear symptoms can be primary otalgia (ear pathology present) or secondary otalgia (ear symptom not caused by primary ear pathology).[172] A source for secondary otalgia is the cervical spine. Once otolaryngologic diseases have been ruled out as the cause of ear symptoms, the focus needs to be on CSD and TMD as sources of secondary ear symptoms.[173] Kuttila and colleagues did an interview and examination of 100 participants with otalgia.[174] In this study, 91 participants had secondary otalgia and 9 participants had primary otalgia. It was determined that the 91 particpants with secondary symptoms had more signs and symptoms related to CSD than of TMD. Neck pain may be a predictor for secondary ear symptoms.[173] Patients with secondary otalgia should routinely have an examination of the cervical spine and TMD.[173,174] Ear symptoms originating from the cervical spine are referred to as *cervicogenic somatosensory ear symptoms (CSES)*.[175] A common source for CSES is myofascial trigger points in the cervical spine muscles, especially the sternocleidomastoid muscle.[176-178]

The pathophysiology for subjective tinnitus, subjective fullness, and subjective hearing loss is more complex. Primary tinnitus (a pathology is present) represents only 1% of cases of tinnitus.[179] Ten percent of the population suffers from subjective tinnitus with a multifactorial etiology.[179] Subjective tinnitus, fullness, and hearing loss may be related to an increase in activity of the tensor veli palatine and tensor tympani. These are muscles of the middle ear and are innervated by the trigeminal nerve. One function of the tensor veli palatine is to open and close the eustachian tubes.[180] This muscle allows air pressure to equalize between the tympanic cavity and the outside air.[180] The tensor tympani originates from the cartilaginous portion of the eustachian tube and crosses the middle ear by a slender tendon and attaches itself to the manubrium of the malleus.[180] This muscle tenses the tympanic membrane by drawing the tympanic membrane medially to dampen noise.[180] Regarding the tensor veli palatine and tensor tympani, Ramirez et al states, "[t]hese are muscles of the middle ear although they are really muscles of mastication because they are modulated by motoneurons coming from the trigeminal motor nucleus."[181] The trigeminal motor neuron system may be modulated by cervical nociceptive afferent information resulting in an increase in muscle activity of the tensor veli palatine and tensor tympani. A high prevalence of somatosensory tinnitus is associated with the cervical spine, which infers cervical spine treatment may reduce tinnitus.[181-183] Abel and Levine demonstrated that patients with subjective tinnitus could change their tinnitus with forceful head and neck contractions.[184] In the same study, about 80% of nonclinical participants, who had ongoing tinnitus at the time of testing, could modulate their tinnitus with head and neck contractions. These findings support the concept of a neural threshold for tinnitus. The cervical spine may be a source for ear pain, subjective tinnitus, subjective fullness, and subjective hearing loss.

Cervical Spine Examination

A negative proviso is not a part of the diagnostic criteria for neck pain. However, if the patient's TMD and HFP (TTH or migraine) is not responding to medications, injections, or an oral appliance and the HFP is not better accounted for by another condition, the cervical spine needs to be considered. Clearly, if the patient is complaining of neck pain, the cervical spine will need to be evaluated and treated. Some patients may not complain of neck pain but instead complain of stiffness and tightness in their neck. The objective of the cervical spine examination is to modify the patient's familiar symptoms (neck, upper extremity, headache, jaw, facial, and/or ear symptoms) through tests of provocation consisting of palpation for active/latent myofascial trigger points, active and passive ROM testing. The clinical examination described in Appendix B is only a portion of a more comprehensive clinical examination that can be performed by the physical therapist. Michiels and colleagues assessed the diagnostic value of passive segmental testing, adapted Spurling test, strength and endurance of the deep flexor neck muscles, and 16 muscle palpation sites for myofascial trigger points to diagnose cervicogenic tinnitus.[185] A group of 17 international physical therapists completed several surveys to arrive at a consensus of 11 most useful physical examination tests to identify cervical musculoskeletal impairments in patients with headaches.[186] Patients with neck pain should have an assessment for psychosocial distress. The PHQ and the GCPS questionnaires recommended in the TMD evaluation would be appropriate to use in a comprehensive evaluation for patients with neck pain.[35,36]

Imaging of the cervical spine is not necessary to diagnose neck pain. Asymptomatic patients have positive imaging findings of cervical spondylitis and cervical disk herniation in 25% of patients less than 40 years old and in 60% of patients greater than 40 years old.[187] Imaging studies of the cervical spine are required if cervical radiculopathy or myelopathy signs and symptoms are present or if red flags are identified (see Table 14-1).

Clinician's should not be quick to conclude a patient has anatomic alignment problems of their cervical vertebrae from visually observing forward head posture or from using surface measurements of head and neck posture. When participants judged to have extreme head and neck posture based on external appearance or surface measurements were then imaged, participants showed vertebral positioning in the upper cervical spine were within the normal population distribution.[188] There are not adequate studies available comparing patients with neck pain to the asymptomatic population in order to make conclusions about any specific physical dimensions of posture related to neck pain (ie, forward head posture).[189,190] Maintaining good posture in a sitting, standing, or sleeping position is important. However, patients are to be encouraged to move frequently their head, neck, and shoulders throughout the day (especially if the patient's occupation involves sitting) vs staying in one static correct posture. Future studies should investigate the dynamics of posture as it relates to neck pain, CGH, CSES, TMD, and HFP.

Treatment Guidelines for Neck Pain

Conservative care for acute or chronic neck pain consists of several treatment strategies tailored to the individual patient. Treatments to the cervical spine will reduce or eliminate CGH and CSES symptoms, and if related, a reduction or elimination of symptoms may be seen in patients diagnosed or misdiagnosed with TTH and migraine.

Conservative care consists of patient education and behavioral modification, especially in sitting and sleeping postures. Manual therapy includes soft tissue massage, facet joint mobilization/manipulation, and dry needling. Therapeutic exercise (strength, condition, and flexibility), modalities, and cervical traction will complete the conventional treatment approach for neck pain. It is beyond the scope of this chapter to discuss in detail, indications, and method of application of all interventions available to the physical therapist. The evidence suggests a combination of the previous treatment strategies provides the best relief for patients suffering from neck pain and associated cephalic symptoms originating from the cervical spine.[191-197]

Should the patient not respond to conventional physical therapy treatments, there are other nonsurgical treatment options available. These treatments may include medication, injections to include lidocaine and botulinum toxin, epidural injections, nerve root injections, facet joint denervation, stellate ganglion block, and sphenopalatine block. These procedures lack Level I and Level II evidence in achieving a positive treatment outcome for neck pain with or without radiculopathy.[198-205] Cervical spine surgery includes laminectomy and fusion. Long-term benefits of surgery when compared to conservative care have similar results. Three studies examined the effects of surgery and conservative care on pain for sensory loss and weakness in patients who had minimal to moderate cervical radiculopathy or myelopathy.[206-208] No differences were found in sensation or motor strength between patients who were treated surgically and those who were managed conservatively in follow-up examinations at 24 and 36 months.[206-208]

CONCLUSION

Many conditions listed by ICHD contribute to HFP.[1] This chapter focused on TMD and CSD as 2 musculoskeletal disorders contributing to HFP. The evidence clearly indicates a conservative and a cost-effective approach is required for nearly all patients diagnosed with common TMD and CSD. Physical therapists, with the necessary knowledge and skills, are best equipped to manage all common diagnostic subsets of TMD and CSD. Patients not responding to physical therapy will require management from the physician, dentist, and/or oral surgeon. Health care professionals working together and recognizing what each profession has to offer will achieve the best outcomes for patients suffering from TMD and CSD.

REFERENCES

1. Headache Classification Committee of the International Headache Society. The International Classification of Headache Disorders, 3rd edition (beta version). *Cephalalgia*. 2013;33(9):629-808. doi:10.1177/0333102413485658

2. American Academy of Orofacial Pain; Klasser GD, Reyes MR. *Orofacial Pain: Guidelines for Assessment, Diagnosis, and Management*. 7th ed. Quintessence Publishing Co; 2023.

3. Dworkin SF, Huggins KH, LeResche L, et al. Epidemiology of signs and symptoms in temporomandibular disorders: clinical signs in cases and controls. *J Am Dent Assoc.* 1990;120(3):273-281. doi:10.14219/jada.archive.1990.0043

4. Schwenk TL. Healthcare expenditures for back and neck pain. *Journal Watch.* 2008:7(2).

5. Fricton JR, Schiffman EL. Epidemiology of temporomandibular disorders. In: Fricton JR, Dubner R, eds. *Orofacial Pain and Temporomandibular Disorders.* Raven Press; 1995.

6. Frymoyer JW, Durett CL. The economic impact of spinal disorders. In: Frymoyer JW, ed. *The Adult Spine: Principles and Practice.* Vol 2. Lippincott-Raven; 1997.

7. Martin BI, Deyo RA, Mirza SK, et al. Expenditures and health status among adults with back and neck problems. *JAMA.* 2008;299(6):656-664. doi:10.1001/jama.299.6.656

8. Marmulla R, Wörtche R, Mühling J, Hassfeld S. Geometric accuracy of the NewTom 9000 Cone Beam CT. *Dentomaxillofac Radiol.* 2005;34(1): 28–31. doi:10.1259/dmfr/31342245

9. Petersson A. What you can and cannot see in TMJ imaging- an overview related to the RDC/TMD diagnostic system. *J Oral Rehabil.* 2010;37(10):771-788. doi:10.1111/j.1365-2842.2010.02108.x

10. Jarvik JG, Deyo RA. Diagnostic evaluation of low back pain with emphasis on imaging. *Ann Intern Med.* 2002;137(7):586-597. doi:10.7326/0003-4819-137-7-200210010-00010

11. Larheim TA, Westesson PL, Sano T. Temporomandibular joint disk displacement: comparison in asymptomatic volunteers and patients. *Radiology.* 2001;218(2):428-432. doi:10.1148/radiology.218.2.r01fe11428

12. Aiken A, Bouloux G, Hudgins P. MR imaging of the temporomandibular joint. *Magn Reson Imaging Clin N Am.* 2012;20(3):397-412. doi:10.1016/j.mric.2012.05.002

13. Greene CS. The Role of Technology in TMD Diagnosis. In: Laskin DM, Greene CS, Hylander WL, eds. *Temporomandibular Disorders: An Evidence-Based Approach to Diagnosis and Treatment.* Quintessence Publishing Co; 2006:193-202.

14. Manfredini D, Favero L, Federzoni E, Cocilovo F, Guarda-Nardini L. Kinesiographic recordings of jaw movements are not accurate to detect magnetic resonance-diagnosed temporomandibular joint (TMJ) effusion and disk displacement: findings from a validation study. *Oral Surg Oral Med Oral Pathol Oral Radiol.* 2012;114(4):457-463. doi:10.1016/j.oooo.2012.04.016

15. Mohl ND, Lund JP, Widmer CG, McCall WD. Devices for the diagnosis and treatment of temporomandibular disorders. Part II: Electromyography and sonography. *J Prosthet Dent.* 1990;63(3):332-336. doi:10.1016/0022-3913(90)90207-s

16. American Association for Dental, Oral, and Craniofacial Research. American Association for Dental Research's Policy Statement on Temporomandibular Disorders (TMD). March 3, 2010. http://www.aadronline.org/i4a/pages/index.cfm?pageid=3465#TMD

17. Costen JB. A syndrome of ear and sinus symptoms dependent upon disturbed function of the temporomandibular joint. *Ann Otol Rhinol Laryngol.* 1934;43(1):1-15. doi:10.1177/000348943404300101

18. Türp JC, Schindler H. The dental occlusion as a suspected cause for TMDs: epidemiological and etiological considerations. *J Oral Rehabil.* 2012;39(7):502-512. doi:10.1111/j.1365-28422.2012.02304.x

19. Cooper BC, International College of Cranio-Mandibular Orthopedics. Temporomandibular disorders: a position paper of the International College of Cranio-Mandibular Orthopedics (ICCMO). *Cranio.* 2011;29(3):237-244. doi:10.1179/crn.2011.034

20. Gremillion HA. TMD and maladaptive occlusion: does a link exist? *Cranio.* 1995;13(4):205-206.

21. Friction J. Current evidence providing clarity in management of temporomandibular disorders: summary of a systematic review of randomized clinical trials for intra-oral appliances and occlusal therapies. *J Evid Base Dent Pract.* 2006;6(1):48-52. doi:10.1016/j.jebdp.2005.12.020

22. Koh H, Robinson PG. Occlusal adjustment for treating and preventing temporomandibular joint disorders. *Cochrane Database Syst Rev.* 2003;(1):CD003812. doi:10.1002/14651858.CD003812

23. Gremillion HA. The relationship between occlusion and TMD: an evidence-based discussion. *J Evid Base Dent Pract.* 2006;6(1):43-47. doi:10.1016/j.jebdp.2005.12.014

24. Klasser GD, Greene CS. The changing field of temporomandibular disorders: what dentists need to know. *J Can Dent Assoc.* 2009;75(1):49-53.

25. Xie Q, Li X, Xu X. The difficult relationship between occlusal interferences and temporomandibular disorder – insights from animal and human experimental studies. *J Oral Rehabil.* 2013;40(4):279-295. doi:10.1111/joor.12034

26. Greene CS. The etiology of temporomandibular disorders: implication for treatment. *J Orofac Pain.* 2001;15(2):93-105.

27. Okeson, JP. *Management of Temporomandibular Disorders and Occlusion.* 7th ed. Elsevier; 2013.

28. Dworkin SF, LeResche L. Research diagnostic criteria for temporomandibular disorders: review, criteria, examination and specifications critique. *J Craniomandib Disord.* 1992;6(4):301-355.

29. Schiffman E, Ohrbach R, Truelove E, et al. Diagnostic criteria for temporomandibular disorders (DC/TMD) for clinical and research applications: recommendations of the International RDC/TMD Consortium Network* and orofacial pain special interest group-dagger. *J Oral Facial Pain Headache.* 2014;28(1):6-27. doi:10.11607/jop.1151

30. Kraus, S. Characteristics of 511 patients with temporomandibular disorders referred for physical therapy. *Oral Surg Oral Med Oral Pathol Oral Radiol.* 2014;118(4):432-439. doi:10.1016/j.oooo.2014.06.005

31. Lobbezoo-Scholte AM, Lobbezzo F, Steenks MH, De Leeuw JR, Bosman F. Diagnostic subgroups of craniomandibular disorders. Part II: symptom profiles. *J Orofac Pain.* 1995;9(1):37-43.

32. Kraus S, Prodoehl J. Disc displacement without reduction with limited opening: a clinical diagnostic accuracy study. *Physiotherap Theory Pract.* 2017;33(3):238-244. doi:10.1080/09593985.2017.1288282

33. Ohrbach R, Larsson P, and List T. The jaw functional limitation scale: development, reliability, and validity of 8-item and 20-item versions. *J Orofacial Pain.* 2008;22(3):219-230.

34. Bardin L, Malfetes N, Newman-Tancredi A, Depoortère R. Chronic restraint stress induces mechanical and cold allodynia, and enhances inflammatory pain in rat: relevance to human stress-associated painful pathologies. *Behav Brain Res.* 2009;205(2):360-366. doi:10.1016/j.bbr.2009.07.005

35. Kroenke, K; Spitzer, R; Williams, JB. The patient health questionnaire-2: validity of a two-item depression screener. *Med Care.* 2003;41(11):1284-1292. doi:10.1097/01.MLR.0000093487.78664.3C

36. Von Korff M. Assessment of chronic pain in epidemiological and health services research: empirical bases and new directions. In: Turk DC, Melzack R, eds. *Handbook of Pain Assessment.* 3rd ed. Guilford Press; 2011:455-473.

37. Kotiranta U, Suvinen T, Kauko T, et al. Subtyping patients with temporomandibular disorder in a primary health care setting on the basis of the research diagnostic criteria for temporomandibular disorders axis II pain-related disability: a step toward tailored treatment planning?. *J Oral Facial Pain Headache.* 2015;29(2):126-134. doi:10.11607/ofph.1319

38. Giesecke T, Gracely RH, Williams DA, Geisser ME, Petzke FWm Clauw DJ. The relationship between depression, clinical pain, and experimental pain in a chronic pain cohort. *Arthritis Rheum.* 2005; 52(5):1577-1584. doi:10.1002/art.21008

39. Kietrys DM, Palombaro KM, Mannheimer JS. Dry needling for management of pain in the upper quarter and craniofacial region. *Curr Pain Headache Rep.* 2014;18(8):437. doi:10.1007/s11916-014-0437-0

40. Hsieh Y-L, Kao M-J, Kuan T-S, Chen S-M, Chen J-T, Hong C-Z. Dry needling to a key myofascial trigger point may reduce the irritability of satellite MTrPs. *Am J Phys Med Rehabil.* 2007;86(5):397-403. doi:10.1097/PHM.0b013e31804a554d

41. Pruim GJ, de Jongh HJ, ten Bosch JJ. Forces acting on the mandible during bilateral static bite at different bite force levels. *J Biomech.* 1980;13(9):755-763. doi:10.1016/0021-9290(80)90237-7

42. Visscher CM, Lobbezoo F, Naeije M. A reliability study of dynamic and static pain tests in temporomandibular disorder patient. *J Orofac Pain.* 2007;21(1):39-45.

43. Kraus SL. Temporomandibular disorders. In: Saunders HD, Ryan RS, eds. *Evaluation, Treatment and Prevention of Musculoskeletal Disorders.* 4th ed. Saunders Group; 2004:173-210.

44. Kraus S. Failure to make the correct diagnosis: part II a physical therapist's perspective. In: Bouloux GF, ed. *Complications of Temporomandibular Joint Surgery.* Springer; 2017: 17-28.

45. Laskin D, Greenfield W, Gale E, et al. *The Presidents' Conference on the Examination, Diagnosis and Management of Temporomandibular Disorders.* American Dental Association; 1982.

46. Kraus S, Bender S, Prodoehl J. Part IV: management principles. In: Gremillion HA, Klasser GD, eds. *Temporomandibular Disorders: A Translational Approach From Basic Science to Clinical Applicability.* Springer; 2018:141-171

47. Fricton J, Look JO, Wright E, et al. Systematic review and meta-analysis of randomized controlled trials evaluating intraoral orthopedic appliances for temporomandibular disorders. *J Orofac Pain.* 2010;24(3):237-254.

48. Fricton J, Heir GM. History of temporomandibular disorders and orofacial pain in the United States. In: Chang Chung S, Friction J, eds. *The Past, Present and Future of Temporomandibular Disorders and Orofacial Pain.* Shinhung International; 2006.

49. Al-Ani MZ, Davies SJ, Gray RJM, Sloan P, Glenny AM. Stabilisation splint therapy for temporomandibular pain dysfunction syndrome. *Cochrane Database Syst Rev.* 2004;(1):CD002778. doi:10.1002/14651858.CD002778.pub2

50. Clark G, Minakuchi H. Oral appliances. In: Laskin DM, Greene CS, Hylander WL. *Temporomandibular Disorders: An Evidence-Based Approach to Diagnosis and Treatment.* CBS; 2006.

51. Kraus SL. *Clinics in Physical Therapy: Temporomandibular Disorders.* 2nd ed. Churchill Livingstone; 1994.

52. Kraus SL. Physical therapy management of temporomandibular disorders. In: Fonesca R, Bays RA, Quinn PD, eds. *Oral and Maxillofacial Surgery: Temporomandibular Disorders.* Saunders Company; 2000:161-193.

53. Kraus SL. Temporomandibular disorders, head and orofacial pain: cervical spine considerations. *Dent Clin North Am.* 2007;51(1):161-193. doi:10.01016/j.cden.2006.10.001

54. Overmeer T, Boersma K. What messages do patients remember? Relationships among patients' perceptions of physical therapists' messages, patient characteristics, satisfaction, and outcome. *Phys Ther.* 2016;96(3):275-283. doi:10.2522/ptj.20140557

55. Klasser GD, Rei N, Lavigne GJ. Sleep bruxism etiology: the evolution of a changing paradigm. *J Can Dent Assoc.* 2015;81:f2.

56. Reissmann DR, John MT, Aigner A, Schön G, Sierwald I, Schiffman EL. Interaction between awake and sleep bruxism is associated with increased presence of painful temporomandibular disorder. *J Oral Facial Pain Headache.* 2017;31(4):299-305. doi:10.11607/ofph.1885

57. Ling C, Rönn T. Epigenetic adaptation to regular exercise in humans. *Drug Discov Today.* 2014;19(7):1015-1018. doi:10.1016/j.drudis.2014.03.006

58. Tick, H. Nutrition and pain. *Phys Med Rehabil Clin N Am.* 2015;26(2):309-320. doi:10.1016/j.pmr.2014.12.006

59. Moldofsky H. Sleep and pain. *Sleep Med Rev.* 2001;5(5);385-396. doi:10.1053/smrv.2001.0179

60. McNeely ML, Armijo Olivo S, Magee DJ. A systematic review of the effectiveness of physical therapy interventions for temporomandibular disorders. *Phys Ther.* 2006;86(5):710-725.

61. Medlicott MS, Harris SR. A systematic review of the effectiveness of exercise, manual therapy, electrotherapy, relaxation training, and biofeedback in the management of temporomandibular disorder. *Phys Ther.* 2006;86(7):955-973.

62. Craane B, Ubele Dijkstra P, Stappaerts K, De Latt A. Methodological quality of a systematic review on physical therapy for temporomandibular disorders: influence of hand search and quality scales. *Clin Oral Investig.* 2012;16(1):295-303. doi:10.1007/s00784-010-0490-y

63. Rodrigues Martins W, Castro Blasczyk J, Furlan de Oliveira MA, et al. Efficacy of musculoskeletal manual approach in the treatment of temporomandibular joint disorder: a systematic review with meta-analysis. *Man Ther.* 2016;21:10-17. doi:10.1016/j.math.2015.06.009

64. Calixtre LB, Moreira RFC, Franchini GH, Alburquerque-Sendin F, Oliveira AB. Manual therapy for the management of pain and limited range of motion in subjects with signs and symptoms of temporomandibular disorder: a systematic review of randomised controlled trials. *J Oral Rehabil.* 2015;42(11):847-861. doi:10.1111/joor.12321

65. Armijo-Olivo S, Pitance L, Singh V, Neto F, Thie N, Michelotti A. Effectiveness of manual therapy and therapeutic exercise for temporomandibular disorders: systematic review and meta-analysis. *Phys Ther.* 2016;96(1):9-25. doi:10.2522/ptj.20140548

66. Milam SB. Pathophysiology and epidemiology of TMJ. *J Musculoskel Neuron Interact.* 2003;3(4):382-390.

67. Westesson P-L, Bronstein SL, Liedberg J. Internal derangement of the temporomandibular joint: morphologic description with correlation to joint function. *Oral Surg Oral Med Oral Pathol.* 1985;59(4):323-331. doi:10.1015/0030-4220(85)90051-9

68. Nitzan DW, Dolwick MF, Heft MW. Arthroscopic lavage and lysis of the temporomandibular joint: a change in perspective. *J Oral Maxillofac Surg.* 1990;48(8):798-801. doi:10.1016/0278-2391(90)90335-y

69. Sato S, Goto S, Kawamura H, Motegi K. The natural course of nonreducing disc displacement of the TMJ: relationship of clinical findings at initial visit to outcome after 12 months without treatment. *J Orofac Pain.* 1997;11(4):315-320.

70. Miernik M, Więckiewicz W. TMJ Disc Displacement without Reduction Management: A Systematic Review. Adv Clin Exp Med 2015; 24 (4): 731–735.

71. Al-Baghdadi M, Durham J, Araujo-Soares V, Robalino S, Errington L, Steele J. TMJ disc displacement without reduction management: a systematic review. *J Dent Res.* 2014;93(7):37S-51S. doi:10.1177/0022034528333

72. Kraus S, Prodoehl J. Outcomes and patient satisfaction following individualized physical therapy treatment for patients diagnosed with temporomandibular disc displacement without reduction with limited opening: a cross-sectional study. *Cranio.* 2019;37(1):20-27. doi:10.1080/08869634.2017.1379260

73. Naeije M, Te Veldhuis AH, Te Veldhuis EC, Lobbezoo F. Disc displacement within the human temporomandibular joint: a systematic review of a 'noisy annoyance'. *J Oral Rehabil.* 2013;40(2):139-158. doi:10.1111/joor.12016

74. Stegenga B. Osteoarthritis of the temporomandibular organ and its relationship with disc displacement. *J Orofac Pain.* 2001;15(3):193-205.

75. Sato S, Goto S, Nasu F, Motegi K. Natural course of disc displacement with reduction of the temporomandibular joint: changes in clinical signs and symptoms. *J Oral Maxillofac Surg.* 2003;61(1):32-34. doi:10.1053/joms.2003.50005

76. Klasser GD, Greene CS. Predoctoral teaching of temporomandibular disorders: a survey of U.S. and Canadian dental schools. *J Am Dent Assoc.* 2007;138(2):231-237. doi:10.14219/jada.archive.2007.0142

77. Commission on Dental Accreditation. Establishment of the commission. American Dental Association. http://www.ada.org/en/coda/accreditation/about-us/

78. Fricton J, Chen H, Shaefer JR, et al. New curriculum standards for teaching temporomandibular disorders in dental schools: a commentary. *J Am Dent Assoc.* 2022;153(5):395-398. doi:10.1016/j.adaj.2021.11.013

79. National Commission on Recognition of Dental Specialties and Certifying Boards. Requirements for recognition of dental specialties. 2023. Accessed February 14, 2023. https://ncrdscb.ada.org/recognized-dental-specialties

80. Yost O, Liverman CT, English R, Mackey S, Bond EC, eds; National Academies of Sciences, Engineering, and Medicine; Health and Medicine Division; Board on Health Care Services; Board on Health Sciences Policy; Committee on Temporomandibular Disorders (TMDs): From Research Discoveries to Clinical Treatment. *Temporomandibular Disorders: Priorities for Research and Care.* National Academies Press (US); 2020.

81. Gadotti IC, Lakow A, Cheung J, Tang M. Physical therapists' self-perceived adequacy of entry-level education and their current confidence levels with respect to temporomandibular disorders: a pilot study. Cranio. 2020;38(5):312-319. doi:10.1080/08869634.2018.1525117

82. Prodoehl J, Kraus S, Klasser GD, Hall KD. Temporomandibular disorder content in the curricula of physical therapist professional programs in the United States. Cranio. 2020;38(6):376-388. doi:10.1080/08869634.2018.1560983

83. American Board of Physical Therapy Specialties. APTA specialist certification- governed by ABPTS. American Physical Therapy Association. June 26, 2018. http://www.abpts.org.

84. American Board of Physical Therapy Specialties. *2019 Orthopedic Specialist Certification Candidate Guide.* American Physical Therapy Association; 2019:13.

85. Shaffer SM, Brismee J-M, Courtney CA, Sizer PS. The status of temporomandibular and cervical spine education in credentialed orthopedic manual physical therapy fellowship programs: a comparison of didactic and clinical education exposure. *J Man Manip Ther.* 2015;23(1):51-56. doi:10.1179/2042618614Y.0000000087

86. Shaffer SM, Stuhr SH, Sizer PS, Courtney CA, Brismée J-M. The status of temporomandibular and cervical spine education in post-professional physical therapy training programs recognized by Member Organizations of IFOMPT: an investigation of didactic and clinical education. *J Man Manip Ther.* 2018;26(2):102-108. doi:10.1080/10669817.2017.1422614

87. Physical Therapy Board of Craniofacial and Cervical Therapeutics. CCTT certification, mission statement, certification development. Physical Therapy Board of Craniofacial and Cervical Therapeutics. www.ptbcct.org

88. Peterson S, Shepard M, Farrell J, Rhon DI. The blind men, the elephant, and the continuing education course: why higher standards are needed in physical therapist professional development. *J Orthop Sports Phys Ther.* 2022;52(10):642-646. doi:10.2519/jospt.2022.11377

89. Development of a Clinical Practice Guideline: Diagnosis and Management of Temporomandibular Disorders for Physical Therapists. Sponsored by the Academy of Orthopedic Physical Therapy, American Physical Therapy Association. Guideline Development Group Janey Prodoehl, PT, PhD, CCTT (lead), Emily Kahnert, PT, DPT, CCTT, Stephen Shaffer, PT, ScD, Josiah Sault, PT, DPT, OCS, FAAOMPT, Giovanni Berardi, PT, DPT, PhD, Isabel Moreno Hay, DDS PhD ABOP ABDSM, Alison Duncombe, PT, DPT, Emily Nicklies, PT, DPT, Donald Nixdorf, DDS, MS, Justin Durham, BDS MFDSRCS FDSRCS (OS) PhD, Christine McDonough PT, PhD. Journal of Orthopedic and Sports Physical therapy with target publication January 2024

90. DiCaprio MR, Covey A, Bernstein J. Curricular requirements for musculoskeletal medicine in American medical schools. *J Bone Joint Surg Am.* 2003;85(3):565-567. doi:10.2106/00004623-200303000-00027

91. Hampton T. Improvements needed in management of temporomandibular joint disorders. *JAMA.* 2008;299(10):1119-1121. doi:10.1001/jama.299.10.1119

92. Greene CS, Bertagna AE. Seeking treatment for temporomandibular disorders: what patients can expect from non-dental health care providers. 2019;127(5):399-407. doi:10.1016/j.oooo.2019.01.007

93. Ciancaglini R, Testa M, Radaelli G. Association of neck pain with symptoms of temporomandibular dysfunction in the general adult population. *Scand J Rehabil Med.* 1999;31(1):17-22. doi:10.1080/003655099444687

94. von Piekartz H, Pudelko A, Danzeisen M, Hall T, Ballenberger N. Do subjects with acute/subacute temporomandibular disorder have associated cervical impairments: a cross-sectional study. *Man Ther.* 2016;26:208-215. doi:10.1016/j.math.2016.09.001

95. Kirveskari P, Alanen P, Karskela V, et al. Association of functional state of stomatognathic system with mobility of cervical spine and neck muscle tenderness. *Acta Odont Scand.* 1988;46(5):281-286. doi:10.3109.00016358809004778

96. Lobbezoo-Scholte AM, de Leeuw R, Steenks M, Bosman F, Buchner R, Olthoff LW. Diagnostic subgroups of craniomandibular disorders. Part 1: self-report data and clinical findings. *J Orofac Pain.* 1995;9(1):24-36.

97. Serrao M, Rossi P, Parisi L, et al. Trigemino-cervical-spinal reflexes in humans. *Clin Neurophysiol.* 2003;114(9):1697-1703. doi:10.1016/s1388-245(03)00132-9

98. Gunduz A, Uzun N, Irem Ornek N, Unalan H, Sahir Karamehmetoglu S, Kiziltan ME. Trigemino-cervical reflex in spinal cord injury. *Neurosci Lett.* 2014;580(19):169-172. doi:10.1016/j.neulet.2014.08.006

99. Xiong G, Matsushita M. Upper cervical afferents to the motor trigeminal nucleus and the subnucleus oralis of the spinal trigeminal nucleus in the rat: an anterograde and retrograde tracing study. *Neurosci Lett.* 2000;286(2):127-130. doi:10.1016/s0304-3940(00)01115-0

100. Bruijn SM, Massaad F, Maclellan MJ, Van Gestel L, Ivanenko YP, Duysens J. Are effects of the symmetric and asymmetric tonic neck reflexes still visible in healthy adults?. *Neurosci Lett.* 2013;556: 89-92. doi:10.1016/j.neulet.2013.10.028

101. Funakoshi M, Amano N. Effects of the tonic neck reflex on the jaw muscles of the rat. *J Dent Res.* 1973;52(4):668-673. doi:10.1177/00220345730520040501

102. Funakoshi M, Fujita N, Takehana S. Relations between occlusal interference and jaw muscle activities in response to changes in head position. *J Dent Res.* 1976;55(4):684-690. doi:10.1177/00220345760550042401

103. Wyke BD. Neurology of the cervical spinal joints. *J Physiother.* 1979;65:72-76.

104. Abrahams VC, Kori AA, Loeb GE, Richmond FJ, Rose PK, Keirstead SA. Facial input to neck motoneurons: trigemino-cervical reflexes in the conscious and anaesthetised cat. *Exp Brain Res.* 1993;97(1):23-30. doi:10.1007/BF00228814

105. Haggman-Henrikson B, Eriksson P-O. Head movements during chewing: relation to size and texture of bolus. *J Dent Res.* 2004;83(11):864-868. doi:10.1177/154405910408301108

106. Zafar H, Nordh E, Eriksson PO. Temporal coordination between mandibular and head-neck movements during jaw opening-closing tasks in man. *Arch Oral Biol.* 2000;45(8):675-682. doi:10.1016/s0003-9969(00)00032-7

107. Zafar H, Nordh E, Eriksson P-O. Spatiotemporal consistency of human mandibular and head-neck movement trajectories during jaw opening-closing tasks. *Exp Brain Res.* 2002;146:70–76.

108. Eriksson P-O, Haggman-Henrikson B, Nordh E, Zafar H. Co-ordinated mandibular and head-neck movements during rhythmic jaw activities in man. *J Dent Res.* 2000;79(6):1378-1384. doi:1177/00220345000790060501

109. Haggman-Henrikson B, Nordh E, Zafar H, Eriksson P-O. Head immobilization can impair jaw function. *J Dent Res.* 2006;85(11):1001-1005. doi:10.1177/154405910608501105

110. Zafar H, Nordh E, Eriksson P-O. Impaired positioning of the gape in whiplash-associated disorders. *Swed Dent J.* 2006;30(1):9-15.

111. Milidonis MK, Kraus SL, Segal RL, Widmer CG. Genioglossi muscle activity in response to changes in anterior/neutral head posture. *Am J Orthod Dentofacial Orthop.* 1993;103(1):39-44. doi:10.1016/0889-5406(93)70102-T

112. Darling DW, Kraus SL, Glasheen-Wray MB. Relationship of head posture and the rest position of the mandible. *J Prosthet Dent.* 1984;52(1):111-115. doi:10.1016/0022-3913(84)90192-6

113. Goldstein DF, Kraus SL, Williams WB, Glasheen-Way M. Influence of cervical posture on mandibular movement. *J Prosthet Dent.* 1984;52(3):421-426. doi:10.1016/0022-3913(84)80460-8

114. Visscher CM, Huddleston Slater JJ, Lobbezoo F, Naeije M. Kinematics of the human mandible for different head postures. *J Oral Rehabil.* 2000;27(4):299-305. doi:10.1046/j.1365-2842.2000.00518.x

115. Mohl ND. The role of head posture in mandibular function. In: Solberg WK, Clark GT, eds. *Abnormal Jaw Mechanics Diagnosis and Treatment.* Quintessence Publishing; 1984:97-111.

116. Miles TS. Postural control of the human mandible. *Arch Oral Biol.* 2007;52(4):347-352. doi:10.1016/j.archoralbio.2006.12.017

117. List, T, Dworkin SF. Comparing TMD diagnoses and clinical findings at Swedish and US TMD centers using research diagnostic criteria for temporomandibular disorders. *J Orofac Pain.* 1996;10(3):240-253.

118. Niemi SM, Levoska S, Rekola KE, Keinanen-Kiukaanniemi SM. Neck and shoulder symptoms of high school students and associated psychosocial factors. *J Adolesc Health.* 1997;20(3):238-242. doi:10.1016/S1054-139X(96)00219-4

119. Mongini F, Ciccone G, Ceccarelli M, Baldi I, Ferrero L. Muscle tenderness in different types of facial pain and its relation to anxiety and depression: a cross-sectional study on 649 patients. *Pain.* 2007;131(1-2):106-111. doi:10.1016/j.pain.2006.12.017

120. Komiyama O, Arai M, Kawara M, Kobayashi K, De Laat A. Pain patterns and mandibular dysfunction following experimental trapezius muscle pain. *J Orofac Pain.* 2005;19(2):119-126.

121. Hu JW, Yu XM, Vernon H, Sessle BJ. Excitatory effect on neck and jaw muscle activity of inflammatory irritant applied to cervical paraspinal muscles. *Pain.* 1993;55(2):243-250. doi:10.1016/0304-3959(93)90153-G

122. Carlson CR, Okeson J, Falace DA, Nitz AJ, Lindroth JE. Reduction of pain and EMG activity in the masseter region by trapezius trigger point injection. *Pain.* 1993;55(3):397-400. doi:10.1016/0304-3959(93)90018-K

123. Tsai C-T, Hsieh L-F, Kuan T-S, Kao M-J, Chou L-W, Hong C-Z. Remote effects of dry needling on the irritability of the myofascial trigger point in the upper trapezius muscle. *Am J Phys Med Rehabil.* 2010;89(2):133-140. doi:10.1097/PHM.0b013e3181a5b1bc

124. Cornelison LE, Hawkins JL, Durham PL. Elevated levels of calcitonin gene-related peptide in upper spinal cord promotes sensitization of primary trigeminal nociceptive neurons. *Neuroscience.* 2016;339:491-501. doi:10.1016/j.neuroscience.2016.10.013

125. Armijo-Olivo S, Fuentes J, Major PW, Warren S, Thie NMR, Magee DJ. The association between neck disability and jaw disability. *J Oral Rehabil.* 2010;37(9):670-679. doi:10.1111/j.1365-2842.2010.02098.x

126. De Laat A, Meulemann H, Stevens A, Verbeke G. Correlation between cervical spine and temporomandibular disorders. *Clin Oral Investig.* 1998;2(2):54-57. doi:10.1007/s007840050045

127. Armijo-Olivo S, Magee D. Cervical musculoskeletal impairments and temporomandibular disorders. *J Oral Maxillofac Res.* 2013;3(4):e4. doi:10.5037/jomr.2012.3404

128. Silveira A, Gadotti IC, Armijo-Olivo S, Biasotto-Gonzalez DA, Magee D. Jaw dysfunction is associated with neck disability and muscle tenderness in subjects with and without chronic temporomandibular disorders. *Biomed Res Int.* 2015;2015:512792. doi:10.1155/2015/512792

129. La Touche R, Fernandez-de-las-Penas C, Fernandez-Carnero J, et al. The effects of manual therapy and exercise directed at the cervical spine on pain and pressure pain sensitivity in patients with myofascial temporomandibular disorders. *J Oral Rehabil.* 2009;36(9):644-652. doi:10.1111/j.1365-2842.2009.01980.x

130. Komiyama, O, Arai M, Kitamura, et al. Effect of posture correction in patients with painful limited mouth opening. *J Dent Res.* 1996;75:434.

131. Komiyama O, Kawara M, Arai M, Asano I, Kobayashi K. Posture correction as part of behavioral therapy in treatment of myofascial pain with limited opening. *J Oral Rehabil.* 1999;26(5):428-435. doi:10.1046/j.1365-2842.1999.00412.x

132. Turp JC, Kowalski CJ, O'Leary N, Stohler CS. Pain maps from facial pain patients indicate a broad pain geography. *J Dent Res.* 1998;77(6):1465-1472. doi:10.1177/00220345980770061101

133. Hagberg C, Hagberg M, Kopp S. Musculoskeletal symptoms and psychological factors among patients with craniomandibular disorders. *Acta Odontol Scand.* 1994;52(3):170-177. doi:10.3109/00016359409027592

134. Sipila K, Ylostalo P, Joukamaa M, Knuuttila ML. Comorbidity between facial pain, widespread pain, and depressive symptoms in young adults. *J Orofac Pain.* 2006;20(1):24-30.

135. Bogduk N. The neck and headaches. *Neurol Clin.* 2004;22(1):151-171. doi:10.1016/S0733-8619(03)00100-2

136. Kerr FW. Structural relation of the trigeminal spinal tract to upper cervical roots and the solitary nucleus in cat. *Exp Neurol.* 1961;4:134-148. doi:10.1016/0014-4886(61)90036-x

137. Biondi DM. Cervicogenic headache: mechanisms, evaluation, and treatment strategies. *J Am Osteopath Assoc.* 2000;100(9 Suppl): S7-S14.

138. Bogduk N. Anatomy and physiology of headache. Biomed Pharmacother. 1995;49(10):435-445. doi:10.1016/0753-3322(96)82687-4

139. Haldeman S, Dagenais S. Cervicogenic headaches: a critical review. *Spine.* 2001;1(1):31-46. doi:10.1016/s1529-9430(01)00024-9

140. Bogduk N. The anatomical basis for cervicogenic headache. *J Manipulative Physiol Ther.* 1992;15(1):67-70.

141. Bogduk N. Cervicogenic headache: anatomic basis and pathophysiologic mechanisms. *Curr Pain Headache Rep.* 2001;5(4):382-386. doi:10.1007/s11916-001-0029-7

142. Sjaastad O, Saunte C, Hovdahl H, Breivik H, Gronbaek E. "Cervicogenic" headache. An hypothesis. *Cephalalgia.* 1983;3(4):249-256. doi:10.1046/j.1468-2982.1983.0304249.x

143. Nilsson N. The prevalence of cervicogenic headache in a random population sample of 20–59 year olds. *Spine.* 1995;20(17):1884-1888. doi:10.1097/00007632-199509000-00008

144. Sjaastad O, Fredriksen TA, Pfaffenrath V. Cervicogenic headache: diagnostic criteria. The Cervicogenic Headache International Study Group. *Headache.* 1998;38(6):442-445. doi:10.1046/j.1526-4610.1998.3806442.x

145. Simons DG, Travell JG, Simons LS. *Myofascial pain and dysfunction: the trigger point manual, volume 1.* 2nd ed. Williams and Wilkins; 1999.

146. Dalessio DJ. Muscles of the head and neck as sources of headache and other pain. In: Dalessio DJ, ed. *Wolff's Headache and Other Head Pain.* 3rd ed. Oxford University Press; 1972:525-60.

147. Phu Do T, Ferja Heldarskard G, Torring Kolding L, Hvedstrup J, Winther Schytz H. Myofascial trigger points in migraine and tension-type headache. *J Headache Pain.* 2018;19(1):84. doi:10.1186/s10194-018-0913-8

148. Sakai F, Ebihara S, Akiyama M, Horikawa M. Pericranial muscle hardness in tension-type headache A non-invasive measurement method and its clinical application. *Brain.* 1995;118(2):523-531. doi:10.1093/brain/118.2.523

149. Ashina M, Bendtsen L, Jensen R, Sakai F, Olesen J. Muscle hardness in patients with chronic tension-type headache: relation to actual headache state. *Pain.* 1999;79(2-3):201-205. doi:10.1016/s0304-3959(98)00167-5

150. Fernández-de-las-Peñas C, Alonso-Blanco C, Luz Cuadrado M, Gerwin RD, Pareja JA. Trigger points in the suboccipital muscles and forward head posture in tension-type headache. *Headache.* 2006;46(3):454–460. doi:10.1111/j.1526-4610.2006.00288.x

151. Caspersen N, Hirsvang JR, Kroell L, et al. Is there a relation between tension-type headache, temporomandibular disorders and sleep?. *Pain Res Treat.* 2013;2013:845684. doi:10.1155/2013/845684

152. Jensen R, Olesen J. Initiating mechanisms of experimentally induced tension-type headache. *Cephalalgia.* 1996;16(3):175-182. doi:10.1046/j.1468-2982.1996.1603175.x

153. Svensson P. Muscle pain in the head: overlap between temporomandibular disorders and tension-type headaches. *Curr Opin Neurol.* 2007;20(3):320-325. doi:10.1097/WCO.0b013e328136c1f9

154. Freund BJ, Schwartz M. Relief of tension-type headache symptoms in subjects with temporomandibular disorders treated with botulinum toxin-A. *Headache.* 2002;42(10):1033-1037. doi:10.1046/j.1526-4610.2002.02234.x

155. Lipton RB, Stewart WF, Diamond S, Diamond ML, Reed M. Prevalence and burden of migraine in the United States: data from the American Migraine Study II. *Headache.* 2001;41(7):646-657. doi:10.1046/j.1523-4610.2001.041007646.x

156. Lipton RB, Dodick D, Sadosky R, et al. A self-administered screener for migraine In primary care: the ID migraine validation study. *Neurology.* 2003;61(3):375-382. doi:10.1212/01.wnl.0000078940.53438.83

157. Blau JN, MacGregor EA. Migraine and the neck. *Headache.* 1994;34(2):88-90. doi:10.1111/j.1526-4610.1994.hed3402088.x

158. Calhoun AH, Ford S, Millen C, Finkel AG, Truong Y, Nie Y. The prevalence of neck pain in migraine. *Headache.* 2010;50(8):1273-1277. doi:10.1111/j.1526-4610.2009.01608.x

159. Kelman L. The triggers or precipitants of the acute migraine attack. *Cephalalgia.* 2007;27(5):394-402. doi:10.1111/j.1468-2982.2007.01303.x

160. Vernon H, Steiman I, Hagino C. Cervicogenic dysfunction in muscle contraction headache and migraine: a descriptive study. *J Manipulative Physiol Ther.* 1992;15(7):418-429.

161. Yi X, Cook AJ, Hamill-Ruth RJ, Rowlingson JC. Cervicogenic headache in patients with presumed migraine: missed diagnosis or misdiagnosis?. *J Pain.* 2005;6(10):700-703. doi:10.1016/j.jpain.2005.04.005

162. Calandre EP, Hidalgo J, Garcia-Leiva JM, Rico-Villademoro F. Trigger point evaluation in migraine patients: an indication for peripheral sensitization linked to migraine predisposition?. *Eur J Neurol.* 2006;13(3):244-249. doi:10.1111/j.1468-1331.2006.01181.x

163. Giamberardino MA, Tafuri E, Savini A, et al. Contribution of myofascial trigger points to migraine symptoms. *J Pain.* 2007;8(11):869-878. doi:10.1016/j.jpain.2007.06.002

164. Shevel E, Spierings EH. Cervical muscles in the pathogenesis of migraine headache. *J Headache Pain.* 2004;5(1):12–14. doi:10.1007/s10194-004-0062-0

165. Fernandez-de-Las Penas C, Cuadrado ML, Pareja JA. Myofascial trigger points, neck mobility and forward head posture in unilateral migraine. *Cephalalgia.* 2006;26(9):1061-1070. doi:10.1111/j.1468-2982.2006.01162.x

166. Giamberardino MA, Tafuri E, Savini A, et al. Contribution of myofascial trigger points to migraine symptoms. *J Pain.* 2007;8(11):869-878. doi:10.1016/j.jpain.2007.06.002

167. Tali D, Menahem I, Vered E, Kalichman L. Upper cervical mobility, posture and myofascial trigger points in subjects with episodic migraine: case-control study. *J Bodyw Mov Ther.* 2014;18(4):569-575. doi:10.1016/j.jbmt.2014.01.006

168. Jensen K, Tuxen C, Olesen J. Pericranial muscle tenderness and pressure-pain threshold in the temporal region during common migraine. *Pain.* 1988;35(1):65-70. doi:10.1016/0304-3959(88)90277-1

169. Gonçalves DAG, Camparis CM, Speciali JG, Franco AL, Castanharo SM, Bigal ME. Temporomandibular disorders are differentially associated with headache diagnoses: a controlled study. *Clin J Pain.* 2011;27(7):611-615. doi:10.1097/AJP.0b013e31820e12f5

170. Franco AL, Gonçalves DAG, Castanharo SM, Speciali JG, Bigal ME, Camparis CM. Migraine is the most prevalent primary headache in individuals with temporomandibular disorders. *J Orofac Pain.* 2010;24(3):287-292.

171. Garrigos-Pedron M, Touche RL, Navarro-Desentre P, Gracia-Naya M, Segura-Orti E. Effects of a physical therapy protocol in patients with chronic migraine and temporomandibular disorders: a randomized, single-blinded, clinical trial. *J Orofac Pain.* 2018;32(2):137-150. doi:10.11607/ofph.1912

172. Paparella MM, Jung TTK. Odontalgia. In: Paparella MM, Shumrik DA, Gluckman JL, eds. *Otolaryngology.* Saunders; 1991:1237–1242.

173. Kuttila SJ, Kuttila MH, Niemi PM, et al. Secondary otalgia in an adult population. *Arch Otolaryngol Head Neck Surg.* 2001;127:401-405

174. Kuttila S, Kuttila M, Le Bell Y, Alanen P, Suonpaa J. Characteristics of subjects with secondary otalgia. *J Orofac Pain.* 2004;18(3):226–234.

175. Oostendorp RAB, Bakker I, Elvers H, et al. Cervicogenic somatosensory tinnitus: an indication for manual therapy? Part 1: theoretical concept. *Man Ther.* 2016;23:120-123. doi:10.1016/j.math.2015.11.008

176. Fernandez-de-Las-Penas C, Galan-Del-Rio F, Alonso-Blanco C, Jimenez-Garcia R, Arendt-Nielsen L, Svensson P. Referred pain from muscle trigger points in the masticatory and neck-shoulder musculature in women with temporomandibular disorders. *J Pain.* 2010;11(12):1295-1304. doi:10.1016/j.jpain.2010.03.005

177. Alonso-Blanco C, Fernández-de-Las-Peñas C, de-la-Llave-Rincón AI, Zarco-Moreno P, Galan-Del-Rio F, Svensson P. Characteristics of referred muscle pain to the head from active trigger points in women with myofascial temporomandibular pain and fibromyalgia syndrome. *J Headache Pain.* 2012;13(8):625-637. doi:10.1007/s10194-012-0477-y

178. Gola R, Chossegros C, Orthlieb JD, Lepetre C, Ulmer E. Otologic manifestations of the pain dysfunction syndrome of the stomatognathic system. *Rev Stomatol Chir Maxillofac.* 1992;93(4):224-230.

179. Rubinstein B. Tinnitus and craniomandibular disorders- is there a link? *Swed Dent J Suppl.* 1993;95:1-46.

180. Schames J, Schames M, Boyd JP, Eurel L. Trigeminal pharyngioplasty: treatment of the forgotten accessory muscles of mastication which are associated with orofacial pain and ear symptomology. *J Pain Manag.* 2002;12:102.112.

181. Ramirez Aristeguieta LM, Sandoval Ortiz GP, Ballesteros LE. Theories on otic symptoms in temporomandibular disorders: past and present. *Int J Morphol.* 2005;23(2):141-156. doi:10.4067/S0717-95022005000200009

182. Ganz Sanchez T, Bezerra Rocha C. Diagnosis and management of somatosensory tinnitus: review article. *Clinics.* 2011;66(6):1089-1094. doi:10.1590/S1807-59322011000600028

183. Levine RA. Somatic (craniocervical) tinnitus and the dorsal cochlear nucleus hypothesis. *Am J Otolaryngol.* 1999;20(6):351-362. doi:10.1016/S0196-0709(99)90074-1

184. Abel MD, Levine RA. Muscle contractions and auditory perception in tinnitus patients and nonclinical patients. *Cranio.* 2004;22(3):181-191. doi:10.1179/crn.2004.024

185. Michiels S, Van de Heyning P, Truijen S, De Hertogh W. Diagnostic value of clinical cervical spine tests in patients with cervicogenic somatic tinnitus. *Phys Ther.* 2015;95(11):1529-1535. doi:10.2522/ptj.20140457

186. Luedtke K, Boissonnault W, Caspersen N, et al. International consensus on the most useful physical examination tests used by physiotherapists for patients with headache: A Delphi study. *Man Ther.* 2016;23:17-24. doi:10.1016/j.math.2016.02.010

187. Schellhas KP, Smith MD, Gundry CR, Pollei SR. Cervical discogenic pain: prospective correlation of magnetic resonance imaging and discography in asymptomatic subjects and pain sufferers. *Spine.* 1996;21(3):300-311. doi:10.1097/00007632-199602010-00009

188. Johnson GM. The correlation between surface measurement of head and neck posture and the anatomic position of the upper cervical vertebrae. *Spine.* 1998;23(8):921-927. doi:10.1097/00007632-199804150-00015

189. Refshauge KM, Goodsell M, Lee M. The relationship between surface contour and vertebral body measures of upper spine curvature. *Spine.* 1994;19(19):2180-2185. doi:10.1097/00007632-199410000-00010

190. Grimmer K. The relationship between cervical resting posture and neck pain. *J Physiother.* 1996;82(1):45-51. doi:10.1016/S0031-9406(05)66998-2

191. Spitzer WO, Skovron ML, Salmi LR, et al. Scientific monograph of the Quebec Task Force on whiplash-associated disorders: redefining "whiplash" and its management. *Spine.* 1995;20(8 Suppl):1S-73S.

192. Blanpied PR, Gross AR, Elliott JM, et al. Neck pain: revision 2017. *J Orthop Sports Phys Ther.* 2017;47(7):A1-A83. doi:10.2519/jospt.2017.0302

193. Gross AR, Hoving JL, Haines TA, et al. Manipulation and mobilization for mechanical neck disorders. *Spine.* 2004;29(14):1541-1548. doi:10.1097/01.brs.0000131218.35875.ed

194. Gross A, Miller J, D'Sylva J, et al. Manipulation or mobilization for neck pain: a Cochrane Review. *Man Ther.* 2010;15(4):315-333. doi:10.1016/j.math.2010.04.002

195. Gross A, Forget M, St George K, et al. Patient education for neck pain. *Cochrane Database Syst Rev.* 2012;(3):CD005106. doi:10.1002/14651858.CD005106.pub4

196. Verhagen AP, Bierma-Zeinstra SMA, Burdorf A, Stynes SM, de Vet HCW, Koes BW. Conservative interventions for treating work-related complaints of the arm, neck or shoulder in adults. *Cochrane Database Syst Rev.* 2013;2013(12):CD008742. doi:10.1002/14651858.CD008742.pub2

197. Gross AR, Paquin JP, Dupont G, et al. Exercises for mechanical neck disorders: a Cochrane review update. *Man Ther.* 2016;24:25-45. doi:10.1016/j.math.2016.04.005

198. Peloso PM, Khan M, Gross AR, et al. Pharmacological interventions including medical injections for neck pain: an overview as part of the ICON project. *Open Orthop J.* 2013;7:473-493. doi:10.2174/1874325001307010473

199. Peloso P, Gross A, Haines T, et al. Medicinal and injection therapies for mechanical neck disorders. *Cochrane Database Syst Rev.* 2007;(3):CD000319. doi:10.1002/14651858.CD000319.pub4

200. Tschopp KP, Gysin C. Local injection therapy in 107 patients with myofascial pain syndrome of the head and neck. *J Otorhinolaryngol Relat Spec.* 1996;58(6):306-310. doi:10.1159/000276860

201. Langevin P, Peloso PMJ, Lowcock J, et al. Botulinum toxin for subacute/chronic neck pain. *Cochrane Database Syst Rev.* 2011;(7):CD008626. doi:10.1002/14651858.CD008626.pub2

202. Carragee EJ, Hurwitz EL, Cheng I, et al. Treatment of neck pain injections and surgical interventions: results of the bone and joint decade 2000–2010 task force on neck pain and its associated disorders. *Spine.* 2008;33(4 Suppl):S153-S169. doi:10.1097/BRS.0b013e31816445ea

203. Manchikanti L, Cash KA, Pampati V, Wargo BW, Malla Y. Management of chronic pain of cervical disc herniation and radiculitis with fluoroscopic cervical interlaminar epidural injections. *Int J Med Sci.* 2012; 9(6):424-434. doi:10.7150/ijms.4444

204. Nikolaidis I, Fouyas IP, Sandercock PA, Statham PF. Surgery for cervical radiculopathy or myelopathy. *Cochrane Database Syst Rev.* 2010;2010(1):CD001466. doi:10.1002/14651858.CD001466.pub3

205. Carragee EJ, Hurwitz EL, Cheng I, et al. Treatment of neck pain: injections and surgical interventions: results of the bone and joint decade 2000–2010 task force on neck pain and its associated disorders. *Spine.* 2008;33(4 Suppl):S153-S169. doi:10.1097/BRS.0b013e31816445ea

206. Persson LC, Carlsson C-A, Carlsson JY. Long-lasting cervical radicular pain managed with surgery, physiotherapy, or a cervical collar. *Spine.* 1997;22(7):751-758. doi:10.1097/00007632-199704010-00007

207. Bednarik J, Kadanka Z, Vohanka S, Stejskal L, Vlach O, Schroder R. The value of somatosensory- and motor-evoked potentials in predicting and monitoring the effect of therapy in spondylotic cervical myelopathy. Prospective randomized study. *Spine.* 1999;24(15):1593-1598. doi:10.1097/00007632-199908010-00014

208. Kadanka Z, Mares M, Bednanik J, et al. Approaches to spondylotic cervical myelopathy: conservative versus surgical results in a 3-year follow-up study. *Spine.* 2002;27(20):2205-2210. doi:10.1097/01.BRS.0000029255.77224.BB

APPENDIX A

HISTORY AND PHYSICAL EXAMINATION FOR COMMON TEMPOROMANDIBULAR DISORDER DIAGNOSTIC SUBSETS

TEMPOROMANDIBULAR DISORDER MYOGENOUS DIAGNOSTIC SUBSETS

MYALGIA

Sensitivity 0.90 and specificity 0.99

History

- Patient reports pain located in the jaw, temple, and/or ear areas.
- Patient reports pain modified with jaw movement, function, or parafunction.

Physical Examination

Familiar pain is modified by

- Palpation of the temporalis and/or masseter muscles (palpation identifies active or latent myofascial trigger point[s]).
- Maximum unassisted active opening (opening may or may not be limited; see Figures 14-2 and 14-3).

HEADACHE ATTRIBUTED TO TEMPOROMANDIBULAR DISORDER

Sensitivity 0.89 and specificity 0.87

History

- Patient reports headache of any type in the temple.
- Patient reports headache, modified with jaw movement, function, or parafunction.

Physical Examination

Familiar pain (headache located in temple area) is modified by

- Positive examination for myalgia (headache felt in the temporalis muscle).
- Positive examination for arthralgia (during the examination, pain is referred from TMJ to temple area).

Clinical Points

- To make a diagnosis of HTMD, requires the patient to complain of a headache in the temple area confirmed by the diagnosis of myalgia of the temporalis muscle(s).
- HTMD can also be referred to the temple area from the TMJ. This requires that the patient's headache, located in the temple(s) area, be modified by the examination directed toward the TMJ and the diagnosis of arthralgia is confirmed. Arthralgia is not as common of a source for HTMD as is myalgia.
- Headache is not better accounted for by another headache diagnosis.

TEMPOROMANDIBULAR DISORDER ARTHROGENOUS DIAGNOSTIC SUBSETS

ARTHRALGIA

Sensitivity 0.89 and specificity 0.98

History

- Patient reports pain located in the jaw, temple, ear, or in front of ear.
- Patient reports pain modified with jaw movement, function, or parafunction.

(continued)

APPENDIX A (CONTINUED)

HISTORY AND PHYSICAL EXAMINATION FOR COMMON TEMPOROMANDIBULAR DISORDER DIAGNOSTIC SUBSETS

Physical Examination

Familiar pain is modified by

- Palpation of the lateral pole or around the lateral pole (done with back teeth together and slightly apart).

- Maximum unassisted or assisted opening, protrusion, and/or right or left lateral excursion (see Figures 14-2 through 14-5).

- Bite test (see Figure 14-1).

(continued)

APPENDIX A (CONTINUED)

HISTORY AND PHYSICAL EXAMINATION FOR
COMMON TEMPOROMANDIBULAR DISORDER DIAGNOSTIC SUBSETS

Clinical Point
The following diagnostic subsets, *dislocation* and *subluxation,* are frequently misused. See Key Terms for the definitions of dislocation and subluxation. DC/TMD uses the term subluxation when their definition is actually describing dislocation.[29] This author has added his version of what the history and physical examination should consist of to diagnosis subluxation.

DISLOCATION
Sensitivity 0.98 and specificity 1.00
History
• Patient reports jaw locking in a wide-open mouth position even for a moment, so they could not close from a wide-open position. Closing could only be done by a self-maneuver or with assistance.
Physical Examination
• No physical examination is necessary if at the time of the examination, the patient is unable to close from a wide-open position. Locking that occurs intermittently can only be diagnosed by what the patient recalls in the history.

SUBLUXATION
No sensitivity or specificity values have been established.
History
• Patient reports when closing from a wide-open mouth position, their jaw catches and/or the patient may report that their jaw feels like it is "going out of place" toward the end of a wide-open mouth position and/or on closing from a wide-open mouth position.
• Patient may report a noise toward the end of a wide-open mouth position and/or a noise at the beginning of closing from a wide-open mouth position.
Physical Examination
Palpating over the lateral pole
• Opening wide and/or on closing from a wide-open mouth position, a judder* is detected.
• An eminence click** is felt at the end of a wide-open mouth position and/or the beginning of closing from a wide-open mouth position.
* Judder is a sudden change in mandibular movement toward the end of a wide-open mouth position and/or from the beginning of closing from a wide-open mouth position. Patient may state they feel their "jaw is going out of place." The more acute the angle is between the articular eminence and the articular tubercle, the more pronounced the judder may be.
** An eminence click occurs as the condyle translates past the articular crest on opening and/or on closing. The articular crest is the anatomical point on the temporal bone between the articular eminence and articular tubercle. The more acute the angle is between the articular eminence and the articular tubercle, the more pronounced the click may be.
Clinical Point
• Without a judder and/or eminence click, subluxation can still occur, but the examination is not sensitive enough to make the diagnosis.

(continued)

APPENDIX A (CONTINUED)

HISTORY AND PHYSICAL EXAMINATION FOR COMMON TEMPOROMANDIBULAR DISORDER DIAGNOSTIC SUBSETS

DISK DISPLACEMENT WITH REDUCTION

Sensitivity 0.34 and specificity 0.92

History

- Patient reports a noise (click) emanating from the TMJ with jaw movement or function.

Physical Examination

- Palpating over the lateral pole of the condyle, a click is detected during jaw opening and/or closing movements (see Figure 14-6).
- Palpating over the lateral pole of the condyle, a click may or may not be detected during protrusive and/or right or left lateral excursion.
- If the first bullet point was positive, the elimination test* is positive.

* Elimination test. Patient opens past the open click, then closes in a protrusive position to bring central incisors end to end. With repeated opening and closing in a protruded position, the opening and closing clicks are eliminated (a positive elimination test).

Clinical Points

- An opening click can be early, intermediate, or late. Regardless where in range the opening click occurs, the closing click (often difficult to detect) occurs toward the end of closing.
- A click detected during protrusion and/or right or left lateral excursions without an opening click seldom occurs. It is the opening click with a closing click and a positive elimination test that confirms the diagnosis of a DDwR.

DISK DISPLACEMENT WITH REDUCTION WITH INTERMITTENT LOCKING

Sensitivity 0.38 and specificity 0.98

History

- Patient reports a noise with jaw movement or function.
- Patient reports jaw intermittently locks closed. Patient is unable to open wide without pressing on their jaw or moving their jaw in a lateral or protrusive manner to get it to unlock.

Physical Examination

- Positive findings for DDwR.
- Intermittent locking on opening is observed. If not observed, a patient will need to report having had intermittent locking within the last 30 days.

DISK DISPLACEMENT WITHOUT REDUCTION WITH LIMITED OPENING

Sensitivity 0.80 and specificity 0.97

History

- Patient reports having had TMJ noise (clicking) with or without intermittent locking.
- Patient reports being limited in mouth opening severe enough to interfere with ability to eat, yawn, brush teeth, etc. Patient may refer to their jaw being locked closed (see Figure 14-8).

Physical Examination

- Maximum active unassisted IO 30 mm or less (see Figures 14-2 and 14-3).

(continued)

APPENDIX A (CONTINUED)

HISTORY AND PHYSICAL EXAMINATION FOR COMMON TEMPOROMANDIBULAR DISORDER DIAGNOSTIC SUBSETS

Clinical Points
What may or may not be observed during active jaw movement
• Deflection during opening to side of the involved joint.
• Deflection during protrusion to side of the involved joint.
• Decrease in lateral excursion to the opposite side of the involved joint.

DISK DISPLACEMENT WITHOUT REDUCTION WITHOUT LIMITED OPENING

Sensitivity 0.54 and specificity 0.79
History
• Patient reports having had a history of TMJ noise (clicking) with or without intermittent locking.
• Patient reports having had limited mouth opening severe enough to interfere with ability to eat, yawn, brush teeth, etc. Over time, their mouth opening improved.
Physical Examination
• Maximum active unassisted IO greater than 30 mm (see Figure 14-2).
Clinical Point
• This diagnosis relies on the patient's memory. This diagnosis cannot be made by the clinical examination if the patient cannot recall having a history as described earlier. Without a clear history, imaging would be required to make the diagnosis. However, imaging is not necessary because this stage of disk displacement is often not painful or limits jaw function.

DEGENERATIVE DISK DISEASE

Sensitivity 0.55 and specificity 0.61
History
• Patient reports a "grinding" noise (crepitus) emanating from their TMJ with jaw movement or function.
Physical Examination
• Palpating over the lateral pole of the condyle, crepitus is detected during jaw opening and closing movements and/or protrusion and/or right or left lateral excursion.
Clinical Point
• Without crepitus being detected, this diagnosis cannot be made, and imaging would be required to make the diagnosis. However, imaging would only be necessary if patient's TMJ pain (diagnosis of arthralgia with or without a diagnosis of a disk displacement) is not responding to physical therapy and an oral appliance. Then imaging with a referral to an oral surgeon is indicated.

Sensitivity and specificity values for TMD diagnostic subsets are from Schiffman et al.[29]

History and physical examination for TMD diagnostic subsets, except for subluxation, are based in part on but with modifications from Schiffman et al.[29]

APPENDIX B

HISTORY AND PHYSICAL EXAMINATION FOR CERVICAL SPINE DISORDER CONTRIBUTING TO HEADACHE AND FACIAL PAIN SYMPTOMS

CLINICAL EXAMINATION FOR CERVICAL SPINE DISORDERS

History

- Patient reports neck symptoms to include pain, stiffness, and/or tightness in the occipital, neck, shoulder, and/or upper extremity areas.
- Patient reports neck symptoms are modified by any one or combination of
  - Static activities involving sitting (eg, computer, driving) and sleeping.
  - Dynamic activities to include pushing, pulling, lifting, and reaching.

Physical Examination

Familiar symptoms are modified by

- Active and/or passive cervical flexion, extension, rotation, and/or side-bending.
- Palpation of the sternocleidomastoid, trapezius, levator scapulae, suboccipitals, and/or posterior midline cervical muscles.

CLINICAL EXAMINATION FOR CERVICOGENIC HEADACHE

History

- Patient reports pain localized in the neck and occipital region to project to the forehead, orbital region, temples, vertex, or ears.
- Patient reports headache is modified by any one or combination of
  - Static activities involving sitting (eg, computer, driving) and sleeping.
  - Dynamic activities to include pushing, pulling, lifting, and reaching.

Physical Examination

- Headache is modified by provocation tests as described in the physical examination for CSD.

Clinical Points

- Depending on tissue irritation, a reproduction or an increase in the CGH may or may not occur during the physical examination, but the patient reports headache has occurred in the past 30 days with the headache being modified by what was described above in the history.
- The headache is not better accounted for by another headache diagnosis.

(continued)

APPENDIX B (CONTINUED)

HISTORY AND PHYSICAL EXAMINATION FOR CERVICAL SPINE DISORDER CONTRIBUTING TO HEADACHE AND FACIAL PAIN SYMPTOMS

CLINICAL EXAMINATION FOR CERVICOGENIC SOMATOSENSORY EAR SYMPTOMS

History

- Patient reports having ear symptoms (pain, tinnitus, fullness, hearing loss) that coincide with neck symptoms and/or a CGH.
- Patient reports ear symptoms are modified by any one or combination of
  - ○ Static activities involving sitting (eg, computer, driving) and sleeping.
  - ○ Dynamic activities to include pushing, pulling, lifting, and reaching.

Physical Examination

- Ear symptoms are modified by provocation tests described in the physical examination for CSD.

Clinical Points

- Depending on tissue irritation, a reproduction or an increase in ear symptoms may or may not occur during the physical examination, but the patient reports ear symptoms have occurred in the past 30 days with ear symptoms modified by what was described above in the history.
- The ear symptoms are not better accounted for by another diagnosis.

APPENDIX C

INTERVENTION STRATEGIES USED IN THE INDIVIDUALIZED TREATMENT PLAN FOR PATIENTS WITH TEMPOROMANDIBULAR DISORDER	
TREATMENT STRATEGY	**DESCRIPTION**
Patient education	Patient education involves many facets. Fundamental to patient education is an explanation of their diagnosis, treatment objectives, expectations of treatment, frequency, cost, and expected number of treatments. Education to reduce unnecessary psychosocial distress due to misinformation is essential to achieve optimal treatment outcomes.
	The patient is educated on other treatment options that are available for TMD. This includes medications, oral appliances, and surgical interventions. Pros and cons of all treatments are discussed based on the available scientific evidence.
Behavioral modification	Behavioral modification is defined as the direct changing of unwanted behavior. Behavioral modification incorporates cognitive awareness exercises such as TUTA and WW. Being mindful to focus on the relaxation of the muscles of mastication will help to reduce diurnal bruxism. TUTA and WW are applied all day, especially when experiencing triggers for bruxism. Triggers include physical, focused, emotional, and psychosocial distress triggers. Eliminating harmful parafunctional activities including gum chewing, chewing ice, and fingernail biting is essential. The patient is to avoid hard/chewy food but to focus on a nonpainful diet. Behavioral modification also includes the correction of poor sitting and sleeping postures.
Therapeutic exercise	Therapeutic exercise is defined as any exercise performed with the aim of improving a single parameter, such as strength, range of motion (ROM), flexibility, or endurance. Depending on the TMD diagnostic subset, therapeutic jaw exercise can consist of active, active assistive, and/or passive jaw exercises with the goal of improving ROM to achieve functional mandibular dynamics. Jaw strengthening exercises are seldom, if ever, needed.
Neuromuscular reeducation	Neuromuscular reeducation is defined as the reeducation of movement, balance, kinesthetic sense, posture, and proprioception. Mandibular kinesthetic and proprioceptive exercises are used to enhance self-awareness of jaw movement and position.
Manual therapy	Manual therapy consists of soft tissue mobilization, joint mobilization, and dry needling.
	Soft tissue mobilization: The movement of contractile or inert tissues in such a way as to effect change in that structure or its related elements. Targeted tissues are the muscles of mastication.
	Joint mobilization: The act of moving articular structures generally performed passively by the physical therapist, with appropriate positioning to facilitate the intended movement. Intraoral techniques directed toward the head of the condyle consist of arthrokinematic techniques to create movement of joint distraction, condylar translation, and lateral glide (a joint play movement). Intraoral joint mobilization may be used for disk displacements or for capsular tightness due to trauma to the mandible and/or immobilization that occurs post-TMJ or post-orthognathic surgery.
	Dry needling: Is the insertion of a solid filiform needle into a latent or active myofascial trigger point.
	(continued)

APPENDIX C (CONTINUED)

INTERVENTION STRATEGIES USED IN THE INDIVIDUALIZED TREATMENT PLAN FOR PATIENTS WITH TEMPOROMANDIBULAR DISORDER

TREATMENT STRATEGY	DESCRIPTION
Modalities	Continuous ultrasound energy is absorbed in tissues with high collagen content. Used to heat tissue that has shortened or scarred down. Stretching can be done during or after to improve flexibility. Primary use is for chronic capsular tightness due to trauma and/or immobilization that occurs after trauma to the TMJ, TMJ arthrotomy, or orthognathic surgery.
	Pulsed ultrasound facilitates healing in the inflammatory and proliferative phase and is used for transdermal transport of anti-inflammatory medications (ketoprofen) referred to as *phonophoresis*. Primary use is for TMJ arthralgia or arthralgia after TMJ arthrocentesis, arthroscopy, and arthrotomy.
	Iontophoresis is the process by which drugs, usually anti-inflammatory in nature, are introduced to a small body part via direct electrical current. It is noninvasive, painless, and eliminates potential side effects and adverse reactions that can occur with medications delivered orally or by injection. Iontophoresis is used primarily for TMJ arthralgia but can be used to treat myalgia of the masseter muscle.
	Interferential stimulation is a type of electrical stimulation used for the control of pain. Interferential stimulation is believed to penetrate to deeper tissues than other forms of electrical stimulation such as transcutaneous electrical nerve stimulation. At higher frequencies, there is a decrease in skin resistance with interferential stimulation allowing the patient to tolerate interferential current better than transcutaneous electrical nerve stimulation, especially when applied over the masseter and/or TMJs. To avoid the crossover effect as with true interferential, premodulated interferential stimulation is used. When applied over the masseter muscles, a premodulated interferential stimulation with an intermittent setting of 10 to 15 seconds on and 10 to 15 seconds off is preferred by the author of this chapter. The intermittent current cues the patient when to perform active, active assistive, passive, and/or cognitive awareness exercises at the same time receiving the benefits from premodulation interferential stimulation of a reduction in pain, edema, and myalgia.

15

Mobilization/Manipulation of the Cervical and Thoracic Spine (Techniques)

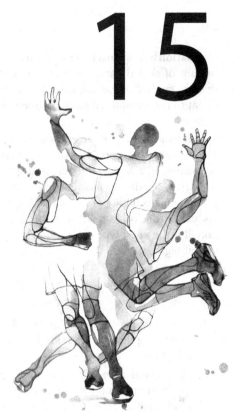

*Alec Kay, PT, DMT, ATC, OCS
and Ola Grimsby, PT*

Coordinative locking: This would be utilized with active mobilization or other active exercise approaches. In this type of locking, we take advantage of the coordination of the patient to control the movement so the mobilization does not exceed the range of motion (ROM) we would like them to work within. If there is a tissue tolerance or reactivity range that is most therapeutic, we would instruct and educate the patient to work in that range and they would use their coordination to perform the desired motion for the desired outcome. An example would be a patient with right facet joint cartilage irritation at C5-C6. We ask the patient to perform right rotation for compression/decompression and gliding of the articular cartilage for optimal stimulation, but only in the range that is pain free and tolerated by the joint. They would stop under their own control. As with all manual therapy approaches, a detailed and comprehensive evaluation is crucial for safe and effective application and outcome. For optimal application of joint mobilization, it is necessary for the provider to develop skill and sensitivity with their handling so that they can grade the joint mobility in the specific spinal segments. This will allow the technique to be most effective. In the case of trying to decrease pain and muscle guarding (ie, neurological influences), specificity of application is less important. With segmental mobility restrictions, specificity of technique is imperative.

Dorsal horn inhibition: The inhibition of pain perception through firing of an inhibitory interneuron, located in the dorsal horn of the spinal cord. This occurs through the stimulation and firing of mechanoreceptors.

Joint mobility: The joint play passively available.

Ligamentous locking: This is using collagen tension to decrease movement in a region of the spine. An example would be using flexion of the lower segments of the lumbar spine in side lying to lock out those segments while applying a rotation or side-bending mobilization to the segments cranial to where the locking has been introduced.

Manipulation: High-velocity, low-amplitude thrust within the range of joint motion aiming to inhibit pain and guarding, normalize ROM, and somatovisceral reflexes.

Mechanoreceptor: Sensory receptors located in collagen and joint capsules that are sensitive to mechanical stress and specific to speed of mechanical stress, location in body, and refractory period. Type IV fires with tissue trauma and relays pain perception.

Wallmann HW, Donatelli R, eds. *Foundations of Orthopedic Physical Therapy* (pp 437-452).
© 2024 Taylor & Francis Group.

Oscillations: A manual therapy technique comprising a continuum of skilled passive movements to the joint complex that are applied at varying speeds and amplitudes with the intent to restore optimal motion, function, and/or to reduce pain.

Spinal locking (also referred to as *coupled forces locking*): This is using the coupled forces in the spine to create facet opposition in a segment or region to prevent that segment from participating in mobilization or manipulation. A discussion and examples of spinal locking are at the end of the discussion on locking. Because this involves facet opposition, it is the safest type of locking when protecting a pathological segment.

CHAPTER QUESTIONS

1. What mobilization technique would be appropriate for improving right cervical side-bending in the mid cervical spine?

2. How could a mobilization technique of left C2-C3 side-bending improve active mobility in other directions such as right C2-C3 side-bending, rotation, or extension?

3. How does manipulation or joint mobilization decrease pain in a spinal segment?

4. What is the difference between an absolute and relative contraindication for manipulation?

5. What is the process for minimizing risk with manipulation?

6. If a patient cannot tolerate mobilization or manipulation directly to a painful segment, what choices does the clinician have in terms of assisting the situation with mobilization or manipulation?

7. Why does manipulation deform collagen less than mobilization?

8. How can manipulation be safer than mobilization when performed properly?

9. How do manipulation and mobilization vary in terms of their affect on pain and muscle guarding utilizing type I and II mechanoreceptor function?

10. What mobilization technique would be appropriate for improving extension of the upper thoracic spine?

11. List the neurological benefits of joint mobilization.

12. List the biomechanical benefits of joint mobilization.

13. In what clinical presentation is specificity of joint mobilization or manipulation very important?

14. In what clinical presentation is specificity of joint mobilization or manipulation less important?

15. What is the rationale for applying locking techniques with mobilization or manipulation?

16. What is the safest type of locking technique?

17. Is it safe to use joint oscillations in a hypermobile joint for pain inhibition if the oscillations are performed in the inner range of collagen tension?

18. What region of the body is it especially important to be aware of any bone weakening disease?

19. How can joint manipulation or mobilization improve vascularity in a region?

20. What may be a likely target for joint mobilization if a patient has a very painful and hypermobile segment at C5-C6?

INTRODUCTION

As long as history has been recorded, there are images and allusions to people helping other people using manual techniques. It comes from the primitive human desire to help another person who is suffering. The following techniques represent a small sample of techniques that have been refined over millennia and chosen for their effectiveness. The effectiveness of the technique depends on detailed evaluation including understanding of patient's anatomy, biomechanics, biopsychosocial presentation, clinical decision making, and skillful application. The rigorous thought and assessment that goes into clinical problem solving determines the benefit of any individual technique. This comes with high-level instruction, reflective mentoring, and countless hours of deep practice. Residency and fellowship programs in orthopedic manual therapy are the most efficient path to learning these techniques at the level of excellence that they deserve.

A thorough understanding of anatomy, biomechanics, neurology, pathology, and psychology is assumed when applying the following techniques. Although the emphasis of this chapter is on the mechanics of manual therapy, one of the clear opportunities we have as physical therapists is to see the patient presentation in a more holistic health view. Clinical practice requires the investigation, understanding, and validation of a patient's biological, social, and psychological status. Any of these aspects can be of great help or be a great obstacle toward improving their status. Master clinicians address these different aspects and this improves outcomes (Figure 15-1).

SPECIFIC MOBILITY TESTING PRINCIPLES FOR "JOINT PLAY"[1]

1. Speed: 5 to 10 oscillations per segment.
2. Grade an average of 3 to 4 segments.
3. Go back and retest.
4. Direction of testing:
   - Flexion
   - Extension
   - Side-bending (x2)
   - Rotation (x2)

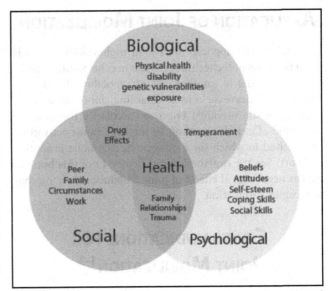

Figure 15-1. The interrelationship between biological, social, and psychological characteristics.

APPLICATION OF JOINT MOBILIZATION

The specific application of joint mobilization depends upon the goals of the technique. Whether the physical therapist is intending to improve collagen mobility directly, decrease pain, decrease muscle guarding, lubricate a joint, improve elastic mobility, improve vascularity through the inhibition of muscle guarding, or improve motor activation, the method in which the mobilization technique is applied will vary. See the explanation in Chapter 12 of this book as well as neurological effects of joint mobilization via mechanoreceptor stimulation.

CONTRAINDICATIONS FOR JOINT MOBILIZATION[1-3]

- Undiagnosed condition
- Psychosis
- Fracture
- Active infection in the joint being mobilized
- Surgical contraindications

UPPER CERVICAL MOBILIZATION TECHNIQUES

Articulation for Flexion Occiput on C1, Supine, and Nonweightbearing

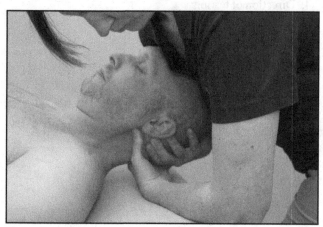

Figure 15-2. Position: The patient is supine with the cranium in a neutral position. The operator is standing at the head of the table with knees slightly flexed. The left hand fixates on the lateral aspect of the transverse processes of C1. The left thumb and index finger do the fixation. The right hand holds under the patient's occiput as the operator's anterior shoulder rests against the patient's forehead. **Mobilization:** The operator moves the cranium into a forward flexion by pressing with the right shoulder over the patient's forehead while rocking the cranium upward and keeping C1 fixated with the right thumb and index finger. **Comments:** Rotation of the cranium occurs at an axis through patient's ears.

Articulation Extension Occiput on C1, Supine, and Nonweightbearing

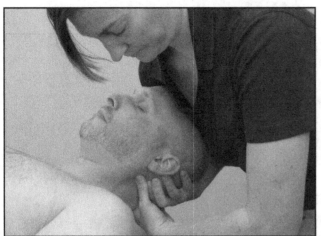

Figure 15-3. Position: The patient is supine with the cranium in a neutral position. The operator is standing at the head of the table with knees slightly flexed. The left hand fixates on the posterior aspect of the transverse processes of C1. The left thumb and index finger do the fixation. The right hand holds under the patient's occiput with the anterior shoulder resting against the patient's forehead. **Mobilization:** The operator moves the cranium into extension by rocking the knees and pressing over the patient's forehead with the right shoulder. This moves the patient's cranium back and downward while the chin moves up and forward. There is no real fixation; however, the left thumb and index finger are placed on the posterior aspect of the transverse processes of C1 for a base to rotate.

Articulation Side-bending Right Occiput on C1, Supine, and Nonweightbearing

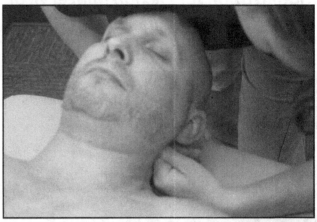

Figure 15-4. Position: The patient is supine with the cranium in a neutral position. The operator is standing at the head of the table with knees slightly flexed. The right hand supports under the occipital area with the right shoulder supporting the forehead. The left thumb is positioned over the lateral tip of the left C1 transverse process. **Mobilization:** The operator moves the cranium into a right side-bending with the right hand and shoulder. The occipital condyles glide to the left while the left thumb fixates the left C1 transverse process. **Comments:** The axis for motion is through the patient's nose.

Articulation Rotation Left Occiput on C1, Supine, and Nonweightbearing

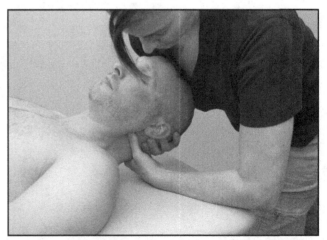

Figure 15-5. Position: The patient is supine at the head of the table, and the operator is standing at the head of the table. The right hand cupping around the occiput. The operator's right shoulder is supporting the patient's head at the left side. His knees are slightly flexed. He is leaning over the table. His right anterior shoulder supports against the patient's head while the right hand controls under the occiput. The left thumb and index fingers are fixating the posterior aspect of the C1 transverse processes. **Mobilization:** The operator carries the cranium, and occipital condyles, into a left rotation by rocking his hips to the right, elevating the right shoulder while maintaining fixation of the transverse processes of C, keeping C1 from following the occipital condyles.

MIDCERVICAL MOBILIZATION TECHNIQUES

Mobilization for Flexion Midcervical Spine (C3-C4), Supine, and Nonweightbearing

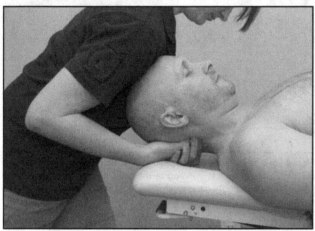

Figure 15-6. Position: The patient lies supine with the head in a neutral position. The operator stands at the head of the table with knees slightly flexed. The operator slides the left hand down so that the web of the hand is fixating over the spinous/transverse processes of C4, while the right upper hand slides down to C3, covering the spinous/transverse processes of C3 in the same manner. **Mobilization:** The operator moves the cranium into a forward flexion by pressing downward and gliding anteriorly with the right shoulder over the patient's forehead. The operator then fixates C4 inferiorly, while the hand over C3 draws the upper 3 vertebrae into flexion.

Mobilization for Extension Midcervical Spine (C3-C4), Supine, and Nonweightbearing

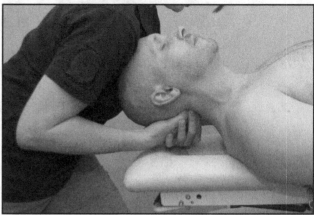

Figure 15-7. Position: The patient lies supine with the head in a neutral position. The operator stands at the head of the table with knees slightly flexed. The operator slides the left hand down so that the web of the hand is fixating over the spinous/transverse processes of C4, while the right upper hand slides down to C3, covering the spinous/transverse processes of C3 in the same manner. **Mobilization:** The operator moves the cranium into backward bending by rocking his knees and pushing the patient's forehead with his right shoulder, moving the cranium back and downward, while the chin moves up and forward. The upper segments including C3 glide posteriorly/inferiorly while the operator's hand provides a counterpressure to C4 in an anterior/superior direction.

Mobilization Side-bending Left Midcervical Spine (C3-C4), Supine, and Nonweightbearing

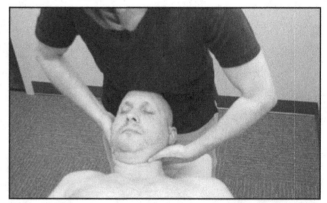

Figure 15-8. Position: The same as testing side-bending left midcervical, except the tip of the left index slides down to the superior articular process of C4 and the radial aspect of the proximal phalanx is placed against the transverse process. The tip of the right index finger slides upward to find the inferior articular process of C3. The operator places the proximal phalanx of the right index finger against it. **Mobilization:** The operator fixates C4 on the left while using the right forearm/hand to carry the head/neck into a left side-bending. The right index finger over C3 specifically moves C3 on C4.

Mobilization for Rotation Right Midcervical Spine (C3-C4), Supine, and Nonweightbearing

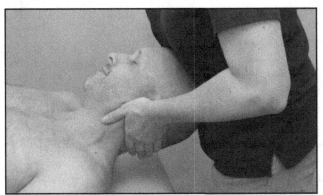

Figure 15-9. Position: The patient is supine. The head is supported under the occiput by the operator's hands with the head resting against the operator's abdomen. The operator slides both hands along the neck so that the radial aspects of the index fingers cover the inferior articular processes of C3 and the thumbs are parallel with the mandible. **Mobilization:** The operator rotates the head to the right with both hands down to C3-C4. The right hand then draws the upper cervical segments, including C3, superiorly by applying a traction force. At the same time the radial aspect of the left index finger applies an anterior/superior directed force to the posterior aspect of the articular process of C3, thus gliding it upward and forward on C4.

CERVICOTHORACIC MOBILIZATION TECHNIQUES

Mobilization for Flexion (C6-C7), Seated, and Weightbearing

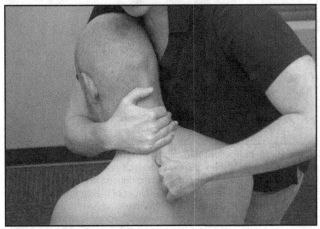

Figure 15-10. Position: The patient sits on a stool or bench. The operator stands to the side of the patient holding the spinous process of C7. The operator's right hand is located on the spinous process of C6. **Mobilization:** The operator flexes the patient's head with his right hand until the slack is taken up down to the level. At the same time, he gives a counter pressure to the spinous process of C7, thus articulating C6-C7.

Mobilization for Extension (C6-C7), Seated, and Weightbearing

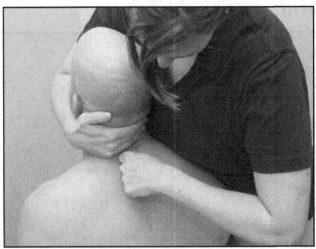

Figure 15-11. Position: The patient sits on a stool or bench. The operator presses with the thumb and index finger of the left hand over the spinous process of C7. He holds around the patient's head and neck with his right arm, and his left hand is located at the spinous process of C6. **Mobilization:** The operator's right arm moves the patient's head and neck backward and down including C6. They hold back C7 with a counter pressure of the left hand.

Mobilization for Side-bending Left (C6-C7), Seated, and Weightbearing

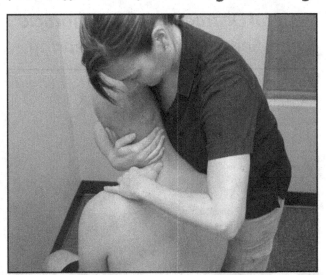

Figure 15-12. Position: The patient sits on a stool or bench. The operator's right arm supports the patient's head, cradling the patient's neck, biceps to forehead. The operator stands behind the patient with his left thumb on the left side of the spinous process of C7. The operator leans the patient's head over the left shoulder. **Mobilization:** The operator side-bends the patient's head to the left with his right hand until the slack is taken up down to C7. At the same time, with his thumb, he gives a counter pressure on the opposite side, against the C7 spinous process.

Mobilization for Rotation Right (C6-C7), Seated, and Weightbearing With Traction

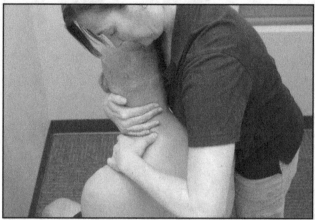

Figure 15-13. Position: The patient sits on a stool or bench. The operator's right arm supports the patient's head, cradling the patient's neck, biceps to forehead. The patient's head is being held between the operator's right arm and chest. The operator places his left thumb on the left side of the spinous process of C7. **Mobilization:** The operator gives distraction to patient's neck by extending his knees and rotates the patient's head to the right until the slack is taken up between C6 and C7. At the same time, he gives a counter pressure with his thumb on the left side of the spinous process of C7 to increase the motion of rotation between C6 and C7 to the right.

THORACIC SPINE JOINT MOBILIZATION

General Distraction of the Thoracic Spine, Seated, and Weightbearing

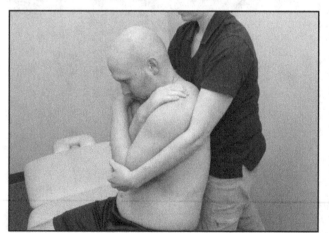

Figure 15-14. Indication: To improve general mobility and to inhibit pain. **Position:** The patient sits at the corner of the table with legs abducted 30 degrees. The patient crosses hands on opposite shoulders. The operator stands behind the patient reaching around to hold on to the patient's elbows. The patient leans back and supports the body against the operator. **Distraction:** The operator pulls the patient against her chest curling the spine into flexion. The operator applies a force through the patient's elbows by extending her knees, thus distracting the spine.

Articulation for Extension T6 With Wedge, Reclined Seated, and Partial Weightbearing

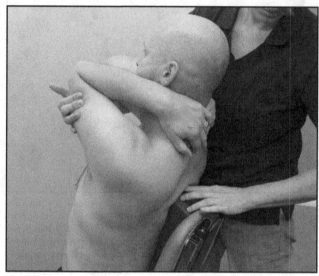

Figure 15-15. Indication: Treatment. **Position:** The same as with forward bending, but the operator holds under the patient's elbows or around the elbows. **Movement:** The operator pulls up on the patient's elbows and applies a downward force throughout the elbows, as she is palpating the space between the T6 and T7 spinous processes. She simultaneously side-bends her trunk to the left.

Articulation for Right Rotation (T6), Prone, and Nonweightbearing

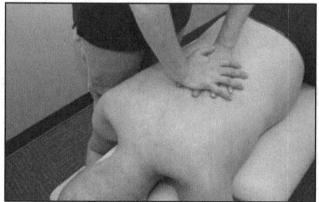

Figure 15-16. Indication: Treatment. **Position:** The patient is in a prone position with arms at the sides. The operator is standing on the left side of the bench. The tip of the index finger of the right hand is placed on the left transverse processes of T6. The middle finger of the right hand is placed on the right transverse process of T7. An alternative hand position is using the pisiforms of both hands on the transverse processes. **Movement:** The operator stabilizes with his left arm and applies the articulation force with his right arm.

Articulation Rotation Right (T7), Side Lying, and Nonweightbearing

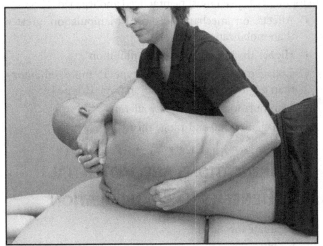

Figure 15-17. Indication: Treatment. **Position:** The patient is side lying at the edge of the table. The patient clasps hands behind the neck. The operator stands in front of the patient. The operator's right arm cradles the head and neck of the patient. The operator's index finger is placed on the left side of the spinous process of T8. **Movement:** The operator applies a rotary force through the patient's neck and forearms.

Articulation Side-bending Left (T7), Side Lying, and Nonweightbearing

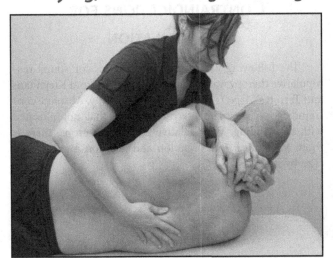

Figure 15-18. Indication: Treatment. **Position:** The patient is side lying at the edge of the table. The patient clasps their hands behind their neck. The operator stands in front of the patient. The operator's left arm cradles the head and neck of the patient. The operator's right thumb is placed on the left side of the spinous process of T8. **Movement:** The operator applies counter pressure with the right thumb on the spinous process of T8 as she side-bends the patient to the left. Side-bending is accomplished by lifting the patient with his right arm.

MOBILIZATION OF THE RIB CAGE

Mobilization of the Left First Rib in a Caudal Direction, Supine, and Nonweightbearing

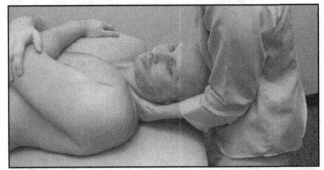

Figure 15-19. Indication: Mobilization. **Position:** The patient is lying supine at the head of the table with the left hand holding the top of the right shoulder. The head is rotated and sidebent to the left, resting on a pillow. The operator stands at the head of the table facing the patient. His right hand is maintaining cervical rotation to the left. The web space of his left thumb and index finger is placed on top of the patient's left first rib pointing in a downward and medial direction. His left ventral forearm is used for support at the cheek. **Mobilization:** The operator presses the left first rib downward, medially and anteriorly in line with the patient's right greater trochanter. He maintains the pressure for 7 to 10 seconds, then releases the pressure slowly. He should follow the respiratory rate of the patient with downward pressure on exhalation.

Testing or Mobilizing the Right Third Ribs Costosternal Spring, Supine, and Nonweightbearing

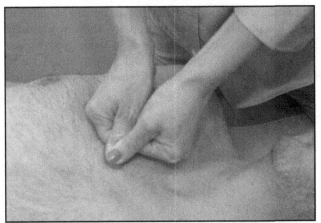

Figure 15-20. Indication: Test. **Position:** The patient is supine with arms along the side. The operator is standing at the head of the table to the right of the patient. He places his right thumb pad horizontally over the right third costosternal joint. His left thumb pad is placed on top of the right thumb. **Test:** The operator applies pressure straight posteriorly through both thumbs in a quick springy motion on the patient's expiration phase as he feels for a springy rebound and the elicitation of tenderness.

Testing Spring or Mobilization of the Costovertebral and the Costotransverse Joints of T8 on the Right

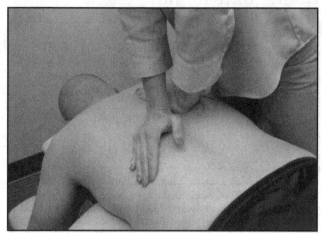

Figure 15-21. Indication: Test or mobilization. **Position:** The patient is lying prone with the cervical spine in a neutral position. A pillow can be placed under the abdomen to reduce lumbar lordosis strain. The operator stands at the patient's left side. The operator's right hypothenar eminence is placed on the patient's left transverse processes of T8. The left hand's hypothenar eminence and little finger are molded on the patient's T8 rib angle located laterally and I 1/2 spinous process interspaces above the T8 spinous process. **Mobilization:** Following the patient's expiration/ inspiration pattern, the operator starts applying pressure with his left hand anteriorly, caudally, and laterally as he applies a counter pressure with his right hand. He springs the rib with a quick pressure and release for testing or maintains a slow gradually increasing stretch pressure for articulation. **Definition of manipulation:** High-velocity, low-amplitude thrust within the range of joint motion aiming to inhibit pain and guarding, normalize ROM, and somatovisceral reflexes.

Because of the glycosaminoglycans present in collagen, there is a powerful dispersion property. This viscoelasticity dispersion of the application of force is much greater when the force is applied rapidly, with high velocity. This leads to less deformation of collagen with manipulation compared to mobilization and can be safer in that respect. Speed is a crucial component of safe, comfortable, and effective joint manipulation. As with all aspects of manual therapy, the development of speed must be practiced and learned.

- Affects on mechanoreceptors: Manipulation greater than mobilization
- Higher the intensity = greater inhibition[4,5]
- Collagen end-range stretch (type I) more inhibitory than beginning range oscillation (type II/type I)[4,5]
- Manipulation high intensity afferent
- Collagen mid to end-range thrust

INDICATIONS AND POTENTIAL BENEFITS OF MANIPULATION

- Facilitate movement
- Inhibit pain
- Increase vascularity
- Decrease muscle guarding
- Release of joint entrapments
- Increase muscle activation
- Improve fluid dynamics
- Psychological effect
- Placebo effect

CONTRAINDICATIONS FOR MANIPULATION

The following list of contraindications for spinal manipulative therapy was updated and adapted from Kleynhans and Terrett's[6] *Aspects of Manipulative Therapy*. Absolute contraindications are to be interpreted just as that, not indicated with this finding. With relative contraindications, there is room for clinical interpretation and decision making on a case-by-case basis.

Absolute

Articular Derangements

- Acute arthritis of any kind
- Rheumatoid arthritis with instability or acute
- Ankylosing spondylitis—Acute
- Dislocation
- Hypermobility of segment
- Ruptured ligaments
- Trauma of recent occurrence—Whiplash
- Advanced degenerative changes
- Congenital generalized hypermobility (Ehlers-Danlos syndrome)

Bone Weakening and Destructive Disease

- Calve's disease
- Fracture
- Malignancy/tumor (primary/secondary)
- Osteomalacia
- Osteoporosis
- Osteomyelitis
- Tuberculosis (Pott's disease)

Circulatory Disturbances

- Aneurysm
- Anticoagulant therapy
- Atherosclerosis
- Visceral arterial disease
- Calcification of aorta

Disk Lesions

- Prolapse with serious neurological changes
- Evidence of more than one spinal nerve root on one side
- Cervical or thoracic joint conditions causing neurological signs in lower limbs
- Acute cervical or lumbar herniation
- Thoracic herniation

Neurologic Dysfunction

- Micturition with sacral root involvement
- Painful movement in all directions
- Transverse myelitis
- Severe root pain
- Malformations of spinal cord including syringomyelia

Unclassified

- Infectious disease
- Uncooperative patient or patient intolerance
- Advanced diabetes when tissue value may be low
- Undiagnosed pain

Relative

Articular Derangements

- Ankylosing spondylitis after acute stage
- Articular deformity
- Congenital anomalies
- Hypertrophic spondyloarthritis
- Osteoarthritis, especially severe or advanced
- Osteochondrosis
- Rheumatoid arthritis—Subacute
- Torticollis
- Inflamed joint

Bone Weakening and Modifying Disease

- Hemangioma
- Paget's disease
- Scheuermann's disease
- Spondylolisthesis/spondylolysis with symptoms

Disk Lesions

- Posterolateral and posteromedial disk protrusions
- Degenerative disease

Neurologic Dysfunction

- Myelopathy
- Nonvertebral pain
- Pyramidal tract involvement
- Radicular pain with disk lesion
- Viscerosomatic reflex pain

Unclassified

- Abdominal hernia
- Asthma
- Dysmenorrhea
- Epicondylitis
- Long-term steroid use
- Low pain threshold
- Peptic ulcer
- Post-spinal surgery
- Pregnancy, especially first trimester
- Scoliosis
- Psychogenic disorders with dependence on therapy
- Patients who have been treated recently by another practitioner
- Signs and symptoms do not match

Manipulation Techniques

Technique: Seated mid Cs unilateral facet distraction on the right (nonphysiological locking).

Patient position: Sitting on corner of table or stool.

Operator position: Standing slightly behind and to the side of the patient.

Hand placement: Operator's arm is loosely positioned around the patient's head and jaw with the ulnar side of the fifth finger on the posterior arch of C6. Operator's other hand is resting on the shoulder of the patient with the thumb fixating the spinous process (or facet) of C7.

- From above, flex to the segment of C6; side-bend to the segment of C6 and rotate to the segment.
- From below, fixate thumb on spinous process or facet and hold steady.

Manipulation thrust: Search for the barrier by adjusting amounts of flexion, side-bending and rotation. When barrier is found apply a high-velocity, low-amplitude technique (HVLAT) of right rotation of C6 with a slight counter rotation with the thumb. It is safer to perform the thrust from the inferior contact because it is a shorter lever.

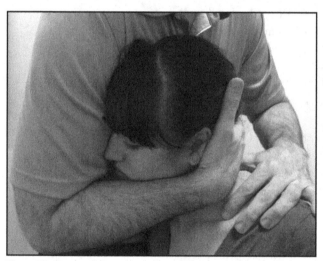

Figure 15-22.

Technique: Rib prone posterior/anterior distraction (gap of costo transverse).

Patient position: Prone.

Operator position: Standing on the side of the table.

Hand placement: The hands are crossed and angled so the ulnar side of the superior hand is placed on the transverse processes of the spinal segments above the rib to be treated. The inferior hand's ulnar border is just lateral to the transverse process on the rib head and shaft on the contralateral side of the patient's body.

Manipulation thrust: Respirations are felt and at the expiratory phase, the barrier is identified and an HVLAT is applied to the rib while holding (pushing) the distal hand anterior thus creating an opposite rotation moment. The thrust is in the direction of the left forearm in the image provided.

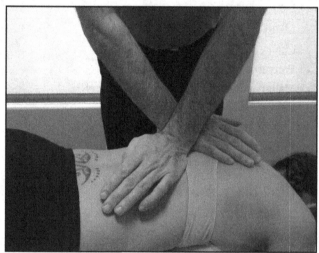

Figure 15-23.

Technique: Rib supine posterior/anterior distraction (gap).

Patient position: Supine close to the edge of the table; arms across the chest or fingers laced behind the neck.

Operator position: Standing to the side of the patient. Operator flexes the patient to the level to be treated.

Hand placement: The operator rotates the patient to access the ribs. One hand reaches around the patient and is placed at the rib so that the finger is touching the spinous process and the thumb is in line with the rib to be treated (salute position) just medial to rib angle. The other arm is placed across the patient's ulnas and controls the amount of flexion, side-bending, and rotation to isolate the barrier.

Manipulation thrust: The operator's arm controls the amount and direction of motion to find the barrier. Near end ROM, an HVLAT through the arms as the operator's torso is directed to the rib perpendicular to the costovertebral surface. Slight counterforce from the bottom via forearm pronation with assist in creating a barrier.

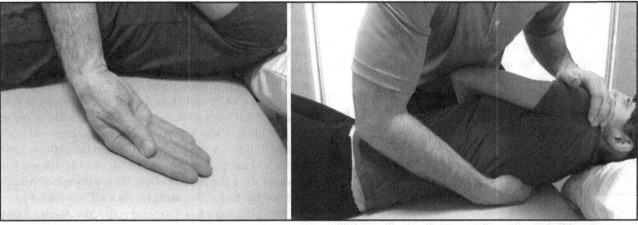

Figure 15-24.

Technique: Occipital-atlanto joint (OA) distraction.

Patient position: Supine close to the edge of the table with body oblique on table to get head closer to corner of table. The patient's cervical spine is side bent toward C2 from below to "lock" mid Cs; rotation of OA away with slight extension of the head to take tension off the alar ligament.

Operator position: Standing toward the top of the table facing superior on the patient's side.

Hand placement: Chin hold position with operator's proximal hand supporting the patient's head by holding under the mandible. The distal hand (second metacarpophalangeal) is under the mastoid process.

Manipulation thrust: Perpendicular to the joint surface of the OA. Thrust is applied with the hand under the mastoid into a cephalad and lateral direction.

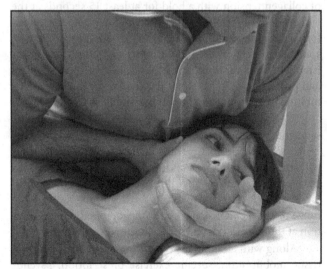

Figure 15-25.

CASE STUDIES

Case Study One

A 38-year-old woman who is a competitive master's level swimmer presented with worsening neck pain over the prior 2-month training cycle. She developed right radicular symptoms in her thumb and forefinger. She has had positive outcomes with physical therapy in the past and came directly to physical therapy in this case with no other imaging or medical workup.

After orthopedic manual physical therapy examination, it was determined that the tissue in lesion is the disk between C5-C6. Other than her subjective report of radiating symptoms, there were no neurological findings that were positive with examination. Compression in neutral and slight flexion was painful and long axis distraction was relieving. There was a positive segmental shear test at C5-C6, and palpation revealed muscle guarding locally with the cervical multifidi and splenius cervicis, levator scapula, and upper trapezius on the right. Hypomobilities were identified in the upper thoracic spine, C2-C3 rotation, and side-bending, as well as right atlanto-axial joint (AA) rotation.

Screening was performed following International Federation of Orthopaedic Manipulative Physical Therapists and American Academy of Orthopaedic Manual Physical Therapists' guidelines for contraindications for joint mobilization and manipulation.

Joint mobilization would be appropriate with the goal of increasing collagen elasticity by performing right AA rotation starting with oscillations in midrange of collagen tension. After some relaxation of muscle guarding and improved elasticity, mobilization could be applied to end range of collagen tension with a hold for at least 15 seconds at the end of the application. The same technique would be applied for rotation and side-bending at C2-C3 and upper thoracic spine. High-velocity, low-amplitude thrust would be administered to facet joints upper thoracic spine with good control and protection of lower cervical spine for the purpose of inhibition of guarding and improving mobility.

With the goal of decreasing pain and muscle guarding, segmental distraction was applied to the facet joints at the spinal segment of C5-C6 with oscillations. The oscillations will stimulate both type I and II mechanoreceptors and inhibit pain and muscle guarding through dorsal horn inhibition. This would be applied in the beginning and middle range of collagen tension along with side-bending and rotation at the same levels and adjacent spinal segments as well.

Along with all other aspects of treatment including soft tissue mobilization, specific exercise prescription, psychological consideration, nutritional education, postural education, ergonomic instruction, swim technique assessment, and education, the prognosis would be good.

It would be very important to assess the patient neurologically each encounter, and if there was any worsening or if the pain was not improving after 2 to 4 weeks, the patient should be referred to the appropriate provider for more testing.

Case Study Two

A 69-year-old man presented with generalized neck pain and occasional headaches. He has had symptoms on and off for 5 years, but they worsened 2 months ago, and he saw his primary care physician who referred him to an orthopedist. The workup included plain films and magnetic resonance imaging, and he was told that he had degenerative disk disease at levels C4-C5, C5-C6, and C6-C7. He was also told he had bone spurring associated with osteoarthritis at multiple levels in his cervical spine, foraminal stenosis on the right at C5-C6, and central canal stenosis worst at C3-C4 and C5-C6 from a broad-based disk bulge. The surgeon told him his neck was "a mess" and eventually he would need surgery. This had a very negative affect on the patient's confidence and self-perception, and he felt that his stiffness has increased since that conversation. He has decreased his activity and has feared that using his neck will worsen his pain.

This gentleman has decreased active and passive ROM in all planes with only 10 degrees of side-bending right and 15 degrees left. All motions were met with a description of dull pain and stiffness. Palpation revealed global muscle guarding and some facet joint thickening of capsular tissue and bony enlargement in the cervical spine. The midcervical spine was hypomobile to joint mobility testing except for left rotation C4-C5 and C5-C6.

He has no contraindication for joint mobilization. He has diabetes, obesity, and hypertension, which make him a poor candidate for cervical manipulation.

An appropriate and productive approach for this gentleman would be the implementation of cervical joint mobilization oscillations for pain inhibition and decreasing muscle guarding in all segments tolerated. End-range holds within the comfort range would be implemented in all restricted planes of motion and not to left rotation C4-C5 and C5-C6. Improving mobility of the upper thoracic spine would assist this patient with functional ROM as well. The upper thoracic spine would be a good target for treatment for its biomechanical contribution to cervical mobility and because it is less painful and irritable in this patient.

In addition to manual techniques, there is some "undoing" of negative thought and imagery that would assist this patient in his improvement. Addressing this biopsychosocial aspect of his pain experience would be part of a comprehensive physical therapy treatment program but is beyond the scope of this chapter.

This patient has good potential for improved comfort and functional ROM with manual physical therapy. Again, this patient needs a global approach and all other aspects of treatment including soft tissue mobilization, education, specific exercise prescription, psychological consideration, nutritional education, postural education, and ergonomic instruction would be indicated. Due to the nocebo effect from his encounter with his physician, biopsychosocial and pain education would need to be a significant part of his treatment as well.

REFERENCES

1. Paris SV. Aspects of manual therapy and assessing bone and joint motion with cineradiography. In: Kaltenborn F. *Proceedings from the International Federation of Orthopedic Manipulative Therapists.* International Federation of Orthopedic Manipulative Therapist Inc; 1977.

2. Grieve GP. *Common Vertebral Joint Problems.* 2nd ed. Churchill Livingstone; 1988.

3. Maitland GD. *Peripheral Manipulation.* 2nd ed. Butterworth; 1977.

4. Wyke B, Polacek P. Articular neurology: the present position. *J Bone Joint Surg Am.* 1975;57(B):40.

5. Wyke B. Articular neurology—a review. *Physiotherapy.* 1972;58(3):94-99.

6. Kleynhans AM, Terrett AGJ. The prevention of injury in spinal manipulative therapy. In: Glasgow EF, ed. *Aspects of Manipulative Therapy.* 2nd ed. Churchill Livingstone; 1985:161-175.

BIBLIOGRAPHY

Beyeler W. Scheuermann's disease and its chiropractic management. *Annals Swiss Chiro Assoc.* 1960;(1):70.

Biller J, Sacco RL, Albuquerque FC, et al. Cervical arterial dissections and association with cervical manipulative therapy: a statement for healthcare professionals from the american heart association/american stroke association. *Stroke.* 2014; 45(10):3155-3174. doi:10.1161/STR.000000000000016

Bollier W. Inflammatory, infections and neoplastic disease of the lumbar spine. *Annals Swiss Chiro Assoc.* 1960.

Boshes LD. Vascular accidents associated with neck manipulation. *JAMA.* 1959;171(11):1602. doi:10.1001/jama.1959.03010290160027

Bourdillon JF. *Spinal manipulation.* 3rd ed. Appleton & Lange; 1982.

Cassidy DJ, Boyle E, Pierre C, et al. Risk of vertebrobasilar stroke and chiropractic care: results of a population-based case-control and case-crossover study. *Spine.* 2008;35(Suppl 4):S176-S183. doi:10.1097/BRS.0b013e3181644600

Cyriax JH. *Textbook of Orthopedic Medicine Volume 2.* 10th ed. Balliere Tindall; 1980.

Dabbert O, Freeman D, Weis A. Spinal meningeal hematoma, warfarin therapy, and chiropractic adjustment. *JAMA.* 1970; 214(11):2058. doi:10.1001/jama.1970.03180110066020

Davidson KC, Weiford EC, Dixon GD. Traumatic vertebral artery pseudoaneurysm following chiropractic manipulation. *Radiology.* 1975;115(3):651-652. doi:10.1148/15.3.651

Dunning J, Mourad F, Giovannico G, Maselli F, Perreault T, Fernández-de-las-Peñas C. Changes in shoulder pain and disability after thrust manipulation in subjects presenting with second and third rib syndrome. *J Manipulative Physiol Ther.* 2015;38(6):382-394. doi:10.1016/j.jmpt.2015.06.008

Dunning JR, Butts R, Mourad F, et al. Upper cervical and upper thoracic manipulation versus mobilization and exercise in patients with cervicogenic headache: a multi-center randomized clinical trial. *BMC Musculoskelet Disord.* 2016; 17(1):17-64. doi:10.1186/s1281-016-0912-3

Droz JM. Indications and contraindications of vertebral manipulations. *Annals Swiss Chiro Assoc.* 1971;5(8).

Dvorak J. Inappropriate indications and contraindications for manual therapy, *J Man Med.* 1991;6(3):85-89.

Dvorak J. Consensus and recommendations as to the side effects and complications of manual therapy of the cervical spine. *J Man Med.* 1991;6(3):117-118.

Good C. Internal forces sustained by the vertebral artery during spinal manipulative therapy. *J Manipulative Physiol Ther.* 2003;26(5):338-339. doi:10.1016/S0161-4754(03)00048-4

Grimsby O. Neurophysiological view points on hypermobilities. *Man Ther.* 1988;2:2-9.

Grillo G. Anomalies of the lumbar spine. *Annals Swiss Chiro Assoc.* 1960;1:56.

Hartman L. *Handbook of Osteopathic Technique.* Hutchinson; 1985.

Hauberg G. Contraindications for the manual therapy of the spine. *Hippokrates.* 1967;38(6):230-235.

Haynes M. Internal forces sustained by the vertebral artery during spinal manipulative therapy. *J Manipulative Physiol Ther.* 2004;27(1):67-68. doi:10.1016/j.jmpt.2003.11.014

Heilig D. Whiplash - mechanics of injury, management of cervical and dorsal involvement. In: Academy of Applied Osteopathy. *1965 Yearbook.* 1965.

Herzog W, Leonard TR, Symons B, Tang C, Wuest S. Vertebral artery strains during high-speed, low amplitude cervical spinal manipulation. *J Electromyogr Kinesiol.* 2012;22(5):740-746. doi:10.1016/j.jelekin.2012.03.005

Hooper J. Low back pain and manipulation. Paraparesis after treatment of low back pain by physical methods. *Med J Aust.* 1973;1(11):549-551.

Hutting N, Verhagen AP, Vijverman V, Keesenberg MDM, Dixon G, Scholten-Peeters GGM. Diagnostic accuracy of premanipulative vertebrobasilar insufficiency tests: a systematic review. *Man Ther.* 2013;18(3):177-182. doi:10.1016/j.math.2012.09.009

Janse J. *Principles and Practice of the Chiropractic: An Anthology.* National College of Chiropractic; 1976.

Jaquet P. *Clinical Chiropractic - A Study of Cases.* Crounauer; 1978.

Jennett WB. A study of 25 cases of compression of the cauda equina by prolapsed intervertebral discs. *J Neurol Neurosurg Psychiatry.* 1956;19(2):109-116. doi:10.1136/jnnp.19.2.109

Johnson EG, Landel R, Kusunose RS, Appel TD. Positive patient outcome after manual cervical spine management despite a positive vertebral artery test. *Man Ther.* 2008;13(4):367-371. doi:10.1016/j.math.2007.12.001

Kaiser G. Orthopedics and traumatology. *J Ortho.* 1973;20:581.

Kaltenborn FM. *Mobilization of the Spinal Column.* New Zealand University Press; 1970.

Kaltenborn FM. *Manual Therapy of the Extremity Joints.* Olaf Norlis Bokhandel; 1976.

Kaltenborn FM. *Mobilization of the Extremity Joints: Examination and Basic Treatment Techniques.* 3rd ed. Olaf Norlis Bokhandel; 1980.

Kaltenborn FM. *Mobilization of the Extremity Joints: Examination and Basic Treatment Techniques.* 4th ed. Olaf Norlis Bokhandel; 1989.

Lindner H. A synopsis of the dystrophies of the lumbar spine. *Annals Swiss Chiro Assoc.* 1960;1:143.

Maigne R. *Orthopaedic Medicine: A New Approach to Vertebral Manipulations.* Thomas Publisher; 1972.

Maitland GD. *Vertebral Manipulation.* 5th ed. Butterworth; 1986.

Maitland GD, Hengeveld E, Banks K, English K. *Vertebral Manipulation.* 7th ed. Elsevier; 2005.

Mehalic T, Farhat SM. Vertebral artery injury from chiropractic manipulation of the neck. *Surg Neurol.* 1974;2(2):125-129.

Miller RG, Burton R. Stroke following chiropractic manipulation of the spine. *JAMA.* 1974;229(2):189-190. doi:10.1001/jama.1974.03230400051034

Mintken PE, Derosa C, Little T, Smith B. A model for standardizing manipulation terminology in physical therapy practice. *J Orthop Sports Phys Ther*. 2008;38(3):A1-A6. doi:10.2519/jospt.2008.0301

Nwuga VCB. *Manipulations of the Spine*. Williams and Wilkins; 1976.

Odom GL. (1970). *Neckache and backache*. Proceedings of the NINCDS Conference on Neckache and Backache, Bethesda, Maryland.

Quesnele JJ, Triano JJ, Noseworthy MD, Wells GD. Changes in vertebral artery blood flow following various head positions and cervical spine manipulation. *J Manipulative Physiol Ther*. 2014;37(1):22-31. doi:10.1016/j.jmpt.2013.07.008

Rade M, Shacklock M, Peharec S, et al. Effect of cervical spine position on upper limb myoelectric activity during pre-manipulative stretch for Mills manipulation: a new model, relations to peripheral nerve biomechanics and specificity of Mills manipulation. *J Electromyogr Kinesiol*. 2012;22(3):363-369. doi:10.1016/j.jelekin.2011.12.006

Rinsky LA, Reynolds GG, Jameson RM, Hamilton RD. A cervical spine cord injury after chiropractic adjustment. *Paraplegia*. 1976;13(4):223-227. doi:10.1038/sc.1976.35

Ritcher RR, Reinking FM. Evidence in practice. *Phys Ther*. 2005;85(6):589-599.

Rushton A, Rivett DA, Carlesso LC, Flynn TW, Hing W, Kerry R. International framework for examination of the cervical region for potential of cervical arterial dysfunction prior to orthopaedic manual therapy intervention. *Man Ther*. 2015;101.

Sandoz R. About some problems pertaining to the choice of indications for chiropractic therapy. *Annals Swiss Chiro Assoc*. 1965;3:201.

Siehl D. Manipulation of the spine under anesthesia. In: Academy of Applied Osteopathy. *1967 Yearbook*. 1967.

Stoddard A. *Manual of Osteopathic Practice*. Hutchinson; 1969.

Symons BP, Leonard T, Herzog W. Internal forces sustained by the vertebral artery during spinal manipulative therapy. *J Manipulative Physiol Ther*. 2002;25(8):504-510. doi:10.1067/mmt.2002.127076

Thomas LC, Rivett DA, Bateman G, Stanwell P, Levi CR. Effect of selected manual therapy interventions for mechanical neck pain on vertebral and internal carotid arterial blood flow and cerebral inflow. *Phys Ther*. 2013;93(11):1563-1574. doi:10.2522/ptj.20120477

Timbrell-Fisher AG. *Treatment by Manipulation in General and Consulting Practice*. 5th ed. HK Lewis; 1948.

Valentini E. The occipito-cervical region. *Annals Swiss Chirop Assoc*. 1969;4:225.

Vaughan B, Moran R, Tehan P, et al. Manual therapy and cervical artery dysfunction: identification of potential risk factors in clinical encounters. *Int J Osteopath Med*. 2016;21:40-50. doi:10.1016/j.ijosm.2016.01.007

Wuest S, Symons B, Leonard T, Herzog W. Preliminary report: biomechanics of vertebral artery segments C1-C6 during cervical spinal manipulation. *J Manipulative Physiol Ther*. 2010;33(4):273-278. doi:10.1016/j.jmpy.2010.03.007

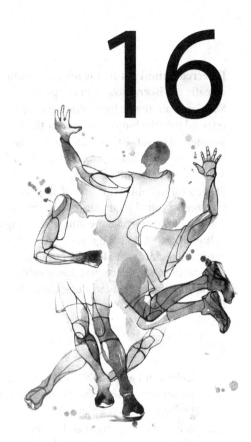

Differential Diagnosis and Manual Therapy of the Lumbar Spine and Pelvis

*Beth Stone Norris, PhD, PT, OCS, E-RYT 500
and Sharon Wang-Price, PT, PhD, OCS*

Aberrant motion: Deviation from expected movement pattern during active trunk flexion and return to upright standing position.

Centralization: Movement of pain or symptoms from a distal to proximal direction toward midline of the spine in response to movement strategies.

Concordant sign: A concordant sign refers to a symptom or symptoms described by the patient that bring the patient to seek physical therapy evaluation and treatment.

Directional preference: A specific movement or posture that decreases pain and/or increases active range of motion (AROM).

Force closure: The mechanism for enhanced pelvic stability that is provided through active tension from muscles extrinsic to the pelvis, passive tension from ligaments, and neural control.

Form closure: Stability of the pelvis that is provided by the shape and structure of the sacroiliac joints (SIJs).

Functional instability: Increased midrange movement of a spinal segment due to loss of neuromuscular control.

Lumbopelvic pain: Pain that is located from the lower costal borders to the ischial tuberosities, central or unilateral, and may give rise to symptomology into the lower extremity.

Mechanical low back pain (LBP): Pain that is reproduced or changed with active and passive movements and positional testing.

Neutral zone: The portion of physiologic range of motion (ROM) of the spinal segment that occurs with minimal internal resistance.

Nonspecific low back pain (NSLBP): LBP that does not have a specific medical diagnosis and is not related to serious pathology. Nonspecific LBP is said to encompass up to 85% of patients presenting with LBP.[1]

Peripheralization: Movement of pain or symptoms from a midline location in the spine to a distal location.

Radicular pain: A type of referred pain that is caused by involvement of a nerve root.

Radiculopathy: Radiating symptoms of paresthesia, numbness, or weakness caused by involvement of a nerve root.

Red flags: Red flags are signs and symptoms that alert the physical therapist to serious conditions that warrant medical referral only.

Wallmann HW, Donatelli R, eds. *Foundations of
Orthopedic Physical Therapy* (pp 453-516).
© 2024 Taylor & Francis Group.

Referred pain: Pain that is felt at a location away from the somatic or visceral source of the pain.

Sciatica: Pain that is localized to the L4-S2 dermatomes and referred into the buttock, posterior thigh, and calf.

Segmental instability: An increase in the size of the neutral zone of the spine due to a disruption in the osseoligamentous and/or neuromuscular tissues.

Structural instability: A loss of ability to maintain the neutral zone of spinal segments under applied loads due to a disruption of the osseoligamentous stabilizing structures.

Yellow flags: Yellow flags are signs and symptoms of psychosocial factors that alert the physical therapist to proceed with caution, consider referral in combination with physical therapy, or incorporate strategies to address modifiable psychosocial factors.

CHAPTER QUESTIONS

1. Understand anatomical and biomechanical features of the lumbar spine and pelvis that contribute to mobility, stability, and pain generation.

2. Identify the structures and connective tissues that contribute to passive, active, and neural subsystems of lumbopelvic stability.

3. Distinguish between structural and functional lumbar segmental instability (LSI). Identify clinical tests can be used to assess each type of LSI.

4. Differentiate between reduced and excessive force closure. Identify clinical tests can be used to assess for each type of force closure impairment.

5. Identify interview questions to establish an understanding of the nature, severity, and irritability of lumbopelvic pain.

6. Evaluate examination findings to determine the appropriateness of physical therapy and need for referral.

7. Identify self-report outcome measures appropriate for determining level of disability associated with lumbopelvic pain.

8. Which instruments may assist in identifying elevated psychosocial distress?

9. What information is obtained at the conclusion of the lower quarter scan examination (LQSE)?

10. Which examination findings would indicate the inclusion of biomechanical tests?

11. Describe the presentation of pelvic girdle pain (PGP), including signs, symptoms, and common functional impairments.

12. Identify provocation tests for SIJ pain.

13. Which passive mobility iliosacral mobility tests assess for an anteriorly rotated innominate and a posteriorly rotated innominate?

14. How is nutation and counternutation mobility of the sacrum assessed?

15. How does disability, severity, irritability, and the relation of pain to active and passive movement testing contribute to establishing symptom acuity of lumbopelvic pain?

16. Outline examination findings that would assist in evaluation of the subgroup classifications of lumbopelvic pain.

17. Identify intervention strategies congruent with clinical diagnosis classification subgrouping.

18. Identify components of the clinical predication rule identifying patients with LBP who may have short-term benefit with thrust manipulation techniques.

19. Recognize when thrust vs non-thrust manipulation techniques are appropriate as interventions for lumbopelvic pain with mobility deficits.

20. Describe recent evidence for use of muscle energy techniques (METs) in restoring mobility and managing lumbopelvic pain.

INTRODUCTION

LBP that arises from musculoskeletal structures in the lumbar spine and pelvis comprises a large percentage of economic and health care costs in the United States.[2] These costs have increased 65% from 1997 to 2005 due primarily to the high prevalence and recurrence rate of LBP and the increasing number of individuals with chronic LBP.[3,4] LBP is the most frequently seen condition by physical therapists practicing in an outpatient environment.[5] Physical therapy management of LBP encompasses multiple components including the differentiation between the appropriateness for physical therapy and the need for referral; the identification of predictors for recurrent LBP and the development of chronic LBP; the utilization of appropriate tests and measures to identify concordant signs and symptoms; the evaluation of clinical examination findings to identify subgroupings of LBP for diagnostic classification; and the provision of physical therapy interventions that are adherent to subgroup classification systems, matched with impairments of body function identified in the clinical examination, inclusive of a biopsychosocial approach. This chapter is divided into 3 sections. Section I provides an overview of clinically relevant anatomy and biomechanics of the lumbopelvic region and outlines examination procedures for the lumbopelvic region. Section II presents evaluation of examination findings for differential diagnosis using a subgrouping classification process. Section III presents manual therapy interventions for lumbopelvic conditions.

Section I: Lumbopelvic Anatomy, Biomechanics, and Examination Process

Clinically Relevant Considerations of Normal and Abnormal Anatomy and Biomechanics

The lumbopelvic region consists of the lumbar spine, the pelvis, and the hips. Understanding the clinically relevant anatomy and biomechanics of the lumbopelvic region contributes to obtaining an effective history, selecting and administering the appropriate clinical tests, and evaluating examination findings for diagnostic classification. This section presents normal and abnormal (dysfunctional) lumbopelvic anatomy and biomechanics regarding considerations of mobility, stability, and pain generation.

Anatomical and Biomechanical Considerations for Lumbopelvic Mobility

Mobility of the lumbar spine occurs through the interbody joints and the zygapophyseal or facet joints. The interbody joint consists of the intervertebral disk (IVD) and the vertebral bodies above and below. The facet joint is the articulation between the superior articular processes of the inferior vertebrae and the inferior articular processes of the superior vertebrae. For each vertebral segment, there is 1 interbody joint and 2 facet joints. The lumbar facet joints lie primarily in the sagittal plane with the superior facet facing medially and the inferior facet facing laterally. At the lumbosacral junction, the orientation of the facets changes toward the frontal plane, which contributes to the stability of L5 on S1. The facet joints guide and limit motion in the lumbar segment while the interbody joints allow segmental movement to occur and absorb and distribute loads.[6,7]

Lumbar spinal motion occurs in 3 movement planes in the directions of flexion/extension, side-bending, and rotation for a total of 6 degrees of freedom. While the individual motion at each lumbar segment is small, the combined motion of all segments produces approximately 40 to 50 degrees flexion, 15 to 20 degrees extension, 20 degrees side-bending, and 5 to 7 degrees rotation.[8] In contrast to the cervical spine, inconsistency exists in the literature regarding coupling of rotation and side-bending motions in the lumbar spine.[9] During sagittal and frontal plane lumbar motions, one side of the vertebral bodies comes together or approximates while the opposite side moves apart or separates. On the side of the approximation, the nucleus pulposus is compressed and the fibers of the annulus slacken or bulge.[6] Compression of the nucleus pulposus causes the nuclear fluid to move toward the side of separation, increasing tension on the annular fibers

on that side. On the side of the vertebral body separation, the annular fibers will lengthen, increasing in passive tension. A biomechanical description of facet motion includes gliding (upgliding, downgliding), approximation, and distraction, which is driven by the orientation of the lumbar facets. Bilateral upgliding occurs during lumbar flexion and bilateral downgliding occurs during lumbar extension. During side-bending, upgliding occurs contralateral to the direction of side-bending, while downgliding occurs ipsilateral to the direction of side-bending. The medial facing of the superior facets and lateral facing of the inferior facets in a lumbar segment contribute approximation of the facets contralateral to the direction of rotation and distraction or separation of the facets ipsilateral to the direction of rotation.[6] A summary of lumbar biomechanics is presented in Table 16-1.

Motion of the pelvis occurs at the SIJ, pubic symphysis, and hips. The SIJ consists of the sacrum and the 2 innominates of the pelvis. SIJ motion is described as movement of the ilium on the sacrum (iliosacral mobility) or movement of the sacrum on the ilium (sacroiliac mobility). Active iliosacral mobility consists of anterior and posterior rotation (tilting) in the sagittal plane with the trunk remaining stationary. During anterior pelvic rotation, the anterior superior iliac spine (ASIS) moves inferior bilaterally, and the posterior superior iliac spine (PSIS) moves superior bilaterally. During posterior pelvic rotation, the ASIS moves superiorly bilaterally, and the PSIS moves inferiorly bilaterally. With the trunk remaining stationary, anterior pelvic rotation increases the lumbar lordosis and posterior pelvic rotation decreases the lumbar lordosis. Sacroiliac motions consist of rotation and translation. The amount of sacroiliac motion is small and has been estimated to be 1 to 4 degrees of rotation and 1 to 2 mm of anteroposterior translation.[10] Rotation occurs in the sagittal plane and is described as nutation and counternutation. Nutation occurs when the base of the sacrum moves anterior and inferior and is considered flexion of the sacrum. Counternutation occurs when the sacral base moves posterior and superior and is considered extension of the sacrum.[11] When the ilia rotate on a fixed sacrum, relative nutation and counternutation occur with anterior rotation creating relative counternutation of the sacrum and posterior rotation creating relative nutation of the sacrum.

Femur on pelvic hip motion is used in the clinical examination to assess iliosacral mobility with hip extension used to assess anterior pelvic rotation and hip flexion used to assess posterior pelvic rotation. Additionally, pelvic on femur motion of anterior and posterior rotation creates hip flexion and extension, respectively.[8] In summary, when the trunk is maintained in an upright position, anterior pelvic rotation increases lumbar lordosis, produces hip flexion, and is associated with relative counternutation of the sacrum. Similarly, posterior pelvic rotation performed while maintaining an upright trunk, decreases the lumbar lordosis, produces hip extension, and is associated with relative nutation of the sacrum.

Table 16-1

LUMBAR BIOMECHANICS

LUMBAR MOTION	INTERBODY JOINT	FACET JOINT
Flexion	Anterior rotation, anterior glide of superior vertebra Anterior compression, posterior separation	Bilateral upglide of superior facets of the vertebral segment
Extension	Posterior rotation, posterior glide of superior vertebra Posterior compression, anterior separation	Bilateral downglide of superior facets of the vertebral segment
Side-bending	Compression on the side of the concavity, separation on the side of the convexity	Contralateral upglide and ipsilateral downglide of superior facets of the vertebral segment
Rotation	Torsion of the IVD	Approximation of contralateral facets, distraction of ipsilateral facets

Data Source: Norris C. Spinal stabilisation: 2. Limiting factors to end-range motion in the lumbar spine—ScienceDirect. *Physiotherapy.* 1995;81(2):64-72.

The pubic symphysis consists of the 2 pubic bones and the fibrocartilage disk. Together, the pubic symphysis and the 2 SIJs form the pelvic ring. There are 2 primary ligaments providing support to the pubic symphysis. The superior pubic ligament is located over the superior pubis as far laterally as the pubic tubercles.[12] The inferior pubic ligament (subpubic or arcuate ligament) attaches to the inferior pubic rami, has fibers that attach to the pubic disk, and is the stronger ligament.[13] Due to the continuity of the pelvic ring, mobility of the pubic symphysis occurs in conjunction with iliosacral motion. Anterior rotation of the ilium is associated with caudal movement of the pubis, whereas posterior rotation of the ilium is associated with cranial movement of the pubis. Similar to the SIJ, the pubic symphysis joint is an inherently stable joint with only small amounts of motion available (2 mm translation, 1 degree of rotation).[13] Mobility of the pubic symphysis increases during pregnancy with the symphysis expanding 2 to 3 mm during the last trimester.[12,13]

Active movement of the lumbopelvic region involves an integrated coordination between the lumbar spine, pelvis, and hips often called lumbopelvic rhythm. This coordination is best appreciated during standing forward bending of the trunk performed with the knees straight. When moving into forward bending, trunk flexion is achieved sequentially by lumbar flexion, anterior pelvic rotation, and hip flexion. The lumbar spine contributes more to trunk flexion during early motion while the pelvis and hips contribute more to trunk flexion during later motion.[14,15] During the return to upright from a forward flexed position, lumbopelvic rhythm consists of hip extension, followed by posterior pelvic rotation, then

lumbar extension. The hips and pelvis contribute more to early trunk extension motion, whereas the lumbar spine contributes more to final trunk extension motion.[15] Deviations in the lumbopelvic rhythm movement sequence are one type of aberrant motion that is assessed during active movement testing.[16]

Anatomical and Biomechanical Considerations for Lumbopelvic Stability

The ROM of a spinal segment is said to consist of a neutral and elastic zone.[17] The neutral zone is the range of physiologic motion that is produced against minimal internal resistance. The elastic zone extends from the end of the neutral zone to the physiologic limit of ROM. Motion that occurs within the elastic zone occurs against high internal resistance. Spine stability is preserved when the size of the neutral and elastic zones is maintained. Panjabi conceptualized that spine stability is a result of the integrated function of 3 subsystems: (1) the passive musculoskeletal subsystem, (2) the active musculoskeletal subsystem, and (3) the neural and feedback subsystem.[18] The passive subsystem consists of the IVD, osseous, and ligamentous structures specific to the spinal segment and provides stabilization near end range of spinal motions in the elastic zone.[17,19] Structures of the passive subsystem contributing to stability of the lumbar spine are listed in Table 16-2. The active subsystem consists of muscles acting on the spine.[17,19] The neural subsystem consists of nerves and the central nervous system that serve as

Table 16-2

STABILIZING STRUCTURES OF THE PASSIVE SUBSYSTEM FOR THE LUMBAR SPINE

LUMBAR MOTION	PASSIVE SUBSYSTEM STABILIZING STRUCTURES
Extension (increased lordosis)	Anterior longitudinal ligament
	Anterior fibers of annulus
	Approximation of inferior facet of superior vertebra against lamina
	Compression of spinous processes
Flexion (reversal of lordosis)	Posterior longitudinal ligament
	Posterior fibers of annulus
	Iliolumbar ligament (posterior band)
	Ligament flavum
	Joint capsules of facet joints
	Supraspinous and interspinous ligaments
	Superior facet against inferior facet
Side-bending	Contralateral iliolumbar ligament
	Contralateral fibers of annulus
	Contralateral intertransverse ligaments
	Ligamentum flavum
Rotation	Contralateral facet joint approximation
	Annular fibers oriented in direction of the rotation
SACRAL MOTION	**PASSIVE SUBSYSTEM STABILIZING STRUCTURES**
Nutation	Interosseous ligaments
	Sacrotuberous ligaments
	Sacrospinous ligaments
	Short posterior sacroiliac ligaments
Counternutation	Long dorsal sacroiliac ligaments

Data Sources: Norris C. Spinal stabilisation: 2. Limiting factors to end-range motion in the lumbar spine—ScienceDirect. *Physiotherapy.* 1995;81(2):64-72; Vleeming A, Schuenke MD, Masi AT, Carreiro JE, Danneels L, Willard FH. The sacroiliac joint: an overview of its anatomy, function and potential clinical implications. *J Anat.* 2012; 221(6):537-567. doi:10.1111/j.1469-7580.2012.01564.x

force and motion transducers to direct and control the active subsystem. The neural and active subsystem provide stabilization of spinal motion near midrange[17,19] and are sometimes considered together as the neuromuscular subsystem. The active subsystem can be divided into local and global muscles (Table 16-3).[20] Local muscles are located deep and originate and insert directly to the lumbar vertebrae, providing segmental stability. Global muscles are more superficial and do not attach directly to the lumbar vertebrae but produce movement of the trunk and spine.

The 3 subsystems interact together to provide lumbar segmental stability and, when functioning optimally, maintain the size of the neutral zone.[20] When disruption in one system occurs, a second subsystem provides compensation to preserve segmental stability. When dysfunction exceeds the limits of compensation provided by the other subsystems, instability develops.[18] LSI refers to excessive motion between spinal segments and can be broadly classified as structural or functional instability.[21,22] Pathoanatomical conditions such as spondylolisthesis and spondylolysis have traditionally been attributed to LSI and the associated LBP.[20] LSI may occur, however, in absence of pathoanatomical conditions due to disruption or imbalances between the 3 subsystems. Disruption of the passive subsystem that is not compensated for by the neural or active subsystems is referred to as *structural LSI*. Structural LSI is also called *radiologic LSI* due to the use of flexion-extension radiographs as a diagnostic standard to identify increased translation and/or angulation of a spinal segment at the end range of flexion or extension.[22] The development of functional LSI is theorized to occur through

Table 16-3

MUSCLES OF THE ACTIVE SUBSYSTEM OF SPINE STABILITY

ACTIVE SUBSYSTEM	MUSCLES
Local muscles	Lumbar multifidus, psoas major, quadratus lumborum, lumbar parts of the lumbar iliocostalis and longissimus, transversus abdominis, diaphragm, posterior fibers of the internal obliques
Global muscles	Rectus abdominus, external obliques, thoracic part of lumbar iliocostalis

Data Source: O'Sullivan PB. Lumbar segmental "instability": clinical presentation and specific stabilizing exercise management. *Man Ther.* 2000;5(1):2-12. doi:10.1054/math.1999.0213

a disruption of the active or neural subsystems.[22,23] While the gold standard for diagnosis of structural LSI is flexion-extension radiographs, clinical examination tests may assist in the diagnosis process. Functional LSI may exist in the absence of positive radiograph findings; therefore, clinical examination tests are necessary for the classification of functional LSI.[22,24] Conservative treatment of LSI commonly utilizes a movement-based approach that incorporates exercises involving both the local and global muscles of spine stabilization with motor learning principles for retraining of the active and neural subsystems.

The function of the SIJ is to provide stability to the pelvis and to transmit forces between the trunk and lower extremities.[25] The SIJ is an inherently stable joint due to its shape, structure of the articular surfaces, and surrounding ligamentous tissues.[11] The sacrum is a wedge-shaped bone that is wider proximally at the base and anteriorly, which allows the sacrum to fit tightly between the 2 ilia.[26] After puberty, the ilia and sacral articular surfaces change from flat to coarse and contain complementary ridges and depressions that increase the friction between the joint surfaces.[26] The coarse surfaces are not considered pathologic but in response to the need for stability driven by the weight of the trunk in upright standing.[26,27] The SIJ is supported by a strong joint capsule and ligaments that are considered to be among the strongest in the body.[11] The anterior sacroiliac ligaments are weaker than the posterior ligaments, which include the deeper interosseous sacroiliac ligament (short dorsal ligament) and the more superficial posterior sacroiliac ligament (long dorsal ligament). Although the sacrotuberous and sacrospinous ligaments do not cross the SIJ, these ligaments also provide reinforcement to the SIJ posteriorly. Together, these features contribute to SIJ stability via form closure.[11,26] A second component of SIJ stability is force closure, which uses ligamentous tension (intrinsic force), muscle contraction (extrinsic force), and motor control (neural activation) to supplement form stability to allow loads to be transferred between the trunk and lower extremities and controlled mobility to occur.[11,28] In upright standing the weight of the trunk creates a nutation torque on the sacrum, and hip joint compression forces create a posterior rotation torque on the ilium (indirectly nutating the

sacrum). As the sacrum nutates in response to these forces, the sacrum compresses into the ilia and passive tension in the posterior stabilizing ligaments develop, lending nutation to be the close-packed position of the SIJ.[11] Passive tension in the SIJ ligaments also develops in response to muscle activity of the gluteus maximus, piriformis, biceps femoris, and/or latissimus dorsi (via the thoracolumbar fascia [TLF]) due to the connections of these muscles to the SIJ ligaments.[11,28] In addition, these aforementioned muscles are considered part of an outer muscle unit that contributes to force closure through functioning in 4 systems that form muscular slings providing stability to the pelvis.[11,28,29] These sling systems are outlined in Table 16-4. As described previously regarding LSI, the transversus abdominis (via connections to the TLF), internal oblique, multifidus, diaphragm, and pelvic floor are deep or inner muscles that play an important role in stability of the lumbosacral region and contribute to force closure of the SIJ. In particular, neural control to these inner muscles is necessary to both initiate lumbopelvic stability in preparation for joint loading (feedforward motor control) and/or movement as well as to adjust stability needs during dynamic activity (feedback motor control).[11,30,31] Muscle length, strength, and recruitment deficits of these muscles may exist and contribute to impairments of force closure and SIJ movement control.

Although not as commonly observed, excessive force closure activity may exist, creating lumbosacral pain. O'Sullivan and Beales[32,p93] describe a type of PGP disorder that develops from "excessive activation of the motor system local to the pelvis (excessive force closure)." The muscles local to the pelvis (pelvic floor, transversus abdominis, multifidus, gluteal muscles, and iliopsoas) are in a state of heightened cocontraction creating altered motor control characteristics that are most commonly related to PGP. Load transfer tests in these individuals would reproduce pain when manual compression is applied to the pelvis. Individuals with this type of PGP may also have anxiety-related psychosocial impairments. Recognition of excessive force closure as the source of an individual's pain will assist in selection of appropriate intervention strategies that detour from the more commonly prescribed stabilization approach.[33]

Table 16-4	
SLING SYSTEMS CONTRIBUTING TO SACROILIAC JOINT STABILITY	
SLING SYSTEM	**MUSCLES**
Anterior oblique system	Contralateral external oblique and internal oblique, transversus abdominis, anterior abdominal fascia
Posterior oblique system	Contralateral latissiumus dorsi and gluteus maximus
Deep longitudinal system	Mulitfidus, long head of biceps femoris, thoracolumbar fascia, sacrotuberous ligaments
Lateral system	Gluteus medius, minimus, and opposing adductors of the thigh

Data Sources: Pool-Goudzwaard AL, Vleeming A, Stoeckart R, Snijders CJ, Mens JMA. Insufficient lumbopelvic stability: a clinical, anatomical and biomechanical approach to "a-specific" low back pain. *Man Ther*. 1998;3(1):12-20. doi:https://doi.org/10.1054/math.1998.0311; Vleeming A, Schuenke MD, Masi AT, Carreiro JE, Danneels L, Willard FH. The sacroiliac joint: an overview of its anatomy, function and potential clinical implications. *J Anat*. 2012;221(6):537-567. doi:https://doi.org/10.1111/j.1469-7580.2012.01564.x; Willard FH, Vleeming A, Schuenke MD, Danneels L, Schleip R. The thoracolumbar fascia: anatomy, function and clinical considerations. *J Anat*. 2012;221(6):507-536. doi:https://doi.org/10.1111/j.1469-7580.2012.01511.x

Anatomical and Biomechanical Considerations of Pain Generation

While LBP is a significant source of disability worldwide, approximately 90% of individuals with LBP have what is called *NSLBP*, which is not attributed to a known pathoanatomical diagnosis.[34,35] This had resulted in a recommendation by current physical therapy guidelines for a focus on the identification of impairments related to LBP symptomology after excluding the presence of "red flags" suggestive of serious pathology and the presence of significant neurological deficits.[36] A large component of the identification of impairments NSLBP is made by assessing symptom response to movement-based tests. In particular, pain response to movement-based tests may assist with the diagnosis classification of LBP with referred or radiating lower extremity pain. Understanding how lumbar movements affect spine anatomy and biomechanics assists in interpreting the findings of movement-based tests and guiding intervention selection.

Lumbar flexion is associated with the increasing size of the spinal canal and intervertebral foramen (IVF), whereas lumbar extension decreases the size of both. Individuals with symptoms of spinal stenosis (LBP with radiating pain into the lower extremity that increases with standing and walking and decreases with sitting) may have pain reduction with lumbar flexion through the widening of the spinal canal and IVF, which reduces the compression on neural tissues. Conversely, symptom reproduction may occur with lumbar extension as the neural tissues are compressed by both the narrowing of the spinal canal and IVF and segmental stenosis.

As mentioned in the discussion of lumbar biomechanics, lumbar flexion compresses the anterior side of the IVD and widens the intervertebral space posteriorly. The anterior compression of the IVD pushes the nucleus pulposus posteriorly against the posterior aspect of the annulus, which is undergoing lengthening due to the widening of the posterior intervertebral space. If the posterior aspect of the annulus is weak or torn, the IVD may distend posteriorly against sensitive neural tissue and increase pain centrally or create radiating pain into the extremity as lumbar flexion is performed. Lumbar extension, given that the annular wall is still intact, compresses the posterior side of the intervertebral space and pushes the nucleus pulposus anteriorly, which may reduce IVD pressure on neural tissues resulting in a centralization effect on pain referred into the lower extremity. This forms the basis of repeated or sustained lumbar extension in the examination and treatment procedures used by McKenzie's mechanical diagnosis and therapy (MDT) approach.[37]

The SIJ has been found to be the pain source in 13% to 30% of individuals with chronic LBP and is a structure that contributes to PGP.[38,39] Pain referral patterns arising from the SIJ are most consistently described to be unilateral, below the L5 spinous process.[25,40] Pain referral patterns resulting from provocative SIJ injections also include the buttock, lower lumbar area, lower extremity, and groin.[25] O'Sullivan and Beales[41] propose 2 mechanisms through which the SIJ can contribute to PGP: inflammation and dysfunction. Inflammation of the SIJ can involve the joint surfaces and/or surrounding connective tissues and is assessed through provocation tests that apply stress to the joint through compression, distraction, torsion, and shear.[38] Although these tests are described under biomechanical examination procedures, it is important to consider the biomechanical and anatomical basis of the provocation tests. The SIJ compression and distraction tests impart gapping and compression to the anterior and posterior aspects of the joints. The compression test gaps the posterior aspect and compresses the anterior aspect, whereas the distraction test gaps the anterior aspect and compresses the posterior aspect of the SIJs. Another SIJ provocation test, Gaenslen's test, imparts torsion to the SIJs through use of overpressure to hip flexion of one lower extremity and hip extension of the other lower extremity. On the side of hip flexion, the ilium posteriorly rotates, while on the side of hip extension the ilium anteriorly rotates. A posteriorly directed shear force to the SIJ is the basis of the thigh thrust test and the sacral thrust test. Dysfunction is assessed through load transfer tests that examine for impairments of form and force closure, through static palpation of bony landmarks, and through motion palpation of SIJ mobility. The biomechanical basis of load transfer tests involves the use of an active straight leg raise to create limb loading of the pelvis. The ability of the pelvis to maintain stability as the limb load is transferred proximally requires a combination of form (sacral nutation) and force closure (neuromotor activation of the deep stabilizing muscles—transversus abdominis, multifidus, pelvic floor). Lastly, the iliac crest, ASIS, PSIS, sacral base, sacral sulcus, sacral apex, pubic tubercle, and pubic symphysis serve as bony landmarks for static palpation of pelvic symmetry and dynamic palpation of pelvic motion during kinetic tests.

Diagnosis

Current research supports the use of a subgroup classification-based approach when establishing a clinical or physical therapy diagnosis for the individual with lumbopelvic pain.[36,42-44] This approach involves dividing the broad diagnosis of mechanical LBP into subgroups that are classified by the loading responses during a movement-based examination, acuity of symptomology, and determination if psychosocial comorbidities exist. While there are many classification systems and practice guidelines available, those with the best evidence recommend use of clinical examination findings to guide the subgrouping process as opposed to basing diagnosis on the identification of pathoanatomical lesions. The diagnosis process presented in this chapter combines information presented in the American Physical Therapy Association (APTA) *Clinical Practice Guideline (CPG)* for LBP with the Treatment-Based Classification System (TBC) for LBP.[42,45] Together, the identified mechanical LBP-related impairments, established acuity, and the assessment of the risk of psychosocial comorbidities will guide the rehabilitation approach.

Examination Overview

The examination process of a patient with LBP consists of subjective examination of patient history, LQSE, passive motion testing, and selected use of special tests. The patient history and scan examination provide 2 avenues for discerning if medical referral is indicated based on the presence of red flags or if the patient is appropriate for physical therapy management. If, from the patient history, no red flags are apparent, the therapist should formulate a working hypothesis that will be tested in the scan examination and, if needed, in the biomechanical examination and special tests. From the scan examination the clinician is able to make further decisions regarding the need for medical referral based on

neurological test findings and the presence of symptoms that are of nonmusculoskeletal origin; ascertain that symptoms are not referred from joints of the lower extremity or thoracic spine, necessitating a focused examination of these areas; determine if a provisional diagnosis can be made upon which treatment can be initiated; or determine the need to conduct passive motion testing of the lumbar spine and/or use special tests localized to the lumbar spine and/or pelvis. Spinal passive motion tests examine for the presence of motion dysfunction in a spinal segment or pelvis that can be broadly classified as hypomobility or hypermobility. Hypomobility is further assessed to determine if the hypomobility is due to articular (joint) or myofascial impairment. Likewise, hypermobility is further assessed to determine if an impairment of lumbopelvic instability exists.

Subjective Examination

Patient report of current symptomology, general health, and past medical conditions are obtained during the subjective component of the examination process. This information is gathered by review of the patient's medical record, review of patient-reported outcome measures (health-related questionnaires and/or outcome measures completed by the patient), and interview of the patient or other caregiver. Through the process of the patient history, rapport can be established with the patient and the process of evaluation is initiated. Information from the subjective examination assists the clinician in identifying the patient's main problem or chief complaint, determining the history of the condition and current medical management, understanding the nature of the patient's pain, establishing the severity and irritability level, and determining contributory factors from past medical history, all of which help guide the objective examination process and determine treatment interventions. Open-ended questions are suggested to best obtain a complete understanding of the primary complaint or condition. Examples of open-ended questions for each component of the subjective examination and their purpose are provided in Table 16-5.

History of the Condition

When first addressing the patient, the clinician should obtain the patient's perspective of the main problem or primary symptoms, how the problem has affected their daily life (presence of activity limitation or disability), and how they have responded to their pain or symptoms (potential fear-avoidance behaviors). Of primary importance is determination of the chief complaint or primary problem and associated symptoms that have led the patient to seek physical therapy. Determining the primary problem and associated symptoms forms the basis for identifying the concordant sign, which will be further defined in the remainder of the subjective examination and investigated throughout the objective examination. Discerning if the symptoms were injury related or associated with predisposing factors such as prolonged positioning, repetitive movements, or exertional activity assists in selecting specific components of the objective

Table 16-5

SUBJECTIVE EXAMINATION COMPONENTS

COMPONENT OF SUBJECTIVE EXAMINATION	SUGGESTED QUESTIONS	PURPOSE
Identification of main problem	What brings you to physical therapy today? What do you have difficulty doing or what are you unable to do because of the pain you are having?	Assists the clinician in determining if the symptoms are movement related and how the problem has affected the patient's function
History of the condition	Are your symptoms related to or the result of an injury? How did your symptoms begin?	Cues the clinician to predisposing factors that may be modifiable to prevent recurrence, such as prolonged positioning, repetitive movements, or exertional activities.
History of the condition	When did you first notice your current symptoms? Is this the first episode of symptoms of this nature?	Assists in determining the acuity of the condition and if the condition is chronic or reoccurring.
History of the condition	What type of treatment have you had for the pain you are currently experiencing? How did this treatment affect your symptoms?	Worsening of symptoms with conservative care may alert the clinician to the possibility of a serious medical condition.
Nature of the condition	Where is your pain located? Describe your current symptoms.	This distinguishes between central vs peripheral symptoms. If symptoms are present in the lower extremity, the type of symptoms assists in distinguishing between referred pain and radiculopathy.
Nature of the condition	Since your symptoms began, have they improved, worsened, or stayed the same?	Provides information about the stability of the condition and, if worsening, may suggest a nonmusculoskeletal condition.
Nature of the condition	Describe your symptoms over the course of a 24-hour time period beginning from when you awake through how you sleep.	Contributes to understanding the stability of symptoms, discerning mechanical vs nonmechanical LBP, the presence of inflammatory conditions, and may necessitate additional questions to the nature of night pain, if present.
Irritability-severity	How would you rate your current pain using a 0 to 10 scale, where 0 is no pain and 10 is the worse imaginable pain? How would you rate your pain over the past 24 hours—At worse and at best?	Provides a baseline level of severity, contributing to understanding the initial irritability level of the patient's symptoms and determining pain persistence.
Irritability	What activities, positions, or movements increase or bring on your symptoms? How long can you perform the activity before your symptoms appear or start to increase? How much time is required for your symptoms to decrease after you cease the activity?	Assists in determining irritability level as nonirritable or irritable.

examination and formulating a hypothesis toward directional preference. Determining when the symptoms began contributes to establishing the acuity level from a temporal perspective as acute, subacute, or chronic. Reviewing current medical management, including medical imaging studies relevant to the current condition, will assist in understanding if there is a potential pathoanatomical diagnosis that may be contributing to the patient's symptoms. Inquiring about previous treatment for the current symptoms will alert the clinician to potential red flags, if there has been failure to improve with conservative care, or to the potential risk for development of chronic LBP.

Nature of the Symptoms

Asking questions to acquire knowledge about the location, type, stability, and behavior of symptoms in relation to activities and through the course of a 24-hour period provides information about the nature of the symptoms or condition. The location and type of pain or symptoms are best obtained through a pain diagram, which will provide a comparison for reassessment after periods of treatment intervention. Within the pain diagram, the patient can notate where symptoms are located and, with the use of symbols, the type of symptoms experienced. The presence of referred pain can be noted and the pattern of the referred pain may assist in forming a provisional differential diagnosis of a lumbar vs pelvic vs hip disorder. For instance, pain that is unilateral, below the level of L5 and radiating into the buttock may be suggestive of SIJ involvement.[11,25] In addition, presence of referred pain should signal the clinician to inquire about movements, positions, or activities that reproduce or increase the symptoms as well as decrease or centralize the symptoms.[37] Based on patient response to movement and position-related questioning, the clinician can plan to include repetitive and/or sustained movement testing during the objective examination. Characteristics of symptoms located distally should be clarified to distinguish between referred pain vs radiculopathy. Symptoms of paresthesia, anesthesia, and weakness may suggest lumbar radiculopathy, indicating the need to highlight the neurological screening tests (eg, sensation, myotome, reflex testing) and neurodynamic testing (eg, straight leg raise, slump testing) during the objective examination. Inquiring about symptomology over a 24-hour period provides information about the effect of rest, daily activity, and sleep tolerance. Mechanical pain may be less upon awakening and increase with daily activity, whereas inflammatory conditions, such as ankylosing spondylitis or osteoarthritis, may be worse upon awakening. The presence of night pain should be investigated in more detail (see section regarding red flags) in consideration of a condition that is of nonmusculoskeletal origin.

Severity and Irritability

Maitland describes the assessment of symptom irritability to include the severity, the intensity of activities to provoke the symptoms, and the time it takes for the symptoms to return to baseline after provocation.[46,47] The irritability status can be used to gage aggressiveness of objective examination procedures and treatment interventions. Severity of symptoms can be assessed using quantifiable measures such as the Numeric Pain Rating Scale (NPRS), an 11-point scale ranging from 0 (no pain) to 10 (worse imaginable pain).[48] The patient provides 3 pain ratings (current, worse, and best level of pain over the past 24 hours), and the average of the 3 ratings is used to provide a measure of pain intensity.[49] A 2-point change on the NPRS has been found to represent a clinically meaningful change for individuals with LBP.[48] The change in severity over a 24-hour period contributes to understanding pain persistence and determining if the pain is constant or intermittent. Constant pain may be indicative of serious medical pathology, whereas intermittent pain is more suggestive of mechanical pain. The next line of questioning distinguishes activities that, when performed, increase the pain and those that help ease or eliminate the pain. Associating the type of movements—flexion vs extension, sustained vs repetitive—with symptom increase and decrease assists in formulating a directional preference that can be tested during the objective examination.[37] Determining the length of time a provoking movement/activity can be performed before symptom onset and the length of time required for symptoms to return to baseline after discontinuing the movement/activity assists in assessing the irritability level.[46] Irritable LBP is considered to be easily aggravated with activity to a moderate to high level of severity and slow to abate after activity cessation. In contrast, nonirritable LBP is considered to be not easily aggravated, has a low severity level, and is quick to abate after activity cessation. Interrater reliability for judgements of irritability using this criterion was found to be moderate (prevalence-adjusted kappa = 0.50).[46,47] Establishing irritability and severity are 2 of the factors that contribute to the diagnosis classifications recommendation by the APTA CPG for LBP[36] and for matching a patient to a rehabilitation approach outlined in the TBC for LBP.[42]

Subjective Examination for Nonmusculoskeletal Pathologies and Psychosocial Factors

The subjective examination is the first step in which the presence or suspension of red and yellow flags may be identified; therefore, the clinician must take care to review intake forms and ask specific questions to screen for these flags.[50,51] The findings of red flags should not be considered in isolation only but in regard to clusters of red flags found to be related to serious medical conditions as described in the following sections.

While the likelihood of lumbopelvic symptoms being related to serious medical pathology is small,[35] clinicians should conduct a systems review to gather the following information during the patient history in consideration of the following serious medical conditions that may give rise to referred pain in the low back or pelvis[52]:

- Red flags for neoplastic conditions
  - Is patient age greater than 50 years?
  - Is there a past history of cancer?
  - Has the patient experienced any unexplained weight loss?
  - Has previous treatment involving rest or physical therapy failed to improve the symptoms?
  - Is the patient awakened with pain at night and unable to return to sleep despite position changes?
  - Does the pain continue to increase?
- Red flags for cauda equina syndrome
  - Does the patient report the presence of bowel or bladder dysfunction including urinary retention, incontinence, and saddle anesthesia?
  - Are there sensory changes in the feet?
  - Does the patient notice weakness in the lower extremities?
- Red flags for spinal fracture
  - Is patient age greater than 70 years?
  - Was pain onset related to history of trauma?
  - Does the patient report prolonged steroid use?
- Red flags for sacral fracture
  - Does the patient report hip pain?
  - Does the patient have diffuse pain throughout the pelvis?
- Red flags for systemic infection
  - Does the patient experience fever, chills, or night sweats?
  - Does the patient have persistent fatigue?

For individuals with LBP, depression and signs of psychosocial distress (fear-avoidance attitudes, beliefs, and behaviors) are prognostic factors that may contribute to poor outcomes, persistent LBP, development of chronic LBP, prolonged disability, or delayed response to treatment, and should be considered as orange and yellow flags, respectfully.[51,53] Both orange and yellow flags may be modifiable when appropriately addressed by mental health specialists (orange flags) or suitably trained health care providers, such as physical therapists, using multimodal treatment (yellow flags).[51,54,55] Given the socioeconomic impact of chronic LBP and associated disability, physical therapists should, in the subjective examination, screen for symptoms of depression and for signs of psychosocial distress such as elevated fear-avoidance attitudes, feelings, and beliefs.

Depression has been found to be associated with poor outcomes, increased pain intensity, persistent pain, and increased disability in individuals with LBP.[56] Two questions taken from the Primary Care Evaluation of Mental Disorders questionnaire[57] have been recommended for inclusion in the medical intake form or during the patient interview to screen for symptoms of depression[56,58]:

- "During the past month have you often been bothered by feeling down, depressed, or hopeless?"
- "During the past month have you often been bothered by little interest or pleasure in doing things?"

Answers to each question are dichotomized ("yes" or "no"). Diagnostic accuracy of these 2 questions for depression is reported as 91.3% sensitivity, 65.0% specificity, negative predictive value of 98.6%, positive predictive value of 21.6%, negative likelihood ratio (-LR) of 0.1, and positive likelihood ratio (+LR) of 2.6 in a sample of primary care patients with at least one physical complaint.[58] Previous research recommended adding a "help" question ("Is this something with which you would like help?") to increase specificity without decreasing sensitivity.[59] Recent research, however, found that the addition of a help question increased specificity from 65.0% to 88.2%, but decreased sensitivity from 91.3% to 59.4%, concluding that the help question is not useful when screening for depression.[58]

Included in the 2015 update to the TBC for LBP[42] and in the APTA CPG for LBP[36] is the use of standard self-report questionnaires in the examination process to evaluate for psychologic distress and/or comorbidities.[36] Suggested self-report questionnaires include the Örebro Musculoskeletal Pain Screening Questionnaire (ÖMPSQ)[60], the Subgroups for Targeted Treatment (STarT) Back Screening Tool,[61] and the Fear-Avoidance Beliefs Questionnaire (FABQ).[62] Findings of elevated psychosocial distress may alert the clinician to the need for inclusion of cognitive behavioral interventions in the treatment plan.[63] Table 16-6 provides an overview of each of the previously mentioned questionnaires available for use by the clinician to assess for the presence of yellow flags and the associated risk.

Patient-reported outcome measures are recommended for the examination of perceived disability and functioning related to LBP. Scores from these measures provide a baseline assessment of LBP-related disability that can be used to evaluate responsiveness to treatment interventions over time. In addition, assessment of disability through the use of outcome measures is a variable used to match the rehabilitation approach in the TBC for LBP.[42] Table 16-7 provides a summary of outcome measures recommended for use when examining a patient with LBP.

Table 16-6

COGNITIVE-AFFECTIVE QUESTIONNAIRES

QUESTIONNAIRE	PURPOSE	DESCRIPTION	SCORING
ÖMPSQ[60]	To identify individuals at risk for persistent pain associated with psychosocial factors	A 25-item questionnaire of which 21 items are scored on a 0 to 10 scale.	Total score ranges from 0 to 210, where higher scores indicate a higher risk of poor outcome.
STarT Back[65]	To subgroup individuals with LBP on the presence of physical and modifiable psychosocial factors	A 9-item questionnaire in which all items except one ("bothersomeness") are answered "agree" or "disagree." The bothersomeness item is answered with a 5-point Likert scale. Four items relate to physical factors and 5 items relate to psychosocial factors.	Total score ranges from 0 to 9, where higher scores indicate high risk. Scoring processes allow subgrouping into 3 groups: high risk (psychosocial subscale score 4 or greater); moderate risk (overall score greater than 3; psychosocial subscale score less than 4); and low risk (overall score 3 or less).
FABQ[62]	To identify patient beliefs related to fear of pain and avoidance of activity due to fear	Consists of 2 subscales and 16 items that are scored on a 7-point Likert scale ("completely disagree" = 0; to "completely agree" = 6). Physical activity subscale (FABQ[PA]) contains 5 items, and the work subscale contains 11 items (FABW[W]).	Physical activity subscale total scores range from 0 to 24. Work subscale total scores range from 0 to 42. Higher scores on both subscales indicate greater fear-avoidance beliefs. Scores greater than 15 on items 2 through 5 of FABQ(PA) and greater than 34 on items 6, 7, 9 through 12, and 15 of FABQ(W) are considered high fear-avoidance behaviors.
Pain Catastrophizing Scale[66]	To assess how individuals experience pain	A 13-item questionnaire in which each item is rated based on the degree to which the person has the feelings or thoughts when they are experiencing pain. A 0-to-4 Likert scale is used, where 0 = not at all and 4 = all the time.	Total scores range from 0 to 52. There are 3 subscale scores related to rumination, magnification, and helpfulness. A total score of 30 represents a high level of pain catastrophizing.

Table 16-7

PATIENT-REPORTED OUTCOME MEASURES

OUTCOME MEASURE	DESCRIPTION	PSYCHOMETRIC PROPERTIES
Oswestry Disability Index (ODI)	The modified ODI contains 10 items, each scored from low to high disability on a 0-to-5 scale. The total score is represented as a percentage. 0% to 20% = minimal disability 21% to 40% = moderate disability 41% to 60% = severe disability	Used primarily for acute LBP Test-retest reliability: 0.84[a] MCID = 6 percentage points[a] MDC90 = 10.5 percentage points[b]
Rolland-Morris Disability Questionnaire	Contains 24 items that provide statements that describe how LBP affects their ability to perform daily activities. Scoring is 0 to 24, with higher scores reflecting greater disability.	Test-retest reliability: 0.86[c] MDC90 = 4 to 5 points[c]
Patient Specific Functional Scale	Patients self-identify up to 5 activities they have difficulty performing or are unable to perform as a result of their pain or condition. Each activity is rated on a scale of 0 to 11, where lower scores indicate more disability.	Test-retest reliability: 0.85 (acute LBP), 0.91 (chronic LBP)[d] MDC90 = 2.5 points MCID = 3.0

MDC = minimum detectable change; MCID = minimal clinically important difference.

Data Sources: [a]Fritz JM, Irrgang JJ. A comparison of a modified Oswestry Low Back Pain Disability Questionnaire and the Quebec Back Pain Disability Scale. *Phys Ther.* 2001;81(2):776-788; [b]Davidson M, Keating JL. A comparison of five low back disability questionnaires: reliability and responsiveness. *Phys Ther.* 2002;82(1):8-24; [c]Stratford PW, Binkley J, Solomon P, Finch E, Gill C, Moreland J. Defining the minimum level of detectable change for the Roland-Morris questionnaire. *Phys Ther.* 1996;76(4):359-365; discussion 366-368; and [d]Horn KK, Jennings S, Richardson G, Vliet DV, Hefford C, Abbott JH. The patient-specific functional scale: psychometrics, clinimetrics, and application as a clinical outcome measure. *J Orthop Sports Phys Ther.* 2012;42(1):30-42. doi:10.2519/jospt.2012.3727

Objective Examination

The objective examination of a patient with lumbopelvic pain begins with an LQSE of the lumbar spine, pelvis, and lower extremity. During the LQSE, clinical tests are utilized to continue screening for red flags that were initiated during the subjective examination, which if present, necessitate consideration for medical referral. If the LQSE is negative for red flags, but positive for reproduction of the concordant sign, the therapist can decide if enough information is present to establish a mechanical diagnosis and begin treatment or if further biomechanical or special tests should be conducted. If the latter is the case, findings from the LQSE can then assist in focusing the biomechanical examination to select regions and tests. The LQSE is performed in a systematic manner using principles of selective tissue tension tests as described by Cyriax[64] and follows the outline as shown in Table 16-8. Components of the LQSE as related to the patient with lumbopelvic pain are highlighted in this section. Patient response to standard components of the LQSE may guide the clinician to perform additional tests to further confirm LQSE

findings. While each of the components of the LQSE contain specific procedures to complete, the scan examination is best conducted in order of position: standing, sitting, supine, prone, side-lying. The summary of the LQSE by position as relevant in the examination of the lumbopelvic region is provided in Table 16-9.

Observation

Observation of patient appearance, behavior, expressions, posture, and movements is conducted throughout the examination process. An informal posture observation is conducted during the subjective examination as the clinician observes the patient's preferred posture in consideration of how comfortable they appear in that posture, are they able to maintain the posture throughout the subjective examination, or are they frequently readjusting to a more comfortable position? General mobility is observed as the patient moves from one position to another, such as sitting to standing or standing to sitting. The patient's gait should be assessed for the presence of antalgia that may exist due to lumbosacral conditions. For example, myotomal weakness from nerve

---

Table 16-8

COMPONENTS OF THE LOWER QUARTER SCAN EXAMINATION

- Observation
- Active movement testing: Lumbar spine, pelvis, lower extremity joints
- Passive movement testing, passive overpressure
- Neurologic testing: L1-S1 dermatone
- Neurologic testing: L1-S1 myotome
- Neurologic testing: Deep tendon reflexes (DTRs)
- Neurologic testing: Pathologic reflexes (Babinski, clonus)
- Neurodynamic testing: Dural mobility
- Stress tests: Lumbar spine, pelvis, hip

---

root involvement may contribute to decreased push-off, toe clearance, or Trendelenburg sign. Similarly, unilateral sacroiliac pain may cause reduced stance on the affected side or shortened step length.

Posture

The posture examination of a patient with lumbopelvic pain should begin with observation of the entire body in standing as a brief general assessment, then a more specific examination of postural presentations that may be associated with lumbopelvic symptomology. The patient should be clothed appropriately to allow both visual inspection and palpation during the posture examination. Before beginning the posture inspection, the patient is asked to point to the area and extent of pain, which should confirm the pain diagram. Fortin's sign, often used to assess for sacroiliac involvement, is when the patient can localize the area of pain with one finger that is placed within 1 cm (2 inches) inferomedial to the PSIS consistently at least 2 times.[67] Postural examination should be performed from the anterior, posterior, and lateral views. Anterior and posterior views provide information related to bilateral symmetry and inspection for frontal plane alignment deviations such as scoliosis or a lateral shift and for pelvic obliquity that may occur with sacroiliac dysfunction or leg length discrepancy. Lateral views provide information related to sagittal plane alignment of the spine and pelvis such as amount of lumbar lordosis or the orientation of the pelvis. From these views, postural deviations should be considered in light of possible contributions to the concordant sign or in adaptation to acute or chronic lumbopelvic pain or dysfunction. Table 16-10 outlines components of a brief postural examination for a patient presenting with lumbopelvic pain.

Sagittal plane deviations in lumbar lordosis are usually graded as increased or decreased based on visual observation. A decreased lordosis, or flattening of the lumbar spine, may be assumed by an individual with lumbar stenosis in an attempt to open the IVF to relieve pressure on the neural tissue. Additional conditions that may result in an assumed flat back posture are disk herniation and SIJ dysfunction.[68] An increased lumbar lordosis may reflect an increased lumbosacral angle associated with the medical diagnosis of spondylolisthesis, suggesting inclusion of palpation for a step-off deformity in the lower lumbar spine and use of instability tests during a biomechanical examination. Deviations from what is considered normal lumbar lordosis should alert the clinician to observe for both the ability to further decrease or increase the lumbar curve during flexion and extension active motion testing, respectively, and for alterations in lumbopelvic rhythm during active movement testing. A lumbar curve that is unchanged during active movement testing or results in altered lumbopelvic rhythm may have associated impairments of muscle length. For example, shortness of the hip flexors and lumbar extensors may be associated with increased lumbar lordosis and reduced curve reversal during active flexion mobility, whereas shortness of the hip extensors and abdominal muscles may be associated with decreased lumbar lordosis and reduction in lumbar lordosis during extension mobility.

After visual observation of posture, palpation of pelvic landmarks is performed to assess symmetry of the ASIS, PSIS, iliac crests, and gluteal folds (Figure 16-1). Palpation should be done at eye level with the patient in standing. If the iliac crest, ASIS, and PSIS are symmetrically higher on one side, a leg length discrepancy or superior innominate (or inferior innominate on contralateral side) may be suspected.

Table 16-9

LUMBOPELVIC EXAMINATION: LOWER QUARTER SCAN

POSITION	EXAMINATION COMPONENT	CLINICAL TEST
Standing	Observation	General appearance
		Posture
		Palpation of bony landmarks
		Gait
	Neurologic testing	Heel walking (L4 myotome)
		Toe rise (S1-2 myotome)
	AROM	Lumbar: flexion, extension, side flexion
	Passive overpressure	Lumbar: flexion, extension, side flexion
Sitting	AROM	Trunk: rotation
	Passive overpressure	Trunk: rotation
	Observation	(Standing palpation +)
	Neurologic testing	DTRs: patella tendon (L3); Achilles tendon (S1-S2)
	Neurodynamic testing	Slump test (radicular symptoms)
	Resisted movements	Trunk flexion, extension, rotation
Supine	Hip passive range of motion (PROM)/ overpressure	Hip flexion, internal rotation, external rotation (both at 90 degrees of hip flexion)
	Neurologic testing	Myotomes: hip flexion (L2, L3); knee extension (L3) ankle dorsiflexion (L4); great toe extension (L5); ankle eversion (L5, S1)
	Neurologic testing	Sensation: L2, L3, L4, L5, S1, S2 dermatomes
	Neurologic testing	Pathologic reflexes (upper motor neuron lesion): Babinski, clonus
	Positional testing	FABER
	Observation/palpation	ASIS, pubic symphysis, leg length (in response to standing bony landmarks)
	Primary stress test-SIJ	Sacroiliac distraction (anterior gapping)
	Stress test-pubis	(If groin pain is present)
Side-lying	Neurologic testing	Hip abduction (L5 myotome)
	Primary stress test-SIJ	Sacroiliac compression (posterior gapping)
Prone	Neurologic testing	Myotomes: knee extension (L3-4); knee flex (L5-S1-2)
	Neurodynamic testing	Prone knee bend (L3 nerve root mobility; if radicular symptoms are present)
	Stress test-lumbar	Posterior-anterior spring test; torsion test
	Stress test-SIJ	(History, standing, +Fortin's sign)

Table 16-10

POSTURAL OBSERVATION EXAMINATION

STRUCTURE	VIEW	DESCRIPTION	LUMBOPELVIC-RELATED CONSIDERATION
Shoulders	Anterior and posterior	• Level bilaterally	• Scoliosis
Inferior angle of scapula	Posterior	• Level bilaterally at about 7th thoracic vertebrae • Equal distance from the spine	• Scoliosis
Spinal curvature	Posterior	• Vertically aligned	• Scoliosis
Iliac crests	Anterior and posterior	• Level bilaterally • In line with shoulders	• Sacroiliac dysfunction • Scoliosis • Leg length discrepancy
PSIS	Posterior	• Level bilaterally	• Sacroiliac dysfunction • Leg length discrepancy
ASIS	Anterior	• Level bilaterally	• Sacroiliac dysfunction • Leg length discrepancy
Lumbar and gluteal muscles	Posterior	• Level gluteal folds • Presence of creases • Symmetric in size bilaterally, atrophy • Muscle spasm	• Sacroiliac dysfunction • Leg length discrepancy • Hypermobility • Inflammatory condition or myopathy • Instability
Lumbar lordosis	Lateral	• Increased • Decreased	• Instability • Stenosis
Knee and patellae orientation	Anterior	• Anterior facing • Level in height	• Hip dysfunction
Foot positioning and arch height	Anterior and lateral	• Amount and symmetry of toe-out • Symmetry in arch height	• Hip dysfunction • Leg length discrepancy

If the iliac crest, ASIS, and PSIS are asymmetrically level on one side, a rotation of an innominate may be suspected. If asymmetry is present in standing, bony landmark palpation is repeated in sitting to discern if the asymmetry is resulting from leg length discrepancy (asymmetry would be present in standing but not sitting) or pelvis dysfunction (asymmetry would be present in both standing and sitting). Although palpation of bony landmarks in the pelvis in theory could provide an indication of pelvic symmetry, most research has found low reliability in static palpation of pelvic landmarks, except for Levangie[69] who utilized equipment to measure the palpated iliac crest, ASIS, and PSIS height (intraclass correlation coefficient = 0.70 to 0.99), which involved procedures not commonly used in the clinic.[69-71] The validity of lumbopelvic landmarks in the diagnosis of SIJ dysfunction is undetermined. Thus, it is recommended to consider a combination of findings, such as palpation assessment of pelvic symmetry and pain presentation, when suspecting SIJ involvement. When present, additional tests to examine motion (kinetic tests) and pain (provocation tests) would be warranted to further examine the SIJ and pubic symphysis for potential pain and/or mobility impairments.

The presence of a lateral shift (the trunk and pelvis are shifted in opposite directions in the frontal plane) in a patient with lumbopelvic pain should be examined to determined its relevance to the patient's symptoms.[72] A shift is considered relevant when correction of the shift alters the location (centralization or peripheralization) or intensity of symptoms.[73] The correction is performed actively by the patient or manually by the clinician with a side glide movement in which the trunk and pelvis are moved in opposite directions to attain vertical alignment (Box 16-1). If this shift is relevant, correction of the shift should be attained prior to performing active movement testing.

Neurologic Testing

The neurologic component of the LQSE consists of standardized testing of the L1-S2 dermatomes, myotomes, and DTRs (patella, hamstring, Achilles), and pathologic reflexes (Babinski, clonus). These are outlined in Table 16-9.

Active Movement Testing

Standard assessment of lumbar AROM consists of cardinal planes of movement with flexion, extension, and side-bending performed in the standing position and rotation performed in the seated position (Figure 16-2). The effect of active movements on patient concordant symptoms is examined with each movement in consideration of reproduction, increase, or decrease of symptoms. Prior to initiating a motion, baseline symptoms should be established to use for comparison during and after each motion tested. For each motion, the therapist should assess the quantity of

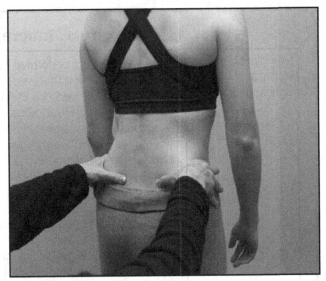

Figure 16-1. Palpation of PSIS landmarks.

motion, quality of motion, and effect of active movements on the patient's symptoms. Quantity of lumbar and pelvic active motion is most often assessed using visual analysis for determination of normal, restricted, or excessive mobility; however, lumbar active motion may be quantified through instrument testing (goniometry, inclinometry procedures, or Schöber technique). Quality of motion includes observation of how the movement is performed, the reversal ability of spinal curves, and if deviations in motion occur outside the expected movement pattern.[74] The identification of clinically positive aberrant movement, defined to involve the presence of 1 or more of 5 types of altered movement patterns, has been shown to have moderate to good interrater reliability (kappa = 0.60 to 0.79), whereas reliability of individual aberrant movements is lower (kappa = 0.00 to 0.61).[24] Hicks et al[16] recommend use of an aberrant movement pattern in which a positive test is the presence of any 1 of the 5 types of aberrant movements. The 5 types of aberrant movement that are observed as the patient performs standing trunk flexion are described in Table 16-11.[16]

Depending upon the irritability and severity of the patient's symptoms, passive overpressure is applied at the end of available AROM to establish end-feel (see Figure 16-2). Normal end-feel for lumbar movement is elastic or soft.[64] The relationship between the ROM in which symptom provocation occurs and/or the relationship between the onset of resistance to passive overpressure and pain can be used to distinguish acute, subacute, and chronic LBP (Table 16-12).[43] Restriction with active movement and/or abnormal end-feels should be further assessed with passive physiologic intervertebral motion (PPIVM) and passive accessory intervertebral motion (PAIVM) testing during the biomechanical examination.

Box 16-1. Lateral Shift Correction

| Side-glide technique for lateral shift correction | The side-glide test is performed by the therapist standing to the side contralateral to the direction the pelvis is shifted. The clinician's shoulder is placed on the lateral aspect of the patient's thorax, and the therapist's hands are interlaced around the lateral aspect of the contralateral pelvis. The therapist performs a side-glide correction by moving the patient's trunk and pelvis in opposite directions while monitoring the patient's symptoms. The lateral shift is considered relevant if the symptoms alter, centralize, or peripheralize during the maneuver. | 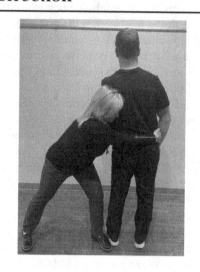 |

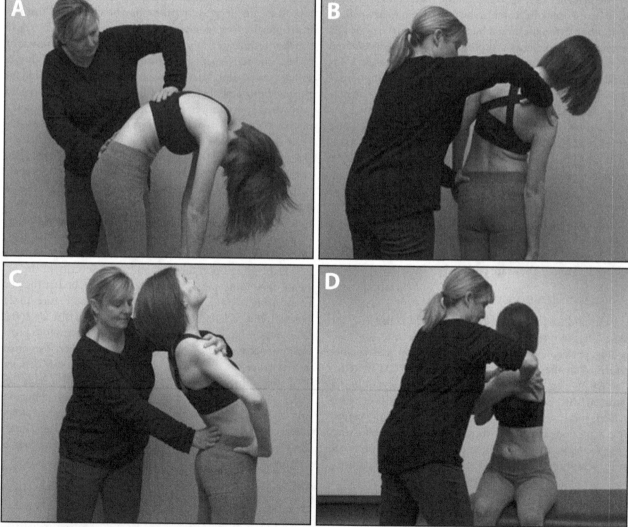

Figure 16-2. AROM with overpressure. (A) Flexion. (B) Side-bending. (C) Extension. (D) Rotation.

Table 16-11

ABERRANT MOVEMENT TEST

MOVEMENT	DESCRIPTION
Reversal of lumbopelvic rhythm	When returning to upright standing from trunk flexion, the knees bend and the trunk shifts anteriorly.
Painful arc in flexion	Pain occurring at one point in the ROM but is absent before or after that point.
Painful arc of return	Pain occurring at one point in the ROM when returning to upright standing from trunk flexion but absent before or after that point.
Gower's sign	Walking the hands up the thighs or pushing the hands on the thighs when returning to upright standing from trunk flexion.
Instability catch	Deviation outside the sagittal plane of motion during trunk flexion.

Positive test = 1 or more movement present.

Data Source: Hicks GE, Fritz JM, Delitto A, Mishock J. Interrater reliability of clinical examination measures for identification of lumbar segmental instability. *Arch Phys Med Rehabil*. 2003;84(12):1858-1864.

Table 16-12

RELATIONSHIP BETWEEN SYMPTOM ONSET, RANGE OF MOTION, AND TISSUE RESISTANCE

	RANGE OF MOTION AND SYMPTOM ONSET	TISSUE RESISTANCE AND SYMPTOM ONSET
ACUTE	Pain during initial and mid-ROM	Pain before resistance
SUBACUTE	Pain occurring at mid- to end ROM	Pain with resistance
CHRONIC	Pain at end ROM or with sustained movements	Pain after resistance

Repetitive and sustained movement testing is an extension of basic active movement testing in the cardinal planes and primary component of the MDT approach to mechanical spinal disorders developed by McKenzie.[37] After symptom response to one movement in a cardinal plane is assessed, the patient performs repetitive movements to the available end range in that motion plane while the clinician observes for motion limitation and inquires about symptom response during movement and immediately after completion of the repetitive movements. Centralization response occurs when symptoms that are distal in nature move proximally with movement testing. A directional preference is established if symptoms are improving or centralizing in one direction and worsening or peripheralizing in the opposite direction. Repetitive movement testing may be performed in standing (loaded) or supine and prone (unloaded) depending upon the symptom irritability. Centralization response

during repeated movements of extension in standing has been found to be associated with diskogenic symptoms (specificity = 0.87; +LR = 2.01).[75] The diagnostic accuracy of centralization during a repeated movement examination as compared to a reference standard of diskography has been reported as specificity of 0.94, sensitivity of 0.40, and +LR of 6.9.[76] Sustained movements or static positioning may also be performed if repetitive movement testing is negative or inconclusive for the patient's concordant sign.

There are 3 main classification syndromes in the MDT approach: derangement, dysfunction, and postural.[73,77-79] Derangement syndrome is characterized by the presence of a directional preference with centralization response to repeated movements. Dysfunction syndrome is characterized by restricted mobility of adaptively shortened structures and pain in one motion direction during single and repeated movement testing. Postural syndrome is characterized by pain reproduction with static positioning during sustained movement testing. Centralization and directional preference components of MDT examination are included in the subgrouping classification of LBP as described by the APTA CPG for LBP[36] and in the TBC.[42] The interrater reliability of MDT examination methods involving repetitive and sustained movement testing for identification of centralization and directional preference was good (kappa = 0.70 and 0.90, respectively).[80] Interrater reliability of classification into the 3 main syndromes of MDT varies from low (kappa = 0.37)[79] to good (kappa = 0.84).[77]

If active movement testing in cardinal planes is negative for symptom provocation, combined movement testing may be performed to provide information regarding pain reproduction through the effect of stretching or compressing structures in movement combinations that produce full ROM. There are 4 basic patterns of combined movements as outlined in Box 16-2. There are 2 patterns that produce movement into flexion quadrants and 2 patterns that produce movement into extension quadrants. The patient actively moves into a quadrant with quantity and quality of movement assessed as previously described. End-feel can be assessed with passive overpressure. Symptoms provoked during the posterior quadrants are usually a result of compression of spinal tissues or the ability of the facet joints to close, whereas symptoms provoked in the anterior quadrants are usually a result of stretching of spinal tissues or the ability of the facet joints to open. Positive findings would indicate inclusion of passive mobility testing of the motions that comprise the implicated quadrant.

If the postural examination has yielded possible pelvic symmetry impairments (eg, alignment of ASIS, PSIS, gluteal folds, iliac crests) combined with pain location and nature that may suggest involvement of the SIJ, the clinician may consider implementing motion (kinetic) tests to assess for sacroiliac dysfunction (Figure 16-3). Active movement of the SIJ cannot be produced independent of the ilium and lumbar spine. Thus, tests that examine motion of the SIJ utilize active movement of the lumbar spine or hip, while palpating landmarks on the pelvis to assess mobility of the SIJ. The standing forward flexion or standing flexion test assesses anterior iliosacral rotation during trunk flexion as the clinician palpates movement at the PSIS bilaterally or palpates one PSIS and S2.[81] A negative test is when both PSIS move symmetrically. A positive test is when one PSIS moves superiorly more than the other. The PSIS that has the furthest upward excursion is considered hypomobile. The seated flexion test is performed and interpreted in the same manner as the standing forward flexion test, but from a seated position, and is considered to examine movement of the sacrum on the ilium.[82] Gillet (marching) test assesses active posterior iliosacral rotation that occurs as one hip is flexed in a marching motion while the examiner palpates movement at the PSIS. The lack of downward movement of the PSIS or superior movement of

the PSIS on the side of hip flexion indicates a positive test.[82] Individual motion palpation tests have been found to have lower reliability than when motion palpation tests were evaluated as a cluster.[82] Positive findings with kinetic testing should be further explored with passive mobility testing of the ilium or sacrum as discussed in the special testing section of this chapter.

The reliability of standing flexion, seated flexion, and Gillet motion palpation tests is fair to moderate for intrarater (kappa = 0.6 to 0.76) and interrater (kappa = 0.44 to 0.84) reliability based on prevalence- and risk-adjusted kappa statistics.[82] When compared to a reference standard of an anesthetic injection in the SIJ, Dreyfuss et al[83] found low sensitivity and specificity for the Gillet motion test. In contrast, Levangie[69] reported high specificity for the seated flexion test (0.93) and Gillet test (0.93) and moderate specificity for the standing flexion test (0.79) when comparing test results to a reference standard of measured innominate torsion.

When diskogenic symptoms such as radiculopathy are suspected from the subjective examination and/or peripheralization of symptoms occurs with active trunk flexion, the scan examination should include tests of neurodynamic mobility. Neurodynamic mobility testing places tension on the dura centrally at the spinal cord and nerve, and on the peripheral nerves to examine the contribution of each to lower extremity symptoms of pain, paresthesia, or spasm. These tests include the slump test, passive straight leg raise (PSLR; Sciatic nerve, L4-S2 spinal nerve roots), and prone knee bend or femoral neurodynamic test (femoral nerve, L2-L4 spinal nerve roots). Each test consists of basic procedure and additional joint movements that act as sensitizers to place further tension on the neural tissue if symptoms are not reproduced with the basic test. When compared to reference standard of magnetic resonance imaging of the lumbar spine in a group of 75 with LBP and/or LBP with leg pain, the sensitive and specificity of the PSLR test was found to be 0.52 (0.42, 0.58) and 0.89 (0.79, 0.95), respectively, while the sensitivity and specificity of the slump test was 0.84 (0.74, 0.90) and 0.83 (0.73, 0.90), respectively.[89] Using these diagnostic accuracy values, +LRs are calculated to be 4.73 for the PSLR test and 4.94 for the slump test, while -LRs are calculated to be 0.54 for the PSLR test and 0.19 for the slump test. Similarly, Ekedahl et al reported moderate to low diagnostic accuracy values for the slump (sensitivity = 0.78, specificity = 0.36) and PSLR test (sensitivity = 0.59, specificity = 0.53) when compared to magnetic resonance imaging–verified disk extrusion.[85] Included in this study were diagnostic accuracy values for the femoral neurodynamic test, which were reported to be 0.43 (sensitivity) and 0.64 (specificity). Because research shows the accuracy of individual neurodynamic tests for lumbar radiculopathy to be low, it is suggested to use a combination of sensory, motor, reflex, and neurodynamic findings when examining for the presence of LBP with radiculopathy.[85-87] Procedures for these tests are provided in Box 16-3.

Box 16-2. Combined Movement Testing

QUADRANT	MOTIONS	TISSUE EFFECT	FIGURE
Right anterior	Flexion, right side flexion, right rotation	Maximal opening on the left side with stretching of left-sided structures	
Left anterior	Flexion, left side flexion, left rotation	Maximal opening on the right side with stretching of right-sided structures	
Right posterior	Extension, right side flexion, right rotation	Maximal closing on the right side with compression of right-sided structures	
Left posterior	Extension, left side flexion, left rotation	Maximal closing on the left side with compression of left-sided structures	

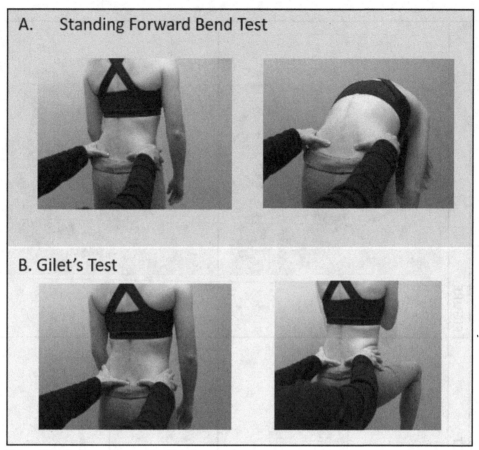

Figure 16-3. Kinetic motion tests for SIJ dysfunction.

Passive Movement Testing

During the LQSE of a patient with pain in the lumbopelvic region, passive movement testing of the hip is performed to assess the contribution of the hip joint to the presenting symptomology. Hip PROM is performed in the directions of flexion and rotation, with internal rotation and external rotation performed in 90 degrees of hip flexion. The quantity of motion available and reproduction of LBP is assessed. Previous research has found hip PROM in the directions of flexion and internal rotation to be limited in individuals with LBP as compared to asymptomatic adults.[88] This same study also found reductions in hip PROM to be significantly associated with high scores (greater disability) on lumbar self-report outcome measures. Hip internal rotation is also used in the clinical predication rule for improvement with lumbopelvic manipulation for acute LBP, with the predictive factor being at least one hip having internal rotation greater than 35 degrees.[89] Passive movement testing of the lumbar spine and pelvis is performed if symptoms are determined to be mechanical in nature but active movement testing has not determined a directional preference that could be used to establish a treatment-based diagnosis. Procedures for lumbar passive movement testing are outlined in the section covering biomechanical tests.

Provocation Stress Testing

The LQSE includes stress or provocation tests that involve manually induced passive forces to the lumbar spine, SIJ, and hip. These tests assist with localizing symptoms to one region of the lumbopelvic complex and can be used to differentiate symptoms arising from the lumbar spine, SIJ, or hips. Provocation testing in the lumbar spine involves application of posterior-anterior pressures, which are applied with the patient in prone, first in a graduated force then using a springing force, over the spinous L1 to L5, while the clinician monitors for provocation of symptoms or muscle spasm (Figure 16-4). A positive posterior-anterior pressure at one or more segmental levels will guide the clinician to performing additional biomechanical tests or assessing the effectiveness of using this technique as a segmental mobilization intervention.

A second group of provocation stress tests targets the SIJ. The decision to use these tests is based on the nature and location of the patient's pain and lack of centralization with repeated movement testing. There are 2 primary SIJ stress tests that can be performed during the scan examination: gapping of the anterior sacroiliac ligaments and compression, which gaps the posterior sacroiliac ligaments. Gapping (or SIJ distraction) is performed in supine as the clinician places the palms of their hands on the opposite ASIS (left palm on the

Box 16-3. Neurodynamic Testing

TEST	DESCRIPTION	INTERPRETATION	FIGURE
Slump	Patient position: Seated Procedure: The patient flexes the thoracic and lumbar spine while the therapist maintains the neck in neutral Sensitizers: • Neck flexion • Knee extension • Ankle dorsiflexion	Positive test: • Symptom reproduction with slump • Symptom reproduction with neck flexion and knee extension that diminishes with neck extension • Symptom reproduction with neck flexion, knee extension, and ankle dorsiflexion that diminishes with knee flexion	
Straight leg raise	Patient position: Supine Procedure: Therapist passively raises the symptomatic lower extremity, keeping the knee straight, creating a caudal traction of the sciatic nerve Sensitizers: • Neck flexion • Ankle dorsiflexion	Positive test: Symptom reproduction from 30 to 70 degrees hip flexion Pain from 0 to 30 degrees: consider acute or serious pathology; malingering	
Prone knee bend	Patient position: Prone Procedure: While stabilizing the patient's pelvis, the therapist passively bends the knee as far as possible Sensitizers: • Hip extension	Positive test: Symptom reproduction from 80 to 100 degrees knee flexion	

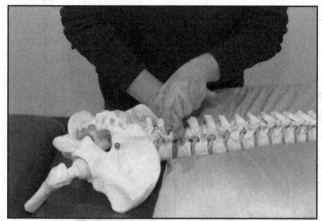

Figure 16-4. Lumbar posterior-anterior pressures for provocation of pain.

right ASIS and right palm on the left ASIS). An outward directed force is applied to the iliac crests, which gaps the anterior ligaments of the SIJ and compresses the posterior aspect. The compression test is performed in side-lying. The clinician places their stacked palms on the lateral aspect of the superior iliac crest and applies a downward force toward the treatment table. In each test, the force is maintained for 30 seconds as symptoms are assessed. Positive test findings are reproduction of pain and pain localized to the SIJ. Box 16-4 presents the primary stress tests for the SIJ. If these tests are positive coupled with a positive Fortin's sign and noncentralization with repeated movement testing, the clinician should proceed with additional primary stress tests contained in the SIJ test cluster to determine the presence of SIJ pain.[38,90] These tests are outlined in Box 16-5 and discussed in the special tests section of this chapter.

The third provocation stress test targets the hip joints. Hip-spine syndrome refers to coexisting dysfunction at the hips and lumbar spine.[91] By passively positioning the hip in motion combinations, stress is applied to the hip joint and the location of symptom provocation can assist in differentiating pain arising from the SIJ or hip. The FABER (flexion abduction external rotation) test is performed with the patient lying supine while the hip of the involved lower extremity is passively flexed, abducted, and externally rotated in a figure-4 position while the opposite ASIS is stabilized. Pressure is applied at the knee to move the hip into more external rotation while symptoms are assessed. Symptom reproduction over the ipsilateral SIJ suggests SIJ pathology and indicates further testing with the SIJ test cluster (described in the special tests section of this chapter).[82] Symptom reproduction in the ipsilateral hip suggests hip pathology and indicates further testing of the hip joint.

First Level Evaluation

At the conclusion of the LQSE, the process of diagnostic triage begins in which medical referral or rehabilitation management is determined. Referral for medical management is indicated based on the presence of red flags suggestive of serious pathology. Rehabilitation management is indicated when examination findings suggest NSLBP or mechanical LBP. If the first level evaluation determines medical management is not needed, the clinician should determine if examination findings gathered thus far support rehabilitation management and can be used to establish a clinical diagnosis, or if rehabilitation management is appropriate. If rehabilitation management is appropriate but a clinical diagnosis cannot be formulated at this point, additional examination tests should be performed to assist in identifying impairments and establishing a clinical diagnosis.

Biomechanical Tests: Passive Intervertebral Motion Testing

If the symptoms are mechanical in nature, biomechanical tests can be used to examine for movement dysfunction in the individual segments of the lumbar spine by assessing for pain provocation, hypomobility, and hypermobility. Positive findings from biomechanical tests can be used to differentiate if hypomobility is due to articular restrictions or extra-articular restrictions, and, if hypermobility is assessed, will guide the clinician to perform special tests for lumbar instability.

There are 2 types of physiologic intervertebral motion (PIVM): PPIVM and PAIVM. PPIVM involves passively moving one vertebra on the other in the physiologic motions of flexion, extension, side-bending, and rotation. PAIVM involves passively producing gliding between joint surfaces of the vertebral segment. PPIVM and PAIVM techniques are interpreted in regard to pain provocation, quantity of motion, and/or end-feel.[92] Pain provocation is considered as either positive (reproduces the concordant symptoms) or negative (does not produce concordant symptoms). Quantity of motion at a vertebral segment is compared to motion of the segment above and below and is characterized as normal, hypomobile, or hypermobile. A 3-point ordinal scale can be used to quantify motion: 0 = hypomobility, 1 = normal mobility, and 2 = hypermobility.[93] End-feel provides an assessment of the quality of motion when the segment is passively moved to end available ROM. End-feel is assessed as normal (capsular) or abnormal. The relationship between pain and end-feel assists in determining irritability. Pain after attainment of end-feel suggests minimal irritability, pain with the attainment of end-feel suggests moderate irritability, and pain before attainment of end-feel suggests high irritability.[64]

PPIVM and PAIVM techniques are commonly used in manual physical assessment of the spine as indicated by a survey of 466 manual physical therapists in New Zealand and the United States in which 66% believed PPIVM to be valid for assessing quantity of segmental motion and 76% believed PAIVM to be valid for assessing quantity of segmental motion.[94] In addition, 98% of the manual therapists used results from these tests to guide treatment decisions. Hypomobility with PAIVM testing in the lumbar spine is a factor included in the clinical prediction rule (CPR) for improvement with lumbopelvic manipulation for acute LBP[89]

Box 16-4. Passive Intervertebral Motion Testing: Passive Accessory Intervertebral Motion

TEST	DESCRIPTION	INTERPRETATION	FIGURE
Central posterior to anterior (CPA)	Patient position: Prone Procedure: The therapist places the ulnar border of the caudal hand perpendicular to the spine so that the pisiform is approximately over the spinous process. The caudal hand is reinforced by the cranial hand. Posterior-anterior pressure are applied with progressive force and motion palpation is compared to the adjacent levels. A spring test can also be performed with the same hand placement.	Positive test: Pain provocation; quantity of motion, end-feel	
Unilateral posterior to anterior (UPA)	Patient position: Prone Procedure: The spinous process is palpated with the finger of one hand while the thumb is placed lateral to the spinous process to locate the approximate area over the transverse process at that spinal level. A thumb over thumb placement can be used to provide the posterior-anterior–directed pressure with progressive force while motion palpation is compared to adjacent levels and to the opposite side at the same level. A spring test can also be performed with the same hand placement.	Positive test: Pain provocation; quantity of motion, end-feel	

Box 16-5. Provocation Tests for Sacroiliac Joint Pain

TEST	DESCRIPTION	INTERPRETATION	FIGURE
Distraction	Patient position: Supine Procedure: The therapist crosses their forearms to place one hand on each ASIS. Steady pressure is applied to each ASIS in a posterior direction to create distraction of the anterior aspect of the SIJs.	Positive test: Pain provocation of the concordant sign	
Compression	Patient position: Side-lying, hips and knees flexed Procedure: The therapist places one hand on the top iliac crest, overlaid by the other hand. A vertical pressure is applied downward through the iliac crest creating compression of the SIJs.	Positive test: Pain provocation of the concordant sign	

(continued)

Box 16-5 (continued). Provocation Tests for Sacroiliac Joint Pain

TEST	DESCRIPTION	INTERPRETATION	FIGURE
Thigh thrust or posterior pelvic pain provocation test	Patient position: Supine Procedure: The therapist flexes the knee and hip of one lower extremity, slightly adducting the thigh. One hand is placed on top of the flexed knee, and the other hand is placed under the patient in the sacrum. A downward directed force is applied through the thigh to create a posterior shear at the SIJ.	Positive test: Pain provocation of the concordant sign	
Sacral thrust	Patient position: Prone Procedure: The therapist places their hand on the sacrum and provides an anterior-directed force to the sacrum to create anterior shearing of the sacrum.	Positive test: Pain provocation of the concordant sign	

(continued)

Box 16-5 (continued). Provocation Tests for Sacroiliac Joint Pain

TEST	DESCRIPTION	INTERPRETATION	FIGURE
Gaenslen's test	Patient position: Supine at the end or side of the table with one lower extremity off of the table and the opposite lower extremity in hip and knee flexion. Procedure: The therapist presses downward on the thigh of the lower extremity off the table while pressing the thigh of the opposite lower extremity toward the patient's chest, creating anterior rotation force and posterior rotation force, respectively.	Positive test: Pain provocation of the concordant sign	
Test item cluster	Gapping, compression, thigh thrust, sacral thrust, Gaenslen's test.	The presence of 3 or more positive primary stress tests suggest SIJ pain	Sensitivity: 0.91 Specificity: 0.78 +LR: 4.16 -LR: 0.12

Data Sources: Laslett M. Evidence-based diagnosis and treatment of the painful sacroiliac joint. *J Man Manip Ther.* 2008;16(3):142-152; Laslett M, Young SB, Aprill CN, McDonald B. Diagnosing painful sacroiliac joints: a validity study of a McKenzie evaluation and sacroiliac provocation tests. *Aust J Physiother.* 2003;49(2):89-97.

and as a predictive factor of failure with lumbar stabilization exercise.[95] Despite the common use of PIVM testing in the lumbopelvic examination, research investigating the reliability and validity of these procedures has produced varied findings (Table 16-13). The diagnostic accuracy of PPIVM testing for lumbar hypomobility has been reported as 0.89 specificity and 0.42 sensitivity (based on flexion PPIVM)[96] and 0.98 to 0.99 specificity and 0.05 to 0.16 sensitivity (based on flexion and extension PPIVM)[93] in the diagnosis of translation lumbar instability. Central PAIVM testing for lumbar instability has higher specificity (0.81 to 0.95) than sensitivity (0.29 to 0.46).[93,97] These findings suggest that both PPIVM and PAIVM are better used for diagnostic testing than screening. Reliability of PAIVM testing is higher for intrarater than interrater[98] and when assessing pain provocation (k = 0.21 to 0.73) as compared to quantity of motion (k = -0.20 to 0.71).[16,98,99] It should be noted that PIVM procedures are evaluated in consideration of multiple components of the lumbopelvic examination and are not considered in isolation as was done in many of the reliability and validity studies. In addition, given the low intrareliability and interreliability for identification of a spinal level, many researchers advise considering PIVM findings relative to regions of the lumbar spine (upper and lower lumbar) instead of the individual spinal segment.[96,100]

PPIVM is performed with the patient in side-lying as the examiner palpates the interspinous space of 2 adjacent vertebrae while inducing passive movement of the vertebral segment in the direction of flexion, extension, side-bending, or rotation (Box 16-6). Palpation of the interspinous space proceeds from L5 and moves cranially as passive lumbar motion is produced. The determination of altered quantity of motion concurrent with pain provocation during PPIVM testing would lead to the use of PAIVM testing.

PAIVM is performed in prone and involves the application of PA pressures on the spinous processes of each vertebra (central PA or CPA) and over the transverse processes (unilateral PA or UPA) as shown in Box 16-4. Contributions for lumbar hypomobility can be considered as articular if motion restriction is found with both PPIVM and PAIVM testing or muscle inextensibility if motion restriction is found with PPIVM testing but PAIVM testing is negative. Muscle inextensibility would warrant utilization of muscle length testing to provide a confirmation. If lumbar hypomobility is suspected from PPIVM testing, further assessment should be conducted with PAIVM testing with which findings of pain provocation, hypermobility, or lack of hypomobility would indicate the need for special tests to examine for lumbopelvic instability.

Special Tests

Based on the findings of the LQSE and/or PIVM biomechanical testing, special tests may be needed to confirm a diagnosis of lumbar instability or to further investigate the presence of PGP. Additionally, if the acuity of the patient is low, special tests of muscle performance may be needed to identify the rehabilitation approach of functional optimization.[42] This section will review examination findings gathered thus far that would warrant the inclusion of special tests for either of these conditions or rehabilitation approach. Then discussion will ensue regarding the special tests best supported by existing evidence to assist in the differential diagnosis process.

Lumbopelvic Instability

Signs and symptoms of instability of the lumbopelvic region are established in the subjective history and LQSE but require the use of special tests to assist in the differential diagnosis process. Subjective signs of instability include complaints of "giving way" or "slipping out," recurrent LBP, pain with transitional movements (eg, sitting more than standing, rolling over in bed), morning pain, and symptoms worsening with the weather.[21] Objective signs of instability during the LQSE and biomechanical examination include aberrant motion, excessive lumbar flexion AROM greater than 53 degrees, pain provocation with PIVM testing, and hypermobility during PPIVM and PAIVM testing.[24,101] Special tests for LSI attempt to examine for both the presence of instability and the contributions of instability that arise from impairments of the neuromotor subsystem (functional instability) or from the passive subsystem (structural instability). The diagnostic standard for structural instability is flexion/extension radiographs that quantify anterior-posterior translation at end ROM.[102] However, a diagnostic reference standard for functional instability does not exist, and functional instability may exist without presence of radiographic instability.[21]

Clinical tests of LSI can be grouped into tests that stress the passive subsystem of spinal stability (structural instability) or tests that assess neuromotor control (functional instability). Clinical tests for structural instability include passive lumbar extension, aberrant motion (see Table 16-11), posterior shear test, the lack of hypomobility with a posterior-anterior PAIVM test, and use of the Beighton hypermobility scale. The diagnostic accuracy of these tests is reported in Table 16-13 and test descriptions are outlined in Box 16-7. Except for the posterior shear test, all tests have higher potential for diagnosis (specificity 0.86 to 0.90) than screening (sensitivity 0.18 to 0.84).[21,103] When considering LRs, the passive lumbar extension test has the strongest +LR (8.8) and -LR (0.2), indicating that there is a moderate but important shift in the probability of LSI being present with a positive test finding or being absent with a negative test finding.[104] Interrater reliability ranged from fair (k = greater than 0.40) to moderate (k = 0.60 to 0.80) for all tests except for the posterior shear test, which had only slight reliability (k = 0.23 to 0.39).[21,22,24,97,105-107]

Clinical tests of functional instability involve cocontraction of the muscles of the active subsystem while the test is performed (Box 16-8). The prone instability test first examines for pain provocation using CPA pressures at each lumbar segment with the patient lying prone over a table with their

Table 16-13

RELIABILITY AND DIAGNOSTIC ACCURACY OF LUMBAR PHYSICAL IMPAIRMENT MEASURES

REFERENCE	PPIVM TEST	RELIABILITY (KAPPA [95% CI])	SENSITIVITY (95% CI)	SPECIFICITY (95% CI)	+LR (95% CI)	-LR (95% CI)
PPIVM of Lumbar Spine						
Abbott & Mercer, 2005[96]	Flexion; lumbar hypomobility	NA	42% (90% CI 19, 71)	89% (90% CI: 71, 96)	3.86 (90% CI: 0.89, 16.31)	0.64 (90% CI: 0.28, 1.04)
Abbott et al, 2005[93]	Flexion; lumbar translation instability	NA	5% (95% CI: 1, 22)	99% (95% CI: 97, 100)	8.73 (95% CI: 0.57, 134.7)	0.96 (95% CI: 0.88, 1.05)
Abbott et al, 2005[93]	Extension; lumbar translation instability	NA	16% (95% CI: 6, 38)	98% (95% CI: 94, 99)	7.07 (95% CI: 1.71, 29.2)	0.86 (95% CI: 71, 1.05)
PAIVM of Lumbar Spine						
Schneider et al, 2008[99]	Central PA spring test	Interrater: k=0.21 (-0.10, 0.53) to 0.73 (0.51, 0.95) for pain provocation; Interrater: k=-0.17 (-0.41, 0.06) to 0.17 (-0.14, 0.48) for motion restriction	NA	NA	NA	NA
Abbott & Mercer, 2005[96]	Central PA: Lumbar hypomobility	NA	0.75 (90% CI: 0.36, 0.94)	0.35 (90% CI: 0.20, 0.55)	1.16 (90% CI: 0.44, 20.3)	0.71 (90% CI: 0.12, 2.75)
Abbott et al, 2005[93]	Central PA: Lumbar segmental instability	NA	0.29 (0.14, 0.50)	0.89 (0.83, 0.93)	2.52 (1.15, 5.53)	0.81 (0.61, 1.06)
Fritz et al, 2005[97]	Central PA	Interrater: k=0.38 95% CI for hypomobility; 0.48 for hypermobility; 0.57 for pain provocation	NA	NA	NA	NA
Fritz et al, 2005[97]	Central PA lack of hypomobility	NA	0.43 (0.27, 0.61)	0.95 (0.77, 0.99)	9.0 (95% CI: 1.3, 63.9)	0.60 (95% CI: 0.43, 0.84)

(continued)

Table 16-13 (continued)

RELIABILITY AND DIAGNOSTIC ACCURACY OF LUMBAR PHYSICAL IMPAIRMENT MEASURES

REFERENCE	PPIVM TEST	RELIABILITY (KAPPA [95% CI])	SENSITIVITY (95% CI)	SPECIFICITY (95% CI)	+LR (95% CI)	-LR (95% CI)
Fritz et al, 2005[97]	Central PA any hypermobility	NA	0.46 (0.30, 0.64)	0.81 (0.60, 0.92)	2.4 (95% CI: 0.93, 6.4)	0.66 (95% CI: 0.44, 0.99)
Landel et al, 2008[184]	Central PA	Interrater: k=0.71 (0.48, 0.94) for lease mobile segment; 0.29 (-0.13, 0.71) for most mobility segment	NA	NA	NA	NA
Hicks et al, 2003[16]	Central PA	Interrater: k=-0.02 (-0.25, 0.28) to 0.26 (-0.01, 0.53) for mobility assessment; interrater: k=0.25 (0.11, 0.40) to 0.55 (0.43, 0.67) for pain provocation	NA	NA	NA	NA
Lumbopelvic Instability Testing						
Hicks et al, 2003[16]	Posterior Shear	Interrater: k=0.35 (0.20, 0.51)	NA	NA	NA	NA
Fritz et al, 2005[97]	Posterior Shear	Interrater: k=0.27 (0.14, 0.41)	NA	NA	NA	NA
Alyazedi et al, 2015[22]	Passive Lumbar Extension Test	Interrater: k=0.46 (0.20, 0.72)	NA	NA	NA	NA
Rabin et al, 2013[107]	Passive Lumbar Extension Test	Interrater: k=0.076 (0.46, 1.00)	NA	NA	NA	NA

(continued)

Table 16-13 (continued)

RELIABILITY AND DIAGNOSTIC ACCURACY OF LUMBAR PHYSICAL IMPAIRMENT MEASURES

REFERENCE	PPIVM TEST	RELIABILITY (KAPPA [95% CI])	SENSITIVITY (95% CI)	SPECIFICITY (95% CI)	+LR (95% CI)	-LR (95% CI)
Alyazedi et al, 2015[22]	Lack of Hypomobility	Interrater: k=-0.020 (-0.22, 0.18)	NA	NA	NA	NA
Fritz et al, 2005[97]	Lack of Hypomobility	NA	0.43 (0.27, 0.61)	0.95 (0.77, 0.99)	9.0 (1.3, 63.9)	0.60 (0.43, 0.84)
Alyazedi et al, 2015[22]	Aberrant Motion	Interrater: k=0.79 (0.39, 1.19)	NA	NA	NA	NA
Rabin et al, 2013[107]	Aberrant Motion	0.64 (0.32, 0.90)	NA	NA	NA	NA
Fritz et al, 2005[97]	Aberrant Motion	Interrater: k=-0.07 (-0.45, 0.31)	NA	NA	NA	NA
Hicks et al, 2003[16]	Aberrant Motion	Interrater: k=0.60 (0.47, 0.73)	NA	NA	NA	NA
Alyazedi et al, 2015[22]	Average Straight Leg Raise > 91 degrees	Interrater: k=0.77 (0.47, 0.98)	NA	NA	NA	NA
Rabin et al, 2013[107]	Average Straight Leg Raise > 91 degrees	0.73 (0.42, 1.00)	NA	NA	NA	NA
Alyazedi et al, 2015[22]	Prone Instability Test	Interrater: k=0.71 (0.45, 0.98)	NA	NA	NA	NA
Rabin et al, 2013[107]	Prone Instability Test	Interrater: k=0.67 (0.29, 1.00)	NA	NA	NA	NA
Fritz et al, 2005[97]	Prone Instability Test	Interrater: k=0.69 (0.59, 0.79)	NA	NA	NA	NA
Hicks et al, 2003[16]	Prone Instability Test	Interrater: k=0.87 (0.80, 0.94)	NA	NA	NA	NA

CI= confidence interval; K = Kappa; LR+ = positive likelihood ratio; LR- = negative likelihood ratio; NA = not assessed; PA = posteroanterior; Sn=sensitivity; Sp=specificity.

Box 16-6. Passive Intervertebral Motion Testing: Passive Physiologic Intervertebral Motion

TEST	DESCRIPTION	INTERPRETATION	FIGURE
Flexion	Patient position: Side-lying, with the spine in sagittal plane neutral Procedure: The patient's knees and hips are passively flexed to induce flexion from L5 cranially to L1. The therapist's caudal hand supports the patient's lower extremities at the lower leg area while palpating the interspinous space for an opening between spinous processes as flexion is passively produced.	Positive test: The amount of separation between spinous processes is compared to the segment above.	
Extension	Patient position: Side-lying, with the spine in sagittal plane neutral Procedure: The patient's knees are flexed while the hips are passively extended to induce extension from L5 cranially to L1. The therapist's caudal hand supports the patient's lower extremities at the lower leg area while palpating the interspinous space for closing between spinous processes as extension is passively produced.	Positive test: The amount of narrowing between spinous processes is compared to the segment above.	

(continued)

Box 16-6 (continued). Passive Intervertebral Motion Testing: Passive Physiologic Intervertebral Motion

TEST	DESCRIPTION	INTERPRETATION	FIGURE
Side-bending	Patient position: Side-lying right to assess left side-bending, with the spine in sagittal plane neutral Procedure: The patient's hips are passively flexed to approximately 90 degrees hip flexion with the knees flexed. The therapist's caudal hand lifts the lower legs upward to induce side-bending to the left. The cranial hand palpates the left lateral aspect of the interspinous space for closing between spinous processes on the side of the concavity.	Positive test: The amount of closing between spinous processes is compared to the segment above.	
Rotation	Patient position: Side-lying right to assess left rotation, with the spine in sagittal plane neutral Procedure: The patient's hips are passively flexed to approximately 90 degrees hip flexion with the knees flexed. The therapist's cranial forearm is placed under the top arm of the patient and used to passively rotate the patient's trunk away in the direction of left rotation. The caudal hand palpates the right lateral aspect of the interspinous space between L1-L2 with one finger at L1, one finger at the interspinous space, and one finger at L2. As rotation is produced, the therapist feels for movement of the superior spinous process toward the tables.	Positive test: Movement of the superior spinous process toward the table as compared to the spinous process below.	

Box 16-7. Special Tests for Lumbopelvic Segmental Instability: Structural

TEST	DESCRIPTION	INTERPRETATION	FIGURE
Passive lumbar extension	Position: Prone Procedure: The therapist passively lifts both lower extremities off of the table about 30 cm.	Positive test: Patient reports LBP and feeling of heaviness in the back.	
Posterior shear	Position: Side-lying, with the spine in sagittal plane neutral Procedure: The patient's hips are passively flexed to approximately 90 degrees hip flexion with the knees flexed, resting against the therapist's hip. The therapist's hands stabilizes the superior segments posteriorly. An anterior to posterior shear is applied by the therapist's hip through the patient's femurs while palpating the movement of the inferior segment.	Positive test: Excessive movement of the inferior segment or symptom provocation.	
Aberrant movement pattern	Position: Standing Procedure: The patient performs standing forward bending and return to upright standing.	Positive test: the presence of any one of the movement patterns instability catch sign, thigh climbing, painful arc of motion, reversal of lumbopelvic rhythm	

Data Source: Alyazedi FM, Lohman EB, Wesley Swen R, Bahjri K. The inter-rater reliability of clinical tests that best predict the subclassification of lumbar segmental instability: structural, functional and combined instability. *J Man Manip Ther.* 2015;23(4):197-204. doi:10.1179/2042618615Y.0000000002

Box 16-8. Special Tests for Lumbopelvic Segmental Instability: Functional

TEST	DESCRIPTION	INTERPRETATION	FIGURE
Prone instability test	Procedure: The patient lies prone over a table with their feet on the floor. The therapist examines for pain provocation using CPA pressures at each lumbar segment. If pain is provoked, the patient lifts their legs off the floor to facilitate activation of the hip extensors and holds the lifted position (cocontraction) as the therapist again provides the posterior-anterior pressure to the painful segment.	Positive test: Reduction in pain with cocontraction as the posterior-anterior pressure is applied.	
Active straight leg raise	Procedure: The patient performs a straight leg raise to about 20 cm off the table for 20 seconds in supine and in prone. The examiner observes movement control of the lifted leg, movement of the pelvis and breathing as the test is performed. The patient is asked to rate their difficulty in performing the test.	Positive test: Difficulty in performing the test is rated on a 6-point scale (not difficult to unable to perform). One point is given for any of the following observations: Breathing difficulty, tremor of the lifting leg, pelvic rotation, or slow speed of lifting the leg, or verbal or nonverbal expression of difficulty. A score of 1 or greater is a positive test.	

feet on the floor. If pain is provoked, the patient lifts their legs off the floor to facilitate activation of the hip extensors and holds the lifted position (cocontraction) as the therapist again provides the posterior-anterior pressure to the painful segment. A positive test is reduction in pain with cocontraction as the posterior-anterior pressure is applied. The active straight leg raise test examines for the deficits in muscles of the active subsystem as the patient performs a straight leg raise with the leg 20 cm off the table, and movement performance is observed. The reliability of the prone instability test is moderate to substantial (k = 0.69 to 0.87), and the reliability of the active straight leg raise is moderate. Although Hicks et al[108] found high specificity for the active straight leg raise (0.92), this was in regard to prediction of success with a stabilization program. Although the prone instability test has been found to have good reliability (k = 0.87),[16] the diagnostic accuracy of the prone instability test was reported to be low.[109] Additional factors potentially contributing to LSI include excessive PSLR test, age, and aberrant movements.

The last group of special tests used to examine for lumbopelvic instability focus on motor control during active movements. These tests are performed in standing, sitting, quadruped, supine, and prone and require sagittal plane or transverse plane control of the lumbar spine as a muscular activation and limb or trunk movement is performed. Luomajoki et al[110] examined the intrarater and interrater reliability of the assessment of motor control ability of individuals with NSLBP during their performance of 10 active movements. The ability of the participant to maintain flexion/extension or rotational control of the lumbopelvic region was rated during the performance of each test. Intrarater reliability ranged from 0.51 to 0.96, whereas interrater reliability ranged from 0.24 to 0.71. Based on reliability calculations, the authors suggest use of the waiters bow and sitting knee extension to examine for flexion motor control, pelvic tilt for extension control, and one leg stance for rotation control.

Pelvic Girdle Pain

PGP is defined as pain that is posterior, unilateral, inferomedial to the PSIS, and below L5 (Fortin's sign).[111] Additional description of symptoms may include referral to the buttock, groin, and posterior thigh, but rarely below the knee. Functional impairments associated with PGP include pain and/or limitation during unilateral weightbearing activities such as stance phase of gait and ascending/descending stairs, transitional movements (eg, sit to stand, rolling over in bed, in/out of car), and prolonged positioning (sitting or standing). PGP is most commonly associated with pregnancy but can occur as a result of trauma or arthritis. Both the lumbar spine and hip can refer pain to the pelvic region; therefore, contributions from the lumbar spine or hip to the patient's symptomology should have been ruled out during the LQSE with negative findings from tests such as absence of centralization, unrestricted and pain free PPIVM of lumbar spine, and absence of hip pain during hip PROM and FABER stress test.[41,112] LQSE findings suggestive of PGP

may include pelvic asymmetry with postural examination and palpation, positive findings with kinetic motion tests (eg, standing forward bend, sitting forward bend, Gillet test), and/or positive primary stress tests of the SIJ (compression and distraction). After excluding the lumbar spine and/or hip as the referral source of the presenting symptomology, clinical tests are conducted to classify the pain as specific or nonspecific. Specific PGP disorders include inflammatory arthritis (eg, ankylosing spondylitis), sacroiliitis and pubic symphysis disorders. Pubic symphysis–related PGP pain is characterized by localized pain to the pubic region or groin. Special tests to further examine the presence of PGP can be grouped into pain provocation tests, load transfer or attenuation tests, and mobility-based tests of the SIJ and pubic symphysis. Of these, pain provocation tests have higher reliability and validity than movement- or palpation-based tests for the pelvic region.

PGP provocation tests can assist in localizing symptoms to the SIJ or pubic symphysis, with positive tests indicating inflammation. Positive findings in each of these tests are reproduction of pain symptoms. SIJ pain provocation tests were initiated in the LQSE with distraction (anterior gapping of the SIJ) and compression (posterior gapping of the SIJ) primary stress tests. If positive, 3 additional SIJ stress tests should be performed: (1) sacral thrust, (2) Gaenslen's test, and (3) thigh thrust (Box 16-5).[112,113] The use of a cluster of tests to examine for the presence of SIJ pain has resulted in increased diagnostic validity and reliability as opposed to just use of a single test.[81,82,114] When 3 or more out of the 5 provocation tests are positive in the absence of centralization, the diagnostic accuracy for SIJ pain is sensitivity (0.91), specificity (0.78), +LR (4.16), and -LR (0.11).[112] Laslett et al[90] revised the test cluster by removing Gaenslen's test because it did not contribute positively to overall diagnostic accuracy and recommended use of distraction, thigh thrust, compression, and sacral thrust for sensitivity of 0.88, specificity of 0.78, and +LR of 4.0. If pain is referred to the groin area, provocation stress test for pubic symphysis is indicated. The test is performed in supine and involves stabilizing the pubis inferiorly on one side while mobilizing caudally on the other side (Figure 16-5A), and stabilizing the pubis superiorly on one side while mobilizing cranially on the other side (Figure 16-5B). Symptom reproduction and quantity of motion is assessed, with pain and/or hypomobility or hypermobility suggestive of pubic symphysis dysfunction. Palpation of boney landmarks and soft tissues may also assist in the diagnosis of SIJ or pubic symphysis pain. Posterior palpation of the sacral sulcus, long dorsal sacroiliac ligament, and sacrotuberous ligament may provoke pain with SIJ involvement. Albert et al[115] found palpation of the pubic symphysis to have high specificity (0.99) and moderate sensitivity (0.88) for classification of pregnancy-related pelvic joint pain.

A second group of special tests for the SIJ examines the ability of the pelvic girdle to transfer loads between the lumbar spine and lower extremities to assess pelvic stability. Stability of the pelvis is achieved through form and force closure of the SIJ.[11] While form closure occurs through the close fitting structure of the joint, force closure occurs through tension in ligaments, thoracolumbar fascia, and muscles to provide compressive forces that stabilize the joint as motion occurs. Load transfer tests involve variations of the active straight leg raise to assess potential impairments of form or force closure. These tests utilize the active straight leg raise test with the addition of manual compression to the pelvis to augment form and force closure or resistance to the muscles of the active subsystem to augment force closure (Figure 16-6). The test can be performed in supine and prone. A positive finding is considered if pain and/or the performance of the active straight leg raise test improves with either form or force closure augmentation. Individuals with PGP may have a less considered impairment of excessive force closure.[32] For these individuals, the active straight leg raise test would be negative, meaning that no pain occurred when the leg was raised, but pain increased when manual compression was applied to the pelvis and/or isometric resistance applied to muscles in the anatomic slings while the straight leg raise is maintained. In addition, high tone or hyperactivity would be present in the pelvic stabilizing muscles, and instruction in relaxation of these muscles would result in pain reduction.[116]

The last group of tests utilizes movement-based tests to examine for SIJ dysfunction. Tests for SIJ dysfunction are initiated with static palpation of pelvic symmetry and motion palpation previously described in the sections about posture and active movement testing, respectively. Additional static palpation tests of the SIJ can be performed including palpation of the sacral sulci, inferior lateral angles, and medial malleoli. Palpation of the sacral sulci, sacral base, sacral apex, and interior lateral angles provides information regarding positional assessment of the sacrum to assess for sacral torsions. Although these palpation-based tests for SIJ dysfunction are commonly performed in the clinic, the reliability of static palpation tests of the sacrum is reported to be poor (kappa = 0.11).[117] The theoretical basis of motion palpation tests for the SIJ utilize hip movement to produce rotation of the innominate, with hip flexion creating posterior rotation of the innominate and hip extension creating anterior rotation of the innominate. Positive findings with static palpation and/or motion palpation tests could be further examined with passive mobility testing of the ilium moving on the sacrum to assess passive physiologic motion and passive accessory motion of the innominate as outlined in Boxes 16-9 and 16-10, respectively. For example, if SIJ palpation tests suggest an anteriorly rotated innominate (ipsilateral ASIS lower and PSIS higher than the contralateral side) with

hypomobility and pain in the direction of posterior rotation (Gillett's test), the therapist would assess mobility and symptom response to passive posterior rotation of the ilium with the patient positioned in side-lying. Passive accessory motion could also be assessed by application of a posterolateral directed pressure to the ASIS on the involved side with the patient lying supine. If repeatedly performed and passive mobility tests positively affect pain, these techniques could then be used for treatment purposes. Passive mobility testing of the sacrum moving on the ilium can also be performed by applying posterior-anterior pressure to the sacral base for assessment of nutation mobility and to the sacral apex for assessment of counternutation mobility.

Muscle Performance Tests

Muscle performance tests can be divided into assessment of motor control of the deep stabilizing muscles and assessment of muscular endurance of global muscles affecting lumbopelvic stability. Impaired function of the deep stabilizing muscles has been found in individuals with LBP. Coactivation of these muscles is assessed using the abdominal drawing in maneuver (ADIM) performed in quadruped, supine, and prone.[31] The ADIM involves "drawing up and in" the pelvic floor, transverse abdominis, and coactivating the lumbar multifidus without activation of the global muscles and while maintaining a neutral lordosis and lateral costal breathing.[20] A pressure biofeedback device (PBD) can be used to quantify the ability to perform the ADIM. Box 16-11 outlines muscle performance tests for the deep stabilizing muscles.

Assessment of the global muscles is performed in consideration of the acuity of the patient and only if the patient can adequately activate the local muscles.[118] McGill et al[119] recommends the use of 3 tests that assess muscular endurance of the trunk flexors (isometric flexion), extensors (isometric extension), and lateral flexors (isometric side bridge). The maximal hold time is recorded, and the ratios are calculated to assess for imbalances in trunk flexion/extension, lateral flexion/extension, and lateral flexion right/left. The reliability of these tests is reported to be excellent (intraclass correlation coefficient = 0.97 to 0.99).[119] Prone bridging and supine bridging are also recommended as muscle performance tests and performance ability of these tests by individuals with chronic LBP has been found to be less when compared to individuals without LBP.[120] Box 16-12 outlines muscle performance tests recommended for use in the lumbopelvic examination.

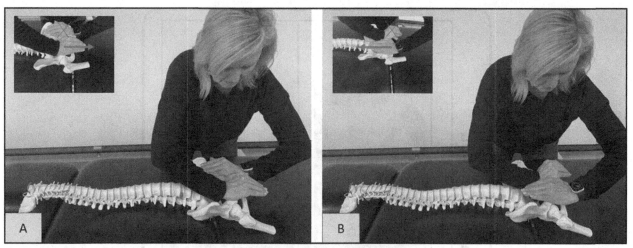

Figure 16-5. Pubic symphysis provocation stress tests. (A) Caudal mobility. (B) Cranial mobility.

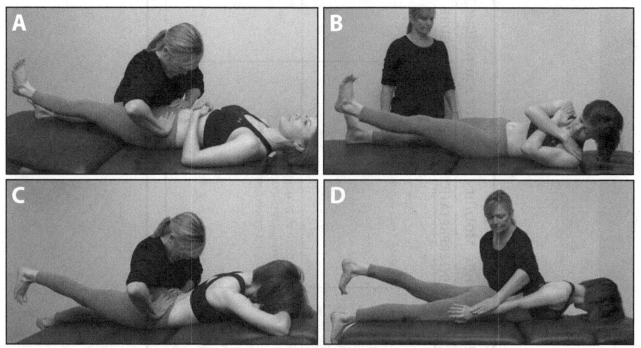

Figure 16-6. Active straight leg raise test. (A) Supine with manual compression. (B) Supine with augmentation of active subsystem. (C) Prone with manual compression. (D) Prone with augmentation of active subsystem.

Box 16-9. Passive Physiologic Mobility Tests for Sacroiliac Joint Dysfunction

TEST	DESCRIPTION	INTERPRETATION	FIGURE
Passive physiologic posterior rotation of innominate	Patient position: Sideyling with the hip in flexion Procedure: Therapist hand placement is on the ASIS and ischial tuberosity to passively posteriorly rotate the innominate of the top lower extremity. Posterior innominate rotation creates nutation of the sacrum.	Positive test: Pain reproduction, movement restriction, response to repeated movement.	
Passive physiologic anterior rotation of innominate	Patient position: Prone with the hip in extension Procedure: Therapist hand placement is on the PSIS to passively anteriorly rotate the innominate. Anterior innominate rotation creates counternutation of the sacrum.	Positive test: Pain reproduction, movement restriction, response to repeated movement.	

Box 16-10. Passive Accessory Mobility Tests for Sacroiliac Joint Dysfunction

TEST	DESCRIPTION	INTERPRETATION	FIGURE
Anterior rotation mobility of ASIS	Patient position: Supine Procedure: The therapist's stabilizing hand is placed on the opposite iliac crest and the mobilizing hand produces an anterior rotation (anteromedial) force on the ipsilateral iliac crest.	Positive test: Pain provocation. Decreased mobility suggests a posteriorly rotated innominate.	
Posterior rotation mobility of PSIS	Patient position: Supine Procedure: The therapist's stabilizing hand is placed on the opposite iliac crest, and the mobilizing hand produces a posterior rotation (posterior lateral) force on the ipsilateral iliac crest.	Positive test: Pain provocation. Decreased mobility suggests an anteriorly rotated innominate.	
Sacral flexion (nutation) mobility	Patient position: Prone Procedure: The therapist places their hand on the sacrum and produces a ventrally directed force to the sacral base.	Positive test: Pain provocation. Decreased mobility suggests an extended or counternutated sacrum.	
Sacral extension (counternutation) mobility	Patient position: Prone Procedure: The therapist places their hand on the sacrum and produces a ventrally directed force to the sacral apex.	Positive test: Pain provocation. Decreased mobility suggests an extended or nutated sacrum.	

Box 16-11. Local Muscle Performance Tests

TEST	DESCRIPTION	FIGURE
ADIM	The following instructions for ADIM is provided to assess local muscle recruitment in quadruped, supine, and prone positions: "Draw in your abdominal wall without moving your spine or pelvis and hold for 10 seconds while breathing normally."	
ADIM Supine	Position: Supine, hooklying with the lumbar spine in neutral lordosis PBD: Place the PBD under the lumbar spine and inflate to 40 mm Hg. As the patient performs the ADIM, the pressure reading should remain the same or slightly increase about 2 to 3 mm Hg. The ADIM is held for 10 seconds. The ability to perform 10 repetitions of the 10-second hold with the PBD is assessed.	
ADIM Prone	Position: Prone PBD: Place the PBD under the lower abdomen and inflate to 70 mm Hg. As the patient performs the ADIM, the pressure reading should decrease by 6 to 10 mm HG. The ability to perform 10 repetitions of the 10-second hold with the PBD is assessed.	

Data Source: Richardson C, Jull G, Hodges PW, Hides JA. *Therapeutic exercise for spinal segmental stabilization in low back pain: scientific basis and clinical approach.* Churchill Livingstone; 1999.

Box 16-12. Global Muscle Performance Tests

TEST	DESCRIPTION	FIGURE
Isometric Trunk Flexion[a]	Position: Semi-reclined with trunk resting against a plinth or bolster inclined 60 degrees from the horizontal. Arms are crossed over their chest, and the knees and hips are flexed with toes held under a strap. The supporting surface is lowered or pulled back to begin the test. The test ends when the trunk lowers below 60 degrees.	
Isometric Trunk Extension[a]	Position: Prone lying on treatment table with the torso off the table from the ASIS cranially. Straps or the examiner secure the lower extremities. The upper extremities are supported on a chair or stool. The patient removes the upper extremities from the support surface to assume a position in which the trunk is parallel to the floor with hands on opposite shoulders. The test ends when the trunk moves below parallel.	
Isometric Lateral Flexion[b]	Position: Side-lying with legs extended, one foot in front of the other, propped on the lower forearm and the top arm across the chest. The patient lifts the lower hip off the floor raising their body until the legs are in line with the trunk. The test ends when the position cannot be maintained.	
Supine Bridge[b]	Position: Supine, hooklying, arms resting at their sides. The patient lifts the hips off the floor until the knees, hips, and torso form a straight inclined line. The test ends when the position cannot be maintained.	
Prone Bridge[b]	Position: Prone on forearms, toes tucked under. The patient lifts their body off the floor until the head, trunk, lower extremities are in a straight, horizontal line. The test ends when the position cannot be maintained.	

Data Sources: [a]Brumitt J, Matheson JW, Meira EP. Core stabilization exercise prescription, part I. *Sports Health.* 2013;5(6):504-509. doihttps://doi.org/10.1177/1941738113502451; [b]McGill SM, Childs A, Liebenson C. Endurance times for low back stabilization exercises: clinical targets for testing and training from a normal database. *Arch Phys Med Rehabil.* 1999;80(8):941-944.

Section II:
Evaluation—Establishing a Clinical Diagnosis for Low Back Pain

Upon completion of the lumbopelvic examination, a second level evaluation is performed in which the clinician establishes the acuity of the symptomology, determines the risk and impact of psychosocial distress, and assesses the objective findings gathered to provide an impairment-based musculoskeletal diagnosis.

Symptom Acuity

The acuity of LBP is traditionally established in relation to temporal components of soft tissue healing using time since onset or duration of symptomology, with symptoms less than 1 month being acute and symptoms greater than 3 months being chronic.[121] Due to the recurring nature of LBP and the increasing prevalence of chronic LBP, the authors of the APTA CPG recommend that tissue irritability, assessed with movement/pain responses to examination procedures, is added to temporal definitions for determination of acuity. For example, acute LBP would have pain and/or mobility restrictions in the initial to mid-ranges of active or passive motions, subacute LBP would have pain and/or mobility restrictions in the mid- to end-ranges of active or passive movements, and chronic LBP would have pain with sustained end-range movements or positions. In the 2015 revision to the TBC, Alrwaily et al[42] use the assessment of irritability to determine clinical status as volatile, stable, or well-controlled as part of the criteria for determining the rehabilitation approach of symptom modulation, movement control, or functional optimization, respectively. The additional criteria used to establish the rehabilitation approach is severity and disability rating. When considering both the recommendations by APTA CPG and the updated TBC, determining the acuity of symptomology requires the evaluation of subjective information related to symptom severity (pain level), irritability (activity tolerance, pain/motion response), and disability (self-report disability outcome scores) as outlined in Table 16-14.

Risk of Psychosocial Distress

Scores from the self-report (ÖMPSQ, STarT) and cognitive-affective questionnaires (Pain Catastrophizing Scale, FABQ) presented in the subjective examination section (see Table 16-6) are interpreted to determine the potential risk for psychosocial distress that may affect prognosis of outcomes related to lumbopelvic pain and assist in guiding the rehabilitation management for these individuals. High scores on the Pain Catastrophizing Scale, FABQ, or ÖMPSQ or medium to high risk on the STarT Back Screening Tool would alert the clinician to include cognitive behavioral intervention strategies or to initiate comanagement with a medical provider trained in cognitive behavioral therapies.[35]

Impairment-Based Subgroup Classification

The APTA CPG for LBP presents a subgroup classification using terminology from the *International Classification of Functioning, Disability and Health* for impairments of body function. The recommended classification subgroups are LBP with mobility deficits, LBP with movement coordination impairments, LBP with related lower extremity pain, LBP with radiating pain, and LBP with related generalized pain. An additional category of LBP with related cognitive or affective tendencies is also included in the CPG to classify individuals with generalized LBP that is influenced by psychosocial comorbidities. In contrast, the TBC by Delitto et al[43] and revised by Fritz et al[45] in 2007 and Alrwaily et al[42] in 2015, classifies subgroups based on primary treatment focus using clusters of examination findings to establish common impairments for each subgroup. Because PGP may present as a distinct disorder independent of referral from the lumbar spine and hips, a classification model for PGP disorders has been proposed by O'Sullivan and Beale.[32,116] Physical therapy diagnosis of lumbopelvic pain presented in this section merges the information from the ATPA CPG, TBC, and PGP classification model to form the following diagnostic classification subgroups:

- Lumbopelvic pain with mobility deficits
- Lumbopelvic pain with movement coordination impairments
- Lumbopelvic pain with referred or radiating lower extremity pain
- Nonspecific PGP
- PGP with reduced force closure
- PGP with excessive force closure

Within each subgroup classification, the rehabilitation approach is guided by evaluation of symptom acuity, disability, and risk of psychosocial distress. Examination findings that would support each subgroup classification are presented in Table 16-15, along with recommended interventions.

Table 16-14

EVALUATING SYMPTOM ACUITY

	DISABILITY: SELF-REPORTED DISABILITY SCORES	SEVERITY: PAIN RATING	IRRITABILITY: ACTIVITY TOLERANCE	IRRITABILITY: RANGE OF MOTION AND SYMPTOM ONSET	IRRITABILITY: TISSUE RESISTANCE AND SYMPTOM ONSET
ACUTE	High	High to moderate	Limited ability to perform activity	Pain during initial and mid-ROM	Pain before resistance
SUBACUTE	Moderate	Moderate to low	Performs activity with some pain	Pain occurring at mid- to end ROM	Pain with resistance
CHRONIC	Low	Low to absent	No limitation to activity	Pain at end ROM or with sustained movements	Pain after resistance

Table 16-15

CLINICAL DIAGNOSIS CLASSIFICATION OF LUMBOPELVIC PAIN

CLASSIFICATION	PRIMARY IMPAIRMENTS	INTERVENTIONS
Lumbopelvic pain with mobility deficits	• Unilateral low back, buttock, or thigh pain • Lumbar AROM deficits and/or pain provocation • Pain and/or hypomobility with PPIVM and PAIVM segmental testing of the lumbar spine	• Manual therapy pain management techniques • Manual therapy mobility techniques • Mobility based therapeutic exercise • Active rest if high acuity, progressing to regular active exercise
Lumbopelvic pain with movement coordination impairments	• Lumbopelvic pain at rest or produced with movement • May have low-back related referred lower extremity pain • Positive aberrant movement testing • Pain and/or hypermobility with PPIVM and PAIVM segmental testing of the lumbar spine • Positive findings with clinical tests for structural and/or functional instability • Decreased ability with muscle performance tests of the trunk and/or pelvis	• Neuromuscular based therapeutic exercise to promote stability using the local and global stabilizing muscles and motor control • Mobility based therapeutic exercise and manual therapy for adjacent areas of hypomobility • Education in utilizing mid-range positions when performing self-care/work tasks • Active rest if high acuity, progressing to regular active exercise
Lumbopelvic pain with referred lower extremity pain	• Low back pain with referred pain into the lower extremity • Postures and/or movements are identified that worsen or peripheralize symptoms • May have postural deformity of reduced lordosis or lateral shift • Lumbar AROM testing with directional preference that centralizes symptoms	• Manual therapy and therapeutic exercises to promote centralization • Education in movements and postures to minimize peripheralization • Restoration of movements that peripheralized symptoms *(continued)*

Table 16-15 (continued)

CLINICAL DIAGNOSIS CLASSIFICATION OF LUMBOPELVIC PAIN

CLASSIFICATION	PRIMARY IMPAIRMENTS	INTERVENTIONS
Lumbopelvic pain with radiating pain	• Low back pain with radiating pain into the lower extremity • Subjective reports of altered lower extremity sensation, numbness or weakness • Pain provocation with lumbar AROM testing • Lower extremity radicular symptoms provoked with neurodynamic tests • May have positive sensory, myotome and/or reflex neurologic tests	• Manual or mechanical traction • Neurodynamic mobilization techniques
Non-specific inflammatory pelvic girdle pain	• Pain with weight bearing loading of the pelvis • Constant pain over the SIJ or referred distally; or pain at the pubic symphysis • Absence of pain with lumbar spine and hip movement testing • Absence of centralization with movement testing of the lumbar spine • Positive SIJ provocation tests • Pain with pelvic compression delivered with SIJ belt • Absence of specific inflammatory disorder	• Controlled rest to minimize stress to the pelvic girdle • Medical referral for anti-inflammatory medications, steroid injections
Pelvic girdle pain with reduced force closure	• Pain with weight bearing loading of the pelvis • Assume postures that "inhibit" local pelvic muscles • Intermittent pain over the SIJ, surrounding muscle structures • Absence of pain with lumbar spine and hip movement testing • Inability to isolate pelvic rotation independent of thoracolumbar spine • Positive SIJ provocation tests • Positive active straight leg raise test (ALSR); symptom decrease with compression or sling activation • Motor control impairment of local pelvic muscles related to reduced force closure • Overuse of thoracolumbar stabilizing muscles • Potentially elevated risk of psychosocial distress	• Neuromuscular based therapeutic exercise focusing on motor control of pelvic stabilizing muscles involved in force closure • Temporary use of SIJ belt • Cognitive behavioral therapy if elevated fear avoidance and/or psychosocial factors • Education for avoidance of postures/movements that inhibit local pelvic muscles • Restorative of independent pelvic mobility

(continued)

Table 16-15 (continued)

Clinical Diagnosis Classification of Lumbopelvic Pain

CLASSIFICATION	PRIMARY IMPAIRMENTS	INTERVENTIONS
Pelvic girdle pain with excessive force closure	• Intermittent pain over the SIJ or surrounding muscle structures • Excessive muscle guarding and cocontraction of trunk and pelvic muscles • Positive SIJ provocation tests • Negative active straight leg raise test; pain with compression during ASLR • Motor control impairment of local muscles related to excessive force closure • Worsening of symptoms with manual compression or use of SIJ belt and performance of stabilization exercises • Short-term relief with stretching, manipulation • Potentially elevated risk of psychosocial distress	• Relaxation techniques and exercises targeting muscles of force closure • Breathing exercises for stress reduction • Postures and movement re-education to avoid excessive cocontraction of lumbopelvic muscles • Manual therapy soft tissue massage and muscle energy techniques to reduce muscle hyperactivity • Cognitive behavioral therapy if elevated fear avoidance and/or psychosocial factors

Data Sources: Alrwaily M, Timko M, Schneider M, et al. Treatment-based classification system for low back pain: revision and update. *Phys Ther.* 2016;96(7):1057-1066. doi:10.2522/ptj.20150345; Delitto A, George SZ, Van Dillen L, et al. Low back pain. *J Orthop Sports Phys Ther.* 2012;42(4):A1-A57. doi:10.2519/jospt.2012.42.4.A1; Fritz JM, Brennan GP, Clifford SN, Hunter SJ, Thackeray A. An examination of the reliability of a classification algorithm for subgrouping patients with low back pain. *Spine.* 2006;31(1):77-82; O'Sullivan PB, Beales DJ. Diagnosis and classification of pelvic girdle pain disorders, part 1: a mechanism based approach within a biopsychosocial framework. *Man Ther.* 2007;12(2):86–97. doi:10.1016/j.math.2007.02.001

Section III: Manual Therapy for the Lumbopelvic Region

Thrust Joint Manipulation (High-Velocity, Low-Amplitude Technique)

Lumbar Spine

A plethora of evidence supports the use of high-velocity, low-amplitude or thrust spinal manipulation for reducing LBP of a musculoskeletal origin.[122-124] A lumbopelvic manipulation (Figure 16-7; also known as the *Chicago roll technique*), originally designed for treating SIJ dysfunction, has been identified as an effective manual therapy technique for reducing acute LBP.[125,126] A CPR was established by Flynn et al in 2002 to identify a subgroup of patients with LBP who are likely to have short-term benefits from this lumbopelvic manipulation. The CPR is satisfied when a patient exhibits 4 out of the 5 following criteria: duration of symptoms less than 16 days, at least one hip with greater than 35 degrees of internal rotation, hypomobility with lumbar spring testing, FABQ work subscale score less than 19, and no symptoms

distal to the knee. The CPR was later validated by Childs et al.[127] Of the 5 criteria of the CPR, duration of symptoms less than 16 days and no symptoms distal to the knee are associated with a good outcome.[128] This manipulation also was found to be effective in pain reduction and disability improvement for patients who had LBP more than 6 months.[129] The recommended dosage of manipulation is 5 to 10 sessions administered over 2 to 4 weeks for acute LBP,[122] and 12 sessions administered over 4 to 6 weeks for chronic LBP.[129,130] Given that no relationship was found between an audible pop during this lumbopelvic manipulation and improvement of ROM, pain, or disability, an audible pop is not necessary for a successful outcome.[129,131] Although this lumbopelvic manipulation was found to be effective for adult patients, this manipulation has not been shown to have the same beneficial effects for adolescents with acute LBP.[132]

Another thrust spinal manipulation technique, performed in side-lying (Figure 16-8) and designed to treat one specific lumbar spinal segment,[133-135] was found to be equally effective for pain reduction and for disability improvement on patients who satisfied the CPR identified by Flynn et al.[89,136] In a recent randomized controlled trial, this side-lying lumbar rotation manipulation was shown to have

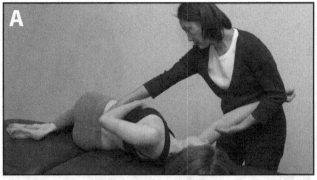
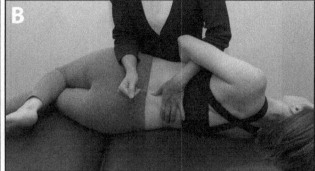

Figure 16-7. Lumbopelvic general manipulation. (A) Setup. (B) End position.

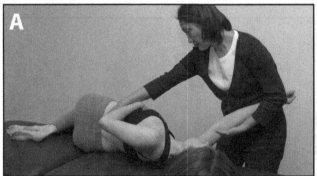
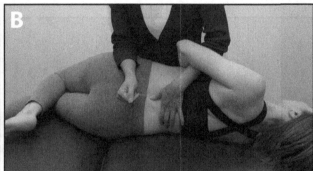

Figure 16-8. Lumbopelvic rotation manipulation. (A) Setup. (B) End position.

greater improvement of disability than a soft tissue technique in patients with chronic LBP.[133] Furthermore, this side-lying lumbar manipulation can be used to improve pain perception and spinal mobility in patients with degenerative disk disease.[137] Patients with a herniated lumbar disk or with lumbar radiculopathy are seldom treated with regional lumbar spinal manipulation. A cohort of patients with acute and chronic low back and leg pain had self-reported improvement up to 1 year following this side-lying lumbar rotation manipulation combined with other treatments, including exercises and modalities, for 2 weeks.[138]

Sacroiliac Joint

Although the lumbopelvic manipulation (see Figure 16-7) was designed originally for treating SIJ dysfunction,[131,139,140] the effectiveness of this manipulation for treating SIJ dysfunction remains lacking, partly due to a lack of valid tests to identify SIJ dysfunction.[141] This manipulation is advocated for treating an anteriorly rotated innominate (ie, posteriorly rotated restriction), when the therapist faces the patient and delivers a thrust on the ASIS in a posteriorly rotated direction (Figure 16-9).[142] The lumbopelvic manipulation described by Flynn et al[89] is used for treating a posteriorly rotated innominate, when the therapist faces away from the patient and delivers a thrust on the ASIS in an anteriorly rotated direction (Figure 16-10).[126,139] Changes such as decreased pressure pain thresholds and α-motoneuron excitability[143] as well as peak plantar pressure redistribution[144,145] were found immediately following an SIJ manipulation. However, there is

conflicting evidence regarding biomechanical changes of the SIJ position following a sacroiliac manipulation. Cibulka et al[139] found improved innominate rotation (tilt) following an SIJ manipulation, whereas Tullberg et al,[146] using roentgen stereophotogrammetric analysis, did not find the changes of the sacrum position relative to the innominate after an SIJ manipulation. One may argue that the conflicting findings were due to different sacroiliac manipulation techniques, the former applied the force on the ilium, whereas the latter applied the force on the sacrum.

Many SIJ manipulation techniques are commonly used by physical therapists despite scarce support from literature. Most of the sacroiliac manipulation techniques originate from osteopathic medicine and are described in detail in several manual therapy textbooks.[135,142,147] In addition, the following SIJ manipulations have been described in the literature. For example, the supine gapping manipulation (Figures 16-11)[148] is used for an anteriorly rotated or a posteriorly rotated innominate, depending on the amount of hip flexion. The prone manipulation (Figure 16-12)[142,147,149] is used for treating a posteriorly rotated innominate. Lastly, the inferior-glide manipulation is used for treating an anteriorly rotated innominate when the patient lies in a supine position (Figure 16-13A),[147,150] and for a posteriorly rotated innominate when the patient lies in a prone position (Figure 16-13B).[151]

Adverse effects, such as cauda equina syndrome, from lumbopelvic manipulation are rare, with 1 in 3.7 million patients presenting with lumbar disk herniation.[152-154] After

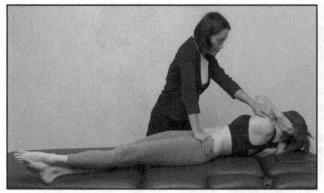

Figure 16-9. SIJ manipulation for anteriorly rotated innominate.

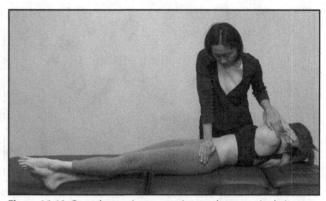

Figure 16-10. Central posterior-to-anterior nonthrust manipulation.

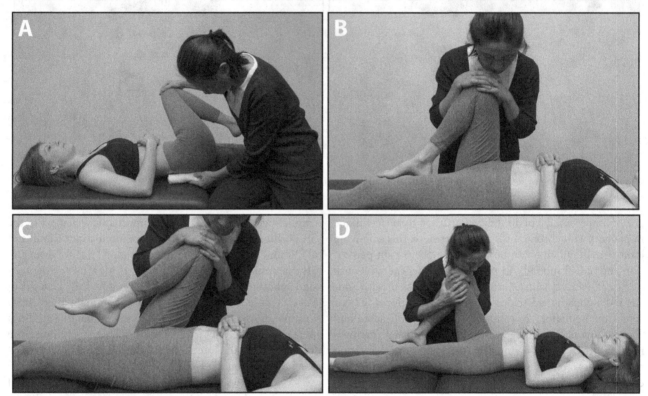

Figure 16-11. SIJ gapping manipulation. (A) Setup. (B) Setup alternate view. (C) Posteriorly rotated innominate. (D) Anteriorly rotated innominate.

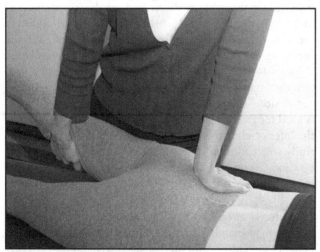

Figure 16-12. SIJ prone manipulation for posteriorly rotated innominate.

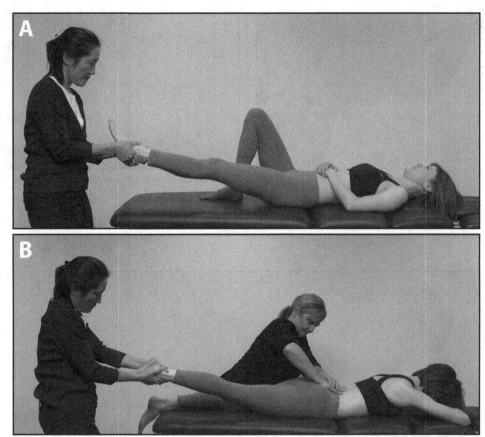

Figure 16-13. SIJ inferior glide manipulation. (A) Upslip and posteriorly rotated innominate. (B) Upslip and anteriorly rotated innominate.

identifying patients who are appropriate candidates for manipulation (eg, by ruling out red flags), a premanipulation hold at the end-range of the manipulation is often used to check the patient's tolerance to the manipulation.[155] Lastly, physical therapists always should obtain consent from patients before a thrust is delivered.[156]

Nonthrust Joint Mobilization

In contrast to high-velocity, low-amplitude thrust manipulation, joint mobilization is performed with low-velocity, rhythmic oscillations[157] or sustained pressures.[158] Maitland's approach of rhythmic oscillations is most often employed by physical therapists for spinal joint mobilization, and it consists of 4 grades: Grade I—small-amplitude oscillations performed at the beginning of the available range of the passive accessory motion; grade II—large-amplitude oscillations within the available range; grade III—large-amplitude oscillations performed from the mid-range to the end of the available range; and grade IV—small-amplitude oscillations performed from at the end of the range to slightly over the limit and into the tissue resistance.[157,159] Grade I and II oscillations are considered appropriate for pain relief in patients with highly irritating LBP, whereas grade III and IV oscillations are advocated for improving joint mobility in patients with less irritating LBP. When thrust manipulation is not appropriate for the patient such as acute inflammation or osteoporosis, joint mobilization should be considered for treating the painful segment or the neighboring segments.

Of the spinal joint mobilizations, posterior-anterior glides, CPA, or UPA (Figures 16-13 and 16-14) are most commonly used by physical therapists. Goodsell et al[160] demonstrated the effectiveness of posterior-anterior glides for reducing pain on worst movement in patients with NSLBP with low irritability. In addition, prone press-ups following posterior-anterior glides (Figure 16-15) were shown to be effective for pain reduction in patients with LBP.[161] The responders who reported a pain reduction of 2 or greater on the 11-point (0 to 10) NPRS immediately following the posterior-anterior and press-up treatment combination (10 minutes) had a greater increased L5-S1 IVD diffusion as compared to the nonresponders. The other commonly performed lumbar mobilization technique is the one described by Maitland and is performed in a manner similar to side-lying lumbar rotation manipulation (see Figure 16-8) but without the thrust component.[147,162] Lastly, distraction with or without using a belt (Figure 16-16) is a sustained lumbar mobilization technique used for increasing lumbar intersegmental space and for pain reduction.[158]

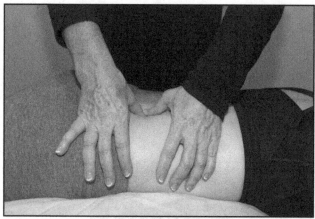

Figure 16-14. Unilateral posterior-to-anterior nonthrust manipulation.

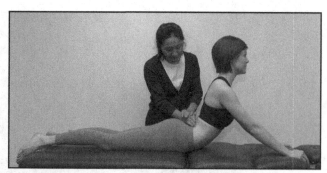

Figure 16-15. Prone press-up with posterior-to-anterior overpressure.

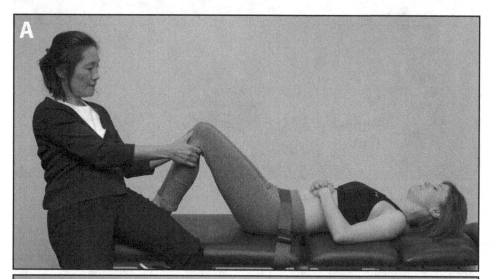

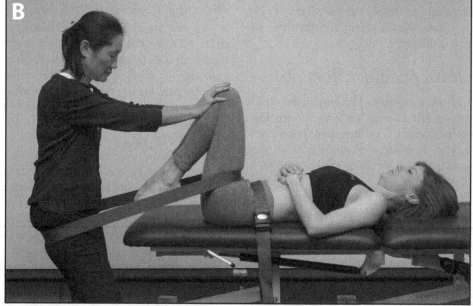

Figure 16-16. Manual traction. (A) Without use of a belt. (B) With use of a belt.

Several research studies[162-164] have shown no differences between thrust joint manipulations and nonthrust joint mobilizations for treating LBP. Cook et al[163] and Learman et al[162] compared nonthrust mobilization, including CPA glides, UPA glides, and side-lying rotation mobilization to supine lumbopelvic manipulation. In addition, Xia et al[164] compared a chiropractic side-lying flexion-distraction mobilization (hold end range for 1 to 3 seconds, 15 cycles) to the side-lying lumbar rotation manipulation.

Hypomobility in nonpainful lumbar segments and in adjacent joints, such as sacroiliac, hip, and thoracic, has long been considered to be a culprit for LBP, particularly in patients with instability or spondylolisthesis.[165,166] It is hypothesized that the lack of hip extension or thoracic or upper lumbar spine extension would increase demands of extension mobility in lower lumbar spine segments, in particular L4-L5 and L5-S1, thus resulting in LBP. Therefore, adding regional manual therapy of the adjacent joints (sacroiliac, hip, and thoracic) to manual therapy of the lumbar spine has been shown to be effective for reducing pain intensity,[167,168] improving function,[167-169] and greater perception of improvement[166] in patients with chronic LBP. In a case series, Burns et al[168] used a series of hip mobilization techniques for treating chronic LBP and had successful outcomes, including long-axis distraction thrust manipulation, supine anterior-posterior mobilization, inferior mobilization and prone posterior-anterior nonthrust mobilization with hip extended, and prone posterior-anterior nonthrust mobilization with the hip in FABER. Both Sung et al[169] and Zafereo et al[166] also demonstrated benefits of adding thoracic manipulations, including sitting and supine thoracic traction manipulations, to regional lumbar manual therapy for patients with chronic LBP. However, the effectiveness of regional manual therapy on adjacent joints has yet to be demonstrated for treating acute or subacute LBP.

Mobilization With Movement or Sustained Natural Apophyseal Glide

Mulligan's movement with mobilization (MWM) or sustained natural apophyseal glide (SNAG) is another common manual therapy approach used by physical therapists for addressing motion deficits and pain.[170] SNAG consists of posterior-anterior glides (central or unilateral) in the direction of the zygapophyseal joint orientation with active or passive physiological motions to a specific lumbar segment. SNAG of the lumbar spine is usually performed with the patient sitting or standing and with a belt to stabilize the pelvis (Figure 16-17). Unlike peripheral MWM to the elbow and ankle, which are well-supported by evidence,[171-174] no randomized clinical trials have been conducted to support the use of MWM or SNAGs to the lumbar spine. Nevertheless, SNAGs are often prescribed for patients with LBP as an additional manual therapy and can be easily converted to self-mobilization techniques for patients to perform independently as a part of a home exercise program. Although Moutzouri et al[175] did not find lumbar mobility improvement in healthy participants following a lumbar SNAG, Exelby[176] reported successful case management for 5 patients with LBP using SNAG techniques, including pain reduction and ROM improvement.

Muscle Energy Technique

The MET was developed by Fred Mitchell Sr, DO, about 50 years ago and is a common manual therapy technique for restoring mobility and improving strength.[177,178] The MET technique consists of 2 components: an isometric contraction and postcontraction relaxation. A recent systematic review[178] concluded that the quality of research for assessing the effects of MET on LBP is poor and that the available evidence is insufficient to determine whether or not MET would be effective for clinical management of LBP. However, this review did not distinguish between lumbar MET and sacroiliac MET, and only included studies in which effect size could be extracted for meta-analysis.

Lumbar Spine

Day and Nitz[179] performed a search of critically appraised topics and found that lumbar METs appeared to be effective in reducing disability for patients with LBP when combined with exercises over a 4-week period as compared to exercise alone. Schenk et al[180] found that the lumbar extension MET (Figure 16-18) significantly improved lumbar extension ROM in asymptomatic individuals. In addition, Wilson et al[181] combined the lumbar flexion MET (Figure 16-19) with supervised motor control and resistance exercises and successfully reduced the disability of patients with acute LBP and motion deficits.

Pelvis

Numerous METs (Figures 16-20 through 16-23) are available for treating sacroiliac and pubic dysfunctions. As with SIJ manipulations, there is a lack of research support for the use of the MET for treating sacroiliac or pubic dysfunctions because the confirmation of the dysfunction mainly relies on the examiner's observation, palpation of certain bony landmarks, and changes of landmarks relative position during movement. Selkow et al[182] found that patients with lumbopelvic pain who received sacroiliac METs had a greater reduction of their worst pain as compared to a group who received a sham treatment. Jonely et al[183] successfully used a multidisciplinary approach including a pubic MET to reduce pain and improve disability for a nulliparous woman with chronic sacroiliac dysfunction.

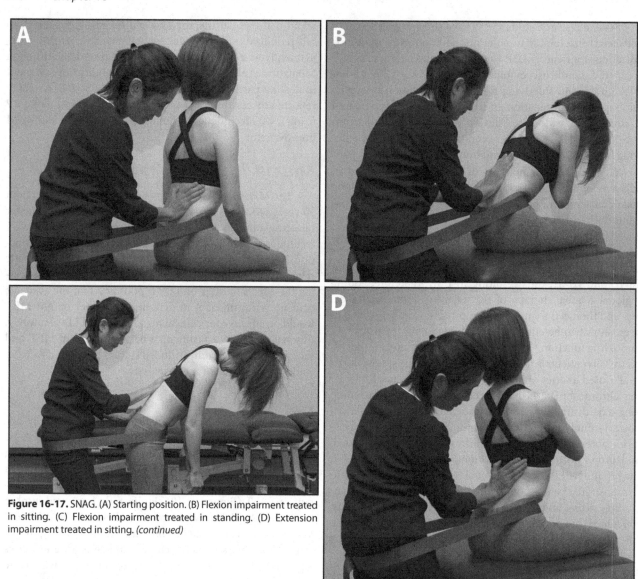

Figure 16-17. SNAG. (A) Starting position. (B) Flexion impairment treated in sitting. (C) Flexion impairment treated in standing. (D) Extension impairment treated in sitting. *(continued)*

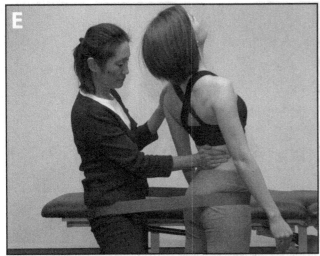

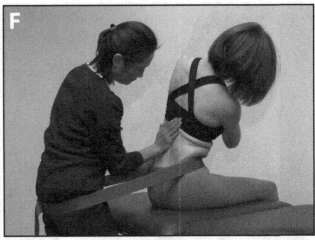

Figure 16-17 (continued). (E) Extension impairment treated in standing. (F) Side-flexion impairment treated in standing. (G) Self-treatment.

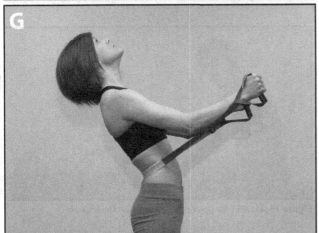

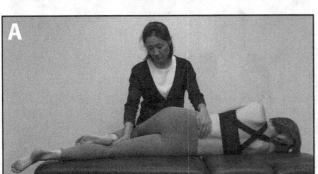

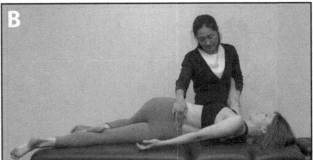

Figure 16-18. MET for lumbar extension. (A) Initial setup positioning into extension with right lower extremity. (B) Initial setup positioning into left rotation. (C) Isometric side-bending resistance provided to left lower extremity.

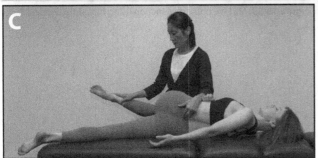

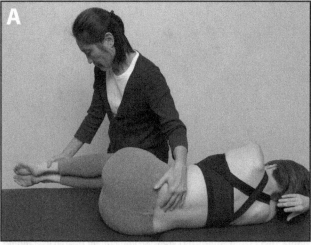
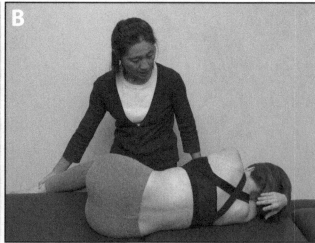

Figure 16-19. MET for lumbar flexion. (A) Initial setup positioning into flexion with bilateral lower extremities. (B) Providing side-bending resistance.

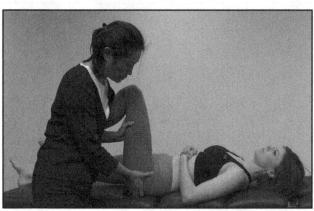

Figure 16-20. MET for anteriorly rotated left innominate.

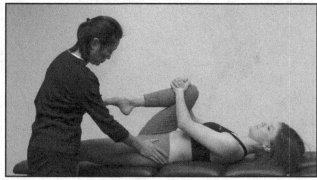

Figure 16-21. MET for posteriorly rotated left innominate.

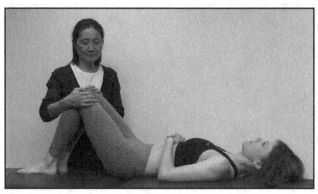

Figure 16-22. MET for pubic dysfunction using hip abduction resistance.

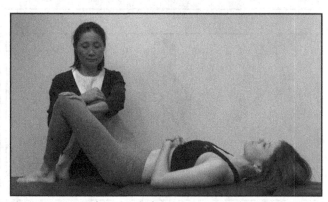

Figure 16-23. MET for pubic dysfunction using hip adduction resistance.

CONCLUSION

Strong evidence has shown that the combination of manual therapy and exercise is most effective in treating LBP.[125] Although thrust manipulation and nonthrust mobilization techniques are most often researched, a variety of manual therapy approaches are available when the thrust manipulation and nonthrust mobilization are not appropriate. It remains debated whether segment-specific lumbar manipulation is more effective than general nonspecific lumbar manipulation.

CASE STUDIES

Case Study One

Subjective Examination

A 37-year-old woman reports to physical therapy with right-sided LBP of insidious onset that occurred gradually over the last 4 months of pregnancy and has increased in intensity over the past 3 weeks. The pain at onset was located to the right buttock region and, over the past week, began radiating into the posterior thigh. Symptoms into the posterior thigh increase within 10 minutes of walking. Sitting is limited to less than 1 hour and standing to less than 15 minutes. She is unable to carry both infant carriers at one time due to pain. Symptom description is dull ache in the right buttock area (constant) and sharp pain into the posterior thigh (intermittent). Sleep is disturbed when rolling over. Pain is better upon awakening and varies throughout the day depending upon activity level. Average pain over the past 24 hours is 5/10 using the NPRS (current 5/10; best 3/10; worse 7/10). The patient denies bowel or bladder dysfunction, paresthesia, lower extremity weakness, or presence of night pain. She delivered (cesarean) twins 3 weeks ago and was on 7 months of bedrest up to the time of delivery. Prior to pregnancy, the patient participated in a regular fitness program 4 to 6 days per week. She is a full-time student in a PhD program. Past medical history is nonsignificant. The patient has not sought medical management for current symptoms; thus, no imaging studies have been conducted.

Patient-Reported Disability Measure

- Modified ODI: 44%

Signs of Depression and Psychosocial Distress

- Negative response to both depression-related screening questions.
- FABQ: 17/24 on FABQ physical activity (questions 2 through 5); 8/42 on work (questions 6, 7, 9 through 12, and 15).

Objective Examination

Observation

Movement from sitting to standing was performed slowly with report of a sharp pain into right low back region. The patient ambulates with a short step length of the right lower extremity and guarded trunk mobility. Pain increases during right lower extremity stance phase.

Posture

Assessed in standing. Pain upon standing from seated position is 5/10. Lumbar lordosis is reduced. Symmetry is present at the shoulders and scapula. Pelvic landmarks are also symmetric. There is no evidence of a lateral shift.

Pain Location

Point identification of pain inferomedial to the right PSIS.

Neurologic Testing

DTRs are 2+. No myotome weakness L2-S2. Sensation intact to light touch L2-S2.

Movement Testing

- Lumbar spine active movement testing: All movements are within normal limits (WNL; flexion is fingertips to ankles), no effect on symptoms, and no pain with overpressure. Noncentralization of symptoms with repeated movement testing.
- Aberrant movements: Painful arc of return and Gower's sign.
- Kinetic tests: Negative; however, pain limits the patient's ability to stand on right lower extremity to perform Gillet test.
- Hip: PROM/overpressure WNL, no effect on symptoms.

Provocation Stress Tests

Pain reproduction with SIJ distraction, decrease symptoms with compression. Right lower extremity FABER increases pain over the right SIJ. Lumbar posterior-anterior pressures have no effect on symptoms.

Neurodynamic Mobility Tests

Negative slump test and PSLR test.

First Level Evaluation

Medical referral is not indicated by the absence of red flags. Examination findings suggest nonspecific lumbopelvic pain; however, additional examination tests are needed to establish a clinical diagnosis.

Biomechanical Tests

PPIVM is normal, no effect on symptoms.

Special Tests

- Active straight leg raise: Positive right lower extremity (tremor of the leg while lifted, verbalized pain); pain decreased with supine compression and augmentation of anterior oblique system sling.
- SIJ cluster: All positive.
- Muscle performance tests: Inability to perform ADIM without holding breath and less than 5 seconds.
- Palpation: Tender with palpation to right sacral sulcus.

Clinical Questions Related to the Case

1. What is the interpretation of the self-report outcome measure?
2. Based on the results of the FABQ, does this patient present with potential psychosocial risk factors?
3. What examination tests support the hypothesis of non-specific lumbopelvic pain?
4. Which examination findings support the decision to perform special tests related to PGP?
5. Which examination findings would contribute to categorizing symptom acuity as acute?
6. What is the most appropriate diagnostic classification subgroup for this patient? Identify the examination findings that lead to this classification.
7. Provide primary intervention principles appropriate for the rehabilitation management of this case.

Case Study Two

Subjective Examination

A 45-year-old man self-referred to physical therapy by his primary care physician with pain radiating into his right lower extremity. Symptom onset was 5 days ago following a weekend cyclocross race competition. The pain at onset occurred immediately when he was dismounting and picking the bike up to cross over a plank barrier. The pain was located to the left low-back region and persisted through the remainder of the race (10 minutes). After returning to his home (a 1-hour drive) the same day, symptoms were radiating into the left posterior thigh. He currently reports pain (in the left low back and posterior thigh) and limited motion when standing upright and leaning to the left. Sitting tolerance is unrestricted; however, there is pain (3/10) when standing upright that decreases to 1/10 within 2 to 3 minutes. Standing pain is 3/10 at greater than 10 minutes. Walking is most painful at 6/10. Prefers to sleep supine with pillow under knees and is unable to lie prone.

Average pain over the past 24 hours is 3/10 using the NPRS (current 3/10; best 0/10; worse 6/10). The patient denies bowel or bladder dysfunction, paresthesia, lower extremity weakness, or presence of night pain. He owns a liquor store and is unable to lift and carry cases of liquor from the storeroom to the display areas without increase in LBP and pain into left thigh. He reports having 3 to 4 prior episodes of similar pain (difficulty standing upright and leaning to the left) over the past year since beginning participating in cyclocross racing. The pain typically resolves within 2 to 3 days after the race, with use of supine lying/feet elevated, use of ibuprofen (Advil) and gentle stretching. He has not received physical therapy for the past episodes of similar pain. Past medical history is nonsignificant. The decision for imaging studies will be made pending physical therapy examination and treatment.

Patient-Reported Disability Measure

- Modified ODI: 42%

Signs of Depression and Psychosocial Distress

- Negative response to both depression-related screening questions.
- FABQ: 9/24 on FABQ physical activity (questions 2 through 5); 10/42 on work (questions 6, 7, 9 through 12, and 15).

Objective Examination

Observation

Movement from sitting to standing was performed cautiously with reports of pain when attempting to attain full upright standing (rated 3/10; no worse). Normal gait pattern, however, walks with slight flexed trunk posture.

Pain Location

Left low back region with pain into left posterior thigh with provoking movements.

Posture

Assessed in standing. Stands in a protective scoliosis with slight flexed trunk posture and right lateral flexion. When in this preferred posture pain is 0/10, and when attempting to correct deviations pain is 3/10 (no worse). There is no evidence of a lateral shift.

Palpation

Left iliac crest high; left PSIS low; left ASIS high; sacral sulci symmetric.

Neurologic Testing

DTR are 2+. No myotome weakness L2-S2. Sensation intact to light touch L2-S2.

Movement Testing

- Lumbar spine active movement testing: Flexion 100% (stiffness); extension less than 10%, pain 4/10; lateral flexion left 50%, pain 3/10; lateral flexion right 100%, pain 0/10; rotation left 100%, no rotation right 90%, pain 1/10. Pain occurred prior to end ROM in extension, lateral flexion left and at end ROM during rotation right. Noncentralization of symptoms with repeated movement testing.
- Lumbopelvic rhythm: Flexion performed with greater hip motion than lumbar during forward bending.
- Aberrant movements: Nonreversal of lumbopelvic rhythm.
- Kinetic tests: Fixation of left ilium in standing forward bend test.
- Hip: PROM/overpressure WNL, no effect on symptoms.

Provocation Stress Tests

Positive lumbar posterior-anterior spring test at L3-L5; negative lumbar torsion test; negative SIJ gapping/compression.

Neurodynamic Mobility Tests

Positive PSLR test left at 50 degrees.

First Level Evaluation

Medical referral is not indicated by the absence of red flags. Examination findings suggest nonspecific lumbopelvic pain with provisional classification as mobility deficit or radicular pain. Additional examination tests are needed to confirm location of mobility deficit to lumbar, pelvis, or sacral regions.

Biomechanical Tests

PPIVM is lumbar extension and left side flexion hypomobile, painful; normal, no effect on symptoms. PAIVM: Lumbar CPA and UPA pressures hypomobile and pain (3/10; abnormal end-feel; pain with tissue resistance) at L4/5, L5/S1.

Pelvic passive accessory motion: Hypomobile anterior rotation left ilium.

Special Tests

- SIJ cluster: Negative.

Clinical Questions Related to the Case

1. Which examination findings would contribute to categorizing symptom acuity as subacute?
2. Based on the results of the FABQ, does this patient present with potential psychosocial risk factors?
3. What examination tests support the hypothesis of lumbar mobility deficits?
4. What examination tests support the hypothesis of pelvic mobility deficits?
5. What examination tests support the hypothesis of radicular pain?
6. Which examination findings support the decision to perform lumbar and pelvic biomechanical tests?
7. What is the most appropriate diagnostic classification subgroup for this patient? Identify the examination findings that led to this classification.
8. Provide primary intervention principles appropriate for the rehabilitation management of this case.

REFERENCES

1. Wong CK, Johnson EK. A narrative review of evidence-based recommendations for the physical examination of the lumbar spine, sacroiliac and hip joint complex. *Musculoskeletal Care.* 2012;10(3):149-161. doi:10.1002/msc.1012
2. Ma VY, Chan L, Carruthers KJ. Incidence, prevalence, costs, and impact on disability of common conditions requiring rehabilitation in the United States: stroke, spinal cord injury, traumatic brain injury, multiple sclerosis, osteoarthritis, rheumatoid arthritis, limb loss, and back pain. *Arch Phys Med Rehabil.* 2014;95(5):986-995.e1. doi:10.1016/j.apmr.2013.10.032
3. Ladeira CE, Cheng SM, Hill CJ. Physical therapists' treatment choices for non-specific low back pain in Florida: an electronic survey. *J Man Manip Ther.* 2015;23(2):109-118. doi:10.1179/20426186 13Y.0000000065
4. Fritz JM, Childs JD, Wainner RS, Flynn TW. Primary care referral of patients with low back pain to physical therapy: Impact on future health care utilization and costs. *Spine.* 2012;37(25):2114-2121. doi:10.1097/BRS.0b013e31825d32f5
5. Gardner K. Physical therapy workforce data. American Physical Therapy Association. Accessed December 21, 2016. http://www.apta.org/WorkforceData/
6. Norris C. Spinal stabilisation: 2. Limiting factors to end-range motion in the lumbar spine. *J Physiother.* 1995;81(2):64-72. doi:10.1016/S0031-9406(05)67047-2
7. Roberts S, Johnson WE. Analysis of aging and degeneration of the human intervertebral disc. *Spine.* 1999;24(5):500-501.
8. Neumann D. *Kinesiology of the Musculoskeletal System. Foundations for Rehabilitation.* 2nd ed. Elsevier; 2010.
9. Legaspi O, Edmond SL. Does the evidence support the existence of lumbar spine coupled motion? A critical review of the literature. *J Orthop Sports Phys Ther.* 2007;37(4):169-178. doi:10.2519/jospt.2007.2300

10. Goode A, Hegedus EJ, Sizer P, Brismee J.-M, Linberg A, Cook CE. (2008). Three-dimensional movements of the sacroiliac joint: a systematic review of the literature and assessment of clinical utility. *J Man Manip Ther.* 2008;16(1);25-38. doi:10.1179/106698108790818639

11. Vleeming A, Schuenke MD, Masi AT, Carreiro JE, Danneels L, Willard FH. The sacroiliac joint: an overview of its anatomy, function and potential clinical implications. *J Anat.* 2012;221(6):537-567. doi:10.1111/j.1469-7580.2012.01564.x

12. Aslan E, Fynes M. (2007). Symphysial pelvic dysfunction. *Curr Opin Obstet Gynecol.* 2007;19(2):133-139. doi:10.1097/GCO.0b013e328034f138

13. Becker I, Woodley SJ, Stringer MD. The adult human pubic symphysis: a systematic review. *J Anat.* 2010:217(5);475-487. doi:10.1111/j.1469-7580.2010.01300.x

14. Esola MA, McClure PW, Fitzgerald GK, Siegler S. Analysis of lumbar spine and hip motion during forward bending in subjects with and without a history of low back pain. *Spine.* 1996;21(1):71-78.

15. Tafazzol A, Arjmand N, Shirazi-Adl A, Parnianpour M. Lumbopelvic rhythm during forward and backward sagittal trunk rotations: combined in vivo measurement with inertial tracking device and biomechanical modeling. *Clin Biomech.* 2014;29(1):7-13. doi:10.1016/j.clinbiomech.2013.10.021

16. Hicks GE, Fritz JM, Delitto A, Mishock J. Interrater reliability of clinical examination measures for identification of lumbar segmental instability. *Arch Phys Med Rehabil.* 2003;84(12):1858–1864.

17. Panjabi MM. The stabilizing system of the spine. Part I. Function, dysfunction, adaptation, and enhancement. *J Spinal Disord Tech.* 1992;5(4):383-389.

18. Panjabi MM. The stabilizing system of the spine. Part I. Function, dysfunction, adaptation, and enhancement. *J Spinal Disord Tech.* 1992;5(4):383-389.

19. Panjabi MM. The stabilizing system of the spine. Part I. Function, dysfunction, adaptation, and enhancement. *J Spinal Disord Tech.* 1992;5(4):383-389.

20. O'Sullivan PB. Lumbar segmental "instability": Clinical presentation and specific stabilizing exercise management. *Man Ther.* 2000;5(1):2-12. doi:10.1054/math.1999.0213

21. Alqarni AM, Schneiders AG, Hendrick PA. Clinical tests to diagnose lumbar segmental instability: a systematic review. *J Orthop Sports Phys Ther.* 2011;41(3):130-140. doi:10.2519/jospt.2011.3457

22. Alyazedi FM, Lohman EB, Wesley Swen R, Bahjri K. The inter-rater reliability of clinical tests that best predict the subclassification of lumbar segmental instability: structural, functional and combined instability. *J Man Manip Ther.* 2015;23(4):197-204. doi:10.1179/2042618615Y.0000000002

23. Beazell JR, Mullins M, Grindstaff TL. (2010). Lumbar instability: an evolving and challenging concept. *J Man Manip Ther.* 2010;18(1):9-14. doi:10.1179/106698110X12595770849443

24. Denteneer L, Stassijns G, De Hertogh W, Truijen S, Van Daele U. Inter- and intrarater reliability of clinical tests associated with functional lumbar segmental instability and motor control impairment in patients with low back pain: a systematic review. *Arch Phys Med Rehabil.* 2017;98(1):151-164. doi:10.1016/j.apmr.2016.07.020

25. Cohen SP. Sacroiliac joint pain: a comprehensive review of anatomy, diagnosis, and treatment. *Anesth Analg.* 2005;101(5):1440-1453. doi:10.1213/01.ANE.0000180831.60169.EA

26. Vleeming A, Stoeckart R, Volkers AC, Snijders CJ. Relation between form and function in the sacroiliac joint. Part I: clinical anatomical aspects. *Spine.* 1990;15(2):130-132.

27. Vleeming A, Volkers AC, Snijders CJ, Stoeckart R. Relation between form and function in the sacroiliac joint. Part II: biomechanical aspects. *Spine.* 1990;15(2):133-136.

28. Pool-Goudzwaard AL, Vleeming A, Stoeckart R, Snijders CJ, Mens JMA. Insufficient lumbopelvic stability: a clinical, anatomical and biomechanical approach to "a-specific" low back pain. *Man Ther.* 1998;3(1):12-20. doi:10.1054/math.1998.0311

29. Willard FH, Vleeming A, Schuenke MD, Danneels L, Schleip R. The thoracolumbar fascia: Anatomy, function and clinical considerations. *J Anat.* 2012;221(6):507-536. doi:10.1111/j.1469-7580.2012.01511.x

30. Arumugam A, Milosavljevic S, Woodley S, Sole G. Effects of external pelvic compression on form closure, force closure, and neuromotor control of the lumbopelvic spine—a systematic review. *Man Ther.* 2012;17(4):275-284. doi:10.1016/j.math.2012.01.010

31. Brumitt J, Matheson JW, Meira EP. Core stabilization exercise prescription, part I. *Sports Health.* 2013:5(6);504-509. doi:10.1177/1941738113502451

32. O'Sullivan PB, Beales DJ. Diagnosis and classification of pelvic girdle pain disorders, part 1: a mechanism based approach within a biopsychosocial framework. *Man Ther.* 2007a;12(2):86-97. doi:10.1016/j.math.2007.02.001

33. O'Sullivan PB. It's time for change with the management of non-specific chronic low back pain. *Br J Sports Med.* 2012;46(4):224-227. doi:10.1136/bjsm.2010.081638

34. Koes BW, van Tulder MW, Thomas S. Diagnosis and treatment of low back pain. *BMJ.* 2006;332(7555):1430-1434. doi:10.1136/bmj.332.7555.1430

35. O'Sullivan PB, Lin IB. Acute low back pain: beyond drug therapies. *P Manag Today.* 2014;1(1):814.

36. Delitto A, George SZ, Van Dillen L, et al. Low back pain. *J Orthop Sports Phys Ther.* 2012;42(4):A1-A57. doi:10.2519/jospt.2012.42.4.A1

37. McKenzie R. *The Lumbar Spine: Mechanical diagnosis and therapy.* 2nd ed. Spinal Publications; 2003.

38. Laslett M. Evidence-based diagnosis and treatment of the painful sacroiliac joint. *J Man Manip Ther.* 2008;16:142-152.

39. Stuber KJ. Specificity, sensitivity, and predictive values of clinical tests of the sacroiliac joint: a systematic review of the literature. *J Can Chiropr Assoc.* 2007;51(1):30-41.

40. Hamidi-Ravari B, Tafazoli S, Chen H, Perret D. Diagnosis and current treatments for sacroiliac joint dysfunction: a review. *Curr Phys Med Rehabil Rep.* 2014;2(1):48-54.

41. O'Sullivan PB, Beales DJ. Diagnosis and classification of pelvic girdle pain disorders, part 1: a mechanism based approach within a biopsychosocial framework. *Man Ther.* 2007b;12(2):86-97. doi:10.1016/j.math.2007.02.001

42. Alrwaily M, Timko M, Schneider M, et al. Treatment-based classification system for low back pain: revision and update. *Phys Ther.* 2016;96(7):1057-1066. doi:10.2522/ptj.20150345

43. Delitto A, Bowling R. (1995). A treatment-based classification approach to low back syndrome: identifying and staging patients for conservative treatment. *Phys Ther.* 1995;75:470-485.

44. Fritz JM, Brennan GP, Clifford SN, Hunter SJ, Thackeray A. An examination of the reliability of a classification algorithm for sub-grouping patients with low back pain. *Spine.* 2006;31(1):77-82.

45. Fritz JM, Cleland JA, Childs JD. Subgrouping patients with low back pain: evolution of a classification approach to physical therapy. *J Orthop Sports Phys Ther.* 2007;37(6):290-302. doi:10.2519/jospt.2007.2498

46. Barakatt ET, Romano PS, Riddle DL, Beckett LA. The reliability of Maitland's irritability judgments in patients with low back pain. *J Man Manip Ther.* 2009;17(3):135-140. doi:10.1179/jmt.2009.17.3.135

47. Barakatt ET, Romano PS, Riddle DL, Beckett LA, Kravitz R. An exploration of Maitland's concept of pain irritability in patients with low back pain. *J Man Manip Ther.* 2009;17(4):196-205. doi:10.1179/106698109791352175

48. Childs JD, Piva SR, Fritz JM. Responsiveness of the numeric pain rating scale in patients with low back pain. *Spine.* 2005;30(11):1331-1334.

49. Jensen MP, Turner JA, Romano JM. What is the maximum number of levels needed in pain intensity measurement? *Pain.* 1994;58(3):387-392.

50. Leerar PJ, Boissonnault W, Domholdt E, Roddey T. Documentation of red flags by physical therapists for patients with low back pain. *J Man Manip Ther.* 2007;15(1):42-49.

51. Nicholas MK, Linton SJ, Watson PJ, Main CJ. Early identification and management of psychological risk factors ("yellow flags") in patients with low back pain: a reappraisal. *Phys Ther.* 2011;91(5):737-753. doi:10.2522/ptj.20100224

52. George SZ, Beneciuk JM, Bialosky JE, et al. (2015). Development of a review-of-systems screening tool for orthopaedic physical therapists: results from the optimal screening for prediction of referral and outcome (OSPRO) cohort. *J Orthop Sports Phys Ther.* 2015;45(7):512-526. doi:10.2519/jospt.2015.5900

53. Pinheiro MB, Ferreira ML, Refshauge K, et al. Symptoms of depression as a prognostic factor for low back pain: a systematic review. *Spine.* 2016;16(1):105-116. doi:10.1016/j.spinee.2015.10.037

54. Alhowimel A, AlOtaibi M, Radford K, Coulson N. Psychosocial factors associated with change in pain and disability outcomes in chronic low back pain patients treated by physiotherapist: a systematic review. *SAGE Open Med.* 2018;6:2050312118757387. doi:10.1177/2050312118757387

55. Sattelmayer M, Lorenz T, Röder C, Hilfiker R. Predictive value of the acute low back pain screening questionnaire and the Örebro musculoskeletal pain screening questionnaire for persisting problems. *Eur Spine J.* 2012;21(Suppl 6):773-784. doi:10.1007/s00586-011-1910-7

56. Haggman S, Maher CG, Refshauge KM. Screening for symptoms of depression by physical therapists managing low back pain. *Phys Ther.* 2004;84(12):1157-1166.

57. Spitzer RL, Williams JB, Kroenke K, et al. Utility of a new procedure for diagnosing mental disorders in primary care. The PRIME-MD 1000 study. *JAMA.* 1994;272(22):1749-1756.

58. Lombardo P, Vaucher P, Haftgoli N, et al. The "help" question doesn't help when screening for major depression: external validation of the three-question screening test for primary care patients managed for physical complaints. *BMC.* 2011;9:114. doi:10.1186/1741-7015-9-114

59. Arroll B, Goodyear-Smith F, Kerse N, Fishman T, Gunn J. Effect of the addition of a "help" question to two screening questions on specificity for diagnosis of depression in general practice: diagnostic validity study. *BMJ.* 2005;331(7521):884. doi:10.1136/bmj.38607.464537.7C

60. Linton SJ, Boersma K. (2003). Early identification of patients at risk of developing a persistent back problem: the predictive validity of the Orebro Musculoskeletal Pain Questionnaire. *Clin J Pain.* 2003;19(2):80-86.

61. Fritz JM, Beneciuk JM, George SZ. Relationship between categorization with the STarT back screening tool and prognosis for people receiving physical therapy for low back pain. *Phys Ther.* 2011;91(5):722-732. doi:10.2522/ptj.20100109

62. Waddell G, Newton M, Henderson I, Somerville D, Main CJ. A fear-avoidance beliefs questionnaire (FABQ) and the role of fear-avoidance beliefs in chronic low back pain and disability. *Pain.* 1993;52(2):157-168.

63. Ikemoto T, Miki K, Matsubara T, Wakao N. Psychological treatment strategy for chronic low back pain. *Spine Surg Relat Res.* 2019;3(3):199-206. doi:10.22603/ssrr.2018-0050

64. Cyriax J. *Textbook of Orthopedic Medicine.* 8th ed. Balliere Tindall and Cassell; 1982.

65. Hill JC, Dunn KM, Lewis M, et al. A primary care back pain screening tool: identifying patient subgroups for initial treatment. *Arthritis Rheum.* 2008;59(5):632-641. doi:10.1002/art.23563

66. Sullivan M, Bishop S, Pivik J. The Pain Catastrophizing Scale: Development and Validation. *Psychol Assess.* 1995;7(4):524-532.

67. Fortin JD, Falco FJ. The Fortin finger test: an indicator of sacroiliac pain. *Am J Orthop.* 1997;26(7):477-480.

68. Cook C. *Orthopedic Manual Therapy: An Evidenced Based Approach.* Pearson Prentice Hall; 2007.

69. Levangie PK. Four clinical tests of sacroiliac joint dysfunction: the association of test results with innominate torsion among patients with and without low back pain. *Phys Ther.* 1999;79(11):1043-1057.

70. Cooperstein R, Hickey M. The reliability of palpating the posterior superior iliac spine: a systematic review. *J Can Chiropr Assoc.* 2016;60(1):36-46.

71. Kilby J, Heneghan NR, Maybury M. Manual palpation of lumbo-pelvic landmarks: a validity study. *Man Ther.* 2012;17(3), 259-262. doi:10.1016/j.math.2011.08.008

72. Donahue MS, Riddle DL, Sullivan MS. Intertester reliability of a modified version of McKenzie's lateral shift assessments obtained on patients with low back pain. *Phys Ther.* 1996;76(7):706-716.

73. Razmjou H, Kramer JF, Yamada R. Intertester reliability of the McKenzie evaluation in assessing patients with mechanical low-back pain. *J Orthop Sports Phys Ther.* 2000;30(7):368-383. doi:10.2519/jospt.2000.30.7.368

74. Biely SA, Silfies SP, Smith SS, Hicks GE. Clinical observation of standing trunk movements: what do the aberrant movement patterns tell us? *J Orthop Sports Phys Ther.* 2014a;44(4):262-272. doi:10.2519/jospt.2014.4988

75. Laslett M, Aprill CN, McDonald B, Oberg B. Clinical predictors of lumbar provocation discography: a study of clinical predictors of lumbar provocation discography. *Eur Spine J.* 2006;15(10):1-12. doi:10.1007/s00586-006-0062-7

76. Laslett M, Oberg B, Aprill CN, McDonald B. Centralization as a predictor of provocation discography results in chronic low back pain, and the influence of disability and distress on diagnostic power. *Spine.* 2005;5(4);370-380.

77. Clare HA, Adams R, Maher CG. Reliability of McKenzie classification of patients with cervical or lumbar pain. *J Manipulative Physiol Ther.* 2005;28(2):122-127. doi:10.1016/j.jmpt.2005.01.003

78. Hefford C. McKenzie classification of mechanical spinal pain: Profile of syndromes and directions of preference. *Man Ther.* 2008;13(1):75-81. doi:10.1016/j.math.2006.08.005

79. Werneke MW, Deutscher D, Hart DL, et al. McKenzie lumbar classification: Inter-rater agreement by physical therapists with different levels of formal McKenzie postgraduate training. *Spine.* 2014;39(3):E182-E190. doi:10.1097/BRS.0000000000000117

80. Kilpikoski S, Airaksinen O, Kankaanpää M, Leminen P, Videman T, Alen M. Interexaminer reliability of low back pain assessment using the McKenzie method. *Spine.* 2002;27(8):E207-E214.

81. Cibulka MT, Koldehoff R. Clinical usefulness of a cluster of sacroiliac joint tests in patients with and without low back pain. *J Orthop Sports Phys Ther.* 1999;29(2):83-89. doi:10.2519/jospt.1999.29.2.83

82. Arab AM, Abdollahi I, Joghataei MT, Golafshani Z, Kazemnejad A. Inter- and intra-examiner reliability of single and composites of selected motion palpation and pain provocation tests for sacroiliac joint. *Man Ther.* 2015;14(2):213-221. doi:10.1016/j.math.2008.02.004

83. Dreyfuss P, Michaelsen M, Pauza K, McLarty J, Bogduk N. The value of medical history and physical examination in diagnosing sacroiliac joint pain. *Spine.* 1996;21(22):2594-2602.

84. Majlesi J, Togay H, Unalan H, Toprak S. The sensitivity and specificity of the Slump and the Straight Leg Raising tests in patients with lumbar disc herniation. *J Clin Rheumatol.* 2008;14(2):87-91. doi:10.1097/RHU.0b013e31816b2f99

85. Ekedahl H, Jönsson B, Annertz M, Frobell RB. (2018). Accuracy of clinical tests in detecting disk herniation and nerve root compression in subjects with lumbar radicular symptoms. *Arch Phys Med Rehabil.* 2018;99(4);726-735. doi:10.1016/j.apmr.2017.11.006

86. Iversen T, Solberg TK, Romner B, et al. Accuracy of physical examination for chronic lumbar radiculopathy. *BMC Musculoskelet Disord.* 2013;14:206. doi:10.1186/1471-2474-14-206

87. Tawa N, Rhoda A, Diener I. Accuracy of clinical neurological examination in diagnosing lumbo-sacral radiculopathy: a systematic literature review. *BMC Musculoskelet Disord.* 2017;18(1):93. doi:10.1186/s12891-016-1383-2

88. Prather H, Cheng A, Steger-May K, Maheshwari V, Van Dillen L. Hip and lumbar spine physical examination findings in people presenting with low back pain, with or without lower extremity pain. *J Orthop Sports Phys Ther.* 2017;47(3):163–172. doi:10.2519/jospt.2017.6567

89. Flynn T, Fritz J, Whitman J, et al. A clinical prediction rule for classifying patients with low back pain who demonstrate short-term improvement with spinal manipulation. *Spine.* 2002;27(24):2835-2843. doi:10.1097/00007632-200212150-00021

90. Laslett M, Aprill CN, McDonald B, Young SB. Diagnosis of sacroiliac joint pain: validity of individual provocation tests and composites of tests. *Man Ther.* 2005;10(3):207-218. doi:10.1016/j.math.2005.01.003

91. Burns SA, Mintken PE, Austin GP. Clinical decision making in a patient with secondary hip-spine syndrome. *Physiother Theory Pract.* 2011;27(5):384-397. doi:10.3109/09593985.2010.509382

92. Meadows J. *Differential Diagnosis in Orthopaedic Physical Therapy: A Case Study Approach.* McGraw-Hill; 1999.

93. Abbott JH, McCane B, Herbison P, Moginie G, Chapple C, Hogarty T. Lumbar segmental instability: A criterion-related validity study of manual therapy assessment. *BMC Musculoskelet Disord.* 2005;6:59. doi:10.1186/1471-2474-6-56

94. Abbott JH, Flynn TW, Fritz JM, Hing WA, Reid D, Whitman JM. Manual physical assessment of spinal segmental motion: intent and validity. *Man Ther.* 2009;14(1):36-44. doi:10.1016/j.math.2007.09.011

95. Teyhen DS, Flynn TW, Childs JD, Abraham LD. (2007). Arthrokinematics in a subgroup of patients likely to benefit from a lumbar stabilization exercise program. *Phys Ther.* 2007;87(3):313-325. doi:10.2522/ptj.20060253

96. Abbott JH, Mercer S. Lumbar segmental hypomobility: criterion-related validity of clinical examination items (a pilot study). *N. Z. J Physiother.* 2005;31(1):3-9.

97. Fritz JM, Piva SR, Childs JD. Accuracy of the clinical examination to predict radiographic instability of the lumbar spine. *Eur Spine J.* 2005;14(8):743-750. doi:10.1007/s00586-004-0803-4

98. Seffinger MA, Najm WI, Mishra SI, et al. Reliability of spinal palpation for diagnosis of back and neck pain: a systematic review of the literature. *Spine.* 2004;29(19):E413-E425.

99. Schneider M, Erhard R, Brach J, Tellin W, Imbarlina F, Delitto A. Spinal palpation for lumbar segmental mobility and pain provocation: an interexaminer reliability study. *J Manipulative Physiol Ther.* 2008;31(6):465-473. doi:10.1016/j.jmpt.2008.06.004

100. Huijbregts PA. (2002). Spinal motion palpation: a review of reliability studies. *J Man Manip Ther.* 2002;10(1):24-39.

101. Alyazedi FM, Lohman EB, Wesley Swen R, Bahjri K. (2015b). The inter-rater reliability of clinical tests that best predict the subclassification of lumbar segmental instability: structural, functional and combined instability. *J Man Manip Ther.* 2015;23(4):197-204. doi:10.1179/2042618615Y.0000000002

102. Knutsson F. The instability associated with disk degeneration in the lumbar spine. *Acta Radiologica.* 1994;25(5-6):593-609. doi:10.3109/00016924409136488

103. Ferrari S, Manni T, Bonetti F, Villafañe JH, Vanti C. A literature review of clinical tests for lumbar instability in low back pain: validity and applicability in clinical practice. *Chiropr Man Ther.* 2015;23:14. doi:10.1186/s12998-015-0058-7

104. Portney LG, Watkins MP. *Foundations of Clinical Research: Applications to Practice.* 3rd ed. Pearson Prentice Hall; 2009.

105. Biely SA, Silfies SP, Smith SS, Hicks GE. Clinical observation of standing trunk movements: what do the aberrant movement patterns tell us? *J Orthop Sports Phys Ther.* 2014b:44(4):262-272.

106. Kasai Y, Morishita K, Kawakita E, Kondo T, Uchida A. A new evaluation method for lumbar spinal instability: passive lumbar extension test. *Phys Ther.* 2006;68:1661-1667.

107. Rabin A, Shashua A, Pizem K, Dar G. The interrater reliability of physical examination tests that may predict the outcome or suggest the need for lumbar stabilization exercises. *J Orthop Sports Phys Ther.* 2013;43(2), 83-90. doi:10.2519/jospt.2013.4310

108. Hicks GE, Fritz JM, Delitto A, McGill SM. Preliminary development of a clinical prediction rule for determining which patients with low back pain will respond to a stabilization exercise program. *Arch Phys Med Rehabil.* 2005;86(9):1753-1762. doi:10.1016/j.apmr.2005.03.033

109. Fritz JM, Piva SR, Childs JD. Accuracy of the clinical examination to predict radiographic instability of the lumbar spine. *Eur Spine J.* 2005;14(8):743–750. doi:10.1007/s00586-004-0803-4

110. Luomajoki H, Kool J, de Bruin ED, Airaksinen O. Reliability of movement control tests in the lumbar spine. *BMC Musculoskelet Disord.* 2007;8:90. doi:10.1186/1471-2474-8-90

111. Vleeming A, Albert HB, Östgaard HC, Sturesson B, Stuge B. European guidelines for the diagnosis and treatment of pelvic girdle pain. *Euro Spine J.* 2008;17(6):794-819. doi:10.1007/s00586-008-0602-4

112. Laslett M, Young SB, April CN, McDonald B. Diagnosing painful sacroiliac joints: a validity study of a McKenzie evaluation and sacroiliac provocation tests. *Aust J Physiother.* 2003;49(2):89-97.

113. van der Wurff P, Hagmeijer RH, Meyne W. Clinical tests of the sacroiliac joint. A systematic methodological review. Part 1: reliability. *Man Ther.* 2000;5(1):30-36. doi:10.1054/math.1999.0228

114. Hancock MJ, Maher CG, Latimer J, et al. Systematic review of tests to identify the disc, SIJ or facet joint as the source of low back pain. *Eur Spine J.* 2007;16(10):1539-1550. doi:10.1007/s00586-007-0391-1

115. Albert H, Godskesen M, Westergaard J. Evaluation of clinical tests used in classification procedures in pregnancy-related pelvic joint pain. *Eur Spine J.* 2000;9(2):161-166. doi:10.1007/s005860050228

116. O'Sullivan PB, Beales DJ. Diagnosis and classification of pelvic girdle pain disorders, part 2: illustration of the utility of a classification system via case studies. *Man Ther.* 2007;12:e1-e12.

117. Holmgren U, Waling K. Inter-examiner reliability of four static palpation tests used for assessing pelvic dysfunction. *Man Ther.* 2008;13(1):50-56. doi:10.1016/j.math.2006.09.009

118. Richardson C, Jull G, Hodges PW, Hides JA. *Therapeutic Exercise for Spinal Segmental Stabilization in Low Back Pain: Scientfc Basis and Clinical Approach.* Churchill Livingstone; 1999.

119. McGill SM, Childs A, Liebenson C. Endurance times for low back stabilization exercises: clinical targets for testing and training from a normal database. *Arch Phys Med Rehabil.* 1999;80(8):941-944.

120. Schellenberg KL, Lang JM, Chan KM, Burnham RS. A clinical tool for office assessment of lumbar spine stabilization endurance: prone and supine bridge maneuvers. *Am J Phys Med Rehabil.* 2007;86(5):380-386. doi:10.1097/PHM.0b013e318032156a

121. Kisner C, Colby LA. *Therapeutic Exercise: Foundations and Techniques.* 6th ed. F. A. Davis; 2012.

122. Dagenais S, Gay RE, Tricco AC, Freeman MD, Mayer JM. NASS contemporary concepts in spine care: spinal manipulation therapy for acute low back pain. *Spine.* 2010;10(10):918-40. doi:10.1016/j.spinee.2010.07.389

123. Ruddock JK, Sallis H, Ness A, Perry RE. Spinal manipulation vs sham manipulation for nonspecific low back pain: a systematic review and meta-analysis. *J Chiropr Med.* 2016;15(3):165-183. doi:10.1016/j.jcm.2016.04.014

124. Cecchi F, Molino-Lova R, Chiti M, et al. Spinal manipulation compared with back school and with individually delivered physiotherapy for the treatment of chronic low back pain: a randomized trial with one-year follow-up. *Clin Rehabil.* 2010;24(1):26-36. doi:10.1177/0269215509342328

125. Delitto A, George SZ, Van Dillen LR, et al. Low back pain. *J Orthop Sports Phys Ther.* 2012;42(4):A1-A57. doi:10.2519/jospt.2012.424. A1

126. Flynn T, Fritz J, Whitman J, et al. A clinical prediction rule for classifying patients with low back pain who demonstrate short-term improvement with spinal manipulation. *Spine.* 2002;27(24):2835-2843. doi:10.1097/00007632-200212150-00021

127. Childs JD, Fritz JM, Flynn TW, et al. A clinical prediction rule to identify patients with low back pain most likely to benefit from spinal manipulation: a validation study. *Ann Intern Med.* 2004;141(12):920-928. doi:10.7326/0003-4819-141-12-200412210-00008

128. Fritz JM, Childs JD, Flynn TW. Pragmatic application of a clinical prediction rule in primary care to identify patients with low back pain with a good prognosis following a brief spinal manipulation intervention. *BMC Fam Pract.* 2005;6(1):29. doi:10.1186/1471-2296-6-29

129. Senna MK, Machaly SA. Does maintained spinal manipulation therapy for chronic nonspecific low back pain result in better long-term outcome? *Spine.* 2011;36(18):1427-1437. doi:10.1097/BRS.0b013e3181f5dfoe

130. Vavrek DA, Sharma R, Haas M. Cost analysis related to dose-response of spinal manipulative therapy for chronic low back pain: outcomes from a randomized controlled trial. *J Manipulative Physiol Ther.* 2014;37(5):300-311. doi:10.1016/j.jmpt.2014.03.002

131. Flynn TW, Fritz JM, Wainner RS, Whitman JM. The audible pop is not necessary for successful spinal high-velocity thrust manipulation in individuals with low back pain. *Arch Phys Med Rehabil.* 2003;84(7):1057-1060. doi:10.1016/s0003-9993(03)00048-0

132. Selhorst M, Selhorst B. Lumbar manipulation and exercise for the treatment of acute low back pain in adolescents: a randomized controlled trial. *J Man Manip Ther.* 2015;23(4):226-233. doi:10.1179/2042618614Y.0000000099

133. Castro-Sánchez AM, Lara-Palomo IC, Matarán-Peñarrocha GA, et al. Short-term effectiveness of spinal manipulative therapy versus functional technique in patients with chronic nonspecific low back pain: a pragmatic randomized controlled trial. *Spine.* 2016;16(3):302-312. doi:10.1016/j.spinee.2015.08.057

134. Cramer GD, Cambron J, Cantu JA, et al. Magnetic resonance imaging zygapophyseal joint space changes (gapping) in low back pain patients following spinal manipulation and side-posture positioning: a randomized controlled mechanisms trial with blinding. *J Manipulative Physiol Ther.* 2013;36(4):203-217. doi:10.1016/j.jmpt.2013.04.003

135. Greeman PE. *Principles of Manual Medicine.* 2nd ed. Williams & Wilkins; 1996.

136. Cleland JA, Fritz JM, Kulig K, et al. Comparison of the effectiveness of three manual physical therapy techniques in a subgroup of patients with low back pain who satisfy a clinical prediction rule. A randomized clinical trial. *Spine.* 2009;34:2720-2729. doi:10.1097/BRS.0b013e31b48809

137. Vieira-Pellenz F, Oliva-Pascual-Vaca A, Rodriguez-Blanco C, Heredia-Rizo AM, Ricard F, Almazán-Campos G. Short-term effect of spinal manipulation on pain perception, spinal mobility, and full height recovery in male subjects with degenerative disk disease: a randomized controlled trial. *Arch Phys Med Rehabil.* 2014;95(9):1613-1619. doi:10.1016/j.apmr.2014.05.002

138. Leemann S, Peterson CK, Schmid C, Anklin B, Humphreys BK. Outcomes of acute and chronic patients with magnetic resonance imaging-confirmed symptomatic lumbar disc herniations receiving high-velocity, low-amplitude, spinal manipulative therapy: a prospective observational cohort study with one-year follow-up. *J Manipulative Physiol Ther.* 2014;37(3):155-163. doi:10.1016/j.jmpt.2013.12.011

139. Cibulka MT, Delitto A, Koldehoff RM. Changes in innominate tilt after manipulation of the sacroiliac joint in patients with low back pain. An experimental study. *Phys Ther.* 1988;68(9):1359-1363. doi:10.1093/ptj/68.9.1359

140. Erhard RE, Delitto A, Cibulka MT. Relative effectiveness of an extension program and a combined program of manipulation and flexion and extension exercises in patients with acute low back syndrome. *Phys Ther.* 1994;74(12):1093-1100. doi:10.1093/ptj.74.12.1093

141. Cibulka MT, Koldehoff R. Clinical usefulness of a cluster of sacroiliac joint tests in patients with and without low back pain. *J Orthop Sports Phys Ther.* 1999;29(2):83-89. doi:10.2519/jospt.1999.29.2.83

142. Gibbons P, Tehan P. *Manipulation of the Spine, Thorax and Pelvis. An Osteopathic Perspective.* 3rd ed. Churchill Livingstone; 2010.

143. Orakifar N, Kamali F, Pirouzi S, Jamshidi F. Sacroiliac joint manipulation attenuates alpha-motoneuron activity in healthy women: a quasi-experimental study. *Arch Phys Med Rehabil.* 2012;93(1):56-61. doi:10.1016/j.apmr.2011.05.027

144. de Oliveira Grassi D, Zanelli de Souza M, Belissa Ferrareto S, Imaculada de Lima Montebelo M, Caldeira de Oliveira Guirro E. Immediate and lasting improvements in weight distribution seen in baropodometry following a high-velocity, low-amplitude thrust manipulation of the sacroiliac joint. *Man Ther.* 2011;16(5):495-500. doi:10.1016/j.math.2011.04.003

145. Méndez-Sánchez R, González-Iglesias J, Sánchez-Sánchez JL, Puente-González AS. Immediate effects of bilateral sacroiliac joint manipulation on plantar pressure distribution in asymptomatic participants. *J Altern Complement Med.* 2014;20(4):251-257. doi:10.1089/acm.2013.0192

146. Tullberg T, Blomberg S, Branth B, Johnsson R. Manipulation does not alter the position of the sacroiliac joint. A roentgen stereophotogrammetric analysis. *Spine.* 1998;23(10):1124-1128. doi:10.1097/00007632-199805150-00010

147. Cook CE. *Orthopedic Manual Therapy: An Evidence-Based Approach.* 2nd ed. Pearson; 2012.

148. Grieve E. Diagnostic tests for mechanical dysfunction of the sacroiliac joints. *J Man Manip Ther.* 2001;9(4):198-206.

149. Ward JS, Coats J, Sorrels K, Walters M, Williams T. Pilot study of the impact sacroiliac joint manipulation has on walking kinematics using motion analysis technology. *J Chiropr Med.* 2013;12(3):143-152. doi:10.1016/j.jcm.2013.05.001

150. Godges JJ, Varnum DR, Sanders KM. Impairment-based examination and disability management of an elderly woman with sacroiliac region pain. *Phys Ther.* 2002;82(8):812-821.

151. Pettman E. *Manipulative Thrust Techniques: An Evidence-Based Approach.* Aardvark; 2007.

152. Haldeman S, Rubinstein SM. Cauda Equina Syndrome in patients undergoing manipulation of the lumbar spine. *Spine.* 1992;17(12):1469-1473. doi:10.1097/00007632-199212000-00005

153. Oliphant D. Safety of spinal manipulation in the treatment of lumbar disk herniations: a systematic review and risk assessment. *J Manipulative Physiol Ther.* 2004;27(3):197-210. doi:10.1016/j.jmpt.2003.12.023

154. Ernst E. Adverse effects of spinal manipulation: a systematic review. *J R Soc Med.* 2007;100(7):330-338. doi:10.1258/jrsm.100.7.330

155. McMorland G, Suter E, Casha S, du Plessis SJ, Hurlbert RJ. Manipulation or microdiskectomy for sciatica? A prospective randomized clinical study. *J Manipulative Physiol Ther.* 2010;33(8):576-584. doi:10.1016/j.jmpt.2010.08.013

156. Carlesso L, Rivett D. Manipulative practice in the cervical spine: a survey of IFOMPT member countries. *J Man Manip Ther.* 2011;19(2):66-70. doi:10.1179/2042618611Y.000000002

157. Maitland GD. *Vertebral Manipulation.* 5th ed. Butterworth-Heinemann; 1986.

158. Kaltenborn FM, Evjenth O, Kaltenborn TB, Morgan D, Vollowitz E. *Manual Mobilization of the Joints: Vol. II, The Spine.* 5th ed. Norli Universitesgaten; 2009.

159. Kisner C, Colby LA. *Therapeutic Exercise: Foundations and Techniques.* 6th ed. F. A. Davis; 2012.

160. Goodsell M, Lee M, Latimer J. Short-term effects of lumbar posteroanterior mobilization in individuals with low-back pain. *J Manipulative Physiol Ther.* 2000;23(5):332-342.

161. Beattie PF, Arnot CF, Donley JW, Noda H, Bailey L. The immediate reduction in low back pain intensity following lumbar joint mobilization and prone press-ups is associated with increased diffusion of water in the L5-S1 intervertebral disc. *J Orthop Sports Phys Ther.* 2010;40(5):256-264. doi:10.2519/jospt.2010.3284

162. Cook C, Learman K, Showalter C, Kabbaz V, O'Halloran B. Early use of thrust manipulation versus non-thrust manipulation: a randomized clinical trial. *Man Ther.* 2013;18(3):191-198. doi:10.1016/j.math.2012.03.005

163. Learman K, Showalter C, O'Halloran B, Donaldson M, Cook C. No differences in outcomes in people with low back pain who met the clinical prediction rule for lumbar spine manipulation when a pragmatic non-thrust manipulation was used as the comparator. *Physiother Can.* 2014;66(4):359-366. doi:10.3138/ptc.2013-49

164. Xia T, Long CR, Gudavalli MR, et al. Similar effects of thrust and nonthrust spinal manipulation found in adults with subacute and chronic low back pain: a controlled trial with adaptive allocation. *Spine.* 2016;41(12):E702-E709. doi:10.1097/BRS.0000000000001373

165. Mitchell T, O'Sullivan PB, Burnett AF, Straker L, Smith A. Regional differences in lumbar spinal posture and the influence of low back pain. *BMC Musculoskelet Disord.* 2008;9:152. doi:10.1186/1471-2474-9-152

166. Zafereo J, Wang-Price S, Roddey T, Brizzolara KJ. Regional manual therapy and motor control exercise for chronic low back pain: a randomized clinical trial. *J Orthop Sports Ther.* 2017;47(1):A28.

167. Aure OF, Nilsen JH, Vasseljen O. Manual therapy and exercise therapy in patients with chronic low back pain: a randomized, controlled trial with 1-year follow-up. *Spine.* 2003;28(6):525-531. doi:10.1097/01.BRS.0000049921.04200.A6

168. Burns SA, Mintken PE, Austin GP, Cleland J. Short-term response of hip mobilizations and exercise in individuals with chronic low back pain: a case series. *J Man Manip Ther.* 2011;19(2):100-107. doi:10.1179/2042618610Y.0000000007

169. Sung Y-B, Lee J-H, Park Y-H. Effects of thoracic mobilization and manipulation on function and mental state in chronic lower back pain. *J Phys Ther Sci.* 2014;26(11):1711-1714. doi:10.1589/jpts.26.1711

170. Mulligan BR. *Manual Therapy: NAGS, SNAGS, MWMS, etc.* 5th ed. Wellington; 2006.

171. Abbott JH, Patla CE, Jensen RH. The initial effects of an elbow mobilization with movement technique on grip strength in subjects with lateral epicondylalgia. *Man Ther.* 2001;6(3):163-169. doi:10.1054/math.2001.0408

172. Collins N, Teys P, Vicenzino B. The initial effects of a Mulligan's mobilization with movement technique on dorsiflexion and pain in subacute ankle sprains. *Man Ther.* 2004;9(2):77-82. doi:10.1016/S1356-689X(03)00101-2

173. Paungmali A, O'Leary S, Souvlis T, Vicenzino B. Hypoalgesic and sympathoexcitatory effects of mobilization with movement for lateral epicondylalgia. *Phys Ther.* 2003;83(4):374-383. doi:10.1093/ptj/83.4.374

174. Vicenzino B, Smith D, Cleland J, Bisset L. Development of a clinical prediction rule to identify initial responders to mobilisation with movement and exercise for lateral epicondylalgia. *Man Ther.* 2009;14(5):550-554. doi:10.1016/j.math.2008.08.004

175. Moutzouri M, Billis E, Strimpakos N, Kottika P, Oldham JA. The effects of the Mulligan Sustained Natural Apophyseal Glide (SNAG) mobilisation in the lumbar flexion range of asymptomatic subjects as measured by the Zebris CMS20 3-D motion analysis system. *BMC Musculoskelet Disord.* 2008;9:131. doi:10.1186/1471-2474-9-131

176. Exelby L. The locked lumbar facet joint: intervention using mobilizations with movement. *Man Ther.* 2001;6(2):116-121. doi:10.1054/math.2001.0394

177. Gibbons P, Tehan P. Muscle energy concepts and coupled motion of the spine. *Man Ther.* 1998;3(2):95-101.

178. Franke H, Fryer G, Ostelo RWJG, Kamper SJ. Muscle energy technique for non-specific low-back pain. *Cochrane Database Syst Rev.* 2015;27(2):CD009852. doi:10.1002/14651858.CD009852.pub2

179. Day JM, Nitz AJ. The effect of muscle energy techniques on disability and pain scores in individuals with low back pain. *J Sport Rehabil.* 2012;21(2):194-198. doi:10.1123/jsr.21.2.194

180. Schenk RJ, MacDiarmid A, Rousselle J. The effect of muscle energy technique on lumbar range of motion. *J Man Manip Ther.* 1997;5(4)179-183. doi:10.1179/jmt.1997.5.4.179

181. Wilson E, Payton O, Donegan-Shoaf L, Dec K. Muscle energy technique in patients with acute low back pain: a pilot clinical trial. *J Orthop Sports Phys Ther.* 2003;33(9):502-512. doi:10.2519/jospt.2003.33.9.502

182. Selkow NM, Grindstaff TL, Cross KM, Pugh K, Hertel J, Saliba S. Short-term effect of muscle energy technique on pain in individuals with non-specific lumbopelvic pain: a pilot study. *J Man Manip Ther.* 2009;17(1):E14-E18. doi:10.1179/jmt.2009.17.1.14E

183. Jonely H, Brismée JM, Desai MJ, Reoli R. Chronic sacroiliac joint and pelvic girdle dysfunction in a 35-year-old nulliparous woman successfully managed with multimodal and multidisciplinary approach. *J Man Manip Ther.* 2015;23(1):20-26. doi:10.1179/2042618614Y.0000000086

184. Landel R, Kulig K, Fredericson M, Li B, Powers CM. Intertester reliability and validity of motion assessments during lumbar spine accessory motion testing. *Phys Ther.* 2008;88(1):43-49. doi:10.2522/ptj.20060179

Evaluation and Rehabilitation of Spinal Stability and Motor Control

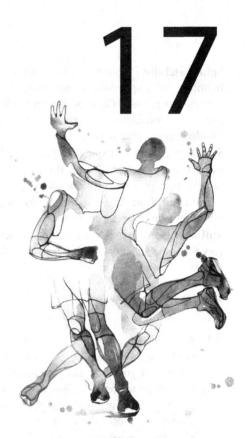

Sonia N. Young, PT, DPT, EdD, MSCS
and Charles Clark, PT, DPT, MHS, MTC, CSCS, CDNT

KEY TERMS

Adaptive motor control: An aspect of motor control where an individual has the ability to change the neuromuscular system in response to external demands[1] while maintaining efficiency and protecting the body.[2]

Control impairment: A functional motor control impairment of the lumbar spine characterized by continual adoption of pain provoking postures into lumbar flexion.[3]

Core stabilization: Training of several trunk and/or hip muscles (often with co-activation of 2 or more of these at once) with the belief that this will increase stiffness, decrease/rehabilitate injuries, and/or improve athletic performance.

Dynamic condition: Any system (eg, the neuromuscular system) that is changing in time in response to internal or external forces.[4]

Global stabilizers: System of muscles with origin on the pelvis and insertion on the thoracic cage that maintain equilibrium of the lumbar spine.[5]

Instability: Inability to maintain or regain stability.[4]

Local stabilizers: System of muscles with origin and/or insertion at the vertebral level that maintain equilibrium of the lumbar spine.[5]

Low back pain (LBP): Neuromusculoskeletal pain occurring between lower thoracic and gluteal areas (often including radiation or concurrent proximal thigh pain) not associated with severe pathology.

Maladaptive motor control: Inability to control or protect the body in response to external demands resulting in impairments.[2]

Motor control: "[T]he ability to regulate or direct the mechanisms essential to movement."[1]

Movement impairment: A functional motor control impairment of the lumbar spine characterized by muscle guarding and an adoption of rigid lumbar extension during movements in an effort to avoid pain provoking positions.[3]

Perturbation: An external force that causes a movement away from original position or trajectory.[4]

Rigidity: Excessive movement restriction beyond that needed to create stability, which can result in a loss of stability and/or poor performance.[3]

Wallmann HW, Donatelli R, eds. *Foundations of Orthopedic Physical Therapy* (pp 517-541).
© 2024 Taylor & Francis Group.

Spinal stability: Ability of the structures of the spine to maintain stable spinal related structures and associated neuromuscular pathways to allow bearing of loads, maintaining position, coordinating movement, and, at the same time, avoiding injury and pain.[4]

Stability: Ability to maintain or regain intended position, movement, or a combination thereof in static or dynamic conditions in preparation for or subsequent to perturbations.[4]

Static condition: Any system (eg, the neuromuscular system) that is in a state of equilibrium.[4]

Stiffness: Construct that trunk muscle activation is necessary for spine stability and that lack of stiffness is associated with injury.[4]

CHAPTER QUESTIONS

1. A patient with impaired motor control of the lumbopelvic region presents at rest with an anterior pelvic tilt and muscle guarding. The patient appears stiff and hesitant during movements. Based on this limited information, which of the following categories of motor control impairment would the patient fit?
   A. Active extension pattern (AEP)
   B. Flexion pattern
   C. Control impairment
   D. Lateral flexion impairment

2. Which of the following is a force that produces a deviation away from the original position or trajectory?
   A. Stability
   B. Vibration
   C. Perturbation
   D. Instability

3. Which of the following is the process of analyzing a functional movement into the component parts?
   A. Lumbopelvic screen
   B. Task analysis
   C. Dynamic analysis
   D. Control process

4. A patient presenting with a movement impairment of the lumbar spine would *most* benefit from which of the following techniques in the beginner stage of rehabilitation?
   A. Neuromuscular reeducation consisting of relaxation training progressing to gentle movements of the lumbar spine
   B. Neuromuscular reeducation consisting of facilitation of abdominal muscles and mobilization away from the restriction
   C. Therapeutic exercise/activities with progressive challenges
   D. Neuromuscular reeducation with perturbations in all directions

5. A practitioner considers the patient's subjective history and environmental factors to be as important as examination findings during an evaluation. Which of the following principles is being applied?
   A. Clinical neuroscience
   B. Biopsychosocial
   C. Social construct
   D. Environmental construct

6. Utilizing the pain mechanism model, pain persistence increasing nervous system sensitivity to same threatening stimuli can result in which of the following?
   A. Decreased pain report from the patient
   B. Overconfidence in functional ability
   C. Fear-avoidance behaviors
   D. More stimuli needed to produce pain than originally

7. Which of the following is a system of muscles with the origin on the pelvis and insertion on the thoracic cage that maintain equilibrium of the lumbar spine?
   A. Global stabilizers
   B. Local stabilizers
   C. Lumbar multifidus and iliocostalis lumborum
   D. Quadratus lumborum and internal oblique

8. Dynamic standing is assessed during a motor examination of the lumbar spine for those patients with nonspecific lumbopelvic pain. Which of the following is considered a cardinal plane trunk movement, a component of this examination?
   A. Standing pelvic tilt
   B. Back bending with hands on hips
   C. Trunk flexion with rotation to the same side
   D. Trunk extension with side-bending to opposite side

9. Which of the following are small trunk muscles that are attached to the lumbar vertebrae and provide stability to the spine?
   A. Global stabilizers
   B. Rectus abdominis and external oblique
   C. Multifidus and transversus abdominis
   D. Iliopsoas and rectus femoris

10. In this motor control strategy, the physical therapist will apply variable perturbations in multiple directions at different speeds on variable surfaces in order to improve which of the following?
    A. Anticipatory balance control
    B. Sensory organization
    C. Dual-task training
    D. Reactive balance control

11. Why should a patient-specific task, such as a recreational or occupational activity simulation, be incorporated into the motor examination for patients with nonspecific lumbar pain?

   A. To allow the physical therapist to see the patient perform a task well

   B. To improve documentation

   C. To identify the patient's motor control during a functional task

   D. To indicate where the patient has mastery of movement

12. Which of the following is the ability of the spine and related neurological structures to bear loads, maintain position, and coordinate movements in order to avoid injury and pain?

   A. Stiffness

   B. Spinal stability

   C. Instability

   D. Maladaptive motor control

13. In this motor control strategy, the patient may be instructed to lift a box while controlling the position of their lumbar spine in order to improve which of the following?

   A. Anticipatory control

   B. Sensory organization

   C. Dual-task training

   D. Reactive control

14. In this area of the pain mechanism model, stressful situations can cause pain reports to increase which of the following?

   A. Processing

   B. Input

   C. Output

   D. Modulating

15. Which of the following represents neuromusculoskeletal pain occurring between lower thoracic and gluteal areas (often including radiation or concurrent proximal thigh pain) not associated with severe pathology?

   A. Structural pain

   B. Nonspecific low back pain (NSLBP)

   C. Combine lumbar pain

   D. Lumbopelvic pain

16. Which of the following approaches allows the clinician to determine an appropriate diagnostic classification and develop an individualized plan of care for those with LBP while attempting to determine the cause of the deficit?

   A. Task analysis

   B. Dual task

   C. Functional assessment

   D. Clinical decision making

17. Which of the following is a system that is changing in time in response to internal or external forces?

   A. Dynamic condition

   B. Static condition

   C. Perturbation

   D. Friction

18. During the motor examination of the lumbar spine, dynamic sitting control is assessed for all of the following *except*:

   A. Compensation patterns

   B. Quality of movement

   C. Reports of pain

   D. Speed of performance

19. A patient with impaired motor control of the lumbopelvic region presents at rest with a posterior pelvic tilt and inability to maintain the spine in a neutral zone. The patient will continually provoke symptoms due to poor awareness of position of the lumbar spine. Based on this limited information, which of the following categories of motor control impairment would the patient fit?

   A. AEP

   B. Flexion pattern

   C. Movement impairment

   D. Lateral flexion impairment

20. Individuals who meet the clinical prediction rule (CPR) indicating they could benefit from spinal stabilization exercises would fall into which of the following motor control impairment categories as a subset?

   A. Control impairment

   B. Movement impairment

   C. Aberrant impairment

   D. Minimal control group

INTRODUCTION

In this chapter, a clinical decision-making model for LBP subtype identification is provided along with rehabilitation techniques designed to improve motor control of the spine. A historical perspective of spinal stabilization theory is provided along with current evidence on motor control, pain science, and a biopsychosocial approach for evaluation and rehabilitation of this population. Building on examination techniques provided in a previous chapter, the practitioner is guided through a motor control examination of the spine using a task analysis approach. Motor control disorders of the lumbar spine are then classified into 2 categories: a movement impairment group (active extension) and a control impairment group (flexion). The practitioner is then guided to develop individualized plans of care based on the specific classification of the motor control disorder. Rehabilitation strategies for patients with these disorders are presented in 3 stages: beginner, intermediate, and advanced.

An overview of spinal control and stability with the process of evaluation and rehabilitation is provided along with supporting evidence.

HISTORICAL PERSPECTIVES

LBP is a complex entity with multiple facets and little consensus on best treatment approach.[3,6] One suggested source of LBP (and ergo treatment focus) is the impairment of the spine to being stable enough to tolerate stressors during performance of functional mobility skills, basic activities of daily living (ADLs), and instrumental activities of daily living (IADLs; eg, sports). Traditional views of spinal stability mirrored those of LBP by focusing on a pathoanatomical-based model, whereby a structural fault is identified and subsequent treatment would attempt to correct that structural fault.[7] As early as 1944, Knutsson[8] associated radiographic findings of excessive intervertebral movements as signs of spinal instability and infers these to be likely causes of LBP. However, most instances of LBP are described as nonspecific as they have no identifiable radiographic findings. Additionally, pathoanatomical findings in the spine will not always produce symptoms as they are often discovered in asymptomatic individuals.[5,9-11] Even when a physical therapist considers a pathoanatomical diagnosis relevant to the patient's presentation, there is a further need to understand the mechanisms that drive the diagnosis in order to prescribe the most suitable treatment plan.[3]

Bergmark[5] laid the initial groundwork for much of what is considered the spinal stability model when he postulated there was a necessary contribution of stiffness from spinal musculature to maintain stability and prevent injury. Panjabi[12,13] further developed this conceptual model with an interdependent stability system consisting of "passive, active, and neural control" of the spine in both end and mid ranges (termed the *neutral zone*) of spinal movement. Panjabi's contribution, in particular, significantly accelerated subsequent research and development of what is now considered core stabilization.[4,12-14] Core stabilization models of treatment have focused on coordinating and controlling trunk posture and associated movement of the spine and associated structures, all within the presence of internal and external forces of increasing complexity.[15,16] This treatment strategy was suggested[4] to be greatly advantageous alone or in concert with other physical therapy interventions. Its therapeutic benefit was suggested to be accomplished by activating, recruiting, and strengthening trunk and abdominal muscles (eg, transversus abdominis and multifidus, which are considered local stabilizers as opposed to global stabilizers [Table 17-1]) to decrease LBP and prevent injury.[5,17,18]

Although there are certainly patients who would benefit from the classic spinal stabilization approach, there are authors and researchers who have challenged this one-size-fits-all approach toward interventions in the LBP population.[3,17,19,20] Current research does not support the intervention approach of cocontraction of local and global stabilizers

for all patients with chronic LBP.[20] In fact, static cocontraction has been shown to require more energy and therefore increase fatigue, cause complaints of pain, and result in instability during dynamic activities.[4] Additionally, co-activation was found to be present in higher levels in those with LBP than with healthy controls.[4,21] This increased cocontraction could be related to impaired motor control. In particular, Lederman challenges several beliefs including the benefit of "core" (local stabilizers) vs global muscle activation and the benefit of training to enhance this recruitment pattern in LBP.[17] O'Sullivan editorialized on the subject extensively and found several contrary study findings (increased cocontraction/hyperactivity and earlier timing onset of core musculature in patients with LBP, as well as lack of superior results with specific stabilization exercises) than those presupposed by conventional core stabilization principles.[20] Smith et al[22] did a systematic review with meta-analyses as well as a comparison with similar meta-analyses and concluded there was strong evidence that stabilization exercises were not more effective than other active exercises in populations with NSLBP.

SUGGESTED APPROACH

The current authors suggest resolving this dilemma by integrating several neuroscience principles into an active rehabilitation approach to this population. First, adoption of biopsychosocial principles is suggested.[20] The biopsychosocial model is a guide to practice that considers an individual's health status as being influenced by multiple components including biological, psychological, and social.[23,24] These components not only influence the diagnosis of a disorder, but also treatment outcomes. In patients with LBP, the physical therapist should therefore consider an individual's subjective history and environmental factors of equal importance to the objective examination findings.[23,24] The World Health Organization's *International Classification of Functioning, Disability and Health (ICF)* model, endorsed by the American Physical Therapy Association, embraces the biopsychosocial model as it provides a framework to classify and measure health and disability.[25] The ICF model, in conjunction with the biopsychosocial model, considers an individual's health status in the context of functioning in their environment and is utilized to guide physical therapy practice and patient/client management.[24] An individualized approach is best utilized with these patients based on clinical decision making within the ICF framework and biopsychosocial perspective. Patients should also be encouraged to manage their own symptoms.[26] While clinicians recognize the need to utilize the biopsychosocial perspective in treatment, they may be unsure how to address the psychological needs of the patient or need training.[27] The current view of spinal stability has been enhanced to include an understanding that multiple systems work together to produce coordinated movements that control motion. Spinal stability is therefore a function of control rather than implying rigidity.

Table 17-1

GLOBAL AND LOCAL SYSTEMS[5,18]

MUSCULOSKELETAL SYSTEM	PROPOSED FUNCTION	MUSCLES INVOLVED
Global system	Large trunk muscles that serve as the primary movers of the spine but without a direct attachment to the lumbar spine	Rectus abdominus External oblique Iliocostalis lumborum*
Local system	Small trunk muscles that are attached to the lumbar vertebrae and provide stability to the spine	Lumbar multifidus^ Internal oblique^ Transversus abdominus^ Psoas major Quadratus lumborum Iliocostalis lumborum**

* Portion.
** Lumbar portion.
^ Main local stabilizers.

PAIN SCIENCE

The second neuroscience principle that needs to be discussed has been termed *pain neuroscience education (PNE).*[27] This education is based on the premise that patients are instructed on the neurophysiology of pain while deemphasizing the focus on the anatomical structural faults.[27] Increased awareness of how the nervous system responds to injury, pain, and perceived threats is necessary along with an understanding of the psychological aspect of pain.[9,28-30] Pain serves to protect the body.[31] However, Gifford[32] and Puentedura and Louw[9] suggest clinicians keep a pain mechanism model in mind with 3 overlapping processes: input, processing, and output (Figure 17-1). With input, stressful situations can negatively affect pain reports. In processing, pain persistence increases nervous system sensitivity to the same threatening stimuli. Therefore, less stimuli are needed to produce pain. As a result, the individual may display fear-avoidance behaviors where they move less in an effort to avoid the positions that increase pain or could cause tissue damage. With output, the body will adopt maladaptive protective responses within various systems.

In the most simplistic way, these principles should serve as the backdrop for all further clinical decision-making choices.[9] For instance, avoidance of same or similar stressful environments would be beneficial at the onset of treatment along with discussion of coping strategies when returning back to the same (perceived) stressful circumstances. Similarly, the patient can be made aware that pain does not necessarily equate to pathoanatomical injury. In one study, PNE combined with therapeutic exercise (which included motor control interventions, strengthening, and aerobic

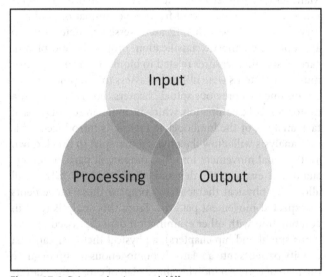

Figure 17-1. Pain mechanism model.[9,32]

exercise) was shown to decrease pain reports better than therapeutic exercise alone.[30] This agrees with a systematic review performed by Louw et al, which explored the use of PNE on individuals with chronic musculoskeletal pain.[27] The authors found that PNE was a viable tool to decrease pain and improve function. Furthermore, a significant reduction of pain occurred when combining PNE with a movement intervention. The clinician should consider a multidimensional approach to nonspecific chronic LBP that includes not only physical interventions but also PNE and treatments to improve cognitive functional sensorimotor control.[33] One such treatment is cognitive functional therapy (CFT), which seeks to influence the emotional response to pain, compensations of movements, and lifestyle modifications to take the focus off of pain.[34] A long-term follow-up of a randomized controlled trial of a CFT group vs a manual therapy and therapeutic exercise group treating nonspecific chronic LBP found that while both groups had similar pain intensities, the CFT group had decreased disability, anxiety, depression, and fear avoidance.[35] Constructs related to PNE will be detailed later in stage I of rehabilitation.

DIAGNOSIS

The O'Sullivan's mechanism–based classification system[3,6,31] (detailed later) will serve as the classification method to identify and treat patients with NSLBP. This system has been found to be effective[6,36-44] and integrates the biopsychosocial and pain science constructs detailed previously. This approach has been found to have more than moderate intertester reliability[45] and excellent face validity.[6]

EVALUATION

Utilizing the Physical Therapist Patient and Client Management Model from the *Guide to Physical Therapist Practice 3.0*,[46] data collected from the examination and history of the patient with LBP are assessed to determine an appropriate diagnostic classification, prognosis, and plan of care. Tests and measures related to biomechanical or neuromuscular systems were utilized to assess this population and are outlined in previous spinal chapters. For this chapter, a motor control examination, which includes an activity-based task analysis of the lumbopelvic region, is introduced. This task analysis will allow the physical therapist to break down a functional movement into the component parts to understand and evaluate the demands of the task.[1,3,6,36] This will allow the physical therapist to compare these movements to expected movement patterns. From this analysis (and in combination with other examination data discussed in previous spinal and hip chapters), a physical therapist can best classify patients into a relatively homogenous group to guide the plan of care. An individualized plan of care is then developed to provide the best treatment strategies to restore best functional movement performance.

MOTOR CONTROL EXAMINATION

From the patient's history, a description of activities that provoke their symptoms can be utilized to map out the specific postures and movements that will be examined during this task analysis. For patients with persistent LBP, a framework for this task analysis (Table 17-2) includes observation of the patient in multiple positions and during functional movements.

The physical therapist should analyze and document the body position (eg, static, dynamic, supine, sitting, standing, patient-specific movements/positions), the specific task tested, the quality of movement, and obvious deviations from the expected performance as noted in Table 17-2. More specifically, abnormal positions or movements of the lumbopelvic area at rest and during movements are identified: position of the lumbopelvic region (anterior tilt/increased lordosis, posterior tilt/decreased lordosis, or neutral); the thoracic spine (increased or decreased thoracic kyphosis); the cervical spine (forward head posture); as well as the provocation of pain, the presence or absence of muscle guarding, fear avoidance, and the quality of movement during static and dynamic functional tasks.[36]

Sitting

A framework for performing the task analysis in sitting is provided in Table 17-2. Within the typical history-taking portion of the physical therapy examination, static motor control of the lumbopelvic region can be assessed by noting above alterations in expected posturing. Static sitting posture assessment can be further refined by having patient seated in a chair with back (less challenge), on a treatment table with foot support (more challenge), or on treatment table without foot support (significant challenge), all while the patient is unaware of the intended observation. The physical therapist can then ascertain if the patient can modify the demonstrated posturing to an optimal strategy.

Dynamic sitting control is assessed by asking the patient to move into and out of varying postures noting the factors listed in Table 17-2. In particular, quality of movement, patient perception of difficulty, and compensation substitution patterns such as use of the upper extremities to return to sit, increased/decreased thoracic kyphosis, and reports of pain at end-range movement should be noted. When the therapist asks the patient to transition into a supine position on the table for further examination tasks, quality of movement and the same characteristics can be assessed.

Table 17-2

TASK ANALYSIS FOR MOTOR EXAMINATION

BODY POSITIONING	TESTED TASK WITH POSSIBLE VARIATIONS
Static sitting	Posture • Usual/demonstrated (during history taking) • With/without back support • Corrective (guided to) best positioning
Dynamic sitting	Slump sitting • Attaining slump sitting • Return to erect sitting Transfer • Sit to stand • Stand to sit
Static standing	Posture • After march in place (typical) • Corrective (guided to) best positioning
Dynamic standing	Cardinal plane trunk movements • Forward bending • Backward bending (with/without hands on hips) • Side-bending • Rotation (with/without pelvic stabilization) Combined trunk movements • Any cardinal trunk movement before another (eg, flexion then side-bending) • Quadrant: Trunk flexion (or extension) combined with rotation/side-bending to same side Gait • Typical • Corrective Combined trunk/extremity movements • Upper or lower extremity movement/positioning combined with trunk movement (eg, reaching overhead with trunk extension) • Squatting movements with different upper extremity positions • Weight shifting movements (eg, marching, unilateral stand, step-ups)

(continued)

Table 17-2 (continued)

TASK ANALYSIS FOR MOTOR EXAMINATION

BODY POSITIONING	TESTED TASK WITH POSSIBLE VARIATIONS
Supine/prone/side-lying	Transfer • Sit to side-lying to supine • Supine to side-lying to sit • Stand to sit Recruitment/facilitation • Pelvic tilt (typical, anterior, posterior, corrective) • Iliopsoas, transverse abdominis, multifidus, gluteals Rolling • Supine to side-lying to prone • Prone to side-lying to supine Hip movement • Internal/external rotation active range of motion (AROM)/passive range of motion (PROM) • Flexion/extension AROM/PROM • Abduction PROM
Patient specific	ADLs/IADLs/occupation/recreation/sport

Standing (Static and Dynamic)

Similar to the dynamic portion of the sitting examination, noted alterations in expected movement patterns can be assessed with noted static and dynamic standing tasks as described in Table 17-2. The improvement or worsening of the patient's capacity/symptoms when similar tasks are done in standing vs sitting are also helpful in understanding the presentation, especially with respect to fear avoidance, volitional guarding, and quality of movement. Similarly, the difficulty of the examination tasks can be ascended in difficulty (from single plane to multiple plane and with addition of extremity movements) to find the current level of tolerance/capability initially or in subsequent sessions. Perhaps less considered in this population than those with lower extremity injuries, observational gait analyses before or after other dynamic standing tasks can add to the physical therapist's knowledge of how the patient functions during this activity. It is useful to observe the patient transitioning from sit to stand to observe compensatory strategies. In Figure 17-2, a patient is being asked to transfer from sit to stand but displays compensatory strategies (ie, using upper extremities to assist in rising). Likewise, cardinal movements along with quadrant movements in all directions are performed (Figure 17-3).

Supine/Prone/Side-lying

Similar to static sitting, the patient may not be aware of the therapist's intent in observing the quality or capability of transfers to or from sit to supine or supine to side-lying to prone. If the patient has difficulty moving into these testing positions, has complaints of pain, or uses compensatory strategies, these should be noted. Similarly, improvement of any or all of these factors with corrective (guided to) technique can be quite enlightening for the patient and provide guidance toward additional patient-specific interventions and education.

During these same noted positions, a variety of tests can be utilized (see Table 17-2) to understand several factors related to the patient's presentation. For instance, the patient demonstrating pelvic girdle/spine positioning in nonweight-bearing or relaxed positions can be compared to prior demonstrated tasks. A patient who demonstrates consistent anterior pelvic tilt only with initial attempts to forward bend may be thought to be less affected by their current symptoms than a patient who maintains this same position during a less provocative positioning like supine or hooklying. Similarly, looking for the patient's full "excursion" of anterior to posterior pelvic tilt along with symptom report and significant

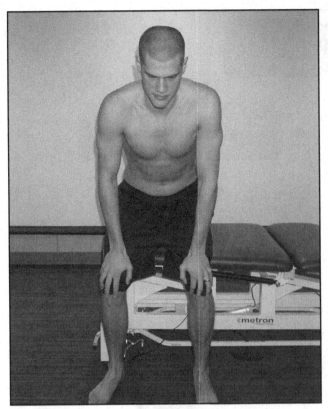

Figure 17-2. Compensatory strategies for sit-to-stand transfer.

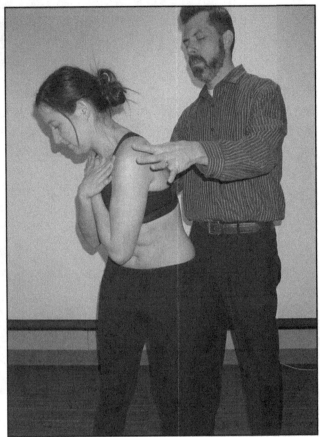

Figure 17-3. Quadrant movement assessment (flexion).

differences between expected range and more focal discomfort during either anterior or posterior tilt motions would be helpful. Lastly, can the patient be guided to and maintain a neutral or preferred pelvic tilt without excessive recruitment of area musculature and/or discomfort?

Beyond examination tasks presented in the hip complex chapter, the authors of this chapter recommend assessment of facilitation of several likely irritable musculature as either a treatment focus and/or as a retest value after other interventions. These could include left vs right palpation of more local musculature such as iliopsoas, gluteal and other hip musculature, abdominals (bracing from rectus abdominis and obliques in particular), and posterior thoracolumbar musculature (erectors and multifidus). Lastly, due to common belief of regional interdependence of hip and lumbar areas,[47-49] hip range of motion (ROM) can be assessed to see what cause can be suggested to be affecting current lumbar symptoms or how relative ROM restrictions might create recurrent compensation in the lumbar spine.

Patient Specific

Any movement or position not assessed by prior examination methods (eg, forklift driver prepositioning upper/lower extremities prior to rotating trunk in usual manner) is performed as needed.

CLINICAL DECISION MAKING

Individuals with persistent and unresolving LBP will often adopt maladaptive strategies of motor recruitment in an attempt to reconcile their need for functional movement requirements while often dealing with the continuation or fear of pain.[3,6,50] These maladaptive strategies can vary by the individual based on frequency; severity; chronicity of noted pain; and, likely, several unique factors such as prior history of same/similar pain, overall health perception, and capacity to cope.[4,9] Similarly, without suggesting to answer cause-effect, these same individuals will often demonstrate unique (or more commonly several) physical impairments (eg, decreased unilateral hip or trunk ROM, specific muscle guarding) concurrently.[9,32,48,49]

Despite this heterogeneity of potential individual and combinations of presentation variables, clinical decision making is an evaluation construct designed to assist the physical therapist to best determine an appropriate or best diagnostic classification with the aim to develop an individualized plan of care for individuals with LBP.[3] This is accomplished by attempting to establish the biomechanical, cognitive, motor control, and/or neuromuscular causes

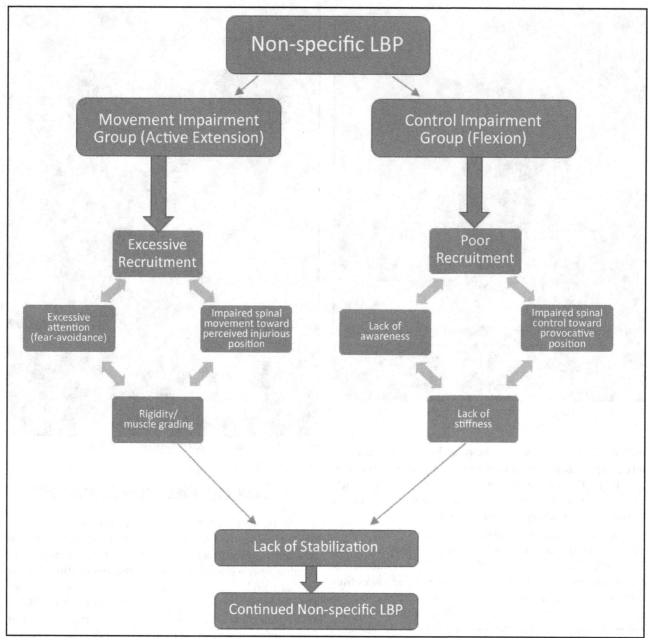

Figure 17-4. Algorithm for motor impairments.

of the deficit and guide the interventions and outcomes of the ongoing treatment.[3] Despite the inference of being done solely at the initial evaluation, the authors suggest clinical decision making will always be individualized and should be changing throughout the episode of care depending on the response to treatment.

Individuals with LBP can be classified into 2 groups (further described later): a movement impairment group (also characterized as a lumbar AEP) and a control impairment group (also characterized as a lumbar flexion pattern).[2,3,6,19,36] The algorithm (Figure 17-4) and information provided later provides the physical therapist with a framework to take examination data and evaluate which classification is most appropriate.

MOVEMENT IMPAIRMENT GROUP (ACTIVE EXTENSION PATTERN)

From the clues provided in the earlier noted examination findings, a broad classification of individuals with lumbopelvic pain who experience apprehension and increased muscle guarding during spinal movements that provoke symptoms are classified as having a movement impairment. This movement impairment classification can be assigned and likely results from the noted apprehension from the individual's attempt to avoid spinal movements that lead to provocation of pain, resulting in decreased spinal mobility in that direction.[3,6] Additionally, the pain or fear of pain leads to

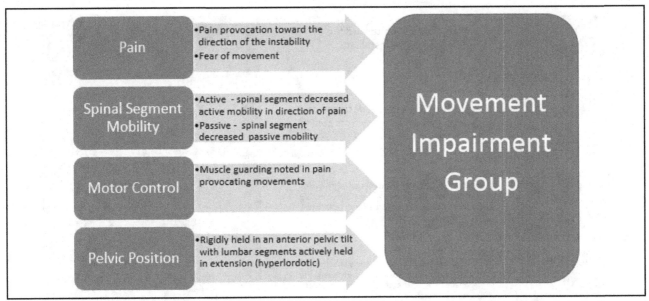

Figure 17-5. Movement impairment (active extension).

alterations in motor recruitment of lumbopelvic muscles[4,51,52] caused by increased muscle guarding in the direction of the pain provocation. As a result, the individual will exhibit decreased passive and active movement of the involved spinal segment due to increased cocontraction and rigidity.[2] The most common pattern for this is termed *AEP*, in which the patient exhibits a postural pattern of lumbar extension, concurrent pelvic anterior tilt, and excessive recruitment of superficial multifidus activity.[2,3,19,31] The patient will also tend to have ongoing (and in some cases exhaustive) strategies to maintain this maladaptive positioning due to fear avoidance of further tissue damage or pain.[2-4] The patient exhibits a postural pattern of lumbar extension in which the pelvis assumes a position of anterior tilt. Individuals are classified as having a movement impairment spinal instability if the examination data reveal the following: rigidly held anterior pelvic tilt with a hyperlordotic curve, cocontraction of core muscles, fear and guarding of movements in all functional positions, and pain provocation toward the direction of instability (Figure 17-5). Figure 17-6 indicates an individual with a movement impairment who has been asked to lie on the treatment table. He exhibits an increased lordosis and decreased ability to relax trunk muscles.

CONTROL IMPAIRMENT GROUP (FLEXION PATTERN)

The most common pattern seen in clinical practice is the control impairment group,[3] also called the *flexion pattern* (Figure 17-7). This group most closely approximates those individuals who meet the instability CPR.[7] The flexion pattern is characterized by a loss of motor control in the lumbar spine resulting in adoption of a posterior pelvic tilt with poor awareness of position during functional movements and

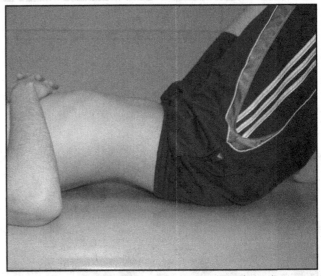

Figure 17-6. Increased lumbar lordosis due to volitional guarding.

classified as a control impairment.[2,3,19,31] This control impairment group is characterized by those individuals who exhibit loss of motor control of spinal segments resulting in poor awareness of position and repetitive adoption of provocative positions. The patient is unable to maintain lumbar extension and therefore remains in a prolonged, flexed position resulting in a kyphotic or decreased lordotic curve. As a result, prolonged lumbar flexion is a risk factor for delayed reflex responses and therefore impaired feedback control.[4] This impaired feedback control can lead to late or inappropriate responses to sudden or unexpected perturbations, placing the patient at risk of injury.[4] These patients have no movement pattern impairment in the direction of pain.[6] The patient will assume a posterior pelvic tilt and will have poor awareness of pelvic position (Figure 17-8).

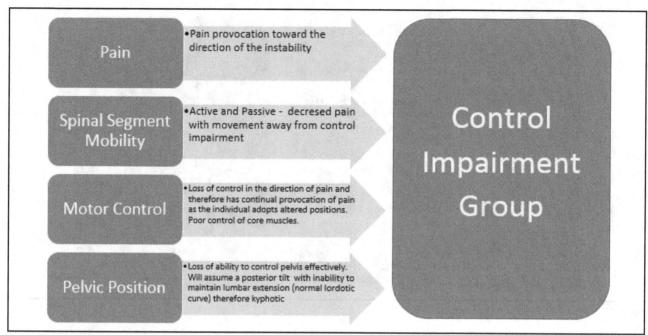

Figure 17-7. Control impairment (flexion pattern).

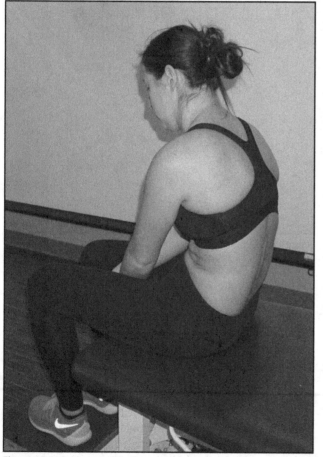

Figure 17-8. Posterior pelvic tilt.

CLINICAL PREDICTION RULE AND SPINAL STABILIZATION EXERCISES

A subset of the control impairment group are those individuals who fit the CPR. This subset group tends to fall within this classification, but there are individuals who might not have all symptoms. Hicks et al[7] predicted which subset of individuals with LBP could benefit from stabilization exercises. This subset is identified by utilizing a CPR in which individuals with at least 3 of the following predictors present have a higher predicted success with stabilization exercises: "positive prone instability test, aberrant movement present, average SLR >91, and age <40y."[7] Rabin et al[53] were unable to validate the CPR, however, it was also not invalidated. This CPR may be more predictive of those who would experience success following lumbar stabilization exercises if aberrant movements and a positive prone instability test are present.[53]

INTERVENTION

Varied strategies are utilized in treating spinal disorders with varied results and outcomes.[53,54] A motor control approach is presented later. This approach will seek to create a construct whereby motor learning in conjunction with balance and coordination activities are integrated to improve static and dynamic control of the spine during functional movements (task oriented). Altered movement patterns occur in individuals with LBP regardless of symptom duration.[55] Additionally, chronic LBP can cause decreased postural awareness and therefore necessitate the use of sensory and motor cues.[56] An individualized plan of care should be established with each patient determined to have a motor or movement control impairment of the lumbopelvic spine. This plan should be developed with the patient's input and should focus on the areas of education, neuromuscular reeducation, and therapeutic exercise/activities with an aim to improving motor control.

Therapy should ideally progress through stages increasing in complexity. Table 17-3 presents a rehabilitation plan based on the type of motor or movement control impairment that aims to increase motor control and decrease maladaptive posturing of the lumbopelvic spine. This is accomplished by utilizing both a physical and cognitive (biopsychosocial) approach. CFT may be appropriate for those individuals with chronic NSLBP who have motor control issues. This approach attempts to decrease and change the patient's perception of pain, decrease muscle guarding and fear, and encourage controlled movements by considering cognitive and other biopsychosocial inputs.[57-61] CFT based on the O'Sullivan classification has been found to have significant outcomes as compared to manual therapy and exercise alone, but it may require advanced training.[62] However, patient education of the neurophysiology of pain in conjunction with sensory and motor training has been found to decrease short-term pain reports in those with NSLBP.[63] Manual therapy may also be used with this population to reduce structural restrictions if found during the examination. For all interventions, patients should be continually monitored and reassessed.

MOVEMENT IMPAIRMENT GROUP (ACTIVE EXTENSION PATTERN)

For patients who fall within the movement impairment group, the goal is to decrease muscle guarding and to restore movement and motor control of the lumbopelvic spine.[3]

Stage One: Beginner

Education

In this stage, the patient is educated on the nature of their pain and the maladaptive positioning of the spine in response. The aim is to decrease fear avoidance of lumbar flexion and to decrease muscle guarding that often opposes this movement. The therapist will explain to the patient that the core muscles do not need to be activated before the patient performs functional movements. Additionally, overactivation of core muscles can increase the pain cycle. A HEP is developed that reinforces techniques performed in the clinic.

Neuromuscular Reeducation

This approach will seek to create a construct whereby motor learning in conjunction with balance and coordination activities are integrated to improve static and dynamic control of the spine during functional movements. Steady-state postural control[1] is encouraged by first cuing the patient into a correct posture and then seeing if the patient can maintain that position while in a static position. The patient is encouraged to relax extensor muscles and slump into a flexed lumbar position while sitting. The patient is then progressed to gentle/small movements of the lumbar spine into flexion by moving from an anterior to a posterior pelvic tilt in various positions.

Balance and coordination activities are introduced with the persistent messaging that relaxation and neutral to posterior pelvic tilt (whichever is more functional for the task instructed) without excessive extended lumbar posturing and/or volitional guarding are all hallmarks of a best strategy while performing nearly all functional activities. This is illustrated in Figure 17-9 as the physical therapist cues the patient into a neutral pelvic tilt and has them stand and maintain this position.

Therapeutic Exercise/Activity

Exercise in this stage will initially focus on deep and diaphragmatic breathing to encourage relaxation and control.

Stage Two: Intermediate

Education

In this stage, concepts introduced in stage 1 are reinforced. The physical therapist will monitor compliance of the HEP and modify as needed.

Neuromuscular Reeducation

Motor control activities move from steady-state to anticipatory postural control in which the patient begins to move the center of mass over a larger area[1] while controlling the position of the spine. A graded movement exposure approach will be employed. Balance and coordination activities are increased in difficulty level with the likelihood of patient

Table 17-3

Intervention Strategies for Movement Impairment and Control Impairment Groups

	MOVEMENT IMPAIRMENT GROUP	CONTROL IMPAIRMENT GROUP

STAGE ONE: BEGINNER	Education
	• PNE
	• Home exercise program (HEP)
	Neuromuscular reeducation
	• Motor control
	  ○ Steady-state postural control[2]
	  ○ Relaxation training
	  ○ Progress to gentle/small movements
	• Balance
	• Coordination
	Therapeutic exercise/activities
	• Breathing
	  ○ Diaphragmatic
		Education
		• PNE
		• HEP
		Neuromuscular reeducation
		• Motor control
		  ○ Steady-state postural control[2]
		  ○ Facilitation
		  ○ Mobilization into restriction
		• Balance
		• Coordination
		Therapeutic exercise/activities
		• Less provocative positions
		  ○ Prone
		  ○ Supine

STAGE TWO: INTERMEDIATE	Education
	• Reinforce stage 1 concepts
	• PNE
	• HEP
	Neuromuscular reeducation
	• Motor control
	  ○ Anticipatory postural control[2]
	• Balance
	• Coordination
	Therapeutic exercise/activities
	• Task oriented/functional
	  ○ Stable
	  ○ Unstable
		Education
		• Reinforce stage 1 concepts
		• PNE
		• HEP
		Neuromuscular reeducation
		• Motor control
		  ○ Anticipatory postural control[2]
		• Balance
		• Coordination
		Therapeutic exercise/activities
		• Task oriented/functional
		  ○ Stable
		  ○ Unstable

(continued)

Table 17-3 (continued)

INTERVENTION STRATEGIES FOR MOVEMENT IMPAIRMENT AND CONTROL IMPAIRMENT GROUPS

	MOVEMENT IMPAIRMENT GROUP	CONTROL IMPAIRMENT GROUP

STAGE THREE: ADVANCES	Education
	• Reinforce stages 1 and 2 concepts
	• HEP
	Neuromuscular reeducation
	• Motor control
	   ◦ Reactive postural control[2]
	• Balance
	• Coordination
	Therapeutic exercise/activities
	• Progressive challenges
	• IADLs
	   ◦ Recreational
	   ◦ Community
		Education
		• Reinforce stages 1 and 2 concepts
		• HEP
		Neuromuscular reeducation
		• Motor control
		   ◦ Reactive postural control[2]
		• Balance
		• Coordination
		Therapeutic exercise/activities
		• Progressive challenges
		• IADLs
		   ◦ Recreational
		   ◦ Community

apprehension occurring, and then worked through on the best coping strategies to mitigate. This is illustrated in Figure 17-10 where the patient is learning to relax into flexed lumbar position with the assistance of a ball while gradually increasing speed and movement.

Therapeutic Exercise/Activity

Task-oriented/functional activities are introduced. For example, the patient is first placed on a stable surface and asked to maintain a relaxed core and then progressed to more unstable surfaces while maintaining this same relaxed position. This is then progressed into Stage 3.

Stage Three: Advanced Stage

Education

The final stage of treatment should focus on reinforcing concepts from the previous stages as the functional task increases in complexity.

Neuromuscular Reeducation

Motor control activities will increase in complexity with reactive postural control encouraged, where the patient is positioned first standing on a stable surface with eyes open and asked to maintain balance while the physical therapist provides small perturbations in each direction to encourage ankle strategies to maintain balance. The patient is then progressed to eyes closed with the same perturbations. The speed and displacement of the perturbations are then

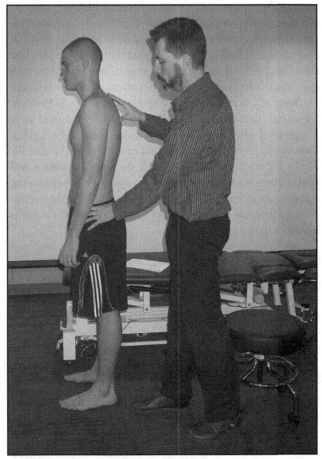

Figure 17-9. Cueing to facilitate neutral pelvis.

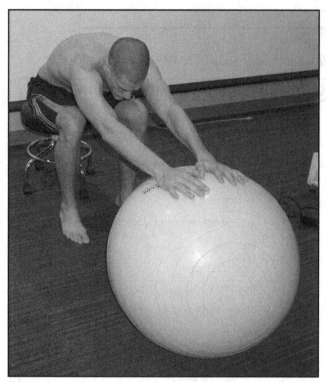

Figure 17-10. Relaxation into lumbar flexion using a ball.

increased in this position with eyes open, which may activate hip strategies as well as ankle strategies. Finally, the patient is placed on a moveable surface and asked to maintain postural control in standing while the physical therapist provides first small and then larger perturbations in all directions with eyes open and then closed. The patient can also perform reaching across midline in all directions or progress to single leg stance.[1] Balance and coordination activities should be at a high level and mimic high-level tasks required for IADLs. Two examples of this are provided in Figures 17-11 and 17-12. In Figure 17-11, the patient is on a stable surface and must maintain control of the lumbar spine while performing a diagonal movement with a ball. In Figure 17-12, the patient is on a moveable structure and performs a squat while maintaining balance.

Therapeutic Exercise/Activity

Interventions should challenge the individual and be related to a functional task that is meaningful to the patient to improve motor control of the lumbopelvic spine during movement.

CONTROL IMPAIRMENT GROUP (FLEXION)

For patients who have been identified to have a control impairment, the goal is to improve motor control of the lumbopelvic region because the lack of control in preventing the provocative positions is stressing structures and increasing pain.[2]

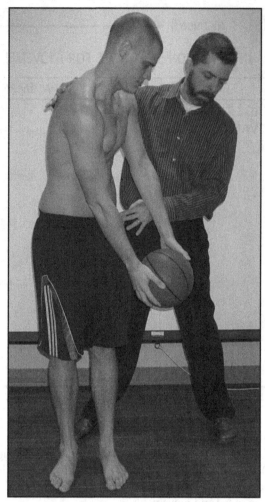

Figure 17-11. Coordination activity in multiple planes of movement.

Stage One: Beginner

Education

In this stage, the patient is educated on the nature of their pain and the relationship to the maladaptive flexed posture in producing the usual pain. The patient is educated on adopting an anterior pelvic tilt and taught to adopt this positioning over the usual posterior pelvic tilt positioning during ADLs. The patient is mobilized into the restriction. An HEP is initiated that reinforces this education.

Neuromuscular Reeducation

Neuromuscular control at this stage focuses on motor control activities to improve steady-state postural control. Core muscle contractions are facilitated through manual cues such as tapping, visual, and verbal cues. In Figure 17-13, the physical therapist is cueing the patient to activate transversus abdominis with manual contact. Mobilization toward the restriction (typically thoracic, lumbar, and/or hip extension) is performed starting passively and progressed to

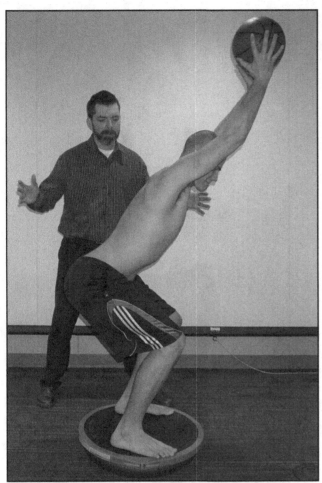

Figure 17-12. Balance activity on an unstable surface.

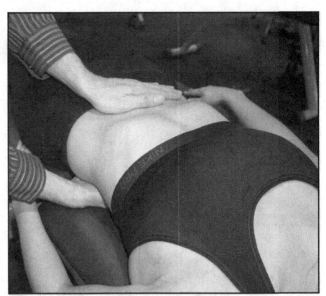

Figure 17-13. Cueing to facilitate transversus abdominus contraction.

active movement. Balance and coordination activities focus on static and dynamic control of the lumbopelvic region during functional tasks.

Therapeutic Exercise/Activity

The patient is placed in a less pain provocative position such as prone and supine with pelvic tilts and pelvic rotation added.

Stage Two: Intermediate

Education

In this stage, concepts from stage 1 are reinforced. The HEP is reviewed for compliance and updated as necessary.

Neuromuscular Reeducation

Motor control activities increase in complexity. Anticipatory motor control is encouraged as the patient activates core muscles and then performs movements at variable speeds in different directions in standing and sitting.[1] Balance and coordination activities likewise increase in complexity moving to a more dynamic control. Figure 17-14

demonstrates the patient activating core trunk muscles while seated on a ball (moveable surface) and marching in place. This skill requires increased motor control.

Therapeutic Exercise/Activity

Task-oriented/functional tasks are introduced starting on stable surfaces and progressing to unstable surfaces as the patient is able to maintain lumbopelvic control. Input should be encouraged from the patient to determine the functional tasks that are most important to them during daily activities.

Stage Three: Advanced Stage

Education

As with the movement impairment group, the final stage of treatment should focus on reinforcing concepts from the previous stages.

Neuromuscular Reeducation

Motor control activities will increase in complexity with reactive postural control encouraged.[1] Balance and coordination activities should be at a high level and mimic high-level tasks required for IADLs. Figure 17-15 demonstrates this as the patient is on a moveable surface while performing a higher-level task. In this case, she is standing on one leg while maintaining an activated core.

Therapeutic Exercise/Activity

Interventions should challenge the individual and be related to a functional task that is meaningful to the patient in order to improve motor control of the lumbopelvic spine during movement.

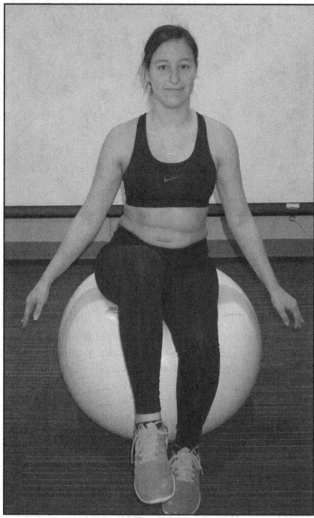

Figure 17-14. Core trunk muscle activation while on a moveable surface.

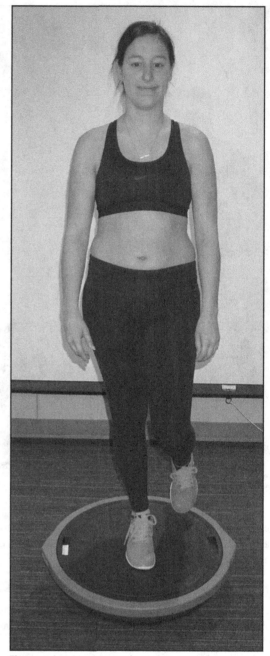

Figure 17-15. Motor control activity in single-leg stance on an unstable surface.

SUBSET OF THE CONTROL IMPAIRMENT GROUP

For a subset of the control impairment group that meet the CPR proposed by Hicks et al[7] and refined by Rabin et al,[53] a more traditional core stabilization program may be warranted in addition to the plan outlined earlier. This program would include a graduated program targeting core muscles, specifically transversus abdominus, erector spinae/multifidus, quadratus lumborum, and oblique abdominals. For each muscle, the individual starts with the first exercise presented and does not progress to the next level of difficulty until the criteria are met. These exercises have been shown to benefit individuals with "segmental instability, clinical instability, and chronic pain."[18]

CONCLUSION

Individuals with motor control impairments of the spine can be classified as having a movement impairment (active extension) or control impairment (flexion). These individuals may benefit from an individualized plan of care that takes into consideration the biopsychosocial aspects of patient care.

CASE STUDIES

The following case studies highlight a motor examination, evaluation, and rehabilitation of 2 individuals with motor impairments of the lumbar spine.

Case Study One: Movement Impairment (Active Extension)

History

A 35-year-old male architect presented with a 3-year history of LBP. Symptoms began soon after moving to a new residence with frequent lifting and carrying of heavy items. Symptoms were initially focal to the lumbar area and became radicular (into the right lower extremity) within the week. Magnetic resonance imaging revealed a herniated L4-5 disk, and after 3 epidurals, radicular symptoms were improved, but low back and gluteal pain was persistent. The patient was then referred to physical therapy and strongly encouraged to avoid forward bending, especially while in standing. Both this initial physical therapy treatment and subsequent chiropractic treatment were unsuccessful. The patient had continued pain after this until the present with ongoing pain

medicine intervention and very consistent compliance with a prior HEP (mostly extension ROM/strengthening exercises). In addition, the patient had been consistently utilizing several strategies to minimize lumbar flexion in his work/home settings and vehicles, including various added lumbar supports. At the time of treatment, the patient was referred to physical therapy by a neurosurgeon in the attempt to avoid lumbar surgery.

Current Symptoms

Right greater than left lumbar and gluteal pain with (at least) daily radiation to posterior hamstring and occasionally proximal calf (right only). He denied any recent altered sensation. Patient reports symptoms worst (tendency to peripheralize) with sitting and static standing tasks while movement, and sleep usually improved symptoms. No reports of bowel or bladder difficulties, but he reported ongoing difficulty with exhaustion and apprehension about unresolved symptoms.

Motor Examination Findings

Static Sitting

Posture. Patient sat at the edge of the examination table with a tight grip and held lumbar area stiffly in extension/increased lordosis with an anterior pelvic tilt (Figure 17-16).

Dynamic Sitting

Slump Sitting. At first, the patient resisted slump sitting and stated he thought it would be harmful. After performing the movement, he reported that slouching did not increase pain.

Transfers. In both sit-to-stand and stand-to-sit transfers, the patient initially refused to lean head over knees and, instead, used his upper extremities to assist with the transfer. He did both of these motions with a grimace and other signs of hypervigilance.

Static Standing

Posture. Continued pattern of lumbar extension/increased lordosis. He demonstrated a side-side weight shift and could not maintain a static position for more than a few seconds.

Dynamic Standing

Cardinal Plane Trunk Movements. Forward bending—Similar to the previous movement, the patient was seemingly upset that the requested movement would be harmful. He then forward bent nearly exclusively with hip flexion and kept the lumbar spine in a lordotic posture throughout. He also used his upper extremities to assist with the return to stand.

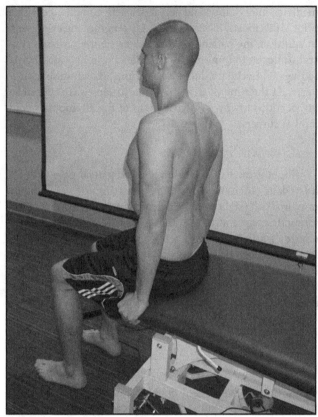

Figure 17-16. Increased lumbar lordosis in sitting.

After much discussion, the patient relaxed his musculature and forward bent with expected loss of lordosis and no pain. He expressed surprise that he had done so with success.

Combined Trunk Movements. After verbal cueing to relax, patient was noted to have good movement within the flexion quadrant to each side and (similar to previous) an ache with movement into the right extension quadrant.

Gait. Typical—Displayed decreased cadence, limited trunk rotation, and decreased arm swing. Corrective—With verbal and tactile (contacts to shoulders) cueing, patient reported ease of motion and increased cadence.

Combined Trunk/Extremity Movements. Backward bending with shoulders flexed was the most painful motion of all. Squatting: Without cueing, patient tended to adopt a hands-on-knees position and avoidance of deepest squat position with lumbar flexion.

Supine/Prone/Side-lying

Transfers. The patient used arms to assist with transfers and had decreased trunk rotation. He held his breath and exhibited stiff and guarded movements during tasks.

Recruitment/Facilitation. The patient required verbal cues to assume a posterior pelvic tilt. When he assumed a neutral pelvis, he reported that he was still in a posterior tilt, but that it was not painful.

Hip Movement. ROM in the right hip was decreased by 25% in internal rotation and extension. Patient noted some apprehension with single hip flexion PROM bilaterally, but negative neural tension signs.

Evaluation/Assessment

Patient presents with signs and symptoms consistent with a physical therapy diagnosis of movement impairment disorder/AEP in the lumbar spine. This was noted from the task-specific analysis examination findings, mostly with fear avoidance into flexion of the lumbar spine and significant focus on adopting an extended spinal posture despite the fact this position was actually uncomfortable. Furthermore, constant adoption of this extended posture led to fatigue, difficulty with accomplishing tasks, and continued provocation of symptoms.

Intervention

Even though the previous findings are listed as belonging to the examination process, stage 1 of his rehabilitative process has already begun. Increasing awareness of prior-held belief strategies that hamper proper function is the hallmark of PNE. Accepting that a change in strategies during ADLs is essential and likely necessary for all other interventions to have any benefit means that the first visit will mostly be PNE in focus. In this patient's case, the breakthrough moment was his realization of no symptom exacerbation (actually improved symptoms than neutral or extension) with forward bending after PNE strategies were adopted. Further education actually occurred throughout the rest of the examination with similar improved (or better than expected) symptoms. From this, physical therapy naturally turned to how to practice allowing flexion to occur in usual tasks.

Outcome

The patient progressed rapidly through stages 1 and 2. The pain and restriction with moving into an extended posture were greatly improved by focused manual therapy to the lower thoracic, lumbar spine, and focused treatment on the right more than the left hip. These were followed up by focused exercises to disassociate these areas with repeated movements into the restricted ROM. Otherwise, exercises within the physical therapy and HEP all sought to reinforce relaxation and gentle recruitment. Progression of neuromuscular reeducation activities included maintaining postural control on a rocker board with small and then large perturbations in all directions with eyes open and then eyes closed (Figure 17-17), single leg stance on the floor with eyes open and then closed, and then while reaching across midline with feedback on relaxation techniques provided. When entering into stage 3, the patient required additional education as he tended to want to revert back to usual patterns of hypervigilance. After 10 physical therapy visits, he was successful at returning to all noted activities with no exacerbation in the end.

Case Study Two: Control Impairment (Flexion)

History

The patient is a 25-year-old woman and the mother of a 6-month-old child. The patient has worsening bilateral lower and middle back pain, especially after the birth of the child. She noted having an occasional ache in the same area prior to pregnancy but reported that the pain would decrease after a workout. During pregnancy, the same symptoms were mild to nonexistent. She denied any trauma or significant stressor otherwise. Patient had returned to working, but mostly at home to allow her to care for her child. This normally entailed her working on a laptop in various positions on a couch or at a dining room table.

Current Symptoms

As noted earlier, the patient reported bilateral thoracic and lumbar pain with the left side mildly worse than right. She denied pain distal to the iliac crest or paresthesia/numbness. Pain tended to occur most with transfers from sitting (especially when working) and with lifting the child carrier from the floor or car. Similarly, car transfers often exacerbated symptoms, especially if she has driven more than 30 minutes. When her symptoms occurred, the discomfort often persisted for 30 minutes or more, but she would walk to decrease symptoms. Weight training was often helpful to minimize symptoms, but treadmill or bicycle use increased symptoms.

Motor Examination Findings

Static Sitting

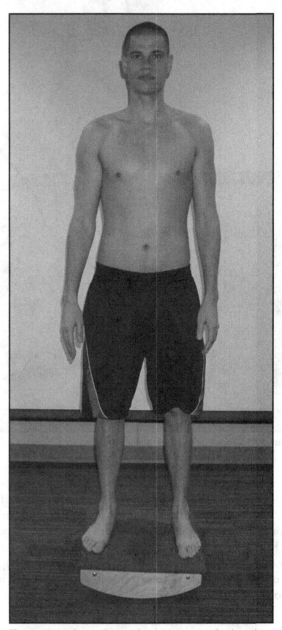

Figure 17-17. Postural control activities on a rocker board.

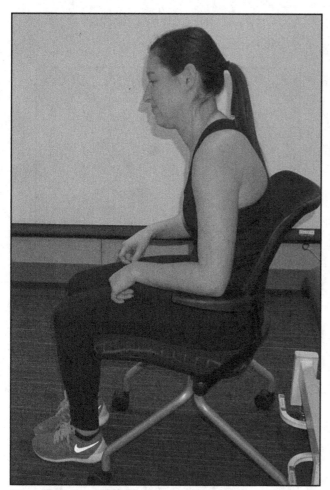

Figure 17-18. Increased kyphotic posture in sitting.

Posture. A kyphotic posture was normally adopted while performing paperwork and during history (Figure 17-18). With tactile cues, the patient was able to attain a neutral spine position but reported fatigue with doing so. After noting her preference for crossing her left leg over the right, she was asked to report what happened if she crossed the right leg over the left. She only noted that it was not painful, but reported it felt "weird."

Dynamic Sitting

Slump Sitting. As noted previously, the patient was able to attain a full slump sit with ease.

Transfers. During sit to stand, she maintained a kyphotic posture and reported usual pain symptoms.

Static Standing

Posture. Noted earlier. Patient was able to attain preferred (neutral) spine positioning but felt she was forcing herself to do so.

Dynamic Standing

Cardinal Plane Trunk Movements. Forward bending—Forward bending ROM was full and without provocation. However, she had difficulty controlling her descent and tended to use her hands to initiate the movement. Repeated movements into forward bending created usual symptoms after returning to stand. Backward bending—Backward bending decreased the symptoms the patient felt in repeated forward bending and was mildly limited.

Side-bending/Rotation. Left side-bending was mildly limited compared to right. Right side-bending tended to cause her to flex forward. She was unable to discern this even after corrective tactile cueing.

Combined Trunk Movements. Repeated flexion quadrant movements were noteworthy for full ROM, but repeated movements into that position reproduced usual symptoms after returning to stand.

Gait. The patient displayed forward flexed posture with arm movement, but no trunk rotation and minimal hip extension.

Combined Trunk/Extremity Movements. Upper or lower extremity movement/positioning combined with trunk movement (eg, reaching overhead with trunk extension).

Supine/Prone/Side-lying

Transfers. The patient tended to flex forward to initiate rolling. Supine-to-sit transfers tended to be the result of using bilateral arm swinging while sit-to-supine transfer was poorly controlled even with verbal cueing to correct.

Recruitment/Facilitation. Posterior pelvic tilt in supine was easy to accomplish and repeated repetitions resulted in usual pain occurrence after return to neutral, but less than when sitting or standing. Anterior pelvic tilt was noteworthy for being very difficult for the patient to accomplish and maintain. The patient displayed fair recruitment of her transversus abdominus, multifidus, and gluteal musculature.

Hip Movement. Most noteworthy was bilateral hip extension ROM loss with the right hip more limited than the left.

Patient Specific

The patient brought her child in to the physical therapy visit. With her child asleep in the usual carrier, she was asked to lift it and simulate placing it in the usual position in the car. She did this with expected flexed lumbar spine and bilateral shoulder shrugging to move into the necessary positions.

Evaluation/Assessment

The patient presented with signs and symptoms consistent with a physical therapy diagnosis of control impairment disorder (flexion pattern) in the lumbar spine. This is noted from the task-specific analysis examination findings, mostly with her habitual positioning into a flexed lumbar position despite the pain reproduction after she did so and her lack of ability to recognize this. Similarly, she also failed to recognize doing repeated activities out of this flexion pattern (eg, weight training, repeated backward bending) actually decreased symptoms. Furthermore, constant adoption of this flexed posture led to difficulty attaining any other postures during usual tasks, which led to continued provocation of symptoms.

Intervention

Stage 1 of her rehabilitative process had already begun with education about the changes in positive/negative symptoms during testing. Increasing awareness of prior-held belief strategies that hamper proper function is the hallmark of PNE. Accepting that a change in strategies during ADLs is essential and likely necessary for all other interventions to have any benefit means that the first visit will mostly be PNE in focus. The patient began to connect symptoms to adoption of prolonged provocative lumbar flexion movements and positions. Similarly, the improvement of symptoms after repeated extended postures (opposite of her favored positioning) supported this assertion. Neuromuscular reeducation focused on cueing adoption of more anterior pelvic tilt in supine and sitting (Figure 17-19). Similarly, ROM exercises promoting thoracic extension were initiated. Stage 1 was also noteworthy for education on specific unavoidable ADLs (childcare tasks in particular) and tactics to improve positioning.

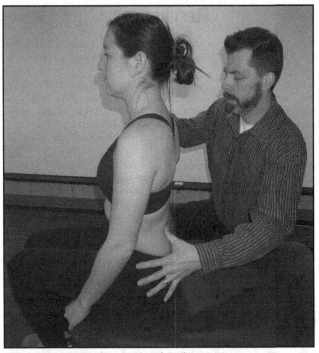

Figure 17-19. Cueing for anterior pelvic tilt in sitting.

Outcome

The patient saw an immediate improvement when adopting physical therapy suggested positions during noted ADLs. However, she frequently noted "failing" when performing functional tasks quickly. Significant time in stages 2 and 3 was spent on improving items like hip extension and thoracic extension/rotation and increasing the difficulty of these tasks with the addition of balance/coordination activities while maintaining optimum positioning. In most cases, progression to a more challenging level required tactile and verbal cues. At the 12-visit mark, the patient was discharged. She felt she was able to attain proper positioning about 80% of the time and only had mild symptom occurrence after failing for a bit on best positioning tactics.

References

1. Shumway-Cook A, Woollacott M. *Motor Control: Translating Research into Clinical Practice*. 4th ed. Lippincott Williams & Wilkins; 2011.

2. O'Sullivan P. Diagnosis, Classification Management of Chronic low back pain - From a mechanism based bio-psycho-social perspective. 2006. file:///C:/Users/WKUUSER/AppData/Roaming/Mozilla/Firefox/Profiles/hw3egrfs.default/zotero/storage/BPPDJ2JP/lumbo-pelvic_workshoplevio7handouts.pdf. Accessed September 16, 2016.

3. O'Sullivan P. Diagnosis and classification of chronic low back pain disorders: maladaptive movement and motor control impairments as underlying mechanism. *Man Ther*. 2005;10(4):242-255. doi:10.1016/j.math.2005.07.001

4. Reeves NP, Narendra KS, Cholewicki J. Spine stability: the six blind men and the elephant. *Clin Biomech Bristol Avon*. 2007;22(3):266-274. doi:10.1016/j.clinbiomech.2006.11.011

5. Bergmark A. Stability of the lumbar spine. A study in mechanical engineering. *Acta Orthop Scand Suppl*. 1989;230:1-54.

6. Dankaerts W, O'Sullivan P. The validity of O'Sullivan's classification system (CS) for a sub-group of NS-CLBP with motor control impairment (MCI): overview of a series of studies and review of the literature. *Man Ther*. 2011;16(1):9-14.

7. Hicks GE, Fritz JM, Delitto A, McGill SM. Preliminary development of a clinical prediction rule for determining which patients with low back pain will respond to a stabilization exercise program. *Arch Phys Med Rehabil*. 2005;86(9):1753-1762. doi:10.1016/j.apmr.2005.03.033

8. Knutsson F. The instability associated with disk degeneration in the lumbar spine. *Acta Radiol*. 1944;25(5-6):593-609.

9. Puentedura EJ, Louw A. A neuroscience approach to managing athletes with low back pain. *Phys Ther Sport*. 2012;13(3):123-133. doi:10.1016/j.ptsp.2011.12.001

10. Nachemson A. Back pain: delimiting the problem in the next millennium. *Int J Law Psychiatry*. 1999;22(5-6):473-490.

11. Dillingham T. Evaluation and management of low back pain: an overview. *Spine State Art Rev*. 9(3):559-774.

12. Panjabi MM. The stabilizing system of the spine. Part I. Function, dysfunction, adaptation, and enhancement. *J Spinal Disord*. 1992;5(4):383-389; discussion 397.

13. Panjabi MM. The stabilizing system of the spine. Part II. Neutral zone and instability hypothesis. *J Spinal Disord*. 1992;5(4):390-396; discussion 397.

14. Hodges PW, Richardson CA. Altered trunk muscle recruitment in people with low back pain with upper limb movement at different speeds. *Arch Phys Med Rehabil*. 1999;80(9):1005-1012.

15. Maaswinkel E, Griffioen M, Perez RSGM, van Dieën JH. Methods for assessment of trunk stabilization, a systematic review. *J Electromyogr Kinesiol*. 2016;26:18-35. doi:10.1016/j.jelekin.2015.12.010

16. Akuthota V, Ferreiro A, Moore T, Fredericson M. Core stability exercise principles. *Curr Sports Med Rep*. 2008;7(1):39-44. doi:10.1097/01.CSMR.0000308663.13278.69

17. Lederman E. The myth of core stability. *J Bodyw Mov Ther*. 2010;14(1):84-98. doi:10.1016/j.jbmt.2009.08.001

18. Biely S, Smith SS, Silfies SP. Clinical instability of the lumbar spine: diagnosis and intervention. *Orthop Pract*. 2006;18(3):11-18.

19. Dankaerts W, O'Sullivan P, Burnett A, Straker L. Altered patterns of superficial trunk muscle activation during sitting in nonspecific chronic low back pain patients: importance of sub-classification. *Spine*. 2006;31(17):2017-2023. doi:10.1097/01.brs.0000228728.11076.82

20. O'Sullivan P. It's time for change with the management of non-specific chronic low back pain. *Br J Sports Med*. 2012;46(4):224-227.

21. van Dieen JH, Cholewicki J, Radebold A. Trunk muscle recruitment patterns in patients with low back pain enhance the stability. *Spine*. 2003;28:834-841. doi:10.1097/00007632-200304150-00018

22. Smith BE, Littlewood C, May S. An update of stabilisation exercises for low back pain: a systematic review with meta-analysis. *BMC Musculoskelet Disord*. 2014;15:416. doi:10.1186/1471-2474-15-416

23. Borrell-Carrió F, Suchman AL, Epstein RM. The Biopsychosocial Model 25 years later: principles, practice, and scientific inquiry. *Ann Fam Med*. 2004;2(6):576-582. doi:10.1370/afm.245

24. Introduction to the guide to physical therapist practice—guide to physical therapist practice. American Physical Therapy Association. http://guidetoptpractice.apta.org/content/1/SEC1.body. Accessed March 11, 2017.

25. *International classification of functioning, disability and health*. World Health Organization. http://www.who.int/classifications/icf/en/. Accessed April 29, 2022.

26. Cowell I, O'Sullivan P, O'Sullivan K, Poyton R, McGregor A, Murtagh G. Perceptions of physiotherapists towards the management of non-specific chronic low back pain from a biopsychosocial perspective: a qualitative study. *Musculoskelet Sci Pract*. 2018;38:113-119. doi:10.1016/j.msksp.2018.10.006

27. Louw A, Zimney K, Puentedura EJ, Diener I. The efficacy of pain neuroscience education on musculoskeletal pain: a systematic review of the literature. *Physiother Theory Pract*. 2016;32(5):332-355. doi:10.1080/09593985.2016.1194646

28. Linton SJ, Shaw WS. Impact of psychological factors in the experience of pain. *Phys Ther*. 2011;91(5):700-711. doi:10.2522/ptj.20100330

29. Foster NE, Delitto A. Embedding psychosocial perspectives within clinical management of low back pain: integration of psychosocially informed management principles into physical therapist practice—challenges and opportunities. *Phys Ther*. 2011;91(5):790-803. doi:10.2522/ptj.20100326

30. Bodes Pardo G, Lluch Girbés E, Roussel NA, Gallego Izquierdo T, Jiménez Penick V, Pecos Martín D. Pain neurophysiology education and therapeutic exercise for patients with chronic low back pain: a single-blind randomized controlled trial. *Arch Phys Med Rehabil*. 2018;99(2):338-347. doi:10.1016/j.apmr.2017.10.016

31. O'Sullivan P, Caneiro JP, O'Keeffe M, O'Sullivan K. Unraveling the complexity of low back pain. *J Orthop Sports Phys Ther*. 2016;46(11):932-937. doi:10.2519/jospt.2016.0609

32. Gifford L. Pain, the tissues and the nervous system: a conceptual model. *Physiotherapy*. 1998;84(1):27-36. doi:10.1016/S0031-9406(05)65900-7

33. Brumagne S, Diers M, Danneels L, Moseley GL, Hodges PW. Neuroplasticity of sensorimotor control in low back pain. *J Orthop Sports Phys Ther*. 2019;49(6):402-414. doi:10.2519/jospt.2019.8489

34. O'Sullivan PB, Caneiro JP, O'Keeffe M, et al. Cognitive functional therapy: an integrated behavioral approach for the targeted management of disabling low back pain. *Phys Ther*. 2018;98(5):408-423. doi:10.1093/ptj/pzy022

35. Vibe Fersum K, Smith A, Kvåle A, Skouen JS, O'Sullivan P. Cognitive functional therapy in patients with non-specific chronic low back pain-a randomized controlled trial 3-year follow-up. *Eur J Pain*. 2019;23(8):1416-1424. doi:10.1002/ejp.1399

36. O'Sullivan PB, Beales DJ. Diagnosis and classification of pelvic girdle pain disorders, part 2: illustration of the utility of a classification system via case studies. *Man Ther*. 2007;12(2):e1-12. doi:10.1016/j.math.2007.03.003

37. Beales DJ, O'Sullivan PB, Briffa NK. Motor control patterns during an active straight leg raise in pain-free subjects. *Spine*. 2009;34(1):E1-E8. doi:10.1097/BRS.0b013e318188b9dd

38. Dankaerts W, O'Sullivan P, Burnett A, Straker L, Davey P, Gupta R. Discriminating healthy controls and two clinical subgroups of nonspecific chronic low back pain patients using trunk muscle activation and lumbosacral kinematics of postures and movements: a statistical classification model. *Spine.* 2009;34(15):1610-1618. doi:10.1097/BRS.0b013e3181aa6175

39. Dankaerts W, O'Sullivan PB, Burnett AF, Straker LM. The use of a mechanism-based classification system to evaluate and direct management of a patient with non-specific chronic low back pain and motor control impairment—a case report. *Man Ther.* 2007;12(2):181-191. doi:10.1016/j.math.2006.05.004

40. O'Sullivan PB, Beales DJ. Diagnosis and classification of pelvic girdle pain disorders—part 1: a mechanism based approach within a biopsychosocial framework. *Man Ther.* 2007;12(2):86-97. doi:10.1016/j.math.2007.02.001

41. O'Sullivan P, Dankaerts W, Burnett A, et al. Evaluation of the flexion relaxation phenomenon of the trunk muscles in sitting. *Spine.* 2006;31(17):2009-2016. doi:10.1097/01.brs.0000228845.27561.e0

42. O'Sullivan PB, Mitchell T, Bulich P, Waller R, Holte J. The relationship between posture and back muscle endurance in industrial workers with flexion-related low back pain. *Man Ther.* 2006;11(4):264-271. doi:10.1016/j.math.2005.04.004

43. Sheeran L, Sparkes V, Caterson B, Busse-Morris M, van Deursen R. Spinal position sense and trunk muscle activity during sitting and standing in nonspecific chronic low back pain: classification analysis. *Spine.* 2012;37(8):E486-495. doi:10.1097/BRS.0b013e31823b00ce

44. Sheeran L, van Deursen R, Caterson B, Sparkes V. Classification-guided versus generalized postural intervention in subgroups of nonspecific chronic low back pain: a pragmatic randomized controlled study. *Spine.* 2013;38(19):1613-1625. doi:10.1097/BRS.0b013e31829e049b

45. Vibe Fersum K, O'Sullivan PB, Kvåle A, Skouen JS. Inter-examiner reliability of a classification system for patients with non-specific low back pain. *Man Ther.* 2009;14(5):555-561. doi:10.1016/j.math.2008.08.003

46. Principles of physical therapist patient and client management — guide to physical therapist practice. American Physical Therapy Association. http://guidetoptpractice.apta.org/content/1/SEC2.body. Accessed March 6, 2017.

47. Porter JL, Wilkinson A. Lumbar-hip flexion motion. A comparative study between asymptomatic and chronic low back pain in 18- to 36-year-old men. *Spine.* 1997;22(13):1508-1513, discussion 1513-1514.

48. Almeida GPL, de Souza VL, Sano SS, Saccol MF, Cohen M. Comparison of hip rotation range of motion in judo athletes with and without history of low back pain. *Man Ther.* 2012;17(3):231-235. doi:10.1016/j.math.2012.01.004

49. Ellison JB, Rose SJ, Sahrmann SA. Patterns of hip rotation range of motion: a comparison between healthy subjects and patients with low back pain. *Phys Ther.* 1990;70(9):537-541.

50. Burnett AF, Cornelius MW, Dankaerts W, O'Sullivan PB. Spinal kinematics and trunk muscle activity in cyclists: a comparison between healthy controls and non-specific chronic low back pain subjects—a pilot investigation. *Man Ther.* 2004;9(4):211-219. doi:10.1016/j.math.2004.06.002

51. Hodges PW, Moseley GL, Gabrielsson A, Gandevia SC. Experimental muscle pain changes feedforward postural responses of the trunk muscles. *Exp Brain Res.* 2003;151(2):262-271. doi:10.1007/s00221-003-1457-x

52. Moseley GL, Nicholas MK, Hodges PW. Does anticipation of back pain predispose to back trouble? *Brain J Neurol.* 2004;127(Pt 10):2339-2347. doi:10.1093/brain/awh248

53. Rabin A, Shashua A, Pizem K, Dickstein R, Dar G. A clinical prediction rule to identify patients with low back pain who are likely to experience short-term success following lumbar stabilization exercises: a randomized controlled validation study. *J Orthop Sports Phys Ther.* 2014;44(1):6-B13. doi:10.2519/jospt.2014.4888

54. Jull G. Discord between approaches to spinal and extremity disorders: is it logical? *J Orthop Sports Phys Ther.* 2016;46(11):938-941. doi:10.2519/jospt.2016.0610

55. Van Dillen LR, Sahrmann SA, Norton BJ, et al. Effect of active limb movements on symptoms in patients with low back pain. *J Orthop Sports Phys Ther.* 2001;31(8):402-413, discussion 414-418. doi:10.2519/jospt.2001.31.8.402

56. Moseley GL. I can't find it! Distorted body image and tactile dysfunction in patients with chronic back pain. *Pain.* 2008;140(1):239-243. doi:10.1016/j.pain.2008.08.001

57. O'Sullivan K, Dankaerts W, O'Sullivan L, O'Sullivan PB. Cognitive functional therapy for disabling nonspecific chronic low back pain: multiple case-cohort study. *Phys Ther.* 2015;95(11):1478-1488. doi:10.2522/ptj.20140406

58. Mannion AF, Junge A, Taimela S, Müntener M, Lorenzo K, Dvorak J. Active therapy for chronic low back pain: part 3. Factors influencing self-rated disability and its change following therapy. *Spine.* 2001;26(8):920-929.

59. Smeets RJEM, Vlaeyen JWS, Kester ADM, Knottnerus JA. Reduction of pain catastrophizing mediates the outcome of both physical and cognitive-behavioral treatment in chronic low back pain. *J Pain.* 2006;7(4):261-271. doi:10.1016/j.jpain.2005.10.011

60. O'Keeffe M, Purtill H, Kennedy N, et al. Individualised cognitive functional therapy compared with a combined exercise and pain education class for patients with non-specific chronic low back pain: study protocol for a multicentre randomised controlled trial. *BMJ Open.* 2015;5(6):e007156. doi:10.1136/bmjopen-2014-007156

61. Synnott A, O'Keeffe M, Bunzli S, et al. Physiotherapists report improved understanding of and attitude toward the cognitive, psychological and social dimensions of chronic low back pain after cognitive functional therapy training: a qualitative study. *J Physiother.* 2016;62(4):215-221. doi:10.1016/j.jphys.2016.08.002

62. Vibe Fersum K, O'Sullivan P, Skouen J, Smith A, Kvåle A. Efficacy of classification-based cognitive functional therapy in patients with non-specific chronic low back pain: A randomized controlled trial. *Eur J Pain.* 2013;17(6):916-928. doi:10.1002/j.1532-2149.2012.00252.x

63. Wälti P, Kool J, Luomajoki H. Short-term effect on pain and function of neurophysiological education and sensorimotor retraining compared to usual physiotherapy in patients with chronic or recurrent non-specific low back pain, a pilot randomized controlled trial. *BMC Musculoskelet Disord.* 2015;16(1):83-93. doi:10.1186/s12891-015-0533-2

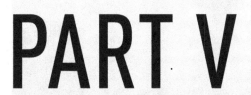

PART V

**Special Topics in
Orthopedic Rehabilitation**

18

Evidence-Based Rehabilitation of Concussion or Mild Traumatic Brain Injury

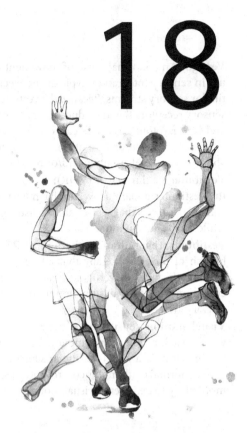

Kenji Carp, PT, OCS, ATC
and Robert Donatelli, PT, PhD

KEY TERMS

Anxiety: A well-recognized psychological condition characterized by a state of heightened unease and apprehension. Anxiety is often associated with the symptoms of concussion, loss of function, and related client self-perception of their impacted social roles. Anxiety is strongly correlated with depression and can result in obsessive behaviors and panic attacks.

Balance: The motor skill of maintaining the body's center of mass over the base of support. Balance is one expression of neuromuscular control (NMC).

Dizziness: A variety of sensations including faint, woozy, and/or unsteady.

Exertion: The expenditure of energy by skeletal and cardiac muscle. Practitioners in the United States commonly refer to this as *aerobic* and *anaerobic* exercise.

Mild traumatic brain injury (MTBI): Also known *concussion*. This consists of diffuse trauma to the brain, which results in transient disruption of numerous brain functions without organic brain damage.

Neuromuscular control (NMC): The process of coordinating movement appropriate to the situation. NMC is achieved by the subconscious integration of sensory input by the central nervous system (CNS) to derive and execute a motor solution through muscle activity.

Nystagmus: Rapid, involuntary movement of both eyes provoked by normal physiological stimuli and in the presence of pathology.

Oculomotor control: The combined actions of the nervous system to coordinate the extra-ocular muscles to move and fixate visual gaze to attain visual sensory input. This is accomplished by orchestration of complex neural pathways in the brainstem, optic nerves, and visual cortex.

Opticokinetic stimuli: Visual images that contain repeating, contrasting striped patterns that induce nystagmus perpendicular to the stripes (opticokinetic nystagmus). This often provokes visual motion sensitivity.

Oscillopsia: A visual illusion of an unstable, oscillating image that occurs when the vestibular ocular reflex (VOR) fails to stabilize gaze.

Sensory integration: In the context of vestibular rehabilitation, sensory integration refers to processing and comparison of visual, somatosensory, and vestibular sensory input to perceive head position and movement.

Wallmann HW, Donatelli R, eds. *Foundations of Orthopedic Physical Therapy* (pp 545-584).
© 2024 Taylor & Francis Group.

Vertigo: An abnormal sense of movement caused by a failure in sensory integration, typically between visual and vestibular sensory streams. Because the vestibular apparatus has sensory receptors that transduce rotary (semicircular canals) and linear (otoliths), errors can occur in the processing of either or both senses of motion. Thus, vertigo refers to an abnormal sense of spinning and/or rocking/drifting.

Vestibular ocular reflex (VOR): A reflexive loop between the vestibular apparatus, vestibular nuclei, and oculomotor control pathways that act to stabilize visual gaze on the target while the head is in motion.

Vestibular rehabilitation therapy (VRT): A specialized branch of physical therapy that addresses conditions such as multiple types of vertigo, imbalance, nausea, and other conditions related to dysfunction in the vestibular and other sensory systems.

Visual motion sensitivity: A type of vertigo that occurs when visual stimuli such as moving backgrounds and optical illusions induce a visual-vestibular sensory conflict. Patients with abnormal oculomotor control and gaze stabilization are more likely to experience visual motion sensitivity.

CHAPTER QUESTIONS

1. What is vertigo and how is it treated?
2. How does MTBI affect the vestibular system?
3. What is the function of the VOR?
4. What is oscillopsia?
5. What is nystagmus and what causes it?
6. What is the function of the otolith system?
7. What is the function of the rods within the retina?
8. What is the function of the cones within the retina?
9. What is the function of the fovea?
10. What is peripheral vertigo?
11. What nerve within the inner ear could be damaged by head trauma?
12. What are the 3 sensory streams are most relevant to our brain for movement and balance?
13. What is vergence?
14. What are saccade eye movements?
15. What is smooth pursuit eye movements?
16. What is optokinetic eye movement?
17. What is the head impulse test (HIT)?
18. What is the dynamic visual acuity test (DVAT)?
19. What is the Balance Error Scoring System (BESS)?
20. What is the Brock's string test?

INTRODUCTION

Some readers of this chapter may wonder why MTBI, also known as *concussion*, is included in a text of orthopedic physical therapy. To begin, MTBI is extremely prevalent as annual estimates for MTBI range from 2 to 3.8 million annually in the United States. This is especially true in people also prone to orthopedic injury such as athletes, military personnel, and drivers.[1-4] Because orthopedic physical therapists are often the first health care provider to encounter clients who have sustained MTBI, it follows that they should have knowledge of the condition for identification, advocacy, and treatment. For example, approximately 20% to 30% (and this is likely underreported) of all high school football players have experienced one or more concussions.[5] Collegiate athletes were shown to be 2.48 times more likely to sustain a lower extremity orthopedic injury in the 90-day period after return to play following an MTBI.[3] So, effective evaluation and treatment of MTBI also provides a means to prevent further orthopedic injury.[6] In addition, studies show testing of balance, measures of oculomotor coordination, and other measures of NMC performed by physical therapists are vital aspects of thorough assessment and triage of MTBI.[1,3,4,6,7,8] While traditionally evaluation of MTBI was in the scope of VRT, new evidence shows a growing role for orthopedic physical therapists in the treatment of concurrent musculoskeletal neck pain, headaches, and sport-specific exertion training.[4,9-12]

PATHOPHYSIOLOGY OF MILD TRAUMATIC BRAIN INJURY

In the uninjured brain, electrochemical signals for thoughts and actions travel through the brain via chains of interconnected neurons. Healthy resting neurons are polarized, meaning they have a negative charge inside and a positive charge outside. The charge is established by the electrical properties of proteins and positively charged potassium ions (K+) inside the neuron membrane against the negatively charged sodium (Na+) and calcium (Ca2+) ions outside the membrane. The natural resting polarity is maintained by pumps in the membrane.[8,13-15]

When a neuron is stimulated, ion channels rapidly open allowing K+ to enter and depolarize the neuron. This change in electrical charge across the membrane propagates down the length of the neuron membrane. At the end of the neuron, the electrical signal triggers the opening of calcium channels, allowing Ca2+ to enter the neuron, releasing the neurotransmitter. The neurotransmitter, or chemical part of the signal, crosses the synapse, binds with receptors in the next neuron, and the process continues.[8,13-15]

The diffuse brain trauma with MTBI is thought to disrupt the neuronal membrane allowing excitatory neurotransmitters, such as glutamate, free to roam the brain. This, in turn, causes a wave of neuronal firing resulting in a mass exodus of K+ and immigration of Ca2+, resulting in a massive degree of neuron depolarization.[13-15] The neuron ion pumps must work overtime to restore the normal resting neuron polarization. To make matters worse, the increased metabolic demand of pumping is accompanied by a transient decrease in cerebral blood flow, thus decreasing available energy to power the pumps.[1,3-5,8,9,11,13-18] So, the concussed brain has a sudden and large metabolic deficit it must pay down before neuronal impulses return to normal. In the meantime, any areas of brain function such as cognitive, emotional, sensory, and motor processing served by the impacted neurons suffer.[4,8-11,14,15,19]

Sensory Integration, Balance, and Vertigo With Mild Traumatic Brain Injury

Sensory integration is the CNS processing and comparison of data from the vestibular, visual, and somatosensory input streams to determine the perception of position.[15,18,20] The vestibular–cochlear organ is housed in the inner ear or "vestibule" of the temporal bone. Most people associate the ear with sensation of sound provided by the cochlea. However, most do not know the vestibular apparatus detects linear and rotational head movements via the otoliths and semicircular canals, respectively. Vestibular input travels to the CNS via cranial nerve VIII, also known as the *vestibulocochlear nerve*.[3,8-10,15] The function of the vestibular apparatus is analogous to that of our smart phone accelerometers and gyroscopes that detect movement of the device and signal the computer processor. Visual perception is discussed in detail in the oculomotor control section later. Somatosensory input refers to the cumulative data from all touch and pressure receptors. Proprioception or joint position sense is one aspect of somatosensory perception.[6,15,20] In the uninjured brain, sensory integration is normally so consistently accurate that perception almost always matches reality.[2,6,8,15,18]

NMC, as defined by Williams et al in 2001, "involves the subconscious integration of sensory information that is processed by the [CNS], resulting in controlled movement through coordinated muscle activity."[21] In plain terms, NMC is the process of producing coordinated movement appropriate to the situational demands. The brain uses sensory integration to perceive head position in space, compares this to the desired goal, and then determines the error signal. Next, it derives and executes a motor solution to achieve the goal. NMC of the head, spine, and extremities is modulated through complex synaptic pathways in the vestibular spinal and colic reflexes.[6,15,18,20,21] Balance is the motor skill of maintaining the center of mass over the base of support and is one of many expressions of NMC.[15,18,20,21]

For example, a gymnast tumbling through the air uses sensory integration of visual, vestibular, and somatosensory inputs to perceive they are underrotated. To correct this, they tighten their body into a smaller package to speed rotation to a vertical orientation at landing (NMC). Upon landing, they use their skill of balance to maintain their center of mass over the base of support to "stick" the landing.

Conversely, an elite baseball hitter must rely nearly exclusively on vision. Hitters have the difficult task of striking a fastball traveling at speeds of 90 to 105 miles per hour. A 95-mile-per-hour fastball takes just 400 milliseconds or roughly the same time as the blink of an eye to reach home plate.[22] Since it takes approximately 180 to 200 milliseconds to swing the bat, that leaves a scant 200 milliseconds to identify the pitch. So, sensory integration of visual input absolutely guides the hitter to execute a feed forward form of NMC, either swing or take the pitch (do not swing). During the swing, the hitter rapidly shifts their weight to transfer energy into the bat while maintaining their center of mass over their base of support (balance).[16,20,22] Thus, the skill of hitting in baseball is a very complex expression of NMC including eye–hand coordination and balance. Due to the fast pitching speeds, the sensory integration necessary for NMC is almost exclusively visually mediated.[16,20-22]

Vertigo is an abnormal perception of motion that is not physically occurring.[16] Vertigo is caused by errors in sensory integration that can occur rarely under normal physiological conditions but very commonly with pathologies affecting sensory perception such as MTBI. An example of physiological vertigo is the perception of persistent spinning movement when a parent or child gets off a playground merry-go-round. In this example, the severe asymmetrical stimulation of the semicircular canals of the vestibular apparatus tricks the brain into a brief period of perceived spinning even though they are off the carousel and have stopped physically moving. The same would be true of a novice figure skater or ballet dancer practicing turns. Thankfully, in the uninjured athlete, the CNS rapidly and accurately processes the sensory input from visual, vestibular, and somatosensory streams to reestablish sensory integration and, in turn, control the vertigo. However, when MTBI affects the CNS neurons that process vestibular input, numerous computational errors occur resulting in faulty sensory integration and thus vertigo of central origin.[2-4,6,7,16,20,23-31] Occasionally, the same head trauma injures the vestibular apparatus and/or vestibulocochlear nerve resulting in altered vestibular sensory input or peripheral vertigo (ie, the damaged inner ear tricks the brain).[2,7,16,23,26-28,32]

Nausea is also common with MTBI and typically correlates with vertigo.[2-4,7,9,16,25,29] This is because the inner ear is also a toxin sensor and thus has reflexive pathways from the vestibulocochlear nerve, through the vestibular brain stem nuclei to the emetic center in the pons, which triggers nausea.[11,15,25] Nausea and vomiting are completely appropriate if a person needs to expel an ingested toxin. Unfortunately, the reflexive pathways to the emetic center are also commonly triggered with central or peripheral vestibular conditions.[1-4,7,11,16,25,29,31,33,34]

OCULOMOTOR CONTROL

Oculomotor control is a specialized form of NMC coordinating eye movements and brief pauses or fixation to capture light on the retina, which the visual cortex uses to form visual perception[16,20,22-30,32] A useful analogy for this is of an old school photographer making a photo mosaic by shooting multiple small photos or a large object and then pasting them together to form one cohesive image. The modern version of this is the panorama feature in smart phone camera applications. Oculomotor control moves the eyes in the same way to capture a series of images on the retina, which the visual cortices process to form a cohesive visual perception of the environment.[3-10,12,14-16,23-30,32]

The retina at the back of the eye holds rods and cones, which transduce photons of light energy into neural impulses. Rods, which react to movement and contrast, are spread across the periphery of the retina.[16,32,24,25] As a result, they provide peripheral visual perception from a great variety of eye positions vs requiring a specific eye movement. For example, a running back breaking through the line of scrimmage can detect an opposing tackler closing in from the side without moving their head or eyes. The running back does not require visual detail, just awareness the tackler is there.

Conversely, cones, which provide the high definition, color, and greatest amount of visual sensory data, reside on the small central fovea of the retina. Consequently, foveal vision, also known as *focal vision*, is correspondingly small (about 4 characters at typical reading distance). So, oculomotor control of foveal vision is normally highly accurate to bring the tiny retinal fovea to the correct location to capture light. This is accomplished by elegant motor programs, which descend from the cortex through the cerebellum, oculomotor, abducens, trochlear brain stem nuclei, and their respective cranial nerves. The efferent neural signals produce combined muscle actions in the 6 extra-ocular muscles, resulting in coordinated eye movement.[15,21-25,32]

The eye movements involved in oculomotor control are further described by the following terms. *Smooth pursuits* track slow moving targets. *Saccades* rapidly move foveal vision from one target to another or catch up to faster moving targets. *Vergence* refers inward eye movements (convergence) to see targets in close and outward eye movements (divergence) to see distant targets. Vergence is a key part of coordination of binocular vision, which provides the depth perception most relevant for balance, eye–hand coordination, and eye–foot forms of NMC. *Fixation of gaze* refers to the cessation of eye movements to capture foveal visual images.[3-10,13-16,21-29] It is important to note we describe these functions of oculomotor control separately to improve understanding, but they interact simultaneously to find and track visual cues of highly varied speed and position in 3-dimensional (3D) space. Because of the relatively large area of the brain devoted to visual processing, oculomotor control is frequently impacted by MTBI.[2-4,8-10,13-16,22-30]

GAZE STABILIZATION AND THE VESTIBULAR OCULAR REFLEX

The VOR is a reflexive loop between the vestibular apparatus, vestibular nuclei, and oculomotor control centers that act to stabilize visual gaze onto a target (ie, maintain visual fixation) while the head is in motion. The net result of a healthy VOR is conjugate eye movement contralateral to the direction of head movement. So, if you move the head left, both eyes will move right to stay on target.[3,4,8-10,13,16,22-29,32]

The typical gain or ratio between head movement and contralateral eye movement produced by the VOR is 0.8, which is why most people get some degree of oscillopsia, or retinal slip at high speeds of oscillating head movement. If the reader does not suffer from vertigo, they should try moving their head side to side as if gesturing, "no" and note the speed at which the text begins to jump. Whereas elite athletes can pose a VOR gain of 1.0 or a one-to-one ratio, which is why an uninjured receiver can see the ball clearly even when running at a full sprint, despite the perturbation of the head. In contrast, clients with impairments in the vestibular system can drop to a VOR gain as low as 0.2 causing massive oscillopsia, which is why they report visual disturbances of "jumpy" or "things look like handheld video," even with minimal head movements.[9,10,14,16,23,26-30]

VISUAL MOTION SENSITIVITY

Visual motion sensitivity is a type of vertigo that occurs when abnormal visual sensory integration creates a visual-vestibular disagreement.[3,4,8-10,16,23-30] A physiological example most of us have experienced is the misperception that our stationary car was rolling backward while viewing a large vehicle pulling forward. Because the other vehicle moving forward provides the same visual stimuli we would receive if our vehicle were rolling backward, it temporarily tricks the brain into the misperception that our vehicle is rolling backward. The misperception feels so real that it even causes the driver to slam on their brakes (misguided NMC and an incorrect motor response). Normally, sensory integration is so rapid and accurate that misperception is rare. However, with MTBI, abnormal oculomotor control can result in visual motion sensitivity with even routine visual stimuli.[2,3,7,9,10,16,23-30]

One example is opticokinetic stimuli that contain repeating high contrast striped patterns that trick the brain into involuntarily moving the eyes perpendicular to the stripes (opticokinetic nystagmus) and induces visual motion sensitivity.[8,12,13,15,16,23-30] Opticokinetic stimuli occur commonly in nature, such as with passing a row of trees or moving crowds. It is also intentionally employed in graphic design to create the illusion of movement and in commercial carpet and fabric design as it manipulates gaze past unsightly stains (Figure 18-1). Visual special effects in media, such as computer-generated animation, camera pans/tilts, jump cuts, and hand-held camera work (oscillopsia), can also provoke visual motion sensitivity. This is why many concussed clients often have symptoms with these types of visual backgrounds.[16,23-30]

EVALUATION, IDENTIFICATION OR PATHOPHYSIOLOGY, AND CLINICAL DECISION MAKING

As previously discussed, the prevalence and impact of MTBI has health care professionals, sports organizations, and society in general yearning for highly predictive clinical measures to both identify MTBI and guide return-to-play/life decisions. Despite our desires this has proved extremely difficult for several reasons. Because MTBI effects multiple areas of brain function including sensory integration, NMC, balance, cognitive, and emotional regulation, clients often have highly variable presentations. Conversely the current literature shows many clinical tests identify only certain aspects of impaired brain function but not others.[1,2,5,7-10,13-17,23,30,34] For example, many balance tests are highly reliable but lack either the sensitivity and/or specificity to accurately identify MTBI when used in isolation.[19,35-46] However, these same balance tests in conjunction with measures of cognitive brain function show markedly improved ability to identify concussed individuals from uninjured.[46-50,51-53]

While many commercial entities advertise a highly predictive "Silver Bullet" test, the published research simply does not support this.[46-50,51-53] Instead the evidence suggests combined testing identifies the different impacted aspects of brain function affected by MTBI. For example, Resch et al demonstrated that the clinical tests ImPACT (cognitive test), Sensory Organization Test (a computerized instrumented balance test), and Revised Head Injury Scale (survey-based symptom catalog) possessed highly variable and in some cases poor sensitivity ranging from 55.0% to 77.5% along with specificity ranging from 52.5% to 100%.[46] Thankfully, when combined as a battery of tests, sensitivity improved to 80% and specificity to 100%. When the cognitive, balance, and symptom scale 3 test battery was interpreted with guidelines, sensitivity further improved to 100%.[46]

Thus, the evidence-based therapist should gather clinical data with the best tests available in our scope of practice namely sensory integration, NMC (including oculomotor control and balance testing), and vestibular tests. This data, when contributed to an interdisciplinary team of physicians, neurologists, neuropsychologists, speech-language pathologists/cognitive therapists, and educational specialists will provide the most comprehensive assessment of MTBI. While laborious, this multidisciplinary-integrated model of care provides the best assessment and management of clients with MTBI.[19,40-46] Historically, assessment of clients with MTBI was conducted by specially trained vestibular physical therapists using high-tech tools, such as infrared video goggle systems, to assess oculomotor control, nystagmus, and computerized posturography to test balance.[1-4,7,8,16] This

Figure 18-1. Opticokinetic stimuli are images containing information alternating high-contrast objects that induce involuntary eye movements and thus the optical illusion of movement.

chapter highlights relevant clinical tests and measures available in most orthopedic settings. Interpretation of the following tests also serves as a guide for referral to a specialized vestibular physical therapist and/or other health professionals in the integrated care model.[8-15,23,24,34,46]

- Dizziness Handicap Inventory (DHI)
- Vestibular Oculomotor Screening (VOMS)
  - Smooth pursuits
  - Saccades
  - Near point convergence (NPC)
  - VOR
  - Visual motion sensitivity
- HIT
- Dynamic visual acuity
- Balance and mobility tests
  - BESS
  - Dynamic Gait Index (DGI)
  - Functional Gait Assessment (FGA)
  - High-Level Mobility Assessment Tool (HiMAT)

Dizziness Handicap Inventory

The DHI is an extremely well-researched outcome measure of balance, mobility, and function relating to limitation from dizziness. The DHI quantifies client limitation secondary to dizziness in a 100-point total scale (higher scores indicate more symptomatic and limited). The survey consists of 25 questions across functional, emotional, and physical domains.[30] The DHI has been shown to be reliable and valid in numerous populations including peripheral and central vestibular dysfunction. Client responses to physical domain questions may guide the clinician to further test sensory integration. For example, questions P1, P11, P13, and P25 all involve head movement and are suggestive of vestibular dysfunction, which would be correlated with additional objective vestibular clinical testing later. Likewise, many patients with MTBI exhibit neuropsychological features and may score higher on the emotional domain questions.[30,31,33]

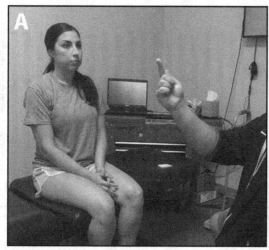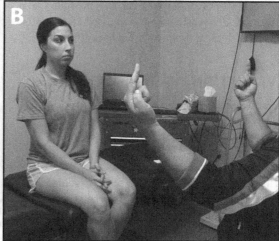

Figure 18-2. VOMS. (A) Horizontal smooth pursuit. (B) Horizontal saccades. *(continued)*

Vestibular Oculomotor Screening

The VOMS has great clinical utility in the assessment of sensory integration of visual and vestibular sensory perception in clients after MTBI. It is highly reliable and positively identifies concussion clients with vestibular and oculomotor dysfunction. It also provides a useful outcomes measure through the analog scoring of symptoms and the objective measurement of NPC. Because the VOMS is not dependent on expensive instrumentation, it can be performed in a variety of settings.[23,54] Clients with abnormal smooth pursuit, saccades, or convergence insufficiency will benefit from referral to vestibular physical therapy.[1,3,4,9,10,15,16,23,34,55] More severe abnormalities in these areas may warrant referral to neuro-opthalmology. Refer to Figure 18-2 for graphic examples of how to perform the VOMS. The VOMS includes the following tests.

Oculomotor

As mentioned earlier, abnormal oculomotor control is common with MTBI secondary to the large areas of the brain involved in visual perception.[8-10,14,16,22,23,27-29,32,55,56] All oculomotor aspects of the VOMS are performed with the client seated and the head still. The client performs the oculomotor tasks described later, while the clinician observes the client's eye movements for abnormalities (see Figure 18-2). Begin by having the client rate their baseline symptoms of headache, dizziness, nausea, and fogginess (referring to cognitive function) on a 0 to 10 analog scale. Symptom scoring is repeated in each area for each of the following components of the VOMS.[23]

To test smooth pursuits the client visually tracks the clinician's single fingertip held at 3 feet from the nose, moving slowly (2 seconds to cover a 3-foot arc), for 2 repetitions in the horizontal and then vertical planes. Catch up saccades or outright loss of target are signs of abnormal smooth pursuit.[23]

Next, the clinician tests saccades by having the client hold their head still and rapidly move visual gaze between 2 fingertips at the same distances, for 10 repetitions horizontally and vertically. Hypo- or hypermetria, also known as *overshoots* or *undershoots* are signs of abnormal saccades.[23]

NPC is tested with the client looking at a single target of 14-point text at about arm's length (relatively distant and divergent). The client then attempts to maintain gaze on the target while moving it toward the nose. The client reports when the target becomes 2 images despite their best efforts. The clinician measures the distance in centimeters with a tape measure and records the best (closest) of 3 trials. Failure of one eye to move inward with the other is abnormal or dysconjugate gaze, also known as *strabismus*, or convergence insufficiency.[21-25,32,34,57,58]

The horizontal and vertical VOR components are performed by having the client focus on a stationary target of 14-point text held 3 feet from the eye. Next, they shake their head through a 20-degree arc of motion for 10 repetitions.[32] Again, rate their symptoms in each area and note any abnormalities such as complaints of oscillopsia.[23,34,55,59] It is also common for clients to close their eyes when oscillopsia occurs as this does temporarily remove the visual misperception and lessens secondary symptoms.[26,29,30,54,58]

To perform the visual motion sensitivity component of the VOMS, instruct the client to stand with feet shoulder width apart while focusing their vision on their thumb held at arm's length while moving the thumb and head in unison through an arc 80 degrees left and right for 5 repetitions.[23] This creates a moving visual background in relation to the focal visual target in the foreground. See Figure 18-2 for graphic demonstration of performance of VOMS. Performing the test in front of more complex visual backgrounds, such as a busy therapy gym, creates higher visual contrast similar to the opticokinetic stimuli depicted in Figure 18-1. This aspect of the VOMS also assesses the patient's ability to cortically suppress the VOR in order to allow the eyes to move in phase with the head.[16]

Mucha et al[23] demonstrated the VOMS possesses excellent internal consistency, Cronbach's alpha of 0.92 for total

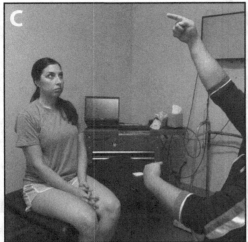
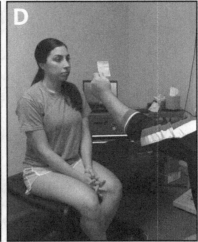
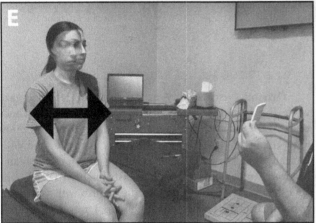
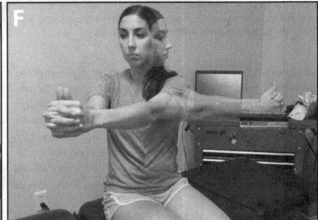

Figure 18-2 (continued). (C) Vertical saccades. (D) NPC. (E) VOR x 1 horizontal (VOR x 1 vertical not depicted). (F) Visual motion sensitivity.

symptom score and NPC distance. Likewise, they demonstrated concurrent validity with other measures of concussion.[23]

In addition, Mucha et al showed the VOMS has been shown highly sensitive and specific. The researchers expressed this in several highly clinically relevant ways. Participants with symptom scores of 2 or higher with any VOMS item showed positive likelihood ratios, from 23.9 with smooth pursuit or vertical saccades to a 42.8 with horizontal VOR. Thus, based on even conservative "bedside estimate," the probability of MTBI is increased by roughly 46% or more with any symptom score of 2 or higher.[23,60] An NPC of 5 cm or greater possessed a positive likelihood ratio of 5.8 or roughly 35% increased probability of MTBI. In actual clinical practice, client history alone provides a high starting index of suspicion for MTBI, and thus, the relative increased probability of MTBI using the 2-point symptom score and 5-cm NPC cutoffs on the VOMS will prove very compelling in ruling in MTBI. They also used area under the receiver operating characteristics to show all VOMS components accurately identified concussed participants. Specific analysis of a predictive model includes abnormal scores; VOR and VOMS symptom scores more than 2 and NPC more than 5 cm achieved an area under the curve of 0.89, meaning this model accurately predicted MTBI roughly 89% of the time.[23]

Subsequent research again showed the VOMS high between trial reliability and determined the minimum detectable change for NPC to be 4 cm.[54] Likewise, research showed the VOMS useful in demonstrating change as patients improve from their higher baseline scores, which becomes increasingly important in demonstrating progress toward positive functional outcomes in current contentious health insurance environments.[58]

Head Impulse Test

The HIT, also known as the *head thrust test,* provides a rapid assessment of VOR function useful to rule out peripheral vestibular loss that can also occur with head trauma.[2,3,7,9,10,16] To perform the HIT, begin by instructing the client to maintain their gaze on a stationary visual target. Next, the clinician gently moves the client's head through a short 5- to 10-degree arc of oscillating capital rotation to relax the cervical musculature and make it difficult for the client to predict the timing or direction of the impending impulse. Now, rapidly thrust or impulse the head from slight rotation back to cervical neutral position (Figure 18-3). Thrusting back into cervical neutral is thought to reduce possible confounding variables from cervical proprioception and cervical vascular insufficiency.[16,59,61] Clients with normal VOR gain

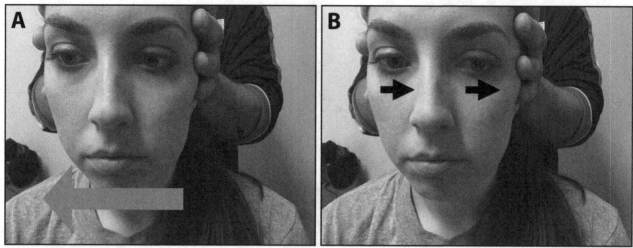

Figure 18-3. HIT. (A) After slow oscillating head movement to relax the patient, the clinician rapidly thrusts the head to the right. Peripheral vestibular hypofunction decreases VOR gain resulting in the eyes moving with the head and off of the target. (B) Observation of saccades to bring the eyes back onto target indicates a positive HIT on the right.

will maintain their gaze on target through the rapid impulse. Conversely, a client with decreased VOR gain will be unable to stabilize gaze on the target, allowing the eyes to drift off target.[7,16,23,34,59,61,62] Once visual fixation is lost, the client's oculomotor control kicks in and executes a saccade to return gaze back onto the target. Observation of this corrective saccade is a positive HIT (see Figure 18-3).[59,61,62] Many clients with a positive HIT do not consciously perceive the loss of visual fixation.[16,59,61]

Noninstrumented HIT was shown to be 71% sensitive in identifying unilateral and 84% for bilateral peripheral vestibular hypofunction, respectively. Specificity of the HIT was found to be 82%.[25,34] This can also be expressed with a positive likelihood ratio of 4.16 or approximately 25% increase in probability of peripheral vestibular hypofunction.[59] Yip et al[61] examined the noninstrumented or bedside HIT compared to the instrumented video HIT. They demonstrated that the bedside HIT had moderate interrater reliability and good sensitivity for detecting peripheral vestibular hypofunction. The beside HIT was shown to have a high negative predictive value meaning a negative HIT strongly tended to rule out peripheral vestibular loss as a source of vertigo.[61] Alasherhi et al[62] demonstrated the video HIT was essentially negative in adult and pediatric participants with MTBI.[42] Additional research showed negative HIT with MTBI and suggested more reflexive aspects of vestibular function not reliant on higher brain processing appear to be spared with MTBI. So, when evaluating a client with vertigo after head trauma, a positive HIT of any kind tends to rule out MTBI and rule in peripheral vestibular loss as a source of vertigo.

Dynamic Visual Acuity Test

Dynamic visual acuity, or the ability to stabilize gaze while the head is in motion, is a measure of VOR function.[3,8-10,12,16,23] The normal gain or ratio of eye to head motion is approximately 0.8.[16,26,59, 61-64] Pathology impacting the VOR typically decreases VOR gain resulting in poor gaze stabilization. Studies have shown the instrumented DVAT reliable in several populations including those with vestibular hypofunction, pediatrics, and high school to college football players.[26,27,55,58,59,61,64] Gottshall et al[55] demonstrated that military personal suffering MTBI had abnormal DVAT, which improved to normal values with vestibular rehabilitation.[55] Landers et al[30] showed that asymptomatic mixed martial arts athletes possessed abnormal scores on DVAT, suggesting a possible link to repetitive head trauma, but acknowledged limitations to their findings as they lacked controls.

For clinicians who do not have access to the equipment, the noninstrumented dynamic visual acuity test (DVAT-NI) has also been shown to have excellent test-retest and intertester reliability (r = 0.94 for yaw or horizontal head movement and r = 0.88 for pitch or vertical head movement in children with bilateral vestibular hypofunction).[63] The DVAT-NI demonstrated high negative predictive values for peripheral vestibular hypofunction, meaning a normal DVAT-NI strongly tends to rule out peripheral vestibular loss.[63] Further research into the reliability and predictive value of DVAT-NI for the MTBI population is needed.

To perform the DVAT-NI, begin with the patient seated, head stationary, and wearing their corrective lenses as necessary. Test static visual acuity by having the client read the lowest line that they can correctly identify all of the letter or ototypes on a standardized optometric eye chart at the specified distance (typically 20 feet for standard Snellen charts). Next, the clinician moves the client's head downward approximately 30 degrees to align the horizontal semicircular canals to the horizontal or yaw plane to be tested. The clinician induces passive horizontal head rotation through a 20- to 30-degree arc. The speed of head movement should be 2.0 Hertz (Hz), meaning 2 cycles of head movement (left to right and back) per second. Metronome smart phone applications can be helpful in maintaining the rapid pace of head movement. Set the metronome to 240 beats per minute to create the corresponding cadence for the clinician to match right and left to one beat each to the desired 2.0-Hz head movement required to maximize test reliability and sensitivity to VOR gain deficit. While maintaining the rapid oscillating head movement, instruct the patient to read the lowest line at which they can correctly identify all the characters. A loss of 3 or more lines is considered abnormal and suggestive of decreased VOR gain.[16,30,63,64]

Balance and Mobility Tests for Mild Traumatic Brain Injury

The authors of this chapter concede that there are numerous excellent reliable and valid tests and measures of balance in the literature. We will discuss those most relevant for the MTBI population, particularly those feasible for therapists in orthopedic settings with limited budgets.

Many clinical balance tests, even computerized posturography, have been shown to have a high incidence of false negatives with athletes who have sustained MTBI.[1,7,8,15,16,19,34-46,54,55,57-62,65-71] This ceiling effect is thought to be explained by the high degree of NMC and balance present in athletes premorbid to concussion and that not every MTBI affects balance. In clinical practice, the authors of this chapter administer the following clinical measures of NMC, balance, and mobility sequentially progressing to more difficult tests as the client reaches a relative ceiling effect for a given test.

Balance Error Scoring System

The BESS is a simple clinical balance test that provides insight into sensory integration and balance, but at a fraction of the cost of high-tech computerized posturography systems as it requires only a timer and foam pad to perform.[35,70,71]

To perform the BESS, the client is instructed to maintain their balance with hands on hips, for 20 seconds each in 3 different positions: feet together, single leg stance, and tandem stance. First, the client stands on a firm surface with their eyes closed to remove visual input and bias toward somatosensory perception. Next, they perform the same procedures but with eyes closed and standing on top of a 10-cm thick medium density foam pad to dampen somatosensory input, which biases for vestibular sensory perception (Figure 18-4). Balance with eyes open is not tested as it was shown to be poorly sensitive in detecting imbalance in controls or concussed individuals.[35,70,71]

During each trial, the clinician thoroughly tallies the errors made by the client in each position and sensory condition for a sample BESS data collection form. The more errors made, the worse the NMC of balance. Healthy controls committed an average of 9 errors across all trials. Errors with firm surface and eyes closed suggest difficulty processing somatosensory input. Errors with compliant foam surface and eyes closed suggest difficulty processing vestibular input common with MTBI.[35,70,71] Research demonstrated the BESS to have moderate to good reliability. The standard BESS was shown to have 60% sensitivity, whereas instrumented or modified BESS had 71.4% sensitivity.

Dynamic Gait Index

The DGI is a widely researched, cost-effective balance test with excellent intrarater and interrater reliability in numerous populations, including clients with vestibular sensory impairment across 8 walking subcomponents.[16,36-38] The clinician scores client performance based on guidelines provided. Scores lower than 19/24 are highly predictive of falling.[16,36-28] Whitney and Hudak[36] demonstrated that clients with vestibular dysfunction with a DGI score of less than or equal to 19/24 were 2.58 times more likely to have fallen over the previous year. Lower scores and/or reproduction of vertigo, dizziness, or nausea with the horizontal head turns, vertical head turns, and pivot turn subcomponents are suggestive of poor vestibular processing.[16,36-38] Studies in adolescents showed a ceiling effect as 50% of nonconcussed participants achieved a maximal score of 24/24.[39]

Functional Gait Assessment

The FGA grew out of the need for a more challenging test when clients reached a ceiling effect on the DGI. The FGA subcomponents are the same as the DGI but with removal of stepping around obstacles and the addition of gait with a narrow base of support, gait with eyes closed, and retro gait. The scoring scale for the FGA is the same as the DGI but with a maximum possible score of 30. The FGA has been shown to be reliable and valid. A cutoff score of 22/30 on the FGA was shown to be effective in predicting falls in community-dwelling older adults.[38] So, it is safe to say any young athletes who scored below 22/30 should be classified as having abnormal balance. Research also demonstrates a ceiling effect in adolescents with the FGA.[39]

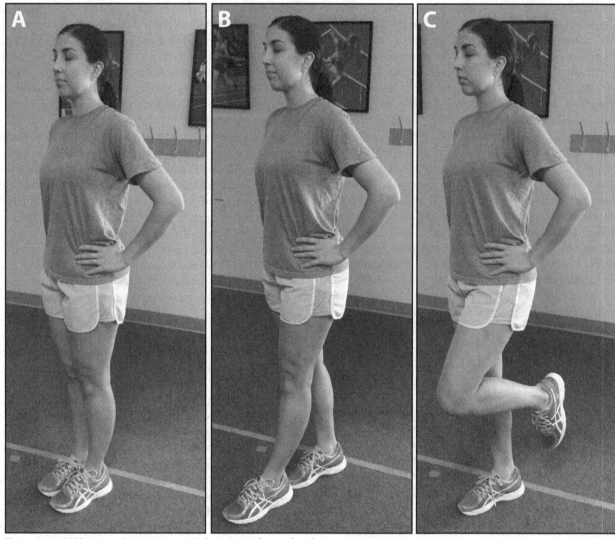

Figure 18-4. BESS test conditions. A, B, and C: Eyes closed, firm surface for somatosensory-biased balance testing in double leg, single leg, and tandem stances. *(continued)*

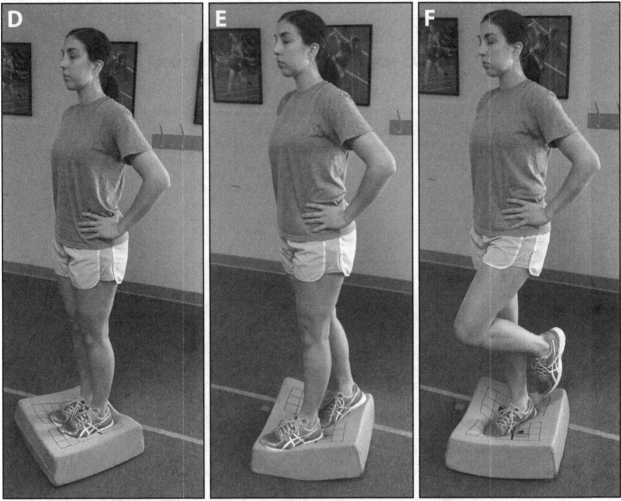

Figure 18-4 (continued). D, E, and F: Same stances with eyes closed on compliant, foam surface for vestibular sensory bias.

High-Level Mobility Assessment Tool

The HiMAT was developed to test highly coordinated individuals such as soldiers and athletes who require a higher relative ceiling for testing. The HiMAT consists of 13 mobility tasks scored by time or distance (Figure 18-5).[19,40-45] The HiMAT was originally developed to examine a client's suffering from traumatic brain injury, which differs from MTBI as it is defined by permanent organic brain damage, visible on imaging.[19,40-45] The HiMAT was also validated for use with MTBI and was shown to have excellent interrater (interclass correlation coefficient = 0.99) and intrarater reliability (interclass correlation coefficient = 0.95). Research showed the HiMAT sensitive and specific enough to discriminate between individuals reporting improvement in their symptoms at 3 months and 6 months post-MTBI. So, the HiMAT is highly responsive to change through the course of treatment but has not been shown to predict MTBI alone.[19,,40-45]

Again, studies have also shown a ceiling effect in the HiMAT as the median scores for young athletic normals were 54/54 for men and 51/54 for women, respectively.[44,45] However, as many symptomatic concussed patients will begin with very low scores, the HiMAT remains an effective measure to demonstrate outcomes of rehabilitation in many patients. In clinical practice many functional tests already used to determine return to play for orthopedic conditions are a logical but not yet researched testing option for those who do reach the ceiling effect with the HiMAT.

Dual Tasking Tests

As mentioned earlier, MTBI often effects cognitive and sensorimotor processing. These have traditionally been assessed separately by neuropsychological tests and NMC tests, respectively. A number of clinical tests for MTBI have high false negative rates, often attributed to ceiling effect with testing of athletic participants who were highly coordinated premorbid to their concussion. Also, researchers have cited the variable effect of MTBI across individuals (ie, some clients have profound dizziness and imbalance but preserved cognitive function or vice versa).[46-49,51]

In response, some researchers have examined the effect of dual tasking balance with a concurrent cognitive challenge and have shown that participants with MTBI exhibit decreased performance as compared to controls.[46-53,72,73] Paradigms for dual tasking can be simple, such as response

A

HiMAT: HIGH LEVEL MOBILITY ASSESSMENT TOOL

PATIENT:

DATE:

Subject suitability: The HiMAT is appropriate for assessing people with high-level balance and mobility problems. The minimal mobility requirement for testing is independent walking over 20m without gait aids. Orthoses are permitted.

Item testing: Testing takes 5-10 minutes. Patients are allowed 1 practice trial for each item.

Instructions: Patients are instructed to perform at their maximum safe speed except for the bounding and stair items.

ITEM	PERFORMANCE	SCORE					
		0	1	2	3	4	5
WALK: The middle 10m of a 20m trial is timed.	sec	X	>6.6	5.4-6.6	4.3-5.3	<4.3	X
WALK BACKWARD: As for walking.	sec		>13.3	8.1-13.3	5.8-8.0	<5.8	X
WALK ON TOES: As for walking. Any heel contact during the middle 10m is recorded as a fail.	sec		>8.9	7.0-8.9	5.4-6.9	<5.4	X
WALK OVER OBSTACLE: As for walking. A house brick is placed across the walkway at the mid-point. Patients must step over the brick without contacting it. A fail is recorded if patients step around the brick or make contact with the brick.	sec		>7.1	5.4-7.1	4.5-5.3	<4.5	X
RUN: The middle 10m of a 20m trial is timed. A fail is recorded if patients fail to have a consistent flight phase during the trial.	sec		>2.7	2.0-2.7	1.7-1.9	<1.7	X
SKIP: The middle 10m of a 20m trial is timed. A fail is recorded if patients fail to have a consistent flight phase during the trial.	sec		>4.0	3.5-4.0	3.0-3.4	<3.0	X
HOP FORWARD (AFFECTED): Patients stand on their more affected leg and hop forward. The time to hop 10m meters is recorded.	sec		>7.0	5.3-7.0	4.1-5.2	<4.1	X
BOUND (AFFECTED): A bound is a jump from one leg to the other with a flight phase. Patients stand behind a line on their less affected leg, hands on hips, and jump forward **landing on their more affected** leg. Each bound is measured from the line to the heel of the landing leg. The average of three trials is recorded.	1) cm 2) 3)		<80	80-103	104-132	>132	X

Figure 18-5. HiMAT. *(continued)*

B

BOUND (LESS AFFECTED): Patients stand behind a line on their more affected leg, hands on hips, and jump forward **landing on their less affected** leg. The average of three trials is recorded.	1) cm 2) 3)			<82	82-105	106-129	>129	X
UP STAIRS DEPENDENT: Patients are asked to walk up a flight of 14 stairs as they normally would and at their normal speed. The trial is recorded from when the patient starts until both feet are at the top. IF: Patient uses rail **OR** not reciprocal gait score for dependent here IF: Patient uses reciprocal gait **AND** no rail automatic score of dependent up stairs at 5 and rate up stairs independent below		sec		>22.8	14.6 - 22.8	12.3 - 14.5	<12.3	
UP STAIRS INDEPENDENT:		sec		>9.1	7.6-9.1	6.8-7.5	<6.8	X
DOWN STAIRS DEPENDENT: As for Up Stairs. IF: Patient uses rail **OR** not reciprocal gait score for dependent here IF: Patient uses reciprocal gait **AND** no rail automatic score of dependent down stairs at 5 and rate independent below		sec		>24.3	17.6 - 24.3	12.8 - 17.5	<12.8	
DOWNSTAIRS INDEPENDENT:		sec		>8.4	6.6-8.4	5.8-6.5	<5.8	X
	SUBTOTAL							

TOTAL HiMAT SCORE   /54

Scoring: All times and distances are recorded in the 'performance' column. The corresponding score for each item is then circled and each column is then subtotaled. Subtotals are then added to calculate the HiMAT score.

Please notify Gavin Williams at gavin@neuro-solutions.net or gavin.williams@epworth.org.au so that the use of the HiMAT can be tracked.

Figure 18-5 (continued). HiMAT. (Reproduced with permission from Gavin Williams.)

to questions (eg, simple math, spelling). The Stroop effect is an interesting mechanism to provide concurrent cognitive challenge in which the patient has to respond to a question with interference in the signal to confuse them. For example, participants that were presented with an audio recording of a word were asked to disregard the meaning of the word (filter it out) and instead process the pitch of the sound signal.[48,49] This may sound straight forward, but one try will quickly show it provides cognitive challenge. The Stroop effect works across numerous sensory streams so long as the interference is present. Initial studies used highly instrumented methods of movement analysis such as computerized posturography, pressure plate measurement of ground reaction forces, and infrared video 3D analysis of movement.[46-53,72,73] Dual or multitasking paradigms are also being examined using high-tech virtual reality simulators to identify MTBI in military personnel.[50] This area holds great promise for identification of MTBI and is deserving of future study.

Physical Exertion Testing

Physical exertion is better known in the United States of America as a combination of any exercise across the spectrum of aerobic to anaerobic energy pathways. Research has shown decreased neurocognitive function in clients with MTBI after physical exertion.[1,4,10,11,13,74-81] Research suggests this may be secondary to abnormal neural regulation of cardiovascular physiology and/or decreased tolerance of the physiological demands of exercise on the body while the brain is in the midst of its metabolic deficit post-MTBI.[4,11,15,74-81]

The Buffalo Concussion Treadmill Test (BCTT) has been shown to have good interrater and intrarater reliability in the MTBI population.[4,77,78,80,81] Haider et al demonstrated the BCTT is 73% sensitive and 78% specific in predicting prolonged recovery (greater than 30 days) from MTBI.[79] To administer the BCTT, have the patient rate their symptoms, heart rate, and Borg Rating of Perceived Exertion (RPE) at rest. Begin walking at approximately 3.3 miles per hour adjusting for client height and ability and record data each minute. Increase treadmill grade by 1 degree each minute and continue this procedure until the client either achieves a fatigue RPE of 19/20 or more likely reports an increase in MTBI symptoms (Figure 18-6). Participants with MTBI were found to have slightly lower resting heart rate as compared to once recovered. In addition, concussed individuals demonstrated abnormally high RPE on the BCTT as compared to once recovered from MTBI.[4,74-81] Clients suffering from vertigo and imbalance often cannot complete the BCTT as it requires enough balance to walk and run and the

associated head movement can provoke vertigo and osscilopsia. Leddy et al have also developed the Buffalo Concussion Bike Test, which controls for these confounds.[80]

TREATMENT OF MILD TRAUMATIC BRAIN INJURY

Evidence-based physical therapy treatment of MTBI can be divided into 4 basic regions:

1. Education to facilitate restoration of normal brain physiology
2. Cervical physical therapy to address neck pain and cervicogenic headaches
3. Vestibular rehabilitation for control of vertigo, dizziness, and balance
4. Exertion training for sport-specific conditioning

Therapists must follow an integrated approach for therapeutic interventions across the 4 regions. For example, vestibular, oculomotor, and balance exercise prescription will prove futile if the client's brain continues to run at a metabolic deficit preventing adaptation to training. Likewise, client tolerance of exertion training will depend largely on vestibular rehabilitation techniques to control vertigo and nausea often provoked with the head movement induced during exertion training. Similarly, physical therapy evaluation of the cervical spine has been shown to differentiate the cervicogenic as aspect headaches and subsequent treatment with joint mobilization and dynamic stabilization training produces favorable outcomes.[9,73] Cervical spine interventions such as manual therapy and neuromuscular training of stabilization will not be discussed here as they are covered in other chapters of this text.

Education to Facilitate Recovery of Brain Function

Effective education of the client and their support network sets the stage for all areas of recovery from MTBI. Therapists should plan on a fair amount of redundancy and simplification of content when educating clients with MTBI as they often have cognitive, anxiety, and/or emotional impairment, which limit their comprehension and compliance. So, when possible, educating their support network such as family members, educators, school administrators, and coaches creates the best possible environment for brain recovery in an imperfect situation.[1-4,7-10,13,14,16,17,48-50,72]

Buffalo Concussion Treadmill Test (BCTT)				
Minute	**Speed /Grade**	**HR**	**RPE**	**Notes**
Resting				
Begin at a brisk walk, approximately 3.3 mph, adjusting for height and ability.				
Increase grade by 1° per minute until either: **• MTBI symptoms increase above baseline** **or** **• Client reaches max HR or RPE or 19 (exhaustion)**				
0				
1				
2				
3				
4				
5				
6				
7				
8				
9				
10				
11				
12				
13				
14				
15				
16				
17				
18				
19				
20				
Post Exercise - slow to 2.5 mph walk at level grade				
1				
2				

Figure 18-6. BCTT sample data collection and instruction form. (Reproduced with permission from Haider MN, Leddy JJ, Wilber CG, et al. The predictive capacity of the Buffalo Concussion Treadmill Test after sport-related concussion in adolescents. Front Neurol. 10:395. doi:10.3389/fneur.2019.00395.)

3 M's Mnemonic device for appropriate brain rest	
Monitor	Clients monitor their MTBI symptoms during activity for an increase above baseline levels.
Modify	Change parameters of activity such as removing cognitive distraction or decreasing intensity of activity.
Move On	If symptoms remain elevated after modification, then discontinue activity, rest the brain, and retrial the same activity at a lower level of intensity later.

Figure 18-7. The 3 Ms mnemonic device to facilitate appropriate brain rest and pacing.

Clinicians should begin by educating the client in the pathophysiology of MTBI and increased metabolic demand in the brain. All areas of recovery of brain function are dependent on overcoming the deficit.[1,3,4,8-12,14] The analogy of balancing a budget through reducing spending (pacing of tasks) and increasing revenue (appropriate brain rest) is often useful in client education.

The previous antiquated concept of total brain rest by sequestering the client from sensory, cognitive, physical, and social stimulation has been shown to have a net negative impact by increasing anxiety, depression, and deconditioning.[4,13,15,17,18,78-85] For some clients, the social isolation of total brain rest appears to create a loop of anxiety, perseveration on symptoms, back to more anxiety, which retards the speed of recovery.[1,4,7-9,16,17,82-85]

Conversely, research supports appropriate brain rest. This means a relative reduction in the level of brain processing that allows the neuron ion pumps to catch up to the metabolic deficit, but without provoking negative effects.[1,4,7-9,16,17] However, educating clients and their support network in this relative concept of appropriate relative brain rest can be challenging. The authors of this chapter employ the mnemonic device monitor, modify, and move on to provide an easy to remember guide to activity during rehabilitation of MTBI (Figure 18-7).

Educating the client in optimal sleep patterns such as establishing a consistent bedtime, avoiding stimulants (eg, caffeine after mid-day), and removing all the numerous forms of media technology (eg, TV, music, tablets, smart phones) prior to bedtime have been shown to be effective strategies to improve sleep. This allows the brain to catch up on the metabolic deficit. Sadly, many clients with MTBI have poor sleep patterns prior to their injury and require further remediation.[1-13,81-84]

The VOMS symptom profile provides clinicians a direct crossover for education. For example, a client with increased headaches and dizziness with the oculomotor aspects of the VOMS requires education as to how MTBI has impacted this area of brain function. Subsequently, the client should be more open to pacing of school activities and complying with related restrictions. Experienced clinicians know underreporting of symptoms and reluctance to modify lifestyle are notorious characteristics of athletes with MTBI. Education also improves patient anxiety provoked by provocation of symptoms, related loss of function, and identity as an athlete, coworker, or other social role.[1-17,81-84]

Vestibular Rehabilitation Therapy

Retrospective studies demonstrated good outcomes with the application of vestibular rehabilitation for clients with MTBI.[3] Likewise, retrospective studies demonstrated favorable outcomes with early physical therapy intervention to address multimodal impairment in sensory integration, imbalance, neck pain, and headaches.[10,74]

In a prospective randomized controlled trial, Schneider and colleagues demonstrated excellent outcomes in participants sustaining MTBI with a 2-pronged intervention of vestibular rehabilitation and cervical spine treatment in physical therapy. After 8 weeks of treatment, 73% of the participants in the intervention group received medical clearance for return to sports participation vs just 7% of controls who received the previous standard care of rest and gentle exertion exercise. Therefore, clients in the vestibular and cervical physical therapy intervention group were 3.91 times more likely to receive medical clearance for return to sports participation than controls. All participants who achieved medical clearance also demonstrated a full recovery and were asymptomatic per additional outcomes measurement with the DHI, FGA, and others.[9] Cervical physical therapy in this study consisted of joint mobilization manual therapy techniques for the cervical and thoracic spine as well as therapeutic exercise for NMC of spinal stabilization, emphasizing upper cervical retraining and sensorimotor techniques. The cervical physical therapy produced favorable outcomes per cervical joint position error, cervical flexor endurance, and rating of neck pain.[9] As mentioned earlier, specific cervical interventions are covered in other chapters of this text.

VRT refers to a specialty branch of physical therapy developed in response to the needs of clients with impaired sensory integration resulting in imbalance, vertigo, nausea, motion sensitivity, oscillopsia, among other symptoms.[3,8-10,14,16] Clinicians skilled in VRT utilize advanced knowledge sensory integration to identify impairments in visual, somatosensory, and vestibular perception. This includes analysis of oculomotor control and nystagmus with instrumented video technologies from which they provide customized interventions to control vertigo, imbalance, and other related symptoms through exercise prescription to promote CNS adaptations and canal repositioning therapies.

VRT is based on applied sensory integration of the visual, somatosensory, as well as vestibular senses. To illustrate this concept, vestibular therapists routinely train visual and somatosensory substitution for clients with impaired vestibular processing.[3,8-10,16,34,55,57,58] Conversely, habituation occurs with repeated doses of stimulation in the problematic sensory stream (typically vestibular and certain visual stimuli). Over time, the CNS learns to recalibrate and decrease the undesirable response.[3,8-10,16] So, clients with impaired vestibular processing will improve with repeated vestibular stimulation and eventually what once provoked vertigo and nausea will no longer do so.

While VRT covers exercise prescription across all 3 streams of sensory integration, we recommend beginning with substitution and then progressing to habituation. Even symptomatic clients can tolerate sensory substitution training and get a rapid control of symptoms. This works to control anxiety and helps to build rapport with clients in the early phase of rehabilitation. In order for habituation to occur, the sensory stimulation must be strong enough to produce an error signal, which drives the CNS adaptations to training.[9,10,16] Unfortunately, this means habituation acutely provokes symptoms. This paradox is very difficult for clients to grasp and can make for a hard sell getting clients to comply. Clients will better tolerate habituation to vestibular and certain visual stimuli following education as to the normalcy of acute symptom provocation. In plain terms, habituation is highly effective, but only if the client feels in control of the process so they continue training.

The majority of clients with MTBI will have difficulty processing vestibular input as evidenced by their complaints of vertigo, nausea, imbalance, and oscillopsia. Likewise, they typically exhibit abnormal testing with vestibular aspects of the VOMS, BESS, DGI, and FGA. Therefore, they are best served by immediate focus on somatosensory substitution. In fact, clients intuitively find somatosensory substitution by touching objects. The therapist should further intervene by instructing the client to increase somatosensory input by using their hands, feet, or face (which have high density of somatosensory receptors) to touch objects or their own body frequently. Somatosensory-biased balance training also provides somatosensory substitution for vestibular loss and is useful in control of vertigo and nausea even in clients who do not have imbalance.

Clients with MTBI often also have difficulty processing visual input, which will declare itself with the oculomotor and visual motion sensitivity components of the VOMS. The therapist should prescribe oculomotor training to remediate this and restore visual sensory processing. Oculomotor training also provides a huge avenue of sensory substitution for vestibular impairment. For example, learned spotting can control vertigo provoked with head movement in walking, shopping, conversing, or sports.

Also, please note the authors of this chapter urge the reader to match exercise prescription to the higher sensory integration, balance, and exertion demands of athletes. Traditional VRT exercise prescription provides an excellent starting point for most athletes. However, this may fall short of stimulating the error signal necessary to meet athletes' hypernormal demands. For example, baseball players have oculomotor and gaze stabilization demands with fielding and hitting tasks that are far greater than the typical client and will require advanced training to match.[8,9,23-30,32,34]

Oculomotor Training

As mentioned earlier, oculomotor training remediates the impaired oculomotor control allowing the client to capture a higher volume of visual cues. It also improves the visual associative cortex's ability to process visual data into meaningful information. The net result is restoration of client perception of their position in relation to the environment. This, in turn, controls their vertigo and visual motion sensitivity, nausea, and imbalance. This is also referred to as *visual sensory substitution* or *sensory reweighting*.[3,4,7-10,16]

If the clinician understands the mechanisms of oculomotor control described with testing, then only a little creativity is required for exercise prescription. As when training any complex movement, begin by simplifying into easier components by training smooth pursuits, saccades, and vergence separately and in a single plane. Then combine mechanisms, planes of target movement, increase speeds, and add sport-specific backgrounds. As the clinician, you should avoid the pitfall of watching the visual target and instead watch the client's eyes for movements other than prescribed such as nystagmus, dysconjugate gaze (one eye off target), inappropriate saccades, and eyes closing.

As oculomotor skill improves, so will balance, vertigo, dizziness, nausea, and visual motion sensitivity. Explicit carryover of oculomotor skill sets to activities of daily living (ADLs) and sports movements will hasten control of symptoms and return to function. For example, a basketball player who gets dizzy rolling off of a pick or turning down a hallway at school should execute saccades prior to the head movement that stimulate the vestibular system and provoke vertigo. This can also be described as teaching an alternate head movement strategy.

We recommend the use of laser pointers with visual training, as they are readily available and provide a small bright foveal target that is visible in nearly all environments. Clients also find the use of laser pointers more game-like, which enhances compliance. In addition, they remove the relative visual movement between a handheld target in the foreground and the background, which can provoke visual motion sensitivity. Also, lasers make for easy changes in target distance necessary to train vergence and visual depth perception. One common client concern when using a laser pointer is that they are cheating with their advanced knowledge of where they are going to point the visual target. Educate them to the effect that you want them to anticipate, which facilitates visual substitution.

Smooth Pursuits

Smooth pursuit is the mechanism for tracking a slow-moving visual target. Any targets moving beyond the ceiling speed for smooth pursuits will trigger saccades. Therefore, cues for tediously slow target movement are key. Watch for catch-up saccades, indicating that they lost the target and need to slow their speed. While evidence for the use of smooth pursuits is not as strong as for the other mechanisms described in later sections, it is often still a useful warm-up of the extra-ocular muscles prior to other drills.[15]

Saccades

Begin with saccades 1 or rapid eye movement onto specific visual targets while the head is stationary. This allows for simpler relearning of oculomotor programming and prevents provocation of vertigo, which can frustrate clients and clinicians alike. Progress to saccades 2, which is rapid eye movement onto targets followed by head movement (Figure 18-8). Initially, train saccades 1 with very deliberate instruction to ensure client success from enhanced visual substitution vs just moving their head and reproducing vertigo. As client saccades skill improves, they will begin spotting more intuitively without conscious knowledge of performance (skilled and autonomous). By the same token, intentional practice of carryover of saccades 1 and 2 skills in anticipation

of head movement will further client control vertigo with head turns with walking, shopping, driving, sports, and even conversation.[3,4,8-10,15]

Vergence

As mentioned previously, many clients with MTBI have convergence insufficiency and will thus benefit from starting with distant (divergent) targets on which they can fixate.[3,9,10,15,32] We recommend against the tradition-based practice of using only handheld visual targets as nearly all sport-specific and many other functional tasks, such as driving, involve visual fixation on targets well beyond arm's length. Instead, train vergence by moving the laser pointer over distant objects and gradually move closer as client skill improves (Figure 18-9).

Control of Visual Motion Sensitivity

Begin by educating clients as to how opticokinetic and other offending visual stimuli induce visual-vestibular sensory conflict so they can understand the phenomenon. Once they can identify the provoking visual stimuli, they can better avoid them. This also helps many patients manage concurrent provocation of anxiety in crowds or other busy visual environments, which they may attribute to other social factors. However, some environments such as schools or big box stores have unavoidable provoking visual stimuli. For these environments, employ carryover of the oculomotor drills discussed earlier. This moves the focal/foveal visual perception from the provoking visual stimuli onto orienting, relevant visual cues. In attentional perception terms this effectively filters out the offending visual stimuli. In lay terms the phrase "out of sight, out of mind" applies.

Set up practice by providing the aforementioned varieties of provoking stimuli: opticokinetic images, computer-generated animation, camera pans/tilts, jump cuts, and handheld camera work (oscillopsia). The authors of this chapter have set up tunable visual training areas in their clinics to provide a variety of practical visual special effects via readily available laser splitters and disco balls. Likewise, open-source internet video media tubes can now be displayed on a variety of monitors, tablets, smart phones, or projected for larger scale to provide virtual images previously available only with expensive virtual reality systems (Figure 18-10).[15,49,85]

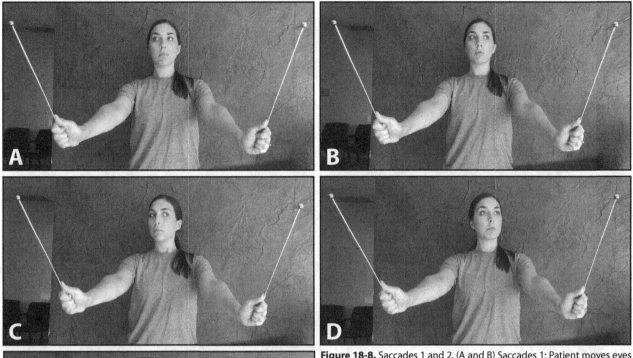

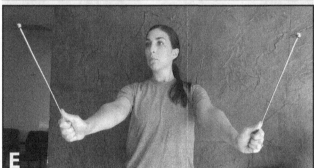

Figure 18-8. Saccades 1 and 2. (A and B) Saccades 1: Patient moves eyes rapidly from target to target while head remains still. (C, D, and E) Patient moves eyes, then head onto target.

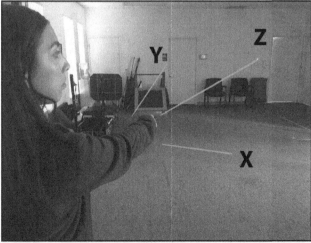

Figure 18-9. Visual training with laser pointer for targeting in 3D. Patient paints targets with laser pointer in environment moving in horizontal (X), vertical (Y), and depth (Z) planes. Patient uses saccades to move to horizontal and vertical targets as well as vergence to change depths, respectively.

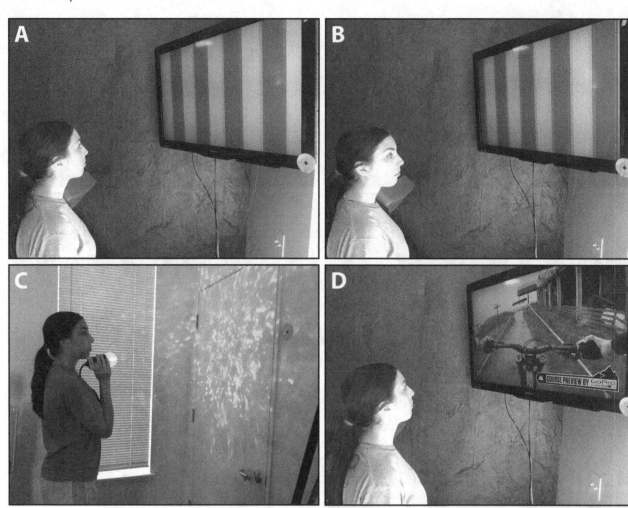

Figure 18-10. Visual motion sensitivity training. Patient views opticokinetic stimulation which provokes visual motion sensitivity (A, C, and D). Patient executes visual saccades to bring gaze onto relevant, orienting, stationary target in lower right of monitor to control visual motion sensitivity (B, C and E).

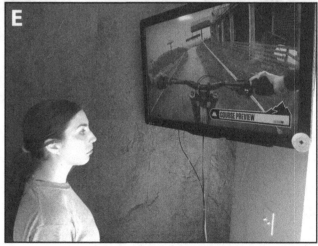

Gaze Stabilization Via Modulation of Vestibular Ocular Reflex Gain

Basic exercise prescription for training of gaze stabilization starts with the VOR x 1 drill, also known as *viewing x 1*. The client maintains visual gaze on a stationary target while oscillating the head back and forth through a tight central arc of cervical motion. To create an error signal and provoke CNS adaptation, the speed of head movement must be fast enough to induce some degree of oscillopsia. For this reason, it helps to use a target with lettering, numbers, or enough detail so that clients can recognize when oscillopsia occurs.[8-10,16] As with all other visual training exercises, VOR x 1 can be performed in horizontal, vertical, and combined planes of motion (Figure 18-11).

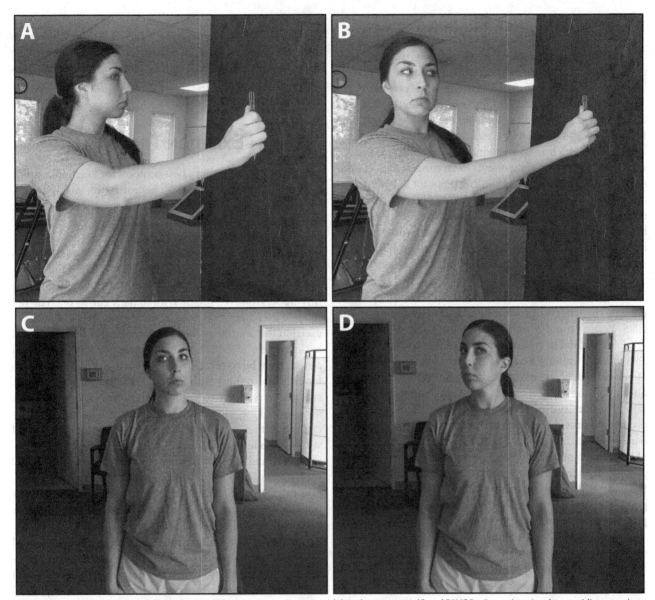

Figure 18-11. VOR x 1 and x 2 drills. (A and B) VOR x 1, stationary target, with head movement. (C and D) VOR x 2, moving visual target (distant swinging pendulum in this case) with head movement in opposite direction of visual target motion.

Progress to VOR x 2 (also known as *viewing x 2*) with the addition of moving the visual target contralateral to head movement, which requires even higher VOR gain. The authors of this chapter find use of a swinging pendulum target allows for performance of VOR x 2 at distances greater than arm's length. This also removes the challenge of coordinating hand movement of the target, allowing the client to concentrate on gaze stabilization (see Figure 18-11). In response to training, the CNS will improve VOR gain, resulting in decreased oscillopsia, improved gaze stabilization, and reduced vertigo. Research also suggests clients learn to interpret images with oscillopsia as an alternate mechanism of adaptation to training. Both mechanisms carryover to improved function with tasks involving head movement such as walking, running, all modes of exertion training, and eventually sports. Highly trained athletes can use a combination

of saccades, gaze stabilization, and even visual memory to orient themselves during high-speed movements. Because gaze stabilization/VOR drills involve head movement, they also provide simultaneous habituation to vestibular input. This also means training for gaze stabilization will provoke acute symptoms, so use this double-edged sword wisely. Simply closing the eyes with rotary head movement further isolates for habituation to vestibular canal input.[3,9,10,16] Some client's abnormal sense of motion may be otolithic or linear in nature, typically described as rocking on a boat, swaying, drifting, or floating. To address this, provide the corresponding provoking head movement by bouncing on a gym ball or the edge of the bed, tilting the head, and then both together.[16] As a general rule, if you can provoke vertigo with a given stimulus, then you can habituate the client to it.

BALANCE TRAINING

Published evidence supports balance training programs that include sensory-specific biasing and perturbation to provide sufficient error signal to provoke CNS adaptations to change.[16] The sensory integration deficits identified with the BESS provide an easy guide to training. For example, somatosensory pathways are typically spared with MTBI, which is why we find less errors and report of symptoms with these components (firm surface, eyes closed) of the BESS. This is a logical starting point for balance training.[3,9,10,16,69,70] Conversely, clients with MTBI typically have difficulty processing vestibular sensory input as evidenced by high errors and provocation of symptoms with vestibular biased condition of the BESS (eyes closed on compliant foam surface).[3,9,10,16,69,70] So, progress to vestibular biased balance training more slowly.

Regardless of the sensory bias, therapists should provide enough challenge to provoke adaptation to training in the CNS. Perturbation or moving the patient out of balance is one easy method to ensure sufficient challenge. Perturbation also induces training feed forward mechanisms of the NMC of balance, which are most relevant to the quick reactions required in sports. Begin clients with static balance on a comfortably wide base of support, narrowing the base as they progress to provide intrinsic perturbation. Then move to dynamic balance tasks by having the client explore the reaches of their limits of stability for greater perturbation[9,10,15,18,20] To provide further extrinsic perturbation the clinician may tap the body and/or balance platform. If the client is not struggling, you are not providing the error signal necessary to promote adaptation.

A variety of balance platforms provide further perturbation. The authors of this chapter favor the Shuttle Balance (Shuttle Systems) as it provides a safe platform to train aggressively as the clinician can arrange the support chains to perturb the platform in the pitch plane and linear translation extrinsically when the therapist jars the platform (Figure 18-12). Add foam on top of the Shuttle Balance, close the eyes, and add head movements to bias for vestibular sensory stimulation. Similar methods of training can be elicited with square, circular, or other shaped boards, foam pads, air filled discs, and creativity.

Dual cognitive tasking was researched as a testing paradigm for clients with MTBI.[47-50,72] Further research is needed into the effect of adapting dual tasking on rehabilitation outcomes. In the meantime, dual tasking can reinforce a synergistic approach with our colleagues in speech-language therapy and neuropsychology by improving the athletes'

understanding of the interconnected nature of cognitive, sensory, and motor processing. Trial dual tasking when an athlete has gained mastery of balance skill by simply asking the client questions. Tablet applications with visual versions of the Stroop effect are readily available in commercial application marketplaces.

EXERTION TRAINING

Research validating a best protocol for exertion training post-MTBI is mixed.[11,13,18,77-81] Recent brain imaging studies suggest there is no increased risk to exertion training with guidance and education as to appropriate intensity.[78] Likewise, experienced clinicians are aware of the role of exertion training for management of concurrent anxiety associated with slower progressing clients.[10,13,15,80-84] If the athlete tolerates treadmill walking with the BCTT, then begin with this mode. However, highly symptomatic clients often do not tolerate even light exertion. In these cases, select a mode of exertion that minimizes head movement and complex visual backgrounds.[1-3,9,10,13,80,81] So, while young athletes might find a stationary bike in a quiet room boring, this setup allows for exertion training with less confounding variables. As clients progress, move to modes with more sensory challenge such as walking, running, and elliptical machines once they can utilize their applied sensory integration tools to control vertigo with head movement. In the later stages of rehabilitation, maximal exertion testing is wise before return to full sports or military service participation. At this point, exertion training and testing will resemble sport-specific functional tests such as shuttle runs and other cutting, jumping, and running drills.

Hinds et al examined the effect of exertion on actual concussed participants using heart rate and RPE to monitor exertion intensity. Heart rate response to exertion did not differ between concussed and nonconcussed participants.[77] Furthermore, the authors find cognitively impaired clients have difficulty calculating maximal and target heart rate. Similarly, heart rate monitors available with smart devices will not work if the client is placed on a beta-blocker medication to treat migraine headaches, which also blunt heart rate response to exercise. Conversely, RPE is reliable, valid, and was shown to be abnormally high in participants with MTBI.[77,80-84] Instruct clients to monitor symptoms while ramping up intensity and then modify down one level of intensity if symptoms increase. If symptoms remain elevated after modification, then "move on" to brain rest and retrial exertion later.

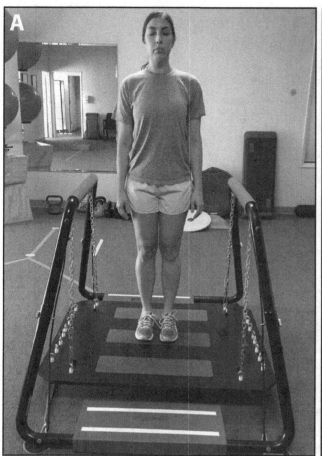

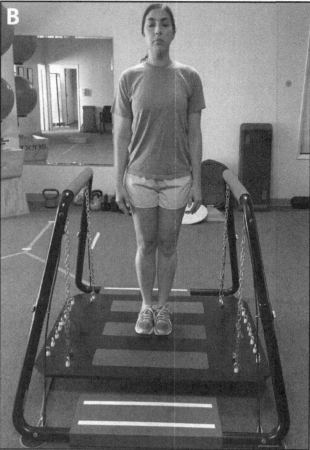

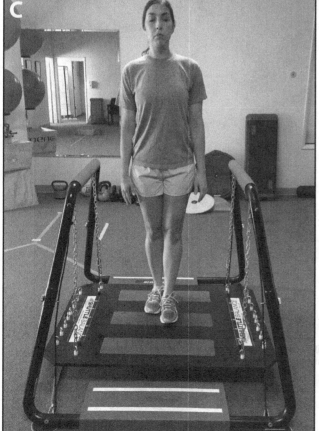

Figure 18-12. Shuttle Balance sample balance training progression. (A) Normal base of support, eyes closed for somatosensory/proprioceptive bias, low challenge. (B) Feet together, eyes closed. (C) Half tandem stance, eyes closed. *(continued)*

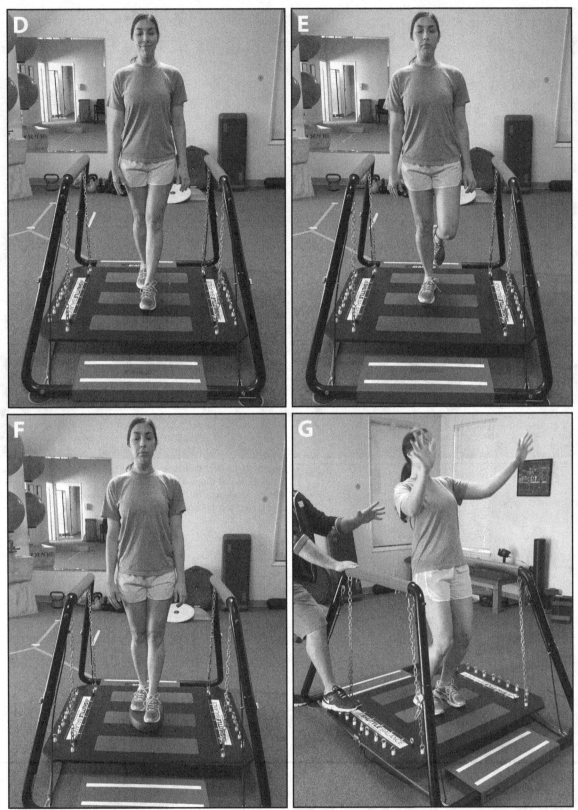

Figure 18-12 (continued). (D) Full tandem stance, eyes closed. (E) Single leg stance, eyes closed. (F) Half tandem stance, with foam cushion between Shuttle Balance platform, eyes closed for vestibular bias, moderate challenge. (G) Extrinsic perturbation of platform for high challenge, feed forward balance training.

CASE STUDIES

Case Study One

The first case study is representative of how evidence-based practice can produce favorable and rapid outcomes for clients with even fairly symptomatic MTBI without complicating factors.[3,9,10] The client was a 17-year-old, semiprofessional hockey defenseman who sustained a concussion when checked into the boards and/or the fisticuffs that followed. His initial evaluation findings are described in tabular format (Table 18-1). As his evaluation findings were all consistent with MTBI, we followed the strong evidence for physical therapy including VRT and cervical joint mobilization and stabilization.[9,10] While evidence for exertion training is not as clear, we included it for the purposes of restoration of normal response to exercise; to avoid deconditioning; to mitigate the increased risk for musculoskeletal injury; for management of anxiety surrounding missed classes, practice, and related feelings of social isolation; as well as to guide decisions on return to hockey.[6,11,80-84] We broke our treatment into tiered phases (see Table 18-1).

The client achieved an excellent outcome with physical therapy post-MTBI. By the end of phase III, he was asymptomatic and maxed out scores on the BESS, DGI, and FGA. By phase IV, he was completely asymptomatic (scores of 0) with all aspects of the VOMS and demonstrated an NPC of 4 cm (within normal limits [WNL]). Likewise, he was symptomatic and scored WNL on the DHI, DVAT, and HiMAT. He also tolerated exertion to 19/20 RPE with maximal treadmill running. Communication of his progress served as the criteria for the physician to approve release to full sports participation. The patient kept one appointment in 30 days' time to confirm no return of MTBI symptoms or limitation with full semiprofessional hockey and was discharged to independent management (see Table 18-1).

Case Study Two

Case Study Two illustrates the complexities of managing clients through protracted recovery from MTBI. The client was a 19-year-old female, collegiate-level, ballroom dance athlete who hit her head on the floor when a novice partner lost his grip during a dip. The dancer was attended by a physician not familiar with MTBI, and she did not receive the typical standard of care for MTBI evaluation. The client and mother reported the patient was diagnosed with MTBI largely based on her report of the mechanism of injury and symptoms of dizziness, vertigo, nausea, imbalance, headaches, light sensitivity, and cognitive impairment. They also reported the client was educated as to the effect that her MTBI would spontaneously resolve with full brain rest in 2 weeks' time. After 12 weeks without improvement, the client sought a second opinion from a member of our local multidisciplinary integrated model for care of MTBI, a fellowship-trained sports medicine internist/board-certified

pediatrician who performed a thorough examination including assessment of coordination and a thorough catalog of MTBI symptoms. Computerized neurocognitive function testing showed marked cognitive impairment. The client was then referred to our clinic and exhibited marked impairment with vestibular, oculomotor, balance, cervical, and exertion testing (Table 18-2).

Both the physician and physical therapy intake forms and subjective interviews included multiple questions pertaining to anxiety, depression, and other psychosocial factors that could impact care. However, the client did not report suffering from anxiety or depression. This is not atypical as those suffering from anxiety and depression often deny the existence of the condition. This appears even more so in athletes as their culture has trained them to be stoic in nature and admission of anxiety/depression is often viewed as a weakness.[5-8,14-17,56,75,81-84]

To fully understand how anxiety affected our client's progress, it helps to understand how arousal impacts sensory integration, NMC, balance, and cognitive brain functions. Appropriate level of arousal is a precursor for optimal attentional focus and cognitive function in sports. For example, an athlete who performs well is described as "in the zone" or at an ideal level of arousal so as to process all of the relevant sensory cues (the rim of the basketball hoop) and simultaneously filter out the irrelevant sensory cues (the hand of the defender trying to block their shot or their parents cheering in the stands). Anxiety is a state of hyper arousal in which the brain becomes so occupied by attempting to process multiple sensory cues that ironically it cannot process any cues successfully. It appears a subpopulation of clients with MTBI and concurrent anxiety enter a positive feedback loop between perception of vertigo and anxiety that ramps up both symptoms and plummets function.[15-17,56,75,81] Researchers have hypothesized this paradoxical state is due to perseveration on perception of symptoms as well as vestibular thalamic pathways. Regardless of the mechanism, this subpopulation struggles greatly when vertigo and anxiety fuel each other. Intervention should focus on control of both vertigo and anxiety simultaneously through coordination of care between physical and cognitive behavioral therapies.

In retrospect, the authors of this chapter wish they had identified the client's premorbid anxiety and depression that would have predicted the client's slow recovery earlier. While open-ended questions allow clients the freedom to communicate more, history remains a place for closed-ended questions specific to anxiety/depression. Earlier identification of anxiety would have led to faster referral to cognitive behavioral therapies and likely faster progress in phases I through III. Instead, we went about applying the evidence for vestibulocervical, also known as *multimodal impairment-based*, physical therapy to control the client's vertigo, nausea, imbalance, headaches, and poor tolerance of exertion. The client showed consistent but excruciatingly slow progress through phases I through III (see Table 18-2).

Table 18-1

TYPICAL RECOVERY FOR CLIENT WITH MILD TRAUMATIC BRAIN INJURY WITH DIZZINESS

INITIAL EVALUATION FINDINGS	HISTORY	DHI	HIT	DVA-NI	VOMS	BALANCE/ MOBILITY TESTING	EXERTION
	A 17-year-old semiprofessional hockey defenseman sustained an MTBI when checked into boards and subsequent fisticuffs	68/100	Negative bilaterally	Abnormal Static visual acuity 20/20 on Snellen eye chart, dropped 3 lines to 20/50 with oscillating horizontal head movement at 2.0 Hz	Abnormal Symptom profile higher than 2 with: • Horizontal saccades • NPC • VOR horizontal • Visual motion sensitivity	BESS: Abnormal 16 errors, reproduction of dizziness, vertigo, nausea with vestibular-biased conditions DGI: Abnormal 16/24, low scores from vestibular-biased components; head movement with reproduction of symptoms	Held at initial evaluation after marked flare of symptoms with other tests
	Referred to sports medicine internist when not spontaneously recovered in 3 weeks			Reproduced complaints noted in history	NPC distance: 15 cm		Subsequent testing visit 2 with recumbent bike, head still showed increased symptoms at intensity of 11/20 or "Light" on Borg RPE
	Complaints include dizziness, vertigo, nausea, mild imbalance, sensitivity to light, headaches, and cognitive fog						

(continued)

Table 18-1 (continued)

TYPICAL RECOVERY FOR CLIENT WITH MILD TRAUMATIC BRAIN INJURY WITH DIZZINESS

PHASE I (WEEK ONE)

Intervention	Education	Cervical	Vestibular (Applied Sensory Integration)	Exertion
	Client, host family, and coaches educated in pathophysiology of MTBI and relationship to increased metabolic demands of the recovering brain. Benefits of optimal sleep. Need for compliance with sports and school restrictions. Educated in concept of appropriate brain rest and pacing of tasks with pneumonic device the 3 Ms: • Monitor symptoms for increase above baseline • Modify activity if symptoms increase • Move on if elevated symptoms persist	Grade IV occipital-atlanto, atlanto-axial, midcervical mobilization. Cervical stabilization training	Visual • Saccades 1 Somatosensory • Balance training easy base of support with eyes closed	Not tolerated visit 1 "Very Light" intensity, 8/20 per Borg RPE on stationary recumbent bike with stable head x 8 minutes
CRITERIA TO PROGRESS	Report of improving sleep cycle Confirmation of appropriate brain rest and pacing of activities at home, school, and team activities (still off all play practice)	Decreased report of cervicogenic component of headaches, cervical active range of motion (AROM) improving	Demonstration of carryover of Saccades 1 and somatosensory substitution for partial control of vertigo, nausea, imbalance with ADLs	Tolerated 8/20 intensity per Borg RPE

(continued)

Table 18-1 (continued)

TYPICAL RECOVERY FOR CLIENT WITH MILD TRAUMATIC BRAIN INJURY WITH DIZZINESS

PHASE II (WEEKS TWO TO THREE)

Intervention	Education	Cervical	Vestibular (Applied Sensory Integration)	Exertion
	Reinforced previous education on appropriate brain rest, pacing of activities, and benefits of optimal sleep Educated in addition of concurrent cognitive challenge with all other forms of training as further progression	Grade V upper thoracic manipulation Self-spinal mobilization Cervical stabilization training	**Visual** • Saccades 1 • Saccades 2 **Visual Motion Sensitivity** • Carryover of saccades drills to move gaze from provoking opticokinetic stimuli; window blinds, iPad applications, hanging mobiles to orienting/relevantly visual cues stickers on wall, laser pointer **Somatosensory** • Balance training narrowing base of support with eyes closed • Extrinsic perturbation with balance on Shuttle Balance **Vestibular** • VOR x 1 at slow speeds just provoking oscillopsia Video game–based balance training combining all of the earlier mentioned items and concurrent cognitive challenge	"Very Light", 9/20 to "Light", 11/20 on Borg RPE Progressed mode of exercise to elliptical machine and treadmill walking as tolerance of head movement improved Increased duration sequentially by 2 minutes as tolerated each bout
CRITERIA TO PROGRESS	Tolerance of school, work, and ADLs with specified restrictions	Cervical AROM WNL Minimal complaint of headaches further rules out migraine headaches if complaints remain severe and limiting	Demonstration of carryover of visual and somatosensory substitution for full control of symptoms with ADLs	Toleration of 11/20 intensity per Borg RPE

(continued)

Table 18-1 (continued)

TYPICAL RECOVERY FOR CLIENT WITH MILD TRAUMATIC BRAIN INJURY WITH DIZZINESS

PHASE III (WEEKS FOUR TO FIVE)

Intervention	Education	Cervical	Vestibular (Applied Sensory Integration)	Exertion
	Emphasis on continued self-management with appropriate brain rest, pacing of activities, and sleep cycle as return to normal activities ramps up	Reinforced cervical stabilization training	Visual • Saccades 2 with increasing speed, complex visual backgrounds, and sport-specific context Visual Motion Sensitivity • Carryover of saccades drills to move gaze off of provoking stimuli; laser splitter projectors for highly opticokinetic images and video media tubes displayed on large format screens onto orienting/relevantly visual cues stickers on wall Somatosensory • Dynamic balance training on Shuttle Balance, sports-specific stances, eyes closed, aggressive extrinsic perturbation by therapist Vestibular • VOR x 1 at progressively faster speeds as tolerated Video game–based balance training combining all of the above and concurrent cognitive challenge in auditory, visual streams	"Somewhat Hard," 13/20 to "Hard," 16/20 on Borg RPE Mode—elliptical and treadmill jog to run Increased duration sequentially by 2 minutes as tolerated each bout
CRITERIA TO PROGRESS	Tolerance of unrestricted school and ADLs	Consistent report of ability to modulate headaches with self-mobilizations and posture and stabilization exercises	Asymptomatic with high level sensory processing and balance drills with concurrent cognitive challenge BESS, DGI, FGA: WNL	Tolerated 16/20 intensity per Borg RPE

(continued)

Table 18-1 (continued)

TYPICAL RECOVERY FOR CLIENT WITH MILD TRAUMATIC BRAIN INJURY WITH DIZZINESS

PHASE IV (WEEKS SIX TO SEVEN)

Intervention	Education	Cervical	Vestibular (Applied Sensory Integration)	Exertion
	Reinforced client understanding of need to complete phase IV prior to return to full sports participation	Repurposing of saccades 2 drill for dynamic cervical stabilization through full range of motion	Visual • Saccades 2 using sport implements; throw, catch, hit, strike at full speeds Visual motion sensitivity • Carryover of saccades drills to move gaze from provoking stimuli in video media tubes; sports point-of-view videos • Large format screens onto orienting/relevantly visual cues within the video image Somatosensory • Plyometrics training on floor and on/off Shuttle Balance • Cutting closed kinetic chain Vestibular • VOR x 1 at high speeds of head movement • VOR x 2 at high speeds of head and target movement Video game–based balance training combining all of the earlier mentioned items and concurrent cognitive challenge	"Very Hard" 17/20 to "Extremely Hard" 19/20 and/or "Maximal Exertion" 20/20 on Borg RPE Mode—treadmill sprinting, Shuttle Run (Shuttle Systems), plyometrics, other functional tests from orthopedic practice Decreased duration of exertion training as intensity approaches maximal Full speed sports conditioning and skills practice without contact
CRITERIA TO PROGRESS	Outcomes measures listed later in the table. Confirmation of effective self-management of symptoms with return to full ADLs, school, work, and skills/conditioning noncontact practice Updated physician upon completion of phase IV as criteria for medical release back to full sports participation	Independent control of headaches with self-management techniques	Asymptomatic with all sports movements, with complex sensory stimulation and concurrent cognitive challenge DHI: 0 to 15 or minimal disability VOMS: WNL per symptoms score 0 to 2 or less and NPC 5 cm or less DVA: WNL per loss of 2 lines or less at 2.0 Hz speed HiMAT: WNL 54/54	Tolerated 60-second sprint to Borg RPE 19 or 20/20 Completion of sport-specific functional tests from orthopedic practice; shuttle run, drop jump, single leg hops, skating lines, etc

(continued)

Table 18-1 (continued)

Typical Recovery for Client With Mild Traumatic Brain Injury With Dizziness

REHABILITATION OUTCOMES	SUBJECTIVE REPORT	DHI	HIT	DVA-NI	VOMS	BALANCE/ MOBILITY TESTING	EXERTION
	Prior level of function and asymptomatic with all ADLs, instrumental ADLs, school, work, and hockey	0/100	Not tested	WNL static acuity 20/20 dropped only 2 lines to 20/40 and asymptomatic	Symptom profile 0 all areas, all components NPC distance: 4 cm	BESS, DGI, FGA all WNL and asymptomatic	Tolerated 60-second treadmill sprint to 19/20 on Borg RPE
						HiMAT WNL and asymptomatic	

Table 18-2

PROLONGED RECOVERY FOR CLIENT WITH MILD TRAUMATIC BRAIN INJURY WITH DIZZINESS

INITIAL EVALUATION FINDINGS	HISTORY	DHI	HIT	DVA-NI	VOMS	BALANCE/ MOBILITY TESTING	EXERTION
	19-year-old female, collegiate ballroom dancer, sustained an MTBI when dropped by partner	93/100	Negative bilaterally	Abnormal Static visual acuity 20/20 on Snellen eye chart, dropped 6 lines to 20/200 with oscillating horizontal head movement at 2.0 Hz	Abnormal Symptom profiles rated 9s and 10s over all areas across all tests	BESS: 21 errors, reproduction of dizziness, vertigo, nausea with vestibular and somatosensory-biased conditions DGI: 15/24, with reproduction of symptoms all subcomponents	Held at initial evaluation after marked flare of symptoms with other tests
	Referred to neurology and then physical therapy when still symptomatic 3 months later			Reproduced complaints noted in history	NPC distance 30 cm Patient also reports strabismus premorbid to MTBI		Subsequent testing in visit 2 with recumbent bike, head still discontinued after 1 minute at 7/20 or "Extremely Light" on Borg RPE
	Complained of dizziness, vertigo, nausea, mild imbalance, sensitivity to light, headaches, and cognitive fog						

(continued)

Table 18-2 (continued)

PROLONGED RECOVERY FOR CLIENT WITH MILD TRAUMATIC BRAIN INJURY WITH DIZZINESS

PHASE I (WEEKS ONE TO FOUR)

Intervention	Education	Cervical	Vestibular (Applied Sensory Integration)	Exertion
	Client and mother were educated in pathophysiology of MTBI and relationship to increased metabolic demands of recovering brain; benefits of optimal sleep; and need for compliance with sports and school restrictions Educated in concept of appropriate brain rest and pacing of tasks with pneumonic device the 3 Ms: • Monitor symptoms for increase above baseline • Modify activity if symptoms increase • Move on if elevated symptoms persist	Grade IV occipital-atlanto, atlanto-axial, midcervical mobilization Neuromuscular training of cervical stabilization; feedback training of longus coli, as well as cervical proprioception training	Visual • Smooth pursuits • Saccades 1 • All visual drills performed with laser pointer for client-controlled distant targets to work around convergence insufficiency Somatosensory • Balance training easy base of support with eyes closed	Not tolerated visit 1 "Very Light" intensity 8/20 per Borg RPE on stationary recumbent bike with stable head x 3 to 8 minutes
CRITERIA TO PROGRESS	Report of improving sleep cycle Confirmation of appropriate brain rest and pacing of activities at home, school, and team activities (still off all play practice)	Decreased report of cervicogenic component of headaches, cervical AROM improving	Demonstration of carryover of saccades 1 and somatosensory substitution for partial control of vertigo, nausea, and imbalance with ADLs	Tolerated 8/20 intensity per Borg RPE

(continued)

Table 18-2 (continued)

PROLONGED RECOVERY FOR CLIENT WITH MILD TRAUMATIC BRAIN INJURY WITH DIZZINESS

PHASE II (WEEKS FIVE TO TEN)

Intervention	Education	Cervical	Vestibular (Applied Sensory Integration)	Exertion
	Reinforced previous education for appropriate brain rest, pacing of activities, and benefits of optimal sleep habits	Client was diagnosed with migraine headaches Transitioned to muscle energy techniques and manual traction for upper cervical spine as these increased cervical motion, pain, and headaches without provocation of migraines	Visual • Saccades 1 • Saccades 2 • Gradual movement of visual targets closer to client to promote convergence Visual motion sensitivity • Carryover of saccades drills to move gaze off of provoking opticokinetic stimuli; window blinds, iPad applications, hanging mobiles, and onto orienting/relevantly visual cues stickers on wall Somatosensory • Balance training narrowing base of support with eyes closed • Extrinsic perturbation with balance on Shuttle Balance Vestibular • VOR x 1 at slow speed that provokes oscillopsia Video game–based balance training combining all of the earlier mentioned and concurrent cognitive challenge	"Very Light" 9/20 to "Light" 11/20 on Borg RPE Progressed mode of exercise to elliptical machine and treadmill walking as tolerance of head movement improved Increased duration sequentially by 2 minutes as tolerated each bout
CRITERIA TO PROGRESS	Tolerance of school, work, and ADLs with specified restrictions	Cervical AROM WNL Minimal complaint of headaches—further rule out migraine headaches if complaints remain severe and limiting	Demonstration of carryover of saccades 1 and somatosensory substitution for partial control of vertigo, nausea, imbalance with rapid head movements with ADLs, driving, and isolated sports movements	Tolerated 11/20 intensity per Borg RPE

(continued)

Table 18-2 (continued)

PROLONGED RECOVERY FOR CLIENT WITH MILD TRAUMATIC BRAIN INJURY WITH DIZZINESS

PHASE III (WEEKS TEN TO EIGHTEEN)

Intervention	Education	Cervical	Vestibular (Applied Sensory Integration)	Exertion
	Identified patient anxiety and referred to further neuropsychology and cognitive behavioral therapy (CBT) Adapted physical therapy education with emphasis on carryover of vestibular rehabilitation sensory processing techniques to control acute symptoms and how this will in turn control anxiety Similar education in use of exertion training for control of anxiety	Reinforced neuromuscular training of cervical stabilization; feedback training of longus coli, as well as cervical proprioception training	Visual • Saccades 2 with increasing speed, complex visual backgrounds, and sport-specific context Visual motion sensitivity • Carryover of saccades drills to move gaze off of provoking stimuli; laser splitter projectors for highly opticokinetic images and video media tubes displayed on large format screens onto orienting/relevantly visual cues stickers on wall Somatosensory • Dynamic balance training on Shuttle Balance, sport-specific stances, eyes closed, aggressive extrinsic perturbation by therapist Vestibular • VOR x 1 at progressively faster speeds as tolerated Video game–based balance training combining all of the earlier mentioned items and concurrent cognitive challenge in auditory, visual streams	"Somewhat Hard" 13/20 to "Hard" 16/20 on Borg RPE Mode—elliptical and treadmill jog to run Increased duration sequentially by 2 minutes as tolerated each bout
CRITERIA TO PROGRESS		Consistent report of ability to modulate headaches with self-mobilizations and posture, stabilization exercises	Asymptomatic with high-level sensory processing and balance drills with concurrent cognitive challenge BESS, DGI, and FGA: WNL	Tolerated 16/20 intensity per Borg RPE

(continued)

Table 18-2 (continued)

PROLONGED RECOVERY FOR CLIENT WITH MILD TRAUMATIC BRAIN INJURY WITH DIZZINESS

PHASE IV (WEEKS SEVENTEEN TO TWENTY-FOUR)

Intervention	Education	Cervical	Vestibular (Applied Sensory Integration)	Exertion
	Reinforced carryover of anxiety control techniques from CBT in general and to enhance tolerance of VRT	Carryover of saccades 2 drill to visual-mediated cervical NMC at full ranges of cervical motion	Visual • Saccades 2 using sport implements; throw, catch, hit, strike at full speeds Visual motion sensitivity • Carryover of saccades drills to move gaze from provoking stimuli in video media tubes; sports point-of-view videos • Large format screens onto orienting/ relevantly visual cues within the video image Somatosensory • Plyometric training on floor and on/off Shuttle Balance • Cutting closed kinetic chain Vestibular • VOR x 1 at high speeds of head movement • VOR x 2 at high speeds of head and target movement Video game–based balance training combining all of the earlier mentioned items and concurrent cognitive challenge	"Very Hard" 17/20 to "Extremely Hard" 19/20 and/or "Maximal Exertion" 20/20 on Borg RPE Mode—treadmill sprinting, shuttle run, plyometrics, other functional tests from orthopedic practice Decreased duration of exertion training as intensity approaches maximal Full-speed sports conditioning and skills practice without contact
CRITERIA TO PROGRESS	See outcomes measures in this table Confirmation of self-management of symptoms with full ADLs, school, work, and dance Updated physician as to patient status to initiate return-to-sport paperwork	Independent control of headaches with self-management techniques	Asymptomatic with all sports movements, with complex sensory stimulation and concurrent cognitive challenge Asymptomatic with VOR x 1 and x 2 DVAT: WNL HiMAT: WNL	Tolerated 60-second sprint to Borg RPE 19 or 20/20 Completion of sport-specific functional tests from orthopedic practice; shuttle run, drop jump, single leg hops, etc

(continued)

Table 18-2 (continued)

PROLONGED RECOVERY FOR CLIENT WITH MILD TRAUMATIC BRAIN INJURY WITH DIZZINESS

REHABILITATION OUTCOMES	SUBJECTIVE REPORT	DHI	HIT	DVA-NI	VOMS	BALANCE/ MOBILITY TESTING	EXERTION
	Prior level of function and asymptomatic with all ADLs, instrumental ADLs, school, work, and dance	11/100—scores accumulated in emotional content	Not tested	WNL static acuity 20/20 dropped only 2 lines to 20/30 and asymptomatic	Symptom profile 0 all areas, all components NPC distance: 4 cm	HiMAT: WNL and asymptomatic	Tolerated 60-second sprint to Borg RPE 18/20
						Asymptomatic and prior level of function with ballet turns on point, through 360-degree arc x 5 repetitions	

Thankfully, mid-phase III, the therapists identified the patterns described earlier when the therapists noted very subtle nonverbal reactions to vestibular and visual motion sensitivity drills. Specifically, the client's face would flush red and/or her eyes would widen slightly. Further closed-ended, explicit questions revealed that the drills were provoking vertigo and concurrent anxiety the client previously denied. The client then volunteered she did not want to "wimp out" and slow progress, so she withheld information about her anxiety premorbid to concussion. The physical therapist updated members of the multidisciplinary team to advocate for referral to a clinical psychologist skilled in CBT to manage anxiety. It is important to note that the client's health insurance carrier was reluctant to cover this vital service, but reference to her anxiety and evidence correlating this to prolonged recovery in the physical therapy record were used to advocate for authorization of services. CBT techniques to control her anxiety included identification of negative thoughts such as, "every time I walk in crowds on campus, I get dizzy and sick." The client replaced these negative thoughts with positive, logical ones such as, "I can prevent my vertigo by applying the visual spotting drill from physical therapy whenever I walk on campus." From a neurocognitive perspective, this facilitated a cortical influence to control the lower regions of the brain from ramping up arousal to the state of anxiety. In full circle, the patient reported that use of self-management techniques for anxiety also seemed to provide enhanced results from her applied sensory integration techniques. We hypothesized that if she achieved normal regulation of emotion and arousal levels, she would then be better able to process relevant sensory cues for effective sensory integration to control vertigo.

The return on investment from identification and referral for treatment of anxiety was remarkable. The client robustly improved tolerance of the vestibular, cervical, and exertion aspects of her physical therapy plan of care. While not a controlled trial, we hypothesized this was the reason for her much faster rate of progression in phase IV. Case Study Two resulted in very favorable outcomes including return to ballroom dance, pursuing undergraduate education, and control of vertigo with all ADLs (see Table 18-2). The authors of this chapter continue to achieve favorable outcomes for difficult cases of MTBI, but now routinely identify predictors of prolonged recovery such as anxiety, depression, and learning disability.[15,17,81,84] Likewise, we now coordinate care with our local multidisciplinary integrated concussion management team including athletic trainers, orthopedists, sports medicine internists, neurologists, neuropsychologists, speech-language therapists, and cognitive behavioral therapists. We advise you to do the same in your area as this will improve your patient outcomes but also therapist quality of life.

REFERENCES

1. Borich MR, Cheung KL, Jones P, Khramova V, Gavrailoff L, Boyd LA, Virji-Babul N. Concussion: current concepts in diagnosis and management. *J Neurol Phys Ther*. 2013:37(3):133-139.

2. Hoffer ME, Gottshall KR, Moore R, Balough BJ, Western D. Characterizing and treating dizziness after mild head trauma. *Otol Neurol*. 2004;25(2):135-138.

3. Alsalaheen BA, Mucha A, Morris LO, et al. Vestibular rehabilitation for dizziness and balance disorders after concussion. *J Neurol Phys Ther*. 2010;34(2):87-93.

4. Leddy, JJ, Sandhu, H, Sodhi, V, Baker, JG, Willer B. Rehabilitation of concussion and post-concussion syndrome. *Sports Health*. 2012; 4(2):147-54.

5. Meier TB, Brummell BJ, Singh R, Neiro CJ, Polanski DW, Bellgowan PS. The underreporting of self-reported symptoms following sports related-concussion. *J Sci Med Sport*. 2015;18(5):507-511.

6. Brooks MA, Peterson K, Biese K, Sanfilippo J, Heiderscheit BC, Bell DR. Concussion increases odds of sustaining a lower extremity injury after return to play among collegiate athletes. *Am J Sports Med*. 2016;44(3):742-747.

7. Corwin DJ, Wiebe DJ, Zonfrillo MR. Vestibular deficits following youth concussion. *Clin Sports Med*. 2011;30(1):89-102.

8. Gurley JM, Hujsak BD, Kelly JL. Vestibular rehabilitation following mild traumatic brain injury. *NeuroRehabilitation*. 2013;32(3):519-528.

9. Schneider KJ, Meeuwisse WH, Nettel-Aguirre A, Barlow K, Boyd L, Kang J, Emery CA. Cervicovestibular rehabilitation in sport-related concussion: a randomised controlled trial. *Br J Sports Med*. 2014;48(17):1294-1298.

10. Grabowski P, Wilson J, Walker A, Enz D, Sijian W. Multimodal impairment-based physical therapy for the treatment of patients with post-concussion syndrome: a retrospective analysis on safety and feasibility. *Phys Ther Sport*. 2017;23:22-30.

11. Baker, JG, Freitas, MS, Leddy, JJ, Kozlowski, KF, Willer, BS. Return to full functioning after graded exercise assessment and progressive exercise treatment of post-concussion syndrome. *Rehabil Res Pract*. 2012;2012:705309. doi:10.1155/2012/705309

12. Storey EP, Wiebe DJ, D'Alonzo BA, et al. Vestibular rehabilitation is associated with visuvestibular improvement in pediatric concussion. *J Neurol Phys Ther*. 2018;42(3):134-141.

13. Schneider KJ, Iverson GL, Emery CA, McCrory P, Herring SA, Meeuwisse WH. The effects of rest and treatment following sport-related concussion: A systematic review of the literature. *Br J Sports Med*. 2013;47(5):304-307.

14. Scherer MR, Schubert MC. Traumatic brain injury and vestibular pathology as a comorbidity after blast exposure. *Phys Ther*. 2009;89(9):980-992.

15. McCrea M, Iverson GL, McAllister TW, et al. An integrated review of recovery after mild traumatic brain injury (MTBI): implications for medical management. *Clin Neuropsychol*. 2009;23(8):1368-1390.

16. Herdman SJ, Clendanial RA. *Vestibular Rehabilitation*. 4th ed. F.A. Davis; 2014.

17. Scopaz, KA, Hatzenbuehler JR. Risk modifiers for concussion and prolonged recovery. *Sports Health*. 2013;5(6):537-541.

18. Silverberg ND, Iverson GL. Is rest after concussion "the best medicine?": recommendations for activity resumption following concussion in athletes, civilians, and military service members. *The J Head Trauma Rehabil*. 2013;28(4):250-259.

19. Williams GP, Robertson V, Greenwood KM. High-Level Mobility Assessment Tool (HiMAT) for traumatic brain injury. Part 1: content validity and discriminability. *Brain Inj*. 2005;19(11):925-932.

20. Shumway-Cook A, Woolacoot M. *Motor Control Theory and Practical Applications*. Williams & Wilkins; 1995.

21. Williams GN, Chmielewski, MA, Rudolph KS, Buchanan TS, Synder-Mackler L. Dynamic knee stability: current theory and implications for clinicians and scientists. *J Ortho Sports Phys Ther.* 2001;31(10):546-566.

22. Higuchi T, Nagami T, Nakata H, Watanabe M, Isaka T, Kanosue K. Contribution about ball trajectory to baseball hitting accuracy. *PLoS One.* 2016;11(2):1-15.

23. Mucha A, Collins M, Elbin RJ, et al. A brief Vestibular/Ocular Motor Screening (VOMS) assessment to evaluate concussions, preliminary findings. *Am J Sports Med.* 2014;42(10):2479-2486.

24. Barnett BP, Singman EL. Vision concerns after mild traumatic brain injury. *Curr Treat Options Neurol.* 2015;17(2):329.

25. Pavlov M, Acheson J, Nicolaou D, Fraser CL, Bronstein AM, Davies R. Effect of developmental binocular vision abnormalities in visual vertigo symptoms and treatment outcomes. *J Neurol Phys Ther.* 2015;39(4):215-224.

26. Schubert MC, Minor LB. Vestibular-ocular physiology underlying vestibular hypofunction. *Phys Ther.* 2004;84(4):373-385.

27. Mohammad MT, Whitney SL, Marchetti GF, Sparta PJ, Ward BK, Furman JM. The reliability and response stability of dynamic testing of the vestibulo-ocular reflex in patients with vestibular disease. *J Vestib Res.* 2011;21(5):277-288.

28. Kaufman DR, Puckett MJ, Smith MJ, Wilson KS, Cheema R, Landers MR. Test-retest reliability and responsiveness of gaze stability and dynamic visual acuity in high school and college football players. *Phys Ther Sport.* 2014;15(3):181-188.

29. Hoffer ME, Gottshall KR. Tracking recovery of vestibular function in individuals with blast-induced head trauma using vestibular-visual-cognitive interaction tests. *J Neurol Phys Ther.* 2010;34(2):94-97.

30. Landers M, Donatelli R, Nash J, Bascharon. Evidence of dynamic visual acuity impairment in asymptomatic martial arts fighters. *Concussion.* 2017;2(3):CNC41. doi:10.2217/cnc-2016-0032

31. Jacobson GP, Newman CW. The development of the Dizziness Handicap Inventory. *Arch Otolaryngol Head Neck Surg.* 1990;116(4):424-427.

32. Samandi U, Ritlop R, Reyes M, et al. Eye tracking detect dysconjugate eye movements associated with structural traumatic brain injury and concussion. *J Neurotrauma.* 2015;32(8):548-556.

33. Jacobson GP, Calder, JH. A screening version of the Dizziness Handicap Inventory (DHI-S). *Am J Otol.* 1998;19(6):804-808.

34. Whitney SL, Sparto PJ. Eye movements, dizziness, and mild traumatic brain injury (mTBI): a topical review of emerging evidence and screening measures. *J Neurol Phys Ther.* 2019;43(Suppl 2):S31-S36.

35. Buckely TA, Munkasy BA, Clouse BP. Sensitivity and specificity of the modified balance error scoring system in concussion collegiate student athletes. *Clin J Sport Med.* 2018;28(2):174-176.

36. Whitney SL, Hudak MT. The Dynamic Gait Index relates to self reported fall history in individuals with vestibular dysfunction. *J Vestib Res.* 2000;10(2):99-105.

37. Wrisley DM, Walker ML, Echternach JL, Strasnick B. Reliability of the Dynamic Gait Index in people with vestibular disorders. *Arch Phys Med Rehabil.* 2003;84:1528-1533.

38. Wrisley DM, Kumar NA. Functional Gait Assessment: concurrent, discriminative, and predictive validity in community-dwelling older adults. *Phys Ther.* 2010; 90(5):761-773.

39. Alsalaheen, BA, Whitney SL, Marchetti GF, et al. Performance of high school adolescents on functional gait and balance measures. *Pediatr Phys Ther.* 2014;26(2):191-199.

40. Williams GP, Robertson V, Greenwood KM. High-Level Mobility Assessment Tool (HiMAT) for traumatic brain injury. Part 2: item generation. *Brain Inj.* 2005;19(1):833-843.

41. Williams GP, Robertson V, Greenwood KM. High-Level Mobility Assessment Tool (HiMAT): integrated reliability, retest reliability, and internal consistency. *Phys Ther.* 2006;86(3):395-400.

42. Williams GP, Greenwood KM, Robertson VJ. The concurrent validity and responsiveness of the High-Level Mobility Assessment Tool for measuring the mobility limitations of people with traumatic brain injury. *Arch Physical Med Rehabil.* 2006;87(3):437-442.

43. Williams GP, Rosie J, DenisenkomS, Taylor D. Normative values for the High-Level Mobility Assessment Tool (HiMAT). *Int J Ther Rehabil.* 2009;16:370-374.

44. Williams GP, Pallant J, Greenwood K. Further development of the High-Level Mobility Assessment Tool (HiMAT). *Brain Inj.* 2010;24(7-8):1027-1031.

45. Kleffelgaard I, Roe, C, Sandvik L, Hellstrom T, Soberg H. Measurement properties of the High-Level Mobility Assessment Tool for mild traumatic brain injury. *Phys Ther.* 2013;93(7):900-910.

46. Resch JE, Brown CN, Schmidt J, Macciocchi SN, Blueitt D, Callum M, Ferrara MS. The sensitivity and specificity of clinical measures of sports concussion: three tests are better than one. *BMJ Open Sport Exerc Med.* 2016;19(2):e000012. doi:10.1136/bmjsem-2015-000012

47. McCulloch K. Attention and dual-take conditions: physical therapy implications for individuals with acquired brain injury. *J Neurol Phys Ther.* 2007;31(3):104-118.

48. Catena RD, Donkelaar PV, Chou L. Cognitive task effects on gait stability following concussion. *Exp Brain Res.* 2007;176(1):23-31.

49. Catena RD, Donkelaar PV, Chou L. The effects of attention capacity in dynamic balance control following concussion. *J Neuroeng Rehabil.* 2011;8:8.

50. Scherer MR, Weightman MM, Radomski MV, Davidson LF, McCullock KL. Returning service members to duty following mild traumatic brain injury: exploring the use of dual-task and multitask assessment methods. *Phys Ther.* 2013;93(9):1254-1267.

51. Alsalaheen BA, Whitney SL, Marchetti GF, et al. Relationship between cognitive assessment and balance measures in adolescents referred for vestibular physical therapy after concussion. *Clin J Sport Med.* 2016;26(1):46-52.

52. Howell DR, Oldham JR, DiFabio M, et al. Single-task and dual-task gait among collegiate athletes of different sports classifications: implications for concussion management. *J Appl Biomech.* 2017;33(1):24-31.

53. Howell DR, Osternig LR, Chou LS. Single-task and dual-task tandem gait performance after concussion. *J Sci Med Sport.* 2017;20(7):622-626.

54. Yorke AM, Smith L, Alsalaheen B. Validity and reliability of the vestibular/ocular motor screening and associations with common concussion screening tools. *Sports Health.* 2017;9(2):174-180.

55. Gotshall K, Drake A, Gray N, McDonald E, Hoffer M. Objective vestibular tests as outcome measures in head injury patients. *Laryngoscope.* 2003;113(10):1746-1750.

56. Whitney SL, Wrisley DM, Brown KE, Furman JM. Is perception of handicap related to functional performance in persons with vestibular dysfunction. *Otol Neurol.* 2004;25(2):139-143.

57. Ventura RE, Balcer LJ, Galetta SL, Rucker JC. Ocular motor assessment in concussion: current status and future directions. *J Neurol Sci.* 2016;361:79-86.

58. Elbin RJ, Sufrinko A, Anderson MN, et al. Prospective changes in vestibular and ocular motor impairment after concussion. *J Neurol Phys Ther.* 2018;42(3):142-148.

59. Schubert MC, Tusa RJ, Grine LE, Herdman SJ. Optimizing the sensitivity of Head Thrust Test for identifying vestibular hypo function. *Phys Ther.* 2004; 84(2):151-158.

60. McGee S. Simplifying likelihood ratios. *J Gen Intern Med.* 2002; 17(8):647-650.

61. Yip CW, Glaser M, Frenzel C, Bayes O, Strupp M. Comparison of the Bedside Head-Impulse Test with Video Head-Impulse Test in a clinical practice setting. A propspective study of 500 outpatients. *Front Neurol.* 2016;7:58.

62. Alasherhi, MM, Sparto PJ, Furman JM, Fedor S, Mucha A, Henry LC, Whitney SJ. The usefulness of video head impulse test in children and adults post concussion. *J Vestib Res.* 2016;26(6):439-446.

63. Rine RM, Braswell J. A clinical test of dynamic visual acuity for children. *Int J Pediatr Otorhinoloaryngol.* 2003;67(11):1195-1201.

64. Paquet N, Chilingaryan G, Fung J. Clinical evaluation of dynamic visual acuity in subjects with unilateral vestibular hypofunction. *Otol Neruotol.* 2009;30(3):368-372.

65. Christy JB, Cochrane GD, Almutairi A, Busettini C, Swanson MW, Weise KK. Peripheral vestibular and balance function in athletes with and without concussion. *J Neurol Phys Ther.* 2019;43(3):153-159.

66. Guskiewicz KM, Perrin DH, Gasneder BM. Effects of mild head injury on postural stability in athletes. *J Athletic Training.* 1996;31(4):300-307.

67. Riemann RL, Guskiewicz KM. Effects of mild head injury as measured through clinical balance testing. *J Athletic Training.* 2000;35(1):19-25.

68. Guskiewicz KM, Bruce SL, Cantu RC, et al. National Athletic Trainer's Association position statement: management of sport-related concussion. *J Athletic Training.* 2004;39(3):280-297.

69. Guskiewicz KM. Balance assessment in the management of sport-related concussion. *Clin Sports Med.* 2011;30(1):89-102.

70. Bell DR, Guskiewicz KM, Clark MA, Padua DA. Systematic review of the balance error scoring system. *Sports Health.* 2011;3(3):287-295.

71. King LA, Horak FB, Mancini M, et al. Instrumenting the Balance Error Scoring System for use with patients reporting persistent balance problems after mild traumatic brain injury. *Arch Phys Med Rehabil.* 2014;95(2):353-359.

72. Howell DR, Osternig LR, Chou LS. Adolescents demonstrate greater gait balance control deficits after concussion than young adults. *Am J Sports Med.* 2015;43(3):625-632.

73. Cheever, K, Kawata K, Tierney R, Galgon A. Cervical injury assessments for concussion evaluation: a review. *J Athl Train.* 2016;51(2):1037-1044.

74. Lennon A Hugentobler JA, Sroka MC, et al. An exploration of the impact of initial timing of physical therapy on safety and outcomes after concussion in adolescents. *J Neurol Phys Ther.* 2018;42(3):123-131.

75. Majerske CW, Mihalik JP, Ren D, et al. Concussion in sports: post-concussive activity levels, symptoms, and neurocognitive performance. *J Athl Train.* 2008;43(3):265-274.

76. Seifert T, Secher NH. Sympathetic influence on cerebral blood flow and metabolism during exercise in humans. *Prog Neurobiol.* 2011; 95(3):406-426.

77. Hinds A, Leddy J, Freitas M, Czuczman N, Willer B. The effect of exertion on heart rate and rating of perceived exertion in acutely concussed individuals. *J Neurol Neurophysiol.* 2016;7(4):388-400.

78. Schmidt J, Rubino C, Boyd LA, Virji-Babul N. The role of physical activity in recovery from concussion in youth: a neuroscience perspective. *J Neurol Phys Ther.* 2018;42(3):155-162.

79. Haider MN, Leddy JJ, Wilber CG, et al. The predictive capacity of the Buffalo Concussion Treadmill Test after sports-related concussion in adolescents. *Front Neurol.* 2019;10:395.

80. Leddy JJ, Haider MN, Ellis ME, Willer BS. Exercise is medicine for concussion. *Curr Sports Med Rep.* 2018;17(8):262-270.

81. Ellis MJ, Ledd J, Willer B. Multi-disciplinary management of athletes with post-concussion syndrome: an evolving pathophysiological approach. *Front Neurol.* 2016;7:136.

82. Lau BC, Collins MW, Lovell MR. Cutoff scores in neurocognitive testing and symptom clusters that predict protracted recovery from concussions in high school athletes. *Neurosurgery.* 2012;70(2):371-379.

83. Lau BC, Kontos AP, Collins MW, Mucha A, Lovell MR. Which on- field signs/symptoms predict protracted recovery from sport-related concussion among high school football players? *Am J Sports Med.* 2011;39(11):2311-2318.

84. Harmon KG, Dresser J, Gammons M, et al. American Medical Society for Sports Medicine position statement: concussion in sport. *Clin J Sport Med.* 2013;23(1):1-18.

85. Rabago CA, Wilken JM. Application of a Mild traumatic brain injury rehabilitation program in a virtual reality environment: a case study. *J Neurol Phys Ther.* 2011;35(4):185-193.

19

Exercises for the Trunk, Shoulder, Hip, and Knee
Electromyographic Evidence

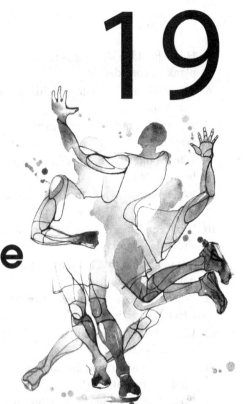

James M. McKivigan, PT

CHAPTER QUESTIONS

1. What are some possible medical uses for the EMG techniques mentioned in this chapter?
2. What is the definition of CLBP?
3. What is considered the body's center of gravity in the anatomical position?
4. What can occur in the spine with high activity of the core muscles?

Wallmann HW, Donatelli R, eds. *Foundations of Orthopedic Physical Therapy* (pp 585-611).
© 2024 Taylor & Francis Group.

5. How should a side support exercise such as the side plank be considered?

6. What is an advantage with active rehabilitation exercising?

7. What is the primary reason for deconditioning syndrome?

8. Why would prescribing Pilates for a patient with CLBP be indicated?

9. What is the significance of internal oblique muscle activation?

10. What can be said about traditional and nontraditional abdominal exercises?

11. Are nontraditional abdominal exercises effective in spinal rehabilitation?

12. What muscles is the power wheel rollout exercise most effective in activating?

13. Why is it important to make small changes in a particular Pilates exercise?

14. How can maximum voluntary isometric contraction be used in rehabilitation?

15. What is the significance of using double-oscillating devices rather than a single-oscillating device in rehabilitation?

16. How should double-oscillating devices be used in rehabilitation?

17. How does motor learning occur?

18. What can be said about the use of unstable surfaces or isometric squats in rehabilitation?

19. Why should shoulder-strengthening programs be included in rehabilitation?

20. What is the effect of hip abduction exercises performed in isolation?

INTRODUCTION

The purpose of this chapter is to provide guidelines for exercises that may be effective for the rehabilitation of the trunk, shoulder, hip, and knee based on evidence gathered from EMG research. Evidence indicates that a substantial relationship exists between the EMG signal amplitude and the amount of force produced by a muscle.[1] Therefore, this chapter discusses studies related to exercises for increasing muscle activity using EMG data related to the trunk, shoulder, hip, and knee.

EMG data from the assessment of neuromuscular activity and neuromuscular demand during high-intensive tasks require normalization to aid interpretation.[2] Normalization provides credibility to EMG studies that look to express the relative neuromuscular capacity of the muscle during an exercise or task, to enable between muscle, between study, and between participant comparisons and to improve the intra-/inter-individual variability of the un-normalized EMG.[2] Muscle contraction is usually an MVIC. Applicability

in clinical practice is gained from analysis of the percentage of MVIC data determined by EMG, which may provide information about muscle activation, recruitment, fatigue, and estimates of muscle force.[1] Researchers indicate that direct measures, such as surface EMG in conjunction with inertial sensors, produce precise, quantitative, and unbiased estimates of exposure to physical risk factors.[3,4]

The use of either traditional or nontraditional exercises have been evidenced with EMG to provide an effective means in the rehabilitation of the trunk, shoulder, hip, and knee in persons suffering from CLBP and other forms of chronic muscle pain. Benefits gained from certain types of exercise programs for influencing rehabilitation in patients suffering from chronic muscle pain has been supported with the use of EMG data. In contrast, some researchers concluded that nontraditional exercises, over that of traditional exercises, were most effective in activating both abdominal and extraneous muscle groups and that clinicians should consider the data and implications for patient rehabilitation.[5,6] However, researchers have suggested that exercise-type interventions ranging from traditional to nontraditional forms of training and/or rehabilitation programs have advantages and play a significant part in patient rehabilitation.[7]

EMG data support one repetition maximum for increasing strength from 0% to 30% MVIC in untrained individuals,[8] indicating that exercises, specific to targeted muscle groups, may signal amplitude in a muscle for increasing overall muscle strength. Exercises producing less than 30% MVIC should be considered by the therapist as exercises suited for motor control and/or endurance training.[8] Better conditioned or advanced individuals in their rehabilitation programs may require increased levels of stimulus to obtain a strength response higher than 30% MVIC. More exercise studies are required before clinicians can make definitive conclusions for determining what types of exercises are most useful for increasing a patient's rehabilitation strength response.

CORE EXERCISE FOR STRENGTH AND ENDURANCE TRAINING

Literature reviews have been performed regarding the effectiveness of exercise for patients with CLBP and chronic muscle pain in general.[9,10] Researchers of these studies indicated that exercise is beneficial for increasing levels of effective treatment in individuals with CLBP.[9,10] However, conclusive thought does not indicate whether one exercise is more effective in reducing pain associated with CLBP or for decreasing timeframes associated with rehabilitation. Researchers concluded that consistent/intensive-type exercises, specifically strengthening exercises, organized aerobic exercises, and general exercises, are more effective for improving the quality of life in patients with CLBP.[11] In contrast, some researchers disagree that intensive exercise is an effective method for reducing rehabilitation timeframes in some patients suffering with other types of chronic pain.[12] Studies provide little evidence to indicate that exercise intensity levels offer more beneficial results when compared to studies conducted on patients suffering from some form of chronic muscular pain.

Literature reviewed has provided evidence on exercise studies involving patients with CLBP and or other forms of chronic muscle pain. However, more exercise studies are required before clinicians can make definitive conclusions for determining what types of exercises are most useful for patients suffering from CLBP and/or other forms of chronic muscle pain. In patients with chronic muscle pain, exercise programs may be most effective in reducing recurring pain rates.

UNDERSTANDING THE CORE

Increasing core strength in an attempt to improve overall health, rehabilitate from injuries, and enhance athletic performance requires an understanding for targeting core stability and balance.[7,13-15] Exercise-type interventions ranging from traditional to nontraditional forms of training and/or rehabilitation programs have been advocated by researchers because each has advantages.[7,13]

Despite much research around the subject, there is confusion in understanding what goes wrong with the core and how to properly train (or retrain) muscle groups. Research outcomes have indicated this confusion relating to the core as trainers and health professionals understand that there is a need to strengthen abdominals utilizing "high-load" (strength/effort) training.[16] In addition, by association, other muscle groups related to the shoulder, hip, and knee that assist in activating abdominals with the use of specific exercises lend to furthering the confusion and misunderstanding on how to train the core properly.

Most people with chronic muscle pain syndromes generally have relatively low-level function and cannot organize fundamental elements for developing the core. Therefore, subjecting them to individual muscle group and high-load training strategies is likely to further aggravate symptoms.[17-19] Therefore, questions regarding the concept and the real value of training the core is required.

HISTORICAL PERSPECTIVE ON CORE

The term *core* is commonly used in the popular media to refer to the trunk.[7] The muscles that are typically associated with the core allow for the transference of torques and angular momentum during performance-type activities, such as kicking or throwing objects,[7] and activities that require use of the legs, knees, hips, and shoulders, in addition to core muscles. Core muscles are those that wrap around and pull in the body's mid-section.[20] The pelvis is the main center of weight shift and load transfer in the body.[20] Increasing core stability will result in a better foundation for force production in the upper and lower extremities.[7,14,21]

CORE STRUCTURE

The pelvis is the main center of weight shift and load transfer in the body.[20] The body's center of gravity is anterior to the second sacral segment (S2) in the standing anatomical position.[20] Therefore, an individual's mechanical core is principally located around the sacrum's front. However, as the diaphragm and anterolateral abdomen are critical for core stabilization and movement control, in whole, the core reaches from the ischial tuberosities up to the midthorax where the diaphragm and transversus abdominis attach.[20] In sum, a balanced postural and functional relationship between the thorax and pelvis affords the ideal condition for promoting core stabilization and strength due to the alignment related to the body's center of gravity.

FUNCTIONAL MECHANISMS

Postural support and spine/pelvic movement are the ability to generate optimal IAP to support both breathing and provision of 3-dimensional (3D) postural and movement control of the trunk, particularly control of the pelvis on the legs.[20,21] Breathing and postural control specifically are linked and important elements common to both mechanisms for generating appropriate levels of IAP.[20]

Breathing is the most fundamental motor pattern. However, postural control mechanisms of the axial column and movement control of the proximal limb girdles are other important factors related to postural support and spine/pelvic movement control. First, postural control mechanisms of the axial column require a balanced but adaptable cooperative activation between the axial flexor and extensor muscle systems,[20] which is helped by appropriate levels of IAP for postural support.[21] Second, postural movement control of the proximal limb girdles, specifically the pelvis for controlling the trunk, assists in controlling spine/pelvic movement and influences postural stability.[20] Coordination of the 3 functional systems (ie, breathing, postural control mechanisms of the axial column, movement control of the proximal limb girdles) results in cooperative activation of many muscles for providing spine/pelvic movement control.[20,21]

The lower pelvic unit contributes significantly to the intrinsic mechanisms of spine/pelvic support and control. The intrinsic system are those muscles found in the abdominal section (ie, the diaphragm, pelvic floor muscles, transversus abdominis) and also the lumbar multifidus, the interspinales and intertransversarii, psoas, medial fibers of quadratus lumborum, iliacus and deep hip rotators, and the internal oblique.[20] Excluding the intrinsic spinal extensors, the deep

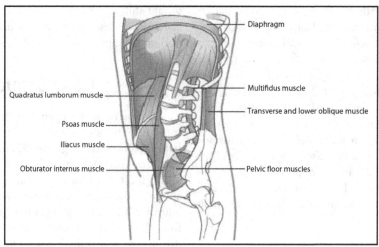

Figure 19-1. Mechanisms of core control.

muscles mentioned form a continuous inner myofascial sleeve surrounding the trunk and pelvic cavity (Figure 19-1). Variable exercise activity within the lower pelvic unit provides the adaptive stability and strength required for achieving and maintaining core control.

TRAINING EXERCISE FOR STRENGTHENING OF THE LOWER BACK

Core stability is defined by 2 terms: *global* and *local stability systems*.[22] Global refers to the larger, superficial muscles (ie, rectus abdominis), which are the main movers for the trunk and hip.[22] Local stability refers to the deep, intrinsic muscles of the abdominal wall (ie, transversus abdominis).[22] This system is responsible for the segmental stability of the spine during whole body activity where movements and postural adjustments are required. Therefore, training exercises for strengthening of the lower back, an area associated with spinal function, is necessary for achieving spinal stability. EMG signal amplitudes ranging from 44.7 ± 19.2 in the rectus abdominis, 54.7 ± 22.9 in the external oblique abdominis, and 36.8 ± 18.6 in percentage of MVIC, respectively, in the abdominal muscles have been recorded during the prone, side, and supine bridge on stable and unstable surfaces, with the highest activity recorded during prone bridge on a stable surface using a Swiss ball amongst a sampled group of 33 healthy volunteers.[22] Implications of this study may provide a foundation for supporting use of these types of exercises for patients suffering from chronic muscle pain associated with the lower back.

Researchers performed an exercise program using surface EMG for recording upper and lower rectus abdominis, external and internal obliques, rectus femoris, latissimus dorsi, and lumbar paraspinal muscle activity.[23] EMG data were collected during 5 repetitions of 10 exercises, then normalized by MVIC. It was determined that upper and lower rectus abdominis activity was generally significantly greater

in the crunch, bent-knee sit-up, and prone position exercises compared with side position exercises.[23] External oblique activity was significantly greater in the prone using a Swiss ball with right hip extension, side crunch on the ball, and side bridge (plank) on toes compared with the prone and side bridge (plank) on knees, the crunch, or the bent-knee sit-up positions.[23] Internal oblique activity was significantly greater in the prone bridge (plank) on ball and prone on ball with left and right hip extension compared with the side crunch on ball and prone and side bridge (plank) on knees positions.[23] Lumbar paraspinal activity was significantly greater in the 3 side position exercises compared with all remaining exercises. Latissimus dorsi activity was significantly greater in the prone on ball with left and right hip extension and prone bridge (plank) on ball and on toes compared with the crunch, bent-knee sit-up, and prone and side bridge (plank) on knees positions.[23] Rectus femoris activity was significantly greater in the prone on ball with left hip extension, bent-knee sit-up, or prone bridge (plank) on toes compared with the remaining exercises.[23] Researchers concluded that the prone position exercises were good alternatives to supine position exercises for recruiting core musculature activity. Side position exercises were better for oblique and lumbar paraspinal muscle recruitment.[23] Implication of the research indicates that because high core muscle activity is associated with high spinal compressive loading, muscle activation patterns should be considered when prescribing trunk exercises to those in which high spinal compressive loading may be harmful.

PRONE POSITION EXERCISE

This exercise is performed with the client face down on a stable surface, such as a plinth, with the clinician ensuring the pelvis is aligned in a neutral position. The exercise can also be done with the body straight, and the legs are aligned with the spine in an unstable position, such as when a person is swimming. Using EMG, distinct contribution of the paraspinal muscle was observed in 3 Pilates exercises: swimming, single leg kick, and double leg kick. Researchers recorded EMG amplitudes of 21% to 52% MVIC during the 3 Pilate prone-type exercises.[24] Muscle activity of the right latissimus dorsi was 46% MVIC, 43% MVIC in the left latissimus dorsi, 52% MVIC for the right multifidus, 49% MVIC in the left multifidus, 21% MVIC in the left gluteus maximus, 22% MVIC in the right gluteus maximus, 49% MVIC in the right semitendinosus, and 53% MVIC in the left semitendinosus.[24] These results may provide basic information for when Pilates exercises are performed in a prone position and may be useful for clinicians prescribing an exercise rehabilitation program.

SIDE SUPPORT EXERCISE

This exercise is performed with the patient on the side and supported on the elbow and feet with the spine aligned in the neutral position. Side position exercises have been determined to be better for oblique and lumbar paraspinal muscle recruitment.[23] Researchers have recorded EMG amplitudes of 40% and 42% MVIC, respectively, in the longissimus thoracis and lumbar multifidus muscles and 69% MVIC in the external oblique muscle on the side of the supporting elbow and feet.[25] Researchers recorded EMG single amplitude levels of 18% MVIC in the rectus abdominis, 45% MVIC in the external oblique, and 25% MVIC in the internal oblique.[22] Other researchers recorded significant increases in EMG signal amplitude levels from 6% to 11% MVIC in the rectus abdominis, 11% to 22% MVIC in the external oblique, and 7% to 27% in the internal oblique.[24] The side support exercise should be considered a good back exercise due to concentration on the abdominal, paraspinal, and quadratus lumborum muscles.

BACK AND ABDOMINAL MUSCLE FUNCTION DURING STABILIZATION EXERCISES

Active rehabilitation has been increasingly advocated as a treatment for CLBP.[26] Under an exercise-based active rehabilitation program, CLBP intensity can be reduced and can also lend to improving back extension strength, endurance, and mobility.[26-28] Therefore, treatment guidelines for encouraging active physical rehabilitation programs should be advocated by clinicians.

CLBP is associated with lumbar paraspinal muscle weakness and poor coordination of these muscles, which results in excessive fatigability.[29-31] Disuse or deconditioning of these muscles results in pain and/or illness, a process called *deconditioning syndrome*.[32,33] Studies suggest that muscle spasms and reflex inhibition of trunk muscles may also contribute to deconditioning syndrome.[34,35]

In active exercise rehabilitation programs, functional limitations can be improved.[26,36] Estimating individual trunk muscle activities is difficult based on simple observation of patient muscle movements and requires an objective strength assessment.[37] Surface EMG can be used to support a quantifiable means for measuring muscle activity and fatigability from an objective perspective.[38,39]

In a recent EMG study, Pilates method-type exercises were shown to increase the strength of trunk stabilizer muscles and consequently reduce CLBP in patients. In this study, the researchers analyzed EMG activity of trunk stabilizer muscles during use of the centering principle of Pilates method-type exercises. Two groups were sampled, a low back pain group (LBPG) and a control group. The centering principle of Pilates method-type exercises was applied only in the control group sample; the researchers compared EMG data between sample groups. In a 2-part test, analysis of root mean square percentage (RMS%), showed a higher stabilizer muscle recruitment amongst the sampled control group (test 1 = 74%; test 2 = 60%) compared to the sampled LBPG (test 1 = 58%; test 2 = 54%) during the performance of Pilates-type exercises.[40] The researchers concluded that impaired lumbar spine stability in patients with CLBP, using the centering principle of Pilates method, is an important finding for physical therapists and should be a prescribed exercise method for increasing trunk muscle strength and reducing CLBP.[40]

In this study, the researchers did not account for load imposed in isometric contraction, as is done in the typical Pilates method practice. Moreover, the occurrence of cross-talk of the EMG signal between internal oblique and transversus abdominis muscle is possible, but in the centering principle, the transversus abdominis contraction must occur, so the EMG signal of internal oblique is accepted as an important indicator of spinal stability, despite the exact contribution of each muscle being unknown.[40] EMG analysis of certain types of nontraditional exercises may provide clinicians a means for measuring a patient's rehabilitation progress compared to traditional forms of exercise methods, as discussed in this study.

ELECTROMYOGRAPHY ANALYSIS OF TRADITIONAL AND NONTRADITIONAL ABDOMINAL EXERCISES

Examining the effectiveness of traditional and nontraditional forms of abdominal exercises may allow for measurement of abdominal muscle activation. Nontraditional abdominal exercises may include the use of devices such as abdominal straps, a power wheel, and/or other marketed exercise equipment/programs for promoting abdominal muscle health and strength.[5] Traditional abdominal exercises may include exercises such as the crunch and bent-knee sit-up,[19,41-43] exercises that do not require equipment for performing, and instead are reliant on an individual's physical

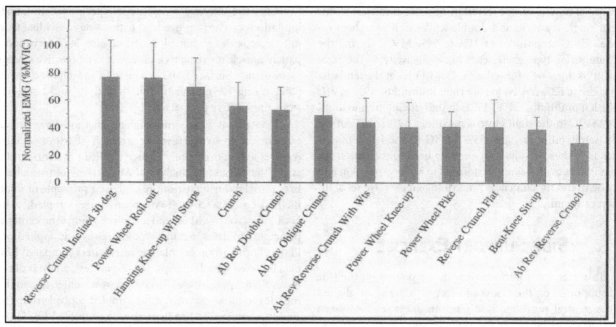

Figure 19-2. Graphical representations of upper and lower rectus abdominis muscle activity (highest to lowest). Upper abdominis.

effort in performing the exercise correctly. Some researchers indicate that traditional forms of abdominal exercises may be problematic for some people with lower back problems.[17-19] These same researchers would advocate the use of nontraditional forms of abdominal exercises for meeting a patient's rehabilitation needs and support this thought with gathered EMG data.[17,18]

In studies comparing the effectiveness of traditional and nontraditional abdominal exercises in activating abdominal and extraneous musculature, surface EMG data gathered by researchers indicated that nontraditional-type exercises were most effective in activating both abdominal and extraneous musculature.[5,6] Surface EMG was used to assess muscle activity from the upper and lower abdominis, external and internal obliques, rectus femoris, latissimus dorsi, and lumbar paraspinal muscles, while both traditional and nontraditional-type exercises were administered.[5] Among exercises tested, the upper rectus abdominis muscle EMG activity was the highest for the power wheel roll-out, hanging knee-up with straps, and reverse crunch inclined 30 degrees and lowest for the Ab-Revolutionizer reverse crunch.[5] EMG data expressing activity in the lower rectus abdominis area were highest for the power wheel roll-out and hanging knee-up with straps and lowest for the Ab-Revolutionizer reverse crunch.[5] Upper and lower rectus abdominis muscle data activity is represented in graphical terms in Figures 19-2 and 19-3 and are ranked from highest to lowest among all exercises. Researchers concluded that nontraditional-type exercises were most effective in activating both abdominal and extraneous muscle groups and that clinicians should consider the data and implications for patient rehabilitation.[5,6] Description of the top 3 exercises demonstrating highest muscle activity, as indicated from EMG data, is offered for increasing the clinician's knowledge on proper technique required for prescribing these highly effective nontraditional types of exercise.

Power Wheel Roll-Out Exercise

A highly effective exercise for activating the upper and lower rectus abdominis and external and internal obliques is the power wheel roll-out. Roll-outs begin from the kneeling position and require the individual performing the exercise to squeeze the abdominals (stomach muscles), which produces a slight posterior pelvic tilt and prevents the abdominal wall from being overly stretched during the exercise. This is important because the power wheel roll-out is an anti-extension core stability exercise that strengthens the spine's ability to resist hyperextension. Individuals performing this exercise for the first time should begin with 3 sets of 3 repetitions and gradually increase sets and repetitions as muscle strength increases.[5]

Hanging Knee-Up With Straps Exercise

Using hanging ab-straps or wrist straps, individuals are required to hang from a bar. Hanging is key because it allows your midsection to fully extend so that contraction of the rectus abdominis, obliquus abdominis, and transversus abdominis can occur. Hanging from a bar without relying on gripping a bar with your hands means you can hang much longer. Once an individual is hanging from a bar and the midsection is fully extended, the individual should exhale and squeeze their abdominal muscles while at the same time lifting both bended knees upward until the knees are 90 degrees with the midsection, pausing at the top to control momentum and then inhaling as the knees are brought back down slowly to the starting position. The hips should remain fixed and motionless as the individual's legs are in motion. Effectiveness of this exercise requires slow and steady movement for avoiding swinging of the body and touching of the feet to the ground in between repetitions.[5]

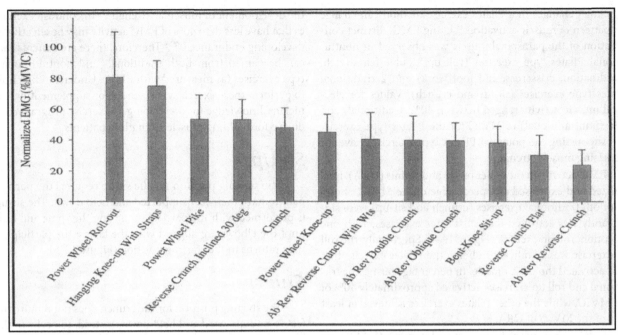

Figure 19-3. Graphical representations of upper and lower rectus abdominis muscle activity (highest to lowest). Lower abdominis.

Reverse Crunch Inclined Thirty Degrees Exercise

The reverse crunch incline is performed on the floor or lying on a flat bench and is performed on an incline of 30 degrees. The individual should orient their body so their head and shoulders are on the higher portion of the inclined source, making the move more effective in working the upper and lower parts of the rectus abdominus, internal obliques, and latissimus dorsi. With hips and knees flexed 90 degrees and the arms positioned either to the side or gripping some form of overhead support, the individual should maximally flex the hips, resulting in 125 to 135 degrees of hip and knee flexion and a posteriorly tilted pelvis. Slow and steady repetitions are recommended by the researcher.[5]

PILATES ABDOMINAL EXERCISES

In a more recent study, researchers compared EMG data when comparing dynamic Pilates abdominal exercises (roll up, double leg stretch, coordination, crisscross, and foot work), against EMG findings of traditional abdominal exercises (sit-up and crunch).[44] Results from the study indicated that Pilates-type exercises promoted greater muscle activation than traditional exercises, mainly in the upper rectus abdominis.[44] Researchers concluded that the nontraditional type of exercises, such as those used in a Pilates exercise program, may have the potential to be prescribed in muscle strengthening programs.[44]

Small changes in a Pilates exercise method can change the pattern of muscle activation.[45] Using EMG, distinct contribution of the paraspinal muscle was observed in nontraditional Pilates-type exercises (roll up, double leg stretch, coordination, crisscross, and foot work) and 2 traditional Pilates-type exercises (sit-up and crunch). Values for electrical muscle activity ranged between 40% (traditional) and 70% (nontraditional) of MVIC for the Pilates-type exercises,[44] supporting the potential Pilates-type exercises have for increasing muscle strength.

EMG activity in the upper rectus abdominis (URA), normalized and expressed as a percentage of the MVIC, shows that both traditional exercises (crunch and sit-up) were significantly less activated than all Pilates exercises, with one exception, roll up exercise (Figure 19-4). Specifically, the roll up exercise was significant in being the Pilates exercise that least activated the URA muscle. In percentage terms, the traditional and roll up exercises activated approximately 40% of the MVIC, while the other Pilates exercises achieved at least 70% of the MVIC of URA.

EMG activity of the lower rectus abdominis (LRA), normalized and expressed as a percentage of the MVIC, showed that only the Pilates exercise crisscross showed significantly greater EMG activity compared to traditional exercises (see Figure 19-4). In the case of the LRA, the EMG activity of the other Pilates exercises was considered similar to the findings of the EMG traditional exercises. In addition, a statistical difference in the percentage of myoelectric activation was observed between the Pilates exercises roll up and crisscross.

In contrast to this study, researchers compared the electrical activity of the abdominal muscles (rectus abdominis and external oblique) during the Pilates exercise roll up with a Swiss ball and elastic band with traditional crunch during the concentric and eccentric phases.[45] Findings showed that the traditional exercise had higher electrical activation of the rectus abdominis than both Pilates exercises.[45] Comparison of study information showed that the roll up and crunch exercises had similar values of the electrical activation (40% of the MVIC, respectively) and showed, together with the sit-up, the least activation.[44] Researchers considered that the lower activation of crunch, sit-up, and roll up exercises was due to 2 main reasons: (1) the maintenance of the lower limbs resting on the ground stabilizes the spine and reduces the demand on the rectus abdominis muscle and (2) the occurrence of one trunk flexion near or above 45 degrees, in the case of the sit-up and roll up exercises. The latter decreases the activation of the rectus abdominis.[44]

In sum, the traditional and the roll up exercises (in percentage terms) activated approximately 40% of the MVIC, whereas the other Pilates exercises achieved at least 70% of the MVIC of URA.[45] Researchers indicated that exercises that have EMG activity higher than 60% of MVIC are considered of high muscle activation and may be more appropriate to the development of muscular strength.[16] In contrast, exercises that have less than 40% of EMG activity may be effective in developing endurance.[8,27,28] Therefore, there are benefits that can be gained from both traditional- and nontraditional-type exercises (as measured with EMG). Understanding how to perform these exercises is essential for supplementing clinicians' knowledge for prescribing an exercise program conducive for building muscle strength in patients.

Sit-Up

The starting position for the sit-up requires the participant to have their feet supported and held down. The sit-up is performed with the participant flexing the spine and hips until the elbows are aligned with the knees; the participant then returns to the starting position (Figure 19-5).

Crunch

The starting position for the crunch does not require the feet to be supported and held down. Instead, to perform the crunch, the participant flexes the spine without hip flexion until both scapulae are off the ground; the participant then returns to the starting position (see Figure 19-5).

Roll Up Exercise

The roll up is performed in a supine position keeping the lower limbs extended, arms internally rotated and flexed overhead at approximately 180 degrees. The participant flexes the spine approximately 90 degrees off the ground and then returns to the starting position (Figure 19-6).

Double Leg Stretch Exercise

The double leg stretch starts in a supine position with a slight neck flexion and flexion of the hips and knees sustained by the hands, returning to extension of upper and lower limbs without touching the ground (see Figure 19-6).

Crisscross

The crisscross starts in a supine position with a slight neck flexion sustained by the hands without contact with the ground, as well as slight hip flexion with knee extended associated with the highest hip abduction. In this exercise, both knees move to touch the opposite elbow during a slight flexion and rotation of the spine (see Figure 19-6).

Coordination Exercise

The coordination exercise is performed similarly to the crisscross except that both lower limbs cross the midline alternately while the right lower limb is superior to the left lower limb. At no time do the feet touch the ground (see Figure 19-6).

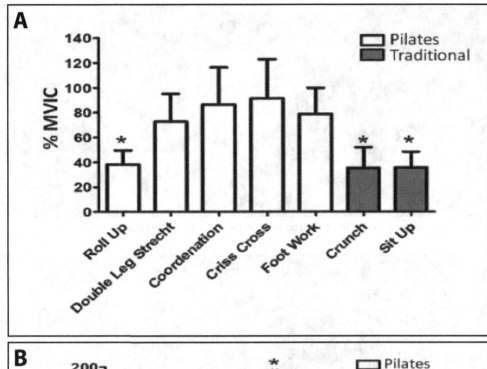

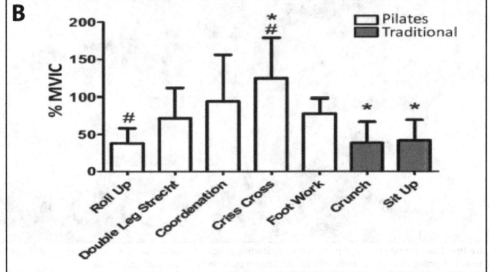

Figure 19-4. Graphical representation of EMG on certain Pilates traditional and nontraditional exercises. (A) Percentage of the MVIC for URA during Pilates and traditional exercises. * Indicates $P < .05$ when compared with other exercises. (B) Percentage of MVIC contraction for LRA during Pilates and traditional exercises. * Indicates the location of statistical differences between Pilates and traditional exercises ($P < .05$). # Indicates the location of statistical differences between the Pilates exercises ($P < .05$).

Footwork Exercise

The footwork exercise is performed starting in the same position as the double leg stretch exercise. The participant then extends both knees with a slight hip flexion and alternately extends the hip until the foot is almost touching the ground. At no time do the feet touch the ground (see Figure 19-6).

It has been indicated that the rectus abdominis muscle is the major flexor of the trunk or torso compared with other muscles in the abdominal wall and plays a significant role in spine stability.[9,10,45] In this sense, it is critical to understand which abdominal muscles are recruited and how active they are while performing a variety of nontraditional and traditional abdominal exercises. Understanding can be helpful for clinicians and other health professionals in developing and prescribing specific abdominal exercises for patients and for facilitating patient rehabilitation.

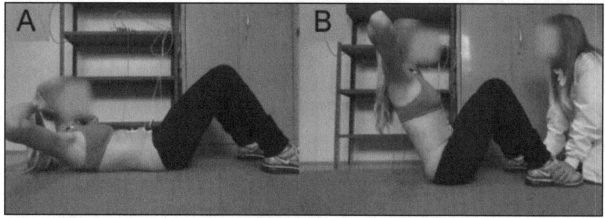

Figure 19-5. Pilates traditional-type exercises. (A) Starting position for the crunch. (B) Starting position for the sit-up.

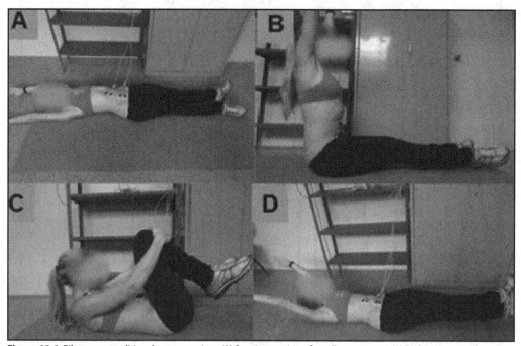

Figure 19-6. Pilates nontraditional-type exercises. (A) Starting position for roll up exercise. (B) Ending position for roll up exercise. (C) Starting position for double stretch. (D) Ending position for double stretch. *(continued)*

TRUNK MUSCLE ELECTROMYOGRAPHIC ACTIVITY WITH UNSTABLE AND UNILATERAL EXERCISES

Strengthening of the core muscles assist in stabilizing the spine.[46,47] Exercise devices have been developed that attempt to activate trunk-stabilizing muscles.[23,46] The objective of these exercise devices is to offer individuals unstable resistance training, which has been shown to increase core muscle activation.[46]

Using surface EMG, 2 types of exercise devices were tested for determining the degree of muscle activation. The Bodyblade,[48] a double-oscillating device (DOD) and Thera-Band's Flexbar, a single-oscillating device (SOD).[49] SOD and DOD exercise equipment are used to induce vibratory stimuli, which coactivates surrounding shoulder and core muscles with the aim of improving muscle strength and endurance.[46]

Bodyblade Exercise Device

Invented by Bruce Hymanson, in 1991, Bodyblade is a flexible blade ranging from 2.5 to 5 feet in length and weighs 1.5 pounds, with a handgrip in the center. The device is engaged either in the sagittal, frontal, or transverse plane and is held at the center. As the user moves the device away and toward their body in an alternating and repetitive sequence, the 2 ends begin to oscillate at a fixed rate with a

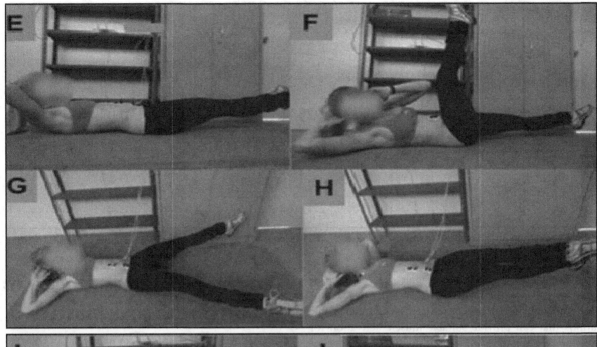

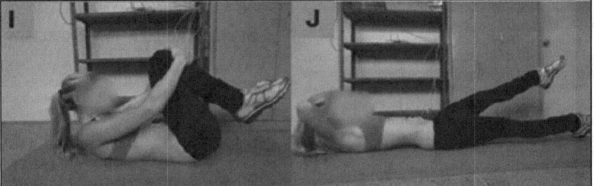

Figure 19-6 (continued). (E) Starting position for crisscross. (F) Ending position for crisscross. (G) Starting position for coordination. (H) Ending position for coordination. (I) Starting position for foot work. (J) Ending position for foot work.

frequency of 4.5 Hertz (Hz).[48] Device oscillation challenges the muscles to keep the joints stable; the more intensely the individual oscillates the device, the greater the resistance must develop within the muscles in response to the DOD's acceleration.[48] This DOD uses inertia to ensure continuous movement of the DOD.[46] Health professionals use DODs to address elements of recovery: power, coordination, endurance, strength, intensity, and stabilization for both patients, athletes, and general populations.[46]

TheraBand Flexbar

TheraBand Flexbar is an SOD that provides muscle resistance, weighs about 0.59 kg, and is 0.3 m in length with a ribbed surface to ensure adequate grasp.[49] The device is used for upper extremity stabilization and to augment grip strength by performing bending, twisting, or oscillating movements.[49] The TheraBand Flexbar provides a variety of resistance levels to match the individual's competency level.[46,49]

Bodyblade Versus TheraBand Flexbar Devices

Researchers compared the EMG data between the Bodyblade (DOD) and TheraBand Flexbar (SOD) exercise devices and determined more benefit was gained in the use of a DOD type of exercise device over that of an SOD type exercise device.[46] Results showed that DOD provided 35.9%, 40.8%, and 52.3% greater anterior deltoid, transverse abdominus/internal oblique, and lumbosacral erector spinae (LSES) activation than that of the SOD. A significant effect for devices showed overall (mean of all muscles), relative (normalized to MVIC) muscle activation for the DOD (58.03% ± 41.53) was 13.4% greater than the SOD (44.6% ± 29.01); the DOD provided 35.9% greater anterior deltoid activation than did the SOD (Figure 19-7).

DOD is an effective tool for the activation of muscles (supported by EMG) incorporated during training and or rehabilitation of the shoulder as compared to traditional means such as weight cuffs and TheraBands.[49,50] Instability

Muscle	DOD	SOD	Effect size	p value
Anterior deltoid	76.99% ± 32.04	49.29% ±17.98	0.86	0.000
Triceps brachii	46.65% ±20.21	43.50% ±14.82	0.16	0.456
Biceps brachii	46.65% ± 28.76	47.13% ±23.73	0.02	0.939
Forearm flexor muscle group	57.88% ±30.31	61.3% ±28.49	0.12	0.625
TA/IO	79.41% ±67.06	47.02% ±43.50	0.48	0.16
LSES	40.57% ± 34.97	19.36% ±17.78	0.61	0.06

Figure 19-7. Effects for DOD and SOD exercise device (Bodyblade vs Thera-Band flexbar).

offered from oscillating or from unstable devices, such as the Bodyblade,[48] provide relatively lower resistive loads or torques compared to the resistance achieved under stable conditions that can provide suitable muscle activation for training or rehabilitation in some individuals.[46,50] In contrast, the unilateral nature of the SOD, namely the Flexbar, was less effective (measured by EMG) for activating transverse abdominis/internal oblique and LSES muscles and thus reduced efficiency for improving the stability of a person's core.[46,49] However, higher activation of the internal oblique has been noted in previous studies using multiple handgrips in performing SOD exercises,[51,52] which may indicate the type of grip used (ie, single/double handed, narrow or wide), could lend to increasing internal oblique muscle activation.

One researcher reported that a wide handgrip position produces a greater latissimus dorsi muscle activation than other handgrip positions.[53] In contrast, researchers indicated that a double-handed grip may provide greater absorption of oscillation by the upper limb musculature,[46] whereas other researchers found that a single-handed grip causes an increase in the oscillation of blades of the SOD and consequently results in absorption to a greater extent by the trunk rather than the limbs.[54] Therefore, variations in handgrips have been shown to promote certain muscle activation processes. Finally, the unilateral nature of the SOD may have led to greater torque asymmetries for promoting greater trunk activation,[46] but it reduces the possibility of strengthening shoulder muscles.[50] Researchers concluded that DOD used in a transverse plane tends to be more effective for activating the trunk and shoulder muscles, while the SOD used in a frontal plane is as effective as a DOD exercise for the arm muscles.[46]

As indicated, strengthening of the core (trunk) muscles assists in stabilizing the spine.[46,47] Although no formal definition of stabilization exercises exists,[55] the approach is aimed at improving the neuromuscular control, strength, and endurance of the muscles that are central to maintaining the dynamic spinal and trunk stability. Therefore, further examination of selected exercises for targeting muscles during dynamic spine stabilization exercises is required.

ELECTROMYOGRAPHIC ACTIVITY OF SELECTED TRUNK MUSCLES DURING DYNAMIC SPINE STABILIZATION EXERCISES

Instability of the lumbar motion segment is considered to be an important cause of CLBP.[21,56] All muscles that traverse the lumbar region are capable of contributing to the stabilization and protection of the lumbar spine.[56] Studies suggest that transversus abdominis muscles and the lumbar multifidus muscles are particularly important for lumbar segmental stability and for control of motion in the trunk.[21,57]

There are several types of trunk stability exercises that have been discussed, specifically Pilates exercises, Swiss ball programs, and floor exercises. These exercise types aim to restore the strength and endurance of the trunk muscles for meeting the demands of lumbopelvic control.[56] However, some researchers claim there is a deficit of stabilization muscles, and incorrect compensation of their activity takes place from the movement muscles if traditional exercise techniques are used in rehabilitation,[7,13-15] and thus, increasing the risk of spinal injury and/or re-injury. Researchers suggest that instead of using a traditional exercise approach, focus should be on specific training of local system muscles, namely transverses abdominis muscles, diaphragm, and multifidus muscles, whose primary role is to be the provisionary source of dynamic stability and segmental control to the spine.[56] Applying principles of motor learning and skill acquisition can assist in this approach.

The purpose of motor learning and skill acquisition is to train the skilled activation of deep muscles and to train the integration of the deep and superficial systems through a dynamic exercise program that varies in environments and contexts to ensure transfer to normal muscle activity.[56] Motor learning occurs in 3 main phases: cognitive, associative, and autonomous.[56] The goal in the cognitive phase of motor learning for CLBP is to contract the deep muscles in a controlled manner by consciously paying attention to the step-by-step execution of the movements. This increases the precision and skill of the contraction of the local muscles. The associative phase involves the isometric cocontraction of the deep abdominal muscles and multifidus muscles. This should be obtained with minimal co-activation of global system muscles. The contraction of the pelvic floor muscles will help to inhibit global muscle substitution.[56] It is critical to provide accurate feedback of contraction quality—this involves either visual (ultrasound imaging) or auditory (EMG) information. Once mastered, intervention shifts to dynamic means for increasing strength and endurance, either by increasing precision, number of repetitions, or holding time. This phase involves performance of the task in increasingly challenging positions, such as using leg-loading tasks or postural challenges[56]; dynamic tasks combined with basic exercise techniques increase muscle strength and endurance.[55] The final stage, the autonomous phase, is achieved after considerable practice and experience. The task becomes habitual or automatic, and the requirement for conscious intervention is reduced.[56]

In a study examining US ballet dancers, researchers explored the effects of training methods using home exercises and a dynamic sling system on core strength, disability, and low back pain.[21] The study did not involve EMG data collection. Instead, conclusions drawn from the study were supported by both subjective and descriptive data. However, data gained from the study support previous studies findings on the importance of strengthening core muscles for increasing spine stability.[21,57] Strong muscles around the trunk, pelvic girdle, and hips are important in the training of ballet students as they form the foundation for the balance, stability, and muscle coordination required to perform basic movements.[21] Regular exercise in addition to dynamic type core stability exercises increases muscle activation and promotes spine stabilization.[57]

Dynamic strengthening exercises consist of added movements (ie, side-to-side movements, jumping, arm swinging, weight loading) to traditional or nontraditional-type exercise activities.[55] An example of this is a study involving 26 healthy adults (13 men and 13 women). Using EMG, effects in selected trunk muscles (normalized by percentage MVIC) was recorded from the rectus abdominis, internal oblique, erector spinae, and multifidus muscles of the dominant side, while the participants performed 3 types of bridging exercises, including bridging alone (bridging 1), bridging with unilateral hip movements (bridging 2), and bridging with bilateral hip movements (bridging 3) in a sling suspension system.[58] The rectus abdominis and internal oblique showed greater EMG activity during bridging 2 and 3 compared to bridging 1, with the greatest internal oblique activity during bridging 3, and the activity of the multifidus appeared to be greater during bridging 3 than during bridging 1 and 2.[58] Researchers further discovered, the internal oblique/ rectus abdominis and multifidus/erector spinae ratios were

significantly higher for bridging 2 (internal/rectus abdominis, 1.89 _ 1.41; multifidus/erector spinae, 1.03 _ 0.19) and bridging 3 (internal oblique/rectus abdominis, 2.34 _ 1.86; multifidus/erector spinae, 1.03 _ 0.15) than bridging 1 (internal oblique/rectus abdominis, 1.35 _ 0.92; multifidus/erector spinae, 0.98 _ 0.16).[58] The internal oblique/rectus abdominis ratio was significantly higher for bridging 3 than for bridging 2. Researchers concluded that adding hip abduction and adduction, particularly bilateral movements, could be a useful method to enhance internal oblique and multifidus EMG activity and their activities relative to global muscles during bridging exercise.[58]

In another study involving 20 healthy young men, an experimental procedure was performed with 2 options: (1) an intervention factor (with and without arm movement) and (2) a bridging factor (on the floor and on a therapeutic ball), during a bridging exercise. EMG data were collected for the rectus abdominis, internal oblique, erector spinae, and multifidus muscles of the dominant side. The researchers' findings showed significant main effects for the intervention factor in the internal oblique and erector spinae and for the bridging factor in the internal oblique.[59] The rectus abdominis and internal oblique showed significant interaction between the intervention and bridge factors. Researchers further found that internal oblique/rectus abdominis ratio during bridging on the floor (without arm movement, 2.05 ± 2.61; with arm movement, 3.24 ± 3.42) and bridging on the ball (without arm movement: 2.95 ± 3.87; with arm movement: 5.77 ± 4.85) showed significant main effects for and significant interaction between the intervention and bridge factors.[59] However, no significant main effects or interaction were found for the multifidus/erector spinae ratio. The researchers concluded from their findings that integrating arm movements (namely, shoulder and elbow) during bridge exercises may be used to provide preferential loading to certain trunk muscle groups and that these effects may be better derived by performing bridge exercises on a therapeutic ball.[59] Implications of this study may contribute to clinicians' prescription of exercise programs that incorporate arm movements, for recruiting certain muscle activity conducive for strengthening, and stabilizing the spine in some patients.

Finally, in a study involving 18 healthy participants (no history of lumbar or trunk muscle problems), assessment of the trunk and leg muscle activities during the trunk tilt exercise was conducted applying a rotation capability. The experiment involved investigation of the anterior, right, posterior, left, anterior right, anterior left, posterior right, and posterior left tilt directions. The trunk tilt device applies forces on the trunk by tilting the whole body from a neutral upright position (Figure 19-8). Participants were fixed at their feet and hips, but the trunk remained unsupported. During the different tilt positions, the participant had to simply stabilize their upper body in the body axis. For this study, participants held their arms crossed against their chests. Exact body and arm positioning throughout the whole study was controlled

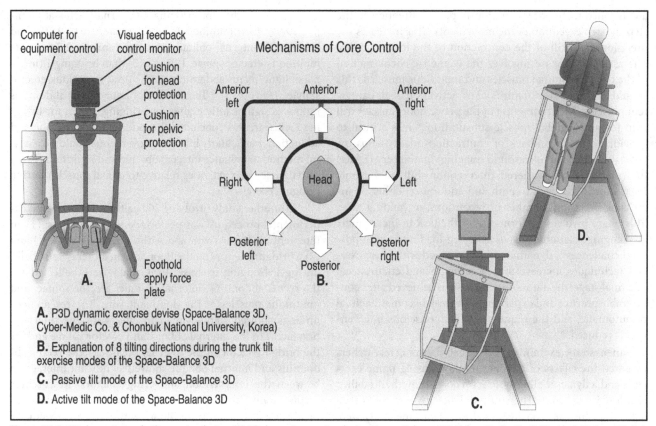

Figure 19-8. 3D dynamic trunk-tilt exercise device. (A) 3D dynamic exercise device (Space-Balance 3D, Cyber-Medic Co. & Chonbuk National Univ.). (B) Explanation of 8 tilting directions during the trunk tilt exercise modes of the Space-Balance 3D. (C) Passive tilt mode of the Space-Balance 3D. (D) Active tilt mode of the Space-Balance 3D.

by the examiner. This 3-dimensional (3D) dynamic equipment was capable of moving 100 degrees in the anterior-posterior direction, 180 degrees in the left-right direction, 100 degrees in the anterior right-posterior left direction, and 100 degrees in the anterior left-posterior right direction because it could be rotated in 3D space.

EMG signals of trunk (rectus abdominis, external oblique, latissimus dorsi, erector spinae) muscles were examined, and RMS values were calculated in both the left and right direction (Figure 19-9). First, findings showed muscle activity in the left rectus abdominis maintaining the active tilt mode in the posterior and posterior left directions being higher than that in the passive tilt mode, and in the case of the right rectus abdominis muscle activity, the active tilt mode in the posterior and posterior right directions were significantly higher.[60] Rectus abdominis muscle activities during the active and passive tilt modes demonstrated significantly higher RMS values in the anterior direction, regardless of whether the muscle was in the active or passive mode (see Figure 19-9). Second, findings showed muscle activity in the left external oblique maintaining the passive tilt mode in the anterior right and anterior left directions being significantly higher, whereas in the case of the right external

oblique muscle activity, the active tilt mode in the posterior left direction resulted in significantly higher values.[60] In terms of external oblique muscle activity in both the active and passive tilt modes by direction, tilting in the posterior right and right directions resulted in higher values of muscle activity than tilting in the posterior left and left directions in the case of the left muscle.[60] In contrast, in the case of the right muscle, the opposite tendency was observed: tilting in the posterior left and left directions caused much higher values than tilting in the posterior right and right directions (see Figure 19-9). Third, according to RMS values of the left and right latissimus dorsi muscle activities in the passive tilt mode showed higher values in all directions except for the anterior and posterior left directions in the case of the left latissimus dorsi.[60] Muscle activity in the passive tilt mode were higher in the posterior, left, and anterior left directions in the case of the right latissimus dorsi. In contrast, there were no significant differences in the muscle activities in different directions (see Figure 19-9).[60] Finally, findings showed no significant muscle activity in the left erector spinae in either the active or passive tilt mode.[60] However, muscle activity in the right erector spinae showed significant activity in the passive and active tilt mode in the anterior direction.[60]

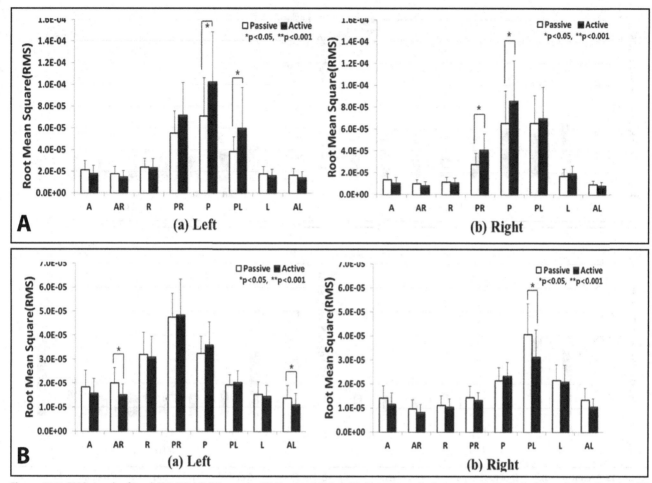

Figure 19-9. EMG signals of trunk (RA, EO, LD, ES) muscles (RMS values). Using 3D-dynamic trunk-tilt exercise device in the left and right direction. (A) RA of RMS in passive and active tilt training in 8 directions. (B) EO of RMS in passive and active tilt training in 8 directions. *(continued)*

Overall, the results of this study indicated that different exercise patterns can be applied depending on the exercise types, which are appropriate and necessary to each user.[60] The researchers believe that the body can be maintained in equilibrium through the interaction between the position and movement execution of the body, which contributes to the improvement of body stabilization.[60] Furthermore, researchers determined that different dynamic exercise patterns can be applied depending on exercise types (traditional or nontraditional) for increasing core strength and spinal stability.

Introduction of dynamic strengthening exercises consisting of added movements to both traditional and nontraditional-type exercises results in trunk muscle activation. Therefore, the researcher believes that having a basic understanding of exercises for increasing trunk muscle strength may allow for adaptation of movements for increasing strength and spinal stability. Analysis of core trunk and hip exercises may provide health professionals fundamental understanding for building an exercise program that may later require adapting dynamic exercise movements for increasing muscle strength and decreasing rehabilitation time for individuals suffering from CLBP or other forms of chronic muscle pain.

ELECTROMYOGRAPHIC ANALYSIS OF THE SHOULDER, HIP, AND KNEE DURING CERTAIN SPORT ACTIVITY

Speed, power, and strength of the knee and hip extensors are vital for success in sports.[61] Steps toward prevention of serious sports injuries like anterior cruciate ligament and CLBP injures require an understanding of training and exercise techniques necessary for reducing incidence.[62] Therefore, examining studies related to sports activities and prevention of injuries is necessary for understanding appropriate exercise programs and the techniques associated with them for decreasing injury.

Muscle activity of leg and trunk muscles in isometric squats executed on stable and/or unstable surfaces may result in increasing muscle activity.[61] Differences in surfaces require specific requirements for promoting muscle activity. For example, increasing the instability of the surface during maximum effort isometric exercise activities may result in muscle activity of the lower limb and superficial trunk muscles.[61]

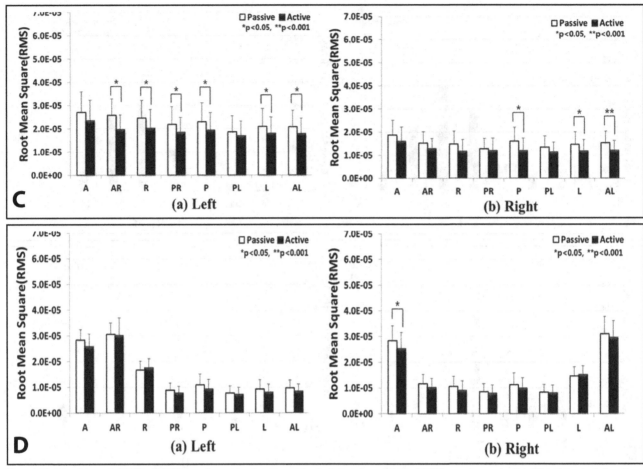

Figure 19-9 (continued). (C) LD of RMS in passive and active tilt training in 8 directions. (D) ES of RMS in passive and active tilt training in 8 directions.

Isometric Squat Exercise

The isometric squat is performed from the standing position, with the participant standing as tall as possible with their feet shoulder-width apart (Figure 19-10). The participant should have their toes pointing forward and push the hips back, bending at the knees and lowering the body until the upper thighs are parallel to the floor or as low as the participant feels comfortable in performing the exercise.

In a study involving 15 healthy men, force output and EMG activities of the rectus femoris, vastus medialis, vastus lateralis, biceps femoris, soleus, rectus abdominis, external oblique, and erector spinae were assessed under conditions of randomized ordering of surfaces. Activity of the leg and trunk muscles in isometric squats executed on stable surfaces (floor), power board, BOSU ball, and balance cone were the surfaces used in this study. Compared with stable surface (749 ± 222 N), the force output using a power board was similar (-7%) but lower for the BOSU ball (-19%) and balance cone (-24%).[61] The force output using the BOSU ball and balance cone was approximately 13% and approximately 18% less than the power board.[61] There were similar EMG activities between the surfaces in all muscles except for rectus femoris, where stable squat provided greater EMG activity than did the other exercises.[61] Lower EMG activity was observed in the rectus femoris using the balance cone compared with the BOSU ball,[61] suggesting that unstable surfaces in isometric squats may be beneficial in rehabilitation and/or increasing the strength and endurance of athletes.[61]

In contrast, researchers determined that there is no discernible benefit of performing the isometric squat in an unstable condition.[63] Assessing the effect of stable vs unstable conditions on force output and muscle activity during an isometric squat, EMG activity during both conditions from the vastus lateralis, vastus medialis, biceps femoris, and medial gastrocnemius muscles were analyzed. Results indicated peak force and rate of force development (RFD) were significantly lower, 45.6% and 40.5% MVIC, in the unstable vs stable condition.[63] Average EMG values for the vastus lateralis and medialis were significantly higher in the stable vs unstable condition.[63] Vastus lateralis and medialis muscle activity was 37.3% and 34.4% less in unstable in comparison to stable conditions.[63] No significant differences were observed in muscle activity of the biceps femoris or gastrocnemius between unstable and stable conditions.[63] In an unstable condition, while performing an isometric squat, significant reduction of peak force, RFD, and agonist muscle activity was concluded from EMG.

Bodyblade Versus Dumbbell Use for Increasing Shoulder Muscle Activation

The shoulder works as a link in the kinetic chain of joint motions and muscle activations to produce optimum athletic function.[64] Throwing objects requires the use of the shoulder muscles. Muscles that are typically associated with the core allow for the transference of torques and angular momentum during the performance-type activities, such as throwing objects.[7]

Shoulder injuries commonly occur in athletics, particularly in sports that involve overhead arm motions (eg, baseball, softball, swimming, tennis).[65] Shoulder-strengthening programs are effective not only in restoring function but also in reducing pain, preventing injury, and improving athletic performance.[65] Therefore, shoulder-strengthening programs are critical in restoring normal function following upper extremity injuries.[65]

Using EMG in the back and shoulder regions, researchers determined that Bodyblade produced greater muscle activity than dumbbell trials.[65] Discussion of the Bodyblade exercise device has already been discussed in this chapter. For this study, EMG activity for the Bodyblade exceeded 50% of the MVIC during both shoulder flexion and abduction.[65] The greatest EMG activity with use of the Bodyblade, relative to MVIC, was recorded in the serratus and infraspinatus. Muscles are responsible for stabilizing the scapula and for facilitating humeral motion by providing a stable base for the prime muscle groups of the humerus (ie, the rotator cuff, deltoid, and long head of the biceps brachii), which offer dynamic stability to the glenohumeral joint.[65] In contrast, for the dumbbell conditions, only the 10-pound trials approached the same effect achieved by the Bodyblade.[65] The implication of this study can offer athletes involved in shoulder intensive usage-type sports a means for training properly and for reducing chance of injury.

Integrating Select Trunk, Shoulder, Hip, and Knee Exercises

In a study for evaluating the level of medial (biceps femoris) and lateral hamstring (semitendinosus) muscle activation during selected exercises, researchers determined that kettlebell swing and Romanian deadlift targeted specifically semitendinosus over biceps femoris[62] with EMG recording very high levels (73%±115% MVIC). In contrast, the supine leg curl and hip extension exercise, specifically targeted the biceps femoris over the semitendinosus, as measured using EMG (75%±87% MVIC).[62] Overall, researchers determined that specific therapeutic exercises for targeting the

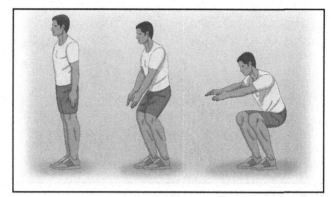

Figure 19-10. Performing the isometric squat.

hamstring can be divided into semitendinosus dominant or biceps femoris dominant hamstring exercises—due to distinct functions of the medial and lateral hamstring muscles.[62] Understanding how these exercises are performed may be critical for use in exercise programs conducive for increasing athletes' muscle strength and endurance and/or for designing a rehabilitation program.

Kettlebell Swing

In performing a kettlebell swing, the participant begins the exercise from a squatting position, with the kettlebell centered in the middle of the feet (Figure 19-11). Grasping hold of the kettlebell and keeping the heels flat, shins vertical, and weight loaded mostly in the heels, the bell should be lifted approximately 5 to 6 inches from the floor. Begin the exercise by driving the hips forward forcefully, making the kettlebell float to the shoulder height. Form a plank with the body at the top of the swing. This will require bracing the abs and creating a straight line from head to heel. Repeat the exercise motion.

Romanian Deadlift

In performing the Romanian deadlift, a participant will hold a bar at hip level with palms facing down grip. The participant's shoulders should be back, the back should be arched, and the knees slightly bent—this is the starting position (Figure 19-12). The participant will lower the bar by moving their butt back as far as possible, while keeping the bar close to the body. The participant's head is looking forward and the shoulders are back. When done correctly, the participant should reach the maximum range of their hamstring flexibility just below the knee. Any further movement will be compensation and should be avoided in the movement. Finally, at the bottom of the participant's range of motion (ROM), the participant returns to the starting position by driving the hips forward to stand up tall.

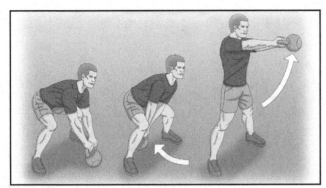

Figure 19-11. Performing the kettlebell exercise.

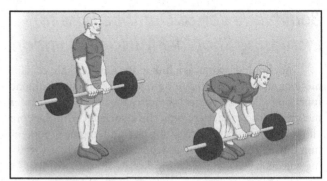

Figure 19-12. Performing the Romanian deadlift exercise.

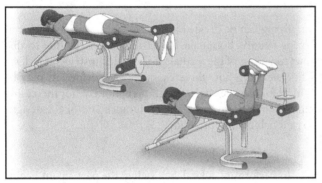

Figure 19-13. Performing the supine leg curl exercise.

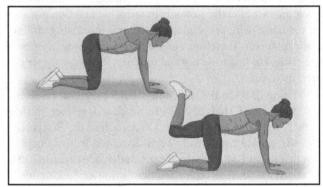

Figure 19-14. Performing the hip extension.

Supine Leg Curl Exercise

In performing this exercise, the participant will require use of a leg curl machine (Figure 19-13). The participant will lie face down on the bench with the knees extending just over the edge of the bench (see Figure 19-13). The participant should adjust the machine so that the padding is on the lower part of the calf muscles. Gripping the machine's handles, the participant will begin the exercise by bending their legs at the knee to bring the padding to touch the back of their legs. The participant will return the weight back to the starting position by using a controlled movement. While performing the exercise, the participant should avoid arching their back.

Hip Extension Exercise

The hip extension exercise can be performed from 2 different positions (standing or kneeling) and may involve the use of stable supporting devices (eg, floor, wall, countertop, chair). From the kneeling position, the participant must kneel on all fours with the hands directly under the shoulders and the knees directly under the hips (Figure 19-14). While maintaining a flat back, extend the right leg until a straight line from the head to the right foot is achieved. The participant will hold this position for 1 second and then return to all fours. The participant will repeat this process with the left leg and continue the process alternating between the right and left leg.

ELECTROMYOGRAPHIC ANALYSIS OF CORE TRUNK AND HIP DURING NINE REHABILITATION EXERCISES

It has been clear that active rehabilitation is essential in the effective long-term resolution of muscle pain. Expanding on this understanding requires interventions from self-stretching targeted muscles, self-mobilization of the joints, muscle activation, core stability, and strength training.[33] Therefore, a logical sequence of rehabilitation is required that allows for clinicians and patients to understand better where they may be in the rehabilitative process and what path they can follow to return to full function. This begins with understanding fundamental exercise routines for increasing muscle strength. The importance of specific trunk, hip, and thigh muscle strengthening and endurance/stabilization exercises is essential in the prevention of injuries.[7,13,15] Weakness and poor endurance of the lumbar extensor, gluteus maximus, and hip external rotator muscles make these muscle groups an important focus requiring attention for individuals suffering with lower extremity injuries and low back pain.[25]

Rehabilitation or performance enhancement training should be regarded on the principle that specific demands on the musculoskeletal system will produce specific adaptations within the system.[25] Exercises designed to increase strength or endurance should target specific muscle groups that are weak or may be important to the activities of athletes

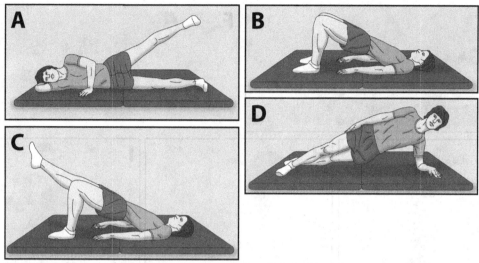

Figure 19-15. Different rehabilitation and training exercises. (A) Active hip abduction in the side-lying position with neutral hip rotation. (B) Bridge exercise to the neutral spine alignment position. (C) Unilateral bridge exercise with one knee extended and the opposite hip extended so that the trunk is in neutral spine alignment. (D) Side bridge exercise with the trunk in neutral spine alignment. (Reprinted with permission from Ekstrom RA, Donatelli RA, Carp KC. Electromyographic analysis of core trunk, hip, and thigh muscles during 9 rehabilitation exercises. *J Orthop Sports Phys Ther.* 2007;37:754-762. https://doi.org/10.2519/jospt.2007.2471. ©*Journal of Orthopaedic & Sports Physical Therapy*®) *(continued)*

and or persons requiring muscle rehabilitation therapy.[7,13-15] Physical therapists should be able to develop a specific exercise program to target Identified muscle impairments. EMG analysis can provide information as to the significant amount of muscular activity an exercise requires to include the optimal positioning for the exercise.

Surface EMG analysis was conducted on 30 participants (19 men and 11 women) in performing 9 exercises. These exercises included the active hip abduction, bridge exercise, unilateral bridge, side bridge, prone bridge on elbows and toes, quadruped arm/lower extremity lift, lateral step-up, standing lunge exercise, and using the dynamic edge (Figure 19-15). The rectus abdominis, external oblique abdominis, longissimus thoracis, lumbar multifidus, gluteus maximus, gluteus medius, vastus medialis obliquus, and hamstring muscles were the focus in this study.

Researchers concluded from EMG analysis that the 9 exercises used for this study could be used for a trunk rehabilitation or performance enhancement program.[25] It should be noted, however, that the conclusion will be based on the individual needs of a patient or athlete, and some exercises may be more beneficial than others for achieving strength.[25]

Hip Abduction Exercise

The active hip abduction exercise is performed in the frontal plane in the side-lying position with neutral hip rotation (see Figure 19-15A). The exercise did not produce significant activation of the core stabilizers, as measured with EMG.[25] However, the exercise was effective in isolating function of the gluteus medius muscle (39% ± 17% MVIC).[25]

In contrast, in a separate study, researchers determined that hip abduction exercise, coupled with bridging exercise, produced greater muscle activation of the abdominal and hip extensor muscles.[66] Results of this study demonstrated that activation of each abdominal and hip extensor muscle (ie, rectus abdominis, external oblique, internal oblique, and gluteus maximus) during bridging exercise and bridging exercise with hip abduction (BEHA) increased with the introduction of the hip abduction exercise as an added exercise coupled with the bridging exercise.[66] EMG signal amplitude (mean ± standard deviation [SD]) showed significant increases during bridging exercise vs BEHA in the rectus abdominis (10.43±9.9% vs 5.59±3.59% MVIC), external oblique (22.11±13.4% vs 11.3±5.06% MVIC), internal oblique (26.97±18.41% vs 7.82±17.63% MVIC), and gluteus medius (26.88±11.04% vs 20.4±8.9% MVIC).

In another study, hip abduction in plank (HAP) with suspension was found to have the strongest potential strengthening effect on core muscles.[67] Muscle activity focusing on 4 trunk muscle groups (rectus abdominis, external oblique, internal oblique/transverse abdominis, and superficial lumbar multifidus [LMF]) was analyzed using EMG during 4 suspension-type exercises (HAP, hamstring curl, chest press, and 45-degree row). EMG signal was significantly different in the 4 trunk muscles during the HAP, hamstring curl, and chest press (20.2%, 10.8%, and 20.3%, respectively).[67] During the HAP, external oblique activation (69.5% [19.3%]) was greater than rectus abdominis and LMF activation. During the hamstring curl, LMF activation (53.6% [27.8%]) was greater than activation of all other abdominal muscles. During the chest press, rectus abdominis

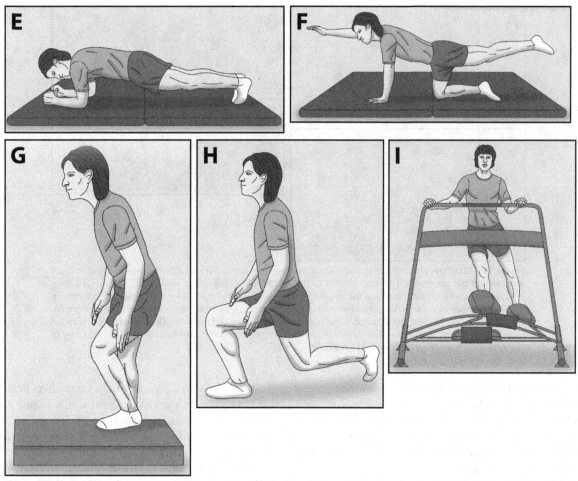

Figure 19-15 (continued). (E) Prone bridge exercise with the trunk in neutral spine alignment. (F) Quadruped arm and lower extremity lift with the trunk in neutral spine alignment. (G) Lateral step-up exercise to a 20.32-cm platform. (H) Standing lunge exercise. (I) Dynamic edge exercise with resistance to side-to-side motions simulating downhill skiing. (Reprinted with permission from Ekstrom RA, Donatelli RA, Carp KC. Electromyographic analysis of core trunk, hip, and thigh muscles during 9 rehabilitation exercises. *J Orthop Sports Phys Ther.* 2007;37:754-762. https://doi.org/10.2519/jospt.2007.2471. ©*Journal of Orthopaedic & Sports Physical Therapy®*)

and external oblique activation were greater than internal oblique and LMF activation, with no difference between rectus abdominis and external oblique activation. There was no significant overall difference in activation of the 4 muscles during the row (20.3%).[67]

Rectus abdominis, external oblique, and internal oblique/transverse abdominis activation was significantly different among the 4 workouts.[67] Rectus abdominis activation during the HAP (39.1 [13.8%]) and chest press (37.3 [21.9%]) was higher than that during the hamstring curl (10.0 [7.5%]) and row (7.9 [5.4%]), but there was no difference between the HAP and chest press or between the hamstring curl and row. External oblique activation was higher during HAP (69.5 [19.4%]) than the chest press (28.6 [19.6%]), hamstring curl (14.7 [10.8%]), or row (10.1 [7.3%]).[67] Internal oblique/transverse abdominis activation was highest during the HAP (61.4 [33.5%]) and lower during the row (18.9 [17.6%]) compared with the chest press (24.8 [13.8%]) and hamstring curl (32.1 [21.0%]).[67] There was no difference in internal oblique/transverse abdominis activation between the chest press and hamstring curl.[67]

EMG data from the studies discussed suggest that the hip abduction exercise alone does not support significant muscle activation,[25] but when introduced in conjunction with other exercise types, significant muscle activation occurs.[66,67]

Bridge Exercise

The bridge exercise is performed in the neutral spine position (see Figure 19-15B). Demonstrating significant EMG values, the longissimus thoracis and LMF showed identical results (mean ± SD; 39% ± 15% MVIC); in conjunction with the external oblique abdominis (22% ± 13% MVIC) muscle group.[25] No significant values were shown for the vastus medialis obliquus (3% ± 3% MVIC). The exercise was effective in isolating function of the gluteus medius muscle (28% ± 17% MVIC).[25] Overall, the correlation between EMG recordings from the muscles during the bridge exercise was at 0.86 (standard error of measurements [SEM], 20.0% MVIC). This indicated that there was good consistency in the EMG recordings.[25]

Unilateral Bridge Exercise

The unilateral bridge exercise is performed in the neutral spine position with the opposite knee extended (see Figure 19-15C). The longissimus thoracis (40%±16% MVIC) and LMF (44%±18% MVIC) demonstrated significant muscle activation in the use of this exercise. In addition, gluteus medius (47%±24% MVIC) and gluteus maximus (40%±20% MVIC) also demonstrated significant muscle activation.[25] In contrast, lesser significance was demonstrated in the vastus medialis obliquus (18%±13% MVIC) and rectus abdominis (14%±13% MVIC) muscle groups.[25] Researchers indicated that to increase abdominal and/or hip extensor muscle activities, using unstable devices, such as a Swiss ball or ball cushion, could be applied in unilateral type exercise conditions.[66]

Side Bridge Exercise

The side bridge exercise is performed with the trunk in neutral spinal alignment (see Figure 19-15D). The gluteus medius (74%±30% MVIC) and gluteus maximus (21%±16% MVIC) demonstrated significant muscle activation in the use of this exercise. In addition, external oblique abdominis (69%±26% MVIC) and rectus abdominis (34%±13% MVIC) also demonstrated significant muscle activation.[25] In contrast, lesser significance was demonstrated in the vastus medialis obliquus (19%±11% MVIC) and hamstring (12%±11% MVIC) muscle groups.[25] Use of nontraditional type of exercise equipment may lend to increasing muscle activation in vastus medialis obliquus and hamstring muscle group when performing this exercise.

Prone Bridge Exercise

The prone bridge exercise is performed with the elbows and toes with the spine in neutral alignment (Figure 19-15E). The external oblique abdominis (47%±21% MVIC) and rectus abdominis (43%±21% MVIC) demonstrated significant muscle activation in the use of this exercise.[25] In contrast, lesser significance was demonstrated in the gluteus medius (27%±11% MVIC) and gluteus maximus (9%±7% MVIC) muscle groups.[25] With even significant lesser results in the longissimus thoracis (6%±4% MVIC), LMF (5%±4% MVIC), and hamstrings (4%±6% MVIC).[25] Researchers indicated that the highest level of muscle activity in the abdominal muscles is achieved during the prone bridge on a Swiss ball.[22]

Quadruped Arm and Lower Extremity Lift

The quadruped arm and lower extremity lift is performed in the neutral spine position (see Figure 19-15F). The gluteus maximus (56%±22% MVIC) and LMF (46%±21% MVIC) demonstrated significant muscle activation in the use of this exercise.[25] In contrast, lesser significance was demonstrated in the rectus abdominis (8%±7% MVIC) and vastus medialis obliquus (16% ± 11% MVIC) muscle groups.[25] Greater significance was recorded in the gluteus medius (42%±17% MVIC) and hamstrings (39%±14% MVIC).[25] The correlation between EMG recordings from the muscles during the quadruped arm and lower extremity lift exercise was at 0.93 (SEM, 20.7% MVIC). This indicated that there was good consistency in the EMG recordings.[25] EMG results suggest that quadruped arm and lower extremity lift exercise with shoulder and hip abduction is more effective to selectively strengthening the lumbar on the side, where the lower extremity is lifted.[68]

Lateral Step-Up Exercise

The lateral step-up exercise begins from the standing position and uses an 8-inch (20.32 cm) platform for performing the exercise (see Figure 19-15G). The step-up activity is conducive to strengthening of the knee joint, which may be instrumental in developing total knee recovery.[69,70] The vastus medialis obliquus (85%±17% MVIC) and gluteus medius (42%±17% MVIC) demonstrated significant muscle activation in the use of this exercise.[25] In contrast, lesser significance was demonstrated in the hamstrings (10%±6% MVIC), external oblique abdominis (15% ± 10% MVIC), and rectus abdominis (5%±3% MVIC) muscle groups.[25]

Standing Lunge Exercise

The standing lunge exercise begins from the standing position and requires the participant to alternate between right and left forward leg movements, without allowing the knee to touch the surface (see Figure 19-15H). The vastus medialis obliquus (76%±19% MVIC) and gluteus maximus (36%±17% MVIC) demonstrated significant muscle activation in the use of this exercise.[25] In contrast, lesser significance was demonstrated in the hamstrings (11%±6% MVIC), external oblique abdominis (17%±11% MVIC), longissimus thoracis (17%±8% MVIC), and rectus abdominis (7%±5% MVIC) muscle groups.[25] Researchers indicated that adding weight to forward lunge exercises increases muscle activation.[71] In contrast, some researchers would argue that proper technique is best for recruitment of muscles when performing lunges,[72] implying that by adding weight when performing lunges, an individual may increase risk of injury if proper technique is not performed.

Dynamic Edge Exercise

The dynamic edge exercise is a resistance machine that employs side-to-side motions for simulating downhill skiing and is performed from the standing position (see Figure 19-15I). Generally, researchers collected EMG signal during exercise activities involving static muscle contractions, except during the dynamic edge exercise.[25] The dynamic edge exercise may be used for endurance training vs meeting a patient's muscle rehabilitation needs.[25] Introduction of dynamic exercise movements may be goal-directed and or individually motivated by a person acting in a particular environment with regard to specific task demands.[73] When patients are able to effectively activate deep muscles, they are progressed to more dynamic exercises in an effort to train the larger stabilizing muscles.[74] Despite claims on the benefits offered from insertion of dynamic exercise movements, EMG data do not indicate extremely high values in use of the dynamic edge device when compared to some of the other simpler exercises already discussed. The vastus medialis obliquus (36% ± 12% MVIC) and gluteus medius (33% ± 16% MVIC) account for the highest values recorded for indicating significant muscle activation in the use of this exercise device.[25] In contrast, greater muscle activation was indicated in the performance of the lateral step-up for the vastus medialis obliquus (85% ± 17% MVIC) and the side bridge for the gluteus medius (74% ± 30% MVIC).[25]

Summary of Electromyographic Analysis of Core Trunk and Hip During Nine Rehabilitation Exercises

The mean EMG activity of each muscle expressed as a percentage of MVIC for each exercise is shown in Tables 19-1 through 19-4. Data are summarized as based on Ekstrom's[25] recorded EMG values. The gluteus medius muscle showed significantly greater activation with the side bridge exercise (mean ± SD; 74% ± 30% MVIC), and the gluteus maximus muscle showed significantly greater activation with the quadruped arm/lower extremity lift exercise (56% ± 22% MVIC) than with any other exercise (see Table 19-1). For the hamstring muscles (see Table 19-2), the quadruped arm/lower extremity lift (39% ± 14% MVIC) and the unilateral bridge (40% ± 17% MVIC) exercises produced the most muscular activity with no significant difference between them. The vastus medialis obliquus muscle showed the greatest activation with the lateral step-up (85% ± 17% MVIC) and lunge exercises (77% ± 19%).

The longissimus thoracis (40% ± 17% MVIC) and LMF (39% ± 15% MVIC to 46% ± 21% MVIC; see Table 19-3) demonstrated similar activity levels with the bilateral bridge, unilateral bridge, side bridge, and the quadruped arm/lower extremity lift exercises. The external oblique abdominis muscle (see Table 19-4) showed the greatest activity with the side bridge exercise (69% ± 26% MVIC). The rectus abdominis muscle activity was greatest with both the prone bridge (43% ± 21% MVIC) and side bridge (34% ± 13% MVIC).

Use of these 9 exercises could be used for a core rehabilitation program—depending on the individual needs of a patient. The exercises that may provide a strengthening stimulus for certain muscles would be the side bridge, the lateral step-up, the lunge, and possibly the quadruped arm/lower extremity lift. Exercises produced EMG signal amplitude markedly greater than the 45% MVIC level, implying that some of the exercises may be more beneficial than others for achieving strength.

CASE STUDIES

Case Study One: Biofeedback for Chronic Low Back Pain

Task Introduction

By chance, you come across Neblett's 2016 review paper entitled "Surface Electromyographic (SEMG) Biofeedback for Chronic Low Back Pain",[75] and you get interested in biofeedback, which—as stated by that author in the abstract— "is a process in which biological information is measured and fed back to a patient and clinician for the purpose of gaining increased awareness and control over physiological domains." You get really interested when you read that "[SEMG], a measure of muscle activity, allows both a patient and clinician to have direct and immediate access to muscle functioning that is not possible with manual palpation or visual observation." And a final click happens to you when you read at the end of the abstract that "SEMG biofeedback can be used to help 'down-train' elevated muscle activity or to 'up-train' weak, inhibited, or paretic muscles," as in your practice you work mainly with patients suffering from CLBP and deconditioned or poorly coordinated muscles may produce CLBP.[29-33]

You shortly acquire the extra equipment, software, and training needed to use SEMG for treatment of your patients with CLBP.

Table 19-1

ELECTROMYOGRAPHY ACTIVITY OF THE GLUTEUS MEDIUS AND GLUTEUS MAXIMUS MUSCLES

EXERCISE	GLUTEUS MEDIUS	GLUTEUS MAXIMUS
1. Side-bridge	74±30[a]	21±16
2. Unilateral-bridge	47±24[b]	40±20[b]
3. Lateral step-up	43±18[b]	29±13
4. Quadruped arm/lower extremity lift	42±17[b]	56±22[a]
5. Active hip abduction	39±17[b]	21±16
6. Dynamic edge	33±16	19±14
7. Lunge	29±12	36±17[b]
8. Bridge	28±17	25±14
9. Prone-bridge	27±11	9±7

* Values expressed as mean ± SD percentage of maximum voluntary isometric contraction (MVIC); n=30; $P < .05$.

[a] For the gluteus medius muscle, exercise 1 produced significantly greater EMG signal amplitude when compared to exercises 2 to 9. For the gluteus maximus muscle, exercise 4 produced significantly greater EMG signal amplitude when compared to all the other exercises.

[b] For the gluteus medius muscle, there was no significant difference in the EMG signal amplitude between exercises 2 to 5, but the EMG signal amplitude was significantly greater in these exercises compared to exercises 7 to 9. For the gluteus maximus muscle, there was no significant difference between exercises 2 and 7, but the EMG signal amplitude was significantly greater for these exercises compared to exercises 1, 3, 5, 6, 8, and 9.

Reprinted with permission from Ekstrom RA, Donatelli RA, Carp KC. Electromyographic analysis of core trunk, hip, and thigh muscles during 9 rehabilitation exercises. *J Orthop Sports Phys Ther.* 2007;37:754-762. https://doi.org/10.2519/jospt.2007.2471. ©*Journal of Orthopaedic & Sports Physical Therapy*®

Table 19-2

ELECTROMYOGRAPHY ACTIVITY OF THE VASTUS MEDIALIS OBLIQUUS AND HAMSTRING MUSCLES

EXERCISE	VASTUS MEDIALIS OBLIQUUS	HAMSTRINGS
1. Lateral step-up	85±17[a]	10±6
2. Lunge	76±19[a]	11±6
3. Dynamic edge	36±12	6±3
4. Prone-bridge	23±13	4±6
5. Side-bridge	19±11	12±11
6. Unilateral-bridge	18±13	40±17[a]
7. Quadruped arm/lower extremity lift	16±11	39±14[a]
8. Active hip abduction	8±8	4±3
9. Bridge	3±3	24±14

* Values expressed as mean ± SD percentage of maximum voluntary isometric contraction (MVIC); n=30; $P < .05$.

[a] For the vastus medialis obliquus muscle, there was no significant difference in the EMG signal amplitude between exercises 1 and 2, but these exercises produced significantly greater EMG signal amplitude when compared to all the other exercises. For the hamstring muscles, there was no significant difference between exercises 6 and 7, but these exercises produced significantly greater EMG signal amplitude when compared to all the other exercises.

Reprinted with permission from Ekstrom RA, Donatelli RA, Carp KC. Electromyographic analysis of core trunk, hip, and thigh muscles during 9 rehabilitation exercises. *J Orthop Sports Phys Ther.* 2007;37:754-762. https://doi.org/10.2519/jospt.2007.2471. ©*Journal of Orthopaedic & Sports Physical Therapy*®

Table 19-3

ELECTROMYOGRAPHY ACTIVITY OF THE LONGISSIMUS THORACIS AND LUMBAR MULTIFIDUS MUSCLES

EXERCISE	LONGISSIMUS THORACIS	LUMBAR MULTIFIDUS
1. Unilateral bridge	40 ± 16[a]	44 ± 18[a]
2. Side-bridge	40 ± 17[a]	42 ± 24[a]
3. Bridge	39 ± 15[a]	39 ± 15[a]
4. Quadruped arm/lower extremity lift	36 ± 18[a]	46 ± 21[a]
5. Lateral step-up	25 ± 10	28 ± 10
6. Dynamic edge	21 ± 10	21 ± 11
7. Active hip abduction	18 ± 14	20 ± 12
8. Lunge	17 ± 8	25 ± 11
9. Prone bridge	6 ± 4	5 ± 4

* Values expressed as mean ± SD percentage of maximum voluntary isometric contraction (MVIC); n = 30; $P < .05$.

[a] For the longissimus thoracis and lumbar multifidus muscles, there was no significant difference in the EMG signal amplitude between exercises 1 to 4, but these exercises produced significantly greater EMG signal amplitude when compared to exercises 5 to 9.

Reprinted with permission from Ekstrom RA, Donatelli RA, Carp KC. Electromyographic analysis of core trunk, hip, and thigh muscles during 9 rehabilitation exercises. *J Orthop Sports Phys Ther.* 2007;37:754-762. https://doi.org/10.2519/jospt.2007.2471. ©*Journal of Orthopaedic & Sports Physical Therapy*®

Table 19-4

ELECTROMYOGRAPHY ACTIVITY OF THE EXTERNAL OBLIQUE ABDOMINIS AND RECTUS ABDOMINIS MUSCLES

EXERCISE	EXTERNAL OBLIQUE ABDOMINIS	RECTUS ABDOMINIS
1. Side-bridge	69 ± 26[a]	34 ± 13[a]
2. Prone-bridge	47 ± 21	43 ± 21[a]
3. Quadruped arm/lower extremity lift	30 ± 18	8 ± 7
4. Unilateral-bridge	23 ± 16	14 ± 13
5. Bridge	22 ± 13	13 ± 11
6. Active hip abduction	18 ± 10	6 ± 4
7. Dynamic edge	18 ± 12	7 ± 5
8. Lunge	17 ± 11	7 ± 5
9. Lateral step-up	15 ± 10	5 ± 3

* Values expressed as mean ± SD percentage of maximum voluntary isometric contraction (MVIC); n = 30; $P < .05$.

[a] For the external oblique abdominis muscle, exercise 1 produced significantly greater EMG signal amplitude when compared to exercises 2 to 9. For the rectus abdominis muscle, there was no significant difference in the EMG signal amplitude between exercises 1 and 2, but these exercises produced significantly greater EMG signal amplitude when compared to exercises 3 to 9.

Reprinted with permission from Ekstrom RA, Donatelli RA, Carp KC. Electromyographic analysis of core trunk, hip, and thigh muscles during 9 rehabilitation exercises. *J Orthop Sports Phys Ther.* 2007;37:754-762. https://doi.org/10.2519/jospt.2007.2471. ©*Journal of Orthopaedic & Sports Physical Therapy*®

Questions

Answer the following questions keeping in mind what you have learned in this chapter.

1. For which of the 3 motor learning main phases would you use the SEMG biofeedback?
2. In order to make the rehabilitation process of your patients with CLBP as efficient and complete as possible, which muscles would you monitor and give feedback on? And, during the performing of which exercises among the ones described in this chapter?

Answers

1. Actually, SEMG biofeedback can be useful in all the 3 phases: (1) cognitive, helping to consciously pay attention to the step-by-step execution of the movements; (2) associative, assisting in minimizing the co-activation of global system muscles and in providing accurate feedback of contraction quality; however, in phase (3), autonomous, the technique starts being less useful, as the task may become automatic and thus the requirement for conscious intervention is reduced.
2. As a matter of fact, we could target any of the exercises and muscles elicited by them that have been described in the sections in which the trunk is studied. We ought to keep in mind, however, that the SEMG of deep muscles may suffer of crosstalk from muscles located above them.

Case Study Two: Consultation About a New Device

Task Introduction

You are a consultant, and an inventor offers you the opportunity to perform a study with a new device that they have invented, designed, and created; it is a quadruple oscillating device (QOD), which is similar to a Bodyblade exercise device (a DOD), in which a couple of variable free weights are placed on the tip of both blade endings. Their hypothesis is that the use of this device will provide more benefits than those obtained with an SOD or even with a DOD, as their device elicits a greater instability. They provide you with one working prototype of their invention, so that you can perform experiments with it. Assume that you have a fully equipped EMG lab.

Questions

1. From what you have read in this chapter, do you believe that they may be right about the importance of the additional vibration generated with their device?
2. Using EMG, how would you compare the effectiveness of this new device against that of an SOD and of a DOD?

Answers

1. Yes, we can guess a priori that they are right because when we induce vibratory stimuli, we provoke co-activation of surrounding shoulder and core muscles.
2. You could perform a study similar to the one displayed in the section on Bodyblade vs TheraBand Flexbar devices, in which the following muscle activity was monitored by EMG during the performance of exercises with the 2 different devices: anterior deltoid, transverse abdominus/internal oblique, and LSES. A comparison of the activity level of those muscles would provide a good estimation of which device elicits higher levels.

As the researchers mentioned in that section, you also could compare the activation levels when the devices are used in a frontal vs transverse plane, in order to check in which way the device is more effective.

You may search in the scientific literature for which other muscles or experiments could be used for this requested task. For example, read the 2016 paper of Escamilla et al.[54] We recommend using Google Scholar for such a search.

REFERENCES

1. Chang DG, Padilla MA, Hargens AR. Surface electromyography: Technical developments and clinical applications in sports medicine. Adaptation Biology and Medicine. 2014. Accessed April 29, 2022. https://www.researchgate.net/profile/Douglas_Chang/publication/264044931_Surface_electromyography_Technical_developments_and_clinical_applications_in_sports_medicine/links/0a85e53caf8f1b2a4e000000.pdf

2. Ball N, Scurr J. Electromyography normalization methods for high velocity muscle actions: review and recommendations. *J Appl Biomech*. 2013;29(5):600-608.

3. Winkel J, Mathiassen S. Assessment of physical work load in epidemiologic studies: concepts, issues and operational considerations. *Ergonomics*. 1994;37(6):979-988. doi:10.1080/00140139408963711

4. Burdorf A, van der Beek A. Exposure assessment strategies for work-related risk factors for musculoskeletal disorders. *Scand J Work Environ Health*. 1999;25(Suppl 4):25-30.

5. Escamilla RF, Hooks TR, Wilk KE. Optimal management of shoulder impingement syndrome. *Open Access J Sports Med*. 2014;5:13-24. doi:10.2147/OAJSM.S36646

6. Ishida H, Watanabe S. Changes in lateral abdominal muscles' thickness immediately after the abdominal drawing-in maneuver and maximum expiration. *J Bodyw Mov Ther*. 2013;17(2):254-258. doi:10.1016/j.jbmt.2012.12.002

7. Haff GG, Triplett NT. *Essentials of Strength Training and Conditioning*. 4th ed. Human Kinetics; 2015.

8. Earp J. The influence of external loading and speed of movement on muscle-tendon unit behavior and its implications for training. Research Online Institutional Repository. 2013. Accessed April 29, 2022. http://ro.ecu.edu.au/theses/533

9. Borges J, Baptista AF, Santana N, et al. Pilates exercises improve low back pain and quality of life in patients with HTLV-1 virus: a randomized crossover clinical trial. *J Bodyw Mov Ther.* 2014;18(1):68-74. doi:10.1016/j.jbmt.2013.05.010

10. Halliday MH, Ferreira PH, Hancock MJ, Clare HA. A randomized controlled trial comparing McKenzie therapy and motor control exercises on the recruitment of trunk muscles in people with chronic low back pain: a trial protocol. *Physiotherapy.* 2015; 101(2):232-238. doi:10.1016/j.physio.2014.07.001

11. Hettinga DM, Jackson A, Moffett JK, May S, Mercer C, Woby SR. A systematic review and synthesis of higher quality evidence of the effectiveness of exercise interventions for non-specific low back pain of at least 6 weeks' duration. *Phys Ther Rev.* 2013;12(3):221-232. doi:10.1179/108331907X222958

12. Harvey LA, Dunlop SA, Churilov L, Galea MP. Early intensive hand rehabilitation is not more effective than usual care plus one-to-one hand therapy in people with sub-acute spinal cord injury ("hands on"): a randomized trial. *J Physiother Phys Rehabil.* 2014; 62(2):88-95. doi:10.1016/j.jphys.2016.02.013

13. Jordan JL, Holden MA, Mason EE, Foster NE. Interventions to improve adherence to exercise for chronic musculoskeletal pain in adults. *Cochrane Database Syst Rev.* 2010;2010(1):CD005956. doi:10.1002/14651858.CD005956.pub2

14. Maeo S, Takahashi T, Takai Y, Kanehisa H. Trunk muscle activities during abdominal bracing: comparison among muscles and exercises. *J Sport Sci Med.* 2012;12(3):467-474.

15. Martuscello JM, Nuzzo JL, Ashley CD, Campbell BI, Orriola JJ, Mayer JM. Systematic review of core muscle activity during physical fitness exercises. *J Strength Cond Res.* 2013;27(6):1684-1698.

16. Escamilla RF, Babb E, DeWitt R, et al. Electromyographic analysis of traditional and nontraditional abdominal exercises: implications for rehabilitation and training. *Phys Ther.* 2006;86(5):656-671.

17. Chang WD, Lin HY, Lai PT. Core strength training for patients with chronic low back pain. *J Phys Ther Sci.* 2015;27(3):619-622. doi:10.1589/jpts.27.619

18. Snarr RL, Esco MR. Electromyographical comparison of plank variations performed with and without instability devices. *J Strength Cond Res.* 2014;28(11):3298-3305.

19. Stenger EM. Electromyographic comparison of a variety of abdominal exercises to the traditional crunch. University of Wisconsin. December 2013. Accessed April 29, 2022. https://minds.wisconsin.edu/handle/1793/67303

20. Key J. The core: understanding it, and retraining its dysfunction. *J Bodyw Mov Ther.* 2013;17(4):541-559. doi:10.1016/j.jbmt.2013.03.012

21. Kline JB, Krauss JR, Maher SF, Qu X. Core strength training using a combination of home exercises and a dynamic sling system for the management of low back pain in pre-professional ballet dancers: a case series. *J Dance Med Sci.* 2013;17(1):24-33. doi:10.12678/1089-313X.17.l.24

22. Czaprowski D, Afeltowicz A, Gębicka A, et al. Abdominal muscle EMG-activity during bridge exercises on stable and unstable surfaces. *Phys Ther Sport.* 2014;15(3):162-168. doi:10.1016/j.ptsp.2013.09.003

23. Escamilla RF, Lewis C, Pecson A, Imamura R, Andrews JR. Muscle activation among supine, prone, and side position exercises with and without a Swiss ball. *Sport Health.* 2016;8(4):372-379. doi:10.1177/1941738116653931

24. Kim BI, Jung JH, Shim J, Kwon HY, Kim H. An analysis of muscle activities of healthy women during Pilates exercises in a prone position. *J Phys Ther Sci.* 2014;26(1):77-79. doi:10.1589/jpts.26.77

25. Ekstrom RA, Donatelli RA, Carp KC. Electromyographic analysis of core trunk, hip, and thigh muscles during 9 rehabilitation exercises. *J Orthop Sports Phys Ther.* 2007;37(12):754-762. doi:10.2519/jospt.2007.2471

26. Haladay DE, Miller SJ, Challis J, Denegar CR. Quality of systematic reviews on specific spinal stabilization exercise for chronic low back pain. *J Orthop Sports Phys Ther.* 2013;43(4):242-250. doi:10.2519/jospt.2013.4346

27. Bliven KCH, Anderson BE. Core stability training for injury prevention. *Sports Health.* 2013;5(6):514-522. doi:10.1177/1941738113481200

28. Lee CW, Hwangbo K, Lee IS. The effects of combination patterns of proprioceptive neuromuscular facilitation and ball exercise on pain and muscle activity of chronic low back pain patients. *J Phys Ther Sci.* 2014;26(1):93-96. doi:10.1589/jpts.26.93

29. Arun B. Effect of myofascial release therapy with motor control exercises on pain, disability and transversus abdominis muscle activation in chronic low back pain. *Research and Reviews.* 2014;3(3): 28-32.

30. Dahlqvist JR, Vissing CR, Thomsen C, Vissing J. Severe paraspinal muscle involvement in facioscapulohumeral muscular dystrophy. *Neurology.* 2014;83(13):1178-1183. doi:10.1212/WNL.0000000000000828

31. Smith N. Gluteus medius function and low back pain; is there a relationship? *Physical Therapy Reviews.* 2013;4(4):283-288. doi:10.1179/ptr.1999.4.4.283

32. Steele J, Bruce-Low S, Smith D. A reappraisal of the deconditioning hypothesis in low back pain: review of evidence from a triumvirate of research methods on specific lumbar extensor deconditioning. *Curr Med Res Opin.* 2014;30(5):865-911. doi:10.1185/03007995.2013.875465

33. Wallden M. Facilitating change through active rehabilitation techniques. *J Bodyw Mov Ther.* 2013;17(4):531-540. doi:10.1016/j.jbmt.2013.09.004

34. Hides JA, Stokes MJ, Saide MJGA, Jull GA, Cooper DH. Evidence of lumbar multifidus muscle wasting ipsilateral to symptoms in patients with acute/subacute low back pain. *Spine.* 1994;19(2):165-172. doi:10.1097/00007632-199401001-00009

35. Richardson C, Jull G, Hodges P, Hides J, Panjabi MM. Therapeutic exercise for spinal segmental stabilization in low back pain. In: *Scientific Basis and Clinical Approach.* Churchill Livingstone; 1999:61-76.

36. Wellington J. Noninvasive and alternative management of chronic low back pain (efficacy and outcomes). *Neuromodulation.* 2014; 17(Suppl 2):24-30. doi:10.1111/ner.12078

37. Harris-Love MO, Fernandez-Rhodes L, Joe G, et al. Assessing function and endurance in adults with spinal and bulbar muscular atrophy: validity of the adult myopathy assessment tool. *Rehab Res Pracy.* 2014;2014:873872. doi:10.1155/2014/873872

38. Engelhardt C, Malfroy Camine V, Ingram D, et al. Comparison of an EMG-based and a stress-based method to predict shoulder muscle forces. *Comput Methods Biomech Biomed Engin.* 2015;18(12):1272-1279. doi:10.1080/10255842.2014.899587

39. Van Damme B, Stevens V, Perneel C, et al. A surface electromyography based objective method to identify patients with nonspecific chronic low back pain, presenting a flexion related movement control impairment. *J Electromyogr Kinesiol.* 2014;24(6):954-964. doi:10.1016/j.jelekin.2014.09.007

40. Marques NR, Morcelli MH, Hallal CZ, Gonçalves M. EMG activity of trunk stabilizer muscles during centering principle of Pilates method. *J Bodyw Mov Ther.* 2013;17(2):185-191. doi:10.1016/j.jbmt.2012.06.002

41. Ellenbecker TS, Wilk KE. Sport-specific rehabilitation after ulnar collateral ligament surgery. In: Dines JS, Altchek WS, eds. *Elbow Ulnar Collateral Ligament Injury.* Springer. 2015;261-277.

42. Justine M, Haron R, Salleh Z, Mohan V. Effects of concentric and eccentric abdominal training on abdominal strength and lumbopelvic stability: a randomized-controlled trial. *Indian J Physiother Occup Ther.* 2013;7(4):131. doi:10.5958/j.0973-5674.7.4.136

43. Peterson DD. Proposed performance standards for the plank for inclusion consideration into the Navy's physical readiness test. *Strength Cond J.* 2013;35(5):22-26. doi:10.1519/SSC.0000000000000003

44. Silva GB, Morgan MM, de Carvalho WRG, et al. Electromyographic activity of rectus abdominis muscles during dynamic Pilates abdominal exercises. *J Bodyw Mov Ther.* 2015;19(4):629-635. doi:10.1016/j.jbmt.2014.11.010

45. Silva MF, Silva MA, Campos RR, et al. A comparative analysis of the electrical activity of the abdominal muscles during traditional and Pilates-based exercises under two conditions. *Revista Brasileira de Cineantropometria e Desempenho Humano.* 2013;15:296-304. doi:10.5007/1980-0037.2013v15n3p296

46. Arora S, Button DC, Basset FA, Behm DG. The effect of double versus single oscillating exercise devices on trunk and limb muscle activation. *Int J Sports Phys Ther.* 2013;8(4):370.

47. Datta A, Sen S. Effects of core strengthening on cardiovascular fitness, flexibility and strength on patients with low back pain. *Journal of Novel Physiotherapies.* 2014;2(202). doi:10.4172/2165-7025.1000202

48. Bodyblade: the complete vibration training system. Bodyblade. 2016. Accessed January 1, 2017. http://www.bodyblade.com

49. Thera-band systems of progressive exercise. Theraband. http://2016. Accessed January 1, 2017. www.theraband.com

50. Da Yeon Choi SHC, Shim JH. Comparisons of shoulder stabilization muscle activities according to postural changes during flexi-bar exercise. *J Phys Ther Sci.* 2015;27(6):1889. doi:10.1589/jpts.27.1889

51. Abdollahi M, Nikkhoo M, Ashouri S, et al. A model for flexi-bar to evaluate intervertebral disc and muscle forces in exercises. *Med Eng Phys.* 2016;38(10):1076-1082. doi:10.1016/j.medengphy.2016.07.006

52. Khalaf K, Abdollahi M, Nikkhoo M, et al. A mechanical model for flexible exercise bars to study the influence of the initial position of the bar on lumbar discs and muscles forces. Paper presented at: 37th Annual International Conference of the IEEE Engineering in Medicine and Biology Society. August 25-29, 2015; Milan, Italy. doi:10.1109/EMBC.2015.7319250

53. Yoo WG. Effect of the foot placements on the latissmus dorsi and low back muscle activities during pull-down exercise. *J Phys Ther Sci.* 2013;25(9):1155-1156. doi:10.1589/jpts.25.1155

54. Escamilla RF, Yamashiro K, Dunning R, et al. An electromyographic analysis of the shoulder complex musculature while performing exercises using the Bodyblade classic and Bodyblade pro. *Inter J Sport Phys Ther.* 2016;11(2):175-189.

55. Moon HJ, Choi KH, Kim DH, et al. Effect of lumbar stabilization and dynamic lumbar strengthening exercises in patients with chronic low back pain. *Ann Rehabil Med.* 2013;37(1):110-117. doi:10.5535/arm.2013.37.1.110

56. Hauggaard A, Persson AL. Specific spinal stabilization exercises in patients with low back pain—a systematic review. *Phys Ther Rev.* 2013;12(3):223-248. doi:10.1179/108331907X222949

57. Aluko A, DeSouza L, Peacock J. The effect of core stability exercises on variations in acceleration of trunk movement, pain, and disability during an episode of acute nonspecific low back pain: a pilot clinical trial. *J Manipulative Physiol Ther.* 2013;36(8):497-504. doi:10.1016/j.jmpt.2012.12.012

58. Park HJ, Oh DW, Kim SY. Effects of integrating hip movements into bridge exercises on electromyographic activities of selected trunk muscles in healthy individuals. *Chiropr Man Therap.* 2014;19(3):246-251. doi:10.1016/j.jbmt.2013.03.012

59. Kim MJ, Oh DW, Park HJ. Integrating arm movement into bridge exercise: effect on EMG activity of selected trunk muscles. *J Electromyogr Kinesiol.* 2013;23(5):1119-1123. doi:10.1016/j.jelekin.2013.07.001

60. Yu CH, Shin SH, Jeong HC, Go DY, Kwon TK. Activity analysis of trunk and leg muscles during whole body tilt exercise. *Biomed Mater Eng.* 2014;24(1):245-254. doi:10.3233/BME-130805

61. Saeterbakken AH, Fimland MS. Muscle force output and electromyographic activity in squats with various unstable surfaces. *J Strength Cond Res.* 2013;27(1):130-136. doi:10.1519/JSC.0b013e3182541d43

62. Zebis MK, Skotte J, Andersen CH, et al. Kettlebell swing targets semitendinosus and supine leg curl targets biceps femoris: an EMG study with rehabilitation implications. *Br J Sports Med.* 2013;47(18):1192-1198. doi:10.1136/bjsports-2011-090281

63. McBride JM, Cormie P, Deane R. Isometric squat force output and muscle activity in stable and unstable conditions. *J Strength Cond Res.* 2006;20(4):915-918.

64. Kibler WB, McMullen J, Uhl T. Shoulder rehabilitation strategies, guidelines, and practice. *Oper Tech Sports Med.* 2012;20(1):103-112. doi:10.1053/j.otsm.2012.03.012

65. Parry JS, Straub R, Cipriani DJ. Shoulder-and back-muscle activation during shoulder abduction and flexion using a Bodyblade Pro versus dumbbells. *J Sport Rehab.* 2012;21(3):266-272. doi:10.1123/jsr.21.3.266

66. Jang EM, Kim MH, Oh JS. Effects of a bridging exercise with hip adduction on the EMG activities of the abdominal and hip extensor muscles in females. *J Phys Ther Sci.* 2013;25(9):1147-1149. doi:10.1589/jpts.25.1147

67. Mok NW, Yeung EW, Cho JC, Hui SC, Liu KC, Pang CH. Core muscle activity during suspension exercises. *J Sci Med Sport.* 2015;18(2):189-194. doi:10.1016/j.jsams.2014.01.002

68. Masaki M, Tateuchi H, Tsukagoshi R, Ibuki S, Ichihashi N. Electromyographic analysis of training to selectively strengthen the lumbar multifidus muscle: effects of different lifting directions and weight loading of the extremities during quadruped upper and lower extremity lifts. *J Man Physio Therap.* 2015;38(2):138-144. doi:10.1016/j.jmpt.2014.07.008

69. Li JS, Hosseini A, Cancre L, Ryan N, Rubash HE, Li G. Kinematic characteristics of the tibiofemoral joint during a step-up activity. *Gait Posture.* 2013;38(4):712-716. doi:10.1016/j.gaitpost.2013.03.004

70. Park KM, Cynn HS, Choung SD. Musculoskeletal predictors of movement quality for the forward step-down test in asymptomatic women. *J Orthop Sport Phys Ther.* 2013;43(7):504-510. doi:10.2519/jospt.2013.4073

71. Jakobsen MD, Sundstrup E, Andersen CH, Aagaard P, Andersen LL. Muscle activity during leg strengthening exercise using free weights and elastic resistance: effects of ballistic vs controlled contractions. *Hum Move Sci.* 2013;32(1):65-78. doi:10.1016/j.humov.2012.07.002

72. Selkowitz DM, Beneck GJ, Powers CM. Which exercises target the gluteal muscles while minimizing activation of the tensor fascia lata? Electromyographic assessment using fine-wire electrodes. *J Ortho Sport Phys Ther.* 2013;43(2):54-64. doi:10.2519/jospt.2013.4116

73. Nassar L. Treatment and rehabilitation of common spine/trunk/head injuries. In: Caine DJ, Russel K, Lim L, eds. *Gymnastics.* International Olympic Committee; 2013:154-169. doi:10.1002/9781118357538.ch13

74. Miller ER, Schenk RJ, Karnes JL, Rousselle JG. A comparison of the McKenzie approach to a specific spine stabilization program for chronic low back pain. *J Man Manip Ther.* 2013;13(2):103-112. doi:10.1179/106698105790824996

75. Neblett R. Surface electromyographic (SEMG) biofeedback for chronic low back pain. *Healthcare (Basel).* 2016;4(2):27.

20

Spinal Manual Trigger Point Therapy and Dry Needling

Johnson McEvoy, BSc, MSc, DPT, MISCP, PT
and Christian Gröbli, PT

KEY TERMS

Active trigger point: A trigger point that causes spontaneous pain. When palpated adequately, it may give rise to a characteristic familiar referred pain pattern.

Dry needling: The insertion of a needle over or into the trigger point for the treatment of myofascial pain. Also known as *trigger point dry needling (TrPDN).*

Latent trigger point: A trigger point that does not cause spontaneous pain and is only painful when palpated.

Local twitch response (LTR): A transit contraction of a group of muscle fibers associated with a trigger point elicited by palpation or needling of the trigger point.

Myalgia: Pain associated with or arising from muscle.

Myofascial pain: The sensory, motor, and autonomic symptoms associated with myofascial trigger points.

Myofascial trigger point (MTrP)/trigger point: A hyperirritable spot in a taut band of skeletal muscle fibers.

Pain pressure threshold (PPT): The minimum mechanical pressure that induces pain.

Taut band: A group of tense muscle fibers.

Trigger point compression release (TrPCR): Sustained manual pressure to a trigger point with the main aim of raising the pain pressure threshold.

CHAPTER QUESTIONS

1. What is the definition of neck pain?
2. What is the definition of low back pain?
3. What are the estimated prevalence rates for neck and low back pain?
4. Is multimodal treatment indicated?
5. Should soft tissue massage be a primary treatment for neck and low back pain?
6. What is a treatment guideline?
7. What are recommended treatment guidelines for low back and neck pain?
8. Define a myofascial trigger point.
9. Define the difference between an active and latent trigger point.
10. What is the integrated hypothesis of trigger point formation?
11. Outline the current understanding of the pathogenesis of trigger points.
12. What is the current understanding of the etiology of trigger points?

Wallmann HW, Donatelli R, eds. *Foundations of Orthopedic Physical Therapy* (pp 613-631).
© 2024 Taylor & Francis Group.

13. What are the 2 main manual techniques used for assessment and treatment of trigger points?

14. Is trigger point palpation reliable?

15. What is trigger point compression release?

16. What is trigger point dry needling?

17. What is the historical context of trigger point dry needling?

18. What are common muscles involved in neck pain?

19. What are common muscles involved in low back pain?

20. What are the basic treatment concepts of myofascial trigger points of the neck?

21. What are the basic treatment concepts of myofascial trigger points of the low back?

INTRODUCTION

Neck pain and low back pain (LBP) are common conditions associated with pain, functional impairment, disability, and psychosocial impacts. People suffering from neck pain and LBP frequently present to physical therapy practice.

Neck pain can include pain and stiffness in the neck area, headache, dizziness, and pain radiating to the shoulder and upper extremities[1]; it can occur insidiously or gradually over time or from posttraumatic onset and will often settle after the acute stage as part of the natural course or perhaps with treatment. Neck pain 1-year prevalence rates range from 4.8% to 79.5% with point prevalence of 0.4% to 41.5%.[2] However, 50% of individuals continue to experience some level of pain or frequent occurrences.[3]

LBP consists of pain and muscle tension or stiffness localized below the costal margin, above the inferior gluteal folds with or without sciatica.[4] Chronic or persistent LBP is very common with 1-year prevalence rates ranging from 0.8% to 82.5% and point prevalence ranging from 1.0% to 58.1%.[5] The vast majority of people will recover within 12 weeks, but similar to neck pain, about 50% will have at least one recurrent episode.

The treatment of neck and back pain is in the context of the biopsychosocial model.[6-8] The management of patients with musculoskeletal pain is complex and physical therapists are strategically guided by the American Physical Therapy Association (APTA) *Guide to Practice*.[9] Patients should undergo a standard physical therapy assessment, which includes subjective history, medical and surgical history, red flag review, current medications, lifestyle factors, objective assessment, and development of a plan of care. Evidence-informed practice should incorporate scientific evidence, clinical reasoning, and judgment coupled with an understanding of patient wish, belief, and values.[10] Treatment should be multimodal in an individualized patient-centered framework.[7,11] Furthermore, patient expectations and preferences play an important role in treatment outcomes and should be considered in the context of treatment delivery.[12]

Due to the complex nature of health care, guidelines have been developed to assist in the application of best practice. Guidelines are defined as "statements that include recommendations intended to optimize patient care that is informed by systematic review of evidence and an assessment of the benefits and harms of alternative care options."[13] The National Institute for Health and Care Excellence (NICE) is a United Kingdom non-departmental public body with the primary aim of setting and improving standards in health care.[14] NICE has published a *Clinical Knowledge Summary for Non-Specific Neck Pain* in 2013 and *Low Back Pain and Sciatica Guidelines* in November 2016.[15,16] These are valuable clinical guidelines in the management of neck and low back disorders. In summary, recommendations are for a multimodal treatment approach including exercise, education, and manual therapy. Although needling therapies (acupuncture) should be considered for chronic neck pain,[15] acupuncture is not currently a guideline recommended for LBP[15,16] and the term *dry needling* was not specifically addressed in the guidelines. Readers are advised to review the NICE guidelines in full. A brief overview of guideline recommendations for neck and back pain are provided in Tables 20-1 and 20-2.

The NICE guidelines recommend a multimodal approach to neck and LBP disorders. A systematic review is a scientific investigation that focuses on a specific question or area and may include a meta-analysis.[13] The Cochrane Library has also published systematic reviews on massage and acupuncture/dry needling for neck and LBP.[17-19]

Cochrane reports that for mechanical neck pain no clear recommendations can be made on the effectiveness of massage.[20] As a standalone treatment, massage provides immediate and short-term effectiveness in both pain and tenderness.[20] In relation to acupuncture and neck disorders, Cochrane published a systematic review in 2016 but withdrew the review in late 2016 to address comments that had arisen from the original review.[21,22] The authors reported that they did not find sufficient studies on dry needling alone to justify separating this needling treatment into a separate review.

However, another recent non-Cochrane systematic review reported that dry needling treatment by physical therapists is more efficient than no treatment, sham dry needling, and other treatments for reducing pain and improving pressure pain threshold in patients presenting with musculoskeletal pain immediately and up to 12 weeks.[23] Dry needling treatment improved functional outcomes when compared to no treatment or sham needling. However, no difference in functional outcomes exists when compared to other physical therapy treatments.[23] Evidence of long-term benefits of dry needling is currently lacking.[23] However, a 2017 Spanish study (n = 130) comparing stretching exercises to stretching exercises and dry needling for neck pain reported favorable outcomes in the dry needling treatment group in terms of pain, function, range of motion (ROM), strength, and pain pressure threshold over muscles. Improvements were present

Table 20-1

NECK PAIN CLINICAL KNOWLEDGE SUMMARY—NICE

NON-SPECIFIC NECK PAIN: CLINICAL KNOWLEDGE SUMMARY (SEPTEMBER 2013)	
< 4 weeks	Provide reassurance Encourage activity and return to a normal lifestyle Firm pillow may provide comfort Simple analgesia

4 to 12 weeks	Same as above measure (< 4 weeks)
	Multimodal treatment strategy
	
	   • Exercise (stretching and strengthening)
	
	   • Some form of manual therapy
	
	   • Acupuncture (dry needling not specifically covered)
	
	   • Addressing any psychological factors
	
	   • Referral to occupational health for work-related neck pain

12 weeks	In addition to above measures (4 to 12 weeks) Trial of amitriptyline or pregabalin (or gabapentin) Referral to pain clinic

Note: Clinicians are recommended to read the full clinical knowledge summary.

Adapted from National Institute for Health and Care Excellence. (2016). *Low Back Pain and Sciatica in Over 16s: Assessment and Management.* Author.

Table 20-2

LOW BACK PAIN AND SCIATICA IN OVER 16. NICE GUIDELINES

LOW BACK PAIN AND SCIATICA IN OVER 16 (NOVEMBER 2016)	
Multimodal Treatment Package	
Exercise Alongside at Least One of the Following:	
1	Self-management Education, advice, and information Information on nature of low back pain and sciatica Encouragement to continue with normal activities as far as possible
2	Consider manual therapy soft tissue therapy only as part of a multimodal treatment package Recommended not to use acupuncture Dry needling was not addressed in this guideline

3	Psychological therapy (eg, cognitive behavioral therapy)
	However, only when:
	
	   • There are significant psychological obstacles to recovery
	
	   • Previous treatments have not been effective

Note: Clinicians are recommended to read the full guideline.

Adapted from National Institute for Health and Care Excellence. (2016). *Low Back Pain and Sciatica in Over 16s: Assessment and Management.* Author.

Table 20-3

TRIGGER POINT CRITERIA

ACTIVE TRIGGER POINT	LATERAL TRIGGER POINT
• Palpable taut band—where accessible	• Palpable taut band—where accessible
• Exquisite spot tenderness on taut band	• Exquisite spot tenderness on taut band (palpation may elicit unfamiliar pain)
• Elicitation of component of patient-recognized pain by palpation	

at discharge and maintained at 3- and 6-month follow-up.[24] The effect size magnitude for pain and function in this study was clinically relevant with pain improvements of almost 80%. This study was not included in the Gattie et al[23] systematic review.

Soft tissue massage has been a traditional keystone of physical therapy practice, and there are more than 80 different forms of massage.[25] Clinical massage is the utilization of various massage techniques, in the therapeutic setting, to achieve a specific outcome such as pain relief, optimizing ROM, function, and quality of life.[25] One such approach in clinical soft tissue therapy is the treatment of MTrPs as described by Travell and later Travell and Simons. Traditionally various techniques were used to treat trigger points including, but not limited to, manual compression release (previously known as ischaemic compression), ice, and stretch and needling therapies including injection therapy and dry needling.[26-28] There has been increasing interest in the treatment of MTrPs in the last 2 decades. Trigger points usually refer pain distally from the muscle and the sensitivity of trigger points to mechanical stimulus, such as manual pressure, has been proposed to be associated with the referred pain. The PPT of trigger points can be measured reliably with a pressure algometer.[29-32] The main rationale for therapeutic soft tissue therapy or dry needling, therefore, is to raise the PPT over the trigger point, which may lead to a reduction in the spontaneous patient pain complaint. Many studies have used the PPT as an experimental measurement and correlated this to the change in patient pain and function.[24,33]

A review of the prevalence of trigger points in patients with neck pain concluded trigger points are a significant clinical entity, most notably in the trapezius, levator scapula, posterior cervical muscles, and sternocleidomastoid.[34] There are less data on the prevalence of trigger points in LBP; however, one study concluded quadratus lumborum, iliocostalis lumborum, and gluteus medius muscles to be the most prevalent, which is in keeping with clinical observation.[35] More quality research is needed on prevalence of trigger points in neck pain and LBP.

This chapter specifically focuses on MTrPs and TrPDN.

MYOFASCIAL TRIGGER POINTS

An MTrP is defined as a hyperirritable spot in skeletal muscle associated with a hypersensitive palpable nodule in the taut band of skeletal muscle fibers.[26,28] Trigger points are defined as being either active or latent; active trigger points give rise to spontaneous pain complaints, whereas latent trigger points are clinically dormant with respect to pain and may give rise to pain if stimulated by muscle contraction, palpation, or needling.[28]

Another characteristic of trigger points is the LTR, which is a transient and rapid contraction of muscle fibers within the taut band elicited by snapping palpation or with insertion of a needle into the trigger point.[28] The jump sign has been used to describe a patient reactionary movement response when a level of pressure is applied to a trigger point.[28] In essence, this is a useful clinical feature to approximate the patient's pain threshold and tolerance. The patient may also verbalize a response. The jump sign should not be confused with the LTR.[28]

The minimum criterion for identification of an active trigger point is an exquisite spot tenderness of a nodule in the taut band that when adequately palpated gives rise to the patient's recognized pain complaint (Table 20-3).[28,36,37] In essence, palpation of an active trigger point reproduces the patient's familiar pain either completely or partially. This technique is a pain provocation test. A latent trigger point due to its lack of pain production is defined as exquisite spot tenderness of a nodule in a taut band. Palpation of a latent trigger point may also produce referred pain, but this is by definition not recognized as the patient symptom.[28,37] Clinically, it is possible that trigger points undulate between latent and active trigger points, responding symptomatically to the loading and lifestyle of the patient.

TRIGGER POINT PALPATION RELIABILITY

The assessment of trigger points relies on the subjective patient complaint, history, and physical examination findings. Clinicians are encouraged to carry out a standard orthopedic physical therapy assessment and include specific

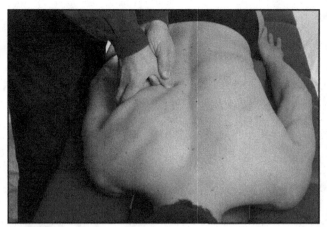

Figure 20-1. Trigger point compression release (flat palpation): Superficial paraspinal muscles thoracic spine. (Reproduced with permission from David G. Simons Academy.)

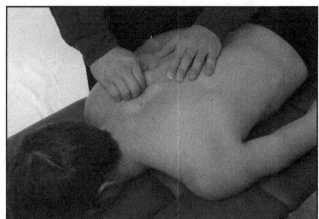

Figure 20-2. Trigger point compression release (pincer grip): Lower trapezius. (Reproduced with permission from David G. Simons Academy.)

palpation examination of muscles suspected to be potential pain generators. MTrP palpation is part of the special tests in the physical examination. Currently, there is no gold standard diagnostic test for MTrPs. Needle electromyography and elastography may have potential diagnostic value in myofascial pain, though these techniques need further research for clinical utility and validity and may not be widely available.[38-50] Current best practice for muscle trigger points relies on palpation.

Due to the reliance on physical examination of muscle palpation, reliability for identification of trigger points is important. Several studies have addressed interrater[36,51-57] and intrarater reliability.[58] In a subsequent systematic review of palpation reliability studies, trigger point palpation reached levels of reliability, but this depended on the specific muscle tested, the level of clinician expertise, training, and consensus on the technique utilized.[37]

Several studies have utilized symptomatic participants with LBP[51,53,55] and neck pain,[36] while 2 studies used asymptomatic participants with latent trigger points in the upper trapezius.[54,56] Gerwin et al stated that features of the trigger point examination should not be assumed to be generally reliable as this can vary from muscle to muscle.[36,37]

McEvoy and Huijbregts[37] reported best evidence synthesis on muscles relating to neck and back pain:

- Sufficient interrater reliability has been established for identification of local tenderness in the upper trapezius and infraspinatus; taut band in the upper trapezius and infraspinatus; referred and the patient's recognized pain and absence or presence of latent or active trigger points in the sternocleidomastoid, upper trapezius, and infraspinatus.

- Sufficient interrater reliability has been established for identification of local tenderness, taut band, recognized pain, and jump sign for both the gluteus medius and the quadratus lumborum muscles, whereas recognition of referred pain has sufficient interrater reliability for the gluteus medius only.[53]

TRIGGER POINT PALPATION TECHNIQUE

Trigger point palpation is a learned skill that involves knowledge of practical muscle anatomy, including muscle location and attachments, muscle fiber direction, and muscle fiber layers.[59] There are 2 basic techniques for trigger point palpation: flat palpation and pincer grip. These are exemplified in Figures 20-1 and 20-2. The 2 different palpation techniques are used for physical assessment and as a method of manual trigger point treatment. They are also employed as part of manual control during trigger point needling techniques. See Figures 20-3 and 20-4 for examples.

Flat palpation (see Figure 20-1): Pressure through the finger(s) or thumb is applied directly to the muscle perpendicular to the muscle fiber. The trigger point is compressed against the underlying tissue or bone. An example of this technique includes pressure on the levator scapula muscle at the attachment of the upper medial border of the scapula or medially directed pressure to the quadratus lumborum toward the transverse processes of L3 or L4 in the lumbar spine.

Pincer grip (see Figure 20-2): Grip is made between the clinician's fingers and thumb with the trigger point compressed in the pincer part of the grip. Essentially, the pressure is perpendicular to the muscle fiber direction. The muscle fibers can be rolled in the grip to allow further examination of the tissues. An example of this technique includes a pincer grip of the upper trapezius muscle.

The patient should be positioned in a relaxed position with the muscle in optimal passive tension. This is a position between passive tension and slack and depends on the individual patient and muscle. The patient with neck pain or LBP is usually treated in the recumbent side lying, supine, or prone position depending on the muscle palpated and the tolerance of the patient for the specific position. Secondly, the patient position should assist in optimizing clinician ergonomics and less demanding palpation technique. Ultimately, the optimal position allows comfort for the patient, ease of

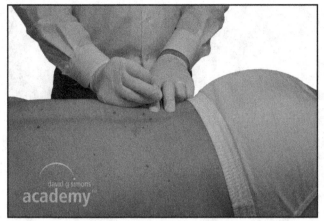

Figure 20-3. Trigger point dry needling: Lumbar superficial paraspinal muscles. (Reproduced with permission from David G. Simons Academy.)

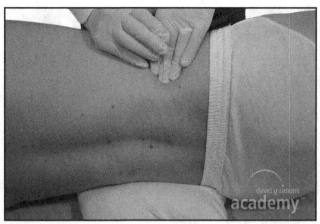

Figure 20-4. Trigger point dry needling: Quadratus lumborum. (Reproduced with permission from David G. Simons Academy.)

access, and allows the clinician to obtain the most useful information from the palpation process.[59]

The clinician palpates perpendicularly to the fibers of the muscle examined. This allows better identification of the taut band in comparison to the relatively relaxed surrounding muscle. The clinician should avoid pressing too deeply during this technique as the relative subtlety of the taut band to the surrounding muscle fibers can be reduced. The taut band is identified as a stiffer region compared to the surrounding muscle. The most sensitive part of the taut band is identified at the trigger point. This is, by definition, the spot tenderness on the taut band as previously described. The taut band will run in the direction of the muscle fibers. Muscle architecture can change depending on the part of the muscle palpated. As an example, consider the difference between the directions of the upper trapezius muscle fibers vs the lower trapezius muscle fibers. Comparison to the opposite side muscle, if asymptomatic, can be helpful.

When the trigger point is accurately located, it is then compressed with firm direct pressure using either the flat or pincer grip technique. The trigger point is compressed to a level that allows elicitation of referred pain or to the patient's tolerance. The muscle is compressed for approximately 15 seconds as it may take some time for the referred pain to arise. If the patient reports referred pain, the quality, nature, and location are discussed. Importantly, it is ascertained if the pain is familiar to the patient. Reproduction of recognized pain is essentially a pain provocation test.

PATHOGENESIS OF TRIGGER POINTS

The integrated hypothesis of trigger point formation by Simons and Travell is a theoretical framework for trigger point development.[28,60] The integrated hypothesis is supported and has been updated in light of new research from a combination of electrodiagnostic, imaging, and histopathologic studies.[60-64] A full review of the pathogenesis of trigger points is beyond the scope of this chapter. Readers are

encouraged to refer to the cited references for further expansion of the integrated hypothesis.

The integrated hypothesis postulates that muscle fiber motor endplates release excessive or sustain increased concentration of acetylcholine. This results in continued sarcomere contraction and subsequent sustained localized muscle fiber tension. Electromyography (EMG) studies have supported this part of the theory.[38,65-68] Another study, utilizing single-fiber EMG, revealed neuroaxonal degeneration and neuromuscular transmission disorders in patients with trigger points.[69] Subsequently, a study by the same authors using single-fiber EMG demonstrated a synaptic delay of motor endplates of motor units leading to suspicion of instability of neuromuscular transmission in the spinal accessory nerves innervating the trapezius muscles of patients.[70]

Stiffness of trigger points has been measured using sono-elastography and magnetic resonance imaging (MRI) elastography.[39-42,50,71,72] Sustained muscle fiber contraction can induce local metabolic demands leading to ischemia and hypoxia, which may activate muscle nociceptors and result in pain.[73-76] Furthermore, stiffened regions of active trigger points demonstrate highly resistive vascular areas when assessed by Doppler imaging.[40] Ultimately, the muscle metabolic stress may result in local fiber irritation, fiber degeneration, energy depletion, and the release of cytokines in the surrounding tissues.[76] This may result in pain and dysfunction of movement.

A study utilizing microdialysis of active trigger points demonstrated significantly increased concentrations of bradykinin, calcitonin gene-related peptide, tumour necrosis factor-α, interleukin-1β, substance P, serotonin, norepinephrine, and acidic conditions consistent with a lowered pH.[77-79] These substances can activate peripheral muscle nociceptors locally in the muscle. Peripheral sensitization of afferent nociceptor sensory nerves can activate dorsal horn neurons and central pain mechanisms.[76,80-83] Sustained nociceptive mechanical stimulation of latent trigger points has been shown to induce central sensitization in healthy participants.[84]

Muscle pain can apparently be inhibited strongly by descending pain modulation pathways, and this may explain in part why muscle pain responds to a broad base of treatment methods.[59,82,85-88]

Neuroimaging research demonstrates that hyperalgesia from trigger points in muscle is processed in similar brain regions as hyperalgesia from other pain conditions.[89,90] Patients with chronic MTrP pain exhibit, in contrast to controls, gray matter atrophy in dorsal and ventral prefrontal brain regions, but it remains unknown if this is associated with the ongoing pain state or peripheral nociceptive input.[91] Essentially, these regional brain changes are associated with areas involved in pain processing and pain modulation. Surprisingly, no evidence was found for the involvement of stress, as assessed by cortisol levels and anxiety questionnaires, in the trigger point participants.[91]

Clinically, trigger points predominately elicit pain[28,92] but may be associated with other sensory phenomena such as paraesthesia.[28,93] Sustained stimulation of latent trigger points in muscle can initiate central sensitization and the spread of pain.[84,94-96] Trigger points may lead to the development of pain and tenderness locally, regionally, and widely and can alter muscle activation patterns,[97,98] accelerate muscle fatigue,[99-101] induce cramp,[102-104] and alter neuromuscular reaction times.[105]

Despite compelling evidence supporting local mechanisms underlying trigger points,[34] the trigger point pathogenesis is still not fully understood.

ETIOLOGY OF TRIGGER POINTS

Different mechanisms have been postulated in the formation of trigger points. These include muscular overload, lifestyle and ergonomic factors, and the presence of metabolic and psychological factors.[27,28,63,106-108]

Trigger point-associated muscle pain is often activated by repeated acute or chronic muscular overload. Chronic muscular overload occurs particularly in postural dysfunctions or repetitive strain injuries.[28,88,109] Acute overloading of the skeletal muscles can be triggered by unaccustomed eccentric muscle work and maximal or submaximal concentric activity. Eccentric contractions cause an irregular and nonuniform extension of the muscle fibers. They result in damage to the cytoskeletal architecture after a short exposure. Eccentric and concentric training and trigger points are associated with local hypoxia. Local hypoxia can be explained by contraction-induced capillary constriction with hypoperfusion. As a result, there is a drop in the pH and release of cytokinins and neurovasoactive substances in the vicinity of trigger points.[77-79]

Metabolic conditions such as hormonal dysfunction and vitamin deficiencies may affect and influence muscle pain. In studies on patients with musculoskeletal pain and trigger points, pathologically altered serum values for vitamin B_{12}, iron, and vitamin D have been detected.[106] In most cases,

a deficiency of the respective vitamin or trace element was present. The extent to which such a deficiency directly affects the development of trigger points has not yet been clarified and further research is needed. Metabolic disorders or nutritional deficiencies are often overlooked or considered clinically nonrelevant.

Increased psychological stress can lead to muscle pain[82] and may also be a negative prognostic factor with treatment of patients with trigger points.[110]

MANAGEMENT OF SPINAL PAIN

Soft Tissue Manual Treatment Focusing on Trigger Points

Trigger Point Compression Release

TrPCR was previously termed *ischemic compression* and was one of the mainstay treatments for trigger points as described by Travell. The patient is appropriately positioned to optimize the target muscle relaxation and its passive tension. Depending on the muscle, various positions can be employed with the focus on the patient's comfort and the clinician's ability to deliver optimal treatment with good ergonomics. Superficial muscles are generally easy to palpate, whereas deep muscles may be challenging or limited in treatment. The muscle is palpated transverse to its muscle fibers or the clinician can use either pincer grip or flat palpation depending on the muscle. When the trigger point is identified, the clinician creates compression by manual palpation. The trigger point is compressed for 20 to 60 seconds.[111] Two techniques have been proposed: nonpainful low pressure for 90 seconds or a higher pain pressure for a shorter duration of 30 seconds.[112] It is usual to complete 3 repetitions. TrPCR may be mixed with stretching and various other techniques including postisometric relaxation (contract/relax), massage, or myofascial release.[28] TrPCR usually leads to an immediate increase in PPT over the muscle; this appears to be an internal reduction in sensitivity in the patient and not due to the reduction of palpation pressure by the clinician.[111] Clinicians need to remain cognizant of surrounding structures such as blood vessels, nerves, and organs to avoid adverse reactions.

Formal soft tissue therapy training in either undergraduate or graduate training or continuing education programs is indicated for clinical technique, knowledge, accuracy, efficiency, and safety.

Trigger Point Dry Needling

TrPDN is an invasive technique where a solid filament needle is inserted into the skin, fascia, and muscle to treat MTrPs. There are 2 main TrPDN techniques: superficial dry needling (SDN) and deep dry needling (DDN). SDN is the insertion of the needle into the skin and fascia overlying a trigger point and was described by UK physician Dr. Peter Baldry in the 1980s.[113,114] The main benefit of this treatment is increased safety in more complicated muscles being needled, such as the scalene, and reduction in posttreatment soreness. In the second technique (DDN), the needle is inserted directly into the muscle and trigger point, and the main aim of the treatment is to elicit LTRs by dynamic needling action. This dynamic technique is directly developed from the original anesthetic injection techniques as described by Travell.[115,116] In a survey of members of the Irish Society of Chartered Physiotherapists (n = 39; 7629 treatments) utilizing TrPDN, 82.7% of treatments were DDN and 17.3% of treatments were SDN.[117]

Originally, TrPDN developed from the intramuscular trigger point injection technique as described by Dr. Janet Travell.[26-28,115,116,118] Travell was influenced by her observations of intramuscular infiltration of local anesthetic into skeletal muscle and proposed that perhaps the physical dry needling technique was responsible for the observed therapeutic effect.[116,119] The first MEDLINE-cited article on dry needling was published by Lewitt in 1979.[119] This was an observatory cohort study of 241 patients with 312 pain sites treated by dry needling. Permanent relief of tenderness of the needled area was observed in 92 cases, relief for several months in 58 cases, several weeks in 63 cases, and for several days in 32 cases out of 288 pain sites followed up. Furthermore, the effectiveness of treatment was related to the intensity of the pain at the trigger point area and the precision of maximal tenderness located by the needle. It was proposed and later supported that the therapeutic effect of needling was related to the mechanical movement of the needle in the muscle and the elicitation of LTRs at trigger points as opposed to the anesthetic or pressure of the fluid injected.[116,119-121]

In more recent times, TrPDN has become popular among physical therapists, and training programs are now popular in many countries. Physical therapy education and training provide practitioners with the anatomy, basic sciences, and clinical foundation to train and employ TrPDN safely and effectively.[122] The first dedicated and authoritative TrPDN textbook was published in 2013.[108] There are varying different dry needling techniques, including TrPDN (SDN and DDN), radiculopathy, trigger point acupuncture, Western acupuncture, and spinal segmental sensitization models.[26,27,108,113-116,123-130]

There is evidence TrPDN is effective for the treatment of pain and dysfunction. Although TrPDN had demonstrated significant efficacy when compared to acupuncture, placebo studies are lacking.[121] Due to the invasive nature of dry needling, placebo trial design is challenging. One novel study demonstrated efficacy of TrPDN in the prevention of pain after total knee arthroplasty in a randomized, double-blinded, placebo-controlled trial.[131] Patients received TrPDN or sham group (no dry needling) while under anesthesia just before total knee replacement. A single double-blinded TrPDN treatment under anesthesia reduced pain in the first month after knee arthroplasty compared to the sham group.

The American Academy of Orthopaedic Manual Physical Therapists (AAOMPT) position statement on dry needling was issued in 2009:

Position: It is the Position of the AAOMPT Executive Committee that dry needling is within the scope of physical therapist practice.

Support statement: Dry needling is a neurophysiological evidence-based treatment technique that requires effective manual assessment of the neuromuscular system. Physical therapists are well trained to utilize dry needling in conjunction with manual physical therapy interventions. Research supports that dry needling improves pain control, reduces muscle tension, normalizes biochemical and electrical dysfunction of motor endplates, and facilitates an accelerated return to active rehabilitation.[132]

Clinicians require training in dry needling for accuracy, efficiency, and safety. Local state and federal laws and rules of scope of practice should be followed. National guidelines can be helpful as a framework for dry needling practice.[133] Because of the invasive nature of dry needling, it poses certain risks not associated with manual therapy. These include, but are not limited to, infection, bleeding and hematoma, and traumatic injury such as pneumothorax.[133-135] In a study of 7629 TrPDN treatments delivered by Irish physiotherapists, no significant adverse events were reported giving an estimated upper-risk rate (using Hanley's rule) for significant adverse events of less than or equal to 0.04%. Common minor adverse events included bruising (7.55%), bleeding (4.65%), pain during treatment (3.01%), and pain after treatment (2.19%). Uncommon adverse events included aggravation of symptoms (0.88%), drowsiness (0.26%), headache (0.14%), and nausea (0.13%). Rare adverse events included fatigue (0.04%), altered emotions (0.04%), shaking, itching, claustrophobia, and numbness (0.01%).[135] Significant adverse events appear to be rare, but have been reported in the literature including pneumothorax and cervical epidural hematoma.[136-138] Formal TrPDN training through continuing education programs is indicated for clinically applicable knowledge, accuracy, efficiency, and safety. The TrPDN techniques in this chapter are for demonstration purposes only and should only be carried out by qualified clinicians who are adequately trained.

TREATMENT

This section presents selected examples of TrPCR and TrPDN of the neck and low back muscles. The main aim in this section is to familiarize the reader with techniques. Practical training in soft tissue and dry needling techniques is required. It is recognized that there are many approaches and that individual clinicians will have varying skills and interests in application of soft tissue therapy. Mixing traditional massage techniques and TrPCR and/or dry needling can be considered. The Swiss combined approach, developed by Swiss physician Dr. Beat Dejung and also taught by the David G. Simons Academy, includes direct trigger point techniques and more general fascial release techniques.[139,140]

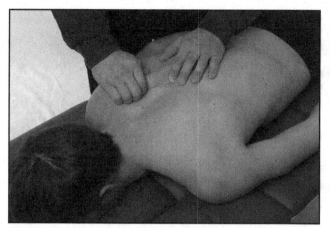

Figure 20-5. Trigger point compression release: Lower trapezius. (Reproduced with permission from David G. Simons Academy.)

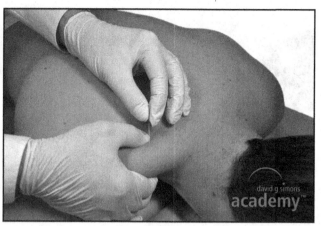

Figure 20-6. Trigger point dry needling: Upper trapezius. (Reproduced with permission from David G. Simons Academy.)

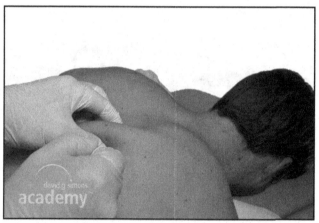

Figure 20-7. Trigger point dry needling: Lower trapezius. (Reproduced with permission from David G. Simons Academy.)

Techniques I and II include local TrPCR and manual stretching. Technique III includes broad manual release of the connective tissue and fascia around the trigger point, and technique IV is manual release of the connective tissue and fascia between 2 muscles (intramuscular mobilization).

It is judicious to also consider patient beliefs, experiences, and expectations in relation to chosen treatments. The addition of education, including pain sciences education, is important and can improve outcomes.[141] As per the guidelines reviewed, clinicians should employ multimodal treatment plans of care as part of the biopsychosocial model.

Prevalence studies indicate common muscles related to neck pain include, but are not limited to, trapezius (upper and lower), levator scapula, and posterior cervical muscles.[34] Data on the prevalence of trigger points in LBP are lacking[34]; however, one study reported quadratus lumborum, iliocostalis lumborum, and gluteus medius muscles were the most prevalent in patients with nonspecific LBP.[35]

SELECTED NECK MUSCLES

Trapezius

The trapezius is one of the most common muscles affected by myofascial pain. This muscle is expansive with 3 sections: upper, middle, and lower (Figures 20-2 and 20-5 through 20-7). It has extensive anatomical attachments from the head and neck, thoracic spine, scapula, and enveloping fascia. Commonly, it is involved in neck pain and tension including tension-type headache. The upper trapezius refers pain to the suprascapular region to the neck and into the head and face. The muscle is involved in direct and indirect movements and stability of the neck–shoulder girdle and upper extremity. The middle trapezius usually refers pain locally and is less common. The lower trapezius usually refers pain to the thoracic region, the suprascapular region, and to the side of the neck. The lower trapezius is a commonly involved area and is often treated for the relief of neck and suprascapular pain.

Positioning: Depending on the part of the muscle to be treated and the technique being used, the patient is treated in prone, side lying, sitting, or supine where the upper trapezius can be easily accessed. The arm is moved into a position allowing optimal passive tension to allow better quality palpation.

Procedure: The upper, middle, and lower part of the trapezius is palpated separately as the muscle fiber directions vary due to the angulation of the muscle. The muscle is superficial under the skin and is the first muscular layer. Flat palpation and pincer grip are used in varying ways to optimize manual treatment.

For TrPDN, a pincer grip is the preferred option for muscle control and also to avoid needling toward the lung. Examples of treatment are presented in Figures 20-2 and 20-5 through 20-7.

Levator Scapula

The levator scapula is an important muscle involved in neck suprascapular and scapular pain (Figures 20-8 through 20-10). It is a thin flat muscle that lies underneath the trapezius and arises from the upper medial angle of the scapula,

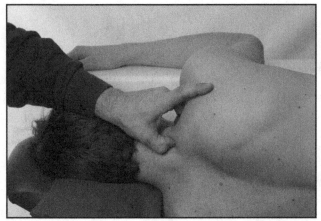

Figure 20-8. Trigger point compression release: Levator scapula. (Reproduced with permission from David G. Simons Academy.)

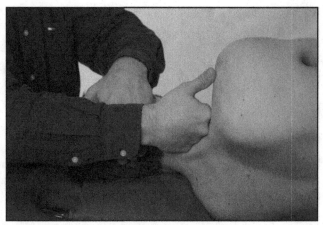

Figure 20-9. Manual myofascial release: Levator scapula. (Reproduced with permission from David G. Simons Academy.)

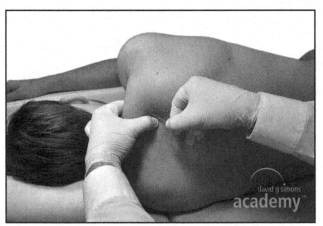

Figure 20-10. Trigger point dry needling: Levator scapula. (Reproduced with permission from David G. Simons Academy.)

attaching to the posterior upper transverse processes. It assists in elevation and downward rotation of the scapula and therefore is both a synergist and an antagonist to the upper trapezius, respectively. With the shoulder fixed, the levator scapula side flexes and rotates the cervical spine. Commonly, the muscle refers pain to the angle of the neck, into the suprascapular region, and scapular region and may be involved in postural syndromes. Furthermore, the muscle may be involved in shoulder dysfunction and clinically is important in subacromial pain syndrome of the shoulder. Often it is treated in conjunction with the trapezius and posterior neck muscles.

Positioning: The patient is treated in varying positions including prone and side lying. The scapula is positioned to place optimal tension on the levator scapula while allowing passive relaxation of the upper trapezius. The levator scapula is palpated through the expansive upper trapezius as it covers it.

Procedure: The muscle is identified as a firmer straplike muscle running upward from the upper medial angle of the scapula. Tenderness is identified along its course by pincer grip or flat palpation. With the pincer grip technique, pressure is placed across the muscle. Flat palpation pressure is applied directly onto the muscle to the ribs below.

For TrPDN, a pincer grip is the preferred option for muscle control and also to avoid needling toward the lung. Examples of treatment are presented in Figures 20-8 through 20-10.

Posterior Cervical Muscles

The posterior cervical muscles consist of 4 layers: (1) trapezius, (2) splenii, (3) semispinalis capitis, semispinalis cervicis, and (4) multifidus and rotatores (Figures 20-11 through 20-14). They form the shape of the back of the cervical area from the transverse process to the spinous process. These muscles assist in combined motions of the neck and stability of the cervical spine. They refer pain to the cervical spine, head, and face. The cervical multifidus commonly refers to the angle of the neck, suprascapular region, and interscapular region, where the referred pain is similar to levator scapula. The muscles are treated as a group.

Positioning: The patient is positioned in prone or side lying.

Procedure: The muscles group of layers 1 to 3 (trapezius, splenii, semispinalis capitis and semispinalis cervicis) are treated with a pincer grip locating the most tender area and applying manual pressure (see Figure 20-11). For the multifidus and rotatores (layer 4), the area of maximal tenderness is located along the cervical segment from C2 to the C7-T1 junction. Direct flat pressure palpation is applied at the tender segment(s) (see Figure 20-12). In reality, to access the multifidus and rotatores, the clinician applies pressure through the superficial layers of muscle (1 to 3) also.

For TrPDN, the superficial muscles of 1 to 3 are treated with a pincer grip technique (see Figure 20-13). For the deeper multifidus and rotatores, flat needling is applied directly medial and caudal, posterior to the transverse process toward the lamina of the cervical spine segment (see Figure 20-14).

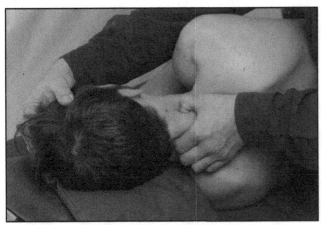

Figure 20-11. Trigger point compression release: Posterior cervical muscles superficial muscle layers with pincer grip treatment. (Reproduced with permission from David G. Simons Academy.)

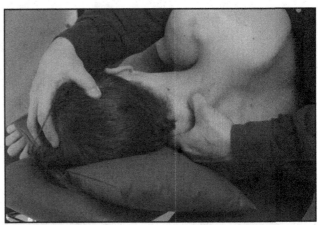

Figure 20-12. Trigger point compression release: Posterior cervical muscles deeper layer of the multifidus with flat palpation treatment. (Reproduced with permission from David G. Simons Academy.)

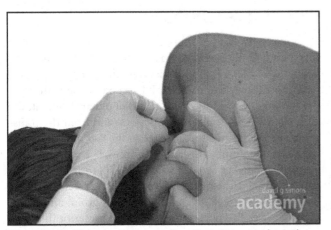

Figure 20-13. Trigger point dry needling: Posterior cervical muscle superficial layer with pincer grip palpation. (Reproduced with permission from David G. Simons Academy.)

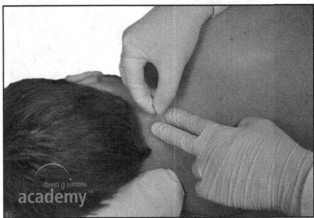

Figure 20-14. Trigger point dry needling: Posterior cervical muscle deeper layer of multifidus flat needling technique. (Reproduced with permission from David G. Simons Academy.)

SELECTED LOW BACK MUSCLES

Superficial and Deep Paraspinal Muscles

The paraspinal extensor muscles are clinically very important in LBP (Figures 20-1, 20-3, and 20-15). The superficial muscles consist of the lateral lying iliocostalis thoracis and lumborum and the more medial longissimus thoracis and semispinalis. The deeper paraspinal muscles consist mainly of the multifidus. The main function of the paraspinal muscles is to extend and assist in rotation of the spine and assist in stability of the thoracic and lumbar spine globally and segmentally. Clinically, the superficial muscles refer distally toward the low back and buttock area. It is important to note that the lower thoracic longissimus and iliocostalis referred distally over the lumbar spine, and it is important to assess these muscles in the lower thoracic area. The multifidus tends to refer locally in the thoracic and lumbar region. However, the L4-L5 S1 segment has a tendency to refer distally in the L4-L5 pattern in the buttock and thigh.[142]

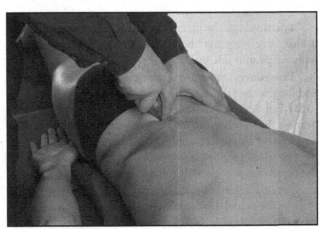

Figure 20-15. Trigger point compression release: Deep paraspinal muscles multifidus of the lumbar spine. (Reproduced with permission from David G. Simons Academy.)

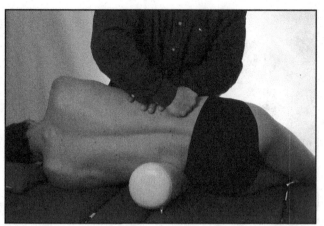

Figure 20-17. Myofascial release: Quadratus lumborum. (Reproduced with permission from David G. Simons Academy.)

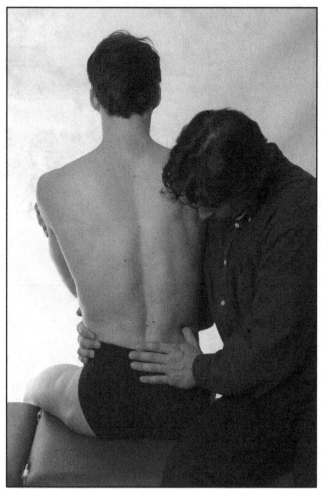

Figure 20-16. Trigger point compression release: Quadratus lumborum in sitting. This can also be carried out in side lying with direct flat palpation from fingers or thumb pressure similar to Figure 20-17. (Reproduced with permission from David G. Simons Academy.)

Positioning: The patient is usually positioned in prone if able. Side lying may be utilized as a secondary position with the painful side up.

Procedure: The superficial muscles of the iliocostalis and longissimus thoracis and iliocostalis lumborum are palpated transversely across the muscles to palpate for local tenderness. In the thoracic region, pressure is applied directly down or on the adjacent underlying rib. In the lumbar spine, the pressure is applied downward or slightly medial toward the transverse process and spinal column.

For the multifidus, this is palpated at the segmental level in the spinal groove between the spinous process and transverse process in both the thoracic and lumbar region. Pressure is applied directly to the muscle through the lumbodorsal fascia and superficial extensors.

Dry needling for the lumbar superficial paraspinal extensors is done directly into the muscle, keeping the needle posterior and medial to the transverse process. In the thoracic region, to reduce the risk of pneumothorax, a very oblique angle is used in a superior to inferior direction to avoid penetrating between the ribs and needling toward the lung.[108]

Quadratus Lumborum

Quadratus lumborum is a small, powerful deep muscle that is commonly overlooked as a source of LBP (Figures 20-4, 20-16, and 20-17). The muscle lies anterior to the superficial lumbar extensor muscles. It has 3 parts: the 12th rib to the top medial part of the ilia and iliolumbar ligament, the 12th rib to L1-L4 transverse processes, and from the transverse process of the lumbar spine to the top medial part of the ilia and iliolumbar ligament. The muscle acts as a lumbar extensor and flexor as well as a stabilizer of the lumbar spine and a hip hiker. The muscle has an extensive referral pattern over the gluteal area, lateral hip, anterior groin, and abdomen and may also refer to the lateral and posterior thigh.[143]

Positioning: The patient is usually treated in side lying for manual and dry needling, but may also be treated in sitting for manual only. Depending on the gap between the rib and the hip, a bolster may be required on the down side to open up the gap on the opposite side to allow optimum access to the muscle.

Procedure: Manual treatment is delivered by thumb or digit pressure directly toward the lumbar transverse processes, below the rib and above the ilium, anterior to the superficial lumbar extensor muscles. The muscle is palpated by direct pressure over the most tender area.

Dry needling technique is carried out with the similar approach to manual therapy aiming to needle toward but not medial to the transverse process. Needling underneath the rib in the vicinity of the L1 vertebrae and the 12th rib is avoided due to the risk of pneumothorax and also anterior into the peritoneum cavity.

Gluteus Medius/Minimus

The gluteus medius and minimus are important muscles for LBP and referred leg pain (Figures 20-18 through 20-20). The gluteus medius arises from the ilium and inserts into the greater trochanter. The gluteus maximus overlies the posterior portion of the gluteus medius about one-third way along

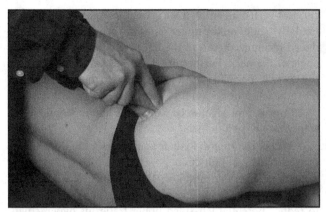

Figure 20-18. Trigger point compression release: Gluteus medius and minimus. (Reproduced with permission from David G. Simons Academy.)

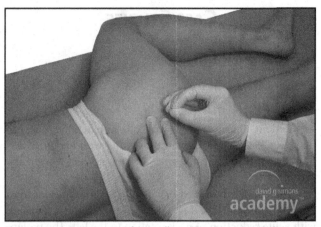

Figure 20-19. Trigger point dry needling: Gluteus medius and minimus posterior section. (Reproduced with permission from David G. Simons Academy.)

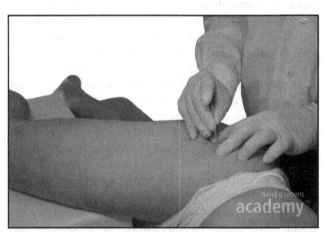

Figure 20-20. Trigger point dry needling: Gluteus medius and minimus anterior section. (Reproduced with permission from David G. Simons Academy.)

the posterior part of the ilium. The gluteus minimus attaches to the anterior portion of the ilium and lies underneath the gluteus medius. The gluteus medius refers pain to the lumbar area, gluteal area, and into the lateral hip and upper posterior thigh. The gluteus minimus, though smaller, has a more extensive referral pain pattern in the thigh and leg. The posterior gluteus minimus refers to the posterior thigh and leg, while the anterior gluteus minimus refers to the lateral hip, thigh, knee, and leg and sometimes to the foot. These muscles are important in abduction of the hip and stability of the hip and lower limb kinetic chain. The significance of these muscles cannot be overemphasized and should be routinely examined in patients presenting with LBP and lower limb disorders.

Positioning: Usually the patient is treated in side lying with the painful side superior. The patient is positioned comfortably, with the hips stacked or the limb can be placed on a bolster for support.

Procedure: With manual therapy, the gluteus medius muscle is palpated transverse to its fibers from the ilium to the trochanter. The gluteus medius is fan-shaped, and the posterior fibers will be more oblique and the anterior fibers less oblique and in a more superior/inferior direction. The muscle is palpated for tenderness and taut bands with direct pressure applied. For the gluteus medius, this is treated anteriorly and deep to the gluteus medius and in front of the iliotibial band through the tensor fascia lata.

Dry needling technique is direct flat needling into the muscle of gluteus medius and minimus needling toward the ilium. Needling below a line between the posterior superior iliac spine and trochanter is avoided due to the presence of the sciatic nerve.

CONCLUSION

MTrP pain is commonly seen in patients with neck and back pain. Myofascial pain can be primary or secondary, and patients should undergo a full regular orthopedic assessment to assist in differential diagnosis. The integrated hypothesis of trigger point formation has been postulated as a theoretical mechanism of myofascial pain from trigger point. Though there is some credible evidence to support the integrated hypothesis, a full understanding is still lacking. Myofascial pain can be diagnosed in certain accessible muscles by trigger point palpation. Palpation reliability is supported for certain muscles. Manual therapy and dry needling are 2 main treatment techniques employed to treat myofascial pain as part of multimodal therapy program, which usually will include exercise and education.

CASE STUDIES

Case Study One

Treatment of Myofascial Trigger Point Neck Pain

Patient characteristics and clinical details: The patient is a 35-year-old woman presenting with left-sided suprascapular pain from the angle of the neck out toward the acromion.

The patient described her pain as an intermittent low-grade tension and ache that at times can lead to muscle spasm with acute reduction of neck rotation to the left. The patient reported the pain can vary from 0/10 to a maximum of 6/10 on a Visual Analog Scale (VAS). This was aggravated by long periods of sitting, driving greater than 45 minutes, and with activities such as lifting heavy files from the shelf or hanging out clothes on the clothesline. She could get relief temporarily with anti-inflammatories and the use of a heat pack. The complaint started 3 months ago insidiously and was associated with an increased workload. The patient works in an office on a computer and telephone and at times requires simultaneous use of both. She does not use a headset. The patient had no medical conditions and no surgical history. She did have an ankle fracture 5 years previously from a fall and recovered with conservative treatment of an orthopedic cast and physiotherapy. The patient was single without children and reported sleeping well and not having significant stress in her life beyond a busy work schedule. She was carrying out aerobic exercise regularly and Pilates up to 3 months ago, but she got out of routine after work became busy. She denied headaches, dizziness, or upper limb symptoms. There were no noted red flags. Neck disability index: 34%.[144]

On examination: The patient was ambulating and transferring normally. Spinal levels were normal. ROM was normal apart from left side rotation where she had a deficit of approximately 10 degrees on the left compared the right. This caused tension-like discomfort in the left upper trapezius and angle of the neck. Passive elevation of the shoulder girdle (reducing upper trapezius length) improved ROM to normal and reduced discomfort. Upper extremity reflexes, manual muscle test, and touch sensitivity were normal. Screen of the left shoulder was normal for ROM, and the Hawkins Kennedy test was normal. Scarf test and acromioclavicular joint palpation were normal. Rotator cuff muscle testing was within normal limits and pain-free. The patient had weakness on upper and lower trapezius on the left compared to the right at 4/5 compared to 5/5 on the Oxford scale. There was some discomfort with the upper trapezius contraction on the left. She was not particularly tender over the cervical vertebrae and left was equal to right. She was particularly tender on the upper outer trapezius, and this reproduced recognized pain in the left suprascapular region and angle of the neck. Furthermore, she was very sensitive over the lower trapezius on the left compared to the right, and this reproduced some discomfort over the upper outer trapezius.

Impression: Myofascial pain of the left upper and lower trapezius.

Aim of treatment: Reduce pain, improve ROM, and improve strength and function.

Treatment: Education on MTrP pain. Discussed ergonomic aspect of work and recommended the use of a headset to reduce potential left-sided upper trapezius hyperactivity from holding the telephone while on the computer.

General exercise recommendations: Restart aerobic style activity in a progressive graded manner to increase central pain modulation for opioid and non-opioid exercise-induced hypoalgesia.

Therapeutic exercise home program: Regular shoulder roll exercises throughout the day to increase upper and lower trapezius perfusion. Chin tuck exercises for deep neck flexor activation. Gentle left-sided upper trapezius stretching exercises in a pain-free manner. Toward the end of her treatment program, the patient was prescribed scapular muscle strengthening exercises using elastic band and also dumbbells.

Manual therapy: TrPCR interspersed with soft tissue massage over the upper and lower trapezius. TrPDN to the left upper and lower trapezius with the elicitation of local twitch responses.

Modalities: Moist heat pre- and posttreatment. Interferential therapy for posttreatment discomfort. Education on supportive treatments.

Outcome: The patient had 6 sessions of physiotherapy over a 10-week treatment period. She had almost complete relief of her pain and was now reporting mostly 0/10 with very irregular 1/10 on VAS. Her neck disability index reduced from 34% to 8%.

The patient was treated with manual trigger point therapy to the left trapezius for one session; this was then coupled with dry needling for 5 sessions. The patient had some posttreatment soreness after the initial dry needling session for 1 to 2 days. She reported the relief after dry needling to be significant and her experience was very positive.

The patient was encouraged to continue with general aerobic activity as part of a healthy lifestyle. She was advised to continue with intermittent therapeutic exercises to maintain scapular and neck muscle strength. Advice and education was completed regarding work, and the patient found the addition of a headset beneficial.

Case Study Two

Treatment of Myofascial Trigger Point Low Back Pain

Patient characteristics and clinical details: The patient was a 60-year-old man who complained of LBP. The pain was located in the right-sided lumbar area radiating to the right-sided buttock. This was intermittent mild-to-moderate and undulating. It was made worse with longer periods of sitting and gardening for more than 1 hour or standing for longer periods. Driving for more than 30 minutes would aggravate him. Walking, lying down, and sleeping were comfortable. He found the use of moist heat and an anti-inflammatory helpful. His symptoms were present for 4 months and were not getting worse. He felt the pain was having a functional impact, and he scored 42% on the modified Oswestry back disability score at initial assessment.[145] He had retired from his teaching job 1 year previously and was walking regularly for at least 40 minutes 5 to 7 times a week. Since his retirement he was also gardening regularly as a hobby. He played golf mostly for the summer months, and this prompted him to attend physiotherapy because golfing season was starting, and he did not want to be limited by back pain. The patient reported attending his general practitioner and was prescribed anti-inflammatories and advice to stay active. He had an x-ray of his lumbar spine, in addition to blood tests. The x-ray showed degenerative joint disease, which was explained as age-related by his general practitioner. His blood tests were normal. He found the anti-inflammatories relieved pain temporarily but had no accumulated effect. The patient had high blood pressure and high cholesterol, and these were both under control along with medication and advice to walk and exercise regularly. There were no noted red flags.

The patient reported the pain initially started after gardening. There was no specific sudden onset; this just started several hours after a prolonged gardening session. The patient reported that in his mid-30s, he had several episodes of acute LBP that lasted less than 6 weeks and he recovered fully.

On examination: The patient was ambulating and transferring independently.

ROM in his low back was within normal limits with discomfort end of range left side flexion reproducing tightness and ache on the right side of the low back over the quadratus lumborum area. He did not have a preferential direction, and there was no centralization of his pain.[146] Extension rotation test was negative. Straight-leg raise was normal and 75 degrees bilaterally. Reflexes at the knees and ankle were normal. Myotomal resisted tests of the lower extremity revealed strength within normal limits. There was no sensory loss. Active straight-leg raise was normal. Hip quadrant test was pain-free with mild restriction of internal rotation at about 30 degrees bilaterally. Laslett's composite sacroiliac joint tests were negative.[147-149]

Palpation of his lumbar spine revealed exquisite tenderness over the right-sided quadratus lumborum that reproduced local pain in the right lumbar and buttock area that was familiar to the patient. Palpation of the right-sided gluteus medius was tender and led to radiated pain around the palpated area but no wider referral.

Further testing revealed single leg balance test reduced on the right compared to the left. Subsequent assessment of hip strength demonstrated right-sided gluteus medius weakness 4/5 on the Oxford scale. Further assessment with a hand-held dynamometer revealed weakness in the posterior gluteus medius on the right side compared to the left with a 25% deficit.

Impression: Myofascial pain of the right-sided quadratus lumborum with active trigger points. Latent trigger points in the right-sided gluteus medius.

Aim of treatment: Educated. Reduce pain in right-sided quadratus lumborum. Improve right-sided hip strength and balance.

Treatment: Education on LBP and MTrP pain and dysfunction. Educated to stay active.

General exercise recommendations: Continue with aerobic activity as tolerated to maintain and increase central pain modulation for opioid and non-opioid exercise-induced hypoalgesia.

Therapeutic exercise home program: The patient was prescribed right-sided gluteal muscle stretches. He was given targeted right-sided hip strengthening exercises for lateral hip muscles in standing abduction with 30 degrees extension to target posterior gluteus medius. He was given bilateral balance exercises with a bias on right side 2-1 repetitions. As he improved, he was prescribed double leg bridge, alternative arm and leg raise supermans, double leg squats, single leg squats, and good morning exercises (modified Romanian dead lifts).

Manual therapy: Targeted TrPCR interspersed with soft tissue massage over para vertebral muscles, quadratus lumborum, and gluteus medius. TrPDN of quadratus lumborum and gluteus medius, with the elicitation of local twitch responses.

Modalities: The patient was given moist heat pre-treatment and moist heat and interferential therapy posttreatment for posttreatment soreness.

Outcome: The patient had 6 sessions of physiotherapy and progressed well. He made substantial gains with the reduction in pain by 90%. His modified Oswestry scored reduced from 42% to 2% by the end of treatment. He was now playing golf pain-free and gardening in shorter bursts interspersed with aerobic exercise. The patient was discharged with a home exercise program to continue 2 to 3 times a week.

REFERENCES

1. International Association for the Study of Pain. *Neck Pain.* Author; 2009.

2. Hoy DG, Protani M, De R, Buchbinder R. The epidemiology of neck pain. *Best Pract Res Clin Rheumatol.* 2010;24(6):783-792.

3. Cohen SP. Epidemiology, diagnosis, and treatment of neck pain. *Mayo Clin Proc.* 2015;90(2):284-299.

4. International Association for the Study of Pain. International Association for the Study of Pain Taxonomy. Accessed 2017 from http://www.iasp-pain.org/Taxonomy?navItemNumber=576.

5. Hoy D, Brooks P, Blyth F, Buchbinder R. The Epidemiology of low back pain. *Best Pract Res Clin Rheumatol.* 2010;24(6):769-781.

6. Engel GL. The need for a new medical model: a challenge for biomedicine. *Science.* 1977;196(4286):129-136.

7. Boyling JD, Jull GA. The future scope of manual therapy. *Grieve's Modern Manual Therapy: The Vertebral Column.* Churchill Livingstone; 2004:xv, 643.

8. Engel GL. The need for a new medical model: a challenge for biomedicine. *Psychodyn Psychiatry.* 2012;40(3):377-396.

9. Sluka KA, International Association for the Study of Pain. *Mechanisms and Management of Pain for the Physical Therapist.* Wolters Kluwer; 2016.

10. Cicerone KD. Evidence-based practice and the limits of rational rehabilitation. *Arch Phys Med Rehabil.* 2005;86(6):1073-1074.

11. Ford JJ, Hahne AJ, Surkitt LD, et al. Individualised physiotherapy as an adjunct to guideline-based advice for low back disorders in primary care: a randomised controlled trial. *Br J Sports Med.* 2016;50(4):237-245. doi:10.1136/bjsports-2015-095058

12. Linde K, Witt CM, Streng A, et al. The impact of patient expectations on outcomes in four randomized controlled trials of acupuncture in patients with chronic pain. *Pain.* 2007;128(3):264-271.

13. Institute of Medicine. *Clinical Practice Guidelines We Can Trust.* National Academies Press; 2011.

14. National Institute for Health and Care Excellence. Accessed 2017. https://www.nice.org.uk/.

15. National Institute for Health and Care Excellence. *Neck Pain: Non-Specific.* Author; 2013.

16. National Institute for Health and Care Excellence. *Low Back Pain and Sciatica in Over 16s: Assessment and Management.* Author; 2016.

17. Furlan A, Tulder M, Cherkin D, et al. Acupuncture and dry-needling for low back pain: an updated systematic review within the framework of the Cochrane Collaboration. *Spine.* 2005;30(8):944-963.

18. Furlan AD, Imamura M, Dryden T, Irvin E. Massage for low back pain: an updated systematic review within the framework of the Cochrane Back Review Group. *Spine (Phila Pa 1976).* 2009;34(16):1669-1684.

19. Furlan AD, Giraldo M, Baskwill A, Irvin E, Imamura M. Massage for low-back pain. *Cochrane Database Syst Rev.* 2015;9: CD001929.

20. Patel KC, Gross A, Graham N, et al. Massage for mechanical neck disorders. *Cochrane Database Syst Rev.* 2012;9:CD004871.

21. Trinh K, Graham N, Irnich D, Cameron ID, Forget M. Acupuncture for neck disorders. *Cochrane Database Syst Rev.* 2016;5:CD004870.

22. Trinh K, Graham N, Irnich D, Cameron ID, Forget M. Withdrawn: acupuncture for neck disorders. *Cochrane Database Syst Rev.* 2016;11:CD004870.

23. Gattie E, Cleland JA, Snodgrass S. The effectiveness of trigger point dry needling for musculoskeletal conditions by physical therapists: a systematic review and meta-analysis. *J Orthop Sports Phys Ther.* 2017;47(3):133-149.

24. Cerezo-Tellez E, Torres-Lacomba M, Fuentes-Gallardo I, et al. Effectiveness of dry needling for chronic nonspecific neck pain: a randomized, single-blinded, clinical trial. *Pain.* 2016;157(9):1905-1917.

25. Sherman KJ, Dixon MW, Thompson D, Cherkin DC. Development of a taxonomy to describe massage treatments for musculoskeletal pain. *BMC Complement Altern Med.* 2006;6:24.

26. Travell JG, Simons DG. *Myofascial Pain and Dysfunction: The Trigger Point Manual.* Williams & Wilkins; 1983.

27. Travell JG, Simons DG. *Myofascial Pain and Dysfunction: The Trigger Point Manual.* Williams & Wilkins; 1992.

28. Simons DG, Travell JG, Simons LS. *Travell and Simons' Myofascial Pain and Dysfunction: The Trigger Point Manual.* Williams & Wilkins; 1999.

29. Fischer AA. Pressure threshold measurement for diagnosis of myofascial pain and evaluation of treatment results. *Clin J Pain.* 1986;2(4):207-214.

30. Fischer AA. Pressure threshold meter: its use for quantification of tender spots. *Arch Phys Med Rehabil.* 1986;67:836-838.

31. Fischer AA. Pressure tolerance over muscles and bones in normal subjects. *Arch Phys Med Rehabil.* 1986;67:406-409.

32. Fischer AA. Reliability of the pressure algometer as a measure of myofascial trigger point sensitivity [letter]. *Pain.* 1987;28(3):411-414.

33. Moraska AF, Schmiege SJ, Mann JD, Butryn N, Krutsch JP. Responsiveness of myofascial trigger points to single and multiple trigger point release massages: a randomized, placebo controlled trial. *Am J Phys Med Rehabil.* 2017;96(9):639-645.

34. Lluch E, Nijs J, De Kooning M, et al. Prevalence, incidence, localization, and pathophysiology of myofascial trigger points in patients with spinal pain: a systematic literature review. *J Manipulative Physiol Ther.* 2015;38(8):587-600.

35. Iglesias-Gonzalez JJ, Munoz-Garcia MT, Rodrigues-de-Souza DP, Alburquerque-Sendin F, Fernandez-de-Las-Penas C. Myofascial trigger points, pain, disability, and sleep quality in patients with chronic nonspecific low back pain. *Pain Med.* 2013.

36. Gerwin RD, Shannon S, Hong CZ, Hubbard D, Gevirtz R. Interrater reliability in myofascial trigger point examination. *Pain.* 1997;69(1-2):65-73.

37. McEvoy J, Huijbregts P. Reliability of myofascial trigger point palpation: a systematic review. In: Dommerholt J, Huijbregts P, eds. *Myofascial Trigger Points: Pathophysiology and Evidenced-Informed Diagnosis and Management.* Sudbury, Jones and Bartlett; 2011.

38. Simons DG, Hong CZ, Simons LS. Endplate potentials are common to midfiber myofacial trigger points. *Am J Phys Med Rehabil.* 2002;81(3):212-222.

39. Sikdar S, Shah JP, Gilliams E, Gebreab T, Gerber LH. Assessment of myofascial trigger points (MTrPs): a new application of ultrasound imaging and vibration sonoelastography. *Conf Proc IEEE Eng Med Biol Soc.* 2008;2008:5585-5588.

40. Sikdar S, Shah JP, Gebreab T, et al. Novel applications of ultrasound technology to visualize and characterize myofascial trigger points and surrounding soft tissue. *Arch Phys Med Rehabil.* 2009;90(11):1829-1838.

41. Ballyns JJ, Shah JP, Hammond J, Gebreab T, Gerber LH, Sikdar S. Objective sonographic measures for characterizing myofascial trigger points associated with cervical pain. *J Ultrasound Med.* 2011;30(10):1331-1340.

42. Ballyns JJ, Turo D, Otto P, et al. Office-based elastographic technique for quantifying mechanical properties of skeletal muscle. *J Ultrasound Med.* 2012;31(8):1209-1219.

43. Shankar H, Reddy S. Two- and three-dimensional ultrasound imaging to facilitate detection and targeting of taut bands in myofascial pain syndrome. *Pain Med.* 2012;13(7):971-975.

44. Barbero M, Cescon C, Tettamanti A, et al. Myofascial trigger points and innervation zone locations in upper trapezius muscles. *BMC Musculoskelet Disord.* 2013;14:179.

45. Muro-Culebras A, Cuesta-Vargas AI. Sono-myography and sono-myoelastography of the tender points of women with fibromyalgia. *Ultrasound Med Biol.* 2013;39(11):1951-1957.

46. Thomas K, Shankar H. Targeting myofascial taut bands by ultrasound. *Curr Pain Headache Rep.* 2013;17(7):349.

47. Turo D, Otto P, Shah JP, et al. Ultrasonic characterization of the upper trapezius muscle in patients with chronic neck pain. *Ultrason Imaging.* 2013;35(2):173-187.

48. Muller CE, Aranha MF, Gaviao MB. Two-dimensional ultrasound and ultrasound elastography imaging of trigger points in women with myofascial pain syndrome treated by acupuncture and electroacupuncture: a double-blinded randomized controlled pilot study. *Ultrason Imaging.* 2015;37(2):152-167.

49. Turo D, Otto P, Hossain M, et al. Novel use of ultrasound elastography to quantify muscle tissue changes after dry needling of myofascial trigger points in patients with chronic myofascial pain. *J Ultrasound Med.* 2015;34(12):2149-2161.

50. Chen Q, Wang HJ, Gay RE, et al. Quantification of myofascial taut bands. *Arch Phys Med Rehabil.* 2016;97(1):67-73.

51. Nice DA, Riddle DL, Lamb RL, Mayhew TP, Rucker K. Intertester reliability of judgments of the presence of trigger points in patients with low back pain. *Arch Phys Med Rehabil.* 1992;73(10):893-898.

52. Wolfe F, Simons DG, Fricton J, et al. The fibromyalgia and myofascial pain syndromes: a preliminary study of tender points and trigger points in persons with fibromyalgia, myofascial pain syndrome and no disease. *J Rheumatol.* 1992;19(6):944-951.

53. Njoo KH, Van der Does E. The occurrence and inter-rater reliability of myofascial trigger points in the quadratus lumborum and gluteus medius: a prospective study in non-specific low back pain patients and controls in general practice. *Pain.* 1994;58(3):317-323.

54. Lew PC, Lewis J, Story I. Inter-therapist reliability in locating latent myofascial trigger points using palpation. *Manual Ther.* 1997;2(2):87-90.

55. Hsieh CY, Hong CZ, Adams AH, et al. (2000). Interexaminer reliability of the palpation of trigger points in the trunk and lower limb muscles. *Arch Phys Med Rehabil.* 2000;81(3):258-264.

56. Sciotti VM, Mittak VL, DiMarco L, et al. Clinical precision of myofascial trigger point location in the trapezius muscle. *Pain.* 2001;93(3):259-266.

57. Bron C, Franssen J, Wensing M, Oostendorp RA. Interrater reliability of palpation of myofascial trigger points in three shoulder muscles. *J Manual Manipulative Ther.* 2007;15(4):203-215.

58. Al-Shenqiti AM, Oldham JA. Test-retest reliability of myofascial trigger point detection in patients with rotator cuff tendonitis. *Clin Rehabil.* 2005;19(5):482-487.

59. McEvoy JJ. Dommerholt Myofascial trigger point of the shoulder. In: Donatelli R, ed. *Physical Therapy of the Shoulder.* Elsevier Churchill Livingstone; 2012:351-380.

60. Simons DG. Review of enigmatic MTrPs as a common cause of enigmatic musculoskeletal pain and dysfunction. *J Electromyogr Kinesiol.* 2004;14:95-107.

61. Gerwin RD, Dommerholt J, Shah JP. An expansion of Simons' integrated hypothesis of trigger point formation. *Curr Pain Headache Rep.* 2004;8(6):468-475.

62. McPartland JM. Travell trigger points—molecular and osteopathic perspectives. *J Am Osteopath Assoc.* 2004;104(6):244-249.

63. Dommerholt J, Bron C, Franssen JLM. Myofascial trigger points: an evidence-informed review. *J Manual Manipulative Ther.* 2006;14(4):203-221.

64. McPartland JM, Simons DG. Myofascial trigger points: translating molecular theory into manual therapy. *J Man Manipulative Ther.* 2006;14(4):232-239.

65. Simons DG, Hong CZ, Simons L. Prevalence of spontaneous electrical activity at trigger spots and control sites in rabbit muscle. *J Musculoskeletal Pain.* 1995;3:35-48.

66. Simons DG, Hong CZ, Simons LS. Nature of myofascial trigger points, active loci (abstract). *J Musculoskeletal Pain.* 1995;3(Suppl 1):62.

67. Simons DG, Hong CZ, Simons LS. Spike activity in trigger points. *J Musculoskeletal Pain.* 1995;3(Suppl 1):125.

68. Hong CZ, Simons DG. Pathophysiologic and electrophysiologic mechanisms of myofascial trigger points. *Arch Phys Med Rehabil.* 1998;79(7):863-872.

69. Chang CW, Chen YR, Chang KF. Evidence of neuroaxonal degeneration in myofascial pain syndrome: a study of neuromuscular jitter by axonal microstimulation. *Eur J Pain.* 2008.

70. Chang CW, Chang KY, Chen YR, Kuo PL. Electrophysiologic evidence of spinal accessory neuropathy in patients with cervical myofascial pain syndrome. *Arch Phys Med Rehabil.* 2011;92(6):935-940.

71. Chen Q, Bensamoun S, Basford JR, Thompson JM, An KN. Identification and quantification of myofascial taut bands with magnetic resonance elastography. *Arch Phys Med Rehabil.* 2007;88(12):1658-1661.

72. Adigozali H, Shadmehr A, Ebrahimi E, Rezasoltani A, Naderi F. Reliability of assessment of upper trapezius morphology, its mechanical properties and blood flow in female patients with myofascial pain syndrome using ultrasonography. *J Bodyw Mov Ther.* 2017;21(1):35-40.

73. Mense S, Stahnke M. Responses in muscle afferent fibres of slow conduction velocity to contractions and ischaemia in the cat. *J Physiol.* 1983;342:383-397.

74. Strobel ES, Krapf M, Suckfull M, Bruckle W, Fleckenstein W, Muller W. Tissue oxygen measurement and 31P magnetic resonance spectroscopy in patients with muscle tension and fibromyalgia. *Rheumatol Int.* 1997;16(5):175-180.

75. Graven-Nielsen T, Mense S. The peripheral apparatus of muscle pain: evidence from animal and human studies. *Clin J Pain.* 2001;17(1):2-10.

76. Mense S, Gerwin RD. *Muscle Pain: Understanding the Mechanisms.* Springer-Verlag; 2010.

77. Shah JP, Phillips TM, Danoff JV, Gerber LH. An in-vivo microanalytical technique for measuring the local biochemical milieu of human skeletal muscle. *J Appl Physiol.* 2005;99:1980-1987.

78. Shah JP, Danoff JV, Desai MJ, et al. Biochemicals associated with pain and inflammation are elevated in sites near to and remote from active myofascial trigger points. *Arch Phys Med Rehabil.* 2008;89(1):16-23.

79. Shah JP, Gilliams EA. Uncovering the biochemical milieu of myofascial trigger points using in vivo microdialysis: an application of muscle pain concepts to myofascial pain syndrome. *J Bodyw Mov Ther.* 2008;12(4):371-384.

80. Hoheisel U, Mense S, Simons D, Yu X-M. Appearance of new receptive fields in rat dorsal horn neurons following noxious stimulation of skeletal muscle: a model for referral of muscle pain? *Neurosci Lett.* 1993;153:9-12.

81. Hoheisel U, Koch K, Mense S. Functional reorganization in the rat dorsal horn during an experimental myositis. *Pain.* 1994;59(1):111-118.

82. Mense S, Simons DG, Russell IJ. *Muscle Pain: Understanding Its Nature, Diagnosis, and Treatment.* Lippincott Williams & Wilkins; 2001.

83. Graven-Nielsen T, Arendt-Nielsen L. Peripheral and central sensitization in musculoskeletal pain disorders: an experimental approach. *Curr Rheumatol Rep.* 2002;4(4):313-321.

84. Xu YM, Ge HY, Arendt-Nielsen L. Sustained nociceptive mechanical stimulation of latent myofascial trigger point induces central sensitization in healthy subjects. *J Pain.* 2010;11(12):1348-1355.

85. Mense S. Descending antinociception and fibromyalgia. *Z Rheumatol.* 1998;57(Suppl 2):23-26.

86. Mense S. (2000). Neurobiological concepts of fibromyalgia—the possible role of descending spinal tracts. *Scand J Rheumatol.* 2000;Suppl 113:24-29.

87. Mense S. The pathogenesis of muscle pain. *Curr Pain Headache Rep.* 2003;7(6):419-425.

88. Dommerholt J, McEvoy J. *Myofascial Trigger Point Approach. Orthopaedic Manual Physical Therapy: From Art to Evidence.* FA Davis; 2015.

89. Niddam DM, Chan RC, Lee SH, Yeh TC, Hsieh JC. Central representation of hyperalgesia from myofascial trigger point. *Neuroimage.* 2008;39(3):1299-1306.

90. Niddam DM. Brain manifestation and modulation of pain from myofascial trigger points. *Curr Pain Headache Rep.* 2009;13(5):370-375.

91. Niddam DM, Lee SH, Su YT, Chan RC. Brain structural changes in patients with chronic myofascial pain. *Eur J Pain.* 2017;21(1):148-158.

92. Travell JG, Rinzler SH. The myofascial genesis of pain. *Postgrad Med.* 1952;11:452-434.

93. Oh S, Kim HK, Kwak J, et al. Causes of hand tingling in visual display terminal workers. *Ann Rehabil Med.* 2013;37(2):221-228.

94. Mense S. [Pathophysiology of low back pain and the transition to the chronic state - experimental data and new concepts]. *Schmerz.* 2001;15(6):413-417.

95. Giamberardino MA. Referred muscle pain/hyperalgesia and central sensitisation. *J Rehabil Med.* 2003;(41 Suppl):85-88.

96. Hidalgo-Lozano A, Fernandez-de-las-Penas C, Alonso-Blanco C, Ge HY, Arendt-Nielsen L, Arroyo-Morales M. Muscle trigger points and pressure pain hyperalgesia in the shoulder muscles in patients with unilateral shoulder impingement: a blinded, controlled study. *Exp Brain Res.* 2010;202(4):915-925.

97. Lucas KR. The impact of latent trigger points on regional muscle function. *Curr Pain Headache Rep.* 2008;12(5):344-349.

98. Lucas KR, Rich PA, Polus BI. Muscle activation patterns in the scapular positioning muscles during loaded scapular plane elevation: the effects of latent myofascial trigger points. *Clin Biomech (Bristol, Avon).* 2010;25(8):765-770.

99. Ge HY, Arendt-Nielsen L, Madeleine P. Accelerated muscle fatigability of latent myofascial trigger points in humans. *Pain Med.* 2012;13(7):957-964.

100. Wang YH, Yin MJ, Fan ZZ, Arendt-Nielsen L, Ge HY, Yue SW. Hyperexcitability to electrical stimulation and accelerated muscle fatiguability of taut bands in rats. *Acupunct Med.* 2014;32(2):172-177.

101. Yu SH, Kim HJ. Electrophysiological characteristics according to activity level of myofascial trigger points. *J Phys Ther Sci.* 2015;27(9):2841-2843.

102. Prateepavanich P, Kupniratsaikul V, Charoensak T. The relationship between myofascial trigger points of gastrocnemius muscle and nocturnal calf cramps. *J Med Assoc Thai.* 1999;82(5):451-459.

103. Ge HY, Zhang Y, Boudreau S, Yue SW, Arendt-Nielsen L. Induction of muscle cramps by nociceptive stimulation of latent myofascial trigger points. *Exp Brain Res.* 2008;187(4):623-629.

104. Vas L, Pai R, Khandagale N, Pattnaik M. Myofascial trigger points as a cause of abnormal cocontraction in writer's cramp. *Pain Med.* 2015;16(10):2041-2045.

105. Yassin M, Talebian S, Ebrahimi Takamjani I, et al. The effects of arm movement on reaction time in patients with latent and active upper trapezius myofascial trigger point. *Med J Islam Repub Iran.* 2015;29:295.

106. Gerwin RD. A review of myofascial pain and fibromyalgia—factors that promote their persistence. *Acupunct Med.* 2005;23(3):121-134.

107. Dommerholt J, Huijbregts P. *Myofascial Trigger Points: Pathophysiology and Evidence-Informed Diagnosis and Management.* Jones and Bartlett Publishers; 2011.

108. Dommerholt J, Fernandez de las Penas C. *Trigger Point Dry Needling: An Evidenced and Clinical Based Approach.* Churchill Livingstone; 2013.

109. Visser B, van Dieen JH. Pathophysiology of upper extremity muscle disorders. *J Electromyogr Kinesiol.* 2006;16(1):1-16.

110. Huang YT, Lin SY, Neoh CA, Wang KY, Jean YH, Shi HY. Dry needling for myofascial pain: prognostic factors. *J Altern Complement Med.* 2011;17(8):755-762.

111. Fryer G, Hodgson L. The effect of manual pressure release on myofascial trigger points in the upper trapezius muscle. *J Bodywork Movement Ther.* 2005;9(4):248-255.

112. Hou CR, Tsai LC, Cheng KF, Chung KC, Hong CZ. Immediate effects of various physical therapeutic modalities on cervical myofascial pain and trigger-point sensitivity. *Arch Phys Med Rehabil.* 2002;83(10):1406-1414.

113. Baldry P. Superficial versus deep dry needling. *Acupunct Med.* 2002;20(2-3):78-81.

114. Baldry PE. *Acupuncture, Trigger Points and Musculoskeletal Pain.* Churchill Livingstone; 2005.

115. Travell J. Basis for the multiple uses of local block of somatic trigger areas (procaine infiltration and ethyl chloride spray). *Miss Valley Med.* 1949;71:13-22.

116. Travell J. *Office Hours: Day and Night. The Autobiography of Janet Travell, MD.* World Publishing; 1968.

117. Brady S, McEvoy J, Dommerholt J, Doody C. *Adverse Events following Trigger Point Dry Needling: A Prospective Survey of Chartered Physiotherapists.* 2012.

118. Travell JG, Rinzler S, Herman M. Pain and disability of the shoulder and arm: treatment by intramuscular infiltration with procaine hydrochloride. *JAMA.* 1942;120:417-422.

119. Lewit K. The needle effect in the relief of myofascial pain. *Pain.* 1979;6(1):83-90.

120. Hong CZ. Lidocaine injection versus dry needling to myofascial trigger point. The importance of the local twitch response. *Am J Phys Med Rehabil.* 1994;73(4):256-263.

121. Cummings TM, White AR. Needling therapies in the management of myofascial trigger point pain: a systematic review. *Arch Phys Med Rehabil.* 2001;82(7):986-992.

122. Halle JS, Halle RJ. Pertinent dry needling considerations for minimizing adverse effects - part one. *Int J Sports Phys Ther.* 2016;11(4):651-662.

123. Gunn CC. *The Gunn Approach to the Treatment of Chronic Pain.* Churchill Livingstone; 1997.

124. Fischer A. New injection techniques for treatment of musculoskeletal pain. In: Rachlin ES, Rachlin IS, eds. *Myofascial Pain and Fibromyalgia - Trigger Point Management.* Mosby; 2002:403-419.

125. Itoh K, Katsumi Y, Kitakoji H. Trigger point acupuncture treatment of chronic low back pain in elderly patients—a blinded RCT. *Acupunct Med.* 2004;22(4):170-177.

126. Dommerholt J, Mayoral O, Gröbli C. Trigger point dry needling. *J Manual Manipulative Ther.* 2006;14(4): E70-E87.

127. Itoh K, Katsumi Y, Hirota S, Kitakoji H. Effects of trigger point acupuncture on chronic low back pain in elderly patients—a sham-controlled randomised trial. *Acupunct Med.* 2006;24(1):5-12.

128. Itoh K, Katsumi Y, Hirota S, Kitakoji H. Randomised trial of trigger point acupuncture compared with other acupuncture for treatment of chronic neck pain. *Complement Ther Med.* 2007;15(3):172-179.

129. White A, Cummings TM, Filshie J. *An Introduction to Western Medical Acupuncture.* Churchill Livingstone/Elsevier; 2008.

130. Itoh K, Hirota S, Katsumi Y, Ochi H, Kitakoji H. Trigger point acupuncture for treatment of knee osteoarthritis—a preliminary RCT for a pragmatic trial. *Acupunct Med.* 2008;26(1):17-26.

131. Mayoral O, Salvat I, Martin MT, et al. Efficacy of myofascial trigger point dry needling in the prevention of pain after total knee arthroplasty: a randomized, double-blinded, placebo-controlled trial. *Evid Based Complement Alternat Med.* 2013;2013:694941.

132. AAOMPT. AAOMPT Position Statements - Dry Needling. Published 2009. Accessed May 22, 2017. http://aaompt.org/Main/About_Us/Position_Statements/Main/About_Us/Position_Statements.aspx?hkey=03f5a333-f28d-4715-b355-cb25fa9bac2c.

133. *ISCP Guidelines for Dry Needling Practice.* Irish Society of Chartered Physiotherapists; 2012.

134. McEvoy J. Trigger point dry needling: safety guidelines. In: Dommerholt J, Fernandez de las Penas C, eds. *Trigger Point Dry Needling: An Evidenced and Clinical Based Approach.* Churchill Livingstone; 2013.

135. Brady S, McEvoy J, Dommerholt J, Doody C. Adverse events following trigger point dry needling: a prospective survey of chartered physiotherapists. *J Man Manip Ther.* 2014;22(3):134-140.

136. Lee JH, Lee H, Jo DJ. An acute cervical epidural hematoma as a complication of dry needling. *Spine (Phila Pa 1976).* 2011;36(13):E891-893.

137. Cummings M, Ross-Marrs R, Gerwin R. Pneumothorax complication of deep dry needling demonstration. *Acupunct Med.* 2014;32(6):517-519.

138. Ronconi G, De Giorgio F, Ricci E, Maggi L, Spagnolo AG, Ferrara PE. [Pneumothorax following dry needling treatment: legal and ethical aspects]. *Ig Sanita Pubbl.* 2016;72(5):505-512.

139. Dejung B, Gröbli C, Colla F, Weissmann R. *Triggerpunkttherapie.* Hans Huber; 2003.

140. DGSA. Manual trigger point therapy: the general trigger point therapy. Accessed May 18, 2017. http://www.dgs-academy.com/en/trigger-point-therapy/manual-trigger-point-therapy/

141. Tellez-Garcia M, de-la-Llave-Rincon AI, Salom-Moreno J, Palacios-Cena M, Ortega-Santiago R, Fernandez-de-Las-Penas C. Neuroscience education in addition to trigger point dry needling for the management of patients with mechanical chronic low back pain: a preliminary clinical trial. *J Bodyw Mov Ther.* 2015;19(3):464-472.

142. Cornwall J, Harris AJ, Mercer SR. The lumbar multifidus muscle and patterns of pain. *Man Ther.* 2006;11(1):40-45.

143. Tucker KJ, Fels M, Walker SR, Hodges PW. Comparison of location, depth, quality, and intensity of experimentally induced pain in 6 low back muscles. *Clin J Pain.* 2014;30(9):800-808.

144. Vernon H, Mior S. The Neck Disability Index: a study of reliability and validity. *J Manipulative Physiol Ther.* 1991;14(7):409-415.

145. Fritz JM, Irrgang JJ. A comparison of a modified Oswestry Low Back Pain Disability Questionnaire and the Quebec Back Pain Disability Scale. *Phys Ther.* 2001;81(2):776-788.

146. Laslett M, Oberg B, Aprill CN, McDonald B. Centralization as a predictor of provocation discography results in chronic low back pain, and the influence of disability and distress on diagnostic power. *Spine J.* 2005;5(4):370-380.

147. Laslett M, Aprill CN, McDonald B, Young SB. Diagnosis of sacroiliac joint pain: validity of individual provocation tests and composites of tests. *Man Ther.* 2005;10(3):207-218.

148. Laslett M. Pain provocation tests for diagnosis of sacroiliac joint pain. *Aust J Physiother.* 2006;52(3):229.

149. Laslett M, Aprill CN, McDonald B. Provocation sacroiliac joint tests have validity in the diagnosis of sacroiliac joint pain. *Arch Phys Med Rehabil.* 2006;87(6):874; author reply 874-875.

21

Yoga for Musculoskeletal Conditions

An Overview and Summary of Evidence

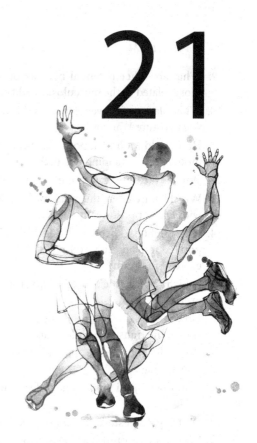

Beth Stone Norris, PhD, PT, OCS, E-RYT 500

KEY TERMS

Asanas: Physical postures performed as a component of yoga practice.

Complementary and alternative medicine (CAM): Non-mainstream therapeutic practices and products that are used in conjunction with conventional medicine.

Dharana: Concentration by fixing the mind on an external object or internal sensation.

Hatha yoga: A style of yoga commonly practiced in the United States and includes physical postures, breathing, concentration or meditation, and mindfulness.

Pranayama: Breath control practices and exercises performed as a component of yoga practice.

Yoga: A mind-body practice that incorporates physical, mental, emotional, and spiritual aspects of health.

CHAPTER QUESTIONS

1. What is the translation of the word "yoga"?
2. How does the mind-body philosophy of yoga compare to the biopsychosocial approach used in the management of subacute and chronic musculoskeletal disorders?
3. When is yoga said to originate?
4. Yoga is most commonly thought to consist of physical postures or poses, which is one of the 8 "limbs" of yoga. What are the 7 other "limbs" of yoga?
5. What is the limb of yoga that focuses on breath control?
6. How can yoga props be used to modify yoga postures to accommodate individuals of differing abilities?
7. What criteria can be used to identify a qualified yoga instructor?
8. How does alignment-based cueing assist in the attainment of steadiness and ease in a yoga posture?

Wallmann HW, Donatelli R, eds. *Foundations of Orthopedic Physical Therapy* (pp 633-662).
© 2024 Taylor & Francis Group.

9. What are other potential benefits of yoga other than those related to the musculoskeletal system?

10. What planes of movement are utilized in the standing yoga posture Warrior I?

11. How could Mountain pose (Tadasana) be used to promote optimal standing posture?

12. What is the importance of utilization of dristhti?

13. Which muscle length impairments may be addressed with Dancer posture?

14. How might backbend postures such as Sphinx be incorporated into an extension-based directional preference exercise program?

15. Which "energy lock" used in yoga is similar to Kegel exercises?

16. How might Uddiyana banda be used to promote activation of the transverse abdominis?

17. What is the 3-part breath used when teaching pranayama?

18. How does Ujjayi pranayama differ from Alternate nostril breathing?

19. Which yoga postures are considered inversions?

20. Which yoga postures can be used to promote relaxation?

Objectives

- Understand the origins of the practice of yoga in the United States.
- Identify the 8 limbs of yoga.
- Describe the main components of Hatha yoga practice.
- Identify categories of yoga postures and the musculoskeletal emphasis and alignment focus of each.
- Provide examples of yoga postures for each posture category.
- Recognize criteria that would identify a yoga instructor qualified to guide yoga practice for an individual with a musculoskeletal condition.
- Be familiar with evidence supporting the use of yoga for common musculoskeletal conditions.
- Describe evidence-based health-related benefits of yoga.
- Identify ways the physical therapist may integrate yoga into health promotion.

Introduction

Musculoskeletal pain conditions affect more than 1.7 billion people worldwide and accounts for more than half of the chronic conditions in people older than 50 years of age in developed countries.[1] A recent report by the US Department of Health and Human Services (the data from the 2012 National Health Statistics Reports) shows that 54.5% (126.6 million) of adults in the United States reported having a musculoskeletal pain disorder, with low back pain (LBP) and arthritic conditions being reported by 22.1% and 20.3% of US adults, respectively.[2] Musculoskeletal pain can contribute to functional impairments, lead to disability, and develop into chronic conditions. From 2009 to 2011, the estimated annual medical costs associated with musculoskeletal conditions was $213 billion, reflecting 5.2% of the national gross domestic product in 2011.[1] Individuals are frequently seeking nonpharmaceutical options from complementary health approaches for health maintenance and symptom management. The National Center for Complementary and Integrative Health (NCCIH) defines "complementary" as non-mainstream approaches to health care that are used in conjunction with conventional, Western medicine.[3] In 2012, 41.6% of individuals with a musculoskeletal pain disorder utilized a CAM health approach as compared to 24.1% of individuals without musculoskeletal pain.[2]

Yoga is 1 of the top 10 CAM health approaches used in the United States.[3] According to the Yoga in America Survey, the number of yoga practitioners in the United States has increased 132% from 15.8 million in 2006 to 36.7 million in 2016.[4] These results also reported that an additional 34% of Americans say they are at least somewhat likely to practice yoga in the next 12 months. The biopsychosocial approach recommended for the management of subacute[5] is similar to the mind-body philosophy of yoga. However, referrals to yoga by health care providers are low.[6] Of individuals using yoga for specific health conditions, only 22% cite having received a referral to yoga from a medical professional.[4] Given the continual rise in yoga popularity in the United States and the increasing preferences for CAM, it is important for health care professionals to expand their knowledge of yoga to best guide, direct, and inform patients seeking yoga as a complementary health approach. In this chapter, an overview of the background of yoga, basic components of yoga practice, and research related to the effects of yoga on the musculoskeletal system and common musculoskeletal conditions are presented. Recommendations for yoga practice to target specific musculoskeletal conditions are provided and 2 sample yoga sessions are outlined.

Yoga Background Overview

Yoga is a mind-body practice that focuses on physical, mental, emotional, and spiritual aspects of health. In Sanskrit, yoga means "to yoke" or "to make one" the mind and body for the purposes of minimizing disease and stress and improving well-being.[7] Yoga originated more than 5000 years ago in India as a meditative spiritual practice and was first introduced in the United States in 1893.[8] While the modern view of yoga is most synonymous with the performance of physical postures (asanas), the physical postures are only 1 of what is described as the 8 paths or limbs of yoga philosophy. This 8-limb path was first presented in a text, *Yoga Sutras of Patanjali*, composed around 200 CE, and consists of ethical behaviors (yamas), self-discipline (niyamas), physical

Table 21-1

COMMON STYLES OF HATHA YOGA

STYLE	DESCRIPTION
Viniyoga	Personalized yoga with therapeutic focus
Hot yoga	Yoga performed in a heated room
Vinyasa	Fluid sequencing yoga linking breath with movement
Restorative	Relaxation-based yoga with use of props to provide body support
Iyengar	Alignment-based yoga with use of props
Integral	Comprehensive, gentle yoga

postures (asanas), breath control (pranayama), inward focus (pratyahara), concentration (dharana), meditation (dyhana), and enlightenment (Samadhi).[9] The evolution of yoga is often thought of as a tree with branches, each of which represents a different approach to yoga. There are 6 main branches of yoga, and of these, Hatha yoga is the branch most commonly practiced in the United States and used most often in yoga-related research. Hatha yoga focuses primarily on physical postures (asanas), breathing (pranayama), and concentration (dharana) or mindfulness (dharana). Just as there are many branches of yoga, there are many styles of Hatha yoga. Table 21-1 outlines the more common styles of Hatha yoga.[10]

COMPONENTS OF YOGA PRACTICE

The term *yoga practice* refers to consistent, intentional, and mindful performance of 1 or more of the 8 paths of yoga. Hatha yoga, the most common style of yoga practiced in the United States, incorporates, at a minimum, asanas (yoga postures), pranayama (breathing), and dharana (concentration). While yoga practice may occur in a group or individual format, those seeking yoga to assist in the management of musculoskeletal pain and/or conditions would benefit by participation first in a private session or group-based practice guided by a qualified yoga instructor before embarking on independent yoga practice. A 2014 Delphi study identifying key components of yoga interventions for musculoskeletal conditions recommends that the instructor should have professional yoga teacher training and experience with teaching yoga to individuals with musculoskeletal conditions.[11] At present, there are no specific state or national licensing or certification requirements for yoga instructors. Organizations that offer yoga certification vary in the background requirements of individuals completing the certification and in the emphasis of the certification. The Professional Yoga Therapy Institute (PYTI), founded by Dr. Ginger Garner in 2000, provides both continuing education courses and certification in medical therapeutic yoga for licensed health care professionals.[12] Medical therapeutic yoga is defined by PYTI as "the

practice of yoga in medicine, rehabilitation, and wellness settings by a licensed health care professional who is completing or has graduated from the [PYTI] program."[12] The PYTI certification program consists of a 15-module curriculum encompassing 145 continuing education credits delivered as a hybrid distance/on-site model. Graduates of the program are credentialed as a Professional Yoga Therapist-Candidate (PYT-c) or Professional Yoga Therapist (PYT) practitioner. The International Association of Yoga Therapists (IAYT) and Yoga Alliance are 2 non-profit, international organizations that have established educational standards for yoga therapist training and yoga teacher training, respectively.[13,14] Certification as a yoga therapist through IAYT requires the completion of a minimum of 800 hours from an IAYT accredited program.[15] Individuals completing a minimum of 200 hours of yoga teacher training from a registered yoga school (RYS) through the Yoga Alliance may apply for credentialing as a registered yoga teacher (RYT) at the 200-hour (RYT 200). In addition, the Yoga Alliance provides advanced credentialing for those completing a 500-hour (RYT 500) yoga teacher training and for those who have completed a minimum of 1000 (E-RYT 200) or 2000 (E-RYT 500) teaching hours, signifying the individual as an experienced yoga teacher.[14] While PYTI requires licensure as a health care professional to pursue credentialing as a PYT, health care licensure is not a prerequisite of the IAYT or Yoga Alliance. PYTI, IAYT, and Yoga Alliance each maintain individual registries of yoga therapists/instructors that physical therapists and the public may access when searching for a qualified yoga instructor.

Evidence supports the biopsychosocial approach in the management of persistent musculoskeletal pain in which interventions encompass physical, psychological, and social factors that can regulate the pain experience.[5,16,17] A well-designed yoga class contains these biopsychosocial elements through the integration of yoga postures with an emphasis on mindfulness, the use of breathing, and relaxation exercises, all delivered in a manner that supports the development of teacher-student and student-student social relationships. Findings from the 2014 Delphi survey of experts in

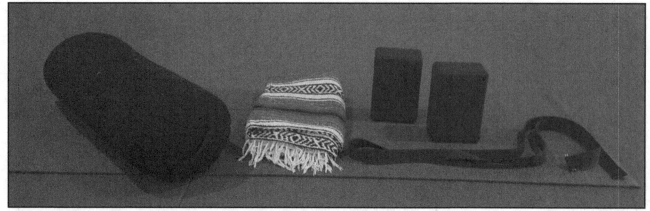

Figure 21-1. Basic yoga props: Blocks, straps, blankets, towels, and bolsters.

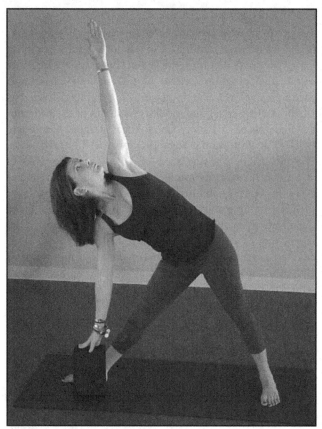

Figure 21-2. Triangle performed with use of a block to bring the ground up to the body.

the design, conduct, and teaching of yoga research related to musculoskeletal conditions suggest that, while the selection of yoga postures should be dependent upon the musculoskeletal condition of interest, the inclusion of mindfulness is an essential component of a yoga intervention to establish the mind-body connection.[11] A brief examination of each of the key components of yoga practice and how they coexist in a yoga class is provided next to assist the reader in understanding the mind-body focus yoga provides.

Yoga Equipment

Equipment and physical space requirements of yoga are minimal, allowing yoga to be cost efficient and readily adaptable to almost any environment. A yoga mat is recommended but not required. The purpose of the yoga mat is to provide protection between oneself and the environmental surface (floor) and to prevent the hands and feet from slipping. An additional use of a mat is to define one's personal space for yoga, especially when yoga is practiced in a group setting. Most yoga mats are rectangular in shape, approximately 24 x 68 inches in size. The thickness of a yoga mat varies and should be considered in regard to the floor surface on which yoga will be performed. A thinner mat, ⅛- to ¼-inch thick, would be best when performing yoga on carpet or a flooring with inherent cushion. The use of a thinner mat in these instances will prevent balance from being dually challenged by mat density and cushioned floor surface. Conversely, when yoga is performed on a hard surface, such as a wood floor, a thicker mat, ½- to 1-inch thick, would contribute to cushioning of bony areas such as the spine.

Yoga props comprise a variety of equipment that are used to modify postures to adjust for individual differences (in mobility and limb length) and to provide support for the body, thus allowing for the attainment of comfortable stillness while in a posture or when performing breathing exercises and meditation. Basic props include yoga blocks, straps, blankets, and/or towels (Figure 21-1). While a yoga block can be made of a variety of materials and sizes, it is generally light in weight, rectangular in shape, and 4 x 6 inches in size. Blocks can be used to bring the ground to the body to prevent connective tissue strain and to assist in obtaining safe alignment while in a yoga posture (Figure 21-2). Straps provide a means to extend the reach between upper extremities and between the upper and lower extremity. Figure 21-3 shows yoga postures performed with use of props to provide individual modifications.

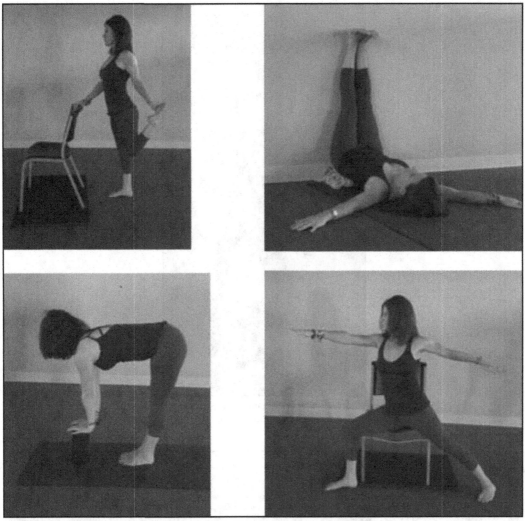

Figure 21-3. Examples of yoga postures performed with props to provide modifications.

Depending upon an individual's physical status, walls and chairs provide additional sources of props. When a student's mobility precludes moving to the floor and balance in standing is impaired, the entire yoga practice can be performed seated in a chair. In addition, chairs or walls provide balance support for standing postures and a surface for the hands or forearms when performing arm support postures. Walls can assist a student in attaining optimal alignment and can provide proprioceptive feedback and stability during a posture. For example, during Warrior I, the foot can be pressed against a wall for either the purpose of stability or to provide feedback of maintaining the lateral border of the foot in contract with the support surface to prevent lowering of the medial arch. Figure 21-4 shows examples of how yoga postures can be modified with the use of a chair or wall. Props such as bolsters and sandbags are often used in restorative style yoga where positioning the body with support to allow complete relaxation is the goal. An example of a restorative yoga posture is shown in Figure 21-5.

Yoga Postures

Yoga postures can be divided into categories that are distinguished by position, movement, and/or anatomical emphasis. These categories consist of standing, forward bending, backward bending, twists, inversions, hip openers, and core awakening.[18] With the exception of standing postures, the remaining categories can be performed in either standing, sitting, or lying on the floor. While each category has distinctive properties, elements of multiple categories may be seen in an individual posture. A misconception held by those unfamiliar with yoga is that yoga postures are performed in a manner that strains the joints and connective tissues by emphasizing the attainment of extreme ranges of motion. An appropriately trained instructor will encourage the student to find the expression of each posture that is in consideration with where they are in the present moment, not in consideration of what others in the class are doing or what the "ideal" posture should look like. The instructor will guide the student with verbal, visual, or manual cues into a posture and, using cues, assist the student to maintain the

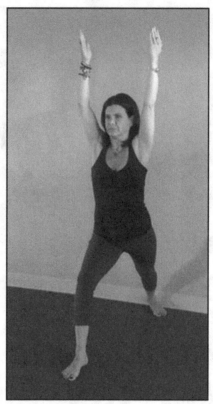

Figure 21-4. Warrior I performed with modifications by placing the foot to wall.

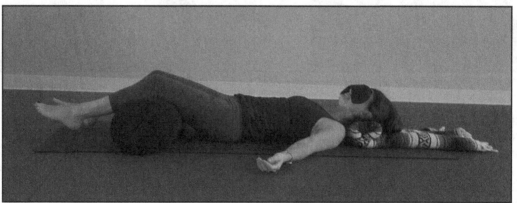

Figure 21-5. Restorative yoga posture.

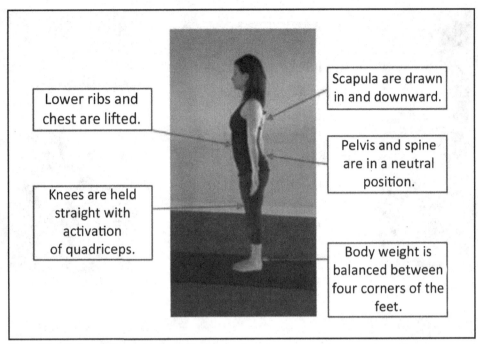

Figure 21-6. Tadasana, Mountain pose, with alignment cues.

posture with steadiness (sthira) and ease or "good space" (sukha). In doing so, yoga postures are performed with attention to segmental alignment and breathing to create "good space," free of strain within the body, and with focus to create "good space," free of strain within the mind. In addition to cues for body positioning and breathing, students are also directed to a point of focus for their eye gaze, called *dristhti*. While the dristhti is cued as an outward point of focus, the result is a deepening internal focus that quiets the mind. An example of these cues can be seen in Mountain pose (Tadasana; Figure 21-6) in which the student is cued to balance their weight between the "4 corners" of each foot so that equal weight is placed on the medial and lateral aspects of the ball of the foot and the heel to prevent collapse of the longitudinal arch. The knees are held straight in through activation of the quadriceps to prevent knee hyperextension. The pelvis is in a neutral position to allow natural curves of the spine, which is supported by a drawing in and up of the abdomen that also creates a lifting of the lower ribs. The shoulder blades are drawn down and back to allow the chest to lift and open. The lifting of the lower ribs and chest creates space for lung expansion as full breaths are encouraged. The gaze is steady and straight ahead.

Yoga postures are maintained in a manner that requires conscious active contraction of some muscles and passive relaxation of other muscles. In addition to affecting the musculoskeletal system, yoga postures also promote circulation, lower autonomic arousal, stimulate the hormonal system, circulate lymph, and reduce inflammatory responses.[19] The yoga postures presented in this section are selected to provide the reader with an idea of basic postures from each category and to introduce the musculoskeletal emphasis and alignment focus of each posture. Examples of how yoga postures can be modified are presented in each posture category.

Standing Postures

Standing postures vary in the base of support and placement of the feet to build strength and balance while moving from simple to complex patterns by utilizing neutral positioning of the lower extremity joints or combinations of horizontal (external and internal rotation), sagittal (flexion and extension), and frontal plane (adduction and abduction) movements. An example of these variations is seen in 4 standing postures: Mountain pose, Chair pose, Warrior I, and Warrior II (Figure 21-7). Mountain pose (Tadasana), a foundational standing posture, involves standing with the feet parallel with the lower extremities in a neutral position at the hips, knees, and ankles. Chair pose (Utkatasana) develops strength in the lower extremities, shoulders, and trunk; increases mobility in the chest and shoulders; and promotes alignment of the spine. Warrior I (Virabhadrasana I) involves standing in semi-tandem position with the forward lower extremity in neutral rotation with hip and knee flexion, while the backward positioned lower extremity is in external rotation with hip and knee extension. Warrior II (Virabhadrasana II) involves standing in hip abduction with the one lower extremity turned out to the side in hip and knee flexion, and the other lower extremity turned in slightly with hip and knee extension. In both Warrior I and II, the arch of the back foot is actively lifted by pressing the lateral border of the foot to the floor.

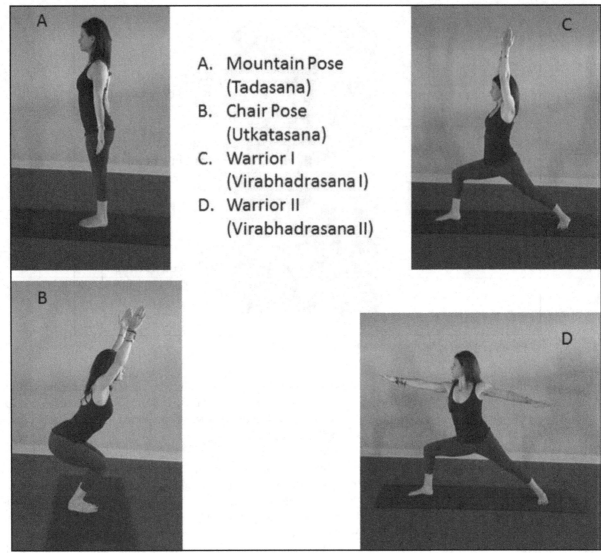

A. Mountain Pose
    (Tadasana)
B. Chair Pose
    (Utkatasana)
C. Warrior I
    (Virabhadrasana I)
D. Warrior II
    (Virabhadrasana II)

Figure 21-7. Examples of standing postures.

Standing postures also include balancing postures that draw upon coordination, focus, and strength. These postures are also performed in variations of hip rotation (neutral, external, or internal) and with incorporations of lower extremity joint mobility and muscle extensibility. Examples of standing balance postures with these variations include Tree (Vrksasana), Dancer (Natarajasana), Eagle (Garudasana), and Warrior III (Virabhadrasana III; Figure 21-8). Tree involves single leg balance in neutral hip rotation while the opposite lower extremity is placed in hip external rotation, knee flexion, and with foot pressed against the inner thigh or medial calf of the supporting lower extremity. Dancer strengthens the standing lower extremity, elongates the muscles along the hip and knee of the lifted lower extremity, and opens the chest and shoulder. Eagle transitions from Mountain to standing on one lower extremity with the opposite lower extremity crossed over the supporting lower extremity to create internal hip rotation with the toes pointing down or the foot wrapped around the supporting calf. Warrior III is performed by lifting one lower extremity backward while bending forward at the hips, maintaining a neutral position of the spine and hips. The standing postures can be performed with the upper extremities by the sides of the body or in variations of elevation, horizontal abduction/adduction, or rotation to create opening of the chest, shoulders, back, or trunk.

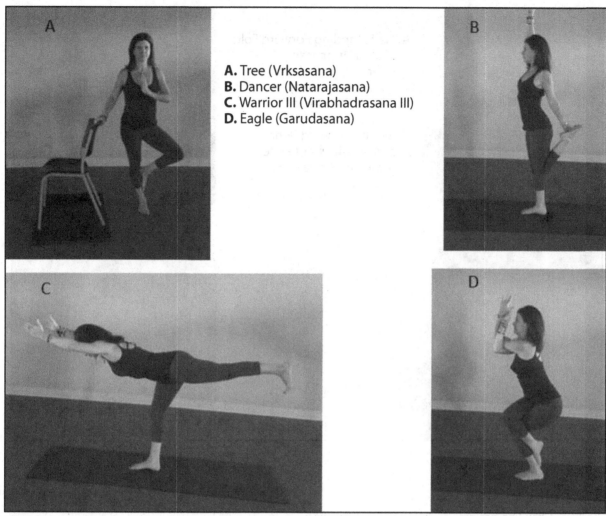

A. Tree (Vrksasana)
B. Dancer (Natarajasana)
C. Warrior III (Virabhadrasana III)
D. Eagle (Garudasana)

Figure 21-8. Standing balance postures with variations in hip rotation.

Forward Bending Postures

Forward bending postures combine folding inward of the anterior aspects of the body (ie, chest to thighs) while opening the posterior aspects of the body (ie, hamstrings, gluteal muscles, spinal muscles). Given that muscles along the posterior chain are often tight or short, forward bends should only be performed after the body is warmed up and with attention to seeking ease in the posture. Breathing is coordinated so that movement into a forward bend occurs on the breath exhalation. As the posture is maintained, tension is slightly released on the breath inhalation and then restored on the breath exhalation. Forward bends can be performed symmetrically, in which both lower extremities are positioned in the same manner, or asymmetrically, in which the lower extremities are in different positions. A basic symmetrical standing forward bend is Half Standing Forward Fold (Adhra Uttanasana), which is part of the sun salutation sequence, while Intense Side Stretch (Parsvottanasana) provides an example of an asymmetrical forward bend. Seated Staff Pose (Dandasana), a symmetrical posture, is the foundational posture for seated forward bends and, for many individuals, achieves the intended focus of opening the hamstrings and calves without inclining the trunk toward the lower extremities as in Paschimottanasana. An asymmetrical seated forward bend posture is Head-to-Knee Forward Bend (Janu Sirsasana). Forward fold postures are shown in Figure 21-9.

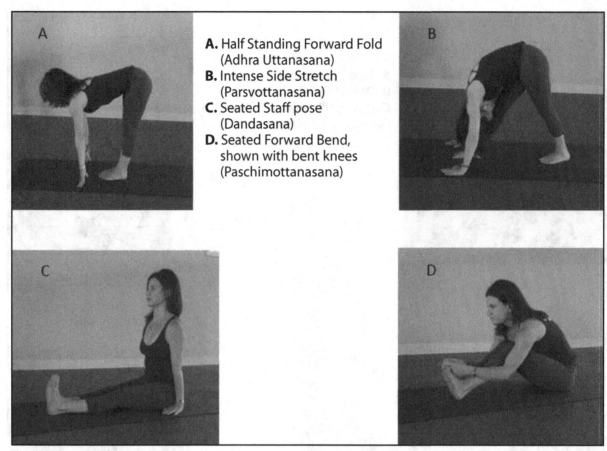

A. Half Standing Forward Fold (Adhra Uttanasana)
B. Intense Side Stretch (Parsvottanasana)
C. Seated Staff pose (Dandasana)
D. Seated Forward Bend, shown with bent knees (Paschimottanasana)

Figure 21-9. Forward fold yoga postures.

Backward Bending Postures

Backward bending postures are intended to open the front of the spine and body, with the emphasis of reversal of the thoracic curve. A secondary goal in select backward bending postures is to strengthen the spine and hip extensors. Backward bending postures are typically performed symmetrically with cues first to create length in the spine with a posterior pelvic tilt before extending and to avoid overextending the lumbar spine by focusing the movement on the thoracic spine. Examples of backward bending postures are Bridge (Setu Bandha Sarvangasana), Sphinx (Naraviralasana), Cobra (Bhujangasana), and Locust (Salabhasana; Figure 21-10). Bridge (see Figure 21-10A) emphasizes pressing the feet, hands, arms, and shoulders to the mat to lift the hips while posteriorly tilting the pelvis and opening the thighs, hips, and chest. This posture can also be performed with the hips supported for a gentle or restorative variation (Figure 21-11). Cobra and Locust (see Figures 21-10B and 21-10D) are considered a spine-strengthening posture series that, when performed sequentially, progressively increases in intensity. Both Cobra and Locust strengthen the muscles along the spine, the hip extensors, scapula depressors, and retractors. Cobra (see Figure 21-10B) involves using the strength of the upper back with assistance from the shoulder depressors to lift the upper back and head from the mat. The upper arms are held next to the sides of the thorax with the palms on the floor, emphasizing retracting and depressing the scapula

and lowering the shoulders from the ears. Locust (see Figure 21-10D) can be progressively performed by lifting one lower extremity at a time with the trunk and head supported on the mat, to lifting the arms, trunk, and head with the hips and legs supported, to the full expression of the posture involving lifting of the lower extremities, upper extremities, trunk, and head. In both Cobra and Locust, the neck is maintained in neutral to avoid overextending the cervical spine. Sphinx is a gentler back bend posture that is performed with the forearms propped on the floor with the elbows either under the shoulders or slightly forward of the shoulders. The scapulae are drawn down and in toward the spine while the forearms pull backward toward the body to bring the chest forward. To avoid overextending the lumbar spine, the pelvis is posteriorly tilted and the lower extremities rotate inward. Sphinx (see Figure 21-10C) can be performed in preparation for Upward Facing Dog posture (Figure 21-12).

While forward bending postures open the posterior aspect of the hips, certain postures performed seated, supine, and prone target additional areas of the hips that are prone to tension from joint compression and/or muscle inextensibility and are known as *hip opening postures*. Bound Angle pose can be performed seated (Baddha Konasana) or supine (Supta Baddha Konasana) and involves positioning the plantar aspect of the feet together with the hips in external rotation and the hips and knees flexed to open the inner thighs (Figure 21-13). In either position, the emphasis is on

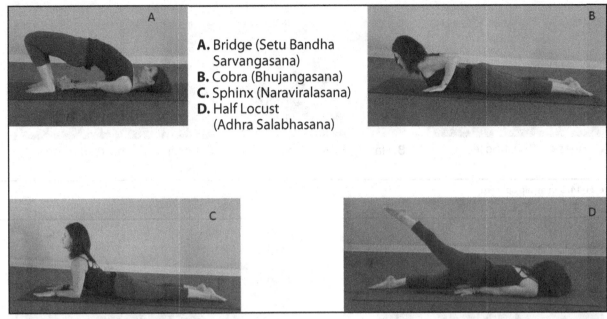

A. Bridge (Setu Bandha
 Sarvangasana)
B. Cobra (Bhujangasana)
C. Sphinx (Naraviralasana)
D. Half Locust
 (Adhra Salabhasana)

Figure 21-10. Backward bend postures.

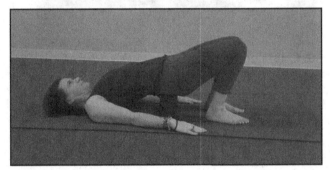

Figure 21-11. Supported Bridge.

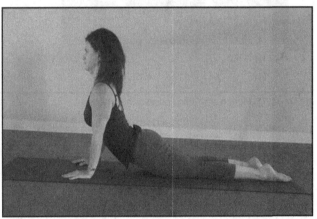

Figure 21-12. Upward Facing Dog posture.

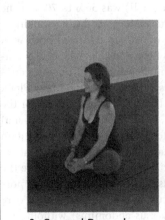
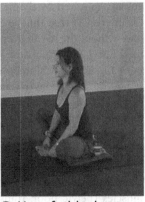
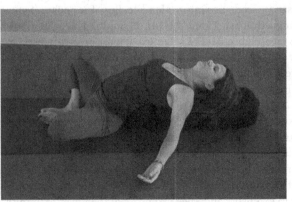

A. Seated Bound
 Angle pose
B. Use of a blanket
 under the hips
C. Supine Bound Angle with bolster

Figure 21-13. Hip opener postures.

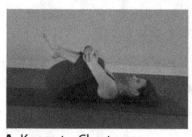
A. Knees-to-Chest pose

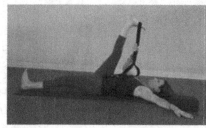
B. Happy Baby pose

C. Reclining Hand-to-Big Toe pose

Figure 21-14. Supine hip openers.

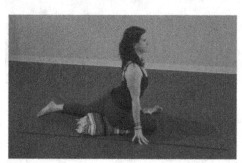
A. Pigeon

B. Child's pose

Figure 21-15. Pigeon and Child's poses as hip openers.

allowing the hips to relax into external rotation on the exhalation breath or to gently contract and relax the external rotators of the hips to reciprocally inhibit the internal rotators as opposed to pressing the knees down with the hands. A folded towel or blanket can be placed under the hips to allow the pelvis to anteriorly rotate and the spine to lengthen (see Figure 21-13B). The supine position allows the spine to be supported while performing hip opening postures such as Knees-to-Chest pose (Apanasana), Happy Baby (Ananda Balasana), and Reclining Hand-to-Big Toe pose (Supta Padangusthasana; Figure 21-14). In supine Knees-to-Chest pose (see Figure 21-14A), the exhalation breath is used to draw the knees to the chest, creating a reversal of the lumbar curve and opening of the posterior hips region. Happy Baby (see Figure 21-14B) is a variation of the Knees-to-Chest pose that involves holding the feet in each hand while bringing the knees to the axilla and the feet toward the ceiling. This posture provides a release to the inner thighs, posterior hips, and low back. During Reclining Hand-to-Big Toe pose (see Figure 21-14C), the intent is to straighten the knee of the lifted lower extremity by contraction of the quadriceps while the hip extensors and knee extensors of the lower extremity remaining on the mat are contracting to straighten the hip and knee, respectively. Pigeon (Eka Pada Rajakapotasana) and Child's poses (Balasana; Figure 21-15) are examples of 2 postures that target the posterior hips.

The attention to posture and alignment contributes to the attainment of core activation, not only in postures for which core activation is the intended goal but also in many common standing postures. A biomechanical analysis of yoga postures contained in the Yoga Empowers Seniors study found that rectus abdominis activity, as measured by electromyography (EMG), in all standing postures contained in the yoga intervention (Mountain, Chair, Tree, One-Leg Balance, Warrior I, and Warrior II) was 50% to 70% of the activity required by the rectus abdominis during walking.[20] Of interest is that this level of activity occurred both with and without the use of props (wall and chair). Ni et al examined EMG activity of core muscles during 11 postures contained in the sun salutation sequence and found Low Plank (Chaturanga Dandasana) to have the highest activity for the external oblique abdominis, High Plank (Kumbhakasana) to have the highest activity for rectus abdominis, Mountain pose with arms overhead (Tadasana) to have the highest activity for longissimus thoracis, and Warrior I to require the highest activity of the gluteus maximus.[21] Specific yoga postures for core activation focus on activating the deep core muscles (pelvic floor, transversus abdominis) without creating excessive tension in the more global muscles (rectus abdominis, obliques) to create space in the spine and ribs allowing the attainment of strength, balance, and mobility when performing postures from the other categories. During

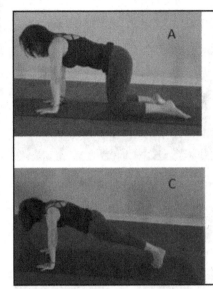
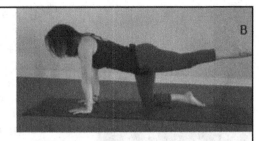
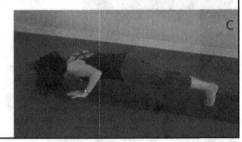

A. Tabletop (Bharmanasana)
B. Tabletop with leg extended
C. High Plank (Kumbhakasana)
D. Low Plank (Chaturanga Dandasana)

Figure 21-16. Core activation postures.

core activation postures, 2 "energy locks" (bandhas) are engaged: Mula bandha and Uddiyana bandha. Mula bandha involves engaging the pelvic floor muscles, similar to Kegel exercises. Uddiyana bandha involves drawing the lower abdomen in and up. The thickness of the transverse abdominis has been found to increase from 10.5 to 17.5 mm during the practice of Uddiyana bandha.[22] Tabletop (Bharmanasana) is a foundational posture that encourages attaining length in the spine from the crown of the head to the sacrum and activating the core with or without extremity movement. Once proficiency of core activation in Tabletop is attained, progression to Plank (Kumbhakasana) can occur. Plank is a component of the sun salutation sequence of yoga postures and can be performed on the hands and toes or hands and knees. Examples of yoga postures for core activation are shown in Figure 21-16.

Twisting Postures

Twisting postures involve rotation of the spine and are performed for the proposed purpose of providing mobility to the spine, creating a massaging action of the internal organs, and stimulating the nervous system. Cueing correct performance of twisting postures is essential to first lengthen the spine on the inhalation breath then initiate movement from the mid thoracic spine on the exhalation. These cues guide a gentle performance of the twisting posture that is not held at an end range of a twist, but instead, ease into and out of the twist with each breath. Standing postures that incorporate twisting include Revolved Triangle (Parivrtta Trikonasana) and Revolved Chair (Parivrtta Utkatasana). Gentle spinal twist is performed in easy sitting posture (seated, knees and hips flexed, heels in line with each other). The contact of the hands on one knee and the floor behind provide an anchor to facilitate activation of the latissimus dorsi, biceps, and pectoralis major and deltoid, which assist the obliques in turning the trunk. Floor Spine Twist (Jathara Parivartanasana)

is performed from Knees-to-Chest pose and involves extending the arms out to the sides at shoulder height with the palms facing up to open the chest and to facilitate the twist to occur in the thoracic spine. The knees can be either stacked together on the floor or a prop can be used to bring the floor to the knees, allowing the shoulders to remain on the floor. Examples of twisting postures are shown in Figure 21-17.

Any posture in which the head is below the heart is considered an inversion posture. Proposed benefits of inversion postures are increased circulation and stimulation of the lymphatic system. Traditional yoga inversions involve contact of the head and/or shoulders with the floor (eg, headstand, shoulder stand); however, these have been found to be the most common postures associated with adverse events in yoga practice.[23] Gentle inversions, such as Legs Up a Wall, Dolphin, and Downward Facing Dog, have been included in research examining effectiveness of yoga for LBP and are recommended in this chapter for consideration in use with individuals with musculoskeletal conditions.[24,25] Legs Up a Wall (Viparita Karani) is a restorative posture and can be performed for an extended length of time, whereas Dolphin (Ardha Pincha Mayurasana) and Downward Facing Dog (Adho Mukha Svanasana) involve arm support and are usually performed for a shorter duration (1 to 5 breaths). Both Dolphin and Downward Facing Dog resemble an inverted V but differ in arm support provided by the forearms (Dolphin) or hands (Downward Facing Dog). Cueing is important to assist the student in activating specific muscles to provide the desired alignment. For example, in both postures, the infraspinatus and teres minor contract to externally rotate the shoulders, and the middle and lower trapezius draw the scapula down and toward midline.[26] The quadriceps and anterior tibialis contract to straighten the knees and lower the heels, respectively. The neck is held in a neutral position to prevent extending the cervical spine. Examples of inversion postures are shown in Figure 21-18.

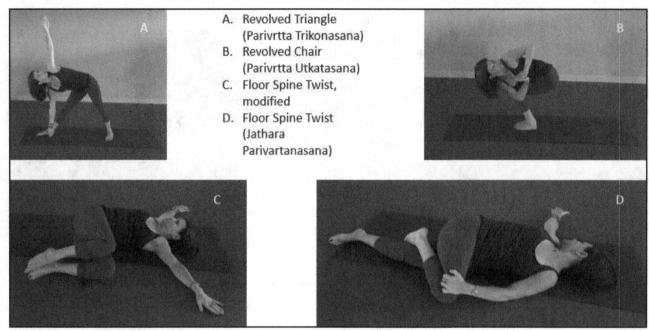

A. Revolved Triangle
   (Parivrtta Trikonasana)
B. Revolved Chair
   (Parivrtta Utkatasana)
C. Floor Spine Twist,
   modified
D. Floor Spine Twist
   (Jathara
   Parivartanasana)

Figure 21-17. Twisting postures.

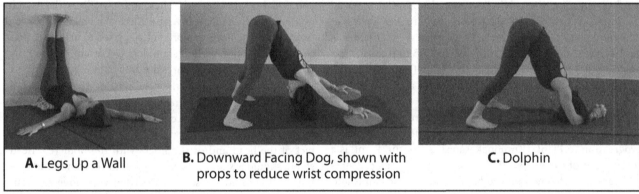

A. Legs Up a Wall   **B.** Downward Facing Dog, shown with   **C.** Dolphin
                             props to reduce wrist compression

Figure 21-18. Inversion postures.

Breathing

While the performance of yoga postures includes the co-ordination of breath when moving in and out of a posture and the continuation of rhythmic breathing when holding a posture, a separate component of yoga practice included in the 8 limbs of yoga is pranayama or breath control. Pranayama consists of yogic breathing techniques or exercises that begin with breath awareness and progress to breath refinement, basic yogic breathing, and breath purification. For most individuals, breathing is an unconscious process. Breath awareness breaks the unconscious pattern of breathing by bringing attention to the breathing cycle and the movements in the body that allow adjustments to breath capacity. Breath refinement involves instruction in how to breathe deeply though the movement of the abdomen (abdominal or belly breathing) or how to take a complete breath to create more space for breath by breathing into the abdomen, rib cage, and chest (3-part breath), both of which will also assist in calming the mind. Breath refinement brings attention to the ratio

of inhalation (Puraka) and exhalation (Rechaka) and teaches how to adjust this ratio to attain relaxation. Basic yogic breathing is known as *ujjayi pranayama,* in which both the inhalation and exhalation occur through the nose, creating a vibrational sound and warming of the breath, which together cultivate an internal awareness and assist with attaining steadiness and ease in the body. Alternate nostril breathing (Nadi [channel] Shodhana [purification]) is an example of breath purification that unites the brain and fingers to channel breath in one nostril and out of the other nostril, with the goal of enhancing intentional focus and creating calmness. Support for alternate nostril breathing (ANB) is found in a study by Telles et al who reported decreased beta wave band activity over the right occipital region recorded by electroencephalography (EEG) after 5 minutes of ANB as compared to 5 minutes of quiet sitting, suggesting the practice of ANB may be calming and reduce arousal.[27] Table 21-2 describes yoga breath techniques that can be incorporated into yoga practice or performed independently of yoga.

Table 21-2

YOGA BREATHING EXERCISES

BREATHING EXERCISE, POSITION	INSTRUCTIONS
Breath Awareness Position: Supine (Savasana) 	• Lie relaxed on your back and bring your awareness to your natural breath. • Do not judge how you breathe, just recognize how you are naturally breathing at this moment. • Distinguish between the inhalation and exhalation. • Where do you feel the air as it flows in? • What parts of your body do you feel moving on the inhalation? • Where do you feel the breath as it flows out? • What parts of your body do you feel moving on the exhalation?
Breath Refinement—Abdomen Breathing Position: Sitting (Easy pose) or lying (Savasana)	• Place one hand on your lower belly. • Breathe slowly and deeply so that your hand rises as you bring air into the deep part of your lungs. • Feel the lungs expand front to back and side to side as you deeply breathe in. • Breathe out completely, feeling your hand lower as the air leaves the deep part of your lungs. • Feel the muscles in your lower belly contract to push the air out.
Breath Refinement—3-Part Breath Position: Sitting (Easy pose) or lying (Savasana)	• Place one hand on your lower belly and one hand on your upper chest. • Breathe into your lower belly (part 1), into your side ribs (part 2), and into your upper chest (part 3). • Breathe out from your upper chest (part 3), from your side ribs (part 2), and from your lower belly (part 1). • As your breath enters and leaves the lower belly, your bottom hand will rise and fall. • As your breath enters and leaves the mid chest region, your side ribs will open and close. • As your breath enters and leaves your upper chest, your top hand will rise and fall.
Breath Refinement—Inhalation and Exhalation Ratios Position: Sitting (Easy pose) or lying (Savasana)	• Begin with 3 to 5 natural breaths. • 1:1 breathing practice—Breathe in for 2 seconds, breathe out for 2 seconds. Gradually progress the length of the inhale and exhale maintaining equal ratio. • 1:2 breathing practice—Breathe in for 2 seconds, breathe out for 4 seconds. If you notice any strain as the exhale lengthens, reduce the length of the exhalation.

(continued)

Table 21-2 (continued)

YOGA BREATHING EXERCISES

BREATHING EXERCISE, POSITION	INSTRUCTIONS
Basic Yogic Breathing—Ujjayi Pranayama (victorious breath) Position: Sitting (Easy pose) or standing (Mountain pose)	• During this exercise, you will breathe in and out with your mouth closed. • Breathe in through your nose across the back of your throat to create an "aahh" sound. Breathe deep from your belly to your rib cage to your chest. • Breathe out through your nose feeling the air across the back of your throat, creating a "hhaa" sound. Exhale completely from your chest to your rib cage to your belly. • Try to keep the inhale and exhale breaths equal length.
Breathe Purification—Alternate Nostril Breathing Position: Sitting (Easy pose)	• Place your right thumb on the outside of your right nostril. • Place your right ring finger on the outside of your left nostril. • Exhale completely. • Close your right nostril with your thumb and breathe in through the left nostril. • Hold your breath briefly as your close your left nostril with your ring finger, maintaining the right nostril closed. • Release your right nostril and breathe out through the right nostril. • Keep the left nostril closed and breathe in through the right nostril. • Hold your breath briefly as your close your right nostril with your thumb, maintaining the left nostril closed. • Release your left nostril and breathe out through the left nostril. • This completes 1 breath cycle. • Complete 5 to 15 cycles, keeping the length of each inhale and exhale equal.

Relaxation

There are specific yoga postures in which the main goal is relaxation of the body and mind. These postures include Corpse pose (Savasana) and Child's pose (Balasana; Figure 21-19). Savasana is performed lying supine with the legs outstretched, the arms slightly away from the body, the back of the hands on the floor, the muscles in the arms and legs completely relaxed, and the eyes closed. This posture may be used between postures, but it is most commonly placed at the end of class and maintained for an extended period of time, at least 5 minutes, to promote total body relaxation. During Savasana, the instructor may provide guided relaxation techniques, such as progressive muscle relaxation or body scan, or direct the instruction toward attainment of an optimal position to facilitate relaxation. Child's pose is another relaxation posture that is used between more challenging yoga postures.

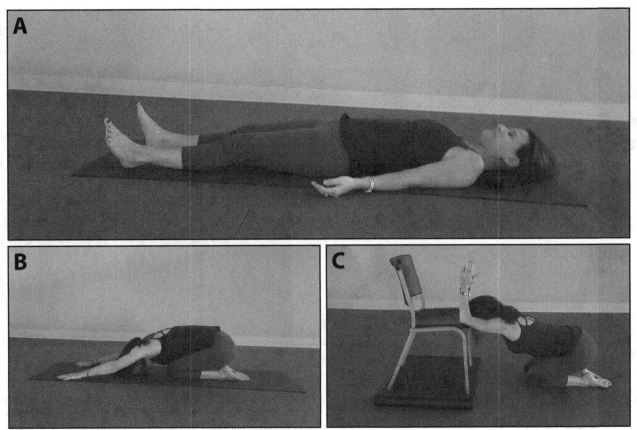

Figure 21-19. Relaxation postures.

This posture is assumed from the hands and knees position by shifting the body weight backward to sit on the heels with the knees apart to allow the trunk to lower between the thighs. The head rests on the floor and the arms rest on the floor beside the legs with the palms up. Restorative yoga postures can also be used to attain relaxation. While restorative postures can be used singularly at the end of class for relaxation, a sequence of restorative yoga postures may be used for the entirety of a class.[28] These postures are performed for a longer period of time (5 to 10 minutes) and involve the use of props to achieve comfort and to support the body. Figure 21-20 shows Child's pose performed as a restorative posture using a bolster under the chest and head, as well as additional restorative yoga postures.

YOGA-RELATED RESEARCH

Yoga research related to the therapeutic benefits of yoga has paralleled the rise in yoga popularity. A bibliometric analysis of trends in research regarding the therapeutic benefits of yoga from 1967 to 2013 identified 486 publications of yoga-related research meeting the definition of a clinical trial. During this time, 76 (16%) of the publications occurred between 2003 and 2008 and 243 (50%) occurred between 2009 and 2013.[29] A second bibliometric analysis of randomized controlled trials (RCTs) investigating the therapeutic

value of yoga interventions published from inception to 2014 found 312 RCTs with a median sample size of 59.[30] The top medical conditions investigated were breast cancer, asthma, depression, type 2 diabetes, LBP, and hypertension. Findings from this analysis highlight quality issues with yoga-related research regarding lack of information regarding the style of yoga examined, what was included in the yoga intervention, and information concerning the comparison interventions. Specifically, the style of yoga was not defined in 38.1% of the RCTs (n = 119). Of those RCTs that specified the yoga intervention, Hatha yoga was used in 11.2% (n = 35) and 9.6% (n = 30) used yogic breathing exercises. Of all the RCTs reviewed, 78.2% (n = 244) included yoga postures, 74.4 % (n = 232) included yoga breathing exercises, and 49% (n = 153) included meditation. The median length of yoga intervention was 9 weeks. Yoga was compared to usual care or no intervention in 55.8% (n = 174) of the RCTs and to exercise in 10.1% (n = 64) of the RCTs. While the number of RCTs investigating the effectiveness of yoga is increasing, systematic reviews frequently cite risk of bias in many of these studies due to lack of blinding of participants, investigators providing the interventions, or outcome assessors. Many reviews acknowledge, however, that the study quality of yoga RCTs may be underestimated because participation in yoga precludes the ability to blind that participant to the intervention they received.

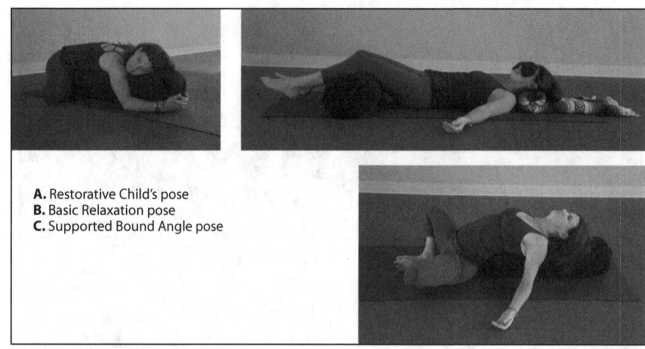

A. Restorative Child's pose
B. Basic Relaxation pose
C. Supported Bound Angle pose

Figure 21-20. Restorative yoga postures.

Adverse Events

An important aspect of yoga-related research is determination of safety or risk of adverse events of those participating in a yoga intervention. A 2017 Cochrane review of yoga as an intervention for LBP found no difference in the risk of adverse events between yoga and exercise controls.[31] Similarly, Cramer et al analyzed the frequency of adverse events in RCTs involving yoga and reported that 94 reported adverse events in 301 identified RCTs published between the years 1975 and 2014, which involved 8430 participants. The authors found no differences in adverse events when comparing yoga and usual care or exercise, concluding that yoga appears to be as safe as usual care and exercise.[32] Of particular concern to many health professionals is the potential risk to the spine when performing yoga. Two research studies involving high-risk spinal conditions, osteoporosis and hyperkyphosis, found beneficial effects of yoga for each musculoskeletal condition without associated adverse events or negative side effects.[33,34]

Health-Related Benefits of Yoga

Yoga has been associated with both physical- and psychological-related benefits in healthy individuals as well as individuals with conditions affecting many body systems. A systematic review of the practice of yoga on physical fitness and function in older adults found improvements in shoulder and hip mobility (measured by range of motion), balance (measured by Berg Balance Scale, single leg stance, and balance confidence), and gait speed (6-minute walk test).[35] A 12-minute daily yoga practice has been found to reverse osteoporotic bone loss in the spine, hips, and femurs as evidenced by increased bone mineral density after the 2-year intervention.[33] While the metabolic level of a Hatha yoga class may be less than the moderate level of physical activity (3.0 MET) recommended by the American College of Sports Medicine for improving and maintaining health,[36] several systematic reviews have found positive effects of yoga practice on the cardiovascular system.[37-39] Results of a systematic review and meta-analysis on the effects of yoga for hypertension found yoga to be associated with a small but significant decline in both systolic and diastolic blood pressure in individuals with prehypertension or hypertension when compared to usual care or no intervention.[37] When the reviewed studies were subgrouped based on the number of components of yoga practice included, larger reductions in systolic and diastolic blood pressure occurred in yoga interventions that included 3 components (postures, meditation, and breathing) as compared to yoga interventions with 2 or 1 component. A meta-analysis by Cramer et al[38] yielded evidence for yoga as compared to usual care on modifiable cardiovascular risk factors of blood pressure, resting heart rate, waist circumference, cholesterol, and insulin resistance in individuals with increased risk of cardiovascular disease as well as healthy individuals. Subgroup analysis found the positive effects of yoga to be most pronounced when a 12-week yoga intervention was utilized. A review and meta-analysis by Chu and colleagues[39] found yoga to be beneficial in improving risk factors for cardiovascular disease and metabolic syndrome when compared to nonexercise controls and as effective as traditional aerobic exercise. The finding of similar benefits of yoga as compared to traditional aerobic activity on cardiovascular disease risk factor reduction is important for individuals, such as those with musculoskeletal pain, who may not be able to tolerate aerobic activity.

Yoga intervention has also been found to result in reduced stress, inflammatory responses, and depression. Novice yoga practitioners have been found to have significantly (41%, $P = .03$) higher levels of interleukin-6 (IL-6), an inflammatory marker, than experienced yoga practitioners,[40] and short-term practice of yoga has resulted in a reduction in stress (decreased cortisol levels) and the inflammatory markers IL-6 and C-reactive protein, suggesting that yoga may have positive benefits for decreasing inflammation.[41,42] A systematic review conducted by Riley and Park found support of yoga in reducing stress through inducing positive affect, self-compassion, inhibition of posterior hypothalamus, and reduction in salivary cortisol.[43] Yoga has been found to increase brain γ-aminobutyric acid (GABA) levels, which is a neurotransmitter that is low in individuals with depression and anxiety disorder.[44,45] The increase in GABA levels was reported after one 60-minute yoga session in experienced yoga practitioners as compared to a control group who read[45] and after 12 weeks of yoga as compared to metabolically matched walking exercise.[44]

Yoga and Back Pain

A 2017 Cochrane Review of yoga treatment for chronic LBP identified 12 RCTs that compared yoga to no intervention or nonexercise intervention (n = 7), to an exercise intervention (n = 3), or to both exercise and nonexercise intervention (n = 2).[31] Yoga intervention was delivered in a group format, 1 to 3 classes per week lasting 45 to 90 minutes per class, 4 to 24 weeks. Nonexercise intervention varied from usual care, waiting list for yoga intervention, self-care education book, or education classes and materials. Yoga intervention was most commonly Hatha yoga style (Iyengar, Viniyoga, British Wheel of Yoga) that included physical postures in addition to breathing, relaxation, or meditation. Exercise interventions were described as therapeutic exercise and consisted of stretching, strengthening, breathing, and relaxation interventions designed and/or led by a physical therapist.[46-48] Outcome assessment included functional disability (ODI, Roland-Morris Disability Questionnaire [RMDQ]), pain (Visual Analog Scale [VAS], Numeric Pain Rating Scale [NPRS], symptom bothersomeness), quality of life (health-related quality of life [HRQL]), depression, and presence of adverse events. For studies comparing yoga to nonexercise controls, yoga resulted in greater improvement in back-related function,[46,47,49-54] pain,[49-51,53,54] and depression.[50] When comparing yoga to exercise controls, one study found greater improvement in back-related function at 12 weeks in a yoga intervention,[46] while another study found both yoga and exercise to have similar improvement in function.[47] Nambi et al[48] found superior improvement in pain and quality of life for yoga as compared to exercise. In all of the studies included in this review, blinding of participants and providers was not performed. The lack of blinding, the use

of self-assessment outcomes, and the heterogeneity between studies resulted in downgrading the evidence to low certainty for yoga compared to nonexercise controls and to very-low certainty when comparing yoga to exercise controls.

Since the publication of the 2017 Cochrane review of yoga treatment for chronic LBP, the effectiveness of yoga for individuals with chronic LBP has been explored through RCTs that have expanded the population to include military veterans. Groessi et al examined the effectiveness of a 12-week bi-weekly 60-minute yoga intervention (physical postures, breathing, attentional focus, and meditation) delivered in a group format.[55] Veterans with chronic LBP (greater than 6 months' duration) were randomly assigned to the yoga group (n = 75) or a delayed yoga treatment group (n = 75). During the 6-month period, both groups continued with usual care related the management of LBP. Low back–related disability assessed with the RMDQ was the primary outcome, while pain intensity assessed with the Brief Pain Inventory Short Version was the secondary outcome. Although there were no differences in disability at 12 weeks, the yoga group had significant differences is RMDQ scores at the 6-month period. Pain intensity was significantly lower for the yoga group at all time periods. In a secondary analysis from the aforementioned study, Groessi et al found veterans who participated in yoga to have significantly greater improvements on secondary health outcomes of pain interference, fatigue, quality of life, self-efficacy, and medication use.[56]

Yoga and Neck Pain

A 2019 systematic review and meta-analysis conducted by Li et al investigated the effects of yoga on chronic nonspecific neck pain (CNNP).[57] Ten RCTs or quasi-RCTs involving adults with CNNP were reviewed. The yoga intervention, consisting of any type of yoga, was compared to exercise, Pilates, or usual care. The duration of the intervention was 10 days to 12 weeks. Primary outcome measures were pain intensity and disability associated with the neck, while secondary outcome measures included cervical range of motion (CROM), quality of life (QOL), and emotional state. For both pain intensity and disability, yoga was superior to the control or alternative intervention. However, subgroup analysis showed significantly greater improvement for yoga as compared to exercise on both primary outcomes with no significant difference between yoga and Pilates or yoga and CAM. The pooled effects of yoga yielded significantly greater improvement than the control or alternative intervention on CROM, QOL, and emotional state.[57]

Of the 10 studies included in the Li et al systematic review and meta-analysis, only 3 examined the effectiveness of a yoga intervention delivered greater than 8 weeks.[58-60] Michalsen et al compared Iyengar yoga to manualized self-care exercise in individuals with CNNP over a 9-week intervention in which yoga was provided in 90-minute sessions once per week.[58] The yoga group had significantly greater reductions in pain, improvements in function (Neck Disability

Index [NDI] and Neck and Pain Disability questionnaire [NAPD]), and improvements in QOL (SF-36). In addition, there were greater improvements in psychological outcomes of depression, fatigue, and anger for the yoga group.

Cramer et al examined the effects of Iyengar yoga compared to home-based exercise in individuals with CNNP.[60] The yoga group received once weekly 90-minute sessions focusing on yoga postures targeting the neck and shoulders supplemented by daily 10-minute home yoga practice. The home-based exercise group was provided a self-care exercise manual with instructions to perform the exercises 10 minutes per day. Primary outcome measures were self-report based and included pain (VAS), function (NDI), and QOL (SF-36) measures at baseline and at 9 weeks. Secondary objective outcome measures included CROM, proprioceptive acuity, and pain pressure threshold (PPT). The yoga groups had significantly less pain, functional disability, and improved QOL as compared to the home-based exercise group. In addition, CROM, proprioceptive acuity, and PPT showed significant improvements for the yoga group. This is one of the few studies that has utilized both self-report outcome measures and objective outcome measures to examine the effectiveness of yoga on neck or back pain. A follow-up study by the same authors was conducted to assess the effects of yoga intervention on CNNP 12 months after completion of the intervention. The findings comparing baseline to 12-month follow-up showed significant improvements in pain, neck-related disability, and bodily pain in the SF-36. In addition, the most important predictor of these improvements was sustained yoga practice over the 12-month period.

Dunleavy et al compared yoga, Pilates, and control in which the exercise intervention (yoga or Pilates) was provided once a week for 12 weeks.[59] Outcomes assessment included function (NDI), pain (NPRS), CROM (composite score), and posture. Participants in both intervention groups, yoga and Pilates, had significantly greater improvements in pain and disability at 6 weeks and 12 weeks, with no differences between the exercise groups. The improvement in pain and disability was sustained 6 weeks after completion of the interventions. There were no improvements in impairment measures of CROM or posture for all groups. The instructors for the exercise interventions were physiotherapists with either certification or advanced training in yoga or Pilates.

Yoga and Osteoarthritis

Research regarding the effect of yoga on osteoarthritis has primarily targeted knee osteoarthritis (KOA) and has been summarized in a focused review,[61] a systematic review,[62] and 2 systematic reviews with meta-analysis.[63,64] These studies included yoga interventions delivered at a frequency of 1 to 6 times per week, 45 to 90 minutes per session, and 6 to 12 weeks in duration. The reviews found positive effects of yoga on pain, mobility, and stiffness while the use of varied outcome measures led to inconclusive findings in the areas of psychosocial function and QOL. In addition to the reviews,

a 2017 Ottawa panel clinical practice guideline concluded that Hatha yoga demonstrated significant improvement for pain relief (Grade B) and physical function (Grade C+) in the management of KOA.[65]

The largest study in the aforementioned reviews was by Ebnezar and colleagues who reported the findings in 3 publications.[66-68] This study involved 250 individuals with KOA (age range 35 to 80) who were randomly assigned to an integrated approach to yoga therapy or a therapeutic exercise intervention. Both interventions were adjunctive to physiotherapy and delivered in 60-minute sessions daily (20 minutes of physiotherapy and 40 minutes of yoga or therapeutic exercise intervention) for 2 weeks followed by independent practice of each intervention at home for 12 weeks. The integrated approach to yoga therapy program combined exercise, yoga asanas, relaxation, breathing, mediation, and education of yoga philosophy for health and lifestyle changes. The therapeutic exercises consisted of "loosening" and strengthening exercises for all major joints followed by knee-specific mobility and strengthening exercises and rest. The physiotherapy delivered to both intervention groups consisted of modalities (transcutaneous electrical nerve stimulation [TENS] and ultrasound). The results were reported in 3 publications.[66-68] Decrease in pain, early morning stiffness, anxiety, blood pressure, and heart rate occurred in both groups with significantly greater reductions in the yoga group after the 2-week intervention and at 3 months after intervention.[66,67] There was significantly greater improvements in the yoga group for pain while walking, knee disability (Western Ontario and McMaster Universities Osteoarthritis Index), active knee flexion range of motion, joint tenderness, joint swelling, and joint crepitus.[68] Similarly, improvements in physical function and general health subscales of the SF-36 occurred for both groups, but were significantly greater in the yoga group.[66]

Less research is available regarding biomechanics of yoga postures and potential impact on KOA symptoms. Brenneman et al included examination of knee adduction moment and EMG during yoga postures used in an investigation of a yoga strengthening program in women with KOA.[69] They reported significant decreases in pain and increases in knee extensor and flexor strength after a 12-week yoga intervention. The knee adduction moment of the yoga postures was less than that during gait and normalized EMG were up to 31% of maximum voluntary isometric contraction. Yoga postures included in the intervention were Chair, Goddess, Kneeling Lunge, Extended Side Angle, Warrior I, Warrior II, and Bridge.

Yoga Compared to Physical Therapy

Only one RCT has compared yoga intervention to physical therapy and involved 320 individuals of low income and high racial diversity with moderate to severe nonspecific chronic LBP.[70,71] Participants were randomly assigned to yoga intervention, physical therapy intervention, or educational intervention. All interventions lasted 12 weeks after which participants were followed over 40 weeks in which "booster" physical therapy or yoga interventions were provided according to study protocol. The yoga intervention consisted of one 75-minute yoga session provided by a trained yoga instructor for 12 weeks and 30 minutes of daily home yoga practice following a DVD and written program. The physical therapy intervention was considered high dosage and consisted of fifteen 60-minute individual physical therapy sessions provided according to the treatment-based classification system for the subgroups of specific exercise or stabilization approach.[72] Each physical therapy session consisted of a reassessment of the subgroup classification with adjustment of exercise interventions, 30 minutes working directly with a physical therapist, and 30 minutes of supervised aerobic activity. Instruction in an individualized home exercise program and supplies to perform the home exercise program were provided to each participant in the physical therapy intervention group. Psychologically informed rehabilitation principles were included with the physical therapy intervention for participants who had elevated fear-avoidance beliefs. The education intervention consisted of a 12-week reading schedule for *The Back Pain Helpbook* and a newsletter delivered every 3 weeks that summarized the main points of the reading chapters. At the conclusion of the 12-week intervention period, the participants in the yoga and physical therapy intervention groups received a 40-week maintenance phase of drop-in yoga sessions, "booster" physical therapy session, or home program of yoga or physical therapy.

Primary outcome measures were function assessed with the RMDQ, pain assessed with the NPRS. Secondary outcome measures were self-report pain medication use and health-related QOL (SF-36). Assessors of the outcome measures were blinded to group assignment, but participants, yoga instructors, and physical therapists were not blinded. Results showed non-inferiority of yoga to physical therapy, indicating that for both function and pain, yoga and physical therapy yielded the same improvement. Both yoga and physical therapy groups had greater reductions in pain medication usage than the education group at 12 weeks. The function and pain-related benefits continued through the maintenance phase for both yoga and physical therapy groups. There was no difference in adverse advents for either yoga or physical therapy. The authors highlighted that these findings relate to a manualized yoga class in which the yoga components were standardized and progressed in a structured manner over the 12-week period, which may differ from community-based yoga classes that are non-manualized. Additional findings from this study regarding work productivity and cost-effectiveness are planned to be reported separately.

Roseen et al conducted a secondary analysis of data from the Saper et al[70] RCT to evaluate the effectiveness of yoga, physical therapy, and education on sleep quality in adults with nonspecific LBP.[71] Sleep quality was assessed with the Pittsburgh Sleep Quality Index (PSQI). Sleep quality significantly improved in both the yoga and physical therapy groups, with no improvement in the education group at 12

weeks and 52 weeks. Immediately following the intervention (12 weeks from baseline) and 40 weeks following intervention completion (52 weeks from baseline), improvement in sleep quality was nonsignificant between all groups except yoga and education. Participants who had 30% or more improvements in pain and physical function at mid-intervention (6 weeks) were more likely to have clinically meaningful improvements in sleep quality at the conclusion of the 12-week intervention.[71] The results of this secondary analysis suggest that both yoga and physical therapy interventions designed for improving chronic LBP and back-related disability may also provide benefit in improving sleep quality.

Cost Effectiveness of Yoga

The cost effectiveness of yoga as an early intervention for nonspecific LBP was investigated by Aboagye and colleagues who compared yoga, exercise, and self-care advice each delivered over 12 weeks.[73] Yoga intervention was described as medical yoga and was provided in group format twice a week for 6 weeks, after which participants continued with a twice weekly home yoga program using a CD and written program. Exercise intervention was provided on an individual basis twice a week for 6 weeks and consisted of a standardized program designed by a physiotherapist with follow-up with the physiotherapist every 2 weeks. The self-care advice group received activity recommendations from a back specialist and a self-care book. HRQL and cost data were measured from baseline to 12-month follow-up. Yoga resulted in significant improvement in HRQL as compared to self-advice but was no different from exercise. A sensitivity analysis based on productivity losses that resulted from sickness absences showed the cost of yoga to be €1887 ($1912.70) and €2761 ($2798.60) less than exercise therapy and self-care advice, respectively, supporting cost-effectiveness of medical yoga.

RECOMMENDATIONS FOR YOGA INTERVENTIONS

Consensus recommendations from a Delphi study identified key components of a musculoskeletal related yoga intervention to be a yoga instructor-guided practice performed 1 to 2 times per week for 60 minutes over an 8-week duration.[11] Although this study recommended 8 weeks to be the minimum duration for yoga practice, which is consistent with the duration utilized in yoga research for arthritis, 12 weeks was the mode of the yoga duration in studies involving LBP.[47,49,50,70,74-77] The Delphi study recommends that yoga instructors should have professional yoga teacher training and experience with teaching yoga to individuals with musculoskeletal conditions.[11] The panelists suggested that yoga for musculoskeletal conditions should integrate physical postures, breathing, and mindfulness and that the instruction of yoga should emphasize safety and postural alignment.

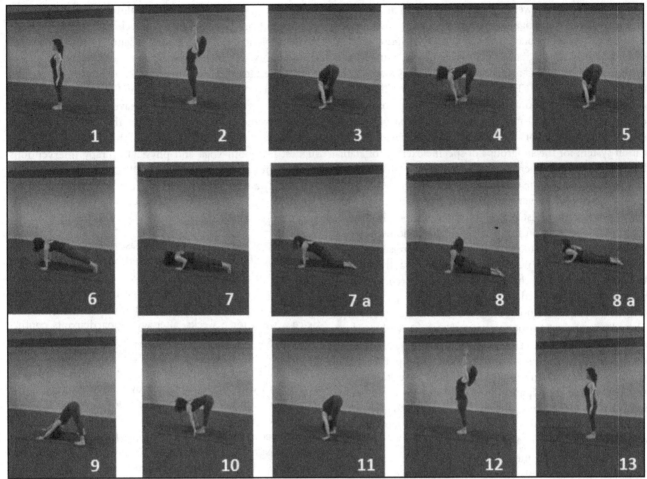

Figure 21-21. Sun Salutation. (1) Mountain. (2) Inhale arms overhead (extended Mountain). (3) Exhale, forward fold. (4) Inhale, half lift. (5) Exhale, fold. (6) Inhale, step back to plank. (7) Exhale, chaturanga OR lower knees (7a). (8) Inhale, Upward Facing Dog OR Cobra (8a). (9) Exhale, Downward Facing Dog. (10) Inhale, step forward to half lift. (11) Exhale, forward fold. (12) Inhale, rise to stand. (13) Exhale, Mountain.

Considerations for the structuring of a yoga session centers around the selection and placement of yoga postures, breathing exercises, and relaxation elements in the class period. Yoga classes are commonly structured in a manner that includes an opening, middle, and closing sequence, where sequence refers to the elements of yoga practice. The opening section typically consists of brief relaxation, breath awareness, and warming yoga postures. An example of a warming sequence of yoga postures is the yoga Sun Salutation (Surya Namaskar) as shown in Figure 21-21. The middle sequence consists of the primary yoga postures selected for the intended purpose of the class. The closing sequence consists of more focused breathing exercises and a longer relaxation component. A sample class for KOA is provided in Table 21-3 and LBP in Table 21-4. Suggested props for modifications are outlined in the table and are encouraged to allow individuals with differing levels of ability to participate and progress with the yoga practice. Cueing for all components of the class should focus on alignment, positioning, breath, and focus.

ROLE OF THE PHYSICAL THERAPIST IN YOGA FOR MUSCULOSKELETAL CONDITIONS

The physical therapist can play an important role in the use of yoga for musculoskeletal conditions. After attaining a working knowledge of yoga and the potential benefits established through yoga-based research, the physical therapist should establish personal experience with yoga by taking classes in their geographic area. This will assist in identifying certified yoga instructors experienced in providing yoga to individuals with musculoskeletal conditions. A collaborative relationship between the physical therapist and qualified yoga instructors can ensue, which may involve screening services, educational trainings, and community workshops. Most yoga studios require potential clients to complete a medical health form prior to beginning yoga, which may identify existing or potential musculoskeletal health conditions. Yoga instructors may then seek screening services of a physical therapist to determine if the individual is safe to begin

Table 21-3

EXAMPLE OF A YOGA PRACTICE FOR OSTEOARTHRITIS

OPENING SEQUENCE	FOCUS	DOSAGE	MODIFICATIONS
Seated Easy pose	Relaxation	2 to 3 minutes	Blanket
Seated Pranayama	Breath awareness	2 to 3 minutes	Blanket
Gentle Spinal Twist	Spine mobility	3 to 5 breaths, each side	Blanket
Seated Bound Angle pose (Baddha Konasana)	Hip opening	3 to 5 breaths	Blanket
Cat Cow (Marjaryasana)	Spine mobility	3 rounds	
Mountain pose (Tadasana)	Standing posture	3 to 5 breaths	Wall or chair assist
Sun Salutation Classic (Surya Namaskar C)	Warming the body	2 rounds	
MIDDLE SEQUENCE	**FOCUS**	**DOSAGE**	**MODIFICATIONS**
Chair (Utkatasana)	Standing posture—strength	3 to 5 breaths	Wall support
Intense Side-Stretch (Parsvottanasana)	Standing posture	3 to 5 breaths, each side	Hands on blocks or chair
One Legged Mountain (Eka Pada Tadasana)	Standing posture—balance	3 to 5 breaths, each side	Wall or chair assist
Tree (Vrksasana)	Standing posture—balance	3 to 5 breaths, each side	Wall or chair assist
Crescent Lunge (Ashta Chandrasana)		3 to 5 breaths, each side	Wall or chair assist
Warrior I (Virabhadrasana I)	Standing posture—strength	3 to 5 breaths, each side	Wall or chair assist
Warrior II (Virabhadrasana II)	Standing posture—strength	3 to 5 breaths, each side	Wall or chair assist
Goddess (Utkata Konasana)		3 to 5 breaths, each side	Chair assist
Extended Side Angle (Utthita Parsvakonasana)		3 to 5 breaths, each side	Wall or chair assist
Bridge (Setu Bandha Sarvangasana)	Floor posture	3 to 5 breaths	
CLOSING SEQUENCE	**FOCUS**	**DOSAGE**	**MODIFICATIONS**
Supine Knees-to-Chest (Apanasana)		3 to 5 breaths	
Reclining Hand-to-Big Toe (Supta Padangusthasana)		3 to 5 breaths, each side	Strap
Seated, Easy pose: Pranayama	Breath refinement: Abdominal breathing	2 to 3 minutes	Blanket
Corpse pose (Savasana)	Relaxation	5 to 10 minutes	

KOA Class is adapted from Brenneman EC, Kuntz AB, Wiebenga EG, Maly MR. A yoga strengthening program designed to minimize the knee adduction moment for women with knee osteoarthritis: a proof-of-principle cohort study. *PloS One.* 2015;10(9):e0136854. doi:10.1371/journal.pone.0136854 and Ebnezar J, Nagarathna R, Yogitha B, Nagendra HR. Effects of an integrated approach of hatha yoga therapy on functional disability, pain and flexibility in osteoarthritis of the knee: a randomized control study. *J Altern Complement Med.* 2012;18(1):1-10.

Table 21-4

EXAMPLE OF A YOGA PRACTICE FOR LOW BACK PAIN

OPENING SEQUENCE	FOCUS	DOSAGE	MODIFICATIONS
Corpse pose (Savasana)	Relaxation, breath awareness	2 to 3 minutes	
Corpse pose (Savasana): Pranayama	Breath refinement— 3-part breath	3 minutes	
Supine Knees-to-Chest (Apanasana)	Spine mobility, hip opener	3 to 5 breaths, each side	
Reclining Spinal Twist (Jathara Parivartanasana)	Twisting posture— spine mobility	3 to 5 breaths, each side	
Mountain pose (Tadasana)	Standing posture	3 breaths	
Mountain pose: Shoulder opener	Standing posture— thoracic and shoulder mobility		Strap
Sun Salutation A (Surya Namaskara A)	Warming the body	2 rounds, 5 breaths in Downward Facing Dog	Hands on block, chair in forward fold and half lift; kneeling plank

MIDDLE SEQUENCE	FOCUS	DOSAGE	MODIFICATIONS
Half Wheel (Ardha Kati Chakrasana)	Standing posture— spine mobility		
Extended hands and feet pose (Utthita Hasta Padasana)	Standing posture— open and chest and upper back		
Intense side-stretch (Parsvottanasana)	Standing posture— forward bend	3 to 5 breaths, each side	Hands on blocks, chair
Triangle (Trikonasana)			
Revolved Triangle (Parivrtta Trikonasana)		3 to 5 breaths, each side	Wall or chair assist
Warrior I (Virabhadrasana I)	Standing posture— strength	3 to 5 breaths, each side	Foot to wall
Baby Dancer	Standing posture— balance, hip opener	3 to 5 breaths, each side	Wall or chair assist
Cobra or Sphinx	Backward bends— spine strengthening	3 to 5 breaths	
Half Locust (Ardha Shalabhasana)	Backward bends— spine strengthening	3 to 5 breaths, each side	
Table (Bharmanasana)	Core activation	3 to 5 breaths	
Child's pose (Balasana)	Relaxation, spine mobility, hip opener	5 breaths	Blanket, block
Reclined chest opener	Chest and upper back opener	5 breaths	Block

(continued)

Table 21-4 (continued)

EXAMPLE OF A YOGA PRACTICE FOR LOW BACK PAIN

CLOSING SEQUENCE	FOCUS	DOSAGE	MODIFICATIONS
Supported Bridge (Setu Bandha Sarvangasana)	Relaxation, front of hip opener	3 to 5 breaths	Block
Legs Up a Wall	Restorative, inversion	5 minutes	Blanket
Pranayama: Alternate nostril breathing	Breath purification: Alternate nostril breathing	2 to 3 rounds	Blanket
Basic relaxation pose	Relaxation	5 to 10 minutes	Bolster, blanket, eye pillow

LBP Class is adapted from Williams K, Abildso C, Steinberg L, et al. Evaluation of the effectiveness and efficacy of Iyengar yoga therapy on chronic low back pain. *Spine*. 2009;34(19):2066-2076. doi:10.1097/BRS.0b013e3181b315cc and Saper RB, Sherman KJ, Delitto A, et al. Yoga vs. physical therapy vs. education for chronic low back pain in predominantly minority populations: study protocol for a randomized controlled trial. *Trials*. 2014;15:67. doi:10.1186/1745-6215-15-67

yoga or if physical therapy or medical referral is indicated. The screening may also provide advice regarding which yoga postures should be modified or avoided to facilitate the safe practice of yoga by an individual with a musculoskeletal condition. As movement specialists with advanced knowledge of anatomy and kinesiology, the physical therapist can offer educational trainings to yoga instructors to supplement yoga certification content. Educational trainings offered to the community by both a yoga instructor and physical therapist may increase the public's awareness of each discipline in the promotion of physical, psychological, and social aspects of health and wellness.

The physical therapist may also choose to complete a credentialed yoga teacher training program to attain a more comprehensive understanding of yoga and to develop an awareness of how select components of yoga may be incorporated in the management of musculoskeletal conditions. For example, utilization of pranayama (breathing) techniques and guided meditation (dhyana) may assist individuals with elevated fear-avoidance beliefs that are limiting their active participation in the management of spinal dysfunction. Similarly, the use of restorative yoga postures may assist in relaxation and stress management in the individual with chronic pain. Incorporation of the alignment-based cueing that accompanies the instruction of yoga postures may assist individuals in attaining more optimal movement patterns for pain and injury prevention. Lastly, the yoga trained physical therapist may develop individualized or group-based yoga classes as a component of health promotion across the lifespan.

CASE STUDY

Yoga for a Young Cross-Country Athlete

A physical therapist, also an E-RYT 500 yoga instructor, was contacted by a parent of a cross-country runner to develop and instruct a yoga practice this runner could use to complement his running training program. The runner (SN), a 16-year-old adolescent boy, had no current musculoskeletal symptoms but had completed the physical therapy provided by this physical therapist for patellofemoral pain of the right knee 3 months prior.

Given the sagittal plane motion of running, yoga postures were selected to create a balance between strengthening and lengthening muscle used in this plane. In addition, side-to-side and twisting postures were also selected to target the less utilized frontal and horizontal planes in running. Based on his prior history of patellofemoral pain, alignment cues during yoga postures were directed toward knee positioning relative to the foot, activation of the quadriceps muscles, and weightbearing distribution to prevent lowering of the medial longitudinal arch of the foot. Throughout the asana component of the yoga practice, SN was cued to maintain a steady eye gaze (dristhti), to promote concentration (dharana) and tuning out of external distractions to maintain an inward focus (pratyahara), both of which are skills he could use to maximize the mental component of cross-country competition. While breathing was cued throughout the yoga asana sequence, the pranayama component of the practice focused on development of the 3-part breath. Legs up the wall was selected as a restorative posture for the closing sequence.

A simple seated meditation was instructed to assist in developing mental focus and relieving stress. While seated, SN focused on even breathing at a pace of 2 to 3 seconds per inhale and exhale. With each inhale and exhale, he mentally counted backward from 20.

A primary component of the yoga practice was use of the sun salutation. The sun salutation, Surya Namaskara, is a series of yoga postures that link movement with breath. An inhale or exhale breath guides movement into each posture in the sequence. A sun salutation sequence was incorporated at the beginning of the asana practice to encourage rhythmic breathing and dynamic warming of the entire body. The sun salutation included kneeling lunge, progressing to low lunge to open the hips. One round of a sun salutation, when lunges are performed, consists of performing the posture series twice, once through stepping back into a lunge with the right leg and once through stepping back into a lunge with the left leg.

SN received 8 yoga sessions as outlined in Table 21-5. A video of his practice was prepared that included verbal instructions from the physical therapist for his use independently. During independent practice, SN was instructed to perform the warming sequence, select 3 standing postures and 3 floor postures from the middle sequence, and to perform the closing sequence. SN was advised to use the sun salutation as a dynamic warm-up prior to running and to use legs up the wall (or tree immediately following practice) as a restorative posture after training. The physical therapist consulted with a local yoga instructor owned studio to establish an 8-week yoga series for cross-country runners. This provided SN the opportunity to continue his yoga practice on a regular basis with other runners.

Table 21-5

YOGA CLASS DEVELOPED FOR A CROSS-COUNTRY RUNNER

OPENING SEQUENCE	FOCUS	DOSAGE
1. Mountain	Weight equally distributed over the 4 corners of each foot (ball of the foot and heel); activation of the thigh, hip, and abdominal muscles; opening the chest	5 to 7 breaths; focus on making the inhale and exhale breaths equal length; progressively increase the length of each inhale and exhale from 2 counts up to 6 counts
2. Sun Salutation	Dynamic warm-up; performed with low lunge to open the hips	2 to 6 rounds; 1 round consists of 2 circuits through the series to all
MIDDLE SEQUENCE	**FOCUS**	**DOSAGE**
3. Half Moon	Stretch the spine in 4 directions; open the ribs	2 breaths each direction
4. Warrior I	Build strength in the thigh of the front leg; increase flexibility in the back leg; strengthen shoulders Emphasize knee over second toe alignment	3 to 5 breaths
5. Warrior II	Build strength in the thigh of the front leg; increase flexibility of the inner thighs; open chest, strengthen upper back Emphasize knee over second toe alignment	3 to 5 breaths
6. Reverse Warrior	Open the ribs	2 breaths
7. Warrior III	Balance; trunk strength; gluteal strength of lifted leg; stretching hamstrings of support leg	2 breaths
8. One Legged Mountain	Balance	2 to 4 breaths
9. High Lunge (crescent lunge)	Build strength in the thigh of the front leg; stretch hip flexors and calf of back leg, strengthen shoulders, mobility of the ankle and toes of back leg	2 to 4 breaths
10. Triangle	Stretch the hamstrings, inner thigh of front leg; stretch hip abductors, ankle evertors of back leg; lengthen the trunk; open the chest	2 to 4 breaths
Repeat postures 5 through 10 on the opposite side		
11. Wide Stance Forward Fold (with hands behind back)	Inner thigh, hamstring, calf stretch; chest and shoulder stretch	2 to 4 breaths
12. Eagle	Balance; outer hip and thigh stretch, upper back stretch	2 to 4 breaths; right and left
13. Malasana	Gluteal stretch, calf stretch, hip mobility	2 to 4 breaths
		(continued)

Table 21-5 (continued)

YOGA CLASS DEVELOPED FOR A CROSS-COUNTRY RUNNER

MIDDLE SEQUENCE	FOCUS	DOSAGE
Savasana	*Transition to Lying on the Floor*	*2 to 4 Breaths*
14. Single Leg lifts	Mobility in the hip, strengthens thighs, stretch hamstrings	6 count leg lift; 6 count leg lower; x 5 each leg
15. Floor Spine Twist	Opens the chest, spine mobility, stretch the outer hip muscles	2 to 4 breaths; each side
16. Cobra	Spine strengthening	3 breaths
17. Half Locust	Strengthen hip extensors	3 breaths each leg
18. Cat/Cow	Spine mobility	3 times
19. Child's pose	Stretch the spine, gluteals, ankle dorsiflexors, and toe extensors	2 to 4 breaths
20. Thunderbolt	Ankle mobility, stretch ankle dorsiflexor and toe extensors	2 to 4 breaths
21. Pigeon	Front leg: hip mobility, stretch deep hip rotators, IT-band Back leg: stretch the hip flexors, ankle dorsiflexors	3 to 5 breaths each side
22. Seated Spine Twist	Spine mobility, outer hip and chest stretch	3 to 5 breaths each side
CLOSING SEQUENCE	**FOCUS**	**DOSAGE**
23. Savasana	Relaxation	3 to 5 breaths
24. Legs Up the Wall	Relaxation, returns blood to the heart	3 to 5 breaths
25. Meditation	Counting meditation—counting down from 20 (1 count per each inhale/exhale)	Breathing at a rate of about 2 to 3 seconds on the inhale and on the exhale

REFERENCES

1. The Big Picture. BMUS: The Burden of Musculoskeletal Diseases in the United States. Accessed December 29, 2016. http://www.bone-andjointburden.org/2014-report/io/big-picture

2. Clarke TC, Black LI, Stussman BJ, Barnes PM, Nahin RL. *Trends in the Use of Complementary Health Approaches Among Adults: United States, 2002-2012.* National Center for Health Statistics; 2015.

3. Complementary, alternative, or integrative health: what's in a name? NCCIH. Published November 11, 2011. Accessed December 30, 2016. https://nccih.nih.gov/health/integrative-health

4. Yoga in America Study. Yoga Journal. Published January 13, 2016. Accessed March 12, 2017. http://www.yogajournal.com/yogainamericastudy/

5. Marin TJ, Van Eerd D, Irvin E, et al. Multidisciplinary biopsychosocial rehabilitation for subacute low back pain. *Cochrane Database Syst Rev.* 2017;6:CD002193. doi:10.1002/14651858.CD002193.pub2

6. Sulenes K, Freitas J, Justice L, Colgan DD, Shean M, Brems C. Underuse of yoga as a referral resource by health professions students. *J Altern Complement Med N Y N.* 2015;21(1):53-59. doi:10.1089/acm.2014.0217

7. Raub JA. Psychophysiologic effects of Hatha Yoga on musculoskeletal and cardiopulmonary function: a literature review. *J Altern Complement Med N Y N.* 2002;8(6):797-812. doi:10.1089/10755530260511810

8. Stephens M. *Teaching Yoga: Essential Foundations and Techniques.* North Atlantic Books; 2010.

9. Satchidananda S. *The Yoga Sutras of Patanjali.* 14th ed. Integral Yoga; 2010.

10. McCrary M. *Pick Your Yoga Practice: Exploring and Understanding Different Styles of Yoga.* New World Library; 2013.

11. Ward L, Stebbings S, Sherman KJ, Cherkin D, Baxter GD. Establishing key components of yoga interventions for musculoskeletal conditions: a Delphi survey. *BMC Complement Altern Med.* 2014;14:196. doi:10.1186/1472-6882-14-196

12. About PYTI. Prof Yoga Ther Institute. Accessed November 10, 2019. https://proyogatherapy.org/about-pyts/

13. About IAYT - International Association of Yoga Therapists (IAYT). Accessed November 11, 2019. https://www.iayt.org/page/AboutLanding

14. Standards | Yoga Alliance. Accessed July 21, 2017. https://www.yogaalliance.org/Designations/Standards

15. Certification Background and Future - International Association of Yoga Therapists (IAYT). Accessed November 11, 2019. https://www.iayt.org/page/Cert_Background

16. Booth J, Moseley GL, Schiltenwolf M, Cashin A, Davies M, Hübscher M. Exercise for chronic musculoskeletal pain: a biopsychosocial approach. *Musculoskeletal Care.* 2017;15(4):413-421. doi:10.1002/msc.1191

17. Stilwell P, Harman K. Contemporary biopsychosocial exercise prescription for chronic low back pain: questioning core stability programs and considering context. *J Can Chiropr Assoc.* 2017;61(1):6-17.

18. Stephens M. *Yoga Sequencing: Designing Transformative Yoga Classes.* North Atlantic Books; 2012.

19. Ross A, Thomas S. The health benefits of yoga and exercise: a review of comparison studies. *J Altern Complement Med N Y N.* 2010;16(1):3-12. doi:10.1089/acm.2009.0044

20. Salem GJ, Yu SS-Y, Wang M-Y, et al. Physical demand profiles of hatha yoga postures performed by older adults. *Evid-Based Complement Altern Med ECAM.* 2013;2013:165763. doi:10.1155/2013/165763

21. Ni M, Mooney K, Harriell K, Balachandran A, Signorile J. Core muscle function during specific yoga poses. *Complement Ther Med.* 2014;22(2):235-243. doi:10.1016/j.ctim.2014.01.007

22. Omkar SN, Vishwas S, Tech B. Yoga techniques as a means of core stability training. *J Bodyw Mov Ther.* 2009;13(1):98-103. doi:10.1016/j.jbmt.2007.10.004

23. Cramer H, Krucoff C, Dobos G. Adverse events associated with yoga: a systematic review of published case reports and case series. *PloS One.* 2013;8(10):e75515. doi:10.1371/journal.pone.0075515

24. Saper RB, Sherman KJ, Delitto A, et al. Yoga vs. physical therapy vs. education for chronic low back pain in predominantly minority populations: study protocol for a randomized controlled trial. *Trials.* 2014;15:67. doi:10.1186/1745-6215-15-67

25. Saper RB, Lemaster CM, Elwy AR, et al. Yoga versus education for veterans with chronic low back pain: study protocol for a randomized controlled trial. *Trials.* 2016;17(1):224. doi:10.1186/s13063-016-1321-5

26. Long R. *The Key Poses of Hatha Yoga.* Bandha Yoga Publications; 2008.

27. Telles S, Bhardwaj AK, Gupta RK, Sharma SK, Monro R, Balkrishna A. A randomized controlled trial to assess pain and magnetic resonance imaging-based (MRI-based) structural spine changes in low back pain patients after yoga practice. *Med Sci Monit Int Med J Exp Clin Res.* 2016;22:3228-3247.

28. Lasater JH. *Relax and Renew.* 2nd ed. Rodmell Press; 2011.

29. Jeter PE, Slutsky J, Singh N, Khalsa SBS. Yoga as a therapeutic intervention: a bibliometric analysis of published research studies from 1967 to 2013. *J Altern Complement Med N Y N.* 2015;21(10):586-592. doi:10.1089/acm.2015.0057

30. Cramer H, Lauche R, Dobos G. Characteristics of randomized controlled trials of yoga: a bibliometric analysis. *BMC Complement Altern Med.* 2014;14:328. doi:10.1186/1472-6882-14-328

31. Wieland LS, Skoetz N, Pilkington K, Vempati R, D'Adamo CR, Berman BM. Yoga treatment for chronic non-specific low back pain. *Cochrane Database Syst Rev.* 2017;1:CD010671. doi:10.1002/14651858.CD010671.pub2

32. Cramer H, Ward L, Saper R, Fishbein D, Dobos G, Lauche R. The safety of yoga: a systematic review and meta-analysis of randomized controlled trials. *Am J Epidemiol.* 2015;182(4):281-293. doi:10.1093/aje/kwv071

33. Lu Y-H, Rosner B, Chang G, Fishman LM. Twelve-minute daily yoga regimen reverses osteoporotic bone loss. *Top Geriatr Rehabil.* 2016;32(2):81-87. doi:10.1097/TGR.0000000000000085

34. Greendale GA, Huang M-H, Karlamangla AS, Seeger L, Crawford S. Yoga decreases kyphosis in senior women and men with adult-onset hyperkyphosis: results of a randomized controlled trial. *J Am Geriatr Soc.* 2009;57(9):1569-1579. doi:10.1111/j.1532-5415.2009.02391.x

35. Roland KP, Jakobi JM, Jones GR. Does yoga engender fitness in older adults? A critical review. *J Aging Phys Act.* 2011;19(1):62-79.

36. Hagins M, Moore W, Rundle A. Does practicing hatha yoga satisfy recommendations for intensity of physical activity which improves and maintains health and cardiovascular fitness? *BMC Complement Altern Med.* 2007;7:40. doi:10.1186/1472-6882-7-40

37. Hagins M, States R, Selfe T, Innes K. Effectiveness of yoga for hypertension: systematic review and meta-analysis. *Evid Based Complement Alternat Med.* 2013;2013:649836.

38. Cramer H, Lauche R, Haller H, Steckhan N, Michalsen A, Dobos G. Effects of yoga on cardiovascular disease risk factors: a systematic review and meta-analysis. *Int J Cardiol.* 2014;173(2):170-183. doi:10.1016/j.ijcard.2014.02.017

39. Chu P, Gotink RA, Yeh GY, Goldie SJ, Hunink MGM. The effectiveness of yoga in modifying risk factors for cardiovascular disease and metabolic syndrome: a systematic review and meta-analysis of randomized controlled trials. *Eur J Prev Cardiol.* 2016;23(3):291-307. doi:10.1177/2047487314562741

40. Kiecolt-Glaser JK, Christian L, Preston H, et al. Stress, inflammation, and yoga practice. *Psychosom Med.* 2010;72(2):113. doi:10.1097/PSY.0b013e3181cb9377

41. Yadav RK, Magan D, Mehta N, Sharma R, Mahapatra SC. Efficacy of a short-term yoga-based lifestyle intervention in reducing stress and inflammation: preliminary results. *J Altern Complement Med N Y N.* 2012;18(7):662-667. doi:10.1089/acm.2011.0265

42. Pullen PR, Nagamia SH, Mehta PK, et al. Effects of yoga on inflammation and exercise capacity in patients with chronic heart failure. *J Card Fail.* 2008;14(5):407-413. doi:10.1016/j.cardfail.2007.12.007

43. Riley KE, Park CL. How does yoga reduce stress? A systematic review of mechanisms of change and guide to future inquiry. *Health Psychol Rev.* 2015;9(3):379-396. doi:10.1080/17437199.2014.981778

44. Streeter CC, Whitfield TH, Owen L, et al. Effects of yoga versus walking on mood, anxiety, and brain GABA levels: a randomized controlled MRS study. *J Altern Complement Med.* 2010;16(11):1145-1152. doi:10.1089/acm.2010.0007

45. Streeter CC, Jensen JE, Perlmutter RM, et al. Yoga Asana sessions increase brain GABA levels: a pilot study. *J Altern Complement Med N Y N.* 2007;13(4):419-426. doi:10.1089/acm.2007.6338

46. Sherman KJ, Cherkin DC, Erro J, Miglioretti DL, Deyo RA. Comparing yoga, exercise, and a self-care book for chronic low back pain: a randomized, controlled trial. *Ann Intern Med.* 2005;143(12):849-856.

47. Sherman KJ, Cherkin DC, Wellman RD, et al. A randomized trial comparing yoga, stretching, and a self-care book for chronic low back pain. *Arch Intern Med.* 2011;171(22):2019-2026. doi:10.1001/archinternmed.2011.524

48. Nambi GS, Inbasekaran D, Khuman R, Devi S, Shanmugananth, Jagannathan K. Changes in pain intensity and health related quality of life with Iyengar yoga in nonspecific chronic low back pain: a randomized controlled study. *Int J Yoga.* 2014;7(1):48-53. doi:10.4103/0973-6131.123481

49. Williams KA, Petronis J, Smith D, et al. Effect of Iyengar yoga therapy for chronic low back pain. *Pain.* 2005;115(1-2):107-117. doi:10.1016/j.pain.2005.02.016

50. Williams K, Abildso C, Steinberg L, et al. Evaluation of the effectiveness and efficacy of Iyengar yoga therapy on chronic low back pain. *Spine.* 2009;34(19):2066-2076. doi:10.1097/BRS.0b013e3181b315cc

51. Cox H, Tilbrook H, Aplin J, et al. A randomised controlled trial of yoga for the treatment of chronic low back pain: results of a pilot study. *Complement Ther Clin Pract.* 2010;16(4):187-193. doi:10.1016/j.ctcp.2010.05.007

52. Galantino ML, Bzdewka TM, Eissler-Russo JL, et al. The impact of modified Hatha yoga on chronic low back pain: a pilot study. *Altern Ther Health Med.* 2004;10(2):56-59.

53. Jacobs BP, Mehling W, Avins AL, et al. Feasibility of conducting a clinical trial on Hatha yoga for chronic low back pain: methodological lessons. *Altern Ther Health Med.* 2004;10(2):80-83.

54. Tilbrook HE, Cox H, Hewitt CE, et al. Yoga for chronic low back pain: a randomized trial. *Ann Intern Med.* 2011;155(9):569-578. doi:10.7326/0003-4819-155-9-201111010-00003

55. Groessl EJ, Liu L, Chang DG, et al. Yoga for military veterans with chronic low back pain: a randomized clinical trial. *Am J Prev Med.* 2017;53(5):599-608. doi:10.1016/j.amepre.2017.05.019

56. Groessl EJ, Liu L, Schmalzl L, et al. Secondary outcomes from a randomized controlled trial of yoga for veterans with chronic low-back pain. *Int J Yoga Ther.* 2020;30(1):69-76. doi:10.17761/2020-D-19-00036

57. Li Y, Li S, Jiang J, Yuan S. Effects of yoga on patients with chronic nonspecific neck pain: a PRISMA systematic review and meta-analysis. *Medicine (Baltimore).* 2019;98(8):e14649. doi:10.1097/MD.0000000000014649

58. Michalsen A, Traitteur H, Lüdtke R, et al. Yoga for chronic neck pain: a pilot randomized controlled clinical trial. *J Pain Off J Am Pain Soc.* 2012;13(11):1122-1130. doi:10.1016/j.jpain.2012.08.004

59. Dunleavy K, Kava K, Goldberg A, et al. Comparative effectiveness of Pilates and yoga group exercise interventions for chronic mechanical neck pain: quasi-randomised parallel controlled study. *Physiotherapy.* 2016;102(3):236-242. doi:10.1016/j.physio.2015.06.002

60. Cramer H, Lauche R, Hohmann C, et al. Randomized-controlled trial comparing yoga and home-based exercise for chronic neck pain. *Clin J Pain.* 2013;29(3):216-223. doi:10.1097/AJP.0b013e318251026c

61. Cheung C, Park J, Wyman JF. Effects of yoga on symptoms, physical function, and psychosocial outcomes in adults with osteoarthritis: a focused review. *Am J Phys Med Rehabil.* 2016;95(2):139-151. doi:10.1097/PHM.0000000000000408

62. Kan L, Zhang J, Yang Y, Wang P. The effects of yoga on pain, mobility, and quality of life in patients with knee osteoarthritis: a systematic review. *Evid-Based Complement Altern Med ECAM.* 2016;2016. doi:10.1155/2016/6016532

63. Wang Y, Lu S, Wang R, et al. Integrative effect of yoga practice in patients with knee arthritis: a PRISMA-compliant meta-analysis. *Medicine (Baltimore).* 2018;97(31):e11742. doi:10.1097/MD.0000000000011742

64. Lauche R, Hunter DJ, Adams J, Cramer H. Yoga for osteoarthritis: a systematic review and meta-analysis. *Curr Rheumatol Rep.* 2019;21(9):47. doi:10.1007/s11926-019-0846-5

65. Brosseau L, Taki J, Desjardins B, et al. The Ottawa panel clinical practice guidelines for the management of knee osteoarthritis. Part one: introduction, and mind-body exercise programs. *Clin Rehabil.* 2017;31(5):582-595. doi:10.1177/0269215517691083

66. Ebnezar J, Nagarathna R, Bali Y, Nagendra HR. Effect of an integrated approach of yoga therapy on quality of life in osteoarthritis of the knee joint: a randomized control study. *Int J Yoga.* 2011;4(2):55-63. doi:10.4103/0973-6131.85486

67. Ebnezar J, Nagarathna R, Yogitha B, Nagendra HR. Effect of integrated yoga therapy on pain, morning stiffness and anxiety in osteoarthritis of the knee joint: a randomized control study. *Int J Yoga.* 2012;5(1):28-36. doi:10.4103/0973-6131.91708

68. Ebnezar J, Nagarathna R, Yogitha B, Nagendra HR. Effects of an integrated approach of hatha yoga therapy on functional disability, pain and flexibility in osteoarthritis of the knee: a randomized control study. *J Altern Complement Med.* 2012;18(1):1-10.

69. Brenneman EC, Kuntz AB, Wiebenga EG, Maly MR. A yoga strengthening program designed to minimize the knee adduction moment for women with knee osteoarthritis: a proof-of-principle cohort study. *PloS One.* 2015;10(9):e0136854. doi:10.1371/journal.pone.0136854

70. Saper RB, Lemaster C, Delitto A, et al. Yoga, physical therapy, or education for chronic low back pain: a randomized noninferiority trial. *Ann Intern Med.* 2017;167(2):85-94. doi:10.7326/M16-2579

71. Roseen EJ, Gerlovin H, Femia A, et al. Yoga, physical therapy, and back pain education for sleep quality in low-income racially diverse adults with chronic low back pain: a secondary analysis of a randomized controlled trial. *J Gen Intern Med.* 2020;35(1):167-176. doi:10.1007/s11606-019-05329-4

72. Fritz JM, Brennan GP, Clifford SN, Hunter SJ, Thackeray A. An examination of the reliability of a classification algorithm for subgrouping patients with low back pain. *Spine.* 2006;31(1):77-82.

73. Aboagye E, Karlsson ML, Hagberg J, Jensen I. Cost-effectiveness of early interventions for non-specific low back pain: a randomized controlled study investigating medical yoga, exercise therapy and self-care advice. *J Rehabil Med.* 2015;47(2):167-173. doi:10.2340/16501977-1910

74. Cox H, Tilbrook H, Aplin J, et al. A randomised controlled trial of yoga for the treatment of chronic low back pain: results of a pilot study. *Complement Ther Clin Pract.* 2010;16(4):187-193. doi:10.1016/j.ctcp.2010.05.007

75. Nambi GS, Inbasekaran D, Khuman R, Devi S, Shanmugananth, Jagannathan K. Changes in pain intensity and health related quality of life with Iyengar yoga in nonspecific chronic low back pain: a randomized controlled study. *Int J Yoga.* 2014;7(1):48-53. doi:10.4103/0973-6131.123481

76. Tilbrook HE, Cox H, Hewitt CE, et al. Yoga for chronic low back pain: a randomized trial. *Ann Intern Med.* 2011;155(9):569-578. doi:10.7326/0003-4819-155-9-201111010-00003

77. Saper RB, Sherman KJ, Cullum-Dugan D, Davis RB, Phillips RS, Culpepper L. Yoga for chronic low back pain in a predominantly minority population: a pilot randomized controlled trial. *Altern Ther Health Med.* 2009;15(6):18-27.

Diagnostic Imaging and Ultrasound

Mohini Rawat, DPT, MS, ECS, OCS, RMSK

KEY TERMS

Anechoic: No energy reflected back. Structure appears black on ultrasound imaging.

Anisotropy: Property of being directionally dependent. On ultrasound imaging, structures like tendons exhibit anisotropy, where they may appear hypoechoic or hyperechoic (darker or brighter) depending on probe orientation or transmitted beam angle.

CT: Computed tomography.

Echogenicity: Amount of energy reflected back to the ultrasound transducer.

Hyperechoic: More energy reflected back. Structure appears white on ultrasound imaging.

Hypoechoic: Less energy reflected back. Structure appears grey on ultrasound imaging.

MRA: Magnetic resonance arthrography.

MRI: Magnetic resonance imaging.

CHAPTER QUESTIONS

1. What are the common types of diagnostic imaging available?

2. What is the use of MRI, CT, radiograph, and ultrasound in musculoskeletal imaging?

3. When did we first start using imaging modalities like x-ray, CT, MRI, and ultrasound in medicine?

4. What is point-of-care diagnostic musculoskeletal ultrasound imaging?

5. What are the basic principles of physics behind diagnostic ultrasound?

6. What are the advantages of musculoskeletal ultrasound over other imaging modalities?

7. Describe and distinguish appearance of different types of connective tissues on ultrasound.

8. What value does musculoskeletal ultrasound add to physical therapy evaluation?

9. What are the limitations of musculoskeletal ultrasound?

Wallmann HW, Donatelli R, eds. *Foundations of Orthopedic Physical Therapy* (pp 663-681).
© 2024 Taylor & Francis Group.

10. Are there any contraindications for diagnostic musculoskeletal ultrasound?

11. What types of transducers are used in diagnostic ultrasound and what are they used for?

12. What frequency range is used in diagnostic musculoskeletal ultrasound imaging?

13. What are the indications for musculoskeletal imaging and when should it be used?

14. Is it safe to use ultrasound in postoperative cases like total knee replacements or other surgeries where hardware is present in the body part?

15. Define anisotropy as it relates to ultrasound imaging and what you can do to improve image quality and prevent misinterpretation.

16. What are the most common types of artifacts on ultrasound imaging?

17. What are the controls that you can utilize to optimize the ultrasound image quality?

18. How do you differentiate tendinosis from tenosynovitis on ultrasound imaging?

19. How do you differentiate tendon tear from tendinosis on ultrasound imaging?

20. How do you differentiate vein from artery on ultrasound imaging?

INTRODUCTION

Diagnostic imaging is an important tool in clinical evaluation for musculoskeletal pathology. When used appropriately, it can boost clinical decision making with a positive impact on patient care. A brief review of the history of various imaging modalities in musculoskeletal evaluation and their basic differences will be discussed. Knowledge of the fundamental principles and how they operate is essential in selecting the most effective and appropriate imaging modality. Ultrasound is safe, easily available, cost-effective, and is a real-time imaging modality, which has a wide range of application in neuromusculoskeletal pathologies.

Basic principles, terminology, probe selection, and image optimization of the ultrasound imaging will be presented. Knowledge of artifacts during imaging is important in identification of true pathology and to be better able to differentiate normal from abnormal tissue and physiology. Artifacts are signals or images that do not represent the actual structures. Knowledge and recognition of artifacts gives a better understanding of the pathology and a better identification of the type of structure. To be able to identify various abnormalities or pathologies on ultrasound, one has to know the normal sonoanatomy and how different tissues present on ultrasound imaging. Point-of-care imaging has great advantages, which include better insight into the

patient's problem, greater satisfaction of patient in the care provided, greater confidence of the patient in the provider, and improved overall efficiency of the system.

Diagnostic imaging is used to aid clinical decision making and follows a thorough clinical examination. The most common types of musculoskeletal imaging used in patient care are MRI, radiographs or x-ray, CT scan, and ultrasound. Appropriate and effective use of the imaging modality requires some basic understanding of the principles of the imaging technique and knowledge of what structure is best visualized with a specific type of imaging modality.

HISTORY OF IMAGING

X-rays are the oldest imaging technique, and their first use was demonstrated in 1895 by Wilhelm Rontgen who later was awarded Nobel Prize in Physics in 1901. The first CT studies were performed in 1971.[1] Six years after the first CT scan, the first human MRIs were published in 1977, and it took 5 hours to acquire the imaging study.[1]

Ultrasound was first used in 1942 by Karl Dussik, neurologist and psychiatrist at the University of Vienna, to visualize brain tumors. In 1948, George Ludwig, an internist, used ultrasound to diagnose gallstones at the Naval Medical Research Institute. The first musculoskeletal ultrasound report was published by Karl Dussik in 1958 measuring acoustic attenuation, describing acoustic anisotropy, and suggesting that the pathological process influences attenuation constants.[2] The first musculoskeletal brightness mode scan study, which is also commonly known as *B mode ultrasound scan*, was published in 1972 by Daniel G. McDonald and George R. Leopold describing the use of ultrasound in differentiating Baker's cyst from thrombophlebitis.[3] B mode ultrasound imaging utilizes the pulse-echo technique, where small pulses of ultrasound are transmitted from transducer to human tissue, and as it passes through the human body echo signals get reflected back from each interface to the transducer to be processed to generate the image.[4]

Use of musculoskeletal ultrasound imaging as an adjunct in the evaluation of the neuromusculoskeletal system is rapidly growing worldwide since its inception 60 years ago by Dussik. Its cost-effectiveness, ability to evaluate structures in real time, easy availability, and portability of the equipment makes it widely popular and one of the most effective tools in clinical imaging. A list of advantages of diagnostic musculoskeletal ultrasound is shown in Table 22-1.

Appropriate selection of the imaging modality depends on structure of interest that is in question and knowledge of what information can be gained from different imaging options. To elaborate this point let us review the basic principles of each imaging technique and what structures are best studied by them.

Table 22-1

ADVANTAGES OF DIAGNOSTIC ULTRASOUND IMAGING

Time saving

Cost saving

Real-time evaluation

Readily available

Greater patient satisfaction with care reported[5]

Can be safely used when other imaging modalities are contraindicated

Comparison of contralateral structures possible

X-RAY

Radiograph or x-ray study utilizes x-rays that pass through the human body or area of interest. As the x-ray passes through the body, some of the rays pass through freely while others get absorbed or scattered (attenuated). For example, dense structures, like bone, cause more attenuation of the x-ray than soft tissue or lung. Due to relative differences in densities of different tissues, the x-ray image gets its pictorial representation of the contrast between those structures or tissues ranging from radio-opaque to radiolucent. Indications for x-ray imaging for the musculoskeletal system includes, but is not limited to, bony deformity, fractures, dislocations, arthritis, and joint pain. X-rays are ionizing radiation and can cause biological changes; therefore, unnecessary exposure should be avoided.[6]

COMPUTED TOMOGRAPHY

CT scans originated from the x-ray modality in 1971. CT image acquisition requires rotation of the x-ray tube and detector row around the patient to obtain a large number of views. These many views are then used to reconstruct the CT image, which is a composition of matrix of picture element or pixels. Unlike x-ray imaging, which is selective imaging of an area with one view taken at a time, CT scan has the capability of whole body scan, which can be viewed in different angles (eg, in polytrauma cases). Musculoskeletal indications include bone disorders, soft tissue tumors, and muscle disorders. Because CT scan utilizes x-rays, there is exposure of ionizing radiation to the body; therefore, unnecessary exposure should be avoided.[7]

MAGNETIC RESONANCE IMAGING

MRI utilizes strong magnetic fields to generate images of the human body. There is no use of ionizing radiations, like in x-ray and CT scan. Simply stated, the patient is placed in a strong magnetic field where radio waves are transmitted; in turn, the patient emits a signal that is received and used to reconstruct the MRI image. We are made up of atoms, which consist of a nucleus and the nucleus contains protons and neutrons with a net positive charge. The hydrogen nucleus possesses a property of "spin" dependent on the number of protons, but does not spin by itself; it induces a magnetic moment generating a local magnetic field with north and south poles. When it is placed in a strong external magnetic field, like the ones in an MRI scanner, the nucleus is aligned in parallel with or perpendicular to the external magnetic field. Depending on its orientation to the magnetic field, the nuclei can be in a high-energy state (oriented perpendicular to the magnetic field direction) or low-energy state (oriented parallel to the magnetic field).[8]

Nuclei within the static magnetic field are excited by the application of a second radiofrequency magnetic field applied perpendicular to the first static magnetic field. The absorption of the energy by the nucleus causes a transition from a high-energy state to a low-energy state and vice versa on relaxation, and the energy absorbed by the nuclei induces a voltage that can be detected by the radio-coil. This voltage is amplified and displayed as free induction decay. The signal averaged free induction decay is then resolved by Fourier transformation into an image (MRI image).[8] Because MRI utilizes strong magnetic fields, a patient with hardware like open reduction internal fixation, joint arthroplasty, or other implanted devices cannot receive MRI imaging.

MRA is a technique of MRI, where dye or contrast agent is injected into the joint to visualize internal joint derangements, labral pathology, meniscal pathology, differentiate type of tendon tears, intra-articular loose bodies, ligament pathology, or other articular defects.[9] Diagnostic accuracy of MRA exceeds that of conventional MRI in visualizing intra-articular structures, capsuloligamentous structures, and for the staging of lesions of cartilage or labrum.[10] Because MRA is a minimally invasive diagnostic procedure, it is reserved for specific intra-articular disorders.

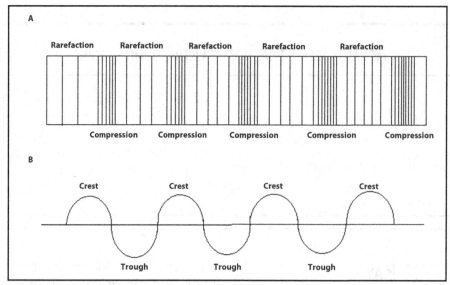

Figure 22-1. (A) Longitudinal wave: movement of particles in the same direction as the direction of wave propagation. (B) Transverse wave: movement of particles perpendicular to the direction of wave propagation.

ULTRASOUND

Ultrasound utilizes sound waves that are transmitted to human tissue and the returning echoes are used to generate the image. The range of human hearing or audible range is between 20 and 20,000 Hz. Anything above 20,000 Hz is considered ultrasound. The frequency range for diagnostic ultrasound imaging is between 2 and 18 MHz.[11]

The transducer is responsible for the generation of the ultrasound beam and also acts as a receiver of the returning echoes, which are then converted into the electrical signal resulting in the ultrasound image on the screen. There are different types of transducers that are used in musculoskeletal ultrasound imaging, and their selection is based on the spatial resolution, penetration, area being studied, and signal-to-noise ratio desired. The basic principle of ultrasound imaging is conversion of mechanical energy into electrical energy and vice versa. This is achieved by the piezoelectric crystals in the transducer, which are arranged in a multilayer arrangement.

Sound waves travel as a sinusoidal longitudinal wave propagating by means of compression and rarefaction of the medium in which it travels. The longitudinal mechanical wave movement of the particles is in the same direction as the direction of wave propagation, resulting in areas of greater density (compression) and areas of lesser density (rarefaction).[12] The difference between a longitudinal and a transverse wave is shown in Figure 22-1. The transmitted ultrasound beam to the human body produces an echo at each tissue interface (Figure 22-2). These returned echoes are used to generate an ultrasound image by converting this mechanical energy into an electrical signal. This is achieved by pulse-echo technique, where the ultrasound beam is transmitted to the human tissue via the transducer in bursts or pulses of 1 microsecond duration spaced 1 millisecond apart with pulse repetition rate of 1000 pulses per second and then returning echoes are used to generate an image.[12] Therefore, the ultrasound beam is not continuously transmitted to the human body or medium. The transducer sends the ultrasound and then stops to listen to the returning echoes. It transmits 1% of the time and spends 99% of the time listening.[12] The duty factor of a diagnostic ultrasound machine usually ranges between 0.1% to 1% depending on the depth of the structure of interest. The transducer spends more time listening to echoes than transmitting ultrasound waves.

Depending on the medium through which ultrasound is traveling, it can have a different velocity or direction. The speed of sound in different tissue mediums is shown in Table 22-2.[13]

Sound waves attenuate as they pass through different tissue mediums. There is greater attenuation of the higher frequency beam than the lower frequency beam. As the ultrasound passes through different tissue interfaces of human tissue it gets reflected, refracted, scattered, and absorbed,[14] which is the basis of why structures appear the way they appear on ultrasound.

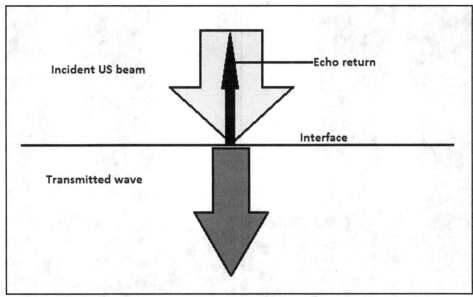

Figure 22-2. Transmitted beam and echo return from each tissue interface.

Table 22-2	
SPEED OF SOUND IN VARIOUS TISSUE MEDIUM	
TISSUE MEDIUM	**SPEED (M/SEC)**
Air	330
Fat	1450
Soft tissue	1540
Bone	4080

Transducer Selection

There are 3 main types of transducers used in musculoskeletal ultrasound imaging: (1) linear, (2) curvilinear, and (3) hockey stick transducer. Figure 22-3 shows these 3 transducers and the images obtained with these transducers.

1. Linear transducer: This transducer is the most commonly used transducer in neuromusculoskeletal imaging and can be used for imaging most of the extremities except for deeper structures or regions like anterior and posterior hip or spine imaging.

2. Curvilinear transducer: This transducer has a wider footprint and provides an extended field of view and greater penetration with some compromise on the resolution. Scans with a curvilinear probe are fan- or pie-shaped as seen in Figure 22-3.

3. Hockey stick transducer: This transducer is essentially a linear transducer but with a smaller footprint. Its shape makes it appropriate for scanning superficial small structures and for areas where adequate skin contact with a linear probe is difficult to achieve, such as digits or around the bony prominences to scan

superficial structures. Another good example is the scan of the medial or lateral aspect of the digit or web space, which requires transducer contact in the web space.

Higher-frequency probes are used for scanning superficial structures or for greater resolution. Higher frequency provides better resolution but does not provide greater penetration for the scanning of deeper structures. Higher frequencies are used for structures like nerves, tendons, ligaments, or other superficial structures around the joint area. Lower-frequency probes, on the other hand, provide greater penetration at the expense of resolution. Lower frequencies are used for deeper structures like anterior or posterior hip or posterior structures of the spine.[15] Ultrasound can resolve much finer details than MRI in nerve or tendon imaging to study the internal architecture. In addition, ultrasound has a flexible plane of view, which is helpful in nerve imaging as the course of a nerve does not follow a specific plane, and with ultrasound, you can follow the tortuous course better than MRI. Important considerations when selecting ultrasound vs MRI as an imaging modality for musculoskeletal pathologies are described in Table 22-3.[16]

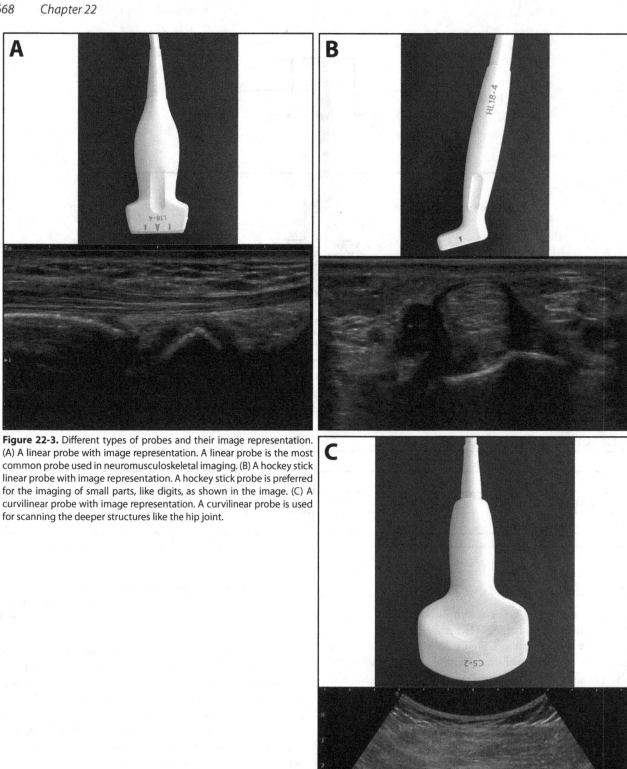

Figure 22-3. Different types of probes and their image representation. (A) A linear probe with image representation. A linear probe is the most common probe used in neuromusculoskeletal imaging. (B) A hockey stick linear probe with image representation. A hockey stick probe is preferred for the imaging of small parts, like digits, as shown in the image. (C) A curvilinear probe with image representation. A curvilinear probe is used for scanning the deeper structures like the hip joint.

Table 22-3

CONSIDERATIONS WHEN PICKING ULTRASOUND VERSUS MAGNETIC RESONANCE IMAGING AS IMAGING MODALITY

1. Ultrasound imaging has no contraindications unlike MRI, which is contraindicated in patients with a pacemaker or metal implants.

2. Ultrasound is real-time evaluation, and the imaging protocol can be modified based on clinical information gained during the patient interaction.

3. Ultrasound is operator dependent, which also means there is a flexible field of view to visualize structures with a tortuous course like nerves and tendons.

4. Ultrasound is a better choice and reveals much finer details of nerves and tendons.

5. It is easy to do a contralateral comparison study with ultrasound.

6. It is easy to obtain physiological information regarding vascularity, neoangiogenesis, or important surrounding blood vessels with just a push of a button on ultrasound imaging.

7. Ultrasound is better able to differentiate fluid from solid soft tissue, and to further enhance this ability, a compressibility test with the probe can be performed.

8. Ultrasound is great for guided diagnostic and therapeutic interventions.

9. Ultrasound imaging is safe, comfortable, and well tolerated compared to MRI where patients may suffer from claustrophobia or be subjected to extended scan times in the MRI scanner.

10. Ultrasound can detect almost all foreign bodies, even the radiolucent wood splinters and much smaller foreign bodies that may be difficult to visualize on MRI.

Getting the Best Image

To obtain the best image, it is important to optimize gain, depth, resolution, and identify image artifacts. Let us look at each component individually.

Gain

Ultrasound machines have an important and powerful amplification control called *time gain compensation (TGC)*. The TGC control can be used to increased output signal at the depth of the structure of interest. There is also an option to increase or decrease overall gain of the entire image.

Depth

Depth can be altered by frequency selection and altering the depth selection feature, which can be used to optimize the depth for scanning. The depth of the scan is displayed as a scale on the left or right side of the screen. Scanning at increased depths results in reduction of the frame rate, which in turn can compromise image quality.

Resolution

There are 2 types of resolution: (1) axial resolution and (2) lateral resolution. The ability to differentiate 2 adjacent structures lying in the direction of the ultrasound beam is called *axial resolution*. For a structure to be visualized, the

distance between them has to be larger than the wavelength of the emitted ultrasound. Wavelength is inversely proportional to frequency, and therefore, higher frequency gives better resolution. However, at higher frequencies there is greater attenuation, and therefore, we are only able to see superficial structures. There is a trade-off between axial resolution and depth of penetration.

The ability to differentiate 2 structures lying side by side in the direction perpendicular to the direction of the ultrasound beam is called *lateral resolution*. Lateral resolution can be improved by focusing the beam using the focal point selection on the machine at the correct level and by correct selection of the transducer.[17]

Artifacts

Artifact is the part of the image that is not the true representation of the structure or physiology.[18] Knowledge of artifacts is vital for the interpretation of the image and successful scanning. The most common types of artifacts are listed below and are shown in Figure 22-4:

- Posterior enhancement: This artifact is most commonly seen in cystic masses like a ganglion cyst. Posterior enhancement is seen as sudden brightening or a hyperechoic signal deeper to the posterior wall of the cystic mass. An example of posterior enhancement can be seen in Figure 22-4.

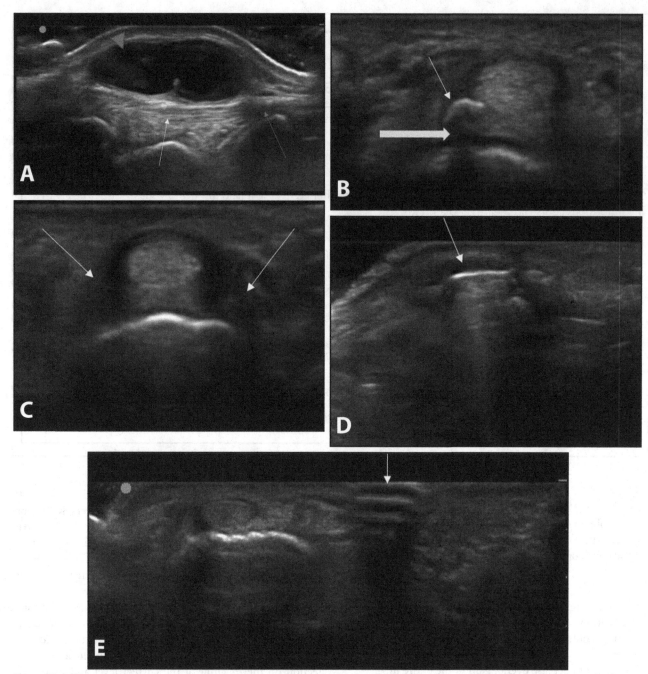

Figure 22-4. (A) Posterior enhancement: Ganglion cyst (arrowhead) on the dorsum of the wrist with underlying tendon. The tendon under the cyst appears bright (thin arrow) compared to the same tendon that continues distally (right thin arrow). This brightness under the cyst is called posterior enhancement. (B) Posterior shadowing: Short axis or transverse view of the flexor tendon of the digit with sesamoid bone (thin arrow). Under the sesamoid bone darker shadow (bold arrow) is posterior shadowing. (C) Lateral cystic shadowing: Short axis or transverse view of the tendon. On either side of the tendon darker areas (thin arrows) are lateral cystic shadowing artifact. (D) Reverberation or comet tail: Metal plate in the digit (arrow) causing reverberation artifact or comet tail artifact underneath it. (E) Contact artifact: Loss of transducer or probe contact at a specific area (arrow), resulting in contact artifact.

- Posterior shadowing: This artifact is seen when a highly reflective interface reflects maximum echo with very little to no transmission through it. The most common example being a big calcific mass or metal or other solid structure. Underneath the highly reflective interface or structure a darker shadow is observed, which is known as *posterior shadowing*. An example of posterior shadowing can be seen in Figure 22-4.
- Lateral cystic shadowing: This artifact is commonly seen in round structures like soft tissue masses or in a short axis/transverse view of the tendon. Due to refraction of sound waves on the edges of the round structure, a darker area is observed on the sides of the round structure, which is referred to as a *lateral cystic shadowing artifact*.
- Reverberation or comet tail: This artifact is seen in highly reflective structures like foreign bodies (eg, metal, needle, calcific deposit). Because the structure is highly reflective, the ultrasound beam bounces back and forth between the structure and the transducer and produces a reverberation or comet tail artifact underneath the reflective structure.
- Contact artifact: This artifact is seen when there is inadequate contact between the probe and the area of the body being examined. Gel is a coupling medium used in ultrasound scanning to increase the transmission of the ultrasound beam into the tissue. An inadequate amount of gel used in the examination results in poor transmission of the ultrasound beam into the tissue and can result in contact artifact. An example of contact artifact can be seen in Figure 22-4.[13]

Terms for Ultrasound Image

Following are some terms that will be used to describe the ultrasound image:

- Echogenicity: This is the amount of energy reflected back from the tissue. The greater the energy reflected back, the brighter the structure appears. For example, bone appears white on ultrasound, whereas an artery appears back.[19]
- Attenuation: This is the loss of amplitude and intensity as the sound (ultrasound) travels through the medium and is a result of reflection and scattering. Some structures cause greater attenuation than others do.[4]

- Transducer footprint: The tip of the transducer head is referred to as the *footprint*. The footprint is the part that is in direct contact with the body during scanning. A larger footprint is desired for a wider field of view and a smaller footprint is more appropriate for smaller areas and structures.[19]
- Acoustic impedance: As the sound wave passes through the human body, different mediums respond differently on the extent to which the medium can resist change. This property to resist change is called *acoustic impedance*. Differences in acoustic impedance of different tissue mediums create reflective interfaces that are represented on the ultrasound image with different echo intensities.[4]

Appearance of Different Tissues on Ultrasound Imaging

Muscle

Muscle appears as a hypoechoic (dark) structure with hyperechoic (white) fascicles, which are tightly packed collagenous structures. In a long axis view, muscle appears as a hypoechoic structure with fusiform, unipennate, or multipennate arrangement of fascicles. In short axis view, muscle appears as a hypoechoic (dark) structure with interspersed hyperechoic (white) fibroadipose septa or perimysium.

Tendon

Tendon appears as a hyperechoic (white) structure. In a long axis view, tendon appears as a cord-like hyperechoic structure with an echogenic fibrillar pattern of collagen arrangement. In short axis view, tendon appears as a round hyperechoic (white) structure with a bristle-like appearance or tightly packed hyperechoic dots. Tendons exhibit anisotropy on ultrasound and therefore utmost care is needed to keep the transducer/probe perpendicular to the tendon being studied. If the ultrasound beam or transducer is not perpendicular to the probe, the tendon may appear hypoechoic (dark), which is associated with pathology. An example of anisotropy can be seen in Figure 22-5.

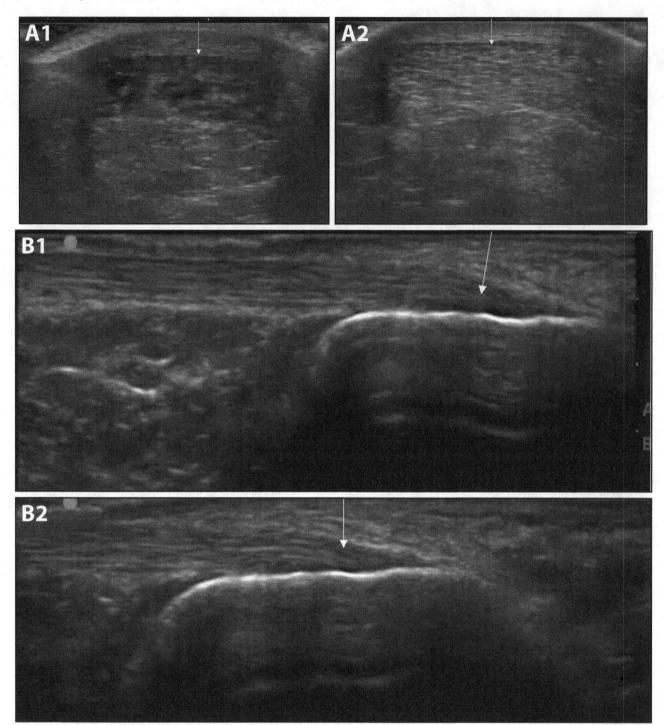

Figure 22-5. Tendon anisotropy. (A1) Short axis or transverse view of the tendon with probe orientation not 90 degrees to the tendon resulting in hypoechoic (dark) tendon. (A2) Upon tilting the probe to strike the ultrasound beam 90 degrees normal tendon bristle-like appearance in short axis view. (B1) Long axis or longitudinal view of the tendon with hypoechoic area in the distal part of the tendon as it attaches to bone. This is due to incident ultrasound beam not striking the distal tendon at a 90-degree angle. (B2) Upon changing the probe placement to be parallel to the distal part of the tendon so that the incident beam strikes the tendon at a 90-degree angle, the darker area disappears.

Table 22-4

HOW TO DIFFERENTIATE AN ARTERY FROM A VEIN

	ARTERY	VEIN
COMPRESSIBILITY TEST	Cannot obliterate with probe pressure.	Can obliterate with probe pressure.
FLOW SIGNAL	Color signal detects pulsatile blood flow.	Color signal shows slow flow and is sensitive of probe positioning.
WALLS	Stronger and thicker walls consist of 3 layers: Tunica intima, tunica media, and tunica adventitia.	Relatively thin walls and larger lumen, can appear bulbous or tortuous, and valves can be seen.

Ligament

Ligaments on ultrasound imaging appear as a hyperechoic band connecting bone to bone. Depending on the angle of sound beam to the ligament, fibers can appear hyperechoic (white) or hypoechoic (dark), and it is for this reason that ligaments are best imaged in a stretched position. The greatest advantage of ultrasound is that it is real time, and therefore, dynamic tests to check the ligament integrity can be done when the integrity of the ligament is in question.

Bone

Bone on ultrasound imaging appears hyperechoic (white). Bone is a highly reflective interface, and therefore, structures deeper to the bone cannot be visualized on ultrasound. It is for this reason that MRI is the first choice for meniscus, cartilage, or labral pathology.

Nerve

Nerves have a variable echo signal and echo texture depending on the location in which they are being studied. In short axis view, nerves exhibit a "honey-comb" fascicular pattern or "starry night appearance." In long axis view, nerves appear hypoechoic (dark) with echogenic lines and enclosed in 2 bold hyperechoic (white) margins.

Blood Vessels

Blood vessels appear anechoic (black) on ultrasound. In short axis view, they appear as round anechoic (black) structures. In long axis view, they appear as cord-like or tube-like structures. On color ultrasound or Doppler ultrasound, color signal or flow signal can be detected. Arteries and veins can be differentiated on ultrasound by a compressibility test, flow signal type, and the appearance of walls as shown in Table 22-4.

Cartilage

Cartilage can have a different echo signal on ultrasound depending on its composition. Articular hyaline cartilage appears anechoic or hypoechoic. Fibrocartilage in meniscus or labrum appears hyperechoic and has a triangular appearance on ultrasound. Figure 22-6 shows the appearance of different tissues on ultrasound.

Common Pathologies on Musculoskeletal Ultrasound

Tendon Pathology

Tendons can be studied in great detail with ultrasound. Ultrasound imaging can be used to differentiate a tendon tear from tendinosis or tenosynovitis. Real-time ultrasound scanning can be used to check tendon instability and to grade the extent of tendon instability, which is not possible with other imaging modalities. Clinical examination and special tests are not sensitive enough to differentiate tendinosis, tenosynovitis, and partial tendon tears, and the clinical presentation may be similar in these pathologies. Appearance of tendinosis, tenosynovitis, and partial tears of tendon on ultrasound imaging can be seen in Figure 22-7.

Muscle Pathology

Normal echotexture of muscle is described in the previous section and shown in Figure 22-6. Normal muscle is hypoechoic with hyperechoic septa or perimysium. When muscle is atrophied, normal muscle tissue is replaced by connective tissue and fat. An ultrasound image of atrophied muscle is hyperechoic compared to healthy muscle tissue, which is hypoechoic. Muscle tears, when acute, appear as focal hypoechoic or anechoic (dark) defect in the muscle tissue. The focal defect can be further enhanced by (1) dynamic maneuvering of the transducer by compressibility test (where pressure is exerted from the transducer to the area being studied) and (2) by actively or passively moving the body part to visualize the defect in the muscle clearly. An example of a muscle tear on ultrasound image can be seen in Figure 22-8.

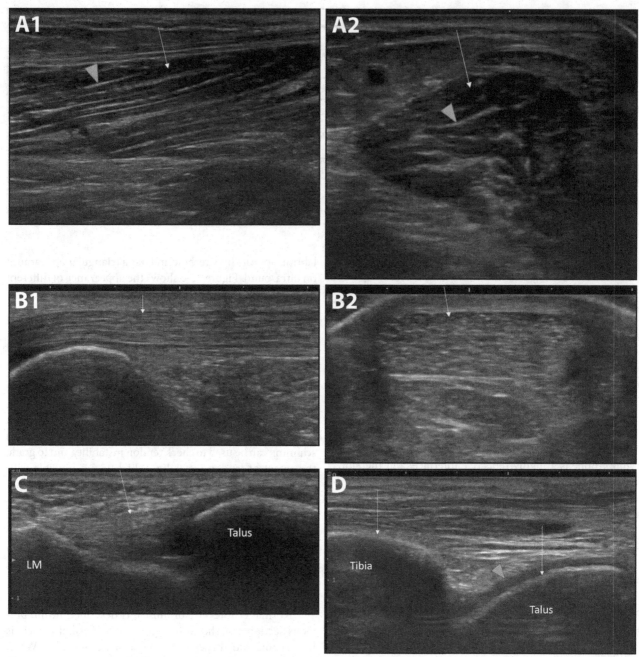

Figure 22-6. Appearance of different tissue on ultrasound. (A) Muscle. (1) Long axis view of the muscle (arrow). Muscle appears hypoechoic with hyperechoic fascicles or perimysium (arrowhead). (2) Short axis view of the muscles (arrow) with hyperechoic fascicles or connective tissue (arrowhead). (B) Tendon. (1) Long axis view of the tendon (arrow). Tendon appears as hyperechoic uniform fibrillar structure. (2) In short axis view, tendon appears hyperechoic with bristle-like appearance. (C) Ligament. Ligament appears as hyperechoic band (arrow). Example shows anterior talofibular ligament as hyperechoic band between lateral malleolus (LM) and talus. (D) Bone. Bone appears hyperechoic (arrows). Image shows distal tibia and talus and (arrowhead) anechoic cartilage lining the talus. *(continued)*

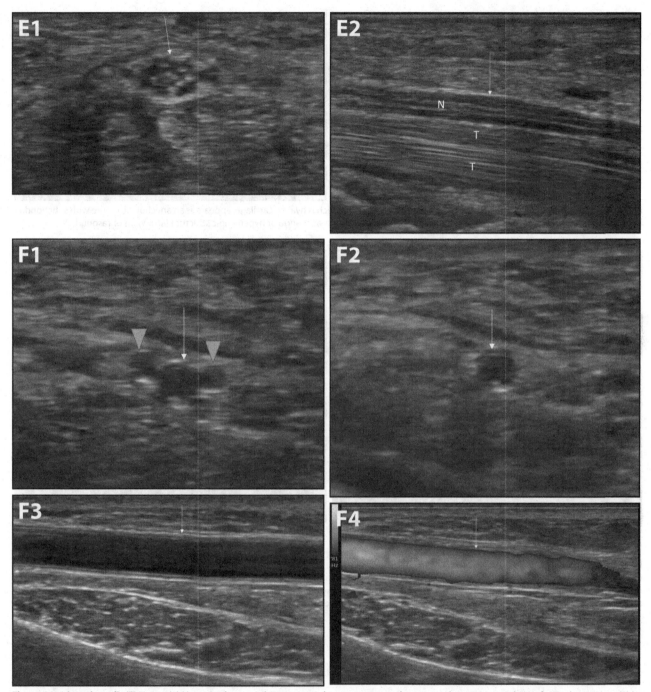

Figure 22-6 (continued). (E) Nerve. (1) Nerve in short axis has starry-night appearance or honey-comb appearance due to fascicular pattern. (2) In long axis view, nerve shows fascicular arrangement of repeating hypoechoic bands between 2 bold hyperechoic lines within the nerve. Compared to tendons (T), the nerve (N) appears hypoechoic. (F) Blood vessels. (1) Short axis view of artery (arrow) and veins (arrowheads). (2) With transducer pressure, veins are obliterated and no longer seen, but arteries can still be seen. (3) In long axis view, the artery or vein appears as an anechoic band. (4) Upon turning the color doppler ultrasound on, flow signal can be seen. *(continued)*

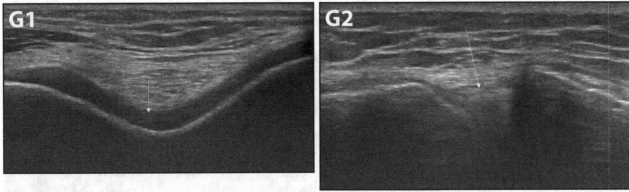

Figure 22-6 (continued). (G) Cartilage. (1) Femoral trochlear cartilage, which is hyaline cartilage, appears as an anechoic structure with subchondral bone. (2) The medial meniscus of the knee is a fibrocartilage and it appears as triangular hyperechoic structure (arrow) on ultrasound.

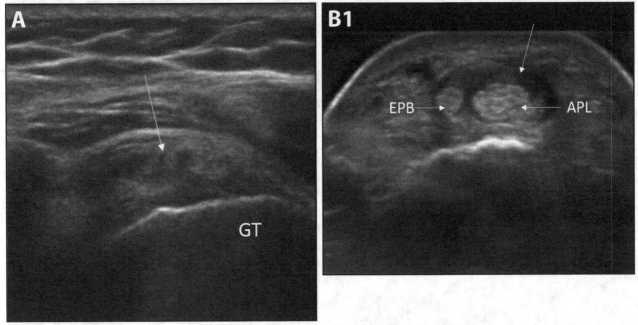

Figure 22-7. (A) Tendinosis. Image shows supraspinatus tendon (arrow) attaching to greater tubercle (GT). Tendon appears hypoechoic, heterogenous with loss of normal fibrillar pattern. (B) Tenosynovitis. (1) Image shows De Quervain's tenosynovitis affecting extensor pollicis brevis (EPB) and abductor pollicis longus (APL). Inflamed tenosynovium is seen as a hypoechoic signal around the tendon (top arrow). *(continued)*

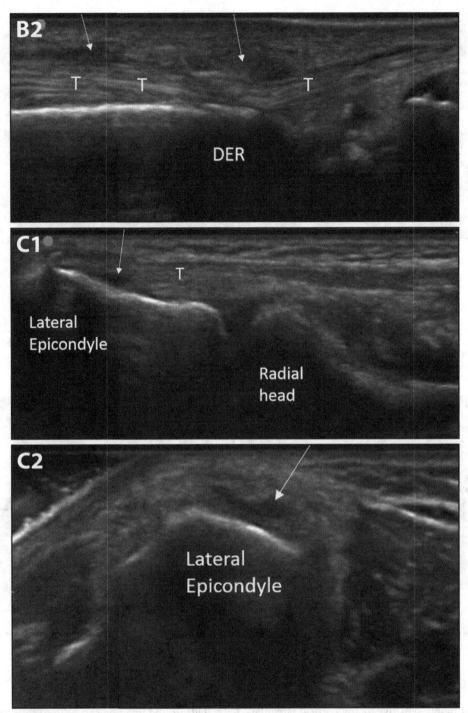

Figure 22-7 (continued). (B) (2) Long axis view of the tendon also shows hypoechoic signal around the tendon (arrows); however, tendon (T) shows normal fibrillar pattern and is uniform in appearance, distal end of radius (DER). (C) Partial tear of tendon. (1) Long axis view of the common extensor tendon (T) attaching to the lateral epicondyle. Partial tear appears as a focal anechoic defect in the tendon (arrow). (2) In the short axis view, partial tear of the tendon can be confirmed as a focal anechoic defect (arrow).

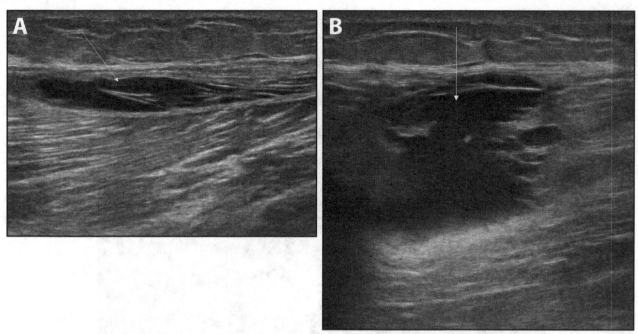

Figure 22-8. Muscle tear. (A) Partial tear of biceps femoris muscle at the level of distal thigh can be seen as a focal anechoic defect (arrow). In this long axis view, intact normal muscle fibers can be seen deeper to the focal defect. (B) Short axis view of the muscle with focal defect in the muscle (arrow) and the resultant hematoma causing posterior enhancement artifact.

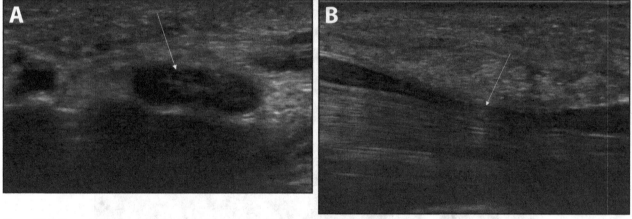

Figure 22-9. Nerve entrapment. (A) Short axis view of the median nerve shows hypoechoic swelling with loss of normal fascicular pattern. Nerve is enlarged and swollen. (B) Long axis view of the nerve shows hypoechoic nerve swelling distal and proximal to the entrapment site with "hour glass deformity" or constriction site (arrow).

Bone Pathology

Ultrasound is highly sensitive to any cortical irregularity, and therefore, it is important to know the normal bony contours and bony protuberances. For example, the bone anatomy of the distal ends of metacarpals and metatarsals may give an appearance of cortical breach where the head meets the neck. Bony abnormalities that can be seen with ultrasound imaging include bony erosion, hypertrophic changes or bony osteophytes, stress fractures, and bony defects. Fractures can be seen as a "step-off deformity" or focal breaks. It is important to note that radiographs and CT scans are the first choice for fracture evaluation because ultrasound imaging does not give complete information about the malalignment, displacement, and overview of the bone and joint anatomy of the region.

Nerve Pathology

Ultrasound imaging can be used to assess nerve entrapment or other peripheral nerve pathology. It is possible to follow the course of the nerve to find out the site of entrapment or to evaluate the integrity of the nerve. Nerve at the site of entrapment shows focal swelling with loss of fascicular pattern and physical deformation of the nerve. An example of nerve entrapment is shown in Figure 22-9. Other abnormalities that have similar presentation as nerve entrapment syndrome include space-occupying lesions such as a ganglion cyst compressing the nerve, extrinsic compression by a soft tissue mass, anomalous muscle compressing the nerve, or peripheral neuropathy.

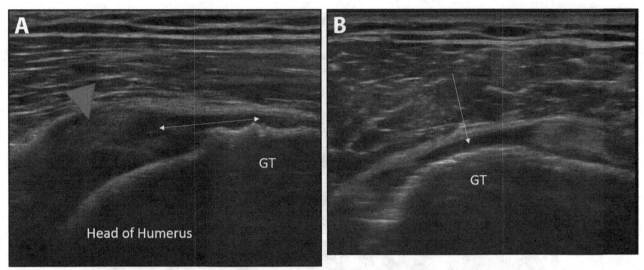

Figure 22-10. Case Study One. (A) A full-thickness tear of the supraspinatus tendon with retracted tendon stump (arrowhead). The double headed yellow arrow shows the distance of retracted stump from bone attachment at greater tubercle (GT). (B) Short axis view of the supraspinatus tendon shows absence of tendon or non-visualization of the tendon over the greater tubercle (GT).

Ligament Pathology

Ultrasound imaging can be used to check the integrity of the ligaments. Real-time assessment of the ligaments in a neutral or stressed position with ultrasound imaging can reveal if the ligament is intact, partially torn, or completely torn. Real-time evaluation of the ligament is of great value in a scenario where there is acute injury resulting in swelling and muscle guarding of the surrounding tissue. A ligament stress test and palpation may be suggestive of ligament tear but not definitive; however, including ultrasound imaging with the stress test can boost the assessment and add more clarity to the examination.[20,21]

CASE STUDIES

Case Study One

A 53-year-old man presented with acute onset pain with an inability to raise the arm, which happened after lifting heavy boxes 2 days ago. On ultrasound scan of the shoulder, a full-thickness tear of the supraspinatus tendon and effusion of the shoulder was seen. Figure 22-10 shows the full-thickness complete tear of the supraspinatus tendon with retracted tendon stump. This patient was then referred for an orthopedic surgeon's consultation.

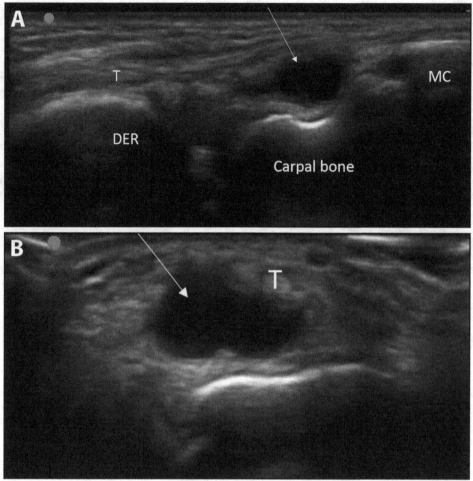

Figure 22-11. Case Study Two. (A) Long axis view of the wrist dorsum shows a ganglion cyst (arrow) that presents as an anechoic structure over the carpal bone. There is overlying fourth dorsal compartment extensor tendon (T). Distal end of radius (DER), metacarpal (MC). (B) Short axis view of the wrist confirms the ganglion cyst (arrow), overlying tendon (T) can be seen as a hyperechoic structure.

Case Study Two

A 36-year-old woman presented with gradual onset of a dull ache on the dorsum of the right wrist. She reported difficulty with activities that require weightbearing on an extended wrist and difficulty with lifting weights as part of her gym workout. There was no evidence of localized tenderness over the extensor tendons of the wrist, and range of motion was full with some discomfort at the end range of wrist extension. On ultrasound examination of the wrist, there was a ganglion cyst on the dorsum of the wrist measuring 1.25 x 0.69 x 1.31 cm as shown in Figure 22-11. This patient was sent for orthopedic consultation. She was advised to wear a wrist brace with possible aspiration of the cyst if the symptoms do not resolve in 3 to 4 weeks with conservative care.

REFERENCES

1. Edelman RR. The history of MR imaging as seen through the pages of radiology. *Radiology*. 2014;273(2 Suppl):S181-S200.

2. Dussik KT, Fritch DJ, Kyriazidou M, Sear RS. Measurements of articular tissues with ultrasound. *American Journal of Physical Medicine*. 1958;37(3):160-165.

3. Kane D, Grassi W, Sturrock R, Balint PV. A brief history of musculoskeletal ultrasound: "from bats and ships to babies and hips." *Rheumatology (Oxford, England)*. 2004;43(7):931-933.

4. Chan V, Perlas A. Basics of ultrasound imaging. In: Narouze SN, ed. *Atlas of Ultrasound-Guided Procedures in Interventional Pain Management*. Springer New York; 2011:13-19.

5. Wheeler P. What do patients think about diagnostic ultrasound? A pilot study to investigate patient-perceived benefits with the use of musculoskeletal diagnostic ultrasound in an outpatient clinic setting. *International Musculoskeletal Medicine*. 2010;32(2):68-71.

6. Lin EC. Radiation risk from medical imaging. *Mayo Clinic Proceedings*. 2010;85(12):1142-1146.

7. Thrall JH. Radiation exposure in CT scanning and risk: where are we? *Radiology*. 2012;264(2):325-328.

8. Grover VP, Tognarelli JM, Crossey MM, Cox IJ, Taylor-Robinson SD, McPhail MJ. Magnetic resonance imaging: principles and techniques: lessons for clinicians. *J Clin Exp Hepatol*. 2015;5(3):246-255.

9. Saupe N, Zanetti M, Pfirrmann CW, Wels T, Schwenke C, Hodler J. Pain and other side effects after MR arthrography: prospective evaluation in 1085 patients. *Radiology*. 2009;250(3):830-838.

10. Hernandez Filho G. Magnetic resonance arthrography: what is its importance in the present day? *Radiol Bras*. 2018;51(2):V.

11. Martin DJ, Wells ITP, Goodwin CR. Physics of ultrasound. *Anaesthesia & Intensive Care Medicine*. 2015;16(3):132-135.

12. Williams D. The physics of ultrasound. *Anaesthesia & Intensive Care Medicine*. 2012;13(6):264-268.

13. Feldman MK, Katyal S, Blackwood MS. US artifacts. *Radiographics*. 2009;29(4):1179-1189.

14. Shriki J. Ultrasound physics. *Crit Care Clin*. 2014;30(1):1-24, v.

15. Enriquez JL, Wu TS. An introduction to ultrasound equipment and knobology. *Crit Care Clin*. 2014;30(1):25-45, v.

16. Nazarian LN. The top 10 reasons musculoskeletal sonography is an important complementary or alternative technique to MRI. *AJR Am J Roentgenol*. 2008;190(6):1621-1626.

17. Ng A, Swanevelder J. Resolution in ultrasound imaging. *Continuing Education in Anaesthesia Critical Care & Pain*. 2011;11(5):186-192.

18. Prabhu SJ, Kanal K, Bhargava P, Vaidya S, Dighe MK. Ultrasound artifacts: classification, applied physics with illustrations, and imaging appearances. *Ultrasound Quarterly*. 2014;30(2):145-157.

19. Ihnatsenka B, Boezaart AP. Ultrasound: basic understanding and learning the language. *Int J Shoulder Surg*. 2010;4(3):55-62.

20. Smith W, Hackel JG, Goitz HT, Bouffard JA, Nelson AM. Utilization of sonography and a stress device in the assessment of partial tears of the ulnar collateral ligament in throwers. *Int J Sports Phys Ther*. 2011;6(1):45-50.

21. Cho JH, Lee DH, Song HK, Bang JY, Lee KT, Park YU. Value of stress ultrasound for the diagnosis of chronic ankle instability compared to manual anterior drawer test, stress radiography, magnetic resonance imaging, and arthroscopy. *Knee Surgery, Sports Traumatology, Arthroscopy*. 2016;24(4):1022-1028.

23

Blood Flow Restriction Training

Implications for Orthopedic Physical Therapy

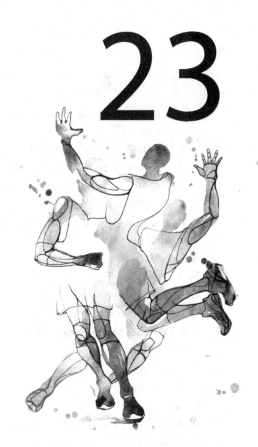

Alyssa M. Weatherholt, PhD; William R. VanWye, PT, DPT, PhD; and Johnny G. Owens, MPT

KEY TERMS

Blood flow restriction (BFR) training: A training tool that applies a tourniquet cuff to the most proximal location on the extremity prior to exercise.

Delayed onset muscle soreness (DOMS): The pain and stiffness felt in muscles several hours to days after unaccustomed or strenuous exercise.

Delfi: A BFR training system that uses pneumatic cuffs to apply pressure to the exercising limb. Unlike the KAATSU system, Delfi systems can automatically measure the patient's limb occlusion pressure (LOP) and recommend a personalized tourniquet pressure (PTP) specific to the patient, to fully occlude venous return without occluding arterial blood flow.

KAATSU: A patented BFR training system developed by Dr. Yoshiaki Sato that uses pneumatic cuffs to apply pressure to the exercising limb.

Limb occlusion pressure (LOP): The minimum pressure required to a patient's limb to reduce or stop the flow of blood into the limb distal to the cuff.

Nerve injury: An acute or permanent damage to the nerve by pressure, stretching, or cutting. Injury to the nerve can result in muscles not working correctly or loss of feeling in the damaged area.

Personalization: A recommended PTP specific to the patient.

Rhabdomyolysis: A potentially life-threatening syndrome resulting from the breakdown of skeletal muscle fibers with leakage of muscle contents into the circulation. The most common causes are crush injury, overexertion, alcohol abuse, and certain medicines and toxic substances.

Wallmann HW, Donatelli R, eds. *Foundations of Orthopedic Physical Therapy* (pp 683-693).
© 2024 Taylor & Francis Group.

CHAPTER QUESTIONS

1. Which of the following is the recommended training intensity for BFR?

   A. 5% to 10% of the individual's 1 repetition maximum

   B. 20% to 30% of the individual's 1 repetition maximum

   C. 40% to 50% of the individual's 1 repetition maximum

   D. 60% to 80% of the individual's 1 repetition maximum

2. BFR entails complete occlusion of which of the following?

   A. Venous flow

   B. Arterial flow

   C. Both venous and arterial flow

   D. Neither venous or arterial flow

3. BFR LOP should be between which of the following?

   A. 10% to 40%

   B. 20% to 50%

   C. 40% to 80%

   D. 60% to 100%

4. Which of the following is the recommended BFR training frequency?

   A. 1 to 2 times per week

   B. 2 to 3 times per week

   C. 3 to 4 times per week

   D. 4 to 5 times per week

5. Which test or measure would be the BEST method for determining BFR LOP?

   A. Pain rating

   B. Perceived tightness

   C. Skin coloration

   D. Doppler

6. Which of the following is equal to 1 SKU?

   A. 1 mm Hg

   B. 5 mm Hg

   C. 10 mm Hg

   D. 50 mm Hg

7. The KAASTU cuffs are typically _____ compared to the Delfi cuffs.

   A. Narrower

   B. Wider

   C. Longer

   D. Shorter

8. During BFR training, which of the following is consistent with an incidence of a deep venous thrombosis (DVT)?

   A. Approximately 0.1%

   B. Approximately 0.5%

   C. Approximately 1%

   D. Approximately 5%

9. True or False—BFR training increases the risk of exercise-induced muscle damage when compared to maximal eccentric exercise.

10. During BFR training, which of the following is consistent with an incidence of transient nerve injury?

    A. About 1% to 2%

    B. About 3% to 4%

    C. About 5% to 6%

    D. About 6% to 7%

11. True or False—An exaggerated exercise pressure reflex is more likely to occur in those with cardiovascular disease?

12. Tennent et al examined the impact of BFR training in individuals 4 weeks after arthroscopic knee surgery and found the incidence of thrombus formation to be which of the following?

    A. 0%

    B. 2%

    C. 4%

    D. 8%

13. Why might BFR training be better tolerated by a patient who has knee osteoarthritis?

14. How would cuff width affect LOP?

15. What is a potential mechanism explaining how BFR training results in muscular adaptations?

16. Which of the following is consistent with a typical volume for BFR training?

    A. 1 to 2 sets of 8 to 12 repetitions, 60-second rest break in-between sets

    B. 4 to 5 sets of 8 to 12 repetitions, 60-second rest break in-between sets

    C. 1 to 2 sets of 15 to 30 repetitions, 30-second rest break in-between sets

    D. 4 to 5 sets of 15 to 30 repetitions, 30-second rest break in-between sets

17. True or False—BFR training results in early hypertrophy with strength gains coming later.

18. BFR training cuffs should be placed on which of the following areas?

    A. Target muscle

    B. Target joint

    C. Distal portion of an extremity

    D. Proximal portion of an extremity

19. What is the physiological effect of occluding venous flow during exercise?

20. What would be the effect of arterial flow occlusion during exercise?

INTRODUCTION

BFR training is gaining in popularity as a method to improve muscular strength and hypertrophy. Although well-established in the exercise physiology literature, BFR training is an emerging modality in physical therapist settings. Health care practitioners are now using BFR for patients with various musculoskeletal conditions for prehabilitation or postoperative rehabilitation.[1-9] BFR training entails applying a tourniquet cuff to the most proximal location on the upper or lower extremity prior to exercise.

The benefit of using BFR training is the ability to achieve muscle hypertrophy with the use of light loads (ie, 20% to 30% of 1 repetition maximum [1RM]). The addition of BFR with low-intensity resistance or aerobic training produces muscular strength and hypertrophy gains comparable to traditional resistance training.[10,11] This is advantageous for individuals working with patients in rehabilitation settings because moderate to high intensity (ie, 65% or greater 1RM) resistance training is often contraindicated. Therefore, physical therapists working in orthopedic settings should have a basic understanding of BFR training.

MUSCULAR ADAPTATIONS FROM BLOOD FLOW RESTRICTION TRAINING

BFR training is thought to induce muscular strength and hypertrophy gains by completely occluding venous blood flow while allowing arterial in-flow (partial arterial occlusion) in the exercising limb. This results in a hypoxic condition to the exercised limb, thus causing high levels of metabolic stress in conjunction with minimal mechanical tension. Metabolic stress induces a hormonal cascade response, cell swelling, production of reactive oxygen species (ROS), increased fast-twitch fiber recruitment, and intramuscular anabolic/anti-catabolic cell signaling.[12] In addition to the effects of hormones, it has been shown that myofiber hypertrophy was stimulated by a marked proliferation of myogenic stem cells after BFR training.[13] The muscular adaptations associated with BFR training can occur within a shorter training period than traditional resistance training (ie, measurable adaptations noticed within 2 weeks vs 8 weeks).[10] This is especially beneficial for patients at risk for significant atrophy (eg, postoperative, injury, nonweightbearing).

HISTORY OF BLOOD FLOW RESTRICTION TRAINING

In the late 1960s, BFR training was developed in Japan as KAATSU training by Yoshiaki Sato.[14] Until the recent decade, BFR training equipment was scarce outside of Japan. In the past 5 years, BFR training equipment has emerged throughout many countries including the United States with multiple types of equipment and updated protocols.[11] Early research for BFR training began as a focus on healthy populations for exercise training in order to understand the physiological adaptations.[15] In recent years, interest for BFR training has expanded to clinical populations, which has led to the use of medical-grade tourniquet instruments and cuffs and the adoption of personalized tourniquet pressures for safe and consistent therapy and patient outcomes.[15] These advancements in both technology and personalization are enabling the rehabilitation of a wide range of clinical populations.

CLINICAL IMPLEMENTATION

There is no official guideline for BFR protocol; however, general practice has been demonstrated through a number of published control trials. A typical training protocol includes the following:

- Apply a cuff pressure between 40% to 80% of the patient's LOP
- Resistance training at 20% to 30% of 1RM
- 75 repetitions over 4 sets of 30, 15, 15, and 15 repetitions with 30-second rest periods between sets
- Training for 2 to 3 days per week
- Recommended prescribed therapy period between 4 to 12 weeks

TYPES OF BLOOD FLOW RESTRICTION EQUIPMENT

Currently, there are several types of devices used to apply BFR therapy to both healthy and clinical populations. Due to the wide range of available BFR devices, ranging from surgical-grade, pneumatic tourniquet systems to homemade elastic bands, inconsistencies exist in methodology, equipment, and in levels of restriction pressure used. These inconsistencies lead to decreased safety and effectiveness of the BFR therapy and prevent the application of a consistent BFR stimulus between patients. In order to select the optimal device to consistently achieve optimal patient outcomes in rehabilitation, it is important to understand factors affecting BFR safety and effectiveness. Research has demonstrated that personalized pressures,[15] medical-grade technology,[16] larger cuff width, limb locations, and stance are important factors when putting together a BFR rehabilitation program.[15]

The most popular BFR brands are Delfi and KAATSU (Figures 23-1 and 23-2).[17,18] While both brands use pneumatic systems to apply BFR, they are quite different in their overall design (Table 23-1).

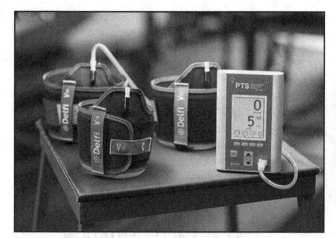

Figure 23-1. Delfi system.

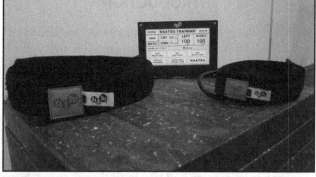

Figure 23-2. KAATSU system.

Table 23-1

DIFFERENCES BETWEEN DELFI AND KAATSU TRAINING DEVICES

DELFI	KAATSU
• Built in Doppler for automatic determination of LOP and PTP specific to the patient, to fully occlude venous return without occluding arterial blood flow	• Manual observation of determination of LOP and PTP by skin coloration, perception of pulsation under the cuff, and muscle failure at the end of the BFR therapy
• Wide pneumatic cuffs	• Narrow pneumatic cuffs
• Application of lower pressure gradients to the limb	• Application of higher pressure gradients to the limb

Delfi

For more than 30 years, members of the Delfi team have been extensively involved in improving automatic tourniquet safety through the development and evaluation of new technologies.[19] This experience led to the development of the Delfi Personalized Tourniquet System for Blood Flow Restriction (PTS for BFR).

The PTS for BFR is a Food and Drug Administration (FDA)–Device Listed, Class I medical device. As such, Delfi complies with US medical device quality management systems and other applicable regulatory requirements to ensure safe and effective products. The PTS for BFR employs proprietary, patented, and clinically proven sensing technology within the unit to automatically measure the patient's LOP, thus allowing the clinician to adjust the desired PTP as a percentage of the individual's LOP, as recommended by recent literature.[15] Delfi's system restricts blood flow by pressurizing and regulating a wide pneumatic cuff, applied to the proximal end of the working limb, at the desired PTP. In order to purchase or use this device on patients, the professional must hold a license in the health care field and have demonstrated understanding of BFR rehabilitation through academic accreditation or certification in a BFR course hosted by Owens Recovery Science, an FDA-registered establishment for

physical therapists, occupational therapists, athletic trainers, doctors of chiropractic, and other medical professionals seeking certification in personalized BFR rehabilitation training. It is essential that BFR rehabilitation is prescribed by a trained practitioner who uses clinical judgment with knowledge of the appropriate protocols and possible contraindications, and who maintains personalized restrictive pressures.[20]

The Personalized Tourniquet System for Blood Flow Restriction

Currently, the literature recommends that the safest and most optimal rehabilitation pressure applied by a BFR training device is between 40% to 80% of the patient's LOP, depending on which limb is being trained, the type of exercise, and the patient comfort levels.[21] In the BFR literature, some devices use a hand-held Doppler to manually measure the patient's LOP. However, this method is not often performed outside of clinical studies due to the additional specialized equipment requiring substantial training and time for accurate measurements. Thus, less accurate and more subjective methods of setting pressures are employed, such as using the following: pain scale, tightness scale, skin coloration, feeling of pulsations, or simply using standard pressures not personalized to the patient. Without measuring the LOP, these methods may result in rehabilitation being performed at too high or too low of BFR, and the safety and effectiveness of the BFR therapy may be compromised.

The Delfi PTS for BFR automatically measures LOP by a novel sensing technology, typically taking less than 1 minute, and determines a personalized restrictive pressure as a percentage of LOP, ensuring the applied pressure is safe and at an appropriate level to achieve the desired effects of muscle strength and hypertrophy. In addition, the PTS for BFR automatically regulates pressure during exercise to remain near the set level during pressure fluctuations of muscle contraction cycles.[16]

In addition, the Delfi system has a BFR pressure application timer, safety alarms, and reperfusion timer for BFR. The BFR application timer allows the setting of a maximum therapy session time, at which point the cuff will automatically deflate to allow reperfusion. After each cuff inflation, there is a reperfusion timer in which the cuff cannot be inflated to ensure reperfusion of the limb. These features minimize the risk of user error and ensure safe and effective BFR application to the patient. The Delfi user interface uses intuitive controls with large texts and symbols on a color LCD screen. The unit is portable, can be plugged into a standard electrical outlet, or run on a rechargeable battery for up to 4 hours (Figure 23-3).

The Easi-Fit Cuffs

The Delfi Easi-Fit for BFR Cuffs are 11.5 cm wide, contoured, surgical-grade tourniquet cuffs with patented variable-fit fasteners. Delfi offers 4 sizes of cuffs covering a limb circumference range from 27.94 cm to 101.6 cm. The contoured shape, variable-fit fasteners, and multiple sizes provide a personalized fit to a wide range of limb tapers and sizes. In contrast, when a cylindrical cuff is applied to a tapered limb, a gap may be present between the limb and the distal end of the cuff. This gap reduces the effectiveness of the pressure transmission to the limb and results in higher pressures and higher pressure gradients. Delfi's contour cuffs eliminate the presence of this gap, ensuring pressure is applied evenly and at the lowest possible, personalized pressure. The wide cuff design is proven to require lower pressure levels and applies lower pressure gradients, decreasing risk of nerve- and other tourniquet-related injuries.[17] Delfi includes matching limb protection sleeves with each Delfi Easi-Fit for BFR Cuff to prevent pinching and wrinkling of the skin beneath the pressurized cuff, thereby increasing patient comfort and improving application of pressure onto the limb.

Operation

A matching limb protection sleeve is applied to the proximal end of the working limb. The matched Delfi Easi-Fit for BFR cuff is applied over the sleeve, and then pneumatically connected to the Delfi PTS for BFR via an air tube. The patient's LOP is automatically measured and the PTP is

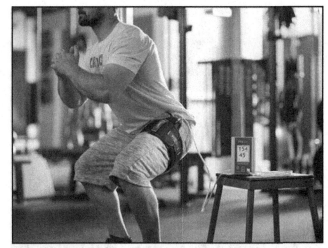

Figure 23-3. Squat with a Delfi system.

determined while the patient is in the supine position. The licensed health care professional selects a suitable therapy duration and inflates the cuff to the PTP. The patient undergoes the BFR therapy, and upon the completion of the BFR therapy, the cuff is deflated.

The PTS for BFR has built-in safety limits for cuff pressure and the duration for a therapy session. The cuff pressure is adjustable between 20 mm Hg and 350 mm Hg. The duration of a therapy session is adjustable between 1 minute and 30 minutes. At the end of each therapy session, the PTS for BFR automatically deflates and prevents subsequent inflation for at least 1 minute to allow time for limb reperfusion.

KAATSU

There are 2 types of KAATSU training units for purchase from KAATSU Global, Inc if one goes through Certified KAATSU specialist training:

1. The KAATSU Master
2. The KAATSU Nano

The main differences between the KAATSU Master and the KAATSU Nano are the size and the maximum settable pressure. The KAATSU Nano is smaller than the KAATSU Master and has a maximum settable pressure of 400 Standard KAATSU units (SKU) compared to 500 SKU for the KAATSU Master (1 SKU equals 1 mm Hg).

The KAATSU Master

The KAATSU Master is a portable touch-screen device that provides compressed air to pneumatic cuffs that are placed around the upper arms and legs of patients or clients. The KAATSU system restricts blood flow to the working limb by applying a cuff pressure at an optimal SKU. Optimal SKU is determined manually by skin coloration, pulsation, and 3-point exercise. Optimal SKU is achieved when the patient's skin color on the training limbs is observed to be pink or beefy red, the patient feels pulsations under the cuff, and muscular failure is met during the final third set. In general,

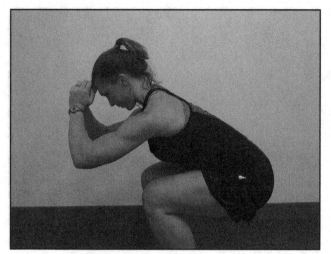

Figure 23-4. Squat with a KAATSU system.

the upper limb achieves optimal SKU at a lower pressure than the lower limb.

The KAATSU Master has several controls in the device for safety purposes to allow immediate cuff deflation. The unit can be plugged into a standard electrical outlet or run on a rechargeable battery for up to 2.5 hours (Figure 23-4).

KAATSU Air Bands

The KAATSU Air Bands or the pneumatic cuffs are 5 cm in width, cylindrical in shape, and come in 6 different sizes. The arm band sizes are as follows: small (18 to 28 cm in circumference), medium (28 to 38 cm in circumference), and large (38 to 48 cm in circumference). The leg band sizes include the following: small (40 to 50 cm in circumference), medium (50 to 60 cm in circumference), and large (60 to 70 cm in circumference). If the patient has a larger leg or arm circumference than the size large, the cuff will have to be special ordered. Each unit comes with a pair of cuffs for both arms and legs. Additional cuff sizes may be ordered at any time.

Compared to the Delfi Easi-Fit for BFR Cuffs, the KAATSU Air Bands are narrow and cylindrical, which may require higher pressures and, thus, higher pressure gradients to achieve the same BFR stimulus. This is relevant due to previous research noting that higher levels of cuff pressure and higher pressure gradients underneath tourniquet cuffs may potentially place the individual at a higher risk for injury.[22,23]

Operation

The KAATSU Air Band is wrapped over clothing, around the proximal end of the exercising limb, and tightened to a base SKU. The recommended base SKU for healthy adults is 30 to 40 SKU and 20 to 30 SKU for clinical populations. The cuff tightness can be measured by connecting an air tube to the KAATSU Master to see how much pressure was applied. Once the base SKU is applied, optimal SKU is administered to the cuff by manually observing skin coloration and pulsation under the cuff. After each BFR session,

the optimal SKU may be adjusted to cause muscular failure during the final third set. Once the cuff is inflated to appropriate training pressure, the KAATSU Air Band can be disconnected from the unit for the workout period. During this period, cuff pressure is not regulated. Upon the completion of the BFR therapy, the cuff is deflated.

SPECIAL CONSIDERATIONS

Previous studies have found that, when properly implemented, BFR training does not add any additional risk when compared to traditional exercise modes.[12,24] Potential concerns of BFR training include blood clots, deleterious cardiovascular responses, muscle/nerve damage, and an abnormal autonomic nervous system response.[20] These potential concerns can be minimized if a trained health care practitioner with knowledge of blood flow restriction therapy performs a thorough subjective and physical examination to identify any potential contraindications and prescribes the therapy with the use of regulated, medical-grade equipment. The contraindications for exclusion from BFR training are included in Table 23-2. Some of the noted negative outcomes associated with BFR training are described later.

Thrombus Formation

A possible safety concern regarding BFR training includes thrombus formation (ie, blood clot) due to the potential for pooling of blood in the extremities. Studies examining BFR training with healthy individuals and older adults with heart disease found no change in blood markers for thrombin generation or intravascular clot formation.[25,26] Furthermore, data from 2 surveys of nearly 13,000 individuals utilizing BFR training found that the incidence of deep venous thrombosis was less than 0.06% and pulmonary embolism was less than 0.01%.[20,27] Proper health screening with training load and personalized restrictive pressure is very important in preventing this negative outcome. However, BFR with light load resistance training or no exercise has been shown to stimulate the fibrinolytic system similar to resistance training without BFR.[26,28,29] This is an important finding because the fibrinolytic system, when activated, inhibits thrombus formation, which is contrary to the potential risk of thrombus formation.

Muscle Damage

Delayed onset muscle soreness, or DOMS, is commonly reported after a bout of BFR training within 24, 48, or even 72 hours after the training period.[30,31] In general, it is well established that unaccustomed exercise results in muscle damage, especially if the exercise involves large muscle groups performing eccentric actions.[32] The amount of muscle damage associated with BFR training is conflicting; however, a comparison between maximal eccentric actions and BFR training to exhaustion in untrained individuals revealed

Table 23-2

CONTRAINDICATIONS FOR BLOOD FLOW RESTRICTION TRAINING

CONDITION
Cardiovascular Disease Signs and Symptoms
• Unstable hypertension
• Venous thrombosis
• Blood clotting disorder
• Chest discomfort
• Syncope
• Heart murmur
• Irregular heart rate
• Sleep apnea
• Ankle swelling
• Shortness of breath
• Intermittent claudication
Lifestyle
• Age
• Smoking
• Sedentary
• Obesity
• Uncontrolled diabetes
Other
• Extremities with dialysis access
• Acidosis
• Extremity infection
• Cancer
• Open fracture
• Skin grafts
• Increased intracranial pressure
• Open soft tissue injuries
• Lymphectomies
• Medication that increases risk for blood clotting

comparable amounts of exercise-induced muscle damage.[33,34] Therefore, DOMS is normal after unaccustomed exercise, with and without BFR, and should return to resting levels within 24 to 72 hours.

DOMS can be associated with several exercise-induced muscle damage markers. These markers in the literature include administering resting and post-test time until back-to-resting values. Some of the tests include maximal force output, muscle swelling, range of motion (ROM), and blood markers. The maximum force output with BFR training does not revert back-to-resting values immediately after and post 24 hours training, while muscle swelling and ROM values return within 24 hours after BFR training.[16,30,35] When measuring blood markers for muscle damage, myoglobin, interleukin-6, and creatine kinase were not found to be elevated immediately after BFR training.[36] Therefore, given this information, it does not appear that BFR training produces muscle damage greater than that of traditional resistance training methods.

Excessive muscle damage (ie, rhabdomyolysis) has been reported in BFR training literature to be less than 0.01%.[20,27] However, it is likely that the reported excess muscle damage was due to unaccustomed exercise and improper use of BFR. As mentioned earlier, if BFR training is administered correctly by a trained professional on properly indicated patients, then it is unlikely a serious adverse event will take place.

Nerve Conduction

Another potential side effect associated with BFR training is the feeling of numbness.[27] This is likely due to modifiable prescription variables such as the width of the cuff, duration of inflation, and inflation pressures. The incidence is low (less than 2%) and cases are transient in nature.[27] However, the correct selection and application of the cuff (ie, size, site, pressure) is essential for preventing peripheral nerve injury. It is well established in the literature that higher levels of tourniquet pressure and higher pressure gradients underneath tourniquet cuffs are associated with a higher risk of nerve-related injury.[22,23] The tourniquet pressure and pressure gradients can be minimized by the adoption of personalized pressure based on a patient's LOP, in conjunction with the use of a wide contoured cuff to further reduce necessary average pressure.[37]

Abnormal Exercise Pressure Reflex

There are concerns that BFR could cause an exaggerated exercise pressure reflex (EPR). It is hypothesized that reduced blood flow to the working muscles could lead to EPR-mediated cardiovascular complications and result in excessive blood pressure elevation. Although an abnormal EPR could occur in the apparently healthy, the hesitation is heightened for at-risk populations such as individuals diagnosed with heart failure, hypertension, or peripheral artery disease. These individuals are predisposed to an exaggerated increase in sympathetic nervous system activity during exercise.[38] However, the risk of an adverse event can be mitigated by using personalized cuff inflation pressures, wider cuffs, and by reducing the BFR pressure (eg, by reducing the percentage of LOP used to determine PTP).[39]

CLINICAL USES OF BLOOD FLOW RESTRICTION

Although BFR training is relatively new in rehabilitation settings, there is promising research for orthopedic physical therapists. Hughes et al conducted a systematic review of 20 studies comparing low-load (LL) resistance training to LL-BFR resistance training. Some of the conditions in this review include anterior cruciate ligament (ACL) reconstruction, knee osteoarthritis, and sarcopenia. The authors found that LL-BFR was more effective and better tolerated by patients, therefore making it a potential clinical rehabilitation tool.[8]

Postoperative Knee Surgery

Hughes and colleagues compared subjective knee pain in 30 ACL patients after ACL surgery undergoing low-level 30% 1RM leg press with BFR vs high-load (HL) 70% 1RM free flow conditions. Immediately after and the following 24 hours the participants in the BFR condition had significantly less knee pain than the HL group. Hemodynamics were also assessed with no differences noted between groups.[40]

A randomized controlled trial (RCT) on military service members comparing BFR plus exercise vs the same exercise under free flow condition for 4 weeks after knee arthroscopy found significant improvements in hypertrophy, self-reported scores, and quadriceps strength in the BFR group. Participants were also tested for thrombus formation at baseline and after 4 weeks of training via Duplex Ultrasound scans with no signs of thrombus formation in either group.[3]

Knee Osteoarthritis

An RCT examined LL-BFR resistance training in women with osteoarthritis. The study included 48 participants who were randomized into 1 of 3 groups: LL resistance training, LL-BFR resistance training, and high-intensity resistance training (ie, 80% 1RM). The authors found that after 12 weeks of training, LL-BFR resistance training produced similar results in lower extremity muscle strength and quadriceps muscle mass when compared to high-intensity resistance training. It is also critical to note that a number of participants in the high-intensity resistance training group were unable to complete the study due to high levels of pain while exercising. In addition, pre- and post-assessment via a disease-specific inventory (Western Ontario and McMaster Universities Index [WOMAC]) revealed that LL-BFR resistance training resulted in similar improvements in physical functioning and pain when compared to high-intensity resistance training and LL resistance training, respectively.[9]

Patellofemoral Pain

Giles and colleagues performed a double-blind RCT of 69 participants with patellofemoral pain (PFP). The individuals were randomized into 2 groups: moderate intensity (ie, 70% 1RM) quadriceps strengthening and LL-BFR (ie, 30% 1RM) quadriceps strengthening. Both groups performed the same quadriceps strengthening exercises. This included leg press (0 to 60 degrees knee flexion) and leg extension (90 to 45 degrees) exercises. After 8 weeks of training, the participants in LL-BFR quadriceps strengthening group had a greater reduction in pain during activities of daily living. However, both groups improved similarly in strength and hypertrophy. The authors hypothesized that individuals with PFP who also experience pain with quadriceps contraction may be unable to engage in moderate- to high-intensity resistance training, thus limiting their ability to tolerate this type of rehabilitation program.[6] Thus, LL-BFR resistance training could be used as an alternative method for quadriceps strengthening in this population.

CONCLUSION

Knowledge of BFR training for physical therapists working in an orthopedic setting is beneficial because of the ability to achieve muscular adaptations comparable to traditional resistance training. This is advantageous for individuals working with patients in rehabilitation settings for whom moderate to high-intensity (ie, greater than or equal to 65% 1RM) resistance training is often contraindicated. Therefore, the physical therapist should have a basic understanding of this training modality.

CASE STUDIES

Case Study One

Patient: 25-year-old man

Diagnosis: Postoperative arthroscopic knee surgery, partial meniscectomy

- Subjective examination
  - Medical history: Right knee meniscus tear
  - Patient interview: Patient was postoperative day 1 right knee partial meniscectomy. The patient had a 2-year history of right knee pain, beginning during a cutting maneuver during an intramural basketball game. He experienced pain and swelling after each game without a change in performance. However, the pain and swelling became chronic, preventing him from playing basketball. Over the past 6 months, it also began affecting his daily function. The patient was referred to an orthopedic surgeon who ordered magnetic resonance imaging, and determined the patient was a candidate for surgery. The patient worked as a middle school science

teacher. His pain ratings were as follows: Current 3/10, at worst a 7/10. His goal was to return to his previous level of function, which included playing intramural basketball.

  - Review of systems: Unremarkable
- Physical examination
  - Systems review
    - Observation including posture: Well-developed male; visible right quadriceps atrophy
    - Cardiovascular and pulmonary: Unremarkable
    - Gait: Bilateral axillary crutches, right lower extremity foot flat weightbearing
    - Gross ROM: See measures later
    - Gross strength: See measures later
    - Neurological
      - Dermatomes: Within normal limits (WNL)
      - Myotomes: WNL
  - Test and measures
    - Active range of motion (AROM): Goniometer
      - Right knee extension to 0 degrees, knee flexion to 90 degrees
      - Left knee extension to 0 degrees, knee flexion to 130 degrees
    - Passive range of motion (PROM) including overpressures: Goniometer
      - Right knee extension to 0 degrees, knee flexion to 95 degrees. Left knee extension to 5 degrees hyperextension and knee flexion to 135 degrees.
    - Manual muscle testing: Left lower extremity and bilateral upper extremities 5/5. Right lower extremity not tested due to pain and limited knee ROM.
    - Circumference measurements: Right midthigh 2.75 cm less than left mid-thigh
- What is the plan of action for this patient (clinical decision-making process)?
  - The main concern was the significant right quadriceps atrophy. The American College of Sports Medicine (ACSM) recommends using greater than or equal to 60% of the individual's 1RM in order to improve muscular strength, power, or endurance. This intensity is needed for adequate recruitment of type II muscle fibers. However, the patient cannot safely perform resistance training at this intensity due to his recent surgery. Therefore, the therapist prescribed BFR training.
    - Frequency: 2 times per week
    - Intensity: 20% of the patient's 1RM, calculated based on the 1RM testing of the left lower extremity

- Type and time: Resistance training exercises per physician protocol with addition of BFR: BFR was applied to the proximal right thigh with 80% limb occlusion pressure
  - Example
    - Straight leg raises in supine with BFR
    - 75 repetitions completed as follows: 30 repetitions, 15 repetitions, 15 repetitions, and 15 repetitions
    - 30-second rest between sets and cuff inflated throughout the set

Case Study Two

Patient: 27-year-old woman
Diagnosis: Patellofemoral pain syndrome

- Subjective examination
  - Medical history: Left knee pain
  - Patient interview: Patient was diagnosed with left patellofemoral pain syndrome 1 week ago. The patient is an office assistant who loves to start her day with a 5-mile run. Over the past 6 months, she has been training for her first mini-marathon. She started to train on flat land, but recently started to train on hilly land. Two weeks ago, the patient began feeling pain in the front of her left knee while running downhill. Last week, she had to stop running after 3 miles because of her knee pain. Her pain ratings were as follows: current 5/10, at worst a 10/10. Her goal is to return to her previous level of function, which included competing in the mini-marathon without pain.
  - Review of systems: Unremarkable
- Physical examination
  - Systems review
    - Observation including posture: Well-developed woman with left quadriceps atrophy
    - Cardiovascular and pulmonary: Unremarkable
    - Gait: Left lower extremity foot flat weightbearing
    - Gross ROM: Lateral tracking of the patella
    - Gross strength: Weak quadriceps, hamstrings, and hip abductors; muscle imbalance between hip internal and external rotators
    - Neurological
      - Dermatomes: WNL
      - Myotomes: WNL
- What is the plan of action for this patient (clinical decision-making process)?
  - The main concern was the significant left quadriceps atrophy, weak hip muscles, flat foot, and lateral tracking of the patella.

- For the lateral tracking of the patella, special tape was placed on the front of her knee to help reduce her pain and allow for proper muscle activation.
- For the flat foot, new footwear.
- The ACSM recommends using greater than or equal to 60% of the individual's 1RM in order to improve muscular strength, power, or endurance. This intensity is needed for adequate recruitment of type II muscle fibers. However, the patient cannot safely perform resistance training at this intensity due to her pain. Therefore, the therapist prescribed BFR training.
  - Frequency: 2 times per week
  - Intensity: 20% of the patient's 1RM, calculated based on the 1RM testing of the left lower extremity
  - Type and time: Resistance training exercises per physician protocol with addition of BFR. BFR was applied to the proximal left thigh with 80% limb occlusion pressure.
    - Example exercises
      - Single leg bridge push-up with BFR and straight leg raises in supine with BFR
      - Each exercise: 75 repetitions completed as follows: 30 repetitions, 15 repetitions, 15 repetitions, and 15 repetitions
      - 30-second rest between sets and cuff inflated throughout the set

REFERENCES

1. Park S-Y, Kwak YS, Harveson A, Weavil JC, Seo KE. Low intensity resistance exercise training with blood flow restriction: insight into cardiovascular function, and skeletal muscle hypertrophy in humans. *Korean Journal of Physiology & Pharmacology.* 2015;19(3):191-196.

2. Franz A, Queitsch FP, Behringer M, Mayer C, Krauspe R, Zilkens C. Blood flow restriction training as a prehabilitation concept in total knee arthroplasty: a narrative review about current preoperative interventions and the potential impact of BFR. *Medical Hypotheses.* 2018;110:53-59.

3. Tennent DJ, Hylden CM, Johnson AE, Burns TC, Wilken JM, Owens JG. Blood flow restriction training after knee arthroscopy: a randomized controlled pilot study. *Clin J Sport Med.* 2017;27(3):245-252.

4. Abe T, Sakamaki M, Fujita S, et al. Effects of low-intensity walk training with restricted leg blood flow on muscle strength and aerobic capacity in older adults. *J Geriatr Phys Ther.* 2010;33(1):34-40.

5. Ladlow P, Coppack RJ, Dharm-Datta S, et al. The effects of low-intensity blood flow restricted exercise compared with conventional resistance training on the clinical outcomes of active UK military personnel following a 3-week in-patient rehabilitation programme: protocol for a randomized controlled feasibility study. *Pilot and Feasibility Studies.* 2017;3(1):71.

6. Giles L, Webster KE, McClelland J, Cook JL. Quadriceps strengthening with and without blood flow restriction in the treatment of patellofemoral pain: a double-blind randomised trial. *Br J Sports Med.* 2017;51(23):1688-1694.

7. Yow BG, Tennent DJ, Dowd TC, Loenneke JP, Owens JG. Blood flow restriction training after achilles tendon rupture. *J Foot Ankle Surg.* 2018;57(3):635-638.

8. Hughes L, Paton B, Rosenblatt B, Gissane C, Patterson SD. Blood flow restriction training in clinical musculoskeletal rehabilitation: a systematic review and meta-analysis. *Br J Sports Med.* 2017;51(13):1003-1011.

9. Ferraz RB, Gualano B, Rodrigues R, et al. Benefits of resistance training with blood flow restriction in knee osteoarthritis. *Med Sci Sports Exerc.* 2018;50(5):897-905.

10. Loenneke JP, Wilson JM, Marín PJ, Zourdos MC, Bemben MG. Low intensity blood flow restriction training: a meta-analysis. *Eur J Appl Physiol.* 2012;112(5):1849-1859.

11. Scott BR, Loenneke JP, Slattery KM, Dascombe BJ. Exercise with blood flow restriction: an updated evidence-based approach for enhanced muscular development. *Sports Med.* 2015;45(3):313-325.

12. Manini TM, Clark BC. Blood flow restricted exercise and skeletal muscle health. *Exerc Sport Sci Rev.* 2009;37(2):78-85.

13. Nielsen JL, Aagaard P, Bech RD, et al. Proliferation of myogenic stem cells in human skeletal muscle in response to low-load resistance training with blood flow restriction. *J Physiol.* 2012;590(17):4351-4361.

14. Sato Y. The history and future of KAATSU training. *International Journal of KAATSU Training Research.* 2005;1(1):1-5.

15. Loenneke JP, Fahs CA, Rossow LM, et al. Effects of cuff width on arterial occlusion: implications for blood flow restricted exercise. *Eur J Appl Physiol.* 2012;112(8):2903-2912.

16. Loenneke J, Thiebaud R, Abe T. Does blood flow restriction result in skeletal muscle damage? A critical review of available evidence. *Scand J Med Sci Sports.* 2014;24(6).

17. Sato Y. Belt for muscle training. Google Patents; 2016.

18. McEwen JA, Owens JG, Jeyasurya J. Why is it crucial to use personalized occlusion pressures in blood flow restriction (BFR) rehabilitation? *Journal of Medical and Biological Engineering.* 2018;39(3):1-5.

19. McEwen JA. Complications of and improvements in pneumatic tourniquets used in surgery. *Medical Instrumentation.* 1981;15(4):253-257.

20. Patterson SD, Brandner CR. The role of blood flow restriction training for applied practitioners: a questionnaire-based survey. *J Sports Sci.* 2018;36(2):123-130.

21. Mattocks KT, Jessee MB, Mouser JG, et al. The application of blood flow restriction: lessons from the laboratory. *Curr Sports Med Rep.* 2018;17(4):129-134.

22. Noordin S, McEwen JA, Kragh Jr CJF, Eisen A, Masri BA. Surgical tourniquets in orthopaedics. *J Bone Joint Surg Am.* 2009;91(12):2958-2967.

23. Ochoa J, Danta G, Fowler T, Gilliatt R. Nature of the nerve lesion caused by a pneumatic tourniquet. *Nature.* 1971;233(5317):265.

24. Pope ZK, Willardson JM, Schoenfeld BJ. Exercise and blood flow restriction. *J Strength Cond Res.* 2013;27(10):2914-2926.

25. Clark B, Manini T, Hoffman R, et al. Relative safety of 4 weeks of blood flow-restricted resistance exercise in young, healthy adults. *Scand J Med Sci Sports.* 2011;21(5):653-662.

26. Madarame H, Kurano M, Fukumura K, Fukuda T, Nakajima T. Haemostatic and inflammatory responses to blood flow-restricted exercise in patients with ischaemic heart disease: a pilot study. *Clin Physiol Funct Imaging.* 2013;33(1):11-17.

27. Nakajima T, Kurano M, Iida H, et al. Use and safety of KAATSU training: results of a national survey. *International Journal of KAATSU Training Research.* 2006;2(1):5-13.

28. Madarame H, Kurano M, Takano H, et al. Effects of low-intensity resistance exercise with blood flow restriction on co-agulation system in healthy subjects. *Clin Physiol Funct Imaging.* 2010;30(3):210-213.

29. Nakajima T, Takano H, Kurano M, et al. Effects of KAATSU training on haemostasis in healthy subjects. *International Journal of KAATSU Training Research.* 2007;3(1):11-20.

30. Thiebaud RS, Yasuda T, Loenneke JP, Abe T. Effects of low-intensity concentric and eccentric exercise combined with blood flow restriction on indices of exercise-induced muscle damage. *Interv Med Appl Sci.* 2013;5(2):53-59.

31. Brandner CR, Warmington SA. Delayed onset muscle soreness and perceived exertion after blood flow restriction exercise. *J Strength Cond Res.* 2017;31(11):3101-3108.

32. Brandner CR, May AK, Clarkson MJ, Warmington SA. Reported side-effects and safety considerations for the use of blood flow restriction during exercise in practice and research. *Techniques in Orthopaedics.* 2018;33(2):114-121.

33. Sieljacks P, Matzon A, Wernbom M, Ringgaard S, Vissing K, Overgaard K. Muscle damage and repeated bout effect following blood flow restricted exercise. *Eur J Appl Physiol.* 2016;116(3):513-525.

34. Takarada Y, Nakamura Y, Aruga S, Onda T, Miyazaki S, Ishii N. Rapid increase in plasma growth hormone after low-intensity resistance exercise with vascular occlusion. *J Appl Physiol.* 2000;88(1):61-65.

35. Loenneke JP, Thiebaud RS, Fahs CA, Rossow LM, Abe T, Bemben MG. Blood flow restriction does not result in prolonged decrements in torque. *Eur J Appl Physiol.* 2013;113(4):923-931.

36. Karabulut M, Sherk VD, Bemben DA, Bemben MG. Inflammation marker, damage marker and anabolic hormone responses to resistance training with vascular restriction in older males. *Clin Physiol Funct Imaging.* 2013;33(5):393-399.

37. Younger AS, McEwen JA, Inkpen K. Wide contoured thigh cuffs and automated limb occlusion measurement allow lower tourniquet pressures. *Clin Orthop Relat Res.* 2004;428:286-293.

38. Spranger MD, Krishnan AC, Levy PD, O'Leary DS, Smith SA. Blood flow restriction training and the exercise pressor reflex: a call for concern. *American Journal of Physiology-Heart and Circulatory Physiology.* 2015;309(9):H1440-H1452.

39. Jessee MB, Buckner SL, Mouser JG, Mattocks KT, Loenneke JP. Letter to the editor: applying the blood flow restriction pressure: the elephant in the room. *Am J Physiol Heart Circ Physiol.* 2016;310(1):H132-H133.

40. Hughes L, Paton B, Haddad F, Rosenblatt B, Gissane C, Patterson SD. Comparison of the acute perceptual and blood pressure response to heavy load and light load blood flow restriction resistance exercise in anterior cruciate ligament reconstruction patients and non-injured populations. *Phys Ther Sport.* 2018;33:54-61.

FINANCIAL DISCLOSURES

Dr. Kristi M. Angelopoulou reported no financial or proprietary interest in the materials presented herein.

Dr. Charles Baycroft has not disclosed any relevant financial relationships.

Dr. Bill Boissonnault has not disclosed any relevant financial relationships.

Dr. Benjamin S. Boyd presents continuing education courses on neurodynamic testing and treatment to clinicians (mainly physical therapists) on behalf of the Neuro Orthopaedic Institute (NOI) Group. They are paid as independent contractors for their teaching. They have no other financial relationships with the NOI Group nor their products. They declare that they have no other known conflicts of interest.

Dr. Blair Bundy reported no financial or proprietary interest in the materials presented herein.

Kenji Carp has not disclosed any relevant financial relationships.

Dr. Charles Clark has not disclosed any relevant financial relationships.

Dr. Jena Cleary reported no financial or proprietary interest in the materials presented herein.

Dr. Michel W. Coppieters presents continuing education courses on neurodynamic testing and treatment to clinicians (mainly physical therapists) on behalf of the Neuro Orthopaedic Institute (NOI) Group. They are paid as independent contractors for their teaching. They have no other financial relationships with the NOI Group nor their products. They declare that they have no other known conflicts of interest.

Georgeta Donatelli has not disclosed any relevant financial relationships.

Dr. Robert Donatelli reported no financial or proprietary interest in the materials presented herein.

Dr. Mary Beth Geiser reported no financial or proprietary interest in the materials presented herein.

Ola Grimsby reported no financial or proprietary interest in the materials presented herein.

Christian Gröbli has not disclosed any relevant financial relationships.

Dr. Chad Hanson reported no financial or proprietary interest in the materials presented herein.

Dr. Corbin Hedt reported no financial or proprietary interest in the materials presented herein.

Matthew L. Holland reported no financial or proprietary interest in the materials presented herein.

Dr. Shain I. Howard has not disclosed any relevant financial relationships.

Dr. Alec Kay reported no financial or proprietary interest in the materials presented herein.

Dr. Tyler Kent reported no financial or proprietary interest in the materials presented herein.

Steven L. Kraus reported no financial or proprietary interest in the materials presented herein.

Dr. Kevin J. Lawrence has not disclosed any relevant financial relationships.

Dr. Graham Linck reported no financial or proprietary interest in the materials presented herein.

Dr. Tammy Luttrell reported no financial or proprietary interest in the materials presented herein.

Dr. Johnson McEvoy reported no financial or proprietary interest in the materials presented herein.

James M. McKivigan has not disclosed any relevant financial relationships.

Dr. Robert J. Nee presents continuing education courses on neurodynamic testing and treatment to clinicians (mainly physical therapists) on behalf of the Neuro Orthopaedic Institute (NOI) Group. They are paid as independent contractors for their teaching. They have no other financial relationships with the NOI Group nor their products. They declare that they have no other known conflicts of interest.

Dr. Beth Stone Norris reported no financial or proprietary interest in the materials presented herein.

Dr. William H. O'Grady reported no financial or proprietary interest in the materials presented herein.

Johnny G. Owens is a medical advisory for Delfi Medical Innovations and CEO of Owens Recovery Science.

Dr. Jeevan Pandya reported no financial or proprietary interest in the materials presented herein.

Janette Powell reported no financial or proprietary interest in the materials presented herein.

Dr. Mohini Rawat reported no financial or proprietary interest in the materials presented herein.

Dr. Rodrigo Miguel Ruivo reported no financial or proprietary interest in the materials presented herein.

Dr. Mike Russell has not disclosed any relevant financial relationships.

Dr. William R. VanWye reported no financial or proprietary interest in the materials presented herein.

Dr. Harvey W. Wallmann reported no financial or proprietary interest in the materials presented herein.

Dr. Sharon Wang-Price reported no financial or proprietary interest in the materials presented herein.

Dr. Alyssa M. Weatherholt reported no financial or proprietary interest in the materials presented herein.

Dr. Sonia N. Young reported no financial or proprietary interest in the materials presented herein.

INDEX

Printed in the United States
by Baker & Taylor Publisher Services